IMAGE-GUIDED RADIATION THERAPY: A CLINICAL PERSPECTIVE

Editors

Arno J. Mundt, MD
Department of Radiation Oncology
University of California San Diego
La Jolla, California, USA

John Roeske, PhD
Department of Radiation Oncology
Loyola University
Chicago, Illinois, USA

2011
PEOPLE'S MEDICAL PUBLISHING HOUSE—USA
SHELTON, CONNECTICUT

People's Medical Publishing House-USA

2 Enterprise Drive, Suite 509
Shelton, CT 06484
Tel: 203-402-0646
Fax: 203-402-0854
E-mail: info@pmph-usa.com

09 10 11 12/PMPH/9 8 7 6 5 4 3 2

ISBN 13: 978-1-60795-042-4
ISBN 10: 1-60795-042-1

Printed in China by People's Medical Publishing House
Copyeditor/Typesetter: Spearhead Global, Inc.
Cover design: Mary McKeon

Library of Congress Cataloging-in-Publication Data
LOC CIP data on file

Notice: The authors and publisher have made every effort to ensure that the patient care recommended herein, including choice of drugs and drug dosages, is in accord with the accepted standard and practice at the time of publication. However, since research and regulation constantly change clinical standards, the reader is urged to check the product information sheet included in the package of each drug, which includes recommended doses, warnings, and contraindications. This is particularly important with new or infrequently used drugs. Any treatment regimen, particularly one involving medication, involves inherent risk that must be weighed on a case-by-case basis against the benefits anticipated. The reader is cautioned that the purpose of this book is to inform and enlighten; the information contained herein is not intended as, and should not be employed as, a substitute for individual diagnosis and treatment.

Sales and Distribution

Canada
McGraw-Hill Ryerson Education
Customer Care
300 Water St
Whitby, Ontario L1N 9B6
Canada
Tel: 1-800-565-5758
Fax: 1-800-463-5885
www.mcgrawhill.ca

Foreign Rights
People's Medical Publishing House
Suzanne Robidoux, Copyright Sales Manager
International Trade Department
No. 19, Pan Jia Yuan Nan Li
Chaoyang District
Beijing 100021
P.R. China
Tel: 8610-59787337
Fax: 8610-59787336
www.pmph.com/en/

Japan
United Publishers Services Limited
1-32-5 Higashi-Shinagawa
Shinagawa-ku, Tokyo 140-0002
Japan
Tel: 03-5479-7251
Fax: 03-5479-7307
Email: kakimoto@ups.co.jp

United Kingdom, Europe, Middle East, Africa
McGraw Hill Education
Shoppenhangers Road
Maidenhead
Berkshire, SL6 2QL
England
Tel: 44-0-1628-502500
Fax: 44-0-1628-635895
www.mcgraw-hill.co.uk

Singapore, Thailand, Philippines, Indonesia
Vietnam, Pacific Rim, Korea
McGraw-Hill Education
60 Tuas Basin Link
Singapore 638775
Tel: 65-6863-1580
Fax: 65-6862-3354
www.mcgraw-hill.com.sg

Australia, New Zealand, Papua New Guinea, Fiji,
Tonga, Solomon Islands, Cook Islands
Woodsland Pty Limited
Unit 7/5 Vuko Place
Warriewood NSW 2102
Australia
Tel: 61-2-9970-5111
Fax: 61-2-9970-5002
www.woodslane.com.au

Brazil
SuperPedido Tecmedd
Beatriz Alves, Foreign Trade Department
R. Sansao Alves dos Santos, 102 7th floor
Brooklin Novo
Sao Paolo 04571-090
Brazil
Tel: 55-16-3512-5539
www.superpedidotecmedd.com.br

India, Bangladesh, Pakistan, Sri Lanka, Malaysia
CBS Publishers
4819/X1 Prahlad Street 24
Ansari Road, Darya Ganj, New Delhi-110002
India
Tel: 91-11-23266861/67
Fax: 91-11-23266818
Email:cbspubs@vsnl.com

People's Republic of China
People's Medical Publishing House
International Trade Department
No. 19, Pan Jia Yuan Nan Li
Chaoyang District
Beijing 100021
P.R. China
Tel: 8610-67653342
Fax: 8610-67691034
www.pmph.com/en/

CONTRIBUTORS

Chapter 1

Arno J. Mundt, MD
Department of Radiation Oncology
University of California San Diego
La Jolla, California, USA

John Roeske, PhD
Department of Radiation Oncology
Loyola University
Chicago, Illinois, USA

Chapter 2

Joshua D. Lawson, MD
Department of Radiation Oncology
University of California San Diego
La Jolla, California, USA

Timothy Fox, PhD
Department of Radiation Oncology
Emory University
Atlanta, Georgia, USA

Chapter 3

Anca Ligia Grosu, MD
Department of Radiation Oncology
University of Freiburg
Freiburg, Germany

Wolfgang Andreas Weber, MD
Department of Nuclear Medicine
University of Freiburg
Freiburg, Germany

Ursula Nestle, MD
Department of Radiation Oncology
University of Freiburg
Freiburg, Germany

Chapter 4

Vincent Khoo, MD, MB, BS, FRANZCR, FRCR
Department of Radiotherapy
Royal Marsden NHS Foundation Trust and
Institute of Cancer Research
University of London
London, United Kingdom

Daryl Lim Joon, MB, BS, FRANZCR
Austin Health Centre and University of Melbourne
Melbourne, Australia

Chapter 5

Judit Boda-Heggemann, MD
Klinik für Strahlentherapie und Radioonkologie
Universitätsmedizin Mannheim/
Universität Heidelberg
Mannheim, Germany

Frank Lohr, MD
Klinik für Strahlentherapie und Radioonkologie
Universitätsmedizin Mannheim/
Universität Heidelberg
Mannheim, Germany

Martin Fuss, MD
Department of Radiation Medicine
Oregon Health & Science University
Portland, Oregon, USA

Chapter 6

Shidong Li, PhD
Department of Radiation Oncology
Temple University Hospital
Philadelphia, Pennsylvania, USA

Chapter 7

Yildirim D. Mutaf, PhD
Department of Radiation Oncology
University of Pittsburgh Medical Center
Pittsburgh, Pennsylvania, USA

Chapter 8

Chang Ming Charlie Ma, PhD
Department of Radiation Oncology
Fox Chase Cancer Center
Philadelphia, Pennsylvania, USA

Chapter 9

Masayori Ishikawa PhD
Research Center for Cooperative Projects
Hokkaido University
Graduate School of Medicine
Sapporo, Japan

Srijit Kamath, PhD
Department of Radiation Oncology
University of Florida
Gainesville, Florida, USA

Cheng Saw, PhD
Division of Radiation Oncology
Penn State Cancer Institute
Hershey, Pennsylvania, USA

Anil Sethi, PhD
Department of Radiation Oncology
Loyola University
Chicago, Illinois, USA

Hiroki Shirato, MD
Department of Radiology
Hokkaido University
Sapporo, Japan

William Y. Song, PhD
Department of Radiation Oncology
University of California San Diego
La Jolla, California, USA

Chapter 10

Thomas Rockwell Mackie, PhD
Morgridge Institute for Research
University of Wisconsin
Madison, Wisconsin, USA

Olivier Morin, PhD
Department of Radiation Oncology
University of California San Francisco
San Francisco, California, USA

Gustavo H. Olivera, PhD
Department of Medical Physics
University of Wisconsin
Madison, Wisconsin, USA

Jean Pouliot, PhD
Department of Radiation Oncology
University of California San Francisco
San Francisco, California, USA

Chapter 11

Laura Cerviño, PhD
Department of Radiation Oncology
University of California San Diego
La Jolla, California USA

Steve B. Jiang, PhD
Department of Radiation Oncology
University of California San Diego
La Jolla, California, USA

Chapter 12

Dale W. Litzenberg, PhD
Department of Radiation Oncology
University of Michigan Hospital
Ann Arbor, Michigan, USA

Chapter 13

James Bowsher, PhD
Department of Radiation Oncology
Duke University
Durham, North Carolina, USA

James F. Dempsey, PhD
Viewray, Inc.
Cleveland, Ohio, USA

Jan J.W. Lagendijk, PhD
Department of Radiotherapy
University Medical Center Utrecht
Utrecht, The Netherlands

Masatoshi Mitsuya PhD
Tohoku University
Graduate School of Medicine
Sendai, Japan

Bas W. Raaymakers PhD
Department of Radiotherapy
University Medical Centre Utrecht
Utrecht, The Netherlands

Richard H. Stark, MS
ViewRay, Inc.
Cleveland, Ohio, USA

Yoshihiro Takai, MD, PhD
Departments of Radiology and Radiation Oncology
Hirosaki University
Aomori, Japan

Fang-Fang Yin, PhD
Department of Radiation Oncology
Duke University
Durham, North Carolina, USA

Chapter 14

Erica Kinsey, PhD
Department of Radiation Oncology
University of California San Diego
La Jolla, California, USA

Daniel J. Scanderbeg, PhD
Department of Radiation Oncology
University of California San Diego
La Jolla, California, USA

Jia-Zhu Wang, PhD
Department of Radiation Oncology
University of California San Diego
La Jolla, California, USA

Trent X. Ning, PhD
Department of Radiation Oncology
University of California San Diego
La Jolla, California, USA

Todd Pawlicki, PhD
Department of Radiation Oncology
University of California San Diego
La Jolla, California, USA

Chapter 15

Ashwatha Narayana, MD
Departments of Radiation Oncology and
Neurosurgery
New York University
New York, New York, USA

Jenghwa Chang, PhD
Department of Radiation Oncology
Cornell University
New York, New York, USA

Chapter 15A

Stefanie Milker-Zabel MD
Department of RadioOncology and Radiotherapy
University Hospital of Heidelberg
University of Heidelberg
Heidelberg, Germany

Angelika Zabel-du Bois MD
Department of RadioOncology and Radiotherapy
University Hospital of Heidelberg
University of Heidelberg
Heidelberg, Germany

Chapter 15B

Åse Ballangrud, PhD
Department of Medical Physics
Memorial Sloan-Kettering Cancer Center
New York, New York, USA

Stella Lymberis, MD
Department of Radiation Oncology
NYU School of Medicine
New York, New York, USA

Kathryn Beal, MD
Department of Radiation Oncology
Memorial Sloan-Kettering Cancer Center
New York, NY

Philip H. Gutin, MD
Department of Neurosurgery
Memorial Sloan-Kettering Cancer Center
New York, New York

Jenghwa Chang, PhD
Department of Radiation Oncology
Cornell University
New York, New York, USA

Chapter 15C

Joseph Stancanello, PhD
Siemens AG Healthcare
Erlangen, Germany

Carlo Cavedon, PhD
Department of Medical Physics
University Hospital of Verona
Verona, Italy

Federico Colombo, MD
Stereotactic Radiosurgery Centre
San Bortolo Hospital
Vicenza, Italy

Paolo Francescon, PhD
Medical Physics Department
San Bortolo Hospital
Vicenza, Italy

Leopoldo Casentini, MD
Stereotactic Radiosurgery Centre
San Bortolo Hospital
Vicenza, Italy

Francesco Causin, MD
Neuroradiology - Endovascular Interventional
Neuroradiology Unit
University Hospital of Padova
Padova, Italy

Chapter 15D

Alan T. Villavicencio, MD
Boulder Neurosurgical Associates
Boulder, Colorado, USA

Lee McNeely, MD
Alpine Radiation Oncology
Rocky Mountain CyberKnife Center
Boulder CO, USA

Chapter 15E

Edward Melian, MD
Departments of Radiation Oncology
and Neurological Surgery
Loyola University Chicago
Maywood, Il, USA

Anil Sethi, PhD
Department of Radiation Oncology
Loyola University
Chicago, Illinois, USA

Chapter 16

Andreas Rimner MD
Department of Radiation Oncology
Memorial Sloan-Kettering Cancer Center
New York, New York, USA

Nancy Lee, MD
Radiation Oncology
Memorial Sloan-Kettering Cancer Center
New York, New York, USA

Chapter 16A

Indira Madani, MD, PhD
Department of Radiotherapy
Ghent University Hospital
Ghent, Belgium

Wilfried De Neve, MD, PhD
Department of Radiotherapy
Ghent University Hospital
Ghent, Belgium

Chapter 16B

Chien-Yu Lin, MD
Department of Radiation Oncology
Chang Gung Memorial Hospital at Linkou
Chang Gung University
Taoyuan, Taiwan

Joseph Tung-Chieh Chang, MD, MHA
Department of Radiation Oncology
Chang Gung Memorial Hospital at Linkou
Chang Gung University
Taoyuan, Taiwan

Chapter 16C

Andreas Rimner MD
Department of Radiation Oncology
Memorial Sloan-Kettering Cancer Center
New York, New York, USA

Nancy Lee, MD
Radiation Oncology
Memorial Sloan-Kettering Cancer Center
New York, New York, USA

Chapter 16D

Xiao-Kang Zheng, MD
Department of Radiation Oncology
Nanfang Hospital of Southern Medical University
Guangzhou, China

Long-Hua Chen, MD
Department of Radiation Oncology
Nanfang Hospital of Southern Medical University
Guangzhou, China

Chapter 16E

Felix Y Feng, MD
Department of Radiation Oncology
University of Michigan
Ann Arbor, Michigan, USA

Scott W. Hadley, PhD
Department of Radiation Oncology
University of Michigan
Ann Arbor, Michigan, USA

Avraham Eisbruch, MD
Department of Radiation Oncology
University of Michigan
Ann Arbor, Michigan, USA

Chapter 16F

Ke Sheng, PhD
Department of Radiation Oncology
University of Virginia
Charlottesville, Virginia, USA

Paul W. Read, MD, PhD
Department of Radiation Oncology
University of Virginia
Charlottesville, Virginia, USA

Chapter 16G

Vivek Krishan Mehta, MD
Department of Radiation Oncology
Swedish Cancer Institute
Seattle, Washington, USA

Tony P. Wong, PhD
Department of Radiation Oncology
Swedish Cancer Institute
Seattle, Washington, USA

Chapter 16H

Joseph K. Salama, MD
Department of Radiation Oncology
Duke University
Durham, North Carolina, USA

Karl Farrey, MS
Department of Radiation and Cellular Oncology
University of Chicago
Chicago, Illinois, USA

Chapter 17

Elizabeth A. Kidd, MD
Department of Radiation Oncology
Stanford University
Stanford, California, USA

Daniel Low, PhD
Department of Radiation Oncology
University of California, Los Angeles
Los Angeles, California, USA

Jeffrey Bradley, MD
Department of Radiation Oncology
Washington University
St. Louis, Missouri, USA

Chapter 17A

Maria Picchio, MD
Department of Nuclear Medicine
San Raffaele Scientific Institute
Milan, Italy

Mariangela Caimi, MD
Department of Radiation Oncology
San Raffaele Scientific Institute
Milan, Italy

Claudio Landoni, MD
Department of Nuclear Medicine
San Raffaele Scientific Institute
University of Milano-Bicocca
Milan, Italy

Cinzia Crivellaro, MD
Department of Nuclear Medicine
University of Milano-Bicocca
Milan, Italy

Filippo Alongi, MD
Department of Radiation Oncology
San Raffaele Scientific Institute
IBFM, National Research Council
Milan, Italy

Nadia Di Muzio, MD
Department of Radiation Oncology
San Raffaele Scientific Institute
Milan, Italy

Cristina Messa, MD
Department of Nuclear Medicine
University of Milano-Bicocca
Milan, Italy

Chapter 17B

Joost Jan Nuyttens, MD, PhD
Department of Radiation Oncology
Erasmus MC-Daniel den Hoed Cancer Center
Rotterdam, The Netherlands

Noelle van der Voort van Zyp, MD
Department of Radiation Oncology
Erasmus MC-Daniel den Hoed Cancer Center
Rotterdam, The Netherlands

Mischa Hoogeman, Msc, PhD
Department of Radiation Oncology
Erasmus MC-Daniel den Hoed Cancer Center
Rotterdam, The Netherlands

Chapter 17C

Jarrod B. Adkison, MD
Department of Human Oncology
University of Wisconsin
Madison, Wisconsin, USA

Ranjini Tolakanahalli, PhD
Department of Human Oncology
University of Wisconsin
Madison, Wisconsin, USA

Deepak Khuntia, MD
Department of Human Oncology
University of Wisconsin
Madison, Wisconsin, USA

Chapter 17D

Ildiko Csiki MD, PhD
Department of Radiation Oncology
Vanderbilt University
Nashville, Tennessee, USA

Misun Hwang BS
Department of Radiation Oncology
Vanderbilt University
Nashville, Tennessee, USA

Wyndee Kirby MS
Department of Radiation Oncology
Vanderbilt University
Nashville, Tennessee, USA

Jostin B. Crass MS
Department of Radiation Oncology
Vanderbilt University
Nashville, Tennessee, USA

George X. Ding, PhD
Department of Radiation Oncology
Vanderbilt University
Nashville, Tennessee, USA

Charles Coffey PhD
Department of Radiation Oncology
Vanderbilt University
Nashville, Tennessee, USA

Bo Lu, MD, PhD
Department of Radiation Oncology
Vanderbilt University
Nashville, Tennessee, USA

Chapter 17E

Ajay P. Sandhu, MD
Department of Radiation Oncology
University of California San Diego
La Jolla, California, USA

Steve B. Jiang, PhD
Department of Radiation Oncology
University of California San Diego
La Jolla, California, USA

Chapter 18

J. Keith DeWyngaert, PhD
Department of Radiation Oncology
NYU School of Medicine
New York, New York, USA

Gabor Jozsef, PhD
Department of Radiation Oncology
NYU School of Medicine
New York, New York, USA

Stella Lymberis, MD
Department of Radiation Oncology
NYU School of Medicine
New York, New York, USA

Stewart J. Becker PhD
Department of Radiation Oncology
NYU School of Medicine
New York, New York, USA

Silvia C. Formenti, MD
Department of Radiation Oncology
NYU School of Medicine
New York, New York, USA

Chapter 18A

Ruth Heimann, MD, PhD
Division of Radiation Oncology
University of Vermont
Burlington, Vermont, USA

Daphne Hard, BS, RTT, CMD
Division of Radiation Oncology
University of Vermont
Burlington, Vermont, USA

Chapter 18B

Yi Rong, PhD
Departments of Human Oncology and
Medical Physics
University of Wisconsin
Madison, Wisconsin, USA

James S. Welsh, MS, MD
Departments of Human Oncology and
Medical Physics
University of Wisconsin
Madison, Wisconsin, USA

Chapter 18C

Leonard Kim, MS, A.Mus.D
Department of Radiation Oncology
William Beaumont Hospital
Royal Oak, Michigan, USA

Yasmin Hasan, MD
Department of Radiation and Cellular Oncology
University of Chicago
Chicago Illinois, USA

Chapter 18D

Douglas A. Miller, M.D
Department of Radiation Oncology
Washington University
St. Louis, MO USA

Eric E. Klein, PhD
Department of Radiation Oncology
Washington University
St. Louis, Missouri, USA

Chapter 18E

Natalya V. Morrow, PhD
Department of Radiation Oncology
Medical College of Wisconsin
Milwaukee, Wisconsin, USA

Julia White, MD
Department of Radiation Oncology
Medical College of Wisconsin
Milwaukee, Wisconsin, USA

X. Allen Li, PhD
Department of Radiation Oncology
Medical College of Wisconsin
Milwaukee, Wisconsin, USA

Chapter 19

Mary Feng, MD
Department of Radiation Oncology
University of Michigan
Ann Arbor, Michigan, USA

Albert C. Koong, MD, PhD
Department of Radiation Oncology
Stanford University
Stanford, California, USA

Edgar Ben-Josef, MD
Department of Radiation Oncology
University of Michigan
Ann Arbor, Michigan, USA

Chapter 19A

Suneel Nagda, MD
Department of Radiation Oncology
Loyola University
Chicago, Illinois, USA

John Roeske, PhD
Department of Radiation Oncology
Loyola University
Chicago, Illinois, USA

Chapter 19B

Charles Cho, MD, MSc
Department of Radiation Oncology
Princess Margaret Hospital
Toronto, Ontario, Canada

Mark T. Lee, MD, MBBS, MSc
Department of Radiation Oncology
Peter MacCallum Cancer Centre
Melbourne, Victoria, Australia

Laura A Dawson, MD
Department of Radiation Oncology
Princess Margaret Hospital
Toronto, Ontario, Canada

Chapter 19C

Daniel Chang, MD
Department of Radiation Oncology
Stanford University
Stanford, California, USA

Albert C. Koong, MD, PhD
Department of Radiation Oncology
Stanford University
Stanford, California, USA

Chapter 19D

Hiroshi Taguchi, MD
Department of Radiology
Hokkaido University
Sapporo, Japan

Masayori Ishikawa PhD
Department of Radiology
Hokkaido University
Sapporo, Japan

Hiroki Shirato, MD
Department of Radiology
Hokkaido University
Sapporo, Japan

Chapter 19E

Chris Lominska, MD
Department of Radiation Oncology
Kansas University
Kansas City, Kansas, USA

Frank Xia, PhD
Department of Radiation Medicine
Georgetown University Medical Center
Washington DC, USA

Nadim Nasr, MD
Virginia Oncology Associates
Norfolk, Virginia, USA

Gregory Gagnon, MD
Radiation Medicine
Georgetown University Medical Center
Washington DC, USA

Chapter 20

Arthur J. Iglesias, MD
Department of Radiation Oncology
University of Miami
Miami, Florida, USA

Dayssy A. Diaz, MD
Department of Radiation Oncology
University of Miami
Miami, Florida, USA

Radka Stoyanova, PhD
Department of Radiation Oncology
University of Miami
Miami, Florida, USA

Alan Pollack, MD, PhD
Department of Radiation Oncology
University of Miami Miller School of Medicine
Sylvester Comprehensive Cancer Center
Miami, Florida, USA

Chapter 20A

Mark K Buyyounouski, MD, MS
Department of Radiation Oncology
Fox Chase Cancer Center
Philadelphia, Pennsylvania, USA

Eric M. Horwitz, MD
Department of Radiation Oncology
Fox Chase Cancer Center
Philadelphia, Pennsylvania, USA

Chapter 20B

Rodney J. Ellis, MD
Department of Radiation Oncology
Case Western Reserve University/ University Hospitals of Cleveland
Cleveland, Ohio, USA

Deborah A. Kaminsky, PhD
Department of Radiation Oncology
Aultman Hospital
Canton, Ohio, USA

Chapter 20C

Fabio L. Cury, MD
Division of Radiation Oncology - Department of Oncology
McGill University
Montreal, Canada

Nicholas J. Rene, MD
Centro de Radioterapia
Rosario, Argentina

William Parker, M.Sc.
Medical Physics
McGill University
Montreal, Canada

Chapter 20D

Irene M. Lips, MD
Department of Radiation Oncology
University Medical Center Utrecht
Utrecht, The Netherlands

Uulke A. van der Heide PhD
Department of Radiation Oncology
University Medical Center Utrecht
Utrecht, The Netherlands

Marco van Vulpen, MD, PhD
Department of Radiation Oncology
University Medical Center Utrecht
Utrecht, The Netherlands

Chapter 20E

Richard Garza, MD
Department of Radiation Oncology
Loyola University
Chicago, Illinois, USA

Anil Sethi, PhD
Department of Radiation Oncology
Loyola University
Chicago, Illinois, USA

Chapter 20F

Christopher King, PhD, MD
Department of Radiation Oncology
University of California Los Angeles
Los Angeles, California, USA

Chapter 20G

John E. Bayouth, PhD
Department of Radiation Oncology
University of Iowa
Iowa City, Iowa, USA

Ryan T. Flynn, PhD
Department of Radiation Oncology
University of Iowa
Iowa City, Iowa, USA

Mark C. Smith, MD
Department of Radiation Oncology
University of Iowa
Iowa City, Iowa, USA

Chapter 20H

Constantine A. Mantz, MD
21st Century Oncology
Fort Myers, Florida, USA

Eduardo P. Fernandez, MD, PhD
21st Century Oncology
Fort Myers, Florida, USA

Chapter 20I

Cesare Cozzarini, MD
Department of Radiation Oncology
San Raffaele Scientific Institute
Milan, Italy

Claudio Fiorino, PhD
Department of Medical Physics
San Raffaele Scientific Institute
Milan, Italy

Sara Broggi, PhD
Department of Medical Physics
San Raffaele Scientific Institute
Milan, Italy

Nadia Di Muzio, MD
Department of Radiation Oncology
San Raffaele Scientific Institute
Milan, Italy

Chapter 20J

Ludvig Paul Muren MSc PhD
Department of Oncology
Aarhus University
Aarhus, Denmark

Jimmi Søndergaard MD
Department of Oncology
Aarhus University
Aarhus, Denmark

Anne Vestergaard MSc
Department of Oncology
Aarhus University
Aarhus, Denmark

Jørgen Petersen MSc
Department of Oncology
Aarhus University
Aarhus, Denmark

Pauliina Wright MSc
Department of Oncology
Aarhus University
Aarhus, Denmark

Ulrik V Elstrøm MSc
Department of Oncology
Aarhus University
Aarhus, Denmark

Cai Grau MD PhD
Department of Oncology
Aarhus University
Aarhus, Denmark

Morten Høyer MD PhD
Department of Oncology
Aarhus University
Aarhus, Denmark

Chapter 20K

Jeffrey Olsen, MD
Department of Radiation Oncology
Washington University
Saint Louis, Missouri, USA

Parag Parikh, BSE, MD
Departments of Radiation Oncology & Biomedical
Engineering
Washington University
Saint Louis, Missouri, USA

Chapter 21

Loren K. Mell, MD
Department of Radiation Oncology
University of California San Diego
La Jolla, California, USA

John Roeske, PhD
Department of Radiation Oncology
Loyola University
Chicago, Illinois, USA

Arno J. Mundt, MD
Department of Radiation Oncology
University of California San Diego
La Jolla, California, USA

Chapter 21A

Alina E. Sturdza, MD
Department of Radiotherapy
Medical University of Vienna
Vienna, Austria

Johannes C. Athanasios Dimopoulos, MD
Department of Radiation Therapy
Metropolitan Hospital
Athens, Greece

Richard Pötter, MD
Department of Radiotherapy
Vienna General Hospital
Medical University of Vienna
Vienna, Austria

Chapter 21B

Perry W. Grigsby, MD
Department of Radiation Oncology
Washington University
St. Louis, Missouri, USA

Chapter 21C

Jennifer F. De Los Santos, MD
Department of Radiation Oncology
University of Alabama at Birmingham
Birmingham, Alabama, USA

Mark C. Langston, MD
Department of Radiology
University of Alabama at Birmingham
Birmingham, Alabama, USA

Janice Carlisle, MEd
Department of Radiation Oncology
University of Alabama at Birmingham
Birmingham, Alabama, USA

Richard Popple, PhD
Department of Radiation Oncology
University of Alabama at Birmingham
Birmingham, Alabama, USA

Chapter 21D

Yun Liang, PhD
Department of Radiation Oncology
University of California San Diego
La Jolla, California, USA

Loren K. Mell, MD
Department of Radiation Oncology
University of California San Diego
La Jolla, California, USA

Chapter 21E

Deidre L Batchelar, PhD, FCCPM
Department of Medical Physics
Sunnybrook Health Sciences Centre
Toronto, Canada

Melanie TM Davidson, PhD, MCCPM
Department of Medical Physics
Sunnybrook Health Sciences Centre
Toronto, Canada

David P D'Souza, MD, FRCPC
Department of Radiation Oncology London Health
Sciences Centre

Chapter 21F

Meritxell Molla, MD
Department of Radiation Oncology
Institut Oncòlogic Teknon.
Barcelona, Spain

Dolors Linero, DSc
Department of Medical Physics.
Institut Oncòlogic Teknon.
Barcelona, Spain

Lluís Escudé, DSc
Department of Medical Physics.
Institut Oncòlogic Teknon.
Barcelona, Spain

Raymond Miralbell, MD
Hôpitaux Universitaries de Genève
Geneva, Switzerland

Chapter 21G

David Bernshaw, MBBS, BMedSci, FRANZCR, FRACP
Division of Radiation Oncology
Peter MacCallum Cancer Centre
East Melbourne, Australia

Sylvia Van Dyk, Dip App Sci MIR
Division of Radiation Oncology
Peter MacCallum Cancer Centre
East Melbourne, Australia

Kailash Narayan, MB,BS, PhD
Division of Radiation Oncology
Peter MacCallum Cancer Centre
East Melbourne, Australia

Chapter 21H

Catheryn M. Yashar, MD
Department of Radiation Oncology
University of California San Diego
La Jolla, California, USA

Brent S. Rose, MD
Department of Radiation Oncology
University of California San Diego
La Jolla, California, USA

William Yashar
Department of Radiation Oncology
University of California San Diego
La Jolla, California, USA

Daniel J. Scanderbeg, PhD
Department of Radiation Oncology
University of California San Diego
La Jolla, California, USA

Chapter 21I

Tracy Bray, MD
Department of Radiation Oncology
Loyola University
Chicago, Illinois, USA

Kevin Albuquerque, MD, MS
Department of Radiation Oncology
Loyola University
Chicago, Illinois, USA

Chapter 22

Michael Spiotto, MD, PhD
Department of Radiation Oncology
Stanford University
Stanford, California, USA

Richard T. Hoppe, MD
Department of Radiation Oncology
Stanford University
Stanford, California, USA

Chapter 22A

Martin Hutchings, MD, PhD
Departments of Oncology and Haematology
Copenhagen University
Copenhagen, Denmark

Deborah Schut, BSc
Department of Radiotherapy
Copenhagen University
Copenhagen, Denmark

Lena Specht, MD, DMSc
Department of Oncology
Copenhagen University
Copenhagen, Denmark

Chapter 22B

Stephanie Terezakis, MD
Department of Radiation Oncology and Molecular
Radiation Sciences
Johns Hopkins University
Baltimore, Maryland, USA

Joachim Yahalom, MD
Department of Radiation Oncology
Memorial Sloan-Kettering Cancer Center
New York, New York, USA

Chapter 22C

Bulent Aydogan, PhD
Department of Radiation and Cellular Oncology
University of Chicago
Chicago, Illinois, USA

Mete Yeginer, PhD
Center for Molecular Biology of Oral Diseases
University of Illinois at Chicago
Chicago, Illinois, USA

Damiano Rondelli, MD
Department of Medicine
University of Illinois at Chicago
Chicago, Illinois,USA

Chapter 22D

Jeffrey Wong, MD
Department of Radiation Oncology and Radiation
Research
City of Hope Cancer Center
Duarte, California, USA

An Liu, PhD, DABMP
Department of Radiation Oncology
City of Hope Cancer Center
Duarte, California, USA

Chapter 22E

Loren K. Mell, MD
Department of Radiation Oncology
University of California San Diego
La Jolla, California, USA

William Y. Song, PhD
Department of Radiation Oncology
University of California San Diego
La Jolla, California, USA

Chapter 23

Thomas E. Merchant, PhD
Division of Radiation Oncology
St. Jude Children's Research Hospital
Memphis, Tennessee, USA

Chris Beltran, PhD
Division of Radiation Oncology
St. Jude Children's Research Hospital
Memphis, Tennessee, USA

Chapter 23A

Joshua D. Lawson, MD
Department of Radiation Oncology
University of California San Diego
La Jolla, California, USA

Jia-Zhu Wang, PhD
Department of Radiation Oncology
University of California San Diego
La Jolla, California, USA

Kevin Murphy, MD
Department of Radiation Oncology
University of California San Diego
La Jolla, California, USA

Chapter 23B

Natia Esiashvili, MD
Department of Radiation Oncology
Emory University
Atlanta, Georgia, USA

Timothy Fox, PhD
Department of Radiation Oncology
Emory University
Atlanta, Georgia, USA

Chapter 24

Kyle Rusthoven, MD
Department of Radiation Oncology
University of Colorado
Aurora, Colorado, USA

Brian D. Kavanagh, MD, MPH
Department of Radiation Oncology
University of Colorado
Aurora, Colorado, USA

Chapter 24A

Francesco Fiorica, MD, PhD
Department of Radiation Oncology
University Hospital
Ferrara, Italy

Francesco Cartei, MD
Department of Radiation Oncology
University Hospital
Ferrara, Italy

Stefano Ursino, MD
Department of Radiation Oncology
University Hospital
Ferrara, Italy

Sara Lappi, PhD
Department of Medical Physics
University Hospital
Ferrara, Italy

Sara Fabbri, PhD
Department of Medical Physics
University Hospital
Ferrara, Italy

Chapter 24B

Joshua D. Lawson, MD
Department of Radiation Oncology
University of California San Diego
La Jolla, California, USA

Sameer K. Nath, MD
Department of Radiation Oncology
University of California San Diego
La Jolla, California, USA

Jia-Zhu Wang, PhD
Department of Radiation Oncology
University of California San Diego
La Jolla, California, USA

Kevin Murphy, MD
Department of Radiation Oncology
University of California San Diego
La Jolla, California, USA

Chapter 24C

Dev R. Puri MD
Department of Radiation Oncology
Memorial Sloan Kettering Cancer Center
New York, New York, USA

Oren Cahlon MD
Department of Radiation Oncology
Memorial Sloan Kettering Cancer Center
New York, New York, USA

Mark H. Bilsky MD
Department of Neurosurgery
Memorial Sloan Kettering Cancer Center
New York, New York, USA

Yoshiya Yamada, MD, FRCPC
Department of Radiation Oncology
Memorial Sloan Kettering Cancer Center
New York, New York, USA

Chapter 24D

Peter C. Gerszten, MD, MPH, FACS
Departments of Neurological Surgery and Radiation Oncology
University of Pittsburgh
Pittsburgh, USA

Steven A. Burton, MD
Department of Radiation Oncology
University of Pittsburgh
Pittsburgh, Pennsylvania, USA

Cihat Ozhasoglu, PhD
Department of Radiation Oncology
University of Pittsburgh
Pittsburgh, Pennsylvania, USA

Chapter 24E

Quynh-Nhu Nguyen, MD
Department of Radiation Oncology
M.D. Anderson Cancer Center
University of Texas
Houston, Texas, USA

Almon S. Shiu, PhD
Department of Radiation Physics
M.D. Anderson Cancer Center
University of Texas,
Houston, Texas, USA

Eric L. Chang, MD
Department of Radiation Oncology
M.D. Anderson Cancer Center
University of Texas
Houston, Texas, USA

Chapter 24F

Chul-Seung Kay, MD
Department of Radiation Oncology
The Catholic University of Korea
Incheon, South Korea

Ji-Yoon Kim, MD
Department of Radiation Oncology
The Catholic University of Korea
Incheon, South Korea

Young-Nam Kang, PhD
Department of Radiation Oncology
The Catholic University of Korea
Seoul, South Korea

Chapter 24G

Fahed Fayad, MD
Cyberknife Center of Miami.
University of Miami
Miami, Florida, USA

William T. Brown, MD
Cyberknife Center of Miami
University of Miami
Miami, Florida, USA

James M. Hevezi, PhD
Cyberknife Center of Miami
University of Miami
Miami, Florida, USA

Xiadong Wu, PhD
Department of Radiology
University of Miami
Miami, Florida, USA

Irene Monterroso, MS
Cyberknife Center of Miami
University of Miami Hospital
Miami, Florida, USA

James G. Schwade, MD
Cyberknife Center of Miami
University of Miami Hospital
Miami, Florida, USA

Chapter 24H

Alan W. Katz, MD, MPH
Department of Radiation Oncology
University of Rochester
Rochester, New York, USA

Praveena Cheruvu, MD
Department of Radiation Oncology
University of Rochester
Rochester, New York, USA

Michael C. Schell, PhD
Department of Radiation Oncology
University of Rochester
Rochester, New York, USA

Abraham Philip, CMD RT(T)
Department of Radiation Oncology
University of Rochester
Rochester, New York, USA

Michael T. Milano, MD, PhD
Department of Radiation Oncology
University of Rochester
Rochester, New York, USA

Chapter 24I

Christopher F. Serago, PhD
Department of Radiation Oncology
Mayo Clinic
Jacksonville, Florida, USA

Laura A. Vallow, MD
Department of Radiation Oncology
Mayo Clinic
Jacksonville, Florida, USA

Ricardo Paz-Fumagalli, MD
Department of Radiology
Mayo Clinic
Jacksonville, Florida, USA

Siyong Kim, PhD
Department of Radiation Oncology
Mayo Clinic
Jacksonville, Florida, USA

Ashley A. Gale, MS
Department of Radiation Oncology
Mayo Clinic
Jacksonville, Florida, USA

Wilza L. Magalhaes, CMD
Department of Radiation Oncology
Mayo Clinic
Jacksonville, Florida, USA

Chapter 24J

Franco Casamassima, MD, PhD
U.O. Clinical Radiobiology
University of Florence
Florence, Italy

Laura Masi, PhD
U.O. Clinical Radiobiology
University of Florence
Florence, Italy

Katia Pasciuti, PhD
U.O. Clinical Radiobiology
University of Florence
Florence, Italy

Claudia Menichelli, MD
U.O. Clinical Radiobiology
University of Florence
Florence, Italy

I. Bonucci, MD
U.O. Clinical Radiobiology
University of Florence
Florence, Italy

Raffaella Doro, PhD
U.O. Clinical Radiobiology
University of Florence
Florence, Italy

Elena D'Imporzano, MD
U.O. Clinical Radiobiology
University of Florence
Florence, Italy

Chapter 24K

Hiroshi Onishi, MD
Department of Radiology
Yamanashi University
Yamanashi, Japan

Masayuki Araya, MD
Department of Radiology
Yamanashi University
Yamanashi, Japan

Kan Marino, MD
Department of Radiology
Yamanashi University
Yamanashi, Japan

Takafumi Komyama M.D
Department of Radiology
Yamanashi University
Yamanashi, Japan

Kengo Kuriyama, MD
Department of Radiology
Yamanashi University
Yamanashi, Japan

Ryo Saito MD
Department of Radiology
Yamanashi University
Yamanashi, Japan

Shinichi Aoki, MD
Department of Radiology
Yamanashi University
Yamanashi, Japan

Yoshiyasu Maehata, MD
Department of Radiology
Yamanashi University
Yamanashi, Japan

Tsutomu Araki, MD
Department of Radiology
Yamanashi University
Yamanashi, Japan

Chapter 25

Daniel R. Simpson, MD
Department of Radiation Oncology
University of California San Diego
La Jolla, California, USA

Sameer K. Nath, MD
Department of Radiation Oncology
University of California San Diego
La Jolla, California, USA

Brent S. Rose, MD
Department of Radiation Oncology
University of California San Diego
La Jolla, California, USA

Loren K. Mell, MD
Department of Radiation Oncology
University of California San Diego
La Jolla, California, USA

Joshua D. Lawson, MD
Department of Radiation Oncology
University of California San Diego
La Jolla, California, USA

Arno J. Mundt, MD
Department of Radiation Oncology
University of California San Diego
La Jolla, California, USA

Chapter 26

Matthew A. Quinn, PhD
Department of Radiation Oncology
Loyola University
Chicago, Illinois, USA

John Roeske, PhD
Department of Radiation Oncology
Loyola University
Chicago, Illinois, USA

Chapter 27

Andre Konski, MD, MBA
Department of Radiation Oncology
Fox Chase Cancer Center
Philadelphia, Pennsylvania, USA

Chapter 28

Bahman Emami, MD
Department of Radiation Oncology
Loyola University
Chicago, Illinois, USA

PREFACE

It was not long after the publication of our first dedicated radiation technology textbook entitled *Intensity Modulated Radiation Therapy: A Clinical Perspective* that we realized that a new technologic revolution was sweeping through the field of radiation oncology. Unlike IMRT, this new revolution of image-guided radiotherapy (IGRT) was quite long in coming, with roots stretching back to the early years of the last century. However, today IGRT permeates nearly every aspect of radiation treatment planning and delivery.

We naturally began to explore the idea of a new comprehensive dedicated textbook focusing on IGRT. In the spirit of our earlier IMRT textbook, we wanted a different type of textbook, one conveying both the "why" and the "how, the art and the science of IGRT. It is our sincere hope that *Image Guided Radiation Therapy: A Clinical Perspective* has achieved these goals.

This text is divided into five separate (but inter-related) parts. The *Introduction* provides an overview of the basic concepts of IGRT and includes a review of its history and present status. *Image-Guided Target Delineation Technologies* presents an in-depth overview of the main imaging modalities used for target delineation, namely computed tomography (CT) including 4-dimensional (4D) CT, magnetic resonance (MR) imaging, and positron emission tomography (PET). *Image Guided Treatment Technologies* systemically introduces the reader to the major in-room IGRT treatment technologies available today, including video, ultrasound, planar, and volumetric-based imaging systems. In addition, overviews of electromagnetic tracking, quality assurance in the IGRT era, and a variety of emerging in-room imaging systems are presented. Organized anatomically, *Clinical Sites and Case Studies* is a comprehensive overview of the clinical applications of IGRT. Within each section, traditional overview chapters are paired with case studies of *actual* treated patients, focusing on image-guided target delineation and image-guided treatment delivery. An effort was made to include not only a wide variety of imaging modalities used for augmenting target delineation but also all the major com-

mercial in-room IGRT systems used in these cases, illustrating their unique features. Selected topics, including adaptive IGRT and the economics of IGRT, are discussed in the *Commentaries* section.

From its conception, it has been our sincere wish to produce a textbook illustrating the depth and breadth of this exciting technology. While some may feel strongly that IGRT *only* refers to in-room imaging technologies, we instead chose to adopt a broader definition which includes the use of sophisticated imaging to augment target and normal tissue delineation. Our goal was to provide an overview of the current level of knowledge in the field in a format accessible to a wide variety of individuals involved in IGRT planning and treatment, including radiation oncologists, medical physicists, radiation therapists and administrators, as well as students and residents.

It was never our intention to produce a textbook focusing on the viewpoint of a single institution or the use of one particular IGRT system. We thus solicited contributors from a wide variety of institutions (both academic and private) with experience in a myriad of IGRT systems and approaches. We also desired to highlight the international flavor of IGRT by including experts from around the globe. In all, there are over 250 contributors from 18 countries, including Argentina, Australia, Austria, Belgium, Canada, China, Denmark, Germany, Greece, Italy, Japan, Korea, Netherlands, Spain, Switzerland, Taiwan, United Kingdom, and the United States. From the United States alone, there are over 157 contributors from 46 institutions, including many of the major cancer centers performing IGRT research.

Such a project as this clearly could not have been accomplished without the help of many individuals. Our gratitude is extended to the many authors who contributed case studies of patients treated in their clinics. We wish to thank the wonderful staff at PMPH including Martin Wonsiewicz and Jason Malley. A special thanks goes out to our project manager, Christine Dodd, for her great attention to detail. Barbara Hanks also deserves recognition for her wonderful secretarial support. Finally, we are truly appreciative to our students, residents, colleagues, and families for their encouragement and endless patience with us over these last two years.

We are extremely pleased with the final product and sincerely hope that it will not only meet the needs of our readers but also contribute to the advancement of the field of radiation oncology as a whole.

Arno J, Mundt, MD
University of California San Diego

John C. Roeske, PhD
Loyola University Medical Center
December 2010

Contents

Chapter 1

Overview

Arno J. Mundt, MD, John C. Roeske, PhD

Image-guided radiation therapy (IGRT) is one of the most popular "buzz words" in radiation oncology today. In almost every new issue of the *International Journal of Radiation Oncology, Biology and Physics* and other academic radiation oncology publications, one finds multiple IGRT articles. Numerous vendors are also promoting an ever-increasing array of novel IGRT technologies. Societies such as the American Society for Radiation Oncology (ASTRO), American College of Radiation Oncology (ACRO), and the American Association of Physicists in Medicine (AAPM) among others all currently offer IGRT symposia and practicums, well attended by physicians and physicists alike.[1,2] Many such professional societies are also releasing position papers and guidelines focusing on IGRT.[3,4]

Despite all this enthusiasm, little consensus exists regarding nearly all aspects of IGRT including its very definition. This is not surprising for the term *image-guided* is itself relatively vague and noninformative, as radiation therapy (RT) has from its inception been guided by images. Various definitions for IGRT can be proposed. A global definition might include *any* aspect of RT involving imaging, including fluoroscopic simulation and port films. However, if asked, most radiation oncologists and medical physicists will typically give a relatively narrow definition of IGRT. Some focus on the use of sophisticated imaging, such as ^{18}F-fluorodeoxyglucose (^{18}F-FDG) positron emission tomography (PET), to guide target delineation. Others choose to focus solely on in-room technologies, such as ultrasound or planar imaging. Others may highlight only select in-room technologies that provide volumetric information, such as megavoltage (MV) computed tomography (CT) or cone beam CT (CBCT).

How should IGRT be defined? Our opinion is that its definition should include *both* major aspects of imaging currently used in modern RT, namely advanced imaging to augment target delineation *and* in-room imaging to optimize patient setup and target localization. In many ways, these two aspects, albeit different, represent two sides of the same coin. Focusing solely on image-guided

target delineation would ignore the revolution occurring as a result of in-room imaging. Conversely, focusing only on in-room imaging would ignore important advancements in treatment planning simply because imaging was performed outside the treatment room. Perhaps these distinctions will become less relevant in the coming years with the development and eventual implementation of novel in-room IGRT technologies, e.g., systems incorporating magnetic resonance (MR) imaging, PET, and even single photon emission CT (SPECT).

For the purposes of this text, we define IGRT as the use of:

(1) advanced imaging modalities, especially those incorporating functional and/or biological information, to augment target and normal tissue delineation; and

(2) in-room imaging to adjust for target motion or positional uncertainty (interfractional and intrafractional), and, potentially, to adapt treatment to tumor response.

All in-room IGRT approaches are included which, for the purposes of this discussion, can be divided into four broad categories, namely ultrasound, video, planar, and volumetric imaging. A summary of the available commercial in-room IGRT systems along with their manufacturers is shown in Table 1-1.

Our *bipartite* definition is reflected throughout this book in which equal weighting is given, whenever possible, to image-guided target delineation and image-guided treatment delivery. This is particularly true in the Clinical Topics and Case Studies where overview chapters are paired with case studies highlighting the use of advanced imaging to augment target delineation and also those illustrating in-room imaging to augment patient setup and target localization.

Historical Perspective

Despite the growing enthusiasm for IGRT in recent years, it is important to recognize that IGRT is not new. In fact, it has now been more than a quarter century since the

TABLE 1–1 In-Room Image-Guided Radiation Therapy (IGRT) Technologies

Product	Vendor	Web Site
Ultrasound-based		
BAT	North American Scientific	http://www.nasmedical.com
SonArray	Varian Oncology Systems	http://www.varian.com
I-Beam	CMS	http://www.cms-stl.com
Restitu	Resonant Medical	http://www.resonantmedical.com
Video-based		
AlignRT	Vision RT	http://www.visionrt.com
Planar imaging-based		
Electronic portal imaging devices		
iView	Elekta	http://www.elekta.com
BeamView	Siemens	http://www.siemens.com
PortalVision	Varian	http://www.varian.com
Cyberknife	Accuracy	http://accuracy.com
Novalis	BrainLab Inc	http://www.brainlab.com
RTRT	Mitsubishi Electronics	http://global.mitsubishielectric.com
Gantry-mounted systems		
OBI	Varian	http://www.varian.com
	Elekta	http://www.elekta.com
Volumetric imaging-based		
Linac-CT systems		
FOCAL	Mitsubishi Electric	http://global.mitsubishielectric.com
Smart Gantry	GE-Yokogawa Medical	http://www.gehealthcare.co.jp
ExaCT	Varian Oncology Systems	http://www.varian.com
Primatom	Siemens	http://www.medical.siemens.com
Helical tomotherapy	Tomotherapy Inc.	http://www.tomotherapy.com
Cone-beam CT	OBI System	http://www.varian.com
	Synergy	http://www.elekta.com
	In-Line	http://www.siemens.medical.com
Cobalt-MR	ViewRay	http://www.viewray.com

Notes. CT = computed tomography; MR = magnetic resonance.

publication of *The Imaging Revolution and Radiation Oncology* by Eli Glatstein and colleagues, an insightful and prescient look into the (then) present and future use of imaging in radiation oncology, including the newly introduced approach of MR.[5] However, image guidance has been used in some form or another for more than a century by radiotherapists for target delineation and treatment delivery.

Image-Guided Target Delineation

Imaging has long been used to delineate and localize tumors that could not be seen or palpated. The mainstay of image guidance in the early years of RT were plain films ("roentgenograms") (Figure 1-1).[6–9] In patients with brain tumors, for example, such films were used to localize brain tumors by identifying areas of bony erosion and calcifications.[10] Oral and other contrast agents were commonly used to increase the sensitivity of plain films for localizing a variety of tumors, including esophageal,[11] kidney,[12] and lung[13] cancers. Interestingly, a popular "contrast" agent was air (Figure 1-2),[14,15] with pneumoencephalography occupying an important role in the localization of central nervous system (CNS) tumors, often

combined with plain films and electroencephalography (EEG),[16] well into the 1970s.[17]

Following World War II, a variety of specialized imaging approaches became increasingly incorporated into RT treatment planning. One of the most popular was lymphangiography for patients with Hodgkin's disease[18] as well as those with other tumors including ovarian,[19] testicular,[20] and cervical[21] cancers (Figure 1-3). Angiography was used in the treatment planning of arteriovenous malformations and primary CNS tumors.[16] Ultrasound was incorporated into the treatment planning of various tumor sites (Figures 1-4 and 1-5).[22–24]

Arguably one of the most important milestones in the history of IGRT was the introduction of CT in the 1970s.[25–27] By today's standards, the quality of early CT scans was extremely poor, but their inherent value in providing direct visualization of deep-seated tumors as well as normal tissues was quickly recognized. Over the subsequent decade, numerous reports using CT-based treatment planning began appearing in the literature in a wide variety of tumor sites including CNS tumors,[28] prostate cancer,[29,30] and lung cancer.[31] As described in Chapter 2, CT simulation is now the mainstay (and often

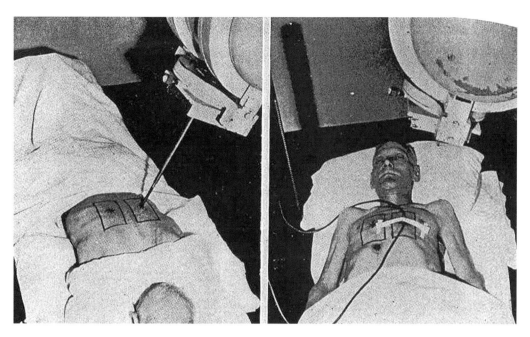

FIGURE 1-1. A patient with esophageal cancer treated on a million-volt roentgen-ray machine, Memorial Hospital, New York (1943). Portals were outlined and the direction of the beams determined by using roentgenograms. Reproduced with permission from Watson WL, et al.[9]

the sole method) of treatment planning in many clinics. Growing interest is also focused on newer CT approaches, notably four-dimensional (4D) CT-based treatment planning in patients with lung cancer (Chapter 17E).[32,33]

The 1980s witnessed the next major milestone in the history of IGRT: the introduction of MR imaging.[34,35] As with CT the decade before, the value of MR-guided

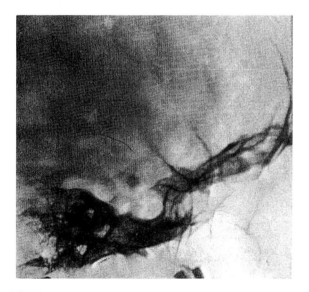

FIGURE 1-2. Pneumoencephalogram in a patient with a brain tumor, Massachusetts General Hospital, Boston (1921). On plain films, an area of calcification was seen. However, the pneumoencephalogram confirms the presence of a mass superior to the mastoid region. Reproduced with permission from Merrill S, et al.[15]

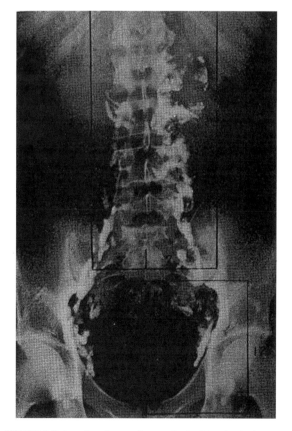

FIGURE 1-3. Lymphangiogram in a patient with a testicular terato-carcinoma involving the paraortic and iliac lymph nodes, Walter Reed Hospital, Washington, DC (1972). The radiation treatment portals based on this image are shown in black. Reproduced with permission from Maier JG et al.[20]

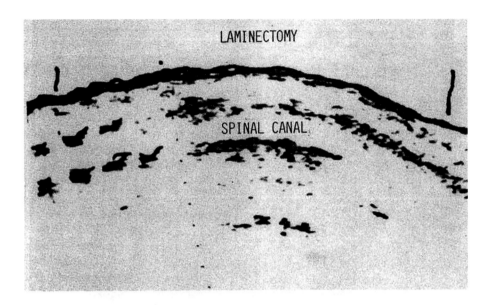

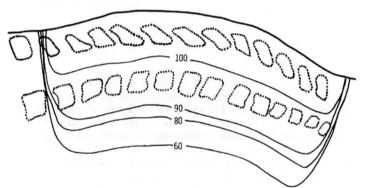

FIGURE 1-4. Localization of the spinal cord with ultrasound in a patient treated following laminectomy. The anterior and posterior margins of the spinal canal are discernible as two continuous lines of echoes. On the left, the spinal canal is seen at points of transmission between the normal neural arches. Isodose contours for a 25 MeV electron beam are shown below. Reproduced with permission from Carson PL et al.[22]

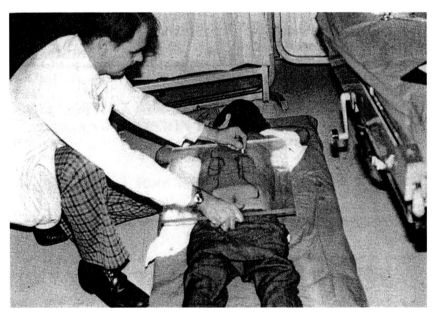

FIGURE 1-5. In a pediatric Hodgkin's disease patient undergoing definitive irradiation, ultrasound is used to localize the kidneys ensuring proper placement of posterior cerrobend blocks during treatment. After the position of the kidneys has been marked on the skin, a transparent plexiglass template is positioned directly against the back of the patient, and the marks are transferred to the plexiglass. Reproduced with permission from Brascho DJ et al.[23]

treatment planning was quickly realized.[36] Today, MR is routinely used in the planning of patients with tumors in the brain and other sites, notably the paranasal sinuses and nasopharynx.[37,38] Magnetic resonance–based treatment planning is also of value in patients with prostate[39] and cervical[40] cancers. Newer MR approaches, notably MR spectroscopy (MRS), provide potentially valuable information in the planning of a variety of tumors.[41,42] See Chapter 4 for an overview of the use of MR in RT treatment planning and Chapters 15B, 15C, 16B, 19B, 20A, 21A, 21D, and 22C for case studies highlighting MR-guided target delineation.

Over the past decade, several novel imaging approaches have been introduced to augment target delineation in patients undergoing RT. ^{18}F-FDG PET and PET/CT imaging have received the most attention and are now routinely used for RT planning in many disease sites, including head and neck cancers,[43] cervical cancers,[44] and lung cancers.[45] Increasing attention is also focused on a number of novel PET tracers.[46,47] An overview of PET-based treatment planning in RT is provided in Chapter 3. See also Chapters 15A, 15C, 16A, 16C, 16D, 17A, 19A, 21B, 21C, 22A, and 22B for case studies highlighting PET-guided target delineation.

Image-Guided Treatment Delivery

The use of in-room imaging technologies to augment patient setup and target localization also has a surprisingly long history. One of the earliest in-room systems was a Cobalt-60 unit paired with an in-room kV imager developed at the Karolinska Institute in the late 1950s (Figure 1-6). At the same time, investigators at the Princess Margaret Hospital in Toronto described their own Cobalt-60 system equipped with kV imaging (Figure 1-7).[48] Another Cobalt system was developed at the Netherlands Cancer

Institute in Amsterdam in the early 1960s (Figure 1-8). Despite this initial enthusiasm, as centers throughout the world moved away from Cobalt to modern linear accelerators, integrated imaging–treatment systems were not developed until the 1990s.

In the 1970s, interest in IGRT arose again, this time focused on video-based systems. Connor and colleagues at the University of Arizona described a video cancellation system for patient repositioning and motion detection.[49] Utilizing live images from a closed-circuit television camera and a stored image on a videodisc, this system could detect repositioning errors and patient movements on the order of a millimeter. As described in Chapter 6, others subsequently developed similar in-room video-based techniques to augment patient setup (Figure 1-9).[50] See Chapters 16H and 18D for case studies illustrating video-based setup in head and neck tumors and breast cancers.

Another important development in the history of IGRT was the introduction of ultrasound-based systems in the mid-1990s. Although enthusiasm quickly became focused on prostate cancer,[51] ultrasound-guidance has been shown to have applications to other tumor sites including breast cancer,[52] gynecologic tumors,[53] and upper abdominal tumors (Figure 1-10).[54] Multiple vendors have developed ultrasound-based systems over the years (Table 1-1). See Chapter 5 for a description of ultrasound-based in-room IGRT systems and Chapters 18A, 20C, 21E, and 21G for case studies highlighting ultrasound-based patient setup and target localization approaches.

The 1990s also witnessed the introduction of a wide array of planar imaging-based in-room IGRT systems. One of the first, and to this day most popular, was electronic portal imaging (EPI). As discussed in Chapter 7, EPI devices (EPIDs) can be used to provide on-line

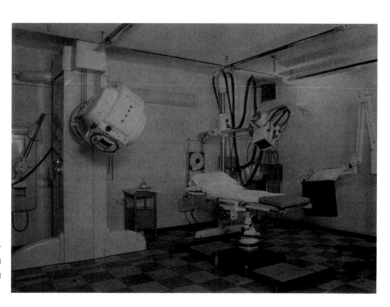

FIGURE 1-6. Early Cobalt-60 unit with in-room kilovoltage (kV) x-ray capability for patient setup. Karolinska University, Stockholm, Sweden (1957). Reproduced with permission.

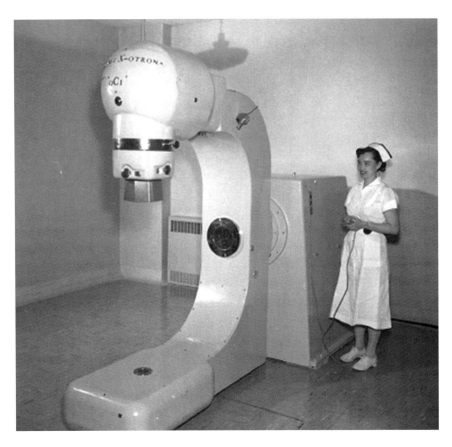

FIGURE 1-7. Integrated Cobalt-60 and in-room kilovoltage (kV) imaging system. Princess Margaret Hospital, Toronto (1959). Reproduced with permission from Johns HE et al.[48]

image-guidance based on alignment of bony landmarks[55] or implanted fiducial markers[56] using the MV treatment beam (see Chapters 16E, 20D, and 24I). More recently, multiple in-room and gantry-mounted kV-planar IGRT systems have been developed that generate higher quality images with less dose to the patient. These systems

are reviewed in Chapter 9. See Chapters 21H and 23B for case studies illustrating the use of gantry-mounted kV planar-imaging IGRT systems for patient setup and target localization.

Several commercial in-room kV planar imaging IGRT systems have been developed in recent years that provide

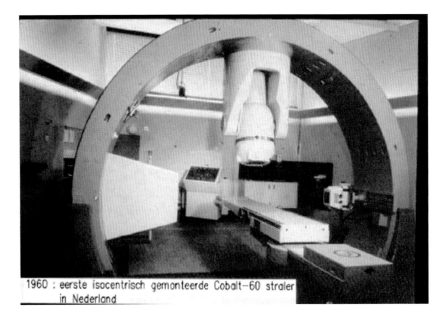

FIGURE 1-8. Integrated Cobalt-60 and in-room kilovoltage (kV) imaging system developed at the Netherlands Cancer Institute, Amsterdam, the Netherlands (1961). A Cobalt-60 treatment head, a small 120-kV diagnostic x-ray unit, an image intensifier coupled to a vidicon camera, and a counter-weight (that also acts as a protection shield) are attached to the inner surface of the ring. Reproduced with permission.

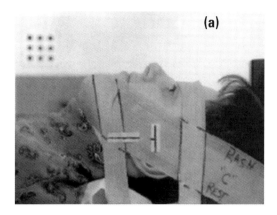
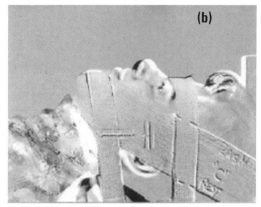
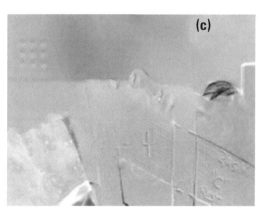

FIGURE 1-9. Clinical use of a video-based patient setup procedure. (a) Reference images acquired on the first day of treatment after physician approval of portal images. On subsequent treatment days, the reference images are retrieved from the image archive and subtracted in real-time from the live video (b). With the aid of a computer monitor in the treatment room, therapists use the live subtraction images to interactively return the patient to the initial position (c). Reproduced with permission from Johnson S et al.[49]

near real-time image-guidance. Adler and colleagues at Stanford University described the Cyberknife (Accuray Inc, Sunnyvale, CA,) in the early 1990s. This novel system consisted of a compact 6-MV linear accelerator mounted on a robotic arm paired with two floor- and ceiling-mounted kV images and detectors.[57] The Novalis system (BrainLAB, Feldkirchen, Germany) was developed later and is comprised of both stereoscopic kV x-ray imagers and infrared cameras for patient positioning and monitoring.[58] The Real-Time Tumor Tracking system (Mitsubishi Electronics Ltd, Tokyo, Japan) consists of four sets of floor- and ceiling-mounted x-ray tubes and imagers that are used to track an implanted fiducial marker and gate the treatment beam when the position of the marker coincides with its planned position.[59] An overview of these and other kV planar-based IGRT systems is provided in Chapter 9. See also Chapters 15D, 15E, 17B, 19D, 19E, 20E, 20F, 24D, 24G, and 24H for case studies focusing on the use of these systems in patients with a variety of tumor sites.

Arguably the most important development in the recent history of IGRT was the introduction of in-room volumetric IGRT systems over the past decade. An early prototype utilizing the MV treatment beam was described in 1982,[60] and commercial systems have been developed utilizing MV[61,62] and, more recently, kV[63–65] imaging. All of the major vendors currently offer volumetric in-room IGRT solutions (Table 1-1). An overview of the available

kV and MV in-room volumetric IGRT systems are provided in Chapters 9 and 10, respectively. See Chapters 16F, 18B, 20G, 20I, 22D, and 24F for case studies highlighting MV volumetric in-room imaging and Chapters 16G, 17D, 17E, 18C, 18E, 20J, 21H, 22E, 24A, 24E, 24J, and 24K for case studies illustrating kV volumetric IGRT techniques.

The evolution of in-room IGRT continues. Numerous investigators are currently exploring a variety of innovative in-room approaches, notably integrated linac-SPECT,[66] linac-MR,[67] and even Cobalt-MR[68] systems, several of which may open the door to true real-time image-guidance. As noted earlier, integration of imaging approaches traditionally performed outside the treatment room may help blur the line between image-guided target delineation and image-guided treatment delivery. These emerging in-room IGRT systems are reviewed in detail in Chapter 13.

Current Status of IGRT

Despite the considerable interest in IGRT, its prevalence and use in the general radiation oncology community remains unclear. In conjunction with our earlier IMRT textbook, we performed a series of nationwide surveys assessing IMRT use.[69,70] We felt it was thus appropriate to perform a similar survey in IGRT as we neared completion of this new textbook. Sent to 1600 radiation oncologists

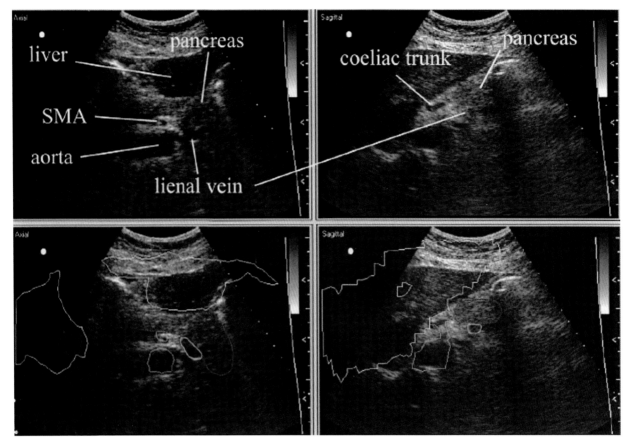

FIGURE 1-10. (Upper) axial and sagittal ultrasound images labeled with anatomically appreciated structures and (lower) with superimposed computed tomography–derived structures after ultrasound acquisition. Note the pancreas outlines in red to better delineate the organ in its positional relation to guidance structures. Reproduced with permission from Fuss M et al.[54]

in the spring of 2009, the survey results were subsequently published in two separate reports: one focusing on image-guided target delineation,[71] the other on image-guided treatment delivery.[72] The overall response rate was 36%, with respondents from 45 states and the District of Columbia, representing academic and private practice physicians alike.

In terms of image-guided target delineation, 94.3% of respondents reported using at least one advanced imaging modality (conventional CT was excluded because of its widespread use). The majority (72.6%) reported, however, using such technologies only rarely or infrequently. The most commonly used technologies were ^{18}F-FDG PET (76%), MR (72%), and 4DCT (44%). The most commonly treated sites were lung (83%), CNS (79%), and head and neck (79%) tumors (Table 1-2). Overall, no difference in the frequency of IGRT use was observed between academic and private physicians (94.7 vs 95.1%, P = .88); however, academics were more likely to use 4DCT, functional MR, and MRS.

Regarding in-room IGRT technologies, 93.5% of respondents reported using some type of in-room imaging. However, most (62%) reported using these technolo-

gies only rarely or infrequently. Nonetheless, nearly 20% reported using in-room IGRT in greater than 75% of their patients.

A wide variety of in-room IGRT technologies were used, with the three most common modalities being MV planar (62.7%), kV planar (57.7%), and volumetric-based approaches (58.8%). The most common disease sites treated were genitourinary (91.1%), head and neck (74.2%), CNS (71.9%), and lung (66.9%) (Table 1-2). Volumetric imaging was most commonly used in patients with lung (59%), head and neck (57%), gastrointestinal (57%), and genitourinary (55%) tumors; kV planar technologies were most commonly used in CNS (63%) tumors. No difference in in-room IGRT use was observed between academic and private practice physicians (94.7 vs 94.8%; P=.78); however, academics were more likely to utilize volumetric imaging and kV planar techniques compared with those in private practice. In addition, academic physicians were more likely to use in-room IGRT technologies frequently (47.5 vs 31.8%, P<.01).

Taken together, these surveys provide a valuable glimpse into the current practice of IGRT (for target delineation and treatment delivery) in the United States.

TABLE 1–2 Use of Image-Guided Target Delineation and Treatment Delivery Technologies: Survey of Practicing American Radiation Oncologists

	CNS, %	H/N, %	Lung, %	Breast, %	GI, %	GYN, %	GU, %	L/L, %	Ped, %
Target delineation									
All modalities	79	80	83	20	53	46	44	56	14
MR	68	37	4	4	7	18	33	4	11
^{18}F-FDG PET	15	3	68	10	40	33	8	47	8
4DCT	2	4	37	5	17	3	3	3	2
Treatment delivery									
All modalities	72	74	67	44	60	58	91	40	24
Video	1	1	0	2	1	1	1	0	1
Ultrasound	0	0	0	2	1	2	23	0	0
MV planar	32	33	30	26	27	27	43	22	11
kV planar	42	37	35	17	28	26	42	17	0
Volumetric	35	38	37	12	33	27	45	15	12

Note. Percentages rounded. ^{18}F-FDG PET = ^{18}F-fluorodeoxyglucose positron emission tomography; 4DCT = four-dimensional computed tomography; CNS = central nervous system (brain); H/N = head and neck; GI = gastrointestinal; GYN = gynecological; GU = genitourinary; kV = kilovoltage; L/L = leukemia and lymphoma; MR = magnetic resonance; MV = megavoltage; Ped = pediatrics. Modified from Simpson DR et al.[70] and Simpson DR et al.[72]

However, it is truly only a snapshot, for it is likely that many (if not all) of these results will change in the coming years as new technologies are introduced and clinical studies are published evaluating the benefits and risks of various approaches.

Numerous interesting and important questions about IGRT were unfortunately not addressed by these surveys, notably the prevalence of IGRT use outside the United States, the motivations for adopting IGRT, the impact IGRT has on clinical practice and patient outcomes, and the quality assurance procedures used for each modality. Moreover, the concept and practice of adaptive IGRT (see "Future Directions" at the end of this chapter) was not addressed. It is hoped that future surveys will help shed light on these and other important questions.

Growing Importance of IGRT

Although it has always been important to accurately delineate and localize targets in patients undergoing RT, the importance of IGRT has increased tremendously in recent years. A major reason for this is the increasing popularity and widespread use of IMRT.[69,70] Unlike conventional techniques, IMRT results in steep dose gradients outside the target tissues requiring a high degree of accuracy during both treatment planning and delivery. IMRT has also provided radiation oncologists with the ability to "dose paint," delivering higher-than-conventional doses to select subregions within the target.[73,74] Such sophisticated approaches can only be fully exploited if these subregions can be precisely indentified during planning and accurately localized during treatment delivery.

Perhaps an even greater impetus for adopting IGRT is the growing interest in stereotactic body radiotherapy (SBRT), whereby high doses are delivered to small to moderate targets throughout the body over a limited number (five or fewer) of high-dose fractions.[75] Various SBRT regimens have become increasingly popular in recent years, many of which utilize previously unimaginable fraction sizes. The latest Radiation Therapy Oncology Group (RTOG) trial of lung SBRT, for example, is exploring 34 Gy in a single fraction. The implementation of such regimens requires not only accurate target delineation but also precise treatment delivery and target localization, if favorable results are to be achieved and the risk of serious adverse sequelae minimized.

A final impetus for IGRT adoption is the increasing importance of minimizing normal tissue toxicities. If current combined chemoradiotherapy approaches are to be further intensified, it is imperative that normal tissues be further spared. Novel imaging approaches not only open the door to better defining tumors (and their subregions), but also to better defining surrounding normal tissues. In fact, novel imaging can be used to identify subregions within normal tissues that may be critical to spare using inverse planning. Examples include highly ventilated regions of the lung in patients with thoracic tumors[76] and hematopoietically active bone marrow sites within the pelvis in patients undergoing pelvic RT and chemotherapy (see Chapter 21D).[77] More such approaches are expected in the future, allowing the development of more intensive but isotoxic treatment regimens in high-risk patients.

Future Directions

In the coming years, IGRT will most likely be expanded beyond its current role to include adaptive IGRT, whereby a patient's treatment plan is modified during treatment based on changes in his/her tumor identified by imaging (both inside and out of the treatment role). Today, adaptive IGRT is performed almost exclusively at select academic institutions within prospective clinical trials, but someday it will most likely be used in the wider radiation oncology community.

Before the routine clinical implementation of adaptive IGRT, however, a host of technical obstacles must first be overcome, including the development of novel deformable image registration algorithms and automated segmentation approaches. Another important obstacle is the time required for the performance of these and other applications, a particular concern when adaptation is to be performed on-line with the patient on the treatment couch. Rapid and effective tools, however, are also needed to allow the widespread implementation of off-line adaptive strategies, particularly if multiple new plans are to be generated. And once such hurdles are overcome, clinical trials are needed to assess the benefits and potential risks of adaptive IGRT.

Fittingly, two of the final chapters of this book are dedicated to adaptive IGRT. Chapter 25 is written from the physician's perspective and focuses on the "why" of adaptive IGRT with a review of the various morphologic and functional changes occurring in tumors and normal tissues throughout treatment. Written from the physicist's perspective, Chapter 26 explores the "how" of adaptive RT with an overview of the technical obstacles that must be overcome and their potential solutions.

References

1. http://www.astro.org. Accessed 17 November 2010.

2. http://www.aapm.org/. Accessed 17 November 2010.

3. Potters L, Gaspar LE, Kavanagh B, et al. American Society for Therapeutic Radiology and Oncology (ASTRO) and American College of Radiology (ACR) practice guidelines for image-guided radiation therapy (IGRT). *Int J Radiat Oncol Biol Phys.* 2010;76(2):319–325.

4. Korreman S, Rasch C, McNair H, et al. The European Society of Therapeutic Radiology and Oncology-European Institute of Radiotherapy (ESTRO-EIR) report on 3D CT-based in-room image guidance systems: a practical and technical review and guide. *Radiother Oncol.* 2010;94(2):129–144.

5. Glatstein E, Lichter AS, Fraass BA, Kelly BA, van de Geijn J. The imaging revolution and radiation oncology: use of CT, ultrasound, and NMR for localization, treatment planning and treatment delivery. *Int J Radiat Oncol Biol Phys.* 1985;11(2):299–314.

6. Holding AF. Roentgen deep therapy in malignant tumors. *Am J Roentgenol.* 1916;3:191–198.

7. Holding AF. Improved cancer prognosis justified by deep roentgen treatment. *Am J Roentgenol.* 1917;4:183–188.

8. Martin CL, Martin JM. Clinical problems in roentgen therapy of deep seated tumors. *Am J Roentgenol.* 1923;10:818–829.

9. Watson WL, Urban J. Million volt roentgen therapy for intrathoracic cancer: palliative effects in a series of sixty-three cases. *Am J Roentgenol.* 1943;49:299–305.

10. Low-Beer BV, Scofield NE, Feldsted ET, Brown RF. Directed beam therapy. II. Multiple small field irradiation of the pituitary gland, pituitary tumors and other intracranial lesions. *Am J Roentgenol Radium Ther Nucl Med.* 1953;69(6):953–968.

11. Smithers DW, Clarkson JR, Strong JA. The roentgen treatment of cancer of the esophagus. *Am J Roentgenol.* 1943;49:606–627.

12. Waters CA. Preoperative irradiation of cortical renal tumors. *Am J Roentgenol.* 1935;33:149–159.

13. Sparks JV. The use of lipiodol as an aid to diagnosis in diseases of the chest. *Br J Radiol.* 1928;1:111–121.

14. Sante LR. The detection of retroperitoneal masses by the aid of pneumoperitoneum. *Am J Roentgenol.* 1921;8:129–134.

15. Merrill AS. The diagnosis of a brain tumor by pneumoventriculography. *Am J Roentgenol.* 1921;8:188–192.

16. Hodges FJ, Holt JF, Bassett RC, Lemmen LJ. Reliability of brain tumor localization by roentgen methods. *Am J Roentgenol Radium Ther Nucl Med.* 1954;71(4):624–631.

17. Salazar OM, Rubin P, McDonald JV, Feldstein ML. High dose radiation therapy in the treatment of glioblastoma multiforme: a preliminary report. *Int J Radiat Oncol Biol Phys.* 1976;1(7-8):717–727.

18. Rubin P, Haluska G, Poulter CA. The basis for segmental sequential irradiation in Hodgkin's disease: clinical experience of patterns of recurrence. *Am J Roentgenol Radium Ther Nucl Med.* 1969;105(4):814–829.

19. De Palo G, Lattuada A, Kenda R, et al. Germ cell tumors of the ovary: the experience of the National Cancer Institute of Milan. I. Dysgerminoma. *Int J Radiat Oncol Biol Phys.* 1987;13(6):853–860.

20. Maier JG, Schamber DT. The role of lymphangiography in the diagnosis and treatment of malignant testicular tumors. *Am J Roentgenol Radium Ther Nucl Med.* 1972;114(3):482–491.

21. Emami B, Watring WG, Tak W, Anderson B, Piro AJ. Para-aortic lymph node radiation in advanced cervical cancer. *Int J Radiat Oncol Biol Phys.* 1980;6(9):1237–1241.

22. Carson PL, Wenzel WW, Avery P, Hendee WR. Ultrasound imaging as an aid to cancer therapy-I. *Int J Radiat Oncol Biol Phys.* 1975;1(1-2):119–132.

23. Brascho DJ, Bryan JM, Wilson EE. Diagnostic ultrasound to determine renal size and position for renal blocking in radiation therapy. *Int J Radiat Oncol Biol Phys.* 1977;2(11-12):1217–1220.

24. Kim RY, Brascho DJ, Wilson EE. Use of ultrasound scan in prostatic I-125 implantation. *Int J Radiat Oncol Biol Phys.* 1984;10(10):1971–1973.

25. DeGinder WL, Mistry V. Enhancement of therapeutic ratio in radiotherapy of brain neoplasms. *Am J Roentgenol Radium Ther Nucl Med.* 1975;123(3):459–470.

26. Stewart JR, Hicks JA, Boone ML, Simpson LD. Computed tomography in radiation therapy (report of the Committee on Radiation Oncology Studies Subcommittee on CT Scanning and Radiation Therapy). *Int J Radiat Oncol Biol Phys.* 1978;4(3-4):313–324.

27. Abadir R, Edwards FM, Larsen G. A feasibility study of computerized tomography radiation therapy treatment planning in transverse, coronal and saggital sections. *Int J Radiat Oncol Biol Phys.* 1978;4(11-12):1107–1109.

28. Abrath FG, Henderson SD, Simpson JR, Moran CJ, Marchosky JA. Dosimetry of CT-guided volumetric IR-192 brain implant. *Int J Radiat Oncol Biol Phys.* 1986;12(3):359–363.

29. Forman JD, Wharam MD, Lee DJ, Zinreich ES, Order SE. Definitive radiotherapy following prostatectomy: results and complications. *Int J Radiat Oncol Biol Phys.* 1986;12(2):185–189.

30. Pilepich MV, Perez CA, Prasad S. Computed tomography in definitive radiotherapy of prostatic carcinoma. *Int J Radiat Oncol Biol Phys.* 1980;6:923–926.

31. Van Houtte P, Piron A, Lustman-Maréchal J, Osteaux M, Henry J. Computed axial tomography (CAT) contribution for dosimetry and treatment evaluation in lung cancer. *Int J Radiat Oncol Biol Phys.* 1980;6(8):995–1000.

32. Louie AV, Rodrigues G, Olsthoorn J, et al. Inter-observer and intra-observer reliability for lung cancer target volume delineation in the 4D-CT era. *Radiother Oncol.* 2010;95(2):166–171.

33. Liu HH, Balter P, Tutt T, et al. Assessing respiration-induced tumor motion and internal target volume using four-dimensional computed tomography for radiotherapy of lung cancer. *Int J Radiat Oncol Biol Phys.* 2007;68(2):531–540.

34. Bydder GM, Steiner RE, Yeung IR, et al. Clinical NMR imaging of the brain: 140 cases. *Am J Neuroradiol.* 1982;3:459–480.

35. Alfidi RJ, Haaga JR, El Yousef SJ, et al. Preliminary experimental results in humans and animals with a superconducting whole-body, nuclear magnetic resonance scanner. *Radiology.* 1982;143(1):175–181.

36. Holland BA, Brant-Zawadzki M, Norman D, Newton TH. Magnetic resonance imaging of primary intracranial tumors: a review. *Int J Radiat Oncol Biol Phys.* 1985;11(2):315–321.

37. Liang SB, Sun Y, Liu LZ, et al. Extension of local disease in nasopharyngeal carcinoma detected by magnetic resonance imaging: improvement of clinical target volume delineation. *Int J Radiat Oncol Biol Phys.* 2009;75(3):742–750.

38. Emami B, Sethi A, Petruzzelli GJ. Influence of MRI on target volume delineation and IMRT planning in nasopharyngeal carcinoma. *Int J Radiat Oncol Biol Phys.* 2003;57(2):481–488.

39. Fonteyne V, Villeirs G, Speleers B, et al. Intensity-modulated radiotherapy as primary therapy for prostate cancer: report on acute toxicity after dose escalation with simultaneous integrated boost to intraprostatic lesion. *Int J Radiat Onol Biol Phys.* 2008;72(3):799–807.

40. Dimopoulos JC, De Vos V, Berger D, et al. Inter-observer comparison of target delineation for MRI-assisted cervical cancer brachytherapy: application of the GYN GEC-ESTRO recommendations. *Radiother Oncol.* 2009;91(2):166–172.

41. Chang J, Thakur SB, Huang W, Narayana A, et al. Magnetic resonance spectroscopy imaging (MRSI) and brain functional magnetic resonance imaging (fMRI) for radiotherapy treatment planning of glioma. *Technol Cancer Res Treat.* 2008;7(5):349–362.

42. van Lin EN, Fütterer JJ, Heijmink SW, et al. IMRT boost dose planning on dominant intraprostatic lesions: gold marker-based three-dimensional fusion of CT with dynamic contrast-enhanced and 1H-spectroscopic MRI. *Int J Radiat Oncol Biol Phys.* 2006;65:291–303.

43. Schwartz DL, Ford EC, Rajendran J, et al. FDG-PET/CT-guided intensity modulated head and neck radiotherapy: a pilot investigation. *Head Neck.* 2005;27(6):478–487.

44. Choi CW, Cho CK, Yoo SY, et al. Image-guided stereotactic body radiation therapy in patients with isolated para-aortic lymph node metastases from uterine cervical and corpus cancer. *Int J Radiat Oncol Biol Phys.* 2009;74(1):147–153.

45. Spratt DE, Diaz R, McElmurray J, et al. Impact of FDG PET/CT on delineation of the gross tumor volume for radiation planning in non-small cell lung cancer. *Clin Nucl Med.* 2010;35(4):237–243.

46. Milker-Zabel S, Zabel-du Bois A, Henze M, et al. Improved target volume definition for fractionated stereotactic radiotherapy in patients with intracranial meningiomas by correlation of CT, MRI, and [68Ga]-DOTATOC-PET. *Int J Radiat Oncol Biol Phys.* 2006;65(1):222–227.

47. Seppälä J, Seppänen M, Arponen E, Lindholm P, Minn H. Carbon-11 acetate PET/CT based dose escalated IMRT in prostate cancer. *Radiother Oncol.* 2009;93(2):234–240.

48. Johns HE, Cunningham JR. A precision cobalt 60 unit for fixed field and rotation therapy. *Am J Roentgenol Radium Ther Nucl Med.* 1959;81(1):4–12.

49. Connor WG, Boone ML, Veomett R, et al. Patient repositioning and motion detection using a video cancellation system. *Int J Radiat Oncol Biol Phys* 1975;1(1–2):147–153.

50. Johnson LS, Milliken BD, Hadley SW, Pelizzari CA, Haraf DJ, Chen GT. Initial clinical experience with a video-based patient positioning system. *Int J Radiat Oncol Biol Phys.* 1999;45(1):205–213.

51. Lattanzi J, McNeeley S, Pinover W, et al. A comparison of daily CT localization to a daily ultrasound-based system in prostate cancer. *Int J Radiat Oncol Biol Phys.* 1999;43(4):719–725.

52. Coles CE, Cash CJ, Treece GM, et al. High definition three-dimensional ultrasound to localise the tumour bed: a breast radiotherapy planning study. *Radiother Oncol.* 2007;84(3):233–241.

53. van Dyk S, Bernshaw D. Ultrasound-based conformal planning for gynaecological brachytherapy. *J Med Imaging Radiat Oncol.* 2008;52(1):77–84.

54. Fuss M, Salter BJ, Cavanaugh SX, et al. Daily ultrasound-based image-guided targeting for radiotherapy of upper abdominal malignancies. *Int J Radiat Oncol Biol Phys.* 2004;59(4):1245–1256.

55. Stroom JC, Olofsen-van Acht MJJ, Quint S, et al. On-line setup corrections during radiotherapy of patients with gynecological tumors. *Int J Radiat Oncol Biol Phys.* 2000;46:499–506.

56. Pouliot J, Bani-Hashemi JA, Chen J, et al. (Non)-migration of radioopaque markers used for on-line localization of the prostate with an electronic portal imaging device. *Int J Radiat Oncol Biol Phys.* 2003;56:862–866.

57. Adler JR Jr, Chang SD, Murphy MJ, Doty J, Geis P, Hancock SL. The Cyberknife: a frameless robotic system for radiosurgery. *Stereotact Funct Neurosurg.* 1997;69(1-4 pt 2):124–128.

58. Yin FF, Zhu J, Yan H, et al. Dosimetric characteristics of Novalis shaped beam surgery unit. *Med Phys.* 2002;29(8):1729–1738.

59. Shirato H, Shimizu S, Kunieda T, et al. Physical aspects of a real-time tumor-tracking system for gated radiotherapy. *Int J Radiat Oncol Biol Phys.* 2000;48(4):1187–1195.

60. Simpson RG, Chen CT, Grubbs EA, Swindell W. A 4-MV CT scanner for radiation therapy: the prototype system. *Med Phys.* 1982;9(4):574–579.

61. Mahan SL, Chase DJ, Ramsey CR. Technical note: output and energy fluctuations of the tomotherapy Hi-Art helical tomotherapy system. *Med Phys.* 2004;31(7):2119–2120.

62. Morin O, Gillis A, Chen J, et al. Megavoltage cone-beam CT: system description and clinical applications. *Med Dosim.* 2006; 31(1):51–61.

63. Kriminski S, Mitschke M, Sorensen S, et al. Respiratory correlated cone-beam computed tomography on an isocentric C-arm. *Phys Med Biol.* 2005;50(22):5263–5280.

64. Jaffray DA, Siewerdsen JH, et al. Cone-beam computed tomography with a flat-panel imager: initial performance characterization. *Med Phys.* 2000;27(6):1311–1323.

65. Guckenberger M, Meyer J, Vordermark D, Baier K, Wilbert J, Flentje M. Magnitude and clinical relevance of translational and rotational patient setup errors: a cone-beam CT study. *Int J Radiat Oncol Biol Phys.* 2006;65(3):934–942.

66. Roper JR, Bowsher JE, Yin FF. On-board SPECT for localizing functional targets: a simulation study. *Med Phys.* 2009;36(5): 1727–1735.

67. Lagendijk JJ, Raaymakers BW, Raaijmakers AJE, et al. MRI/linac integration. *Radiother Oncol.* 2008;86(1):25–29.

68. Dempsey J, Dionne B, Fitzsimmons J, et al. A real-time MRI guided external beam radiotherapy delivery system. *Med Phys.* 2006;33:2254–2254.

69. Mell LK, Roeske JC, Mundt AJ. A survey of intensity-modulated radiation therapy use in the United States. *Cancer.* 2003;98(1):204–211.

70. Mell LK, Mehrotra AK, Mundt AJ. Intensity-modulated radiation therapy use in the U.S., 2004. *Cancer.* 2005;104(6):1296–1303.

71. Simpson DR, Lawson JD, Nath SK, Rose BS, Mundt AJ, Mell LK. Utilization of advanced imaging technologies for target delineation in radiation oncology. *J Am Coll Radiol.* 2009;6(12):876–883.

72. Simpson DR, Lawson JD, Nath SK, et al. Survey of image-guided radiation therapy use in the United States. *Cancer.* 2010 Aug 15;116(16):3953–60.

73. Niyazi M, Bartenstein P, Belka C, Ganswindt U. Choline PET-based dose-painting in prostate cancer: modelling of dose effects. *Radiat Oncol.* 2010;5:23.

74. Seierstad T, Hole KH, Saelen E, Ree AH, Flatmark K, Malinen E. MR-guided simultaneous integrated boost in preoperative radiotherapy of locally advanced rectal cancer following neoadjuvant chemotherapy. *Radiother Oncol.* 2009;93(2):279–284.

75. Lo SS, Fakiris AJ, Chang EL, et al. Stereotactic body radiation therapy: a novel treatment modality. *Nat Rev Clin Oncol.* 2010;7(1):44–54.

76. Munawar I, Yaremko BP, Craig J, et al. Intensity modulated radiotherapy of non-small-cell lung cancer incorporating SPECT ventilation imaging. *Med Phys.* 2010;37(4):1863–1872.

77. Mell LK, Liang Y, Bydder M, et al. Functional MRI-guided bone marrow-sparing intensity modulated radiotherapy for pelvic malignancies. *Int J Radiat Oncol Biol Phys.* 2009;75:S121.

Chapter 2

COMPUTED TOMOGRAPHY

JOSHUA D. LAWSON, MD, TIM FOX, PHD

With the development of commercial computed tomography (CT) simulators, CT simulation has emerged as the cornerstone of radiation therapy (RT) treatment planning. In fact, many RT clinics have abandoned conventional simulators entirely, performing all treatment planning on CT image sets.

The modern CT simulator grew out of the work of Goitein and Abrams who originally described the "beam's-eye-view" planning concept.[1] Additional work by Sherouse and colleagues resulted in the development of a simulator-like system that uses digital information from an imaging data set.[2,3] Virtual simulation, synonymous with CT simulation, allowed for treatment planning by using a virtual patient model created from a three-dimensional (3D) imaging set, as well as produced digitally reconstructed radiographs (DRRs) to be used in conjunction with treatment delivery. Through CT simulation, the 3D treatment planning process soon eclipsed the previous 2D planning process, and became well-established in the radiation oncology community.

Intensity-modulated RT (IMRT) treatment planning followed the establishment of 3D conformal RT, using dose-volume constraints and a computer-aided planning process to arrive at an optimal treatment plan. Computed tomography simulation plays a critical role in IMRT, providing the required segmentation of both target structures and critical neighboring organs at risk (OARs). In addition to CT, other imaging modalities such as magnetic resonance (MR) imaging, positron emission tomography (PET), or single photon emission computed tomography (SPECT) can be registered with the CT simulation scan of the patient to provide more anatomical or functional information to be used in the treatment planning process.

Today, treatment planning relies heavily on information obtained through CT simulation. In this chapter, the CT simulation technology and process, as well as the integration of CT simulation information with image-guided RT (IGRT) systems and emerging uses of CT simulation are discussed.

CT Simulation Technology and Process

The three components of a CT simulator are (1) a CT scanner with flat table top, (2) an integrated laser marking system, and (3) a virtual simulation and visualization software system. As described in the American Association of Physicists in Medicine (AAPM) Task Group (TG)-66 report, treatment polices and planning target volumes should account for the differences between the treatment machine table and the simulator table.[4] The CT scanner itself also differs from a scanner used for diagnostic imaging; whereas most conventional CT scanners use a 70-cm-bore opening, large-bore (85-cm) scanners have been developed expressly for radiation oncology uses. These large-bore scanners increase flexibility for both patient size/positioning and immobilization devices.[5] Large-bore scanners also have an increased scan field of view, 60 cm, compared with 48 cm on most 70-cm-bore units. The other unique component in the simulation suite is an in-room laser marking system. The lasers may be fixed or mobile, with a particular need for mobility in the sagittal laser as the CT table (unlike the table in the treatment room) does not move laterally.

Computed tomography scanners have evolved from conventional scanners acquiring singular axial images step-wise with the table advanced after each image to spiral or helical CT scanners by using simultaneous imaging and table motion. These spiral CT scanners greatly reduce the scan time required, and can reduce motion artifacts. More recently, multislice CT scanners have been increasingly used in CT simulation, allowing simultaneous acquisition of imaging data from multiple axial slices.[6-9] The multiple rows of detectors used by these scanners further reduce the time required as well as the tube heat loading for imaging. Such scanners are especially beneficial when one is simulating the thorax, as breathing artifacts can be minimized with faster acquisition times. Fourdimensional (4D) simulation, as will be discussed in further detail, allows for precise tracking of structure motion throughout the respiratory cycle.

The CT simulation process has been divided into three major categories by the AAPM TG-66 report.[4] Methods for simulating specific anatomical sites have been described by several authors.[1,10]

CT Scan, Patient Positioning, and Immobilization

Prior to scanning, patients are placed in the treatment position. Various immobilization devices may be used to ensure reproducibility of positioning. The immobilization device selected should ideally be indexed to the treatment table. With the use of an immobilization device that is indexed to the table, the record-and-verify system can monitor treatment table coordinates and tighter tolerance limits can also be used. It also allows for therapists to preposition the patient consistently on a daily basis. Contrast agents may also be used to improve visualization of the patient's anatomy. However, for heterogeneity-based calculations in treatment planning, contrast can cause dose-distribution errors because of artificial CT numbers and corresponding tissue densities. To resolve this issue, some centers obtain an additional CT scan without contrast, and others may assign a bulk tissue density, within the planning software, to these regions.

Image acquisition or scanning is performed using preset clinical protocols depending on the body part, treatment technique, or region of interest. Parameters that may be adjusted include kVp, mAs, slice thickness, slice spacing, and total scan time. A small slice thickness and spacing are desirable for producing high-quality DRR images. Figure 2-1 illustrates the impact of slice spacing on automatically generated lung contours. The graph shows the volume error at several slice thicknesses and with several Hounsfield unit (HU) thresholds for contouring. With increasing slice thickness (moving left to right on the x-axis), the errors at a range of HU increase dramatically. It is our practice to use the smallest slice thickness available for each CT simulation. In addition to the scan protocols, scan limits should be specified by the physician and should encompass volume long enough to create DRRs with enough anatomical information. The AAPM TG-66 report recommends that the scan volume should be at least 5 cm or greater in the superior and inferior direction from the anticipated treatment volumes and that longer volumes may be necessary for special situations.[4]

Treatment Planning and CT Simulation

The treatment planning portion of the CT simulation process begins with target and normal structure deline-

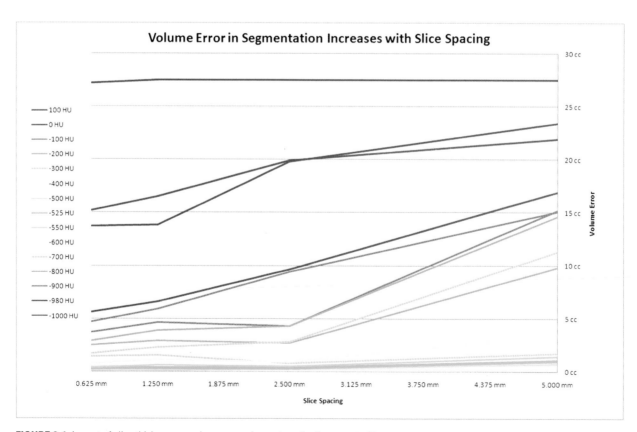

FIGURE 2-1. Impact of slice thickness on volume error of an automatically generated lung contour.

ation. Other imaging studies such as MR and PET/CT may be registered to the planning CT scan to improve target or normal structure delineation. After delineation of the target volumes, a treatment isocenter is created either manually or automatically in the CT study. The automated isocenter placement is performed by the software by computing the centroid of the target volume. After the isocenter has been identified in the virtual simulation software, these coordinates must be transferred to the external laser marking system for localizing on the patient's skin. These marks on the patient's skin are required to ensure a daily reproducible setup at the treatment machine.

Treatment Positioning

On the treatment machine, the patient is positioned according to instructions created from the CT simulation software. Port films are acquired and compared with CT simulation DRRs. In some cases, the patient may undergo treatment setup verification on a conventional simulator before the treatment. However, with the recent development of IGRT, this process is being phased out at many clinics. The conventional simulator may be used for the final step of the planning process, which does not take dedicated time at the treatment machines. The treatment verification process is more time-consuming than typical treatments, and this process saves valuable time during the day. In addition, the conventional simulator can also be used for verifying intrafraction motion of the target volume or critical structures. This can be important for treatment sites in the thorax and abdomen, for example, because of the inability of the CT simulation process to display breathing motion. In such cases, the physician may wish to observe patient breathing on a conventional simulator using fluoroscopic imaging. A well-designed CT simulation process for IMRT planning and delivery can result in all of these steps appearing relatively seamless and the duration of the entire process is relatively short.

Integration of CT Simulation With IGRT Treatment Delivery Systems

Computed tomography imaging data obtained at simulation are used more than any other imaging information for the delineation of target structures, including gross tumor volume (GTV), clinical target volume (CTV), and planning target volume (PTV). The expansions from the GTV to CTV and the CTV to PTV are site-specific and additionally depend on the perceived uncertainty in daily patient positioning. Computed tomography data were used to usher in the era of IMRT, with head and neck[11-14] and prostate[15-28] tumors having the largest amount of available clinical data. The use of IMRT and IGRT has evolved more slowly in some disease sites, particularly those in the female pelvis. However, recent work has been focused on establishing the role of this technology in treatment planning for gynecologic patients.[19-27]

Successful incorporation of these new treatment technologies provides the practitioner with the opportunity to potentially increase the therapeutic ratio with better localization of targets while simultaneously improving the sparing of nearby OARs. Critical to accomplishing this goal, however, is the adequate and appropriate delineation of these targets and the OARs at the time of simulation. With this in mind, the simulation process becomes possibly the most important component of treatment. The importance of the simulation procedure is further amplified in IGRT—the very nature of IGRT is to compare, either visually or automatically, images obtained at or near the time of treatment delivery to images obtained at simulation. Patient shifts and other changes are applied in an attempt to match the images from treatment to the images obtained at simulation. Because the CT images will, therefore, form the reference image set for any image guidance to be employed during treatment, these images become paramount.

Quality Assurance

The AAPM TG-66 report provides a comprehensive quality assurance (QA) program for CT scanners used for simulation, CT simulation software, and the overall CT simulation process.[4] Depending on the CT scanner location and primary use, acceptance testing, commissioning, and QA can be the responsibility of a therapy medical physicist or a diagnostic physicist, or it could be a joint responsibility. The commissioning and periodic QA of the accompanying software and the QA of the CT simulation process is always the responsibility of the therapy physicist. The AAPM TG-66 report establishes a set of QA procedures that are applicable to scanners used for CT simulation regardless of their location and primary purpose. The report breaks the QA tests into three main areas: (1) QA for CT scanners used for CT simulation, (2) QA for CT simulation software, and (3) evaluation of CT simulation process.

QA for CT Scanners Used for CT Simulation

The AAPM TG-66 report addresses QA procedures for CT scanners to ensure consistent operation and a successful CT simulation process. One of the important performance components for daily and monthly testing of the CT scanner is the external laser marking system. These laser systems are used to position the patient in the correct treatment position as well as to place positioning marks on the patient. The accuracy of the lasers affects the reproducibility of patient positioning from CT scanner to the treatment delivery machine. The external laser marking system for the CT scanner consists of three separate components: gantry lasers, wall-mounted lasers, and an overhead mobile sagittal laser. Besides the laser marking system, the other electromechanical components such as the couch and tabletop, gantry tilt, and scan localization from scout image should be part of a comprehensive QA program.

QA for CT Simulation Software

In addition to the CT scanner QA, the AAPM TG-66 report discusses testing features of the CT simulation software for verifying its accuracy. The QA program should verify the following features: image input test, structure delineation, multimodality image registration, machine definition, isocenter calculation and movement, and image reconstruction. One of the final products from the CT simulation process is the generation of DRR images used for verifying the patient positioning at the treatment machine. These DRRs are the reference images for most of the IGRT techniques discussed. The use of poor-quality DRRs can affect the patient positioning process because of the inability to visualize anatomical details.

Evaluation of the CT Simulation Process

After testing the CT scanner components and virtual simulation software, the overall simulation process should be evaluated by the clinical team members. A CT simulation program should include a written set of procedures and be reviewed annually by the clinical staff. Procedures should be written for each treatment site to identify the scan protocol, scan limits, contrast, special instructions, and, possibly, beam arrangements.

Emerging Uses of CT Simulation

Target Motion Management—4D CT Simulation

Fully embracing IGRT demands that the radiation oncologist consider the fact that any singular "image" represents only an instantaneous representation of the patient's anatomy. Single-slice CT scans consist of multiple planar images acquired over a period of several seconds; these images are then used to create a 3D reconstruction with interpolation applied between images. Although there are multiple locations within the body that do not demonstrate appreciable motion, there are several sites with large known variations in structure location, such as the thorax[28–30] and abdomen.[31–33] For treating tumors located in these regions, one must be aware that conventional CT imaging will not be accurate in its display of both target location and shape. This uncertainty is attributable to variability in structure location throughout the respiratory cycle, with static CT images obtained only at several points throughout this cycle.

There are two broad groups of techniques used to accommodate structure motion during the simulation process, and by extension during treatment delivery; these groupings are based on the relationship between the tar-

get and the treatment beams. The first group does not restrict target motion relative to the treatment beams, but accounts for this motion with either geometric or dosimetric considerations. The most basic technique employs the uniform addition of margins based on averages derived from patient populations, ie, arbitrarily adding 1 cm in all directions in all cases. In most cases, this population-derived margin is larger than necessary, resulting in treatment of an unnecessarily large volume of normal tissue. A refinement of this method involves the addition of patient-specific margins as determined by fluoroscopic monitoring of target location, 4D CT scanning, or by obtaining both end-inspiration and end-expiration imaging and creating a PTV that encompasses the extreme end points. The second group of techniques attempts to maintain constancy of target location, either through physical means to restrict motion (abdominal compression,[34] deep inspiratory breath hold,[35] or forced shallow breathing[36]), or through treatment delivery modification (respiratory gating,[37,38] beam tracking,[39,40] or couch-based motion compensation[41]).

Respiratory gating requires use of a modern CT simulation machine able to obtain data in 4D. An example of such a system is a CT simulator equipped with the Real-Time Position Management (RPM) respiratory gated system (Varian Medical Systems, Palo Alto, CA, USA). This 4D CT simulation system creates image sets at specific phases of the respiratory cycle (typically every 10%) and uses these image sets to produce a time-dependent 4D CT study. A small block containing two passive reflective markers is placed on the patient's chest or upper abdomen. An illuminator is used, and the markers reflect infrared light that is detected by a video camera. The two markers are used to track the respiratory movement. A desktop workstation processes the video signals to create a respiratory waveform. This signal can be used prospectively to turn the radiation beam on and off during simulation (as well as treatment) or more commonly, retrospectively, to bin the CT images into the respective phases.

Gated signals are produced with the RPM system by using the phased-based mode. In the prospective mode, the physician specifies a phase interval of the breathing waveform to perform the gated simulation. In the retrospective mode, the patient breathes normally and the CT images are binned based on when they were obtained, relative to the breathing signal. This mode allows for target and normal structure visualization throughout the respiratory cycle. These images can be subsequently used to create patient-specific target structure margins by using the internal target volume concept. Moreover, the same planning set can be used for gating on the linac by selecting an appropriate range of phases for treatment planning and delivery. At the time of treatment, the patient's respirations can be monitored via the RPM reflective box placed on the midsection and the treatment beam can be selectively turned off and on at the predetermined phases of respiration. This technique has been especially useful in treating tumors of the lungs[38,42–44] and liver.[44–46] Its use is expected to increase as the role of hypofractionated radiation or stereotactic body RT continues to expand (see Chapter 17E).

Automated Segmentation

Increasingly complex treatment planning and delivery systems such as IMRT have required increasingly intricate and time-consuming segmentation. Automated segmentation of normal tissues, target structures, or both holds the allure of both decreasing time required for contouring and potentially increasing standardization of contoured structures. Automated segmentation can be broadly divided into two groups—one based on specific imaging characteristics such as the HU and using predetermined thresholds and the other based on sets of atlases, or predeveloped structure sets that may be applied to any particular patient.

Threshold-based segmentation is most commonly used in the delineation of structures with distinctive imaging characteristics. The two most common automatically segmented structures are lung and bone. Threshold-based techniques apply a preset HU threshold to determine a structure's edges. The two variables associated with the

quality of segmentation are the HU threshold and slice thickness. In a phantom study, the evaluation of an air cavity within the phantom demonstrated that, in uniform regions, a significant variation in HU can occur (Figure 2-2). This variation would be amplified in the case of an actual human lung. Figure 2-3 shows the impact of HU threshold selection as well as CT slice thickness on an automatically contoured air cavity.

Intensity-modulated RT requires specified target volumes to be specified for treatment planning. The sharp dose gradients present at the edges of these targets highlight the importance of both meticulous contouring and accurate handling of motion uncertainties. Though standardized volumes do exist for some treatment sites,[47–49] there is still much interuser variability.[50] In response to the time constraints as well as the variability in contoured structures, several commercial systems have been developed that aim to standardize contoured volumes and reduce the time requirement for the delineation of targets and OARs. These systems use structure set templates, or atlases, which can be applied to a specific patient's image set.

Automated segmentation is still in its infancy but offers the potential for improved standardization of contoured structures as well as decreasing the time required of the radiation oncologist or dosimetry staff.

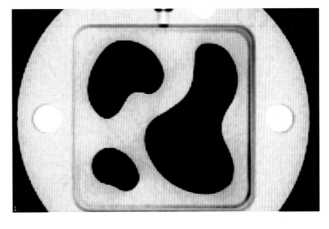

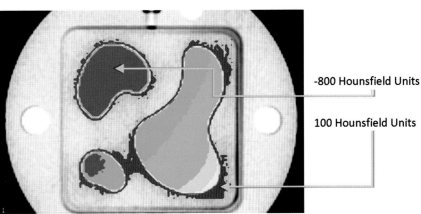

-800 Hounsfield Units

100 Hounsfield Units

FIGURE 2-2. Variation in Hounsfield units across a uniform air cavity within a phantom.

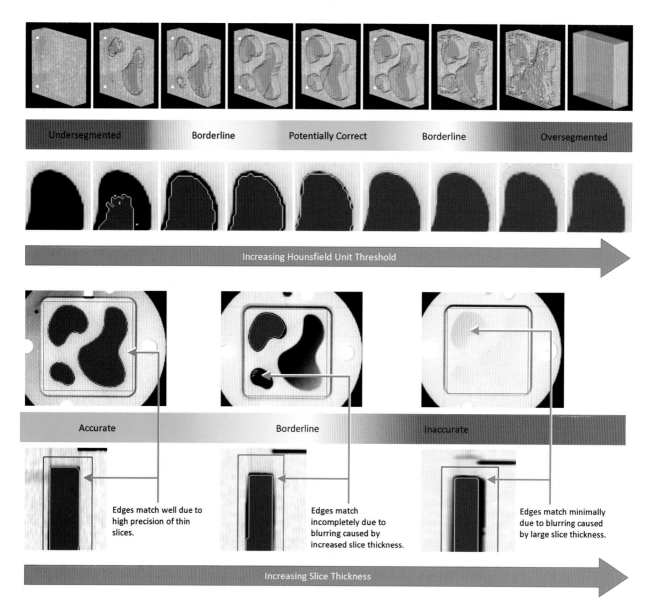

FIGURE 2-3. Impact of Hounsfield unit threshold selection and CT scan slice thickness on automatically generated contours. The effect of increasing the selected Hounsfield unit threshold on an automatically contoured air cavity, progressing from under- to oversegmented from left to right. The increase in error seen with increasing slice thickness from 0.625 mm to 5.0 mm.

Incorporation of Multiple Imaging Modalities

In addition to CT simulation, some departments are using MR or PET/CT scanners with virtual simulation software to create multiple modality simulation systems. Typically, CT scans have been used for providing a tomographic data map of the patient's anatomy; additionally, it provides electron density data for dose calculations. If additional imaging is obtained for improved anatomic or functional detail, these image sets are registered to the CT simulation for treatment planning. Several systems are available to provide automated image registration across multiple modalities. Still, CT remains the cornerstone of the simulation process, in part because of the availability of heterogeneity information for treatment planning as well as the fact that portal films or other IGRT maneuvers are matched to DRR obtained from CT simulation.

For many radiation oncology centers that use multimodality imaging during the CT simulation process, an image registration method will be used to incorporate one image study into another image study for improved decision-making. The aim of registration is to establish an exact point-to-point correspondence (coordinate system transformation) between the voxels of the different modalities, making direct comparison possible. Transformations are either rigid or nonrigid (sometimes called deformable). A rigid coordinate transformation is when only translations in three orthogonal directions and rotations in three directions are allowed. Nonrigid transformations are more complex with nonlinear scaling or warping of one data set as well as rotation and translations. The image that is being matched is typically called the fixed or target image. The image that is moving its coordinate system to match the fixed image is called the moving or floating image.

Some of the most difficult cases of image registration with CT simulation are when multimodality imaging is used such as PET/CT, MR/CT, and PET/MR. Over the past 5 years, automated image registration methods have increasingly used volume-matching or intensity-based matching algorithms.[51,52] Volume-based image registration methods are different than others because they operate directly with the image intensity values (gray values) without user interaction. A popular similarity measure using the voxel intensity histogram for multimodality image registration is mutual information (MI) method. This method is based on the assumption that there is a correlation between groups of voxels that have similar values. Mutual information measures how much information one random variable (image intensity in one image) tells about another random variable (image intensity in the other image). An automated MI algorithm searches for a transformation between the fixed images and the moving images at which identical anatomical landmarks of both images are most closely overlapping. In multimodal image registration, the MI technique has become a standard reference in medical imaging with the implementation in commercial treatment planning systems.

Many image registration methods assume that the two image sets could be registered by using rigid registration. However, this is not always the case as the patient can be positioned differently between imaging scans and the internal organs can change position and shape. This may be because of respiration for the lungs or degree of bladder filling. Deformable or nonrigid registration methods can be employed for these situations but it is not a trivial matter. An active area of image registration methods addresses the deformable image registration methods.[53-56] Deformable image registration extracts structures from one image and elastically deforms them to fit the second image. With the deformable registration methods, the optimization algorithm is locally defined and calculated in small iterative steps by using splines to mathematically represent the surfaces. A drawback of deformable models is that they often need a good initial position to properly converge, which is generally realized by (rigid) preregistration of the images involved.

Conclusions

From the initial use of virtual simulation software for treatment plan creation to target localization for treatment delivery, CT simulation is a fundamental cornerstone of the IGRT process. Over the years, CT simulation has evolved

in the treatment planning process. The use of other imaging modalities with sophisticated image registration methods provides physicians with improvements to the target delineation process. Automated anatomical contouring methods such as atlas-based segmentation are using CT simulation images to identify normal tissue structures to improve efficiencies in the clinic. With the use of CT simulation image studies and onboard volumetric imaging, target localization has progressed from laser-based marking systems with external anatomy to image-guided matching methods with internal anatomy. Combining IMRT and IGRT, CT simulation will become an important element in adaptive radiation therapy. As new treatment planning and delivery systems change, the process of CT simulation will evolve and adapt to provide the clinician with accurate representations of patient anatomy.

References

1. Goitein M, Abrams M, Rowell D, Pollari H, Wiles J. Multidimensional treatment planning: II. Beam's eye-view, back projection, and projection through CT sections. *Int J Radiat Oncol Biol Phys.* 1983;9(6):789–797.
2. Sherouse GW, Bourland JD, Reynolds K, McMurry HL, Mitchell TP, Chaney EL. Virtual simulation in the clinical setting: some practical considerations. *Int J Radiat Oncol Biol Phys.* 1990;19·(4)1059–1065.
3. Sherouse GW, Novins K, Chaney EL. Computation of digitally reconstructed radiographs for use in radiotherapy treatment design. *Int J Radiat Oncol Biol Phys.* 1990;18(3):651–658.
4. Mutic S, Palta JR, Butker EK, et al. Quality assurance for computed-tomography simulators and the computed-tomography-simulation process: report of the AAPM Radiation Therapy Committee Task Group No. 66. *Med Phys.* 2003;30(10):2762–2792.
5. Fuchs T, Kachelriess M, Kalender WA. Technical advances in multi-slice spiral CT. *Eur J Radiol.* 2000;36(2):69–73.
6. Butker EK, Helton DJ, Keller JW, Hughes LL, Crenshaw T, Davis LW. A totally integrated simulation technique for three-field breast treatment using a CT simulator. *Med Phys.* 1996;23(10):1809–1814.
7. Hu H. Multi-slice helical CT: scan and reconstruction. *Med Phys.* 1999;26:5–18.
8. Kalender WA, Polacin A. Physical performance characteristics of spiral CT scanning. *Med Phys.* 1991;18(5):910–915.
9. Klingenbeck-Regn K, Schaller S, Flohr T, Ohnesorge B, Kopp AF, Baum U. Subsecond multi-slice computed tomography: basics and applications. *Eur J Radiol.* 1999;31(2):110–124.
10. Mah K, Danjoux CE, Manship S, Makhani N, Cardoso M, Sixel KE. Computed tomographic simulation of craniospinal fields in pediatric patients: improved treatment accuracy and patient comfort. *Int J Radiat Oncol Biol Phys.* 1998;41(5):997–1003.
11. Lawson JD, Otto K, Chen A, Shin DM, Davis L, Johnstone PA. Concurrent platinum-based chemotherapy and simultaneous modulated accelerated radiation therapy for locally advanced squamous cell carcinoma of the tongue base. *Head Neck.* 2008;30(3):327–335.

12. Lee N, Xia P, Quivey JM, et al. Intensity-modulated radiotherapy in the treatment of nasopharyngeal carcinoma: an update of the UCSF experience. *Int J Radiat Oncol Biol Phys.* 2002;53(1):12–22.

13. de Arruda FF, Puri DR, Zhung J, et al. Intensity-modulated radiation therapy for the treatment of oropharyngeal carcinoma: the Memorial Sloan-Kettering Cancer Center experience. *Int J Radiat Oncol Biol Phys.* 2006;64(2):363–373.

14. Lee N, Xia P, Fischbein NJ, Akazawa P, Akazawa C, Quivey JM. Intensity-modulated radiation therapy for head-and-neck cancer: the UCSF experience focusing on target volume delineation. *Int J Radiat Oncol Biol Phys.* 2003;57(1):49–60.

15. Cahlon O, Zelefsky MJ, Shippy A, et al. Ultra-high dose (86.4 Gy) IMRT for localized prostate cancer: toxicity and biochemical outcomes. *Int J Radiat Oncol Biol Phys.* 2008;71(2):330–337.

16. Ashman JB, Zelefsky MJ, Hunt MS, Leibel SA, Fuks Z. Whole pelvic radiotherapy for prostate cancer using 3D conformal and intensity-modulated radiotherapy. *Int J Radiat Oncol Biol Phys.* 2005;63(3):765–771.

17. Zelefsky MJ, Fuks Z, Hunt M, et al. High-dose intensity modulated radiation therapy for prostate cancer: early toxicity and biochemical outcome in 772 patients. *Int J Radiat Oncol Biol Phys.* 2002;53(5):1111–1116.

18. Burman C, Chui CS, Kutcher G, et al. Planning, delivery, and quality assurance of intensity-modulated radiotherapy using dynamic multileaf collimator: a strategy for large-scale implementation for the treatment of carcinoma of the prostate. *Int J Radiat Oncol Biol Phys.* 1997;39(4):863–873.

19. Jhingran A. Potential advantages of intensity-modulated radiation therapy in gynecologic malignancies. *Semin Radiat Oncol.* 2006;16(3):144–151.

20. Mundt AJ, Lujan AE, Rotmensch J, et al. Intensity-modulated whole pelvic radiotherapy in women with gynecologic malignancies. *Int J Radiat Oncol Biol Phys.* 2002;52(5):1330–1337.

21. Mundt AJ, Roeske JC, Lujan AE. Intensity-modulated radiation therapy in gynecologic malignancies. *Med Dosim.* 2002; 27(2):131–136.

22. Nadeau S, Bouchard M, Germain I, et al. Postoperative irradiation of gynecologic malignancies: improving treatment delivery using aperture-based intensity-modulated radiotherapy. *Int J Radiat Oncol Biol Phys.* 2007;68(2):601–611.

23. Roeske JC, Lujan A, Rotmensch J, Waggoner SE, Yamada D, Mundt AJ. Intensity-modulated whole pelvic radiation therapy in patients with gynecologic malignancies. *Int J Radiat Oncol Biol Phys.* 2000;48(5):1613–1621.

24. Salama JK, Mundt AJ, Roeske J, Mehta N. Preliminary outcome and toxicity report of extended-field, intensity-modulated radiation therapy for gynecologic malignancies. *Int J Radiat Oncol Biol Phys.* 2006;65(4):1170–1176.

25. Salama JK, Roeske JC, Mehta N, Mundt AJ. Intensity-modulated radiation therapy in gynecologic malignancies. *Curr Treat Options Oncol.* 2004;5(2)97–108.

26. Mell LK, Roeske JC, Mundt AJ. A survey of intensity-modulated radiation therapy use in the United States. *Cancer.* 2003;98(1):204–211.

27. Mell LK, Tiryaki H, Ahn KH, Mundt AJ, Roeske JC, Aydogan B. Dosimetric comparison of bone marrow-sparing intensity-

28. Ruschin M, Sixel KE. Integration of digital fluoroscopy with CT-based radiation therapy planning of lung tumors. *Med Phys.* 2002;29(8):1698–1709.

29. Sher DJ, Wolfgang JA, Niemierko A, Choi NC. Quantification of mediastinal and hilar lymph node movement using four-dimensional computed tomography scan: implications for radiation treatment planning. *Int J Radiat Oncol Biol Phys.* 2007; 69(5):1402–1408.

30. Zhang Q, Pevsner A, Hertanto A, et al. A patient-specific respiratory model of anatomical motion for radiation treatment planning. *Med Phys.* 2007;34(4):4772–4781.

31. Fitzpatrick MJ, Starkschall G, Balter P, et al. A novel platform simulating irregular motion to enhance assessment of respiration-correlated radiation therapy procedures. *J Appl Clin Med Phys.* 2005;6(1):13–21.

32. Ramsey CR, Scaperoth D, Arwood D, Oliver AL. Clinical efficacy of respiratory gated conformal radiation therapy. *Med Dosim.* 1999;24(2):115–119.

33. Ringash J, Perkins G, Brierley J, et al. IMRT for adjuvant radiation in gastric cancer: a preferred plan? *Int J Radiat Oncol Biol Phys.* 2005;63(3):732–738.

34. Murray B, Forster K, Timmerman R. Frame-based immobilization and targeting for stereotactic body radiation therapy. *Med Dosim.* 2007;32(2):86–91.

35. Mageras GS, Yorke E. Deep inspiration breath hold and respiratory gating strategies for reducing organ motion in radiation treatment. *Semin Radiat Oncol.* 2004;14(1):65–75.

36. Keall PJ, Mageras GS, Balter JM, et al. The management of respiratory motion in radiation oncology report of AAPM Task Group 76. *Med Phys.* 2006;33(10):3874–3900.

37. Jiang SB, Wolfgang J, Mageras GS. Quality assurance challenges for motion-adaptive radiation therapy: gating, breath holding, and four-dimensional computed tomography. *Int J Radiat Oncol Biol Phys.* 2008;71(1 suppl):S103–S107.

38. Berson AM, Emery R, Rodriguez L, et al. Clinical experience using respiratory gated radiation therapy: comparison of free-breathing and breath-hold techniques. *Int J Radiat Oncol Biol Phys.* 2004;60(2):419–426.

39. Giraud P, Yorke E, Jiang S, Simon L, Rosenzweig K, Mageras G. Reduction of organ motion effects in IMRT and conformal 3D radiation delivery by using gating and tracking techniques. *Cancer Radiother.* 2006;10(5):269–282.

40. Harada T, Shirato H, Ogura S, et al. Real-time tumor-tracking radiation therapy for lung carcinoma by the aid of insertion of a gold marker using bronchofiberscopy. *Cancer.* 2002;95(8):1720–1727.

41. Woo MK, Kim B. An investigation of the reproducibility and usefulness of automatic couch motion in complex radiation therapy techniques. *J Appl Clin Med Phys.* 2002;3(1):46–50.

42. Timmerman RD, Park C, Kavanagh BD. The North American experience with stereotactic body radiation therapy in non-small cell lung cancer. *J Thorac Oncol.* 2007;2(7 suppl 3):S101–S112.

43. Fox T, Simon EL, Elder E, Riffenburgh RH, Johnstone PA. Free breathing gated delivery (FBGD) of lung radiation therapy:

analysis of factors affecting clinical patient throughput. *Lung Cancer*. 2007;56(1):69–75.

44. Wurm RE, Gum F, Erbel S, et al. Image guided respiratory gated hypofractionated Stereotactic Body Radiation Therapy (H-SBRT) for liver and lung tumors: initial experience. *Acta Oncol*. 2006;45(7):881–889.

45. Beddar AS, Kainz K, Briere TM, et al. Correlation between internal fiducial tumor motion and external marker motion for liver tumors imaged with 4D-CT. *Int J Radiat Oncol Biol Phys*. 2007;67(2):630–638.

46. Wagman R, Yorke E, Ford E, et al. Respiratory gating for liver tumors: use in dose escalation. *Int J Radiat Oncol Biol Phys*. 2003;55(3):659–668.

47. Grégoire V, Levendag P, Ang KK, et al. CT-based delineation of lymph node levels and related CTVs in the node-negative neck: DAHANCA, EORTC, GORTEC, NCIC, RTOG consensus guidelines. *Radiother Oncol*. 2003;69(3):227–236.

48. Sidhom MA, Kneebone AB, Lehman M, et al. Post-prostatectomy radiation therapy: consensus guidelines of the Australian and New Zealand Radiation Oncology Genito-Urinary Group. *Radiother Oncol*. 2008;88(1):10–19.

49. Available at: http://www.rtog.org/atlases/contour.html. Accessed 9/14/2010

50. Chao KS, Bhide S, Chen H, et al. Reduce in variation and improve efficiency of target volume delineation by a computer-assisted system using a deformable image registration approach. *Int J Radiat Oncol Biol Phys*. 2007;68(5):1512–1521.

51. Maes F, Collignon A, Vandermeulen D, Marchal G, Suetens P. Multimodality image registration by maximization of mutual information. *IEEE Trans Med Imaging*. 1997;16(2):187–198.

52. Wells WM, Viola P, Kikinis R. Multi-modal volume registration by maximization of mutual information. In: *Second Annual International Symposium on Medical Robotics and Computer Assisted Surgery*. New York, NY: John Wiley & Sons; 1995: 52–62.

53. Thirion JP. Image matching as the diffusion process: an analogy with Maxwell's demons. *Med Image Anal*. 1998;2(3):243–260.

54. Gee J, Reivich M, Bajcsy R. Drastically deforming 3D atlas to match anatomical brain images. *J Comp Assist Tomogr*. 1993;17:225–226.

55. Bajcsy R, Kovacic S. Multiresolution elastic matching. *Comput Vis Graphics Image Processing*. 1989;46:1–21.

56. Thompson P, Toga AW. A surface-based technique for warping three-dimensional images of the brain. *IEEE Trans Med Imaging*. 1996;15(4):402–417.

Chapter 3

Positron Emission Tomography

Anca-Ligia Grosu, MD, Wolfgang A. Weber, MD, Ursula Nestle, MD

In radiation oncology, treatment planning and monitoring is generally based on computed tomography (CT) and magnetic resonance (MR) imaging. These radiological investigations were the basis for the development of three-dimensional (3D) radiation therapy (RT), stereotactic RT, intensity-modulated RT (IMRT), 3D image-guided brachytherapy, and image-guided RT (IGRT). Therefore, traditional CT and MR, also called *anatomical* or *morphological* imaging, have had a significant impact on the development of the entire field of RT.

Over the years, however, we have come to understand not only the advantages but also the limitations of these imaging modalities. Contrast enhancement on CT and T1-MR are not always a true indicator for tumor extension. Hyperintense areas on T2-MR images correlate with a higher water concentration (edema), but are not a specific measure for tumor extension. Moreover, after treatment (surgery, chemotherapy, immunotherapy, or RT), therapy-related changes cannot be reliably differentiated from persistent tumor or tumor recurrence. Last, but not least, traditional CT and MR provide information about the morphology but not the biology of tumors. Therefore, because high precision in the delineation of the target volume is crucial for the success of RT, the integration of newer imaging modalities, with higher sensitivities and specificities for tumor tissue to improve the planning and monitoring of the RT, is mandatory.

In this chapter, the role of positron emission tomography (PET) in the delineation of the gross tumor volume (GTV), for visualization of tumor biology, for treatment monitoring, and for determining the optimal window for RT is presented. The role of PET imaging for staging purposes will not be reviewed.

Tumor Mass Detection and Gross Tumor Delineation

The first rationale for using PET in the target delineation process in patients undergoing RT is its higher sensitivity and specificity for tumor tissue compared with that of CT

and MR in some tumor sites. This has been well demonstrated in many studies that have compared the results of PET with those that are based on other radiological investigations. The hypothesis tested in these reports was that using PET in addition to CT and/or MR increases the accuracy of tumor tissue detection. The ideal PET tracer in this situation should be taken up homogenously from all the cells of the entire tumor and the intensity of the PET uptake should be directly proportional to the density of tumor cells. We will discuss this issue based on two tumor examples, namely brain and lung cancers.

Brain Tumors

[11]C-labeled methionine (MET), ^{123}I-labeled alpha-methyltyrosine (IMT), and ^{18}F-labeled O-(2-fluoroethyl)-L-tyrosine (FET) are the most important radiolabeled amino acids used in the diagnosis of brain tumors. All three tracers have shown a very similar uptake intensity and distribution in brain tumors.[1,2] Currently available amino acid–PET tracers are accumulated by L and A amino acid transporters. Tumor cells take up radiolabeled amino acids at a high rate, whereas there is only a relatively low uptake in normal cerebral tissue. At the level of the blood–brain barrier (BBB), they are independent from the BBB disturbance.

In a review of the literature based on a PubMed (http://www.ncbi.nlm.nih.gov/sites/entrez) search (using the key words: methionine, PET, and brain tumors), we found 45 clinical trials published between 1983 and 2008, including 1721 patients. In 11 studies investigating 706 patients, the data were analyzed by using MET-PET–guided stereotactic biopsies. Between 2000 and 2008, 12 trials (361 patients) evaluated the role of FET-PET in the diagnosis of brain gliomas. In three studies (126 patients), the results were based on PET/MR/CT stereotactic biopsies. The main message of these trials is that the sensitivity and the specificity of MET-PET for both tumor detection and tumor tissue extension are significantly higher than for MR, CT, or fluoro-deoxyglucose (FDG)-PET.[3]

We have earlier evaluated the impact of MET-PET in target volume delineation for RT planning, compared with MR imaging, in 39 patients with brain gliomas following tumor resection.[4,5] Uptake of MET corresponded to the gadolinium (Gd) enhancement in only 13% of the cases. In 74%, the MET volume extended beyond the contrast-enhancing regions, indicating residual tumor. In 69% of the cases, Gd enhancement could be outlined beyond the volume of MET uptake, suggesting postoperative BBB disturbance (Figure 3-1).

Similar results were also reported evaluating the impact of ^{123}I-alpha-methyl-L-tyrosine (IMT)–single-photon emission CT (SPECT) on target volume delineation in nonresected[6] and resected[7] glioma patients. Focal IMT uptake after tumor resection was highly correlated with poor survival, suggesting that amino acids are specific markers for residual tumor tissue.[2]

The first study evaluating the outcome of patients treated with MET-PET or IMT-SPECT–based target delineation was performed in 44 patients with recurrent gliomas re-irradiated with stereotactic fractionated RT.[8] A prospective nonrandomized trial has shown that in patients treated based on amino acids-PET or -SPECT, the median survival time was significantly higher (9 months) compared with patients treated based on CT/MR alone (5 months; $P = .03$). The results of this pilot study have yet to be verified in a randomized trial.

In a recent publication, Lee and coworkers showed that increased uptake on MET-PET imaging obtained before RT and temozolomide was associated with the side of subsequent failure in newly diagnosed glioblastoma (Figure 3-2).[9]

Lung Cancer

FDG-PET was first integrated into RT treatment planning approximately 10 years ago.[10,11] The primary motivation was the clear superiority in diagnostic accuracy of FDG-PET compared with CT in the staging of non–small cell lung cancer (NSCLC), which has meanwhile been accepted by the scientific community and has led to the standard use of FDG-PET with this indication in clinical practice (see Chapter 17A).

The diagnostic accuracy of FDG-PET is only between 85% and 90%. Although it is used for diagnostic purposes, the aim is the optimization of the overall accuracy, compromising on the side of false-positive as well as on that of false-negative findings. For the use of FDG-PET for RT treatment planning, false-negative findings must be minimized to include any suspect tissue.[12,13] This means that a more sensitive interpretation of image data, for example, concerning mediastinal lymph node involvement, is mandatory for RT planning.

In an earlier review, the integration of FDG-PET in RT treatment planning of NSCLC was surveyed. To date, more than 20 studies in more than 600 patients have shown that the use of FDG-PET image data may be advantageous, primarily because of improved coverage of the primary tumor and better protection of healthy tissue. In this context, it is interesting that the FDG-PET–based target volumes may be smaller or larger compared with CT-based ones. However, on the basis of the surgical data regarding the specificity of FDG-PET for tumor staging, it can be assumed that FDG-based target volumes do include the tumor tissue more accurately than

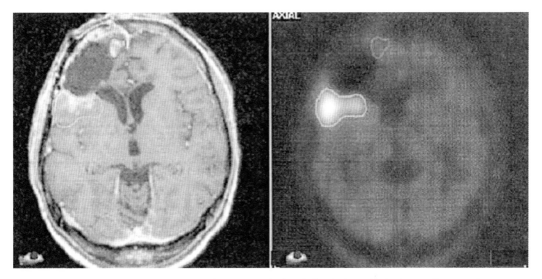

FIGURE 3-1. Grade III astrocytoma is shown 2 weeks postoperatively and 4 days before radiation therapy: T1-magnetic resonance (MR) scan with gadolinium (Gd) contrast (left) and ^{11}C-labeled methionine (MET)-positron emission tomography (PET) (right). The MR and PET data sets were coregistered with commercial software. Areas with both Gd and MET enhancement located in the right temporal lobe (outlined in green) correspond to the residual tumor and represent the gross tumor volume (GTV). Small Gd enhancement area located in the right temporal lobe (pink) shows no MET uptake on PET, indicating blood–brain barrier disturbance from surgery and is not included in the GTV. Printed with permission from Grosu et al.[5]

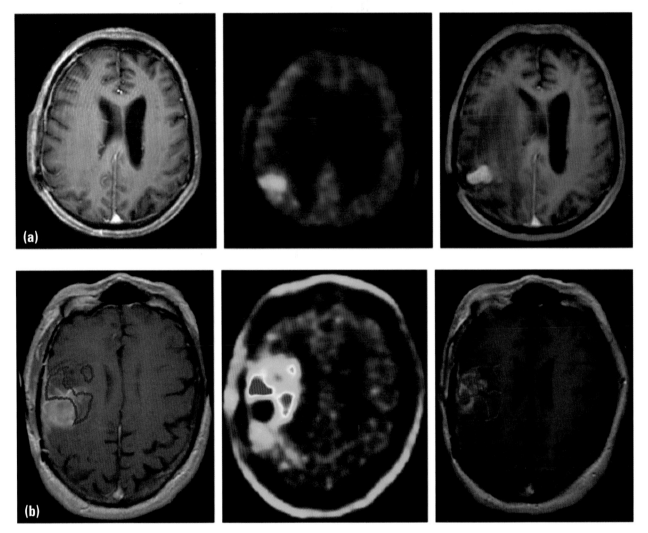

FIGURE 3-2. A patient with a distinct nodule on ^{11}C-methionine positron emission tomography (MET-PET) that was not fully encompassed in the radiotherapy plan **(a)**. Gadolinium-enhanced, T1-weighted magnetic resonance (MR) image (left) shows no appreciable contrast-enhancing lesion in the corresponding area of high uptake in the right parietal region on pretreatment MET-PET (center). An MR image taken 1 month after completion of RT (right) shows a new contrast-enhancing nodule in the area of initial MET-PET uptake (green). The subsequent clinical course confirmed disease progression. Images from a representative patient with a PET gross tumor volume extending beyond the enhancing lesion on MR are shown **(b)**. Pretreatment gadolinium-enhanced, T1-weighted MR (left) shows enhancement along the resection cavity. There is a focus of increased MET-PET (center) uptake directly above the resection cavity. Subsequent MR including MR spectroscopy and PET imaging performed 10 months following therapy shows tumor progression above the resection cavity that overlaps with but is not fully encompassed by the PET-clinical target volume. Printed with permission from Lee et al.[9]

do CT-based volumes. The high percentage of changes in target volumes by FDG-PET reported (20% to 100%) in the literature concerning various parameters of the planning process, such as field sizes, GTV, clinical target volume (CTV), planning target volume (PTV), and normal tissue complication probability, is mainly attributable to two factors: the ability to distinguish the tumor from collapsed lung tissue (atelectasis) and the higher accuracy of FDG-PET in lymph node staging compared with CT. However, because inflammation in the collapsed lung may also lead to FDG accumulation, PET does not help for GTV definition in these cases.

Various methods are currently used for the delineation of FDG accumulations for GTV contouring. One method is the visual contouring by the physician, which is analogous to the method used with CT-based contouring. However, a significant interobserver variability remains.[14] To reduce interobserver variability, clinical protocols have been applied and have succeeded in a significant convergence of FDG-based GTVs contoured by different observers.[15] However, visual contouring remains observer-dependent and by further distribution of the method into clinical practice, the varying experience of the radiotherapist with PET will influence the quality of visual GTV-based contouring. Therefore, other methods for automatic and/or semiautomatic threshold contouring of the often high-contrast FDG accumulations have been investigated.

An example of a relatively simple contrast-oriented method is the "Homburg algorithm"[13,16]:

$$I_{threshold} = A \times I_{lesion} + B \times I_{background} \qquad 1)$$

Here, I_{lesion} is the mean FDG accumulation (standardized uptake value [SUV] or Intensity) of a 3D-isocontour, e.g., 70% of the maximum intensity of the lesion, and $I_{background}$ is the mean FDG accumulation in the surrounding normal tissue. A and B are parameters, which mainly depend on the imaging characteristics of the PET system, which have to be determined by phantom measurements. Other contrast-oriented algorithms lead to similar contouring results; however, they need to be calibrated by phantom measurements. In our experience, other than absolute or relative SUVs, contrast-oriented algorithms are quite robust under clinical conditions. However, calibration to the PET and RT-planning systems is mandatory.[13,16,17] As technical factors such as the methods of reconstruction, attenuation correction of PET images, and data transfer do influence PET imaging, they have to be defined before and kept constant after calibration.

Crucial points in this context are patient positioning and image coregistration. A FDG-PET acquisition for RT treatment planning must be done in the treatment position. It is mandatory to use the same positioning aids as at the other steps of treatment planning and application. Here, photo documentation and laser systems are of considerable help. Irrespective of the kind of scanner used (PET or PET/CT), the correct coregistration of PET data with the CT data set used for RT treatment planning must be verified and corrected, if needed. It should be kept in mind that patient position may change, not only between acquisition on stand-alone PET and CT-scanners, but also during PET/CT acquisition. Failing to correct for the consequent differences in tumor localization may lead to a geographical miss, if PET-derived GTVs are transmitted to CT data sets without critical evaluation of the quality of coregistration. This is best done by comparing anatomical landmarks detectable by both imaging techniques, including the carina, lung apices, spine, sternum, thoracic wall, and—with care because of breathing mobility—the diaphragm. Although nonrigid coregistration algorithms may solve a part of the positioning problem, at the moment, rigid coregistration algorithms are the method of choice. The deformation of image data caused by nonrigid algorithms may result in geometrical inexactnesses or geographical misses, especially in tumors, which are not clearly depicted by the morphological method. Unfortunately, these are the cases in which the integration of FDG-PET into RT treat-

ment planning is most helpful. Further research is clearly needed in this area.

The greatest possible benefit for lung cancer patients from FDG-based treatment planning can only be gained, if, because of the exact depiction of tumor localization by PET, the large irradiation of normal tissues can be omitted. In these patients, this would mean abandoning the concept of the "elective nodal irradiation" (ENI), namely irradiation of large, macroscopically normal parts of the mediastinum.[18] Omitting ENI could lead to a significant improvement in the protection of highly radiosensitive lung tissues with the consequence of permitting higher radiation doses to the tumor. Preliminary clinical data with[19] and even without FDG-PET[20] have suggested that the risk of "out field" recurrences after targeting of the macroscopic tumor alone is small, considerably smaller than the risk for local ("in field") tumor progression. However, prospective randomized clinical studies are needed to show that this approach is truly safe and beneficial.

Visualization of Tumor Biology and Dose Painting

The second rationale for integrating PET into the treatment planning process is the ability of PET to visualize biological pathways, which can be targeted by RT. The imaging of processes including hypoxia, angiogenesis, proliferation, and apoptosis, leads to the identification of different subregions within an inhomogeneous tumor mass that can be individually targeted.

Hypoxia

Clinically, hypoxia, for example, in patients with head and neck tumors, has been shown to be associated with a poor prognosis after RT.[21] Although the underlying mechanisms of radioresistance are still subject to investigation,[22-24] it is potentially valuable to image hypoxia in vivo to increase radiation doses to radioresistant subregions. Several bioreductive substances have been evaluated as hypoxia tracers: [18F]-fluoromisonidazole ([18F]-FMISO), [123I]-iodoazomycin arabinoside ([123I]-IAZA), and [18F]-azomycin arabinoside ([18F]-FAZA) or [60Cu]-labeled methylthiosemicarbazone ([60Cu]-ATSM).

The feasibility of a dose painting concept based on imaging of hypoxic subregions has been investigated by several groups.[25-29] (see Chapter 16C). We have demonstrated that in a significant group of patients with bulky head and neck tumors, the hypoxic volume can be visualized by FAZA-PET (Figure 3-3).[28] In other patients, the hypoxic areas were diffusely distributed in the whole tumor mass and in another subgroup no FAZA uptake could be visualized. However, crucial questions concerning the correlation between hypoxia and perfusion,[30] about the geometrical distribution of the hypoxia over the time,[31] and the response under treatment[30] need to be solved before one can initiate a clinical trial evaluating the impact of incorporating this imaging modality into the radiation treatment planning process.

Proliferation

The proliferation of tumor cells is the basic mechanism for malignant growth. Therefore, attempts have been made to image this parameter, which is thought to be more specific for malignancy compared with glucose consumption. [18F]-fluorine–labeled thymidine analog 3'-deoxy-3'-[18F]-fluorothymidine (FLT) is retained in the cell after phosphorylation by thymidine kinase-1, whose levels correlate with cell proliferation. The FLT uptake in malignant tissue, measured by SUV, appears to be generally lower than the [18F]-FDG uptake. The sensitivity seems to be higher for primary tumors than for lymph node metastases.[32]

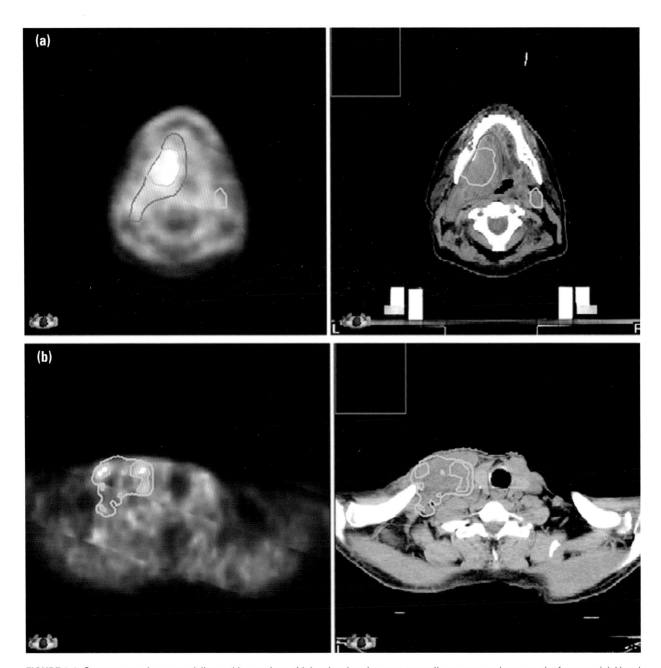

FIGURE 3-3. Gross tumor volume was delineated in a patient with head and neck cancer manually on computed tomography for tumor (pink) and lymph nodes (green). The hypoxic subvolume was delineated automatically on the [18F]-azomycin arabinoside positron emission tomography scan (orange) in a single confluent hypoxic area **(a)** or in multiple diffuse hypoxic areas **(b)**. Reproduced with permission from Grosu et al.[28]

Angiogenesis

The αvβ3 integrin is an important receptor for cell adhesion involved in tumor-induced angiogenesis and metastasis. It mediates migration of activated endothelial cells through the basement membrane during formation of new blood vessels. Particularly interesting is that this integrin is expressed only on the cell surface of tumor cells or activated endothelial cells, and not on normal endothelial cells of established vessels. Haubner et al.[33] and Beer et al.[34] have described noninvasive imaging of αvβ3 integrin expression using ^{18}F-labeled glycosylated Arg-Gly-Asp peptide (^{18}F-Galacto-RGD)–containing glycopeptide and PET. In squamous cell carcinoma of head and neck, for example, αvβ3 integrin appears to be expressed on the endothelial cells and not on the tumor cells, suggesting that RGD-PET could serve as a surrogate for the visualization and evaluation of tumor angiogenesis.[34]

Treatment Monitoring

The third rationale for integrating PET into the treatment planning process is based on the observation that PET can potentially provide a means to differentiate early on treatment responders from nonresponders. Researchers in Munich have investigated in a prospective study patients with esophageal cancer treated with neoadjuvant radiochemotherapy.[35] FDG-PET was performed before and 2 weeks after the start of treatment (0 Gy and 20 Gy). A large decrease in FDG uptake was correlated with a favorable tumor response, whereas a small decrease in SUV was associated with a worse treatment response. Therefore, earlier than CT or MR, FDG-PET could select responders from nonresponders and may aid in the development of highly individualized treatment strategies.[35] Similar results have been reported for cervical cancer, lung cancer, or high grade lymphomas.

Detection of the Optimal Window for the Delivery of Radiation Therapy

The property of PET to visualize the biology of the tumors could be used to show the optimal time for the delivery of the RT. A targeted specific therapy, with vascular growth factor receptor inhibitors, for example, could change a hypoxic tumor into a normoxic one. This would be the optimal window for the delivery of radiation and chemotherapy, a window that could be defined by PET imaging.[36]

References

1. Langen KJ, Ziemons K, Kiwit JC, et al. 3-[123I]iodo-alpha-methyltyrosine and [methyl-11C]-L-methionine uptake in cerebral gliomas: a comparative study using SPECT and PET. *J Nucl Med.* 1997;38(4):517–522.

2. Weber WA, Wester HJ, Grosu AL, et al. O-(2-[18F]fluoroethyl)-L-tyrosine and L-[methyl-11C] methionine uptake in brain tumours: initial results of a comparative study. *Eur J Nucl Med.* 2000;27(5):542–549.

3. Weber WA, Grosu AL, Czernin J. Technology insight: advances in molecular imaging and an appraisal of PET/CT scanning. *Nat Clin Pract Oncol.* 2008;5(3):160–170.

4. Grosu AL, Lachner R, Wiedenmann N, et al. Validation of a method for automatic image fusion (BrainLAB System) of CT data and 11C-methionine-PET data for stereotactic radiotherapy using a LINAC: first clinical experience. *Int J Radiat Oncol Biol Phys.* 2003;56(5):1450–1463.

5. Grosu AL, Weber WA, Riedel E, et al. L-(methyl-11C) methionine positron emission tomography for target delineation in resected high-grade gliomas before radiotherapy. *Int J Radiat Oncol Biol Phys.* 2005;63(1):64–74.

6. Grosu AL, Weber W, Feldmann HJ, et al. First experience with I-123-alpha-methyl-tyrosine SPECT in the 3-D radiation treatment planning of brain gliomas. *Int J Radiat Oncol Biol Phys.* 2000;47(2):517–526.

7. Grosu AL, Feldmann H, Dick S, et al. Implications of IMT-SPECT for postoperative radiotherapy planning in patients with gliomas. *Int J Radiat Oncol Biol Phys.* 2002;54(3):842–854.

8. Grosu AL, Weber WA, Franz M, et al. Reirradiation of recurrent high-grade gliomas using amino acid PET (SPECT)/CT/MRI image fusion to determine gross tumor volume for stereotactic fractionated radiotherapy. *Int J Radiat Oncol Biol Phys.* 2005;63(2):511–519.

9. Lee IH, Piert M, Gomez-Hassan D, et al. Association of 11C-methionine PET uptake with site of failure after concurrent temozolomide and radiation for primary glioblastoma multiforme. *Int J Rad Oncol Biol Phys.* 2009;73(2):478–485.

10. Munley MT, Marks LB, Scarfone C, et al. Multimodality nuclear medicine imaging in three-dimensional radiation treatment planning for lung cancer: challenges and prospects. *Lung Cancer.* 1999;23(2):105–114.

11. Nestle U, Walter K, Schmidt S, et al. 18F-deoxyglucose positron emission tomography (FDG-PET) for the planning of radiotherapy in lung cancer: high impact in patients with atelectasis. *Int J Radiat Oncol Biol Phys.* 1999;44(3):593–597.

12. Nestle U, Hellwig D, Schmidt S, et al. 2-Deoxy-2-[18F]fluoro-D-glucose positron emission tomography in target volume definition for radiotherapy of patients with non-small-cell lung cancer. *Mol Imaging Biol.* 2002;4(3):257–263.

13. Nestle U, Kremp S, Schaefer-Schuler A, et al. Comparison of different methods for delineation of 18F-FDG PET-positive tissue for target volume definition in radiotherapy of patients with non-small cell lung cancer. *J Nucl Med.* 2005;46(8):1342–1348.

14. Pötzsch C, Hofheinz F, van den Hoff J. Vergleich der Inter-Observer-Variabilität bei manueller und automatischer Volumenbestimmung in der PET. *Nuklearmedizin.* 2006;45:A42.

15. MacManus MP, Bayne M, Fimmell N, et al. Reproducibility of "intelligent" contouring of gross tumor volume in non-small cell lung cancer on PET/CT images using a standardized visual method. *Int J Radiat Oncol Biol Phys.* 2007;69:S154–S155.

16. Nestle U, Schaefer-Schuler A, Kremp S, et al. Target volume definition for (18)F-FDG PET-positive lymph nodes in radiotherapy of patients with non-small cell lung cancer. *Eur J Nucl Med Mol Imaging.* 2007;34(4):453–462.

17. Nestle U, Kremp S, Grosu A. Practical integration of [(18)F]-FDG-PET and PET-CT in the planning of radiotherapy for non-small cell lung cancer (NSCLC): the technical basis, ICRU-target volumes, problems, perspectives. *Radiother Oncol.* 2006; 81(2):209–225.

18. Kiricuta IC. Selection and delineation of lymph node target volume for lung cancer conformal radiotherapy. Proposal for standardizing terminology based on surgical experience. *Strahlenther Onkol.* 2001;177(8):410–423.

19. De Ruysscher D, Wanders S, van Haren E, et al. Selective mediastinal node irradiation based on FDG-PET scan data in patients with non-small-cell lung cancer: a prospective clinical study. *Int J Radiat Oncol Biol Phys.* 2005;62(4):988–994.

20. Rosenzweig KE, Sura S, Jackson A, Yorke E. Involved-field radiation therapy for inoperable non-small-cell lung cancer. *J Clin Oncol.* 2007;25(35):5557–5561.

21. Nordsmark M, Bentzen SM, Rudat V, et al. Prognostic value of tumor oxygenation in 397 head and neck tumors after primary radiation therapy. An international multi-center study. *Radiother Oncol.* 2005;77(1):18–24.

22. Troost EG, Bussink J, Kaanders JH, van Eerd J, et al. Comparison of different methods of CAIX quantification in relation to hypoxia in three human head and neck tumor lines. *Radiother Oncol.* 2005;76(2):194–199.

23. Williams KJ, Telfer BA, Xenaki D, et al. Enhanced response to radiotherapy in tumours deficient in the function of hypoxia-inducible factor-1. *Radiother Oncol.* 2005;75(1): 89–98.

24. Yaromina A, Hölscher T, Eicheler W, et al. Does heterogeneity of pimonidazole labelling correspond to the heterogeneity of radiation-response of FaDu human squamous cell carcinoma? *Radiother Oncol.* 2005;76(2):206–212.

25. Rasey JS, Koh WJ, Evans ML, et al. Quantifying regional hypoxia in human tumors with positron emission tomography of [18F]fluoromisonidazole: a pretherapy study of 37 patients. *Int J Radiat Oncol Biol Phys.* 1996;36(2):417–428.

26. Chao KS, Bosch WR, Mutic S, et al. A novel approach to overcome hypoxic tumor resistance: Cu-ATSM-guided intensity-modulated radiation therapy. *Int J Radiat Oncol Biol Phys.* 2001;49(4):1171–1182.

27. Eschmann SM, Paulsen F, Reimold M, et al. Prognostic impact of hypoxia imaging with 18F-misonidazole PET in non-small cell lung cancer and head and neck cancer before radiotherapy. *J Nucl Med.* 2005;46(2):253–260.

28. Grosu AL, Souvatzoglou M, Roper B, et al. Hypoxia imaging with FAZA-PET and theoretical considerations with regard to dose painting for individualization of radiotherapy in patients with head and neck cancer. *Int J Radiat Oncol Biol Phys.* 2007;69(2):541–551.

29. Lee NY, Mechalakos JG, Nehmeh S, et al. Fluorine-18-labeled fluoromisonidazole positron emission and computed tomography-guided intensity-modulated radiotherapy for head and neck cancer: a feasibility study. *Int J Radiat Oncol Biol Phys.* 2008; 70(1):2–13.

30. Thorwarth D, Eschmann SM, Scheiderbauer J, Paulsen F, Alber M. Kinetic analysis of dynamic 18F-fluoromisonidazol PET correlates with radiation treatment outcome in head and neck cancer. *BMC Cancer.* 2005;5:152.

31. Nehmeh SA, Lee NY, Schröder H, et al. Reproducibility of intratumor distribution of (18)F-fluoromisonidazole in head and neck cancer. *Int J Radiat Oncol Biol Phys.* 2008;70(1):235–242.

32. Buck AK, Hetzel M, Schirrmeister H, et al. Clinical relevance of imaging proliferative activity in lung nodules. *Eur J Nucl Med Mol Imaging.* 2005;32(5):525–533.

33. Haubner R, Wester HJ, Weber WA. Noninvasive imaging of alpha(v)beta3 integrin expression using 18F-labeled RGD-containing glycopeptide and positron emission tomography. *Cancer Res.* 2001;61(5):1781–1785.

34. Beer AJ, Grosu AL, Carlsen J, et al. Feasibility of (18F)galacto-RGD PET for imaging of αvβ3 expression on neovasculature in patients with squamous cell carcinoma of head and neck. *Clin Cancer Res.* 2007(22 pt 1);13:6610–6616.

35. Weber WA. Assessing tumor response to therapy. *J Nucl Med.* 2009;50(suppl 1):1S–10S.

36. Jain RK, Duda DG, Clark JW, Loeffler JS. Lessons from phase III clinical trials on anti-VEGF therapy for cancer. *Nat Clin Pract Oncol.* 2006;3(1):24–40.

Chapter 4

Magnetic Resonance Imaging

Vincent Khoo, MD, FRACR, Daryl Lim Joon, MB, BS, FRACR

The development of cross-sectional imaging with computed tomography (CT) has enabled the introduction of conformal radiation therapy (CRT) and, subsequently, intensity-modulated radiation therapy (IMRT) with other advanced planning techniques such as helical tomotherapy and volumetric arc therapies. To realize the potential benefits of such advanced planning techniques, it is important to ensure that target volumes for treatment are defined appropriately by using the most relevant imaging modalities. The standard imaging modality is CT but other imaging modalities such as magnetic resonance (MR) imaging and positron emission tomography (PET) are now being utilized for target volume definition in radiation therapy (RT) treatment planning and as part of image-guided RT (IGRT) or biological targeting strategies.

Magnetic resonance imaging is being increasingly used for oncologic disease staging. For many anatomical regions such as in the central nervous system (CNS), head and neck, and pelvis, MR is now considered to be the imaging modality of choice for staging and tumor assessment. The diverse imaging capabilities of MR provide for better soft tissue characterization as well as the ability to assess functional/biological information. This greater functionality can be utilized in RT treatment planning and the IGRT process. Magnetic resonance imaging can improve morphological target volume delineation as well as provide four-dimensional (4D) information.[1] In this manner, 4D data can estimate the positional variability of the intended target and its surrounding normal structures during a fractionated RT course. This has direct benefits for any sophisticated planning technique including IGRT.

In recent years, there have been many advances in the field of MR from new contrast media to developments in hardware technology. Many previous research-based MR techniques and sequences are now commonplace that can provide characterization of tumor regions and tissue function. Ultra-fast volumetric and three-dimensional (3D) cine sequences offer the opportunity to assess target/organ motion and deformation, which can be used to optimize treatment margins and provide more reliable treatment delivery. Together, the functionality of MR provides immense scope to improve the therapeutic ratio for both external beam RT and brachytherapy.

In this chapter, the basis and rationale for the use of MR in target volume delineation as well as pertinent issues regarding its use in RT treatment planning will be discussed. In addition, recent and forthcoming developments in MR and their impact on RT with attention to target volume definition and IGRT will be reviewed.

MR Methodology

Magnetic resonance measures the radiofrequency energy emitted when tissue hydrogen atoms (protons) in the presence of strong external magnetic fields transition between nuclear spin states. The main MR imaging parameters used to characterize tissue contrast depend on the relative timings of the applied pulse(s), magnetic field gradients, and signal acquisition in relation to the proton density structure of the imaged tissue. Magnetic resonance sequences are often designed toward a particular relaxation time, which may be T1-weighted (spin-lattice) or T2-weighted (spin-spin). The possibility of having a extensive set of potential combinations of possible timings (i.e., varying values of echo [TE] and repetition [TR] times) and arrangements for the various sequencing parameters even within any particular weighted sequence permits imaging of the same tissue with variable subtle differences in contrast, thus enabling better morphological characterization relative to CT. In addition, there is a choice of contrast agents as well as functional information that can be used to demonstrate different structural and biological tissue features. The main difference between MR and CT is that the relative pixel intensities in MR images remain a function of proton densities and different proton spin relaxation times with different tissues whereas CT images depend on x-ray attenuation by tissues that are a function of atomic number and electron density.[2] Thus, MR does not use ionizing radiation.

Rationale of MR Use in Treatment Planning

The standard process in RT treatment planning is to use CT data as they provide geometrically stable images with the direct correlation of the Hounsfield units into measures of x-ray attenuation for dose calculation. Although CT images can easily discriminate between anatomical structures with substantially different Hounsfield units such as air, tissue, and bone, it is more difficult to distinguish between soft tissue structures that possess similar x-ray attenuation properties such as in the pelvis or abdomen. Often, diagnostic radiologists need to rely on the presence of fatty planes or organ boundary interfaces lined with adequate fascia as well as their understanding of normal anatomy to distinguish between normal and abnormal tumor regions. As such, the parameters for CT imaging are more limited compared with the range of imaging parameters available in MR.

The inherent extensive imaging flexibility of MR enables the different soft tissues of very similar Hounsfield units within the same anatomical region to be imaged with the production of varying signal intensities and different imaging contrasts that is exploited for improved diagnosis. Tumors often have similar Hounsfield units or electron densities as their adjacent soft tissue structures.

When different MR sequences are used, the tumor and normal tissue regions can be better characterized such that boundary discrimination between the tumor and normal structures are better defined. In this manner, MR can optimize target volume delineation (Table 4-1).

Other advantages of MR include the ability to avoid bony and metal artifacts typically present when one is imaging with CT. Large, thick cortical bone can attenuate x-rays and reduces the adjacent soft tissue quality, often obscuring the identification of tumors located close by as well as critical organs at risk (OARs). Improved OAR definition can be utilized in both IMRT and IGRT for conformal avoidance schemes. Magnetic resonance imaging can also be used to evaluate for disease recurrence in previously irradiated sites by distinguishing between posttreatment fibrotic changes and recurrent cancer, allowing the initiation of earlier retreatment if appropriate. Magnetic resonance imaging also has true multiplanar capability allowing imaging in any oblique plane, potentially avoiding the partial volume effect seen with conventional axial CT images or when the tumor geometry changes substantially between imaged slices. However, modern spiral CT can now provide high-resolution slicing and reasonable 3D reconstruction to overcome this limitation. Using parasagittal and/or paracoronal views together with 4D information can also provide improved

TABLE 4–1 Advantages and Disadvantages of Magnetic Resonance (MR) Imaging for Radiotherapy Treatment Planning

Features	Advantages	Disadvantages
Patient	• Noninvasive or minimally invasive • Minimal patient risks • Nonionizing (particularly beneficial for children and pregnant women)	• Claustrophobia • Contraindicated in patients with some pacemakers or internal loose metal foreign bodies particularly in the orbits
Imaging	• Wide range and functionality of imaging parameters • Superior soft tissue imaging • Excellent spatial resolution • True multiplanar capability • Improved definition of tumor extent and delineation for treatment volumes because of better imaging of soft tissue structures and tissue planes especially postsurgery • May distinguish between posttreatment fibrosis and tumor recurrence • Can avoid image artifact from metal prostheses and large bony regions • Able to reduce inter- and intraobserver variability • Can provide functional and biological information for functional avoidance or biological targeting • Ultrafast volumetric and cine mode acquisitions to assess temporal–spatial variations for target motion or deformation • Can be coregistered with CT data for radiotherapy treatment planning	• Lack of electron density information for dosimetry • Lack of cortical bone information to create digitally reconstructed radiographs • Image distortion (systems and object-induced distortions) • May have longer scan times than CT with potential for motion artifacts • Need for specific training to comprehend and understand MR imaging • Radiotherapy systems can only import transverse MR images and cannot take full advantage of sagittal and coronal in-plane MR images • Most immobilization devices may not be MR compatible
Contrast agents	• New contrast agents (i.e., USPIO) for nodal assessment • Less incidence of allergic reactions to gadolinium than iodine-based contrast agents	
Machine	• Scanner bore flange openings can lessen patient claustrophobia • Open systems for easier patient access, tolerance, and positioning for RT	• Smaller bore than CT (52 cm vs 82 cm to 85 cm) • Less available and accessible than CT • Curved table top

Notes. Adapted from Khoo V et al.[139] CT = computed tomography; MR = magnetic resonance; RT = radiotherapy; USPIO = ultrasmall paramagnetic iron oxide.

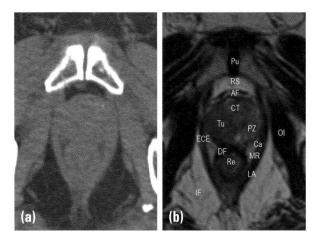

FIGURE 4-1. A case example in prostate cancer of a transaxial view with computed tomography (CT) (a) and magnetic resonance (MR) imaging (b) is shown. The prostatic capsule is better visualized with MR and the tumor and extracapsular extension is visible on the right side of the peripheral zone of the prostate gland, which is not seen on CT. In addition, internal prostate zonal architecture can be seen in the MR image but not on CT. AF = prostate anterior fibromuscular layer; Ca = capsule; CT = prostate central and transition zone; DF = Denonvilliers fascia; ECE = extracapsular extension; IF = ischiorectal fossa; LA = levator ani; MR = mesorectum; OI = obturator internus; Pu = pubis; PZ = prostate peripheral zone; Re = rectum; RS = retropubic space; Tu = tumor.

appreciation of both 3D anatomy and temporal-spatial variations for OARs and tumor and aids target volume delineation for both treatment planning and design of IGRT schemes (Figures 4-1 to 4-3).

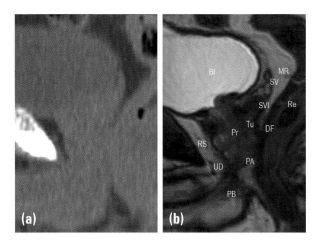

FIGURE 4-2. A case example in prostate cancer of a sagittal view with computed tomography (CT) (a) and magnetic resonance (MR) imaging (b) is shown. The tumor and seminal vesicle invasion are seen on MR but are not visualized on CT. There is also better distinction between the prostate, notably the apex and its adjacent structures such as the urogenital diaphragm, penile bulb, rectum, and bladder, with MR compared with CT. BI = bladder; DF = Denonvilliers fascia; MR = mesorectum; PA = prostate apex; PB = prostate base; Pr = prostate; Re = rectum; RS = retropubic space; SV = seminal vesicle; SVI = seminal vesicle invasion; Tu = tumor; UD = urogenital diaphragm.

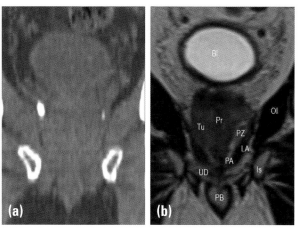

FIGURE 4-3. A case example in prostate cancer of a coronal view with computed tomography (CT) (a) and magnetic resonance (MR) imaging (b) is shown. There is better definition of the prostate gland boundaries and the adjacent structures on MR than on the CT images. Is = ischium; LA – levator ani; PA – prostate apex; PB – penile bulb; Pr = prostate; PZ = prostate peripheral zone; OI = obturator internus; Tu = tumor; UD = urogenital diaphragm.

Another important aspect of improved tissue visualization with MR is that it provides for increased reliability and consistency in target volume definition, reducing both interobserver and intraobserver variability. This is particularly important for the quality assurance (QA) of clinical trials, whether it is a local or multicenter study as substantial interobserver variability can impact trial outcomes. However, the greatest opportunity with MR is that functional and biological information can be obtained with MR, further improving target volume delineation and permitting new opportunities for novel strategies such as simultaneous integrated boosts and IGRT.

The use of MR for RT requires appropriate understanding and training. For radiation oncologists whose main focus is target volume definition, specific and supervised training is needed enabling the planner to understand the principles of MR, what individual MR sequences are designed to demonstrate, and the caveats in its use.[3] It is still beneficial to interact closely with experienced diagnostic MR radiologists and MR physicists, particularly if functional MR imaging or 4D data are being utilized. In the United Kingdom, the Royal College of Radiologists has endorsed the concept of a multidisciplinary team approach for the definition of RT target volumes.[4] In the ideal situation, the diagnostic MR radiologist and the radiation oncologist would sit together to perform target delineation. In certain situations, it may also be advisable to have the attending surgeon or any other relevant specialist(s) in attendance. The increasingly widespread use of Picture Archiving and Communication Systems can facilitate coordination between busy team members, avoiding the need for the simultaneous physical presence of the specialists as each specialist can contribute individually and at different times. For this process to be efficient, the clinical case in question will need to be adequately discussed such that the intended aim of treatment is apparent to all members. This can also be extended to the IGRT approach for adaptive and predictive strategies where the input of the MR physicist and treatment planning team would be invaluable.

Clinical Applications of Conventional MR Imaging

Many centers have incorporated some form of MR imaging into the planning process of CNS tumors because of reported quantitative improvements in target volume definition in up to 80% of cases.[5-7] Magnetic resonance imaging can also provide complementary information.[8] In a study of base-of-skull meningiomas, MR improved tumor visualization compared with CT because of x-ray attenuation secondary to bone, obscuring soft tissue detail on CT images. However, CT provided different and complementary information on bony erosion that was not available with MR (Figure 4-4).[9] The use of CT-MR fusion is becoming routine for treatment planning in CNS tumors and is aided by automated and atlas-based segmentation algorithms.[10,11] Interest is also focused on

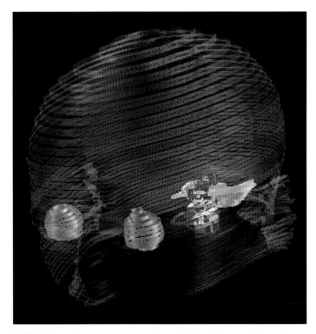

FIGURE 4-4. An example case of a patient with a skull-based meningioma illustrating differences between magnetic resonance (MR) imaging and computed tomography (CT) assessment of the clinical target volume (CTV) is shown. The three-dimensional reconstructed view of the CT-defined CTV (yellow) and MR-defined CTV (red) illustrates the spatial and complementary differences in CTV definition by the two different imaging modalities; in particular, the MR-defined CTV demonstrates tumor extending laterally along the petrous ridge that was not seen with CT. Reproduced with permission from Khoo V et al.[9]

the integration of functional information for biological targeting (see Chapter 15C).[12]

Magnetic resonance imaging is useful in head and neck RT by defining (1) tumor infiltration along the upper aero-digestive tract and adjacent fascial planes, (2) tumor infiltration of adjacent soft tissue structures and tissue planes, (3) perineural infiltration and intracranial extension (particularly with nasopharyngeal tumors), and (4) nodal metastases. In nasopharyngeal cancer, MR has been shown to alter disease staging in 50% of cases.[13,14] A study of more than 250 nasopharyngeal cases detected up to 40% of intracranial infiltration on MR that was missed by CT.[15] Illustration of the use of MR for target delineation in a patient with nasopharyngeal cancer is shown in Chapter 16B. Magnetic resonance segmentation algorithms based on contrast enhancement and signal intensity ratios of MR sequences may also aid the planning process.[16] Current studies are exploring PET combined with MR/CT imaging[17] and pathologic validation of imaging with provides valuable insight for treatment planning and biological IGRT.[18,19]

Magnetic resonance imaging provides excellent evaluation for pelvic cancers and is considered the imaging method of choice at some centers.[20,21] For prostate cancer, MR provides improved local staging and overcomes the limitations of CT such as defining the prostatic apex and the prostatic–rectal boundaries.[22,23] Often, the prostatic capsule, which cannot be distinguished from adjacent tissues on CT, can be seen as a thin rim of low-signal intensity on T2-weighted MR (Figures 4-1 to 4-3).[24] Comparison of coregistered CT-MR planning data sets have noted that CT overestimates the treatment volume in prostate cancer patients by as much as 27% to 43% because of the soft tissue uncertainty in CT delineation.[25-28] Magnetic resonance imaging can also be useful where the internal pelvic anatomy has been substantially altered because of previous surgery.[29] It is also beneficial when severe CT metal artifacts from hip prostheses obscure relevant anatomy.[30] See Chapter 20A for an illustration of the use of MR-based treatment planning in prostate cancer.

The use of MR-based treatment planning in prostate cancer patients may improve target volume delineation by taking into account prostate motion and deformation.[31] This can lead to better shaping and delivery of treatment fields reducing unnecessary dosing to important adjacent normal structures such as the rectum and penile bulb.[32,33] This has implications when proton therapy is being used.[34] Magnetic resonance–compatible and novel markers are also available for prostate IGRT and increase the utility of MR for RT.[35,36] Coregistration of CT and MR images has been used in prostate brachytherapy for both high- and low-dose rate regimens, providing better target definition, reducing delineation uncertainty, and aiding needle localization and postimplant dosimetry.[37,38] Methods of MR-based perineal implantation of the prostate that use automated systems within standard and 3T MR scanners as well as with open MR scanners are being devised but will need clinical validation.[39-41] Similar benefits are noted for MR-based brachytherapy treatment planning in other tumor sites such as head and neck, sarcomas, and gynecology.[42] The Gynecological GEC-ESTRO Working Group has strongly advocated the use of MR for brachytherapy[43] (see Chapter 21A).

There is also developing support for the use of MR in gynecologic external beam RT as well as brachytherapy.[43,44] For locally advanced cervical cancer, the use of MR for a combined adaptive RT and brachytherapy program has improved local control rates.[45] It also has applications for IGRT and its potential use with an MR linear accelerator to optimize IMRT has been described.[46] In rectal cancer, MR can improve assessment of disease infiltration longitudinally along the rectal wall and its extent into the mesorectum and anal sphincter.[47-49] This can aid treatment decision and RT planning for sphincter-sparing approaches, tumor boosting, and dose escalation with or without concurrent chemotherapy.

Considerations for Using MR in RT Planning

Although MR is quite attractive for RT planning, there are certain issues that need to be considered when one is utilizing MR for target volume delineation, treatment planning, or target verification. Such aspects include the lack of electron density information, potential MR image distortion, and specific patient considerations with MR scanners. Several in-depth reviews have been published on these subjects.[2,50]

Dose Calculation

The use of any images for RT treatment planning necessitates geometrically accurate images with electron density information that is needed for tissue inhomogeneity assessment and calculation of dose distributions. Both of these parameters are available from CT data where the Hounsfield units can be directly calibrated with electron density values. However, MR images provide signal intensities but not electron density information. Furthermore, image distortion may occur limiting spatial accuracy. Such issues need to assessed and evaluated before MR images can be used in RT either alone or in combination with CT data.

One method to overcome the lack of electron density information is to manually assign x-ray attenuation coefficient values to the different signal intensity regions within the MR image. However, this would be a laborious and time-consuming process. In regions where the internal anatomy is homogenous and without substantial attenuation variation such as the brain, then simple automated segmentation for the skull and brain may be easily achieved and assigned a homogenous CT attenuation value for dose calculation. Investigators have compared the dosimetry between CT- and MR-alone–based CNS treatment plans and reported equivalent results to within 2%.[51,52] Using similar methods for prostate irradiation, some studies have reported reasonable dosimetric correlation between CT-based and MR-based dose calculations (within 2% to 3%); however, others have found differences in dosimetry of greater than 2% if bone and water CT number bulk-assigned values were not assigned to the pelvic MR images.[53] It is more difficult to assign a single CT attenuation value to anatomical regions such as the head and neck or thorax where there are significant air, bone, and tissue regions, which can alter dose computation. The development of patient-based anatomical atlas sets and improved segmentation software programs for MR images may provide improved means for region allocation of attenuation factors and lead to using MR alone for treatment planning in complex anatomical regions.

The other method of utilizing MR images with CT is image registration of the two modalities, creating a common image set where the information from both modalities is available. This method is more commonly used than the previous method as it permits the correlation of both image sets within the treatment planning system. Once QA of the image registration has been performed, the user can easily use either data set to optimize visualization of the target volume and have this volume automatically registered within the CT data set for subsequent production of digital reconstructed radiographs (DRRs) and dose calculation. The methodology for autosegmentation and image coregistration is outside the scope of this chapter and the reader is referred to standard medical physics textbooks.[2]

Image Distortion

One of the main issues that limits the widespread use of MR images in RT is image distortion. In general terms, MR image distortions can be classified into two main categories, namely system-related or object-induced (Figure 4-5).

System-related MR distortions have several inter-related factors and can be attributed to imperfections of the magnet, the operating system, and imaging procedures.[50] Contributing factors include the presence of inhomogeneities within the magnet field, nonlinearities of the applied gradient fields, and eddy currents, which occur when applied gradients are turned on and off. In general, the effects of system-related distortion are least at the center of the magnet where the magnetic field is most homogenous. As the homogeneity of the magnetic field decreases with distance, the magnitude of the distortion may increase and is largest at the periphery of the image field-of-view (FOV), potentially a concern for

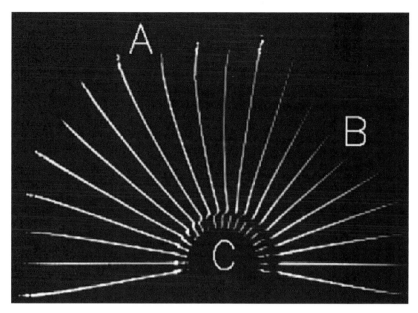

FIGURE 4-5. Illustration of various forms of distortion in magnetic resonance (MR) imaging with a phantom consisting of a coplanar array of water-filled tubes embedded within in a circular solid plastic (PMMA) block is shown. System distortion effects are seen in the apparent curvature of the tubes at A and their disappearance at B, which was attributable to warping distortion of the imaging plane. Magnetic susceptibility differences because of the presence of the plastic support block at C give rise to object-induced distortions in the form of discontinuities at the point where each tube enters the support block. Reproduced with permission from Khoo V et al.[50]

image coregistration if the registration process relies on fiducials placed on the skin as the distortion will cause spatial misplacement of the fiducials and subsequent misregistration.

When any object is placed within a magnetic field, effects from magnetic susceptibility and chemical shift may give rise to object-induced distortions.[50] Different tissues will have different intrinsic magnetic susceptibilities. The effects of this can be pronounced at tissue boundaries such as between air cavities and soft tissues or bone as in the sinuses of the face or within the thorax. Chemical shift effects result from the different behavior of protons in fat and tissue. Fat protons "precess" at a slower rate than do water protons and this results in a chemical shift effect where the positions of fat and water protons are shifted from their true spatial locations. This effect may also occur where there are substantial fatty regions such as in the abdomen and pelvis.

Such image distortions need to be assessed, minimized, and/or corrected before being used alone or with image coregistration to avoid introducing a systematic error in spatial position of the target or OARs into the planning process. Many methods exist to address these issues with most commercial MR systems and some RT treatment planning vendors providing distortion correction software modules for their systems. In principle, the aim is to quantify the presence and extent of any MR distortion. We have previously described an integrated process for the evaluation and correction of both system-related and object-induced distortions as well as the formation of QA programs.[54–57]

System-related distortion should be quantified and mapped. This can be achieved by using a specially designed phantom (the so-called linearity test object, LTO) with a preset geometrical array of markers in 3D, providing 3D spatial assessments of the imaging volume used for treatment planning. In addition, a similar array of 3D markers are placed within a specially designed flat MR couch and a patient reference frame to provide another set of marker positions that covers the periphery of the entire FOV during MR imaging. The LTO or the patient can be housed within this reference marker setup. There is also a separate set of markers placed on the patient's surface to provide assessment of object-induced effects. In brief, the positions of all markers are mapped within the imaging volume by using a dedicated automated algorithm. It is important that the same MR scanner and imaging sequence used for mapping are also used to image the patient. System-related distortion should be quantified for the individual MR scanner and sequence used. This method can then be used for both correction and QA of stability of the system. The use of read-out gradient reversal imaging and postprocessing image corrections can account for object-induced effects. Distortional shifts of up to 5 mm can be corrected.[54–57] Other correction methods have been reported to reduce distortions by a factor of two.[58] There are also site-specific phantoms with air cavities to assess the use of MR for thoracic RT.[59]

Other MR Considerations

As noted previously, the effect of distortion is least within the center of the magnet. Where possible, the patient should thus be arranged such that the volumes of interest are located as close as possible to this region. When larger FOVs are used, the potential distortion at the periphery may be avoided by extracting the central imaged region alone for subsequent coregistration with CT.

Protocols for MR imaging need to address the aim, which may differ if the data are needed for temporal–spatial information instead of morphological or functional

TABLE 4–2 Potential Questions to be Addressed When One Is Determining the Use of Magnetic Resonance (MR) Imaging for Radiotherapy Treatment Planning

- It is important to clarify the aim of MR imaging for the radiotherapy process. What is the MR going to demonstrate? Is morphological or functional information needed? What is the best MR sequence needed to provide the information? Are 3D or 4D data needed?
- Will there be a need to use contrast agents and what type of contrast agents are needed?
- What is the relevant volume or anatomical region to be imaged?
- What degree of image resolution is needed?
- What are the parameters for image acquisition (i.e., slice orientation, slice thickness, and slice gaps)?
- What is the influence of various body coils or internal body MR probes on the MR images for coregistration?
- What is the extent of MR image distortion associated with the MR sequence, FOV used, and in the anatomical region being imaged with the particular MR machine?
- What is the appropriate quality assurance program to ensure reliability of image quality and data transfer?

Notes. Adapted from Khoo V et al.[139] 3D = three-dimensional; 4D = four-dimensional; FOV = field of view; MR = magnetic resonance.

target volume delineation. It is also important to evaluate for the best sequence that will offer the optimal combination of image quality/resolution with minimal image distortion as these sequences will differ depending on the disease process and anatomical site. Some of the issues that will need to be addressed are outlined in Table 4-2.

Utilization of MR in RT planning should mimic the standard CT planning scenario and set-up procedures, including the use of a flat bed insert and scanning the patient in the treatment position. If immobilization devices are used, they should be MR-compatible. Patient instructions should be kept the same such as keeping a full or empty bladder or rectum. In the ideal situation, the CT and MR scans should be timed as close as possible to each other. Attention is needed to ensure that all protocols that use MR images are optimized to maintain the best use of its functionality.

Hardware Developments and Clinical Applications

Higher Tesla (3T) MR Scanners

Since the initial development of MR, field strengths have been increasing from 0.5T (Tesla) to 1.5T scanners with subsequent improvements in image quality. Image quality (or resolution) is related to the signal-to-noise ratio with image quality increasing when the signal is strengthened and the noise reduced. As the signal-to-noise ratio increases approximately in a linear manner with field strength, the use of higher field strengths provide higher resolution images with improved tissue contrast. In addition, acquisition times may also be reduced,

potentially reducing associated motion artifacts from physiological activity. The development of 3T MR scanners can improve the imaging quality by using external phase array coils. Some investigators have reported that in prostate MR, the image quality from external phase array coils using 3T are comparable to endorectal coils at 1.5T[60] and in some cases exceeding them.[61] This approach can avoid internal organ deformation and the need for sophisticated coregistration software to deal with deformation. 3T MR scanners can also improve the resolution for assessed metabolites in MR spectroscopy (MRS) and applications of functional MR for better definition of tumor regions such as for brain[62] and prostate[63] RT. There are some issues that may limit the use of 3T MR scanners in RT, including the potential exacerbation of magnetic susceptibility effects, doubling of the chemical shift effect, patient safety, and engineering challenges. Currently, higher than 3T MR scanners are being developed and the clinical utility of such scanners for RT treatment planning remains to be defined.

Several potential imaging issues exist with higher-Tesla scanners. Magnetic susceptibility effects are usually located at tissue boundaries and higher field strengths may exacerbate such effects leading to increased signal intensities.[64] In turn, this may result in misdiagnosis when one is using contrast studies, leading to misidentification of abnormal areas and erroneous target volumes. It is important to have pre- and postcontrast studies for appropriate comparison. There is also an impact on chemical shift effects, which may be either a disadvantage or advantage. The chemical shift effect is doubled with 3T fields causing misregistration of fat and water tissues if these MR images are not corrected when they are coregistered with CT. However, this pronounced chemical shift effect is utilized in MRS to increase the resolution of identifying tissue metabolites for example in brain and prostate cancer.[62,65,66]

The energy deposited within the patient when one is using 3T machines is a potential concern as it may be up to four times that of 1.5T scanners. This may result from the opportunity to use faster or more intensive pulse sequences with the 3T scanners. However, this energy can be modified appropriately by changing the pulse sequence protocols or reducing the imaged volume of tissue. A smaller scanning bore diameter will also restrict the scanning of larger patients and may increase the effects of claustrophobia. Of note, these higher-Tesla scanners are currently substantially more expensive than 1.5T machines but this may change as they become more widely available.

In prostate cancer, the use of 3T-based MR sequences may aid selective biopsy of suspicious regions for disease mapping.[67] Magnetic resonance spectroscopy (using 3T scanners) citrate-choline assessment may permit better localization of biological tumor regions for boosting with IMRT and IGRT as well as with brachytherapy.[65,66]

The use of 3T-based dynamic contrast-enhanced MR (dcMR) and diffusion-weighted MR (dwMR) may also provide better assessment of disease recurrence post-RT.[68] Similarly, MRS can be used for primary brain cancer RT planning and to assess for residual disease (see the following section on MRS).[62]

MR Simulators

Open- and low-field MR scanners can be utilized as RT simulators similar to the CT simulator. Some of the advantages of MR simulation include greater soft tissue image contrast, particularly T1-weighted images, reduced vessel flow and ghosting artifacts, and the opportunity to use immobilization devices that can be size-restricted with conventional MR scanners. Systems-related distortions can be larger with open low-field MR scanners but these can be easily corrected and object-induced distortion effects are generally much less because of the lower magnetic field strength.[42,69] One study has reported negligible distortion within radial distances less than 12 cm when one is planning RT in CNS tumor patients.[70] Some of the limitations of low-field MR include potentially longer time to complete individual MR sequences but this can be minimized by appropriate sequence selection. Another limitation is the lack of bone definition to create DRRs for treatment verification, which can be overcome by delineation software to highlight bony regions.

The lower signal-to-noise ratio may limit high-quality diagnostic images but relatively good-quality images have been obtained with low-field 0.2T MR in regions of interest such as the prostate that can be used for prostate treatment planning.[71] In a study of 243 cases patients with prostate, lung, and brain tumors, it was reported that open low-field MR simulation provided appropriate treatment planning images in up to 95% of cases.[42] The investigators reported improved tumor volume definition with MR for two thirds of the cases studied, leading to 40% reduction of organ and clinical target volume. For the prostate patients, this led to a 15% reduction in mean rectal dose and for the brain tumor patients, MR image quality was considered superior to CT in 87% of cases.

MR Linear Accelerators

The integration of a MR system and a linear accelerator is analogous to the incorporation of CT with a linear accelerator (i.e., the helical tomotherapy system) and represents a very exciting development. Such a system combines the superior imaging capabilities of MR with RT and may provide further opportunities to optimize IMRT and IGRT strategies.[72] There are a few approaches to this concept.[73,74] Such combined systems are still in development as there are many technical issues to be overcome before they become a practical reality. A fully functioning prototype still remains to be built at the time of writing but progress is encouraging. See Chapter 13 "Emerging In-Room Technologies" for a description of a prototype MR Linear Accelerator system.

MR Contrast Agents

Regional lymph nodes are often included in the clinical target volume in the radiotherapeutic treatment of many cancer sites. It is thus important to appropriately define nodal volumes to ensure optimal local control. However, the elucidation of pathologically involved lymph nodes is poor when one is using morphological imaging techniques as clinical involvement is only denoted with simple size criteria. This methodology cannot accurately account for microscopic and subclinical disease involvement and surgery remains the gold standard in establishing lymph node involvement. Up to 20% of normal-size lymph nodes can be positive for microscopic disease and up to 30% of enlarged lymph nodes may only show inflammation and no tumor. With standard MR methods, the signal intensity and degree of contrast enhancement between benign and malignant lymph nodes is not reliable enough to provide satisfactory discrimination between normal and abnormal lymph nodes.

Ultrasmall Superparamagnetic Iron Oxide Particles

Recently, ultrasmall superparamagnetic iron oxide (USPIO) particles have been used as contrast agents in MR to identify and discriminate between normal and abnormal lymph nodes. These particles are injected into the bloodstream and are taken up by macrophages and subsequently transported via the lymphatic system to lymph nodes. In the reticuloendothelial system, these macrophages with ingested USPIO particles result in a reduction in signal intensity within a node because of the negative enhancement from the iron oxide particles. When the patient is scanned 24 to 26 hours later allowing time for the macrophages to accumulate in the nodal system, this lowering of signal intensity caused by the presence of macrophages laden with USPIO particles within normal nodes produces a negative enhancement image. In nodes that are involved or replaced by tumor, macrophages with ingested USPIO particles are prevented from occupying the node by the tumor and the MR signal intensity in pathologically involved nodes is preserved.

Studies evaluating USPIO particles have reported a relatively high sensitivity and specificity of up to 90% in detecting small-volume disease involvement in lymph nodes.[75,76] A recent pilot study comparing the clinical assessment of nodal appearance using ferumoxtran-10 versus nodal resection confirmed a sensitivity of 100% and specificity of 96% in patients with renal cancers.[77] This method can also be used with 3D sequences to map lymph nodes along blood vessels and provide accurate surgical templates for treatment planning rather than the traditional use of nodal volumes based on regional and bony landmarks. It is imperative to avoid inadequate nodal coverage that may compromise disease control or unnecessarily nodal irradiation that may increase treatment toxicity.[78,79] The obvious benefit of reliable subclinical disease detection is to permit individualization of treatment fields with involved nodes selected for dose escalation and uninvolved nodal regions may have reduced prophylactic nodal doses or be avoided completely. Optimizing the irradiated nodal volumes may also permit better patient tolerance of concurrent therapies with systemic agents such as chemotherapy, radiosensitizers, or biological agents and allow dose intensification.

The treatment of head and neck tumors exemplifies this management challenge. Imaging with USPIO has been used to aid in the planning of head and neck surgery.[76] It may also be used to complement the recommendations for CT-defined nodal volumes in head and neck RT.[80] For nodal coverage in a variety of pelvic cancers, it was reported that 3D margins of 12 mm around the distal para-aortic vessels, 10 mm for the common iliac, 9 mm for the external iliac, and 10 mm for the internal iliac with a 22 mm margin anterior to the sacrum and 22 mm margin medial to the pelvic sidewalls would adequately encompass the majority of pelvic nodes.[81] Although USPIO detection of subclinical disease may be an important advancement, it remains a morphological imaging method with certain limitations. For example, the threshold size for detecting pathological involvement may be 2 mm to 3 mm in a 5-mm to 10-mm node and false positives may occur if there is fibrosis or fatty replacement of the nodes.[82] However, USPIO particles may be combined with other imaging methods such as PET to further increase its sensitivity and specificity.

Developments in MR Sequences and Techniques

MR Sequences

There is a diverse array of MR sequences that have applications in RT treatment planning such as ultrafast imaging, volumetric sequences, and cine-mode acquisition. Such sequences provide 4D data on target motion and OAR displacement, which can be used to modify planning margins and to initiate IGRT strategies. Ultrafast imaging can be obtained by MR sequences such as echo planar imaging. This type of imaging has several applications particularly when one is evaluating targets or structures affected by rapid motion effects including respiration and cardiac motion. The 4D data obtained may also be used to model patterns of change for IGRT, evaluate gated images, or even to compare the impact of different IGRT strategies.[83] An MR-compatible–based active breathing control device has been developed.[84] More recently, a magnetization transfer method has been relatively well

correlated with PET to evaluate issues of atelectasis near tumor tissue and can be used for RT planning.[85] Ultrafast, volumetric, and cine MR sequences provide noninvasive means to evaluate not only variability in target volume positioning during RT but also the temporal variation in target volume deformation that may occur inter- and intrafractionally. These are pertinent issues that currently limit RT prevision and have justified the development of IGRT.

The regional anatomical 4D data providing by volumetric and cine-mode MR information is useful for determining appropriate site-specific planning margins and to aid in the design of IGRT strategies. In lung irradiation, cine MR can evaluate intrathoracic tumor mobility for patient individualization of treatment margins[86,87] and to determine the efficacy of free-breathing gating techniques.[88] When one is considering potential benefits for soft tissue delineation, MR can provide better visualization of cardiac structure (myocardium and ventricular space) compared with CT for heart dose–volume assessment by breath hold in left breast RT.[89] It has also been used to assess thoracic spinal cord motion, which can aid extracranial stereotactic RT.[90]

In prostate cancer, cine MR has been used to evaluate the magnitude of intrafraction organ motion.[91,92] Similar studies have been undertaken for cervical cancer.[93] Such intrafraction data can be used to determine the potential impact of rectal volume changes for planning margins as well as the degree of target deformation that may occur during irradiation.[94] Target volume deformation has also been investigated for bladder cancers where the whole organ usually forms the target. In an IGRT program termed "POLO" or predictive organ localization, cine MR studies are obtained to characterize a priori the individual patient's bladder temporal–spatial changes as it fills such that the appropriate treatment plan can be selected to compensate for the degree of bladder deformation occurring during this period.[95] In this manner, anistropic and reduced planning margins may be used while minimizing potential geographical misses.[96]

Developments in MR Techniques

Magnetic resonance can also be used to evaluate tissue pathophysiology and tumor response providing functional and biological information in addition to simple morphological assessments. This information can be used to define appropriate active tumor regions for IGRT. Features of cancer growth including vascular neoangiogenesis, excessive cellular growth, and tissue biochemistry are exploited by MR techniques such as dynamic contrast-enhanced MR (dcMR), diffusion weighted MR (dwMR), and MRS. Although these techniques have been used mainly for research, they are now being evaluated in clinical studies with promising results.

Dynamic Contrast-Enhanced MR

Dynamic contrast-enhanced MR imaging is a method that can examine the vascular dynamics of tumor neoangiogenesis. Different tissue enhancement curves can be recognized for normal, tumor, and irradiated tissues[97] such that normal tissues can be distinguished from cancerous tissue, and local active tissue regions can be identified for RT targeting or dose boosting, as well as permitting monitoring of tumor response or recurrence. This technique uses fast MR sequences to characterize tissue or organ vascular perfusion by following the sequential passage of injected low-molecular-weight contrast agents. Vascular perfusion changes are subsequently represented as qualitative time-dependent enhancement curves for different tissue regions. Various MR sequences can be used to assess the passage of the low-molecular-weight contrast agents through the tissues. T2-weighted sequences, being more sensitive to the vascular phase, can better display tissue perfusion and have been used widely for brain tumors.[98] T1-weighted sequences can better demonstrate microvessel perfusion, permeability, and extracellular leakage effects[99] and have been reported to be useful in breast, musculoskeletal, and pelvic cancers.[68,100–103]

In a clinical–pathological correlation study of 42 prostate cancer patients imaged by dcMR prior to prostatectomy, dcMR has been reported to be more sensitive than simple T2-weighted MR imaging in detecting disease regions.[104] It has also been used to optimize IMRT regimes in cervical cancer.[72] In prostate cancer patients failing external beam irradiation, dcMR can identify and localize residual disease, potentially permitting early salvage therapy such as high-intensity focused ultrasound (HIFU) ablation if the disease remains localized.[105] The use of both dcMR and dwMR has been reported to be applicable in defining local prostate cancer progression following HIFU.[106]

Tumor recurrence can also be detected with dcMR in the previously irradiated breast[107] and prostate.[108,109] In addition, dcMR has been used to predict response to RT in head and neck,[110] rectal,[111] and cervical cancers.[102] With appropriate tumor enhancement curves, the status of lymph nodes may also be assessed for microscopic involvement, but only a small anatomical area can be assessed at a time and not the entire nodal drainage region.

Diffusion Weighted MR

Diffusion weighted MR is a method that assesses the imaged tissues' diffusion capacity. In tumor regions where there is cellular proliferation producing increased cellular density, the diffusion of water molecules through this abnormal region is reduced and apparent diffusion coefficient (ADC) maps can be generated from various anatomical regions of interest. Tumor regions are more likely to have a lower ADC than normal regions.

Clinical Applications of dwMR

Early studies suggest that dwMR may help distinguish between malignant and benign lesions in patients with brain,[112] rectal,[113,114] prostate,[115,116] and cervical[117] cancers. However, dwMR studies in some cancer types such as soft tissue sarcomas were not found to be as helpful because of substantial overlap in ADC values.[118,119] The use of dwMR tumor–defined areas may permit the assessment of tumor response during a course of therapy and regions of poor response may be selected for radiation boosts. In prostate cancer, dwMR has been used to define seminal vesicle involvement to optimize irradiation[120] and may identify foci of disease within the either the peripheral or transitional zone for additional boosting.[121] It may also be used to define more aggressive tumor subtypes.[122] In rectal cancer, studies suggest that ADC values may provide indicators of tumor response to chemoradiation,[123,124] which can be used to alter and optimize treatment strategies.

Diffusion Tensor Imaging

Diffusion tensor MR (DTI) is a method that assesses white matter abnormalities based on cerebral tissue anisotropy. The metric feature of anisotropy provides a measure of tissue disorganization. It can provide better information on disease involvement of white matter tracts and can be a useful method of assessing subclinical tumor infiltration in white matter[125] as well as early disease progression following therapy[126] and radiation effects.[127]

Clinical Applications of Diffusion Tensor Imaging

Diffusion tensor imaging has been reported to identify larger white matter tract abnormalities than T2-weighted imaging in a small series of high-grade gliomas together with detection of unrecognized contralateral involvement in four out of 13 of these cases[128] and has been useful in planning craniospinal irradiation in children.[129] It may also be used to clarify patterns of disease recurrence or progression following stereotactic RT.[130] Although these findings need confirmation in larger studies, it has the potential to aid RT treatment planning.

Diffusion tensor imaging can also be used with magnetoencephalography to design treatment plans to limit doses to relevant functional white matter regions or white tracts. This method can offer treatment plan individualization and reduce relevant neurological dysfunction for the patient.[131] It can also be complementary to other imaging techniques including PET that are being assessed for target volume delineation in brain RT treatment planning to ensure there is appropriate target coverage.

MR Spectroscopy

The assessment of tissue metabolites such as choline, creatine, lactate, lipids, and citrate can be used to profile normal and tumor tissue regions within organs by using MRS. The nuclei of different metabolites produce distinct characteristic peaks when subjected to magnetic fields and permit different biochemical compounds within tissue to be evaluated and distinguished.[132] Magnetic resonance spectroscopy has advantages over radio-labelled methods as it does not require specific labelling of compounds and utilization pathways. The pattern of the spectra of these examined tissue metabolites can then be used to assess for metabolically active disease regions for specific targeting or boosting, and to distinguish between fibrosis, necrosis, and recurrence as well as to evaluate disease responses.

There are some limitations in the use of MRS for RT treatment planning. First of all, the signal with standard MR scanners for MRS remains relatively small and signal-to-noise ratio may limit adequate assessment. Spatial resolution remains coarse in the order of 6 mm to 10 mm with current 1.5T scanners and can restrict full utilization. This may improve with the use of higher-Tesla scanners although there are other limitations when one is using these scanners as noted in the previous section. Coregistration of MRS with MR and CT images is still required for both assessment and application in treatment planning. Magnetic resonance spectroscopy has been investigated in several cancers but its use is mainly limited to larger institutions and research centers and it is still not widely available. The applications of MRS remain under active research and have not been fully quantified. Other reasons for limited use may also exist including available expertise and cost of the software, as well as the extra time needed to perform these examinations and subsequently its integration for treatment planning.

Clinical Applications of MRS

The use of MRS in the brain has been intensively studied. Magnetic resonance spectroscopy has been used to distinguish between different tumor types with brain cancers.[133] Recently, investigators have reported that MRS may help to identify more disease presence based on the choline-to-creatine ratio compared with the morphological tumor volumes outlined by MR-based planning.[134] The information from MRS can be used with functional MR information to initiate a program of IMRT dose escalation.

Multimodality imaging with MRS and PET has been described to distinguish disease recurrence from radiation injury and to aid in the RT decision-making.[135,136] The changing patterns of the MRS spectra of relevant brain metabolites following therapy in malignant glioma have also been reported to be potentially useful for prognosis.[137,138] This may offer opportunities for adaptive IGRT strategies.[138]

Conclusions

Many advantages exist for incorporating MR in RT treatment planning. The main benefit is the superior soft tissue characterization that can aid target volume delineation. More recent MR developments have offered improved resolution of disease extent and functional/biological tumor information with advances in higher-Tesla scanners, MR contrast agents, sequences, and techniques. Moreover, MR can identify tumor recurrence and distinguish between disease and fibrosis/normal tissues. Magnetic resonance can offer disease response assessment on a morphological and biochemical/biological basis and provide dosimetry assessment with MR gel systems. However, it is imperative to ensure appropriate QA procedures are in place for its use. Some of the newer MR techniques will need correlation against histopathology to provide validation. Clinical studies using MR-assisted or MR-based RT are still needed to define benefits in patient outcomes. Close collaborations are needed between all the different medical specialities and will be best achieved through a dedicated multidisciplinary team approach.

References

1. Khoo VS. MRI—"magic radiotherapy imaging" for treatment planning? *Br J Radiol.* 2000;73(867):229–233.
2. Khoo V. Magnetic resonance imaging in treatment planning. In: Mayles P, Nahum A, Rosenwald JC, eds. *Handbook of Radiotherapy Physics: Theory and Practice.* 1st ed. Boca Raton, Florida: CRC Press; 2007: 657–668.
3. Sundar S, Symonds RP. Diagnostic radiology for radiotherapist: the case for structured training in cross-sectional imaging (CT and MRI). *Clin Oncol (R Coll Radiol).* 2002;14(5):413–414.
4. Board-of-the-Faculty-of-Clinical-Oncology. Imaging for oncologists: collaboration between clinical radiologists and clinical oncologists in diagnosis, staging and radiotherapy planning. London, England: Royal College of Radiologists; 2004.
5. Thornton AF, Sandler HM, Ten Haken RK, et al. The clinical utility of magnetic resonance imaging in the 3-dimensional treatment planning of brain neoplasms. *Int J Radiat Oncol Biol Phys.* 1992;24(4):767–775.
6. Heester MA, Wijrdeman HK, Struikmans H, Witkamp T, Moerland MA. Brain tumor delineation based on CT and MR imaging. Implications for radiotherapy treament planning. *Strahlenther Onkol.* 1993;169(12):729–733.
7. Sultanem K, Patrocinio H, Lambert C, et al. The use of hypofractionated intensity-modulated irradiation in the treatment of glioblastoma multiforme: preliminary results of a prospective trial. *Int J Radiat Oncol Biol Phys.* 2004;58(1):247–252.
8. Ten Haken RK, Thornton AF, Sandler HM, et al. A quantitative assessment of the addition of MRI to CT-based, 3-D treatment planning of brain tumors. *Radiother Oncol.* 1992;25(2):121–133.
9. Khoo VS, Adams EJ, Saran F, et al. A comparison of clinical target volumes determined by CT and MRI for the radiotherapy planning of base of skull meningiomas. *Int J Radiat Oncol Biol Phys.* 2000;46(5):1309–1317.

10. Mazzara GP, Velthuizen RP, Pearlman JL, Greenberg HM, Wagner H. Brain tumor target volume determination for radiation treatment planning through automated MRI segmentation. *Int J Radiat Oncol Biol Phys.* 2004;59(1):300–312.

11. Bondiau PY, Malandain G, Chanalet S, et al. Atlas-based automatic segmentation of MR images: validation study on the brainstem in radiotherapy context. *Int J Radiat Oncol Biol Phys.* 2005;61(1):289–298.

12. Levivier M, Massager N, Wikler D, Goldman S. Modern multimodal neuroimaging for radiosurgery: the example of PET scan integration. *Acta Neurochir Suppl.* 2004;91:1–7.

13. Manavis J, Sivridis L, Koukourakis MI. Nasopharyngeal carcinoma: the impact of CT-scan and of MRI on staging, radiotherapy treatment planning, and outcome of the disease. *Clin Imaging.* 2005;29(2):128–133.

14. Emami B, Sethi A, Petruzzelli GJ. Influence of MRI on target volume delineation and IMRT planning in nasopharyngeal carcinoma. *Int J Radiat Oncol Biol Phys.* 2003;57(2):481–488.

15. Chung NN, Ting LL, Hsu WC, Lui LT, Wang PM. Impact of magnetic resonance imaging versus CT on nasopharyngeal carcinoma: primary tumor target delineation for radiotherapy. *Head Neck.* 2004;26(3):241–246.

16. Lee FK, Yeung DK, King AD, Leung SF, Ahuja A. Segmentation of nasopharyngeal carcinoma (NPC) lesions in MR images. *Int J Radiat Oncol Biol Phys.* 2005;61(2):608–620.

17. Nishioka T, Shiga T, Shirato H, et al. Image fusion between 18FDG-PET and MRI/CT for radiotherapy planning of oropharyngeal and nasopharyngeal carcinomas. *Int J Radiat Oncol Biol Phys.* 2002;53(4):1051–1057.

18. Daisne JF, Duprez T, Weynand B, et al. Tumor volume in pharyngolaryngeal squamous cell carcinoma: comparison at CT, MR imaging, and FDG PET and validation with surgical specimen. *Radiology.* 2004;233(1):93–100.

19. Geets X, Tomsej M, Lee JA, et al. Adaptive biological image-guided IMRT with anatomic and functional imaging in pharyngo-laryngeal tumors: impact on target volume delineation and dose distribution using helical tomotherapy. *Radiother Oncol.* 2007;85(1):105–115.

20. Barentsz JO, Engelbrecht MR, Witjes JA, de la Rosette JJ, van der Graaf M. MR imaging of the male pelvis. *Eur Radiol.* 1999;9(9):1722–1736.

21. Heenan SD. Magnetic resonance imaging in prostate cancer. *Prostate Cancer Prostatic Dis.* 2004;7(4):282–288.

22. Khoo VS, Padhani AR, Tanner SF, Finnigan DJ, Leach MO, Dearnaley DP. Comparison of MRI with CT for the radiotherapy planning of prostate cancer: a feasibility study. *Br J Radiol.* 1999;72(858):590–597.

23. Wachter S, Wachter-Gerstner N, Bock T, et al. Interobserver comparison of CT and MRI-based prostate apex definition. Clinical relevance for conformal radiotherapy treatment planning. *Strahlenther Onkol.* 2002;178(5):263–268.

24. Cheng D, Tempany CM. MR imaging of the prostate and bladder. *Semin Ultrasound CT MR.* 1998;19(1):67–89.

25. Roach M III, Faillace-Akazawa P, Malfatti C, Holland J, Hricak H. Prostate volumes defined by magnetic resonance imaging and computerized tomographic scans for three-dimensional conformal radiotherapy. *Int J Radiat Oncol Biol Phys.* 1996;35(5):1011–1018.

26. Kagawa K, Lee WR, Schultheiss TE, Hunt MA, Shaer AH, Hanks GE. Initial clinical assessment of CT-MRI image fusion software in localization of the prostate for 3D conformal radiation therapy. *Int J Radiat Oncol Biol Phys.* 1997;38(2):319–325.

27. Rasch C, Barillot I, Remeijer P, Touw A, van Herk M, Lebesque JV. Definition of the prostate in CT and MRI: a multi-observer study. *Int J Radiat Oncol Biol Phys.* 1999;43(1):57–66.

28. Sannazzari GL, Ragona R, Ruo Redda MG, Giglioli FR, Isolato G, Guarneri A. CT-MRI image fusion for delineation of volumes in three-dimensional conformal radiation therapy in the treatment of localized prostate cancer. *Br J Radiol.* 2002;75(895):603–607.

29. Lau HY, Kagawa K, Lee WR, Hunt MA, Shaer AH, Hanks GE. Short communication: CT-MRI image fusion for 3D conformal prostate radiotherapy: use in patients with altered pelvic anatomy. *Br J Radiol.* 1996;69(828):1165–1170.

30. Rosewall T, Kong V, Vesprini D, et al. Prostate delineation using CT and MRI for radiotherapy patients with bilateral hip prostheses. *Radiother Oncol.* 2009;90(3):325–330.

31. Kerkhof EM, van der Put RW, Raaymakers BW, van der Heide UA, van Vulpen M, Lagendijk JJ. Variation in target and rectum dose due to prostate deformation: an assessment by repeated MR imaging and treatment planning. *Phys Med Biol.* 2008;53(20):5623–5634.

32. Steenbakkers RJ, Deurloo KE, Nowak PJ, Lebesque JV, van Herk M, Rasch CR. Reduction of dose delivered to the rectum and bulb of the penis using MRI delineation for radiotherapy of the prostate. *Int J Radiat Oncol Biol Phys.* 2003;57(5):1269–1279.

33. Buyyounouski MK, Horwitz EM, Price RA, Hanlon AL, Uzzo RG, Pollack A. Intensity-modulated radiotherapy with MRI simulation to reduce doses received by erectile tissue during prostate cancer treatment. *Int J Radiat Oncol Biol Phys.* 2004;58(3):743–749.

34. Yeung AR, Vargas CE, Falchook A, et al. Dose-volume differences for computed tomography and magnetic resonance imaging segmentation and planning for proton prostate cancer therapy. *Int J Radiat Oncol Biol Phys.* 2008;72(5):1426–1433.

35. Carl J, Nielsen J, Holmberg M, Højkjaer Larsen E, Fabrin K, Fisker RV. A new fiducial marker for image-guided radiotherapy of prostate cancer: clinical experience. *Acta Oncol.* 2008;47(7):1358–1366.

36. Frank SJ, Stafford RJ, Bankson JA, et al. A novel MRI marker for prostate brachytherapy. *Int J Radiat Oncol Biol Phys.* 2008;71(1):5–8.

37. Ménard C, Susil RC, Choyke P, et al. MRI-guided HDR prostate brachytherapy in standard 1.5T scanner. *Int J Radiat Oncol Biol Phys.* 2004;59(5):1414–1423.

38. Citrin D, Ning H, Guion P, et al. Inverse treatment planning based on MRI for HDR prostate brachytherapy. *Int J Radiat Oncol Biol Phys.* 2005;61(4):1267–1275.

39. Fischer GS, DiMaio SP, Iordachita II, Fichtinger G. Robotic assistant for transperineal prostate interventions in 3T closed MRI. *Med Image Comput Comput Assist Interv.* 2007;10(pt 1):425–433.

40. Muntener M, Patriciu A, Petrisor D, et al. Transperineal prostate intervention: robot for fully automated MR imaging—system description and proof of principle in a canine model. *Radiology.* 2008;247(2):543–549.

41. Lakosi F, Antal G, Vandulek C, et al. Technical feasibility of transperineal MR-guided prostate interventions in a low-field open MRI unit: canine study. *Pathol Oncol Res.* 2009;15(3):315–322.

42. Krempien RC, Daeuber S, Hensley FW, Wannenmacher M, Harms W. Image fusion of CT and MRI data enables improved target volume definition in 3D-brachytherapy treatment planning. *Brachytherapy.* 2003;2(3):164–171.

43. Pötter R, Haie-Meder C, Van Limbergen E, et al. Recommendations from gynaecological (GYN) GEC ESTRO working group (II): concepts and terms in 3D image-based treatment planning in cervix cancer brachytherapy-3D dose volume parameters and aspects of 3D image-based anatomy, radiation physics, radiobiology. *Radiother Oncol.* 2006;78(1):67–77.

44. Barillot I, Reynaud-Bougnoux A. The use of MRI in planning radiotherapy for gynaecological tumours. *Cancer Imaging.* 2006; 6:100–106.

45. Pötter R, Dimopoulos J, Georg P, et al. Clinical impact of MRI assisted dose volume adaptation and dose escalation in brachytherapy of locally advanced cervix cancer. *Radiother Oncol.* 2007;83(2):148–155.

46. Kerkhof EM, Raaymakers BW, van der Heide UA, van de Bunt L. Online MRI guidance for healthy tissue sparing in patients with cervical cancer: an IMRT planning study. *Radiother Oncol.* 2008;88(2):241–249.

47. Blomqvist L, Holm T, Nyrén S, Svanström R, Ulvskog Y, Iselius L. MR imaging and computed tomography in patients with rectal tumours clinically judged as locally advanced. *Clin Radiol.* 2002;57(3):211–218.

48. Beets-Tan RG, Lettinga T, Beets GL. Pre-operative imaging of rectal cancer and its impact on surgical performance and treatment outcome. *Eur J Surg Oncol.* 2005;31(5):681–688.

49. Ferri M, Laghi A, Mingazzini P, et al. Pre-operative assessment of extramural invasion and sphincteral involvement in rectal cancer by magnetic resonance imaging with phased-array coil. *Colorectal Dis.* 2005;7(4):387–393.

50. Khoo VS, Dearnaley DP, Finnigan DJ, Padhani A, Tanner SF, Leach MO. Magnetic resonance imaging (MRI): considerations and applications in radiotherapy treatment planning. *Radiother Oncol.* 1997;42(1):1–15.

51. Schad LR, Blüml S, Hawighorst H, Wenz F, Lorenz WJ. Radiosurgical treatment planning of brain metastases based on a fast, three-dimensional MR imaging technique. *Magn Reson Imaging.* 1994;12(5):811–819.

52. Wang C, Chao M, Lee L, Xing L. MRI-based treatment planning with electron density information mapped from CT images: a preliminary study. *Technol Cancer Res Treat.* 2008;7(5): 341–348.

53. Lee YK, Bollet M, Charles-Edwards G, et al. Radiotherapy treatment planning of prostate cancer using magnetic resonance imaging alone. *Radiother Oncol.* 2003;66(2):203–216.

54. Finnigan DJ, Tanner SF, Dearnaley DP, et al. Distortion-corrected magnetic resonance images for pelvic radiotherapy treatment planning. In: Faulkner K, Carey B, Crellin A, Harrison RM, eds. *Quantitative Imaging in Oncology.* London, England: British Institute of Radiology; 1997: 72–76.

55. Tanner SF, Finnigan DJ, Khoo VS, Mayles P, Dearnaley DP, Leach MO. Radiotherapy planning of the pelvis using distor-

56. tion corrected MR images: the removal of system distortions. *Phys Med Biol.* 2000;45(8):2117–2132.

56. Doran SJ, Charles-Edwards L, Reinsberg SA, Leach MO. A complete distortion correction for MR images: I. Gradient warp correction. *Phys Med Biol.* 2005;50(7):1343–1361.

57. Reinsberg SA, Doran SJ, Charles-Edwards EM, Leach MO. A complete distortion correction for MR images: II. Rectification of static-field inhomogeneities by similarity-based profile mapping. *Phys Med Biol.* 2005;50(11):2651–2661.

58. Petersch B, Bogner J, Fransson A, Lorang T, Pötter R. Effects of geometric distortion in 0.2T MRI on radiotherapy treatment planning of prostate cancer. *Radiother Oncol.* 2004;71(1): 55–64.

59. Koch N, Liu HH, Olsson LE, Jackson EF. Assessment of geometrical accuracy of magnetic resonance images for radiation therapy of lung cancers. *J Appl Clin Med Phys.* 2003;4(4): 352–364.

60. Sosna J, Pedrosa I, Dewolf WC, Mahallati H, Lenkinski RE, Rofsky NM. MR imaging of the prostate at 3 Tesla: comparison of an external phased-array coil to imaging with an endorectal coil at 1.5 Tesla. *Acad Radiol.* 2004;11(8):857–862.

61. Bloch BN, Rofsky NM, Baroni RH, Marquis RP, Pedrosa I, Lenkinski RE. 3 Tesla magnetic resonance imaging of the prostate with combined pelvic phased-array and endorectal coils; Initial experience(1). *Acad Radiol.* 2004;11(8):863–867.

62. Pirzkall A, Li X, Oh J, et al. 3D MRSI for resected high-grade gliomas before RT: tumor extent according to metabolic activity in relation to MRI. *Int J Radiat Oncol Biol Phys.* 2004;59(1): 126–137.

63. Pickett B, Vigneault E, Kurhanewicz J, Verhey L, Roach M. Static field intensity modulation to treat a dominant intra-prostatic lesion to 90 Gy compared to seven field 3-dimensional radiotherapy. *Int J Radiat Oncol Biol Phys.* 1999;44(4):921–929.

64. Mack A, Wolff R, Scheib S, et al. Analyzing 3-tesla magnetic resonance imaging units for implementation in radiosurgery. *J Neurosurg.* 2005;102 suppl:158–164.

65. DiBiase SJ, Hosseinzadeh K, Gullapalli RP, et al. Magnetic resonance spectroscopic imaging-guided brachytherapy for localized prostate cancer. *Int J Radiat Oncol Biol Phys.* 2002;52(2): 429–438.

66. van Lin EN, Fütterer JJ, Heijmink SW, et al. IMRT boost dose planning on dominant intraprostatic lesions: gold marker-based three-dimensional fusion of CT with dynamic contrast-enhanced and 1H-spectroscopic MRI. *Int J Radiat Oncol Biol Phys.* 2006;65(1):291–303.

67. Hambrock T, Fütterer JJ, Huisman HJ, et al. Thirty-two-channel coil 3T magnetic resonance-guided biopsies of prostate tumor suspicious regions identified on multimodality 3T magnetic resonance imaging: technique and feasibility. *Invest Radiol.* 2008;43(10):686–694.

68. Kim CK, Park BK, Park W, Kim SS. Prostate MR imaging at 3T using a phased-arrayed coil in predicting locally recurrent prostate cancer after radiation therapy: preliminary experience. *Abdom Imaging.* 2010;35(2):246–252.

69. Mizowaki T, Nagata Y, Okajima K, et al. Development of an MR simulator: experimental verification of geometric distortion and clinical application. *Radiology.* 1996;199(3):855–860.

70. Kristensen BH, Laursen FJ, Logager V, Geertsen PF, Kraup-Hansen A. Dosimetric and geometric evaluation of an open low-field magnetic resonance simulator for radiotherapy treatment planning of brain tumours. *Radiother Oncol.* 2008;87(1):100–109.

71. Deasy NP, Conry BG, Lewis JL, et al. Local staging of prostate cancer with 0.2 T body coil MRI. *Clin Radiol.* 1997;52(12):933–937.

72. Yamashita Y, Harada M, Torashima M, et al. Dynamic MR imaging of recurrent postoperative cervical cancer. *J Magn Reson Imaging.* 1996;6(1):167–171.

73. Lagendijk JJ, Raaymakers BW, Raaijmakers AJ, et al. MRI/linac integration. *Radiother Oncol.* 2008;86(1):25–29.

74. Kirkby C, Stanescu T, Rathee S, Carlone M, Murray B, Fallone BG. Patient dosimetry for hybrid MRI-radiotherapy systems. *Med Phys.* 2008;35(3):1019–1027.

75. Harisinghani MG, Saini S, Weissleder R, et al. MR lymphangiography using ultrasmall superparamagnetic iron oxide in patients with primary abdominal and pelvic malignancies: radiographic-pathologic correlation. *AJR Am J Roentgenol.* 1999;172(5):1347–1351.

76. Mack MG, Balzer JO, Straub R, Eichler K, Vogl TJ. Superparamagnetic iron oxide-enhanced MR imaging of head and neck lymph nodes. *Radiology.* 2002;222(1):239–244.

77. Guimaraes AR, Tabatabei S, Dahl D, McDougal WS, Weissleder R, Harisinghani MG. Pilot study evaluating use of lymphotrophic nanoparticle-enhanced magnetic resonance imaging for assessing lymph nodes in renal cell cancer. *Urology.* 2008;71(4):708–712.

78. Portaluri M, Bambace S, Perez C, et al. Clinical and anatomical guidelines in pelvic cancer contouring for radiotherapy treatment planning. *Cancer Radiother.* 2004;8(4):222–229.

79. Martin J, Joon DL, Ng N, et al. Towards individualised radiotherapy for stage I seminoma. *Radiother Oncol.* 2005; 76(3):251–256.

80. Grégoire V, Coche E, Cosnard G, Hamoir M, Reychler H. Selection and delineation of lymph node target volumes in head and neck conformal radiotherapy. Proposal for standardizing terminology and procedure based on the surgical experience. *Radiother Oncol.* 2000;56(2):135–150.

81. Dinniwell R, Chan P, Czarnota G, et al. Pelvic lymph node topography for radiotherapy treatment planning from ferumoxtran-10 contrast-enhanced magnetic resonance imaging. *Int J Radiat Oncol Biol Phys.* 2009;74(3):844–851.

82. Kim JY, Harisinghani MG. MR imaging staging of pelvic lymph nodes. *Magn Reson Imaging Clin N Am.* 2004;12(3):581–586.

83. Rohlfing T, Maurer CR Jr, O'Dell WG, Zhong J. Modeling liver motion and deformation during the respiratory cycle using intensity-based nonrigid registration of gated MR images. *Med Phys.* 2004;31(3):427–432.

84. Arnold JF, Mörchel P, Glaser E, Pracht ED, Jakob PM. Lung MRI using an MR-compatible active breathing control (MR-ABC). *Magn Reson Med.* 2007;58(6):1092–1098.

85. Arnold JF, Kotas M, Pyzalski RW, Pracht ED, Flentje M, Jakob PM. Potential of magnetization transfer MRI for target volume definition in patients with non-small-cell lung cancer. *J Magn Reson Imaging.* 2008;28(6):1417–1424.

86. Plathow C, Ley S, Fink C, et al. Analysis of intrathoracic tumor mobility during whole breathing cycle by dynamic MRI. *Int J Radiat Oncol Biol Phys.* 2004;59(4):952–959.

87. Cai J, Read PW, Larner JM, Jones DR, Benedict SH, Sheng K. Reproducibility of interfraction lung motion probability distribution function using dynamic MRI: statistical analysis. *Int J Radiat Oncol Biol Phys.* 2008;72(4):1228–1235.

88. Liu HH, Koch N, Starkschall G, et al. Evaluation of internal lung motion for respiratory-gated radiotherapy using MRI: Part II-margin reduction of internal target volume. *Int J Radiat Oncol Biol Phys.* 2004;60(5):1473–1483.

89. Krauss DJ, Kestin LL, Raff G, et al. MRI-based volumetric assessment of cardiac anatomy and dose reduction via active breathing control during irradiation for left-sided breast cancer. *Int J Radiat Oncol Biol Phys.* 2005;61(4):1243–1250.

90. Cai J, Sheng K, Sheehan JP, Benedict SH, Larner JM, Read PW. Evaluation of thoracic spinal cord motion using dynamic MRI. *Radiother Oncol.* 2007;84(3):279–282.

91. Padhani AR, Khoo VS, Suckling J, Husband JE, Leach MO, Dearnaley DP. Evaluating the effect of rectal distension and rectal movement on prostate gland position using cine MRI. *Int J Radiat Oncol Biol Phys.* 1999;44(3):525–533.

92. Ghilezan MJ, Jaffray DA, Siewerdsen JH, et al. Prostate gland motion assessed with cine-magnetic resonance imaging (cine-MRI). *Int J Radiat Oncol Biol Phys.* 2005;62(2):406–417.

93. Chan P, Dinniwell R, Haider MA, et al. Inter- and intrafractional tumor and organ movement in patients with cervical cancer undergoing radiotherapy: a cinematic-MRI point-of-interest study. *Int J Radiat Oncol Biol Phys.* 2008;70(5):1507–1515.

94. Khoo VS, Bedford JL, Padhani A, et al. Prostate and rectal deformation assessed using cine magnetic resonance imaging (MRI) during a course of radical prostate radiotherapy. *Radiother Oncol.* 2002;64(S1):285.

95. Mangar SA, Scurr E, Huddart RA, et al. Assessing intrafractional bladder motion using cine-MRI as initial methodology for predictive organ localization (POLO) in radiotherapy for bladder cancer. *Radiother Oncol.* 2007;85(2):207–214.

96. Lalondrelle S, Hansen V, McNair H, et al. Adaptive-Predictive Organ Localisation (A-POLO): evaluation of a novel adaptive planning methodology. *Radiother Oncol.* 2008;88(S2):98.

97. Padhani AR, Husband JE. Dynamic contrast-enhanced MRI studies in oncology with an emphasis on quantification, validation and human studies. *Clin Radiol.* 2001;56(8):607–620.

98. Sugahara T, Korogi Y, Kochi M, et al. Correlation of MR imaging-determined cerebral blood volume maps with histologic and angiographic determination of vascularity of gliomas. *AJR Am J Roentgenol.* 1998;171(6):1479–1486.

99. Neeman M, Provenzale JM, Dewhirst MW. Magnetic resonance imaging applications in the evaluation of tumor angiogenesis. *Semin Radiat Oncol.* 2001;11(1):70–82.

100. Yabuuchi H, Matsuo Y, Okafuji T, et al. Enhanced mass on contrast-enhanced breast MR imaging: lesion characterization using combination of dynamic contrast-enhanced and diffusion-weighted MR images. *J Magn Reson Imaging.* 2008;28(5):1157–1165.

101. De Vries A, Griebel J, Kremser C, et al. Monitoring of tumor microcirculation during fractionated radiation therapy in patients with rectal carcinoma: preliminary results and implications for therapy. *Radiology*. 2000;217(2):385–391.

102. Mayr NA, Yuh WT, Arnholt JC, et al. Pixel analysis of MR perfusion imaging in predicting radiation therapy outcome in cervical cancer. *J Magn Reson Imaging*. 2000;12(6):1027–1033.

103. Zhang XM, Yu D, Zhang HL, et al. 3D dynamic contrast-enhanced MRI of rectal carcinoma at 3T: correlation with microvascular density and vascular endothelial growth factor markers of tumor angiogenesis. *J Magn Reson Imaging*. 2008; 27(6):1309–1316.

104. Girouin N, Mège-Lechevallier F, Tonina Senes A, et al. Prostate dynamic contrast-enhanced MRI with simple visual diagnostic criteria: is it reasonable? *Eur Radiol*. 2007;17(6):1498–1509.

105. Haider MA, Chung P, Sweet J, et al. Dynamic contrast-enhanced magnetic resonance imaging for localization of recurrent prostate cancer after external beam radiotherapy. *Int J Radiat Oncol Biol Phys*. 2008;70(2):425–430.

106. Kim CK, Park BK, Lee HM, Kim SS, Kim E. MRI techniques for prediction of local tumor progression after high-intensity focused ultrasonic ablation of prostate cancer. *AJR Am J Roentgenol*. 2008;190(5):1180–1186.

107. Dao TH, Rahmouni A, Campana F, Laurent M, Asselain B, Fourquet A. Tumor recurrence versus fibrosis in the irradiated breast: differentiation with dynamic gadolinium-enhanced MR imaging. *Radiology*. 1993;187(3):751–755.

108. Hawnaur JM, Zhu XP, Hutchinson CE. Quantitative dynamic contrast enhanced MRI of recurrent pelvic masses in patients treated for cancer. *Br J Radiol*. 1998;71(851):1136–1142.

109. Rouvière O, Valette O, Grivolat S, et al. Recurrent prostate cancer after external beam radiotherapy: value of contrast-enhanced dynamic MRI in localizing intraprostatic tumor—correlation with biopsy findings. *Urology*. 2004;63(5):922–927.

110. Tomura N, Omachi K, Sakuma I, et al. Dynamic contrast-enhanced magnetic resonance imaging in radiotherapeutic efficacy in the head and neck tumors. *Am J Otolaryngol*. 2005; 26(3):163–167.

111. Devries AF, Griebel J, Kremser C, et al. Tumor microcirculation evaluated by dynamic magnetic resonance imaging predicts therapy outcome for primary rectal carcinoma. *Cancer Res*. 2001;61(6):2513–2516.

112. Rees J. Advances in magnetic resonance imaging of brain tumours. *Curr Opin Neurol*. 2003;16(6):643–650.

113. Hosonuma T, Tozaki M, Ichiba N, et al. Clinical usefulness of diffusion-weighted imaging using low and high b-values to detect rectal cancer. *Magn Reson Med Sci*. 2006;5(4):173–177.

114. Rao SX, Zeng MS, Chen CZ, et al. The value of diffusion-weighted imaging in combination with T2-weighted imaging for rectal cancer detection. *Eur J Radiol*. 2008;65(2):299–303.

115. Kim JH, Kim JK, Park BW, Kim N, Cho KS. Apparent diffusion coefficient: prostate cancer versus noncancerous tissue according to anatomical region. *J Magn Reson Imaging*. 2008;28(5): 1173–1179.

116. Van As N, Charles-Edwards E, Jackson A, et al. Correlation of diffusion-weighted MRI with whole mount radical prostatectomy specimens. *Br J Radiol*. 2008;81(986):456–462.

117. McVeigh PZ, Syed AM, Milosevic M, Fyles A, Maider MA. Diffusion-weighted MRI in cervical cancer. *Eur Radiol*. 2008; 18(5):1058–1064.

118. Einarsdóttir H, Karlsson M, Wejde J, Bauer HC. Diffusion-weighted MRI of soft tissue tumours. *Eur Radiol*. 2004;14(6): 959–963.

119. Tamai K, Koyama T, Saga T, et al. The utility of diffusion-weighted MR imaging for differentiating uterine sarcomas from benign leiomyomas. *Eur Radiol*. 2008;18(4):723–730.

120. Kim CK, Choi D, Park BK, Kwon GY, Lim HK. Diffusion-weighted MR imaging for the evaluation of seminal vesicle invasion in prostate cancer: initial results. *J Magn Reson Imaging*. 2008;28(4):963–969.

121. Yoshizako T, Wada A, Hayashi T, et al. Usefulness of diffusion-weighted imaging and dynamic contrast-enhanced magnetic resonance imaging in the diagnosis of prostate transition-zone cancer. *Acta Radiol*. 2008;49(10):1207–1213.

122. deSouza NM, Riches SF, Vanas NJ, et al. Diffusion-weighted magnetic resonance imaging: a potential non-invasive marker of tumour aggressiveness in localized prostate cancer. *Clin Radiol*. 2008;63(7):774–782.

123. Dzik-Jurasz A, Domenig C, George M, et al. Diffusion MRI for prediction of response of rectal cancer to chemoradiation. *Lancet*. 2002;360(9329):307–308.

124. Kremser C, Judmaier W, Hein P, et al. Preliminary results on the influence of chemoradiation on apparent diffusion coefficients of primary rectal carcinoma measured by magnetic resonance imaging. *Strahlenther Onkol*. 2003;179(9): 641–649.

125. Verma R, Zacharaki EI, Ou Y, et al. Multiparametric tissue characterization of brain neoplasms and their recurrence using pattern classification of MR images. *Acad Radiol*. 2008; 15(8):966–977.

126. Weber MA, Giesel FL, Stieltjes B. MRI for identification of progression in brain tumors: from morphology to function. *Expert Rev Neurother*. 2008;8(10):1507–1525.

127. Haris M, Kumar S, Raj MK, et al. Serial diffusion tensor imaging to characterize radiation-induced changes in normal-appearing white matter following radiotherapy in patients with adult low-grade gliomas. *Radiat Med*. 2008;26(3): 140–150.

128. Price SJ, Burnet NG, Donovan T, et al. Diffusion tensor imaging of brain tumours at 3T: a potential tool for assessing white matter tract invasion? *Clin Radiol*. 2003;58(6):455–462.

129. Nazmy MS, Attalla EM, Refeat A. Effect of magnetic resonance myelography on the target volume in craniospinal irradiation in children. *Clin Oncol (R Coll Radiol)*. 2009;21(1):14–18.

130. Krishnan AP, Asher IM, Davis D, Okunieff P, O'Dell WG. Evidence that MR diffusion tensor imaging (tractography) predicts the natural history of regional progression in patients irradiated conformally for primary brain tumors. *Int J Radiat Oncol Biol Phys*. 2008;71(5):1553–1562.

131. Aoyama H, Kamada K, Shirato H, et al. Integration of functional brain information into stereotactic irradiation treatment planning using magnetoencephalography and magnetic resonance axonography. *Int J Radiat Oncol Biol Phys*. 2004;58(4): 1177–1183.

132. Govindaraju V, Young K, Maudsley AA. Proton NMR chemical shifts and coupling constants for brain metabolites. *NMR Biomed.* 2000;13(3):129–153.

133. Preul MC, Caramanos Z, Collins DL, et al. Accurate, noninvasive diagnosis of human brain tumors by using proton magnetic resonance spectroscopy. *Nat Med.* 1996;2(3): 323–325.

134. Narayana A, Chang J, Thakur S, et al. Use of MR spectroscopy and functional imaging in the treatment planning of gliomas. *Br J Radiol.* 2007;80(953):347–354.

135. Zeng QS, Li CF, Zhang K, Liu H, Kang XS, Zhen JH. Multivoxel 3D proton MR spectroscopy in the distinction of recurrent glioma from radiation injury. *J Neurooncol.* 2007;84(1): 63–69.

136. Seo YS, Chung TW, Kim IY, Bom HS, Min JJ. Enhanced detectability of recurrent brain tumor using glucose-loading F-18 FDG PET. *Clin Nucl Med.* 2008;33(1):32–33.

137. Kuznetsov YE, Caramanos Z, Antel SB, et al. Proton magnetic resonance spectroscopic imaging can predict length of survival in patients with supratentorial gliomas. *Neurosurgery.* 2003;53(3):565–574; discussion 574–576.

138. Alexander A, Murtha A, Abdulkarim B, et al. Prognostic significance of serial magnetic resonance spectroscopies over the course of radiation therapy for patients with malignant glioma. *Clin Invest Med.* 2006;29(5):301–311.

139. Khoo VS, Joon DL. New developments in MRI for target volume delineation in radiotherapy. *Br J Radiol.* 2006;79 Spec No 1:S2–S15.

Chapter 5

Ultrasound Systems

Judit Boda-Heggemann, MD, Frank Lohr, MD, Martin Fuss MD

Regardless of the fact that verification of radiation treatment setup through port films and early adaptations of in-room computed tomography (CT)-on-rails represent valid forms of image guidance, it was the clinical introduction of ultrasound-based image guidance that truly initiated the current era of image-guided radiation therapy (IGRT). Initially designed for image guidance of prostate cancer radiation therapy (RT), this technology has been adopted for upper abdominal radiation treatment among other treatment sites in recent years.

Conceptually, the use of ultrasound for RT image guidance is intriguing and promises several advantages over the use of other image-guidance modalities. Ultrasound image guidance is a nonionizing imaging technology that can be used on a daily basis without adding any additional radiation dose. Moreover, ultrasound renders real-time images, and can depict anatomy with high soft-tissue contrast. Image data can be rendered in two-dimensional (2D) or three-dimensional (3D) modes, allowing one to either select freeze-frames in one or more imaging planes, or acquire a 3D volume imaging cube. The limitations of ultrasound, however, are largely related to the fact that radiation target volumes located posterior to bony structures or air cavities may not be easily depicted for image guidance.

Ultrasound-based target localization and positioning as represented by the Nomos BAT device (B-mode acquisition and targeting device; Nomos Inc, now BestNomos, Pittsburgh, PA; Figure 5-1) constituted the first commercially available image-guidance technology that integrated with almost any commercial RT planning software, and defined a clinically efficient workflow for online image guidance. Critical to the clinical acceptance of this novel image-guidance process was a clearly defined, user-friendly, and intuitive workflow. Through virtual user alignment of target and organs at risk (OARs) outlines to the ultrasound anatomy, an automated output of corrective linear accelerator table shifts in x-, y-, and z-coordinates are generated, allowing for adjustment of

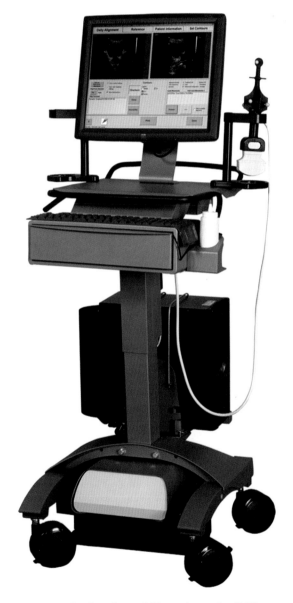

FIGURE 5-1. The B-mode acquisition and targeting (BAT) system is shown.

the patient's position through treatment table translations or shifts.[1–3]

Workflow and Systems

With the original BAT system and other ultrasound-based image-guidance systems, images of the target volume and OARs are acquired and matched with superimposed contours. These are referenced by a calibrated ultrasound transducer to the corresponding linear accelerator isocenter, after having been imported from a RT planning system. Following virtual structure to anatomy alignments, translational corrective shifts can be made to optimize the patient and target setup online before initiation of beam delivery. Though technically feasible, rotational data for setup adjustment are not typically provided.

As previously mentioned, the first commercially available transabdominal ultrasound image-guidance system was the Nomos BAT-system, which allows for daily 3D soft-tissue repositioning. The BAT system accepts DICOM RT import of the 3D contours of targets, OARs, or other guidance structures as generated during the RT planning process. Those structures are manually matched to a real-time planar image (2D imaging plane); the imaging plane can be freely chosen and changed in real time, effectively allowing for a 3D structure match. Two imaging planes (often approximately axial and sagittal) are captured for optimal structure-to-anatomy registration, documentation, and optional offline physician review of the setup at a later time.[1–4]

Localization of the transducer was initially performed mechanically through an encoder-arm mounted ultrasound transducer. This solution allowed for a fully self-contained and mobile system that could be used in multiple linear accelerator vaults, but the arm had limited reach, and the mechanical design also restricted the choice of imaging planes. Other solutions used optical tracking through transducer-mounted active or passive reflectors or light sources, and ceiling-mounted camera systems in the linear accelerator room. These solutions required camera systems in all rooms intended for ultrasound image-guidance use.

To overcome the potential limitations of 2D ultrasound imaging and to avoid the risk of poor image plane choice for target alignment, select systems acquired an ultrasound data volume, which allowed for the review and registration of structure outlines in 3D (SonArray, Varian Medical Systems, Palo Alto, CA; Restitu, Resonant Medical, Montreal, Canada).[5,6] Common to these systems, as well as other commercially available units (ExacTrac Ultrasound Module, BrainLAB, Feldkirchen, Germany, and I-Beam System, Elekta-CMS, Maryland Heights, MO) is the output of table translations along the main room axes for patient positioning optimization. Notably, the Restitu system can operate in a mode

that registers daily ultrasound images with other imaging modalities, specifically CT. Its registration process allows for automatic CT to ultrasound image registration, thereby providing comprehensive anatomical information by combining imaging modalities.[7] The ExacTrac 3D ultrasound software reconstructs CT images in different planes based on the simulation-acquired CT data cube. Planes are chosen in correspondence with the ultrasound plane and, thus, matching of ultrasound images with CT reconstructions is possible. The time requirement for the daily ultrasound-based image guidance procedure is approximately 5 minutes.[1–6,8–10]

Training

Diagnostic ultrasound imaging is not part of the educational curriculum for radiation oncology in most countries. Thus, the implementation of this novel image-guidance modality poses challenges and requires additional training, specifically hands-on training in use of the ultrasound units, and quality image acquisition using the hand-held ultrasound transducer. The key challenge is the real-time imaging mode inherent to modern ultrasound imaging systems. The user has to recognize anatomy, and must select appropriate freeze-frames to achieve optimal target positioning, or else acquire an appropriate ultrasound image data volume. As evident from the controversies surrounding the use of ultrasound image guidance in radiation oncology, training and its impact on the quality of the image-guidance procedure are critical components of successful integration into the daily clinical workflow.

It is recommended to consult with diagnostic ultrasound technologists or radiologists to establish clinical training. Vendor-supported training is typically directed toward technical use of the respective ultrasound units and the workflow to assess the radiation target's position once ultrasound image data are acquired. Soliciting hands-on training by formally trained diagnostic ultrasound imaging personnel will ensure that the RT team acquires the necessary skills in using an ultrasound transducer to depict the actual target region. Under ideal circumstances, such training may be staged over several weeks or even months to track and further improve the process and quality of ultrasound-based image-guidance.

Clinical Integration of Ultrasound-Based Image Guidance

As the CT data sets for RT planning also provide the reference data for daily ultrasound-based image guidance, CT simulation data should be acquired with a maximum slice thickness of 3 mm for prostate, and no more then 5 mm for abdominal targets.[1,2,8] To facilitate prostate image guidance, the treatment planning CT should be performed with an empty rectum, optimally with use of an enema immediately before CT imaging, and a moderately filled bladder.[11,12] This setup approach will help ensure an ultrasound "imaging-window" through the bladder onto the prostate. The empty rectum does not yield better ultrasound visualization, but already increases the likelihood for more reliable daily prostate setup, as rectum filling is typically reduced during the course of radiation administration. The clinical target volume (CTV) and OARs are contoured manually or automatically in a treatment planning system (TPS), and are transmitted to the ultrasound system as 3D structures in DICOM RT format. These reference structures provide the basis for stereotactic organ localization. For treatment of prostate cancer, the prostate, seminal vesicles, anterior rectal wall and bladder should be contoured. To facilitate alignment with the ultrasound-depicted anatomy, an accurate rendering of the anatomic prostate and seminal vesicles as compared to a potentially more generous CTV is preferable. Ultrasound can reliably depict intraprostatic calcifications, and implanted gold markers or operative clips. Thus, such guidance structures can also be delineated, and exported to the ultrasound image-guidance system.

For IGRT of abdominal targets, in addition to an actual target or macroscopic tumor, delineation of surrogate structures such as organ outlines, major blood vessels, anterior surface of vertebral bodies, operative clips, and others can guide treatments of pancreatic and hepatobiliary target volumes. For these organ sites, the respective CTVs may contain macroscopic tumor, as well as normal tissues at risk for subclinical tumor involvement.

Ultrasound image acquisition as the basis for the image-guidance procedure requires some basic device settings appropriate to the region to be visualized. Often, these settings are preprogrammed into ultrasound image-guidance units. It is recommended to involve an experienced, ideally diagnostic ultrasound user to optimize these standard settings. Ultrasound imaging requires gel between skin and transducer to provide optimal transducer-to-tissue sound-coupling, and to minimize ultrasound reflections from the transducer–skin interface. Although a small amount of ultrasound gel or even a small amount of fluid may suffice, a generous administration of gel will more likely provide clinically sufficient imaging quality. Even though it appears that especially the untrained user favors increased transducer probe pressure to obtain a subjectively better ultrasound image, in reality this action is not likely to actually improve tumor depiction. In fact, such pressure has the potential to move a target away from the transducer, most likely posterior relative to the natural resting position of the organ. It is advised to first increase the amount of ultrasound gel, as this will more likely result in improvement of ultrasound imaging quality. A gentle hand providing only the necessary amount of contact between transducer and skin is actually critical to acquiring ultrasound imaging of high quality, and is also more comfortable for the patient.

Quality Assurance

Quality assurance (QA) should be performed for all commercially available systems on a regular and often daily basis.[13,14] The BATCAM system (third-generation BAT), for example, must undergo daily QA with a vendor-provided phantom: the phantom has to be aligned to the linear accelerator room isocenter with a laser setup first. The position of the phantom is tracked by a ceiling-mounted camera system, with an accuracy of 0.5 mm. The reference phantom position is then stored in the system (isocenter calibration). Monthly QA should include checking the position of internal phantom structures, as ultrasound phantoms are prone to volume loss over time (Figure 5-2),

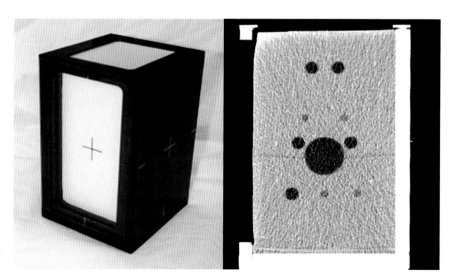

FIGURE 5-2. The B-mode acquisition and targeting (BAT) phantom for calibration and quality assurance, photo, and computed tomography image, respectively, is shown.

and also the accuracy of tracking of the relative phantom and table movements.

Clinical Experience

Prostate Cancer

In clinical use, image guidance for external beam RT of prostate cancer has been the predominant application of ultrasound image guidance (Figure 5-3). Ultrasound-based image guidance for delivery of conformal radiation treatments to the prostate is widely employed and has been well documented over the past decade. The initial report on the use of this image-guidance modality introduced the concept and workflow, and reported comparative target localization data with daily CT-based image guidance with ultrasound-based image-guidance in 10 patients.[2] Compared with the more elaborate daily CT guidance procedure, ultrasound image guidance was judged to be both simple and expeditious. The provided image guidance was found to be functionally equivalent to CT, with significantly positive correlation of derived shifts between the modalities in three dimensions. Interestingly, remain-

ing discrepancies between ultrasound and CT-assessed setup were largely attributed to limitations of CT imaging, rather than associated with the use of the ultrasound device. See Chapter 20C for a discussion of ultrasound-based image guidance in a patient with prostate cancer.

A later update of the Fox Chase Cancer Center (FCCC) experience in 35 patients reconfirmed a high correlation between CT and ultrasound-based image guidance in all three dimensions.[15] Also in 2000, the Cleveland Clinic group reported on ultrasound-guided short-course intensity-modulated radiotherapy (IMRT) (70 Gy in 28 fractions of 2.5 Gy each) in 51 patients.[3] Although no data on actual daily prostate alignment shifts were reported, the authors elected to use the Nomos BAT system to avoid random as well as systematic setup errors based on the favorable findings in the previously quoted papers. As an indirect indicator of the capability of ultrasound-based image guidance to achieve its desired goal of positioning the prostate and related organs at risk accurately relative to the radiation beam geometry, no increase in acute radiation toxicities was observed when compared with patients treated conformally to 78 Gy in conventional fractionation.

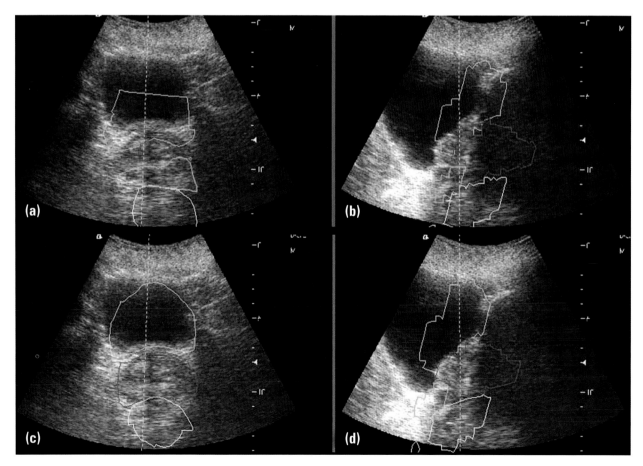

FIGURE 5-3. Ultrasound-based prostate localization: Axial (left) and sagittal (right) ultrasound images with superimposed organ and target structures from the simulation computed tomography scan are shown. Structures displayed are prostate (red), bladder (orange), and rectum (yellow). Upper figures represent the setup before, and lower figures after, B-mode acquisition and targeting (BAT) position correction.

In subsequent years, clinical experiences from multiple centers were reported. Morr and colleagues reported on 23 patients, of which the BAT system was capable of producing images of sufficient quality for daily image guidance in 19.[9] As potential planning target volume (PTV) underdosage was avoided in 63% of 185 image-guidance procedures, the modality was considered a useful tool in the application of IMRT for prostate cancer. In one of the largest series reported, researchers from the MD Anderson Cancer Center analyzed 3509 BAT ultrasound-guidance procedures.[4] Image quality was judged to be acceptable for image guidance in almost 95% of attempted procedures. Shifts larger than 5 mm were encountered in 28.6% in anterior–posterior (AP), 23% in superior–inferior (SI), and 9% in right–left (RL) directions, with no systematic shift error encountered along any of the main axes. Alignment errors larger than 5 mm by the performing therapist were detected during offline physician review in less than 3% of image-guidance attempts. At the Nebraska Medical Center, 7825 treatments in 234 patients resulted in an average 3D shift vector length of 7.8 mm with a standard deviation of 6.6 mm, with motion correction predominantly in an oblique superior–posterior direction.[8] Although no numeric frequency of occurrence is provided in the paper, 3D vector shifts of larger than 15 mm and even 20 mm were routinely observed. Other reports support the findings in the aforementioned studies.[3,10] As a general consensus, ultrasound-based image guidance was perceived to greatly facilitate IGRT for prostate carcinoma, and to improve prostate positioning accuracy over skin markers or portal imaging.[4,10,15,16]

Of interest is a series of reports by researchers from the University of Chicago analyzing the impact of ultrasound-based image guidance on acute and late RT-related toxicity.[17,18] In 49 patients each in two cohorts, treated with and without ultrasound guidance, a retrospective outcome analysis revealed similar acute and late genitourinary (GU) toxicities, but slightly lower gastrointestinal (GI) toxicity rates in the BAT group. Although these observations did not reach statistical significance in the regression analysis, a prospective clinical analysis was suggested to clarify the potential of ultrasound-based image guidance to reduce the rates of late, chronic GI toxicity in prostate cancer.

Ultrasound-based image guidance has also been tested in the postprostatectomy setting.[19] When the SonArray image-guidance system was used, setup shifts in six postprostatectomy RT patients were comparable to shifts in 10 patients with intact prostate with mean corrective shift vectors of 5 mm versus 4 mm. The bladder neck, an adequate surrogate reference structure for the prostatic fossa, was readily visualized. However, judging by the lack of additional reports, it appears that postprostatectomy ultrasound image guidance has not found wide clinical adoption.

Upper-Abdominal Tumors

Daily ultrasound-based image guidance for conformal RT of upper-abdominal targets was first reported by the San Antonio group in 2004.[1] Radiation targets included hepatobiliary tumors, pancreatic carcinoma, and other abdominal target volumes. In 62 patients, 1337 image-guidance target localizations were attempted. In 4.2% of attempts, no useful imaging information was provided by ultrasound imaging. Obscured view of the target region by overlying intestinal air content was identified as the main cause. In addition, obese body habitus compromised target visualization when targets were located deeper than 10 cm from the patient's surface. Mean 3D vector shift magnitude from skin marks was 11.4 mm, with about 50%, 25%, and 13% of alignments shifted by a magnitude larger than 10 mm, 15 mm, and 20 mm, respectively. Ultrasound image-guidance shifts were validated in the simulation CT suite in 15 patients, with an average initial setup error reduction of 54%.

On the basis of this favorable experience, subsequent reports document feasibility and outcomes of ultrasound-based IGRT of pancreatic and gallbladder cancer.[20,21] The mean 3D vector magnitude of table correction was 11.7 mm in 39 pancreatic patients (1011 IGRT sessions), with 27% of corrective shifts larger than 15 mm.[21] The vector 3D shifts were slightly larger in 261 daily alignments in nine patients with gallbladder cancer (mean shift vector length 13.9 mm), and, accordingly, 32% of setups were corrected by 3D shifts larger than 15 mm.[20] These reports not only document the feasibility of daily ultrasound-based image guidance for IMRT of abdominal tumors, but also constituted the first reports of combining modern conventionally fractionated RT planning and delivery methods (e.g., IMRT) with daily IGRT. Although no improvement in outcomes over conventional radiation techniques was suggested, this treatment concept did compare favorably to historic data with regard to acute treatment toxicity and survival.

A more recent series retrospectively compared ultrasound-based IGRT for 24 patients with biliary malignancies, with a cohort of matched patients treated with conventional or conformal radiation treatment, but without image guidance.[22] Image-guided radiation therapy afforded delivery of significantly higher radiation doses (mean IGRT 58.3 Gy vs 47.5 Gy in conformal RT; $P = .0001$). Although a nominal increase in acute treatment toxicities was observed in the IGRT cohort, the lack of a statistically significant increase of upper- and lower-GI toxicities is suggestive of the safety of an image-guided approach to realize modest dose escalation in the absence of substantial dose-limiting toxicity.

When abdominal target volumes are treated with IGRT, direct sonographic imaging of the whole target volume is frequently not possible. Organ outlines, large blood vessels, the anterior margin of spinal vertebrae, and operative clips can, however, be used as guidance structures. Most recently, researchers from the University Medical Center Mannheim assessed the accuracy of abdominal ultrasound-based IGRT in large volume IMRT for predominantly gastric malignancies, compared with daily cone-beam CT (CBCT) acquisition.[23] With CBCT assumed as the gold standard, the residual 3D setup error after ultrasound image guidance in patients with good sonographic image quality was 5.8 mm, compared with 7.9 mm in patients with satisfactory image quality. Although the initial setup error was improved upon in both groups, it was concluded that in patients with limited visualization by ultrasound, CBCT would provide the superior means of daily image guidance.

Thus, careful patient selection may be necessary. One factor that was already noted in the first report on abdominal ultrasound-based image guidance was patient body habitus. Choi and coworkers from the San Antonio group analyzed daily setup shifts in relation to body mass index (BMI).[24] Image-guidance data from 86 patients were analyzed, of which 49 patients had a BMI (weight in kg divided by height in meters squared) of at least 25, and were therefore considered as being at least overweight, or falling under the obese category (BMI ≥30). Daily shifts from skin marks showed statistically significant differences in the systematic error components between BMI <25 and BMI ≥25 groups.

According to the reported data, ultrasound-based image guidance in the upper abdomen is clearly feasible and provides for an excellent means of IGRT in select patients. It appears prudent to suggest validation with an alternate image-guidance modality if available. Patient selection is critical to success and accuracy in the abdomen, with slender patients and tumors located in the liver or the retroperitoneum constituting the population most likely to benefit from this image-guidance modality.

Other Sites

As hepatobiliary tumor location has been identified as favorable for ultrasound target position assessment, the utility of this modality for image guidance of liver malignancies treated with stereotactic body RT (SBRT) has been explored in the clinical setting (Figure 5-4).[25–27]

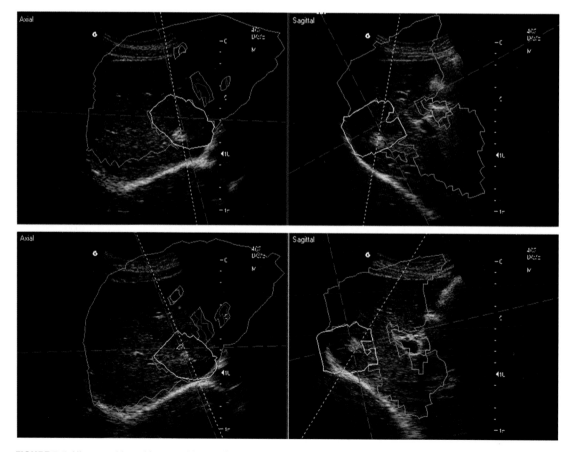

FIGURE 5-4. Ultrasound-based image guidance of a colorectal liver metastasis: Imaging was acquired in breath hold. Axial (left) and sagittal (right) ultrasound images are shown with superimposed organ and target structures from the simulation computed tomography. Structures displayed: target volume (yellow), liver (orange), portal vein (green), and liver veins (red). Upper figures represent the setup before, and lower figures after, B-mode acquisition and targeting (BAT) position correction.

Also, ultrasound-based image guidance for SBRT of adrenal metastases has been documented.[26] For thoracic target localization, the use of ultrasound-based image guidance would be limited to the positional assessment of pleural tumors and tumors extending to the chest wall, as the location of targets in the lung parenchyma could not be readily assessed by this modality. Although the clinical utility of ultrasound-based image guidance for chest wall tumors has been clinically explored, no peer-reviewed data on its utility and benefit or limitations have been made available. Image-guided treatment of localized metastatic spinal disease with stereotactic ultrasound was described for a dedicated system in combination with pretreatment CT.[28]

Pediatric Cancers

Especially for RT of childhood malignant diseases, narrow normal tissue PTV margins yield better acute and chronic radiation tolerance, and reduce the long-term probability of RT-induced secondary malignant neoplasm (SMN). In a recent study of 446 children treated for childhood cancer by RT, 8.3% developed SMN, most of them occurring within or bordering the original radiation field.[29] An additional 5% of these children developed benign neoplasms, some of which also occurred within the radiation fields, making reduction of the high-dose radiation volume a principal goal.

For childhood RT, ionizing imaging modalities have been critically assessed, as their use adds radiation exposure to often large normal tissue volumes. Kudchadker and colleagues recently assessed the radiation dose from portal films acquired during courses of pediatric RT.[30] Total doses accumulated in 11 children through weekly port films acquired during RT for abdominal tumors averaged 31 cGy, with maximum observed doses of 64 cGy. The open-field exposure accounted for more than 80% of the total accumulated dose. Even though no clinical evidence exists to link such low additional radiation doses with a heightened risk for the development of SMN, the potential for such an increase in risk cannot be neglected. On the other hand, the value of image guidance is obvious. Missing the target volume will predictably lead to a decrease in tumor control probability and tumor recurrence will place the children at higher risk than small amounts of additional radiation dose.

For image guidance of childhood abdominal tumors, ultrasound targeting may assume a more relevant role in the future. In a small series of children treated in San Antonio, all ultrasound-based image-guidance attempts were successful and provided clinically sufficient information for setup optimization (data unpublished). Small abdominal diameter and lack of a significant subcutaneous fat layer of the young children constitutes a favorable imaging scenario. A representative case is displayed in Figure 5-5.

Controversies

Image Quality

From the first report describing the use of ultrasound-based image guidance, the actual image quality, usefulness, and accuracy of this unfamiliar imaging modality has been discussed. A sufficient body of data has been generated to suggest the validity of using ultrasound image guidance for both prostate and abdominal target volumes; however, its utility has clearly been dependent on the achieved image quality or ability to depict the target region.

Sonographic image quality is a controversial issue in the discussion of ultrasound-based examinations as it is system-, patient- and user-dependent. The quality of ultrasound images is highly dependent on correct patient preparation, selection of correct system presets, and user technique (Figure 5-6). The initial FCCC experience detailed the utility of ultrasound image guidance even in patients with a large pannus.[2] However, for the data collection of the second report, two patients were excluded owing to inferior imaging quality, without providing detail as to the cause of inferior imaging quality.[15] The MDACC group found the quality of the daily ultrasound images for prostate targeting acceptable in almost 95% of image-guidance attempts.[4]

Similar data have been reported by other groups. Chandra and coworkers reported how inferior imaging quality was dealt with in the actual clinical setting.[4] In 0.6% of attempts the technologists did not make a corrective setup shift owing to poor imaging quality of the ultrasound image-guidance device, and instead aligned according to bony pelvic anatomy. However, in 4.5% of IGRT attempts, a shift was derived based on ultrasound imaging that was later considered inadequate by the reviewing physician. Arguably, this may be one of the main limitations in the clinical integration of ultrasound image guidance. Because of patient-specific anatomical situations, adequate ultrasound target visualization may not be achieved in certain patients. Overlying air content in the bowel or bony ultrasound reflections may lead to insufficient visualization of the target region. Instead of attempting to base clinical decision making on inferior imaging, such patients need to be excluded from this form of daily image guidance. Recognizing such issues and identifying patients suited for ultrasound image guidance can be addressed with ongoing training, and periodic case review in a team discussion, as such cases may not necessarily be encountered among the first patients treated.

As already discussed, ultrasound image quality and patient suitability for ultrasound image guidance is even more critical in targeting abdominal target volumes. In the initial San Antonio series, 4.2% of setups did not allow the derivation of meaningful imaging information for target setup.[1] Following the institutional protocol, those patients were treated according to laser alignment to skin

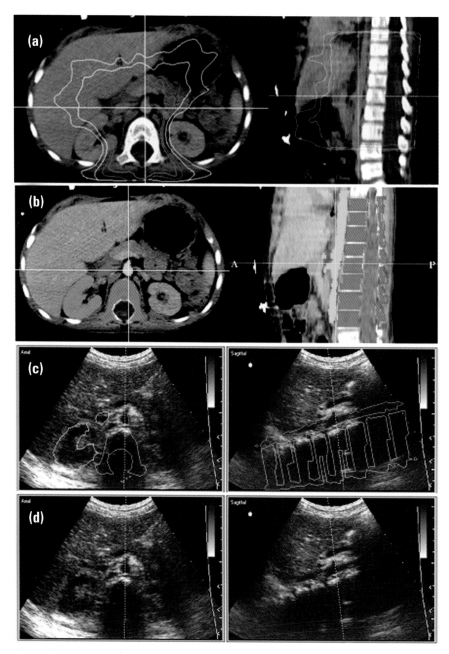

FIGURE 5-5. Ultrasound-based image guidance of pediatric abdominal malignancy (neuroblastoma): The upper figures represent axial and sagittal simulation computed tomography (CT) slices with target volume and corresponding dose distribution **(a)**, as well as anatomical guidance structures delineated for export into the ultrasound-based image-guidance system **(b)** (right kidney [dark green], vena cava [blue], aorta with offspring of the superior mesenteric artery [light green], and vertebral bodies that are part of the clinical target volume [purple]). The lower figures represent real-time acquired axial and sagittal ultrasound freeze frames **(c/d)** with superimposition of structure outlines as derived from the simulation CT scan (In c, please note that the anatomical structure outlines are coded in different colors than those depicted on the CT simulation scan with right kidney [yellow], vena cava [blue], aorta [orange], and vertebral bodies [green]). To match actual ultrasound anatomy with structure outlines in this particular setup, table translations of 3.8 mm to anatomical right, 5.2 mm table up, and 1.1 mm table out were performed (3D magnitude vector of translation 6.5 mm).

marks. Owing to continued problems visualizing the target region, the initially attempted ultrasound image guidance was discontinued in two patients. As a result, less than 1% of clinically used ultrasound-based setups were later judged to have failed qualitatively to provide the nec-

essary imaging content for image-guided targeting. The Mannheim group similarly identified three of 15 patients with poor imaging quality in a trial comparing ultrasound with CBCT targeting for abdominal target volumes, and excluded them from evaluation.[23]

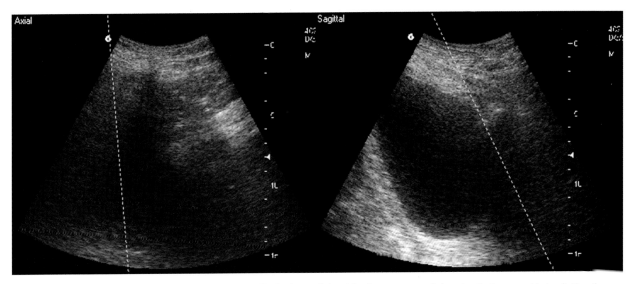

FIGURE 5-6. Ultrasound image with inadequate image quality is shown. It is advised not to use such imaging for image-guided radiation therapy (IGRT).

Accuracy

The accuracy of ultrasound systems or of their derived treatment position is an even more controversial subject.[31,32] Initial clinical reports compared ultrasound-based target setups with CT-derived target localization information, and found the resulting setup to be clinically valid for both prostate and abdominal targeting, although discrepancies between modalities were observed.[1,2,15] In a more recent prospective trial, Feigenberg and colleagues found a strong correlation between BAT and in-room CT-derived shifts, with systematic differences smaller than 1 mm.[33]

Comparative studies of ultrasound-based positioning and x-ray based positioning have rendered more variable results. Besides studies finding a high degree of agreement between assessment of implanted markers in port films with ultrasound alignment,[19] others found that ultrasound guidance did not provide positional improvement over a program that does not provide position adjustment.[34] Of particular concern was an observed correlation between ultrasound-guidance shifts and the residual setup error after those shifts, with larger shifts being correlated with larger residual setup error in cranio-caudal direction, and increasing systematic errors. On the basis of those observations, the investigators raised concern about the clinical implementation in their department.

An early technology adoption study conducted at the University of California San Francisco (UCSF) also compared ultrasound-based prostate positioning with port film analysis for fiducial marker setup in eight patients.[35] Multiple users were asked to align structure outlines to ultrasound anatomy, which was provided by a vendor-trained technologist. All users were new to the technology at the beginning of the study, with no formal information exchange as to their experience in using the device during the study. Although in 92 alignments an initial

AP target setup error of larger than 5 mm was improved by a factor of 2, no improvements were recorded along the cranio-caudal or lateral direction. Between users, alignments of structure outlines with ultrasound anatomy varied, with 50% of alignments showing discrepancies of up to 2 mm; 75% of alignments were within 4 mm. No improvement of this interuser variability was observed over the course of the study. In conclusion, the authors found value in use of ultrasound guidance for the reduction of the AP setup error, for which the penalty of misalignment is greatest, but observed substantial interuser variability.

These experiences highlight compounding sources affecting the accuracy of ultrasound-based image guidance. The impact of uniform training on interuser variability was assessed by the San Antonio group.[36] Based on data from 20 patients treated for prostate cancer, the variation in setup shifts based on one supposedly optimal set of images that was provided to all users was analyzed. Also, all ultrasound-derived shifts were validated against CT imaging as the gold standard. All users underwent hands-on formal training provided by a radiologist experienced in ultrasound imaging. This reference user was able to achieve mean residual setup errors between 1.1 mm and 2.6 mm along the principal room axes. Although experienced typical users, such as a radiation oncologist, a medical physicist, and radiation therapists did not quite match this excellent performance, they achieved on average a 63% improvement in prostate setup over the initial setup error. In contrast, users in early stages of training improved the initial setup on average by 35%. The observed difference was statistically significant. Only five of 194 virtual setups would have introduced a residual setup error larger than the initial setup error, but those errors were all recorded by inexperienced users.

It was concluded that an ultrasound image-guidance system yields immediate positive impact on patient setup. Even users relatively new to the system and still undergoing formal training did improve upon patient setups on a regular basis. There was a clear learning curve, which potentially affords smaller PTV margins when sufficient clinical experience has been gained. Experience in this study was arbitrarily assigned when users had undergone formal hands-on training by both vendor and an ultrasound expert, and had attempted ultrasound image guidance in 10 complete prostate radiation therapy treatment courses (roughly 300 alignments) with daily critical feedback by an already experienced user.

Additional studies assessing the accuracy and inter-user variability using this image-guidance modality have been published, with results largely matching the range of previously detailed observations.[37] Unfortunately, none of these studies described the level of training of the personnel executing the ultrasound targeting.

However, even in programs that had a longer history in the use of ultrasound image guidance, discrepancies between ultrasound-assessed target location, and verification by an alternate imaging modality were observed. The group from the MIMA Cancer Center in Melbourne, Florida retrospectively analyzed 1019 comparative measurements between ultrasound and fiducial-marker assessed prostate setup using the SonArray system.[38] Data collection for this large study included the time frame from approximately 6 to 12 months after the initiation of routine ultrasound-guidance use. As a key finding, the mean absolute vector shift lengths between modalities were observed to be different, with ultrasound-derived shifts revealing significantly more variability than the fiducial marker-derived vectors. Systematic setup errors were observed following ultrasound based setup in the longitudinal direction, with prostate displacement toward the patient's feet. It was concluded that ultrasound and fiducial marker positional assessment are not similar and that the discrepancy is larger than 5 mm. Comparable observations favouring nonultrasound image-guidance modalities were made by the Allegheny Hospital Group, also a group with long-standing ultrasound-based image-guidance experience, as well as researchers from the Medical College of Wisconsin and the University of Victoria.[5,39–41]

All of these studies, however, suffer to some degree from common methodological shortcomings. In all assessments, no real-time correlation between ultrasound and a secondary imaging modality could be performed. Ultrasound targeting and second image modality targeting were performed sequentially, with some time elapsed between imaging, although the actual time window was not reported. From the Mannheim and San Antonio experience, it is deduced that time elapsed between imaging acquisitions ranges from between 5 and 10 minutes, but with longer intervals in individual cases. These data

are likely representative of the above-summarized experiences as all authors reported that ultrasound image guidance requires about 5 minutes in an experienced clinical setting, with more time requirement at earlier stages of implementation. Also there is a varying time-requirement for x-ray-based imaging acquisition.

As systematic discrepancies between ultrasound and other imaging modalities predominantly refer to an oblique anterior–superior to posterior–inferior direction, the notion of systematic prostate motion in this time window cannot be entirely dismissed. Interestingly, this represents the direction of prostate movement with bladder-filling over time (unpublished data from the San Antonio group). Other groups observed rectal gas-filling to be most predictive of short-term, or intrafraction, prostate motion, with the predominant direction of motion again being the superior–anterior to posterior–inferior direction.[42] Over as little as 2 to 4 minutes, the likelihood of the prostate to move more than 2 mm is already almost 9% in a supine setup without rectal balloon immobilization.[43] The authors concluded that a stable prostate position could be only obtained for 4 minutes or less. In patients undergoing hypofractionated RT who were instructed in diet and were provided prophylaxis to reduce bowel gas, the prostate motion error over an average 19-minute interval between two sets of CBCTs, was assessed as 95% within 3.1 mm.[44] In the initial report on continuous real-time prostate motion tracking, 3D prostate shifts of up to 6.6 mm were observed over approximately 10 minutes.[45] Average maximum motion in longitudinal and vertical direction was 3.6 mm and 3.9 mm, respectively. Peak motion was observed to approach or exceed 10 mm in all principal room axes, with some motion lasting longer than 1 minute. Other series have also observed large intrafractional positional changes of greater than 10 mm.[46,47] In another series analyzing real-time electromagnetic prostate motion tracking over an average of 10 minutes, target displacement by more than 3 mm was documented in 13.2% of the time.[48]

There is obviously some difficulty of extending these data to the scenario of comparing two imaging modalities. There appears a clear systematic prostate shift with time, which may or may not explain observed systematic differences between imaging modalities. Also there is obvious randomness in the timing of the secondary positional assessment. Although on average, continuous real-time prostate tracking reveals rather small systematic shifts, it is not uncommon to observe motion spikes during which the prostate is displaced by more than 5 mm for some period of time. If image guidance by an electronic portal imaging device (EPID) assessing for fiducial marker setup is acquired during such motion spikes, a discrepancy between modalities and resulting prostate positional assessment will likely result, and potentially compound data in smaller series.

Also there have been technical issues detected that specifically relate to early generation encoder arm–based BAT systems, which are likely related to some degree to the systematic errors reported.[34,35] A deterioration of encoders may not have been detectable by the initial vendor-recommended QA procedures. This issue has been subsequently identified, and changes in vendor recommendations for QA procedures prevent further encounters with such problems. With the newer, infrared-based systems, no calibration problems have been encountered to date.

None of the available commercial ultrasound image-guidance systems account for tissue inhomogeneity, which was first discussed as a potential source of systematic errors by Fung et al. in 2006.[8] Ultrasound image-guidance systems are typically calibrated for soft-tissue applications with a fixed ultrasonic wave velocity of 1540 meters per second, thus introducing errors in depth-from-transducer representation when used in media with a different speed of sound propagation. Salter and coworkers recently utilized a standard ultrasound phantom to demonstrate the existence of the speed artifact when images were acquired through layers of simulated body fat.[48] It was shown that the presence of fat causes the target to be aliased to a depth greater than it actually is. It was suggested that spatial inaccuracies introduced by this artifact should be considered by the physician during the formulation of the treatment plan.

Lastly, the process of acquiring ultrasound images could contribute to discrepancies. As discussed earlier, a target could be displaced by the pressure exerted by the ultrasound probe. This is an obvious issue for image guidance of abdominal target volumes, but may also affect targeting of the prostate. Although a pressure dislocation effect can be readily demonstrated in a phantom setup,[49] in clinical use and with respect for the patient's comfort level, the impact should be minimal. Serago and others assessed the impact of pressure using a mock probe strapped to the patient's abdomen during CT acquisition.[10] Of 16 patients included in the study, the prostate was displaced to some degree in nine. The direction of displacement was posterior and/or inferior. With one exception, the displacements were less than 3 mm in any direction.

In another report on a volunteer study, the average prostate displacement observed was 3.1 mm, with increasing probe pressure positively correlated with increased prostate displacement. At assumed clinically relevant probe pressure, the magnitude of prostate motion averaged up to 6.3 mm.[50] In a prospective clinical study with synchronous ultrasound and x-ray acquisition in prostate cancer patients that had previously been implanted with iodine seeds, typical clinically required probe pressure was found to induce a shift in prostate position by up to 2.3 mm, and a rotational setup change of up to 2.5 degrees. However, when pressure was applied that was higher than needed for quality ultrasound imaging, prostate displacements of up to 10 mm could be induced.[51]

New and Future Applications

In many anatomical sites, intrafraction motion and deformation attributable to respiratory or cardiac motion, peristalsis, and changing organ filling can be observed.[52] Most IGRT modalities in clinical use are not capable of tracking such changes in real time. Respiration has obvious impact on upper abdominal target motion for target volumes in or around the liver, adrenal glands, pancreas, and other organs.

Ultrasound-based real-time target tracking holds promise for the upper-abdominal region.[53-55] With measurements on various stationary and moving phantoms, transabdominal ultrasound-based tracking has been shown to be feasible for real-time monitoring of target motion during a RT fraction.[56] Ultrasound-based real-time target tracking offers the possibility of a noninvasive, real-time, and low-cost method of tracking target motion during a treatment fraction. Motion of various structures can be followed, for example, by tracking the interference pattern, referred to as speckle tracking, which is already used routinely in heart imaging,[53,57] or a so-called active contours approach.[58] Motion-tracking algorithms and dedicated ultrasound devices are being currently developed. Several problems, however, await a solution including the effect of the ultrasound probe on the dose distribution,[59] QA procedures in cases of moving targets,[60] and elastic matching of deformed structures.[61-62]

Conclusions

When ultrasound-based image guidance became available commercially, it paved the way for the then new concept of IGRT, which benefits thousands of RT patients on a daily basis today. However, there is, with certainty, no other image-guidance modality that has polarized the opinions of the medical community as much as ultrasound image guidance. No other modality appears to be similarly user-dependent, with one faction finding value in its application while the other rejects it emphatically because of concerns of providing no better care for their patients than treating them according to skin mark setup.

The data summarized in this chapter cannot resolve the debate or provide a generalized assessment. It is certainly reasonable to state that ultrasound-based image guidance has to be considered a useful tool in the hands of trained professionals, and for a select patient population. Without a doubt, other volumetric imaging modalities such as CBCT, megavoltage CT, or in-room diagnostic-grade CT imaging can provide for more consistent, less user-dependent means of image guidance, and have found rapid and broad acceptance by the radiation oncology community.

Ultrasound image guidance may still deserve a future in our discipline. Commercially available systems are now technically highly reliable, and are comparatively cost-effective. Truly noninvasive image guidance can be performed without any added ionizing radiation exposure. Thus, the treatment of those patients who are treated with curative intent with a long life expectancy warrants at least consideration of using this form of image guidance, provided the treatment team has become proficient in its use, and the program is applying stringent QA criteria.

References

1. Fuss M, Salter BJ, Cavanaugh SX, et al. Daily ultrasound-based image-guided targeting for radiotherapy of upper abdominal malignancies. *Int J Radiat Oncol Biol Phys.* 2004;59(4):1245–1256.

2. Lattanzi J, McNeeley S, Pinover W, et al. A comparison of daily CT localization to a daily ultrasound-based system in prostate cancer. *Int J Radiat Oncol Biol Phys.* 1999;43(4):719–725.

3. Mohan DS, Kupelian PA, Willoughby TR. Short-course intensity-modulated radiotherapy for localized prostate cancer with daily transabdominal ultrasound localization of the prostate gland. *Int J Radiat Oncol Biol Phys.* 2000;46(3):575–580.

4. Chandra A, Dong L, Huang E, et al. Experience of ultrasound-based daily prostate localization. *Int J Radiat Oncol Biol Phys.* 2003;56(2):436–447.

5. Johnston H, Hilts M, Beckham W, Berthelet E. 3D ultrasound for prostate localization in radiation therapy: a comparison with implanted fiducial markers. *Med Phys.* 2008;35(6):2403–2413.

6. Peignaux K, Truc G, Barillot I, et al. Clinical assessment of the use of the Sonarray system for daily prostate localization. *Radiother Oncol.* 2006;81(2):176–178.

7. Wein W, Röper B, Navab N. Automatic registration and fusion of ultrasound with CT for radiotherapy. *Med Image Comput Comput Assist Interv.* 2005;8(pt 2):303–311.

8. Fung AY, Ayyangar KM, Djajaputra D, Nehru RM, Enke CA. Ultrasound-based guidance of intensity-modulated radiation therapy. *Med Dosim.* 2006;31(1):20–29.

9. Morr J, DiPetrillo T, Tsai JS, Engler M, Wazer DE. Implementation and utility of a daily ultrasound-based localization system with intensity-modulated radiotherapy for prostate cancer. *Int J Radiat Oncol Biol Phys.* 2002;53(5):1124–1129.

10. Serago CF, Chungbin SJ, Buskirk SJ, Ezzell GA, Collie AC, Vora SA. Initial experience with ultrasound localization for positioning prostate cancer patients for external beam radiotherapy. *Int J Radiat Oncol Biol Phys.* 2002;53(5):1130–1138.

11. Ghilezan MJ, Jaffray DA, Siewerdsen JH, et al. Prostate gland motion assessed with cine-magnetic resonance imaging (cine-MRI). *Int J Radiat Oncol Biol Phys.* 2005;62(2):406–417.

12. Stasi M, Munoz F, Fiorino C, et al. Emptying the rectum before treatment delivery limits the variations of rectal dose - volume parameters during 3DCRT of prostate cancer. *Radiother Oncol.* 2006;80(3):363–370.

13. Bissonnette JP. Quality assurance of image-guidance technologies. *Semin Radiat Oncol.* 2007;17(4):278–286.

14. Tomé WA, Meeks SL, Orton NP, Bouchet LG, Bova FJ. Commissioning and quality assurance of an optically guided three-dimensional ultrasound target localization system for radiotherapy. *Med Phys.* 2002;29(6):1781–1788.

15. Lattanzi J, McNeeley S, Donnelly S, et al. Ultrasound-based stereotactic guidance in prostate cancer—quantification of organ motion and set-up errors in external beam radiation therapy. *Comput Aided Surg.* 2000;5(4):289–295.

16. Boda-Heggemann J, Köhler FM, Küpper B, et al. Accuracy of ultrasound-based (BAT) prostate-repositioning: a three-dimensional on-line fiducial-based assessment with cone-beam computed tomography. *Int J Radiat Oncol Biol Phys.* 2008;70(4):1247–1255.

17. Jani AB, Gratzle J, Muresan E, Farrey K, Martel MK. Analysis of acute toxicity with use of transabdominal ultrasonography for prostate positioning during intensity-modulated radiotherapy. *Urology.* 2005;65(3):504–508.

18. Jani AB, Gratzle J, Muresan E, Martel MK. Impact on late toxicity of using transabdominal ultrasound for prostate cancer patients treated with intensity modulated radiotherapy. *Technol Cancer Res Treat.* 2005;4(1):115–120.

19. Chinnaiyan P, Tomée W, Patel R, Chappell R, Ritter M. 3D-ultrasound guided radiation therapy in the post-prostatectomy setting. *Technol Cancer Res Treat.* 2003;2(5):455–458.

20. Fuller CD, Thomas CR Jr, Wong A, et al. Image-guided intensity-modulated radiation therapy for gallbladder carcinoma. *Radiother Oncol.* 2006;81(1):65–72.

21. Fuss M, Wong A, Fuller CD, Salter BJ, Fuss C, Thomas CR. Image-guided intensity-modulated radiotherapy for pancreatic carcinoma. *Gastrointest Cancer Res.* 2007; 1(1):2–11.

22. Fuller CD, Dang ND, Wang SJ, et al. Image-guided intensity-modulated radiotherapy (IG-IMRT) for biliary adenocarcinomas: initial clinical results. *Radiother Oncol.* 2009;92(2):249–254.

23. Boda-Heggemann J, Mennemeyer P, Wertz H, et al. Accuracy of ultrasound-based image guidance for daily positioning of the upper abdomen: an online comparison with cone beam CT. *Int J Radiat Oncol Biol Phys.* 2009;74(3):892–897.

24. Choi M, Fuller CD, Wang SJ, et al. Effect of body mass index on shifts in ultrasound-based image-guided intensity-modulated radiation therapy for abdominal malignancies. *Radiother Oncol.* 2009;91(1):114–119.

25. Boda-Heggemann J, Walter C, Mai S, et al. Frameless stereotactic radiosurgery of a solitary liver metastasis using active breathing control and stereotactic ultrasound. *Strahlenther Onkol.* 2006;182(4):216–221.

26. Fuss M, Boda-Heggemann J, Papanikolau N, Salter BJ. Image-guidance for stereotactic body radiation therapy. *Med Dosim.* 2007;32(2):102–110.

27. Fuss M, Thomas CR Jr. Stereotactic body radiation therapy: an ablative treatment option for primary and secondary liver tumors. *Ann Surg Oncol.* 2004;11(2):130–138.

28. Ryken TC, Meeks SL, Traynelis V, et al. Ultrasonographic guidance for spinal extracranial radiosurgery: technique and application for metastatic spinal lesions. *Neurosurg Focus.* 2001;11(6):e8.

29. Gold DG, Neglia JP, Dusenbery KE. Second neoplasms after megavoltage radiation for pediatric tumors. *Cancer.* 2003 97(10):2588–2596.

30. Kudchadker RJ, Chang EL, Bryan F, Maor MH, Famiglietti R. An evaluation of radiation exposure from portal films taken during definitive course of pediatric radiotherapy. *Int J Radiat Oncol Biol Phys*. 2004;59(4):1229–1235.

31. Boda-Heggemann J, Köhler FM, De Meerleer G, et al. Image-guided radiation therapy: many roads lead to Rome? *Int J Radiat Oncol Biol Phys*. 2008;70(2):646–647; author reply 647.

32. Scarbrough TJ, Ting JY, Kuritzky N. Ultrasound for radiotherapy targeting. *Int J Radiat Oncol Biol Phys*. 2007;68(5):1579; author reply 1579–1580.

33. Feigenberg SJ, Paskalev K, McNeeley S, et al. Comparing computed tomography localization with daily ultrasound during image-guided radiation therapy for the treatment of prostate cancer: a prospective evaluation. *J Appl Clin Med Phys*. 2007;8(3):2268.

34. Van den Heuvel F, Powell T, Seppi E, et al. Independent verification of ultrasound based image-guided radiation treatment, using electronic portal imaging and implanted gold markers. *Med Phys*. 2003;30(11):2878–2887.

35. Langen KM, Pouliot J, Anezinos C, et al. Evaluation of ultrasound-based prostate localization for image-guided radiotherapy. *Int J Radiat Oncol Biol Phys*. 2003;57(3):635–644.

36. Fuss M, Cavanaugh SX, Fuss C, Cheek DA, Salter BJ. Daily stereotactic ultrasound prostate targeting: inter-user variability. *Technol Cancer Res Treat*. 2003;2(2):161–170.

37. McNair HA, Mangar SA, Coffey J, et al. A comparison of CT- and ultrasound-based imaging to localize the prostate for external beam radiotherapy. *Int J Radiat Oncol Biol Phys*. 2006;65(3):678–687.

38. Scarbrough TJ, Golden NM, Ting JY, et al. Comparison of ultrasound and implanted seed marker prostate localization methods: implications for image-guided radiotherapy. *Int J Radiat Oncol Biol Phys*. 2006;65(2):378–387.

39. Gayou O, Miften M. Comparison of mega-voltage cone-beam computed tomography prostate localization with online ultrasound and fiducial markers methods. *Med Phys*. 2008;35(2):531–538.

40. Lin SH, Sugar E, Teslow T, McNutt T, Saleh H, Song DY. Comparison of daily couch shifts using MVCT (TomoTherapy) and B-mode ultrasound (BAT System) during prostate radiotherapy. *Technol Cancer Res Treat*. 2008;7(4):279–285.

41. Peng C, Kainz K, Lawton C, Li XA. A comparison of daily megavoltage CT and ultrasound image guided radiation therapy for prostate cancer. *Med Phys*. 2008;35(12):5619–5628.

42. Adamson J, Wu Q. Inferences about prostate intrafraction motion from pre- and posttreatment volumetric imaging. *Int J Radiat Oncol Biol Phys*. 2009;75(1):260–267.

43. Vargas C, Salta AI, His WC, et al. Cine-magnetic resonance imaging assessment of intrafraction motion for prostate cancer patients supine or prone with and without a rectal balloon. *Am J Clin Oncol*. 33(1):11–6(2010)

44. Willoughby TR, Kupelian PA, Pouliot J, et al. Target localization and real-time tracking using the Calypso 4D localization system in patients with localized prostate cancer. *Int J Radiat Oncol Biol Phys*. 2006;65(2):528–534.

45. Li HS, Chetty IJ, Enke CA, et al. Dosimetric consequences of intrafraction prostate motion. *Int J Radiat Oncol Biol Phys*. 2008;71(3):801–812.

46. Mah D, Freedman G, Milestone B, et al. Measurement of intrafractional prostate motion using magnetic resonance imaging. *Int J Radiat Oncol Biol Phys*. 2002;54(2):568–575.

47. Langen KM, Lu W, Willoughby TR, et al. Dosimetric effect of prostate motion during helical tomotherapy. *Int J Radiat Oncol Biol Phys*. 2009;74(4):1134–1142.

48. Salter BJ, Wang B, Szegedi MW, et al: Evaluation of alignment error due to a speed artifact in stereotactic ultrasound image guidance. *Phys Med Biol*. 2008;53(23):N437–N445.

49. McGahan JP, Ryu J, Fogata M. Ultrasound probe pressure as a source of error in prostate localization for external beam radiotherapy. *Int J Radiat Oncol Biol Phys*. 2004;60(3):788–793.

50. Artignan X, Smitsmans MH, Lebesque JV, Jaffray DA, van Her M, Bartelink H. Online ultrasound image guidance for radiotherapy of prostate cancer: impact of image acquisition on prostate displacement. *Int J Radiat Oncol Biol Phys*. 2004;59(2):595–601.

51. Dobler B, Mai S, Ross C, et al. Evaluation of possible prostate displacement induced by pressure applied during transabdominal ultrasound image acquisition. *Strahlenther Onkol*. 2006;182(4):240–246.

52. Watanabe M, Isobe K, Takisima H, et al. Intrafractional gastric motion and interfractional stomach deformity during radiation therapy. *Radiother Oncol*. 2008;87(3):425–431.

53. Krupa A, Fichtinger G, Hager GD. Real-time tissue tracking with B-mode ultrasound using speckle and visual servoing. *Med Image Comput Comput Assist Interv, Int Conf Med Image Comput Comput Assist Interv*. 2007; 10(pt 2):1–8.

54. Kuo J, von Ramm OT. Three-dimensional motion measurements using feature tracking. *IEEE Trans Ultrason Ferroelectr Freq Control*. 2008;55(4):800–810.

55. Li G, Citrin D, Camphausen K, et al. Advances in 4D medical imaging and 4D radiation therapy. *Technol Cancer Res Treat*. 2008;7(1):67–81.

56. Hsu A, Miller NR, Evans PM, Bamber JC, Webb S. Feasibility of using ultrasound for real-time tracking during radiotherapy. *Med Phys*. 2005;32(6):1500–1512.

57. Notomi Y, Lysyansky P, Setser RM, et al. Measurement of ventricular torsion by two-dimensional ultrasound speckle tracking imaging. *J Am Coll Cardiol*. 2005;45(12):2034–2041.

58. Kühl HP, Papavasiliu TS, Beek AM, Hofman MB, Heusen NS, van Rossum AC. Myocardial viability: rapid assessment with delayed contrast-enhanced MR imaging with three-dimensional inversion-recovery prepared pulse sequence. *Radiology*. 2004;230(2):576–582.

59. Wu J, Dandekar O, Nazareth D, Lei P, D'Souza W, Shekhar R. Effect of ultrasound probe on dose delivery during real-time ultrasound-guided tumor tracking. *Conf Proc IEEE Eng Med Biol Soc*. 2006 1:3799–3802.

60. Boctor EM, Iordachita I, Fichtinger G, Hager GD. Real-time quality control of tracked ultrasound. *Med Image Comput Comput Assist Interv*. 2005;8(pt 1):621–630.

61. Foroughi P, Abolmaesumi P. Elastic registration of 3D ultrasound images. *Med Image Comput Comput Assist Interv*. 2005; 8(pt 1):83–90.

62. Foroughi P, Abolmaesumi P, Hashtrudi-Zaad K. Intra-subject elastic registration of 3D ultrasound images. *Med Image Anal*. 2006;10(5):713–725.

Chapter 6

VIDEO SYSTEMS

SHIDONG LI, PHD

Daily patient repositioning in conventional radiotherapy (RT) relies on skin markers and body immobilization devices.[1-3] It is fast and convenient to check source-to-skin distance (SSD) with the optical distance indicator (ODI) and to align skin markers with room lasers. In-room live-video cameras allow monitoring of patient movements during irradiation. These one- and two-dimensional (2D) optical systems help to avoid gross setup errors. However, they cannot reveal the internal target displacements or changes in body shape. Thus, setup or portal radiographs are also taken to verify the internal anatomy.[4-8]

Optical-marker–based patient repositioning and monitoring are being investigated for three-dimensional (3D) repositioning.[9-17] Laser scanners have also been used for making tissue compensators as well as patient repositioning using scanned surfaces.[18,19] More recently, fast stereo-ovisions (or 3D-video images)[20-23] have been introduced for image-guided RT (IGRT). All 3D-video–guided techniques are noninvasive, efficient, accurate, and may provide real-time surface-based target repositioning, monitoring, and adaptive dose delivery. Results from early pilot studies[24-27] have already shown that such stere-

ovision guidance could potentially eliminate unnecessary ionization radiation in patient position verification and reduce the need for rigid immobilization. The stereovision technique can also be combined with volumetric imaging techniques for future four-dimensional (4D) IGRT.

Geometric Optics in Radiotherapy

Light Ray and Its Reflection

In geometric optics, a light ray as a narrow beam formed by photons or electromagnetic waves travels in a straight line until mostly reflected, absorbed, or refracted by a bright, dark, or transparent obstacle, respectively. The laws of light reflection are: (a) the incident ray, reflected ray, and the normal to the surface element are all in the same plane and (b) the angle of incidence equals the angle of reflection.[28] If a ray incidents on a plane mirror (or light reflector) that has a common normal, then specular (or mirror) reflection occurs; i.e., an incident ray is reflected as a single ray. However, if a light ray strikes a rough surface such as the skin of a human body, then diffuse reflection results. In diffuse reflection, an incident ray is

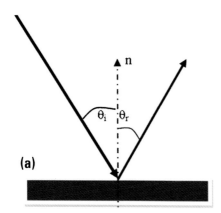 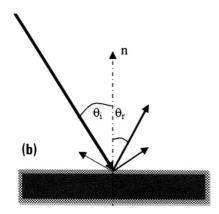

FIGURE 6-1. (a). Specular reflection of a light ray with the angle of incidence, θ_i, equals to the angle of reflection, θ_r. Incidence and reflection rays as well as the normal of the surface, n, are in the same plane. **(b).** Diffuse reflection with reflection angle over 2π. The light intensity is varied with the angles of incidence of θ_i and reflection of θ_r. The length and thickness of a ray represents its luminous intensity.

seemingly reflected over the surface that has surface elements pointing to various directions. Figure 6-1 illustrates the mirror reflection and diffuse reflection. If one considers the reflection light intensity, the Fresnel equation can be used to estimate the reflection coefficient (the reflected fraction of the incident light) that varies significantly on the human skin (surface).[29]

Mirror and diffuse reflections have both been useful in RT. For example, the outline of the radiation field can be projected onto a patient by using the mirror reflection of the light beam that is perpendicular to the x-ray beam. The thin in-field mirror that is 45° to the central axis (CAX) of the x-ray beam will reflect the light beam in the same direction as the x-ray beam. The reflected light beam is then collimated by the beam-shaping devices so that the light emerges from the linac head having the same shape as the x-ray (or electron) portal. The field coordinates and CAX of the broad light beam are demonstrated by the shadow of the crosshairs from the transparent window on the linac head. Figure 6-2 illustrates the optical system built within a typical linac. Note that some of the field light can be reflected back by the leaf-bank reflectors, by the in-field mirror, and by another adjustable mirror. The light travels back and reaches a charged coupled device (CCD) camera that provides the live video view of individual leaf positions and the field shapes.

Another built-in optical system is the ODI, which projects multiple "short-line" rays, with desired angles, to intersect with the CAX crosshair at the specific distances (e.g., 80 cm, 81 cm, 82 cm, ..., 120 cm) from the virtual source. When a patient is on the treatment table, the CAX crosshair, an ODI line, and the number along the ODI line will coincide at the same spot on the patient's skin. The diffuse reflection of the light field and ODI will allow the therapists to visualize the field intersection with the patient and the SSD on the skin from different angles. In case of less-diffuse reflection on very dark skin, the therapist may have to place a ruler or a piece of paper on the skin to show the SSD. These optic systems have been routinely used and are periodically checked for the light field congruence with the radiation field, the ODI agreement with the front pointer, and accuracy of the multileaf collimator (MLC) leaf-bank positions.

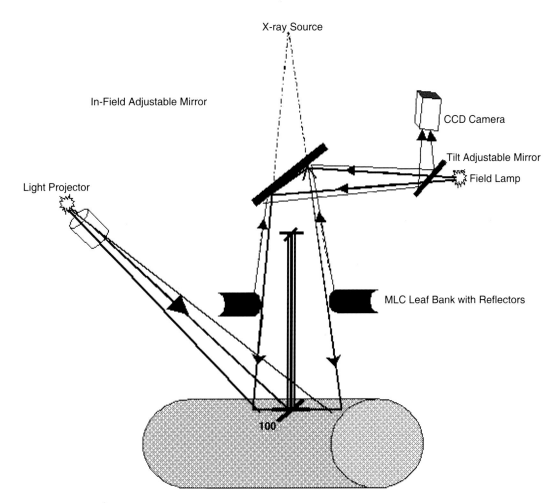

FIGURE 6-2. Illustration of the optics located in the head of the linear accelerator. *Note.* CCD = charge-coupled device; MLC = multileaf collimator.

Refraction, Lens, and Optical Images

A real image of an object refers to an image that can be formed on a screen placed at the position where light rays from a point on the object pass through a common point on the screen. A virtual image refers to an image without the light rays passing through it. Although the virtual image of the light source (dashed lines) in Figure 6-2 is useful in demonstration of the x-ray source position, video imaging generally utilizes real images formed through optical lenses.

The word "lens" is based on the Latin word *lentil* because a double-convex lens is lentil-shaped. A light ray passing through a lens obeys Snell's Laws of Refractions.[30] That is, the product of the sine of the ray angle and the refractive index in the medium is unchanged when light passes through the interface between two media (see Figure 6-3). The surface of a lens can be convex (bulging outward from the lens), concave (depressed into the lens), or planar (flat). A parallel beam of light travelling along the lens axis and passing through a convex lens will be focused on a spot on the axis at the focal length, f. In this case, the lens is called a converging (or positive) lens. The plane perpendicular to the lens axis at the focal length f from the lens is called the focal plane. For a thin lens shown in Figure 6-4, one can use the thin lens formula of $1/f = 1/d_o + 1/d_i$, where d_o and d_i are the object and image distances to the lens geometric center, respectively.

If the object is moved (d_o varied), the image will become blurred and the phenomenon is referred as the depth aberration. Thus, most cameras use an adjustable lens to acquire clear pictures. The lens magnification, M, is given by $-d_i/d_o$ and a negative M will show a real image upside-

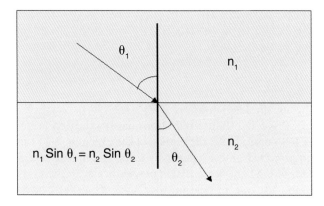

FIGURE 6-3. Snell's Laws of Refraction.

down with respect to the object. This can be corrected at the image display on a screen. The largest size of an object visible through the optical system defines its field of view (FOV). The range of the object distance with clear images defines its depth of field (DOF). Some depth, dispersion, and chromatic aberrations can be minimized through use of a compound lens consisting of multiple low dispersion lenses or special coatings.[31] For a compound lens (or a multilens optical system) in air or vacuum, the thin-lens formulas can be used, but d_o and d_i are measured from the front and rear principal planes, respectively. For simplicity, one can use the single-lens geometry to represent the complex optical system.

Optical Imaging Systems

Video-based imaging has been used for patient repositioning. Researchers at the University of Chicago[32,33] and

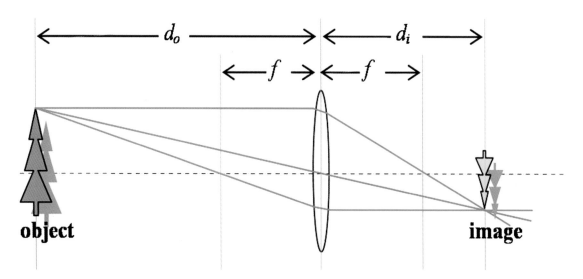

FIGURE 6-4. Real-image of object formed through a thin lens.

Stanford University[34] have used a pair of live video *sub-traction* images to reproduce a patient's position in the treatment room. Two video cameras mounted to the walls and ceiling of the treatment room are directed toward the isocenter. On the first day of treatment, images of the patient from the two cameras are saved for use as a reference for future sessions. When one compares live video with the reference images by using image subtraction, one can interactively move the patient until a null image is produced, thus reproducing the previous position. This technique has been shown to be fast and easy to implement, and has reduced patient repositioning errors. However, the 2D video system requires consistent lighting conditions and lacks 3D or DOF information.

The University of Florida infrared-LED-guided technique[9–12] and the German Cancer Research Center photogrammetric technique[35] can track 3D patient's head movement with an accuracy of less than 0.1 mm. Such systems (including infrared-reflector–based commercial systems) are based on a triangulation localization of the 3D points, as described in the next subsection.

Triangulation Principle

The triangulation principle is shown in Figure 6-5. The angles of alpha (α), beta (β), and the length of the baseline (L) between two cameras can uniquely define the triangle for the surface point of **Q**. Given α, β, and L, the range R from camera 1 to the point **Q** can be calculated according to the formula.

$$R = L\frac{\sin(\beta)}{\sin(\alpha + \beta)} \qquad (1)$$

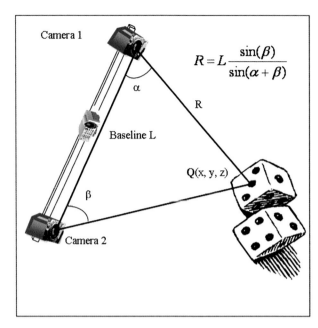

FIGURE 6-5. Illustration of the triangulation principle.

By having the fixed lenses, the video imaging coordinates are fixed in which the baseline of L and the angles α and β can be easily determined.

Figure 6-6 illustrates the imaging geometry for any 3D point **Q** in the scene of the two cameras. The image coordinates relative to the machine coordinates and the baseline L can be previously calibrated. The vector from C_1 to I_1 is within the light ray from **Q** to I_1 such that the α equals arcos($C_1I_1 \cdot L$). Similarly, one can have the light ray from **Q** to I_2 in the second camera with β = arcos

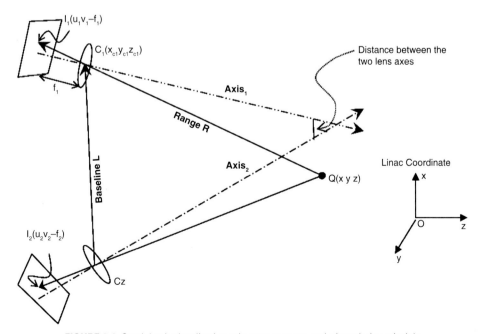

FIGURE 6-6. Spatial point localization using two cameras and triangulation principle.

$(-C_2 I_2 \cdot L)$. With the image plane at the focal distance of f_1 behind the lens center C_1, the image location $I_1 = (u_1, v_1, -f_1)$ in the first camera coincides with the lens axis as its third principle axis, and the predefined transformation matrix from the first camera coincides with the machine coordinates, so that one can calculate the surface point $Q(x, y, z)$ by

$$
\begin{pmatrix} x_Q \\ y_Q \\ z_Q \\ 1 \end{pmatrix} = \begin{bmatrix} r_{11} & r_{12} & r_{13} & x_{C1} \\ r_{21} & r_{22} & r_{23} & y_{C1} \\ r_{31} & r_{32} & r_{33} & z_{C1} \\ 0 & 0 & 0 & 1 \end{bmatrix} \begin{pmatrix} -u_1 R / \sqrt{u_1^2 + v_1^2 + f_1^2} \\ -v_1 R / \sqrt{u_1^2 + v_1^2 + f_1^2} \\ f_1 R / \sqrt{u_1^2 + v_1^2 + f_1^2} \\ 1 \end{pmatrix}. \quad (2)
$$

Here, $C_1(x_{c1}\ y_{c1}\ z_{c1})$ is the effective lens center of the first camera in the machine coordinate system (MCS) that is assigned as the origin of the first camera coordinates. The Q in the first camera coordinate system is given by $Q = -I_1 R / |C_1 I_1|$. The transformation matrix consists of nine rotation parameters r_{ij} and 3D translation from the C_1 to the O. Notice that the two camera axes neither intersect with each other, nor do they have to pass through the machine isocenter, O. Thus, equations (1) and (2) are the general solutions for any 3D point.

A common usage of the infrared marker guidance is for head or body repositioning and tracking in stereotactic RT (SRT). In this case, multiple infrared markers may be attached to the mouthpiece with dental caulk or simply on the surface of interest at the computed tomography (CT) simulation. At each treatment setup, the target position is adjusted by aligning all infrared markers to the simulation markers' locations. A rigid body displacement in six degrees of freedom would require locations of at least three markers. Five or more markers are generally used to improve the accuracy and precision of daily repositioning. Users should ensure proper marker placement so that no markers are blocked or near blocked from the camera views. The markers are usually made as spherical balls with the size of ~1 cm in diameter because the center of such a sphere is uniquely and easily identified from all camera views. Commercial systems such as Novalis ExacTrac (BrainLAB Inc, Feldkirchen, Germany) and CyberKnife (Accuray Inc, Sunnyvale, CA) have combined such an optic system with biplane radiographs for patient positioning and monitoring. Figure 6-7 illustrates the Cyberknife system.

Stereovision (3D-Video Imaging) Systems

The optical marker guidance described previously cannot deal with possible body shape changes and uncertainties

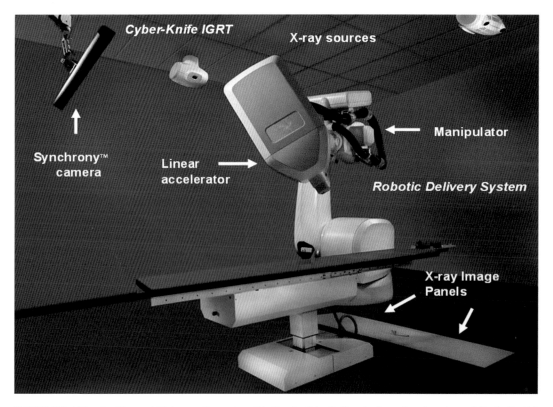

FIGURE 6-7. Video tracking and biplane radiograph verification in CyberKnife robotic system (courtesy of Dr A. Rashid, Georgetown University). *Note.* IGRT = image-guided radiation therapy.

from repeated marker attachments to the patient. Thus, a real-time 3D video guidance has been introduced for patient refixation.[36] In such a system, a 3D video camera captures the patient surface on the treatment table as a snapshot without using any marker or device. The real-time surface image with high spatial resolution of 1 mm or less is then automatically aligned with the reference surface to determine the patient displacements, allowing an accurate and precise online correction. Several commercial and investigational systems are currently available but all have the common features of full-frame reconstruction, quick and reliable image acquisition, and automatic surface alignment.

Full-Frame Reconstruction

A basic property of a stereovision system is the capability of 3D reconstruction of the human body surface from a 3D video camera. The triangulation principle described previously is the operation principle for all 3D video systems except for some laser scanners that may use the time-of-flight method. The Rainbow camera (Genex Technologies, Kensington, MD)[37] is used at our institution and serves as an example to describe the full frame reconstruction. The speckle-based 3D camera such as AlignRT camera (VisionRT Ltd, London, United Kingdom)[38,39] uses the triangulation principle and projecting speckles to define the corresponding points between the two camera views. A laser scanner or topography reconstructs the detail surface through a moving strip of the fan-beam laser similar to the light strips used by a Rainbow camera.

The Rainbow camera is composed of one (or two) color CCD camera(s), a light projector, and a computer.[22,40] The video camera captures an image of specific light patterns projected onto the surface of the patient. From this image, a "range image" is quickly computed according to the modified triangulation principle. For this camera system, the angle β is the angle between the projection light ray and the baseline L, the distance from the light source of the projector to the CCD camera lens center, C_1. The angle α for a given image point in the camera and the baseline L are predetermined as described in the previous section. The key to this 3D video system is the determination of the projection angle, β. A task that is even more challenging is to determine all β angles corresponding to all of the visible points on object's surface, therefore, to obtain a full frame of stereovision in one snapshot. The technique of using individual light strips for the Rainbow camera that can be used for laser topography is described in detail here.

Let us define a new 3D camera coordinate in Figure 6-8 with the origin at the camera optical center C_1, the u'-axis along the baseline, the v'-axis parallel to the projection light fringes (the intersection strips between the image plane and fan beams), and w'-axis following the right-hand coordinate toward the object. In this coordinate system, the focal image plane of the camera is usually not parallel to the C_1-$u'v'$ plane. An image point, $\mathbf{I}(u_i\ v_i\ -f_1)$, in the image plane would be transformed as $(u'_i, v'_i, w'_i) = \mathbf{RotM}(\mathbf{Axis}_1\text{-to-}w') \otimes (u_i\ v_i\ -f_1)^T$ and have two projection points $\mathbf{J}$ and $\mathbf{K}$ onto the C_1-$u'v'$ plane and the u'-axis, respectively. Any surface point $\mathbf{Q}$ also has two projection points $\mathbf{N}$ and $\mathbf{P}$ onto the u'-axis and the C_1-$u'w'$ plane, respectively. Since $tg(\alpha) = |\mathbf{I} - \mathbf{K}| / |\mathbf{K} - \mathbf{C1}|$ and $ctg(\beta) = |\mathbf{S} - \mathbf{N}|/|\mathbf{Q} - \mathbf{N}|$, and $|\mathbf{I} - \mathbf{K}|/|\mathbf{Q} - \mathbf{N}| = |\mathbf{I} - \mathbf{J}|/|\mathbf{N} - \mathbf{P}|$ according to the similar ΔNPQ and ΔIJK, we would have $tg(\alpha)\ ctg(\beta) = (-w'_i/u'_i)\ (|\mathbf{S} - \mathbf{N}|/|\mathbf{N} - \mathbf{P}|) = (-w'_i/u'_i)\ ctg(\beta_o)$. Here, the β_o represents not only the ray of $\mathbf{SQ}$ but also all rays in the fan-beam of the SPQ (or the

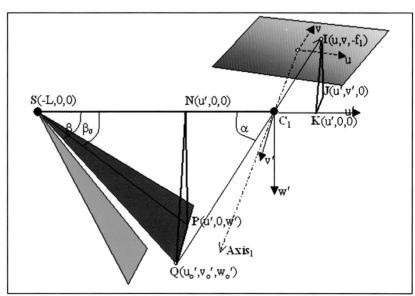

FIGURE 6-8. A point registration in full-frame reconstruction using fan-beam fringes (strips).

light strip of PQ). Now, the 3D coordinates (u′, v′, w′) for any surface point Q in the fan beam can be analytically determined by

$$u'_Q = \frac{u'_i \cdot L}{w'_i \cdot ctg(\beta_o) - u'_i}, v'_Q = \frac{v'_i \cdot L}{w'_i \cdot ctg(\beta_o) - u'_i},$$

$$and \; w'_Q = \frac{w'_i \cdot L}{w'_i \cdot ctg(\beta_o) - u'_i}. \tag{3}$$

Because the baseline L, rotation angle from lens' **Axis1** to the w′-axis, and any image point $I(u_i, v_i, -f_1)$ are available, the only unknown is the projection angle β_o of the corresponding fan beam. For a laser scanner, the fan-beam angle is controlled by the laser scanning angle as function of scanning time, t_{scan}, that is $\beta_o(t_{scan})$. A Rainbow 3D camera can capture the full frame with a snapshot by using an off-the-shelf video projector that projects rainbow light to illuminate 3D objects in the scene simultaneously without using any moving parts as shown in Figure 6-9. Here, the light spectrum distribution (β_i) is uniquely defined by the primary colors red, green, and blue. The proportions of the three primary colors are directly obtained from the three color channels of an off-the-shelf color CCD camera. One can then precisely determine all of the fan-beams' (strips) angle β_i. To increase accuracy, Multiple Rainbow Projections (MRP) can be used.

In clinical applications, the camera is usually mounted on the ceiling of treatment room and views objects at a distance of 150 cm to 220 cm (DOF = 60 cm) with a large

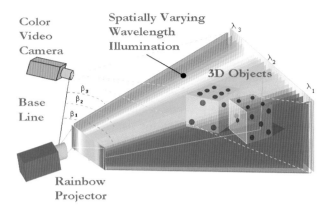

FIGURE 6-9. Illumination of three-dimensional objects with well-defined rainbow fan-beams (or light strips).

FOV of ~50 cm² × 70 cm². The MRP pattern possesses a high rate of variation that helps to differentiate small projection angles and also to minimize the room light effect on the quality of surface images. The room light is relatively uniform and treated as a uniform background. Therefore, there is no effect on surface reconstruction by turning on or off the room light. Figure 6-10 is the screen capture on a Rainbow camera computer at the imaging of a flat phantom (calibration template) in a treatment vault at Johns Hopkins University. The window contains two Rainbow camera views and a 2D live video view on the top row. A plot of the surface movement (red curves) detected by a motion sensor ray showing the phantom

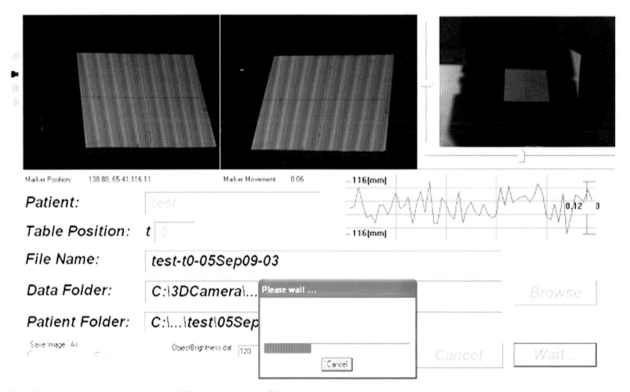

FIGURE 6-10. Screen capture at taking MRP stereovision of a QA phantom on a linac table.

with surface displacements 0.12 mm in the last 10 seconds is also shown, as well as information for the reference file and captured stereovision. The processing bar (pink) in the bottom pop-up window indicates the progress of reconstruction. One third of the reconstruction had been accomplished within a second with a Pentium 4 PC in the year 2003. Full frame reconstruction at less than 0.1 second is possible with high-speed GPU and would provide a cine view by capturing sequential images at a rate of 10 frames per second.

Quick and Reliable Stereovision Acquisition

Reliable surface imaging is important for accurate representation of the body position and shape at the time of treatment. Two common optic image artifacts are the shadow casting caused by the lack of reflecting light at the obstacle shadows and the overexposure holes caused by the strong specular reflection on the polished surface. The latter can be easily eliminated if the polished surface areas are covered by white cotton tapes. The artifacts of shadow casting can be removed by setting a threshold of jumps at the neighboring facets of the reconstructed surface. The 3D camera should be installed with a good view of the surface of interest that would have enough overlapping area with the reference surface.

To take into account an unstable surface caused by unanticipated body movement (such as deep respiration motion for chest or abdomen imaging or facial expression for head and neck imaging), Li et al. have built a motion sensor into the 3D camera system by using a fixed light ray intersected with the moving surface.[26]

Figure 6-11 conceptually illustrates this method and results for monitoring abdominal movement of a patient with lung cancer. The surface movement was represented by the plot of the intersection point displacement (in vertical direction) versus time. This case shows electronic noise in the first 3 seconds after the initiation of the 3D camera followed by a deep respiration at 6 to 12 seconds. Reliable surface images were not taken at the initial noise or during irregular body motion. To use such a novel motion sensor, the sensor ray should point to the area that is sensitive to the motion of interest such as the inferior surface of the chin for mouth movement or the upper abdomen for respiration. The motion sensor ray is adjustable by two orthogonal scroll bars on the side and bottom of the live video view in Figure 6-10. When the displacement plot becomes stable (with the range of displacement of 0.5 mm or less in the last second, a reliable surface image was almost ensured by a snapshot within 0.1 second.

Automatic Surface Alignment

Surface mapping is the process of bringing two 3D data sets into the best possible alignment. The 3D surface image, S, is a 3-tuples, i.e.,

$$S = (V, E, F), \qquad (4)$$

where bold-font V is the vertex set, E is the edge set, and F is the face set. The neighborhood structure of a triangle mesh (the faces and edges) is called the topology of the mesh, and the coordinates of the vertices describe its geometry.[41] With a 3D reference surface, S_R, and treatment surface, S_T, respectively acquired with the patient in the CT-based plan position and with the patient at each treatment, the task is to align S_R and S_T, and quickly estimate

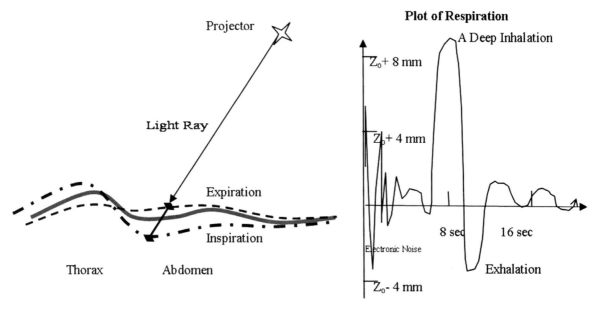

FIGURE 6-11. A ray intersecting with the abdominal surface (left) and a plot of motion versus time (right).

the patient's displacements. There are number of surface-matching algorithms.[42,43] We chose the well-known Iterative Closest Points (ICP)[44] algorithm, which treats the closest points on other data set as corresponding points. Starting from an initial estimate of the unknown parameters, the ICP algorithm recursively refines the closest point pairs and pose estimation. The ICP algorithm also requires a robust criterion to perform corresponding point finding when the pose is poor. We have found that in most clinical situations, the patient has been already set up in the treatment position and automatic alignment can be directly used. Even if the S_T is largely deviated from S_R, one can simply overlap the two surface images S_R and S_T by manually selecting three feature points. Then, ICP automatic alignment can be applied. In any iteration, the S_T has been transformed as

$$S_{T,n} = RotM\,(t_n, \alpha_n) \otimes S_{T,n-1}, \qquad n = 1, 2, 3, \ldots \qquad (5)$$

where n is the number of the iterations and S_{T_0} is the original captured surface data set without transformation. The t_n and α_n are the 3D translational vector and 3D rotation vector, respectively. Both surface images have been registered in the MCS. The rotation matrix may be expressed as a quaternion and the multiplication of the matrices in the iteration process become the addition of multiple quaternions.[45] A k-d tree structure is employed to speed up the computation of finding closest points. The termination of the iteration process is given by the minimal root mean squared (RMS) distance defined as

$$RMS = \left\{ \sum_{i=1}^{n} \| V_T^i - V_R^i \|^2 \right\}^{1/2} / n. \qquad (6)$$

The RMS is usually less than 2.0 mm in patients with good matches.

Clinical Applications

The goal of any IGRT system is to increase the accuracy and precision in delivery of the planned dose distribution to the patient without increasing treatment time and patient inconvenience. Figure 6-12 illustrates an Integral Stereovision-Guided Adaptive Radiotherapy (ISGAR) system that has linked the CT simulator, CT-based treatment plan, daily patient setup, and adaptive dose delivery through stereovision guidance. Such an integral system requires an accurate reference image, precise calibration to correlate the CT image coordinates with the treatment MCS, and accurate dose delivery under stereovision surveillance.

Generation of Reference Surface

The origin of the planning coordinates can be set at the beam isocenter or the treatment machine isocenter. The approved treatment plan data are exported as DICOM data set. Current DICOM RT standard[46] includes five objects: RT Image, RT Dose, RT Structure Set, RT Plan, and RT Treatment Record. The DICOM RT Structure Set, which contains contour structures, markers, and isocenter(s), is crucial to the reference image generation. Most planning systems provide a function to export the DICOM RT structure set. One may use a simple surface reconstruction algorithm described by Biossonnat and others[47] to first triangulate the contours and compute the medial axes and then joint contours on adjacent cross-sections to create a denser mesh surface. The complexity of the branching regions formed by the extremities or position devices is avoided and a reference surface

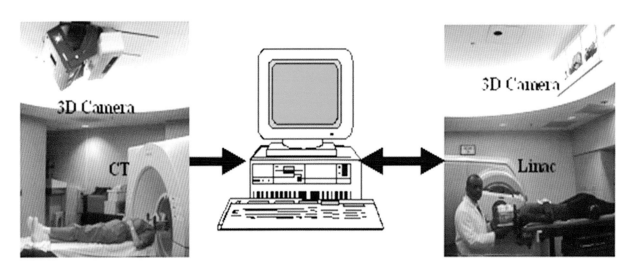

FIGURE 6-12. An Integrated Stereovision-Guided Adaptive Radiotherapy system at Johns Hopkins University with a three-dimensional (3D) camera mounted on the ceiling of the computed tomography–simulation room and another 3D camera mounted on the ceiling of the linac vault for daily patient head reposition and position monitoring.

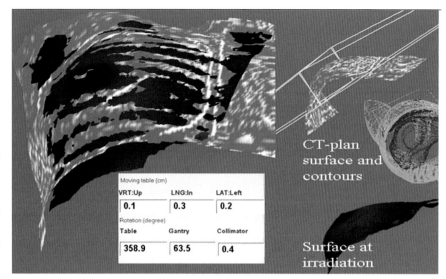

FIGURE 6-13. Illustration of a reference surface in light gray with planned tangential beams and a real-time stereovision in dark gray taken during the medial beam irradiation for the patient. The insert table shows the calculated adaptive isocenter shifts and adapted beam, and table angles based on the surface mapping of the two surface areas shown (left-upper images).

with the same format as the optical surface (0.5-mm or 1-mm interval between neighboring points) can be easily registered in the MCS. Any differences between the CT-simulator image coordinates and treatment MCS should be corrected through a template-based calibration (described later). For optimal surface alignment, the reference surface should be restricted to the target surface area plus a margin for possible setup errors. This reference surface would ensure that body-shape changes far away from the target would not affect the accuracy of ISGAR. Figure 6-13 represents the screen capture of an ISGAR application for a right breast irradiation that uses segmented tangential beams for a patient accrued in a clinical trial at Henry Ford Hospital. One can clearly see the detail of the surface differences between the reference CT scan (light gray with wire and respiration effects) and real-time image on a particular treatment day (dark gray). The global target displacements may be compensated by the adaptive table and beam adjustment shown in the pop-up window.

Template-Based Calibration of CT and Treatment MCS

The calibration template with a printed grid shown in Figure 6-10 is designed to correlate the treatment MCS to the 3D camera image coordinate system. The calibration template is carefully placed on the top of the treatment table and precisely aligned with the corresponding machine axes. A rigid frame transformation is determined by three translational parameters and three rotational parameters. Given the three point locations in the MCS and their locations in the camera system, an analytical solution exists to find transformational parameters. In our study, there are situations where digitization errors and noise on the 3D surface images may be significant. By using a least-squares estimation algorithm, one can minimize these errors. A total of nine points can be digitized on the 3D

surface image of the calibration plate, and their coordinate values in both the camera coordinate system and the MCS are used to compute transformational parameters via the multipoint registration.[48] This template-based calibration is also used for CT simulators so that any small differences between the images are corrected through the calibration to the same coordinate system (i.e., MCS). Markers in CT and MCS will be verified with x-ray images.

Stereovision-Guided Setup and Dose Delivery

Real-time stereovisions after initial patient setup on the treatment table are captured with a 3D camera mounted on the ceiling of a linac vault. The real-time surface is then automatically matched with the reference surface and the measured 3D shifts and rotations may be manually adjusted or remotely corrected through the remote table control. After the table adjustments, surface images can be recaptured and realigned with the reference surface to determine any further corrections needed until there is no significant displacement. The volumetric cone-beam CT (CBCT) images or portal radiographs may also be taken to verify the internal target position and shapes. Significant anatomic changes or deformation may require modification of the treatment plan and the subsequent generation of a new reference surface. During external beam irradiation, surface images may also be captured and matched with the reference surface to confirm the target position. If there was a significant movement, the beam would be interrupted and the displacement would be corrected and verified with real-time stereovisions. Real-time image-guided beam setup for specific treatment sites can be implemented but require further investigation.[49]

Clinical Results

Before clinical implementation, tests on a RANDO (The Phantom Laboratory, Salem, NY) head phantom and a custom breast phantom have achieved submillimeter and subdegree accuracy and precision with ISGAR. The IS-GAR system developed by the author and colleagues at Johns Hopkins University and Henry Ford Hospital had not only detected those unknown displacements but also verified the results with postcorrection images. The results of 20 volunteers with various skin colors have proved the feasibility of unfolding topographic changes of human body.

Figure 6-14 shows the improvement of a daily stereovision-guided head refixation for a patient under stereotactic thermal-plastic cast for Fractionated Stereotactic Radiotherapy (SRT). The reference surface and stereovisions (solid gray) were matched to show the detail surface changes and displacements (shifts and rotations). The submillimeter and subdegree accuracy and precision

are a significant improvement over conventional radiograph-based head repositioning (accuracy of 0.5 mm; precision of 2.0 mm).

The results on 70 SRT/ZMPT patients treated at Johns Hopkins University from 2000 to 2005 have shown improved patient head refixation accuracy (in direction with the largest errors) from 0.4 mm ± 2.3 mm to 0.0 mm ± 1.0 mm in the inferior–superior direction for patients wearing stereotactic facemasks or from 0.8 mm ± 4.3 mm to 0.4 mm ± 1.7 mm in the posterior–anterior direction for patients wearing a flexible head and neck mask, respectively. Figure 6-15 illustrates the results and automatically matched stereovisions for a patient head repositioning for a flexible facemask. The accuracy and precision are comparable among the 61 patients wearing the stereotactic masks and nine patients wearing the flexible masks.

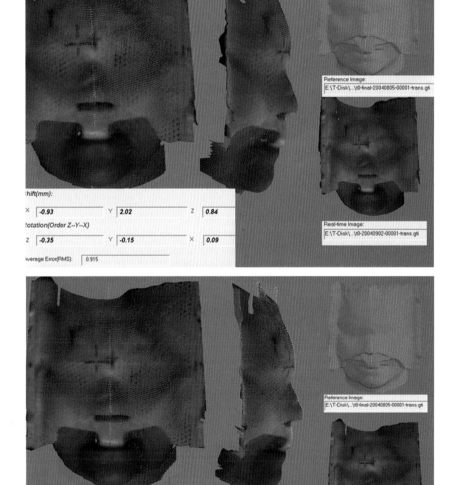

FIGURE 6-14. The front and right lateral views of S_R (blue) and S_T (gray) with shifts of (−0.9, 2.0, 0.8) mm at conventional setup (upper) and (−0.5, 0.4, 0.6) at stereovision-guided reposition (lower).

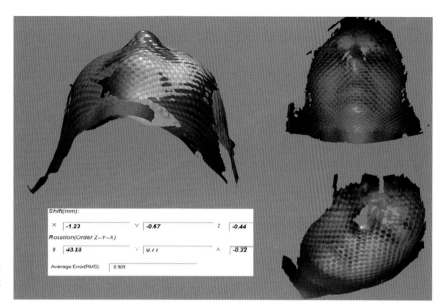

FIGURE 6-15. Stereovision verification of a patient head position for a 45°-couch-kick beam.

This is important because it demonstrated that stereovision guidance could potentially eliminate the use of tight stereotactic masks or even flexible masks that sometimes cause discomfort and even treatment cancelation or resimulation if the patient is unable to tolerate them.

We have shown that small thorax motion is detectable with the fixing-ray motion sensor technique in Figure 6-11. Figure 6-16 illustrates the detection of the small mouth movement for another patient during

stereovision-guided radiotherapy that could be useful for monitoring the target motion during dose delivery for patients with head and neck cancer.

With the ISGAR system, one can also measure the setup marker errors during CT or other volumetric simulation scanning. The marker errors may introduce systematic errors in conventional daily patient repositioning. Figure 6-17 shows the measured results of the simulation setup marker errors for 20 patients receiving

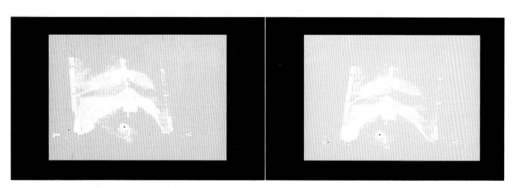

Two CCD camera views of the mask, laser lines, head surface, and ray-skin intersection (dot) on the chin of a patient undertook 3D-video-guided SRT of a brain tumor

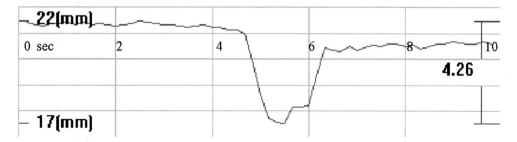

A 4.26-mm chin movement was detected prior to capture a reliable surface image in IGRT

FIGURE 6-16. Mouth motion detected with a ray pointing to the chin (top views) over a 10-second time period.

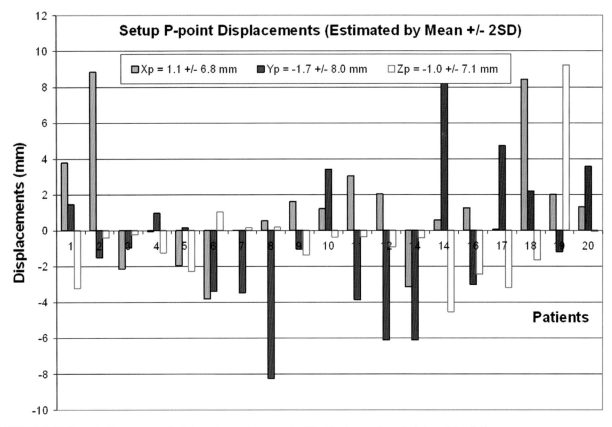

FIGURE 6-17. Computed tomography simulator setup marker errors for 20 patients receiving whole breast irradiation.

whole breast irradiation. Without quick imaging and registration techniques, it is difficult to distinguish the marker errors from organ motion or from daily breast repositioning uncertainties. Figure 6-18 illustrates such a CT-based planning reference surface and a simulation stereovision with setup marker.

Conclusions

The basic principles and clinical use of optical systems such as the light field, ODI, MLC encoder, infrared marker–

aided 3D positioning and tracking, and the ISGAR system are all presented in this chapter. The triangulation principle used for the 3D markers and novel reconstruction of full frame of surface in the 3D video camera and laser topography are emphasized and their clinical applications were discussed. The technique has proven to be useful for many sites of treatment through clinical trials.[50-52] In the future, the real-time stereovision system will be improved as the 4D camera or sensor is integrated with near real-time image-guided adjustment of the treatment beam.[53-55] This surface-based adaptive or gated RT

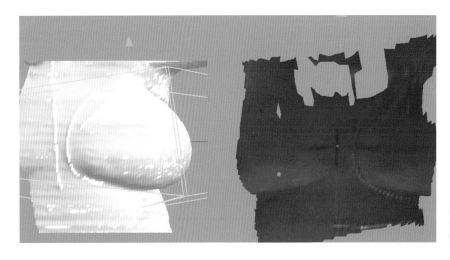

FIGURE 6-18. Reference computed tomography surface and stereovision surface used for setup marker check.

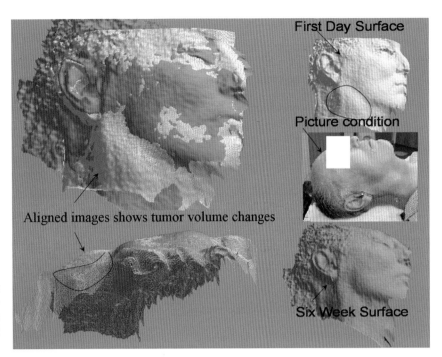

FIGURE 6-19. Matched stereovisions on the first day and during the sixth week of treatment for a head and neck patient with the tumor volume shrinkage from 26.7 cc to 11.2 cc within the defined area.

would provide more accurate information of patient-target motion than current marker-based or air flow-based gating.[56]

Perhaps the most important issue now in the clinical application of the stereovision guidance is how to integrate the new video imaging techniques with other volumetric IGRT techniques. Besides the technical improvements needed for precise and accurate correlation of the surface images with volumetric images, more clinical investigations are required in the near future. For example, on-line image-based target repositioning and verification as well as monitoring during irradiation, adaptive beam (or leaf sequence) setup, treatment modification or on-line planning, and comprehensive clinical validations of the stereovision-guidance are needed for various treatment sites. Some anatomic models for correlation of the surface shape and motion with internal target-structure deformation or motion are desired for the detection through the stereovisions.

Real-time stereovision as an efficient and accurate IGRT approach also provides a useful tool to check the clinical outcomes. Figure 6-19 illustrates that the target volume (surface volume with tumor base outlined by the black curve) changes during the course of treatment can be measured and the results of the volume changes with the delivered doses may immediately be available, thus providing clinicians more time to modify treatment.

In summary, optical systems have traditionally been useful for patient positional verification, beam setup checking, and leaf control in MLC for intensity-modulated RT (IMRT). With the emerging stereovision techniques, 3D and 4D video systems will play an important role for advanced IGRT particularly for 4D

images, gated RT, and efficient and real-time IGRT. The integration of the stereovision guidance with a volumetric imaging system such as CBCT would provide the optimal IGRT system that can not only increase efficiency, accuracy, and precision, but also ensure the accurate target position during the dose delivery.

References

1. Bentel GC, Marks LB, Sherouse GW, et al. The effectiveness of immobilization during prostate irradiation. *Int J Radiat Oncol Biol Phys.* 1997;31(1):143–148.
2. Lyman JT, Phillips MH, Frankel KA, et al. Stereotactic frame for neuroradiology and charged particle Bragg peak radiosurgery of intracranial disorders. *Int J Radiat Oncol Biol Phys.* 1989;16(6):1615–1621.
3. Hunt MA, Kutcher GJ, Burman C, et al. The effect of setup uncertainties on the treatment of nasopharynx cancer. *Int J Radiat Oncol Biol Phys.* 1993;27(2):437–447.
4. Denham JW, Dally MJ, Hunter K, et al. Objective decision-making following a portal film: the results of a pilot study. *Int J Radiat Oncol Biol Phys.* 1993;26(5):869–876.
5. Herman MG, Abrams RA, Mayer RR. Clinical use of on-line portal imaging for daily patient treatment verification. *Int J Radiat Oncol Biol Phys.* 1994;28(4):1017–1023.
6. Yan D, Wong JW, Gustafson G, et al. A new model for "accept or reject" strategies in off-line and on-line megavoltage treatment evaluation. *Int J Radiat Oncol Biol Phys.* 1995;31(4):943–952.
7. Hunt MA, Schultheiss TE, Desobry GE, et al. An evaluation of setup uncertainties for patients treated to pelvic sites. *Int J Radiat Oncol Biol Phys.* 1995;32(1):227–233.
8. Balter JM, Sandler HM, Lam K, et al. Measurement of prostate movement over the course of routine radiotherapy using implanted markers. *Int J Radiat Oncol Biol Phys.* 1995;31(1):113–118.

72 / Image-Guided Radiation Therapy: A Clinical Perspective

9. Bova FJ, Buatti JM, Friedman WA, et al. The University of Florida frameless high-precision stereotactic radiotherapy system. *Int J Radiat Oncol Biol Phys.* 1997;38(4):875–882.

10. Buatti JM, Bova FJ, Friedman WA, et al. Preliminary experience with frameless stereotactic radiotherapy. *Int J Radiat Oncol Biol Phys.* 1998;42(3):591–599.

11. Tome WA, Meeks SL, Buatti JM, et al. A high-precision system for conformal intracranial radiotherapy. *Int J Radiat Oncol Biol Phys.* 2000;47(4):1137–1143.

12. Meeks SL, Bova FJ, Wagner TH, et al. Image localization for frameless stereotactic radiotherapy. *Int J Radiat Oncol Biol Phys.* 2000;46(5):1291–1299.

13. Liu H, Yu Y, Schell MC, et al. Optimal marker placement in photogrammetry patient positioning system. *Med Phys.* 2003;30(2):103–110.

14. Meeks SL, Tomé WA, Willoughby TR, et al. Optically guided patient positioning techniques. *Semin Radiat Oncol.* 2005; 15(3):192–201.

15. Tao S, Wu A, Wu Y, et al. Patient set-up in radiotherapy with video-based positioning system. *Clin Oncol (R Coll Radiol).* 2006;18(4):363–366.

16. Jin JY, Yin FF, Tenn SE, et al. Use of the BrainLAB ExacTrac X-Ray 6D system in image-guided radiotherapy. *Med Dosim.* 2008;33(2):124–134.

17. Lyatskaya Y, James S, Killoran JH, et al. Infrared-guided patient setup for lung cancer patients. *Int J Radiat Oncol Biol Phys.* 2008;71(4):1124–1133.

18. Andrew JW, Aldrich JE, Hale ME, Berry JA. A video-based patient contour acquisition system for the design of radiotherapy compensators. *Med Phys.* 1989;16(3):425–430.

19. Berry JA, Aldrich JE. Surface topography for patient repositioning. *Med Dosim.* 1991;16(2):71–77.

20. Li S, Frassica D, DeWeese T, et al. A real-time image-guided intraoperative high-dose-rate brachytherapy system. *Brachytherapy.* 2003;2(1):5–16.

21. Li S, Geng J. Real-time three-dimensional video image–guided radiation therapy: emerging technology. In: Mundt AJ, Roeske JC, eds. *Intensity Modulated Radiation Therapy: A Clinical Perspective.* Lewiston, NY: BC Decker Inc; 2005: 407–413.

22. Li S, Liu D, Yin G, et al. Real-time 3D-surface-guided head re-fixation useful for fractionated stereotactic radiotherapy. *Med Phys.* 2006;33(2):492–503.

23. Bert C, Metheany KG, Doppke KP, et al. Clinical experience with a 3D surface patient setup system for alignment of partial-breast irradiation patients. *Int J Radiat Oncol Biol Phys.* 2006; 64(4):1265–1274.

24. Schöffel PJ, Harms W, Sroka-Perez G, et al. Accuracy of a commercial optical 3D surface imaging system for realignment of patients for radiotherapy of the thorax. *Phys Med Biol.* 2007;52(13):3949–3963.

25. Brahme A, Nyman P, Skatt B. 4D laser camera for accurate patient positioning, collision avoidance, image fusion and adaptive approaches during diagnostic and therapeutic procedures. *Med Phys.* 2008;35(5):1670–1681.

26. Li S, Kleinberg, LR, Rigamonti D, et al. (2010). Clinical Results of a Pilot Study on Stereovision-Guided Stereotactic Radiotherapy and Intensity Modulated Radiotherapy. Technol Cancer Res Treat, Dec. in press.

27. Li S, Walker E, Liu D, et al. Assessments of feasibility and accuracy of daily reposition and dose delivery for an integrated stereovision guided adaptive radiotherapy (ISGAR) of breast cancer. *Int J Radiat Oncol Biol Phys.* In press.

28. Giancoli DC. Reflection; image formation by a plane mirror. In: Giancoli DC, ed. *Physics Principles With Applications.* 5th ed. Upper Saddle River, NJ: Prentice Hall; 1998: 684–688.

29. Hecht E. *Optics.* 2nd ed. Reading, Mass.: Addison Wesley; 1987: 100–102.

30. Giancoli DC. Refraction: Snell's Law. In: Giancoli DC, ed. *Physics Principles With Applications.* 5th ed. Upper Saddle River, NJ: Prentice Hall; 1998:696–714.

31. Lens [Wikipedia, the free encyclopedia Web site]. Available at: http://en.wikipedia.org/wiki/Optical_lens. Accessed January 3, 2009.

32. Johnson LS, Milliken BD, Hadley SW, et al. Initial clinical experience with a video-based patient positioning system. *Int J Radiat Oncol Biol Phys.* 1999;45(1):205–213.

33. Milliken BD, Rubin SJ, Hamilton RJ, et al. Performance of a video-image-subtraction-based patient positioning system. *Int J Radiat Oncol Biol Phys.* 1997;38(4):855–866.

34. Yan Y, Song Y, Boyer AL. An investigation of a video-based patient repositioning technique. *Int J Radiat Oncol Biol Phys.* 2002;54(2):606–614.

35. Menke M, Hirschfeld F, Mack T, et al. Photogrammetric accuracy measurements of a head holder system used for fractionated radiotherapy. *Int J Radiat Oncol Biol Phys.* 1994;29:1147–1155.

36. Li S, Geng J, Williams J, Chen G. A novel 3D-video-based re-fixation technique for fractionated stereotactic radiotherapy. *Med Phys.* 2000;27:1433.

37. Geng ZJ. Rainbow 3-D camera: new concept of high-speed three dimensional vision system. *Opt Eng.* 1996;35:376–383.

38. Bert C, Metheany KG, Doppke K, Chen G. A phantom evaluation of a stereo-vision surface imaging system for radiotherapy patient setup. *Med Phys.* 2005;32(9):2753–2762.

39. Schöffel PJ, Harms W, Sroka-Perez G, et al. Accuracy of a commercial optical 3D surface imaging system for realignment of patients for radiotherapy of the thorax. *Phys Med Biol.* 2007;52:3949–3963.

40. Huang PS, Zhang C, Chiang FP. High-Speed 3-D shape measurement based on digital fringe projection. *Opt Eng.* 2003; 42:163–168.

41. Greiner G. Representation and processing of surface data. In: Girod B, Greiner G, Niemann H, eds. *Principles of 3D Image Analysis and Synthesis.* Boston, MA: Kluwer Academic Publishers; 2000: 141–152.

42. Shum HY, Szeliski R. Construction of panoramic image mosaics with global and local alignment. *Int J Comput Vis.* 2000;36: 101–130.

43. Dorai C, Weng J, Jian AK. An optimal registration of object views using range data. *IEEE Trans Pattern Analysis Mach Intel.* 1997;19:1131–1138.

44. Sharp GC, Lee SW, Wehe DK. ICP registration using invariant features. *IEEE Trans Pattern Analysis Mach Intel.* 2002;24:90–102.

45. Horn BKP. Close-form solution of absolute orientation using unit quaternions. *J Opt Soc Amer.* 1987;4:629–642.

46. Riddle WR, Pickens DR. Extract data from a DICOM file. *Med. Phys.* 2005;32:1537–1541.

47. Biossonnat JD. Three dimensional reconstruction of complex shapes based in the delaunay triangulation. *INRIA Research Reports.* 1992;1697.

48. Liu D, Li S. Accurate calibration of a stereo-vision system in image-guided radiotherapy. *Med Phys.* 2006;33:4379–4383.

49. Djajajutra D, Li S. Real-time 3D surface-image-guided beam setup in radiotherapy of breast cancer. *Med Phys.* 2005;32:65–76.

50. Krempien R, Hoppe H, Kahrs L, et al. Projector-based augmented reality for intuitive intraoperative guidance in image-guided 3D interstitial brachytherapy. *Int J Radiat Oncol Biol Phys.* 2008;70(3):944–952.

51. Gierga DR, Riboldi M, Turcotte JC, et al. Comparison of target registration errors for multiple image-guided techniques in accelerated partial breast irradiation. *Int J Radiat Oncol Biol Phys.* 2008;70:1239–1246.

52. Cerviño L, Yashar C, Jiang S. Improvement of the stability and reproducibility of deep-inspiration breath hold for left breast irradiation using video-based visual coaching and 3D surface imaging. *Med Phys.* 2008;35:2703.

53. Brahme A, Nyman P, Skatt B. 4D laser camera for accurate patient positioning, collision avoidance, image fusion and adaptive approaches during diagnostic and therapeutic procedures. *Med Phys.* 2008;35(5):1670–1681.

54. Jesson DE, Pavlov KM, Morgan MJ, et al. Imaging surface topography using Lloyd's mirror in photoemission electron microscopy. *Phys Rev Lett.* 2007;99,016013.

55. Posada R, Daul C, Wolf D, et al. Towards a noninvasive intracranial tumor irradiation using 3D optical imaging and multimodal data registration. *Int J Biomed Imaging.* 2007;62030:1–14.

56. Noel CE, Klein EE, Moore KL. A surface-based respiratory surrogate for 4D imaging. *Med Phys.* 2008;35(6):2682.

Chapter 7

ELECTRONIC PORTAL IMAGING DEVICES

YILDIRIM D. MUTAF, PhD

The radiotherapy (RT) planning process requires a geometrical representation of the patient anatomy.[1–3] This information is usually obtained via three-dimensional (3D) radiographic simulators such as computed tomography (CT) imagers in conjunction with magnetic resonance[4,5] (MR) or positron emission tomography[6–8] (PET) imagers. The treatment machine parameters are aligned and dosimetric calculations are performed with respect to a baseline patient geometry, which is hypothesized to be valid for the entire duration of treatment. Therefore, differences between the simulation geometry and the patient geometry during the actual treatment could potentially have dramatic impact[9,10] on the overall care of the patient and in some cases can lead to misadministrations.[11–13]

A simple way of preserving the correlation of patient geometry between the simulation and treatment is to use optical guides such as alignment of superficial landmarks on the patient with in-room coordinates or matching collimated light field shape with drawings on the patient's skin.[14] However, the fundamental problem with these approaches is in the assumption that the landmarks on patient's skin are a valid representation of the internal anatomy. In many RT departments today, this assumption is always put to the test with verification of internal anatomy by using radiographic imaging techniques.[15–19] Although the process termed as portal imaging refers to radiographic imaging of radiation fields (or ports), it is broadly used as radiographic confirmation of simulation geometry at the time of the treatment.

Since the inception of portal imagers, their development has paralleled the technological developments in diagnostic imaging applications. A common approach was to adopt an existing radiographic imaging technology and modify it for the need and environment specific to megavoltage (MV) RT conditions. Therefore, in-room radiographic imaging was historically performed with film cassette technology. Typically sandwiched between two metal plates (acting as build-up layer and generating high-energy electrons), radiographic film provided good

spatial resolution and contrast for in-room treatment verification purposes.[20–23] However, despite good image quality characteristics, the film technology introduced serious disadvantages to clinical operations. In radiographic film, irradiation creates a latent image within the sensitive medium of the film that requires a separate chemical development process. This additional processing creates inefficiency in clinical flow and more importantly introduces a considerable time delay after which the image information may no longer be a representative of the patient geometry because of the possibility of patient movement. Furthermore, film is a disposable material, which requires that the entire procedure needs to be repeated for as many images as necessary for sufficient treatment verification. The verification process, which typically requires a comparison with baseline images, is also cumbersome with films because they are usually reviewed side-by-side on light-boxes. Digital tools and computer systems make this task more practical, but any digital analysis requires the additional step of scanning the film. These shortcomings of film cassette technology promoted the development of electronic radiographic detectors and their incorporation in RT treatment as electronic portal imaging devices (EPIDs).

Although the clinical use of EPIDs started in the early 1980s,[24] its widespread implementation expanded during the 1990s following commercialization by linac manufacturers. Today, EPIDs are considered indispensible clinical tools and their applications have reached far more areas than their original utilization.[25–32] In this chapter, the clinical use of the EPIDs as well as some of the image quality metrics and technology behind these devices will be described.

Clinical Use of Electronic Portal Imagers

Although EPIDs were initially introduced as replacement for the conventional film and cassette technology, their capabilities quickly surpassed those of their predecessor. Today, EPIDs are being utilized not merely as pretreatment verification devices but are also regarded as a major component in RT processes and part of the overall quality assurance (QA) efforts in the clinic.

Patient Positioning and Localization

The necessity for in-room imaging devices stems from the need to verify the correlation between the patient anatomy and the treatment geometry and to apply proper corrections to match the conditions that existed during the treatment simulation. Deviations can be corrected either by simple repositioning of the patient with respect to the treatment coordinate system or by more involved interventions such as requiring consistent bladder or rectal filling during pelvic treatments. There may also be cases where no immediate corrective action is possible such as substantial changes in patient anatomy attributable to tumor shrinkage or weight loss. Such changes may necessitate an alteration in patient's overall treatment strategy.

Patient positioning and field placement errors, collectively termed setup errors,[33–35] can be categorized according to their pattern of occurrence, i.e., random and systematic errors. Random errors imply that amount and the direction of the geometric miss because of setup errors *change* throughout the treatment of the patient.[36–38] Variations in patient's positioning because of the limited accuracy provided by patient's external marks or the changes in anatomy attributable to physiological functions of the patient are all examples of random setup errors. Systematic errors, on the other hand, usually happen once and their amount and direction do not change when uncorrected.[39–42] Examples include geometrical errors caused by the discrepancy of the external laser system with the coordinate system of the treatment machine or miscalculated patient shift instructions.

Both random and systematic setup errors can be detected by using localization provided by portal imaging. If a discrepancy is observed in the patient's anatomy with respect to the expectations, a correction is applied either before the treatment or for subsequent treatment sessions if it requires more thorough analysis. Depending on the required logistics (time, personnel, and availability of tools), observed deviations may be filtered with a predetermined action threshold. The main difference between the correction strategies for random and systematic error is in the frequency of imaging required. Systematic errors, such as the miscalculated patient shifts, can be corrected once and for all remaining treatments when detected. However, random errors cannot be eliminated because the amount of variations can vary significantly from day to day and require more frequent imaging and correction strategies to eliminate them. Despite their persistence, the varying nature of random errors often produces neutralizing dosimetric effects.[35]

Although traditional port films can be used to assess geometrical errors, fast processing and digital image analysis tools provided by EPIDs enable seamless integration of these imaging technologies within the clinical operations. Portal imagers also allow several acquisition modes that aid in identifying various setup errors. Several of these acquisition modes are described in the next section.

Single-Exposure Verification Image

In this acquisition mode, a single image is generated from multiple (typically two or four) image frames. These images are useful for radiographic localization of the treatment isocenter within the anatomy as well as for discovering substantial variations in patient's position (e.g., angle of the neck). As with most MV images, the anatomy visible in such images is limited mostly to bony anatomy and airways.

During setup verification, EPID images are often compared with the digitally reconstructed radiographs (DRR) from the simulation CT images. Isocenter location is superimposed on DRRs and matched to the actual treatment isocenter. The treatment isocenter therefore needs to be identified on the portal imagers and this may be done by using the calibrated pixel coordinates of the imager[43] (virtual reticule) or a physical reticule made up of radio-opaque markers, mounted on the accelerator head. Alternatively, an edge-finding algorithm may be used to detect the collimation size and corresponding coordinate system. Examples of such images are illustrated in Figure 7-1.

Because of decreased differentiation between tissue types at MV energies, localization is typically performed based on bony anatomy such as the spinal column or pelvic bones. However, it is well demonstrated that bony anatomy is not a good surrogate for a large number of treatment sites.[44–47] Therefore, localization based on bony anatomy also could potentially introduce setup errors. Because of their pronounced visibility under MV radiation, metallic markers are occasionally implanted in soft tissue target volumes (e.g., prostate or lung tumors) to reduce the magnitude of these errors.[48,49]

Double-Exposure Verification Image

Double-exposure verification images are primarily used to verify the position and shape of the radiation field. First, a single image is acquired by using the parameters of an actual treatment field with its associated multileaf collimator (MLC). Because of the relatively small size of the irradiated area, localization is limited on the basis of these images alone and, therefore, a second image is acquired with treatment collimation removed and using a larger field size. The two images are normalized and overlaid, producing a single image that depicts the larger patient anatomy as well as the size and shape of an actual

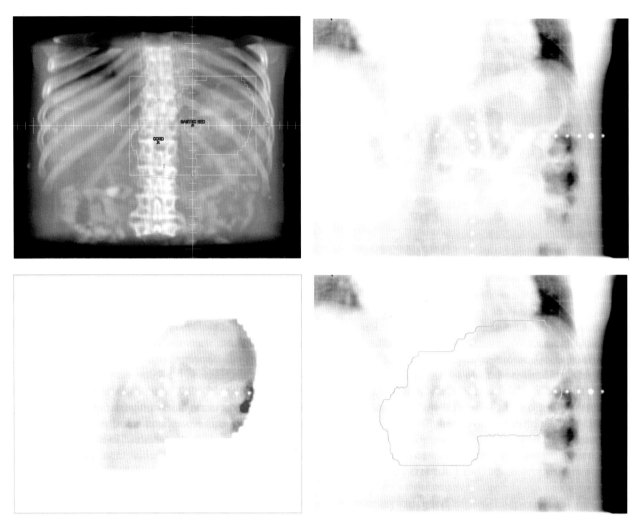

FIGURE 7-1. Digitally reconstructed radiography showing the treatment field collimation (top-left) compared with verification portal images. A single-exposure film (top-right) is acquired with the physical reticule attached to the gantry head. A blocked (bottom-left) field image is acquired for field shape verification and detected field edge from this image is overlaid on the open field image to simulate a double-exposure image (bottom-right).

treatment field. Similarly, edge-finding algorithms are also used to outline the shape of the collimated field. In these images, instead of overlaying two images, only the extracted outline of the collimated field is overlaid on the second larger image.[50–52] An example of double-exposure film with the outline of the collimated field is shown in Figure 7-1.

Treatment Verification

Single- and double-exposure films are mostly used for patient setup and, thus, are acquired before the patient's treatment. However, monitoring of the patient's position during the treatment is also essential in verifying that no patient motion or changes in anatomy (e.g., intestinal gas or changes in respiration) occurred while the patient was continuing the treatment. Such verifications are especially necessary for longer treatments during which it is more difficult for patients to maintain their fixed position.

Because of the mechanical flexibility and digital processing capabilities of modern EPIDs, verification images are taken and analyzed while the patient is undergoing treatment. Positioned at the exit side of the beam, these images are acquired by using the patient's treatment fields at predetermined intervals. An example of this would be the verification of prostate position via the implanted markers and pausing treatment when the development of rectal gas is detected during the patient's treatment.

Organ Motion

Physiological motion of organs increases the degree of complexity in localization of the target volume. Depending on the underlying physiology, this motion can be periodic such as respiratory and cardiac motions or arrhythmic such as swallowing or bowel movement (peristalsis, intestinal gas, etc). According to extensive investigation, organ motion has been demonstrated to result in significant dosimetric consequences if not properly accounted for during treatment.[52-58] In general, three classes of solutions exist to manage organ motion during RT: motion-limiting strategies (e.g., gating or increased immobilization), motion incorporation strategies (e.g., larger margins), and, finally, motion-adaptation strategies (e.g., motion tracking). Although they differ considerably in terms of their clinical implementation, all such approaches share the necessity for an anatomical verification of organ motion. The aim in these verification procedures is to confirm that the pattern and magnitude of motion observed during treatment is the same as it was during pretreatment simulation.

Because of the required processing time and lack of analysis tools, conventional port films were only used as tools to represent the patient's anatomy at a specific moment in time. These snap-shot images seriously limited evaluations of organ motion. However, the introduction of digital radiography and EPIDs has enabled much shorter processing times and superior analysis tools for the evaluation of organ motion. For motion verification, images are acquired continuously in a *cine-mode* and displayed as a movie loop to reveal anatomical motion. To improve the temporal resolution of the displayed images (or refresh rate), these images are usually acquired in very short times and typically without any frame averaging. Additionally, the characteristics of motion could also be observed from a *motion average image,* which is created by a weighted sum of individual snap-shot images and displays the effects of motion as a blur.

Volumetric Imaging

Planar images created by EPIDs naturally limit the evaluation of 3D anatomy of the patient to the two dimensions (2D) of the imager matrix. Despite the acquisition of multiple images from orthogonal directions, these images are evaluated separately and do not provide the full 3D viewing flexibility as observed with CT images. Additionally, because of the averaging effect of ray summing that occurs in such radiographs, the contrast between similar tissue types is greatly reduced.

The limitations of 2D images are eliminated with the development of volume imaging acquisition techniques[59-61] and associated reconstruction algorithms. These 3D images are reconstructed via back projection of multiple planar images acquired at different angles around the patient, which will be discussed in more detail in subsequent chapters. Typical reconstruction requires a complete rotation of the imager around the patient and acquisition of hundreds of planar images.

Three-dimensional imaging while the patient is in treatment position opens up the possibility for verification of individual organ and tumor contours with respect to those encountered at simulation. Additionally, volumetric images could be used to perform 3D dose calculations[62-64] and, hence, to evaluate dosimetric differences with respect to the original treatment plan.[62-64]

Transit Dosimetry

Having outstanding linearity, reproducibility, and dark signal characteristics, modern EPIDs are also used as transit dosimetry detectors.[65-68] Requiring a separate dosimetry calibration and extensive commissioning of dosimetric characteristics of its detectors, these imagers can operate in integrated imaging mode to create a so-called *dose image.* Although such transit dosimetry can be utilized as an in vivo verification tool, EPID dosimetry found greater use for pretreatment plan verifications of intensity modulated fluences.[69-71]

Quality Assurance

As imaging devices that can double as a dosimeter, EPIDs have also been incorporated into the general QA process in many RT departments. Their introduction replaced virtually all quality control tests performed with the help of a radiographic film. Some examples of these tests include light and radiation field congruence tests,[72,73] isocenter stability tests,[74,75] block checks, MLC calibration,[76,77] and MLC performance under dynamic delivery. With these added capabilities, EPIDs are considered to be a versatile clinical tool beyond their main function as patient localization imagers.

Although EPIDs can be very flexible for many applications, their use for QA purposes should be executed carefully. The interplay between the operation characteristics for the imager and the precision needed for a specific test must be clarified before its implementation. For example, the scanning mode acquisition of flat panel portal imagers creates residual motion artifacts for dynamic MLC motion. Hence, these artifacts can introduce systematic errors in the interpretation of MLC performance. Additionally the positioning uncertainty of the imager at oblique angles could create problems when one is using it for very precise mechanical calibrations.[78]

Image Calibration and Preparation

Before an image is presented to the user for any type of evaluation, it is preprocessed to remove the portion of the signal attributable to the device itself. The parameters for this preprocessing are calibrated for each imager separately at an appropriate frequency recommended by the manufacturer.

The EPID pixels may have small variations in their gains and, hence, can cause image artifacts if they are not equalized. Additionally, the nonuniformity of the x-ray beam, such as horns in megavoltage beams, can create

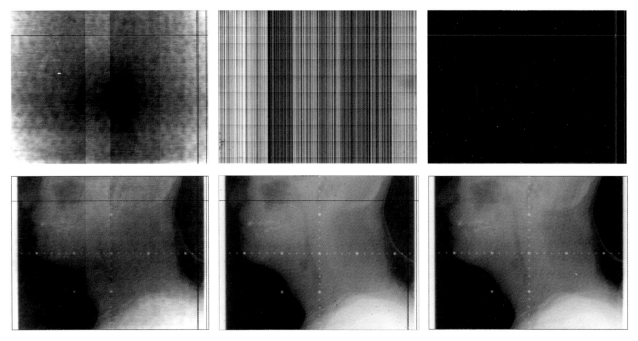

FIGURE 7-2. Flood (top-left), dark (top-middle), and defective pixel map (top-right) images used for image calibration in the PortalVision (Varian Medical Systems, Palo Alto, CA) imaging system are displayed in the upper row. Bottom row of images illustrates the steps of image processing before an image is presented to viewer. Raw portal image (bottom-right) is corrected for gain and background signal of the imager pixels and an intermediate image is created (bottom-middle). This image is further processed to mask the defective pixels of the imager and a final image is created (bottom-right).

similar variations in the raw signal of the imager. These artifacts are corrected by calibrating the imager for pixel gains and a flood image (using a large unobstructed radiation field) is used to create a gain map for each pixel of the imager: $S_{gain}(x, y)$. In addition, a background calibration is also used to remove the system noise from the raw pixel signal generates. Background calibration requires acquisition of a set of dark images (no radiation) that is used to generate a background value for each pixel of the imager: $S_{back}(x, y)$. A simplified calibration algorithm can be formulated as:

$$S_{image}(x, y) = \frac{s_{raw}(x, y) - s_{back}(x, y)}{s_{gain}(x, y) - s_{back}(x, y)} \qquad (1)$$

In addition, in case the EPID may have a damaged element, blank areas can exist in the reconstructed images. To produce better-looking images, these areas may be masked by using a defective pixel map. With these masks, an artificial signal is generated for the location of the defective pixel typically by averaging of the neighboring pixel signals. The dark and flood images as well as the pixel defect map used for calibration of an EPID as described previously are illustrated in Figure 7-2 for the PortalVision portal imaging system (Varian Medical Systems, Palo Alto, CA). Figure 7-2 also depicts the raw and processed portal images through this image development process.

Image Quality in Digital Radiography

A quantitative evaluation of digital radiographic images obtained by EPIDs requires an introduction to commonly used measures of image quality. Therefore, in this section, we will investigate a set of key image quality indicators such as image contrast, spatial resolution, noise, signal-to-noise ratio, and quantum detective efficiency. In the following description and derivations, we adopt the formalism outlined by Motz and Danos[79] and described by several others.[25,28,80]

Image Contrast

An x-ray image is simply formed by the attenuation of the incident x-ray fluence through an object (e.g., the patient) and detection of transmitted fluence via suitable x-ray detectors. The incident fluence carries primary and scatter x-ray contributions, which are then modulated by the response of the detector. Thus, an ideal imager is considered to be one that can transfer the full image information contained in the incident x-ray fluence. Accordingly for an ideal imager, the difference in the image signal registered for two regions of the anatomy will be proportional to the difference of the transmitted x-ray fluence through these regions. Because the images are frequently used to identify specific anatomical features in front of a more familiar background (e.g., bones, air-

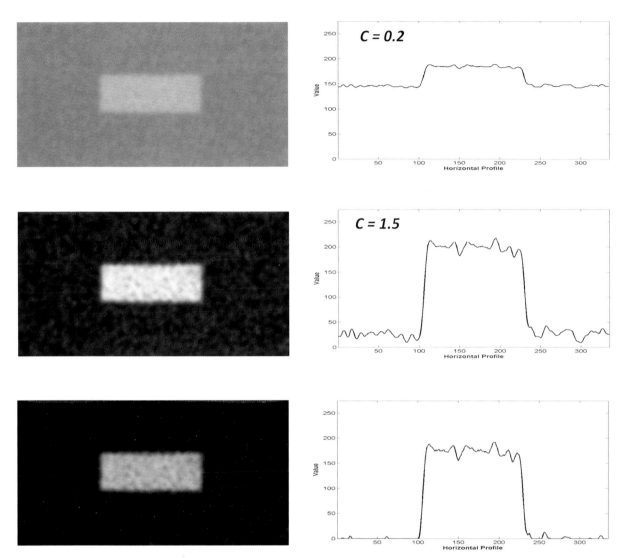

FIGURE 7-3. Simulation of a gray-scale image with varying levels of image contrast (low, medium, and high, from left to right, respectively) and corresponding line profiles across the embedded feature of interest.

ways, any type of anomaly, etc.), a notion of *contrast* is inherently realized, which reflects how an object (imager signal S_{roi}) stands out from its surroundings (imager signal S_{bckg}). For quantitative evaluations, image contrast, C, is expressed as follows:

$$C = \frac{s_{roi} - s_{bckg}}{(s_{roi} + s_{bckg})/2} \qquad (2)$$

In Figure 7-3, a gray-scale image is simulated for varying levels of object contrast to demonstrate its effect on the visibility and identification of image features.

For ideal imagers, image signal, S is proportional to transmitted primary photon fluence, ψ, in addition to a fraction of fluence because of scatter within the anatomy. Thus, the image signal can be expressed as $S \sim \psi_{trans} = \psi_{pri} + \psi_{sca}$ where the scatter contribution is considered to be a fraction of the total transmitted fluence $\psi_{sca} = F \cdot \psi_{trans}$ or $\psi_{sca} = \psi_{pri} \cdot F/(1 - F)$. Because of the dispersive nature of the scatter, the scatter contributions to both background regions of the image and the investigated region of interest is considered to be similar. Therefore, equation 2 for contrast becomes

$$C = 2 \cdot \frac{\left(\psi_{pri}^{roi} + \psi_{sca}\right) - \left(\psi_{pri}^{bckg} + \psi_{sca}\right)}{\left(\psi_{pri}^{roi} + \psi_{sca}\right) + \left(\psi_{pri}^{bckg} + \psi_{sca}\right)} \qquad (3)$$

or

$$C = 2 \cdot \frac{\left(\psi_{pri}^{roi} - \psi_{pri}^{bckg}\right)}{\left(\psi_{pri}^{roi} - \psi_{pri}^{bckg}\right) + \psi_{pri}^{roi} 2F/(1-F)} \qquad (4)$$

In equation 4, the image contrast difference is reduced to differences in primary transmissions through the region of interest and the surrounding background within

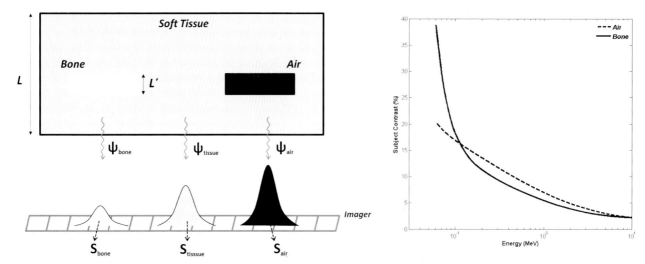

FIGURE 7-4. Generation of imager signals through a hypothetical object embedded with bone- and air-equivalent features is illustrated on left panel. Because of variations in attenuation of the primary beam, regions of the imager beneath the objects register varying magnitudes of imager signal, contributing to the contrast visible in generated images. The input contrast between the embedded feature and the background is also calculated and shown on right as a function of varying x-ray energy (mono-energetic photons).

the imaged object. To facilitate a more straightforward understanding of the concept of contrast, one can refer to a simple homogeneous phantom object made mostly with material radiologically equivalent to soft tissue (thickness of L, and linear attenuation coefficient of μ) as demonstrated in Figure 7-4. The primary attenuations through a homogeneous region of this phantom (background) and through the embedded feature of interest (of length L' and having attenuation coefficient of μ') are given in equations 5 and 6, respectively.

$$\psi_{pri}^{bckg} = \psi_o \cdot e^{-L\alpha} \tag{5}$$

$$\psi_{pri}^{roi} = \psi_o \cdot e^{-(L-L')\alpha} \cdot e^{-L'\alpha'} \tag{6}$$

Inserting these formulas into equation 4, we obtain that the contrast difference between the background soft-tissue and embedded anatomical feature of interest as:

$$C = \frac{2 \cdot (1 - e^{-\Delta})}{\left[1 + e^{-\Delta} + \dfrac{2F}{(1-F)} \right]} \tag{7}$$

where $\Delta \equiv L'(\mu' - \mu)$. Equation 7 indicates that the contrast between the background and a specific signal increases if the size of the feature or the difference between the linear attenuation coefficients increase. The calculation of contrast for 1-cm-thick bone- and air-equivalent materials embedded inside the soft-tissue equivalent phantom (ignoring effects of scatter) is also illustrated in Figure 7-4. Because of the dominance of photoelectric interactions at the lower end of the

kilovoltage (kV) x-ray spectrum and its strong atomic number dependence, the contrast between the soft-tissue ($Z_{eff} \approx 7.1$) and bone ($Z_{eff} \approx 11.6$) or soft-tissue and air ($Z_{eff} \approx 7.3$) is large compared with the contrast produced by higher-energy x-rays. As the energy of x-rays increases, the dominant process for x-ray interactions becomes Compton scattering, and attenuation differences between these materials diminish significantly. For example, even though the contrast between bone and tissue is about 18% for 100 kV x-rays, the contrast drops to 2.5% for 6-MV photons.

Spatial Resolution and Modulation Transfer Function

The spatial resolution of the imaging system has an influence on how accurately the objects can be identified in the spatial dimensions of an image. The ability of the system to resolve two objects while the distance between them gets closer is a measure of its spatial resolution. Although the same term is commonly used to refer to the digitization of the images or the intrinsic pixilation of the imaging detector, spatial resolution describes a broader image property and it also depends on other factors such as scatter within the object and imager, magnification of the object, or the effective size of the x-ray source.

A standard way to describe the spatial resolution of a detector system is to characterize its response to a single point input. The output of the system for such an input, called a point spread function, is modulated because of the interaction of the photons within the imager as well as the intrinsic detector element size of the imager. The net result is a blurring of the image (Figure 7-5). It is difficult to produce a proper single point input, such as a very small

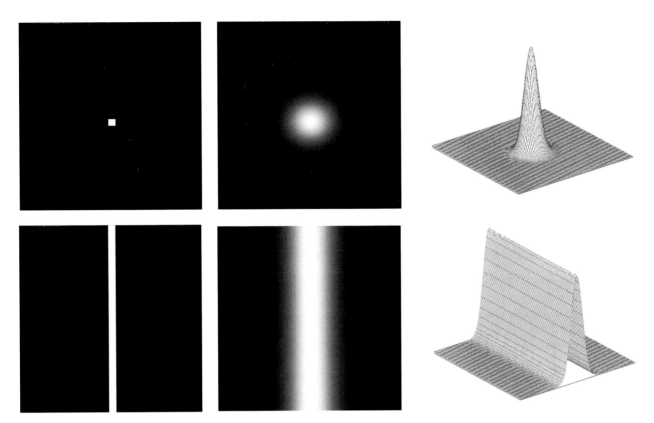

FIGURE 7-5. The concepts of point-spread function and line-spread functions are illustrated respectively on upper and lower panels. Simulated responses of an imager to an ideal point or a line source are shown.

hole aligned in front of a light source; therefore, other spread functions are also used to evaluate imager spatial resolution. The line spread function (LSF) measuring the imager response to a narrow slit is a typical alternative (alignment is only needed in one direction). A hypothetical LSF is illustrated in Figure 7-5. In conventional portal imagers, the dominant source of signal spread is the phosphorescent screen where high-energy x-rays (and electrons) are converted to light photons. Therefore, development of new screens with light-spread–limiting designs (such as phosphor material with columnar structure) and elimination of screens with more efficient image sensors receive substantial attention in the improvement of radiographic imagers.

Rather than working in the spatial domain, spatial resolution of imaging systems is often analyzed in the frequency domain to evaluate system response. In the frequency domain, the response of multiple systems can be represented with a simple product compared with a complicated convolution required in the spatial domain. Within the context of digital imaging, spatial frequency is usually expressed in units of line pairs per millimeter and lower frequencies reflect larger object sizes and higher frequencies are attributed to smaller objects. The modulation transfer function (MTF) describes the quality of the imaging system with respect to its spatial

resolution or its ability to transfer the input contrast of an object as a function of its size (spatial frequency). The MTF is calculated[81-83] as the modulus of the Fourier transform of the spread function, such as LSF and expressed as:

$$MTF(f) = |FT\{LSF(x)\}| \qquad (8)$$

The MTF of an imaging system is the product of the individual MTFs of its components (such as converter, optic elements, detector, etc.) and, hence, can be used to understand the role and performance of each component in the imaging chain. It is also used to compare competing imaging systems for their ability to resolve objects with different spatial frequencies. A simulated image of a bar pattern incorporating features with varying spatial frequencies is shown in Figure 7-6 along with the corresponding MTF calculated for this imager's response.

Image Noise

Noise in radiographic images is another key indicator affecting the image quality. There are several potential sources of noise in reconstructed images, but they are basically classified in two main categories. The first source of noise, called quantum noise or mottle, is attributable

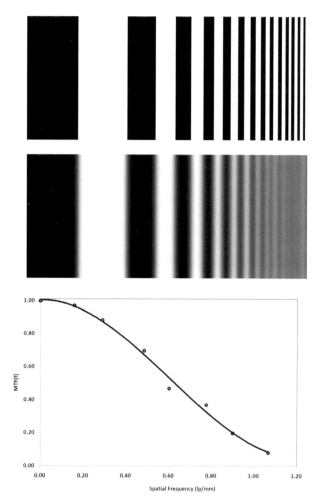

FIGURE 7-6. The concept of modulation transfer function (MTF) and spatial resolution frequency is demonstrated with an input bar pattern (top) and a simulated imager response (middle). Corresponding MTF for the imager response is also plotted (bottom) as a function of input spatial frequency for the pattern.

to the statistical uncertainty in the detection of photons. For a perfect detector, the number of quanta collected in its sensitive volume varies as the measurement is repeated in subsequent times. Therefore, this variability causes differences in image signal attributed to different regions of a radiographic imager and contributes to a sense of noise in the final image. Quantum mottle is usually represented as the standard deviation of the measured quanta, σ_s, and relative noise is defined as the ratio of the measurement standard deviation to the measurement value, σ_s/S. In Figure 7-7, a gray-scale image is shown with varying levels of image noise to demonstrate its effect on the visibility and identification of image features.

Other sources of image noise are attributed to the imaging components and are classified as the system noise. This type of noise may be caused by variations in the sensitivities of the detector elements, fluctuations in the electronic gains applied at individual amplifiers,

or other random design problems. Noise of an imaging system is often described by noise power spectrum represented as a function of spatial frequency (f), and is calculated as the variance (σS^2) of the image signal.

Signal-to-Noise Ratio

Although useful quantities, neither contrast nor noise is solely responsible for object detectability in radiographic images. It is apparent from Figures 7-3 and 7-7 that these two metrics have different roles in assessing image quality. For example, the detectability is perceived to be low when the amount of noise in the image is large even if the image contrast is high. Conversely, high detectability is achieved in images with high contrast and low image noise. Therefore, a hybrid metric is a more suitable figure of merit. The signal-to-noise ratio (SNR) is thus introduced as the most important parameter in evaluations of image quality. The SNR is defined as the ratio of the difference in object and background signals to the statistical noise associated with the detection of photons forming the image signal. The statistical noise is basically the standard deviation in the detection of the incident photons, which is the square root of the measured signal. Hence, the SNR for an object of interest and its background is defined as:

$$ SNR = \frac{s_{roi} - s_{bckg}}{\sqrt{(s_{roi} + s_{bckg})}} \qquad (9) $$

The SNR of the image increases if the overall imager signal increases by collection and subsequent detection of more photons. In radiographic imaging, improving image SNR is limited because of the concerns of increased radiation dose with increased number of incident photons. Therefore, for a perfect imager, SNR is restricted solely by the quantum noise and such systems are said to be "x-ray quantum limited" imagers. Inefficiencies in the detection of incident quanta or introduction of significant system noise beyond the statistical noise will both degrade image SNR.

Using the SNR of an image, Motz and Danos[79] define a detectability threshold less than which objects in corresponding images will not be discernable from the background. They state that a detectability threshold of SNR = 5 is a suitable choice for this threshold but caution that this value could depend on other factors such as the prior knowledge regarding the pattern of the imaged object or presence of additional system noise.

Quantum Detector Efficiency

Because SNR increases as the number of detected photons increases, it is important to have imager systems that account for all available x-ray fluence in the process of forming the digital image. However, realistic imaging systems are far from perfect detectors and a figure of efficiency is

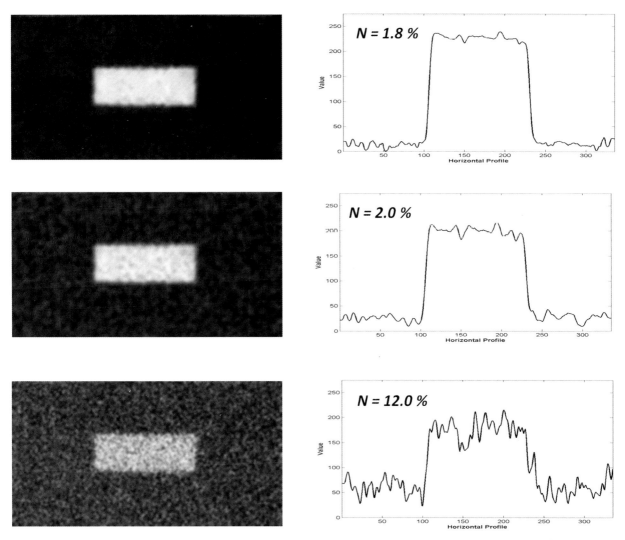

FIGURE 7-7. Simulation of a gray-scale image with varying levels of image noise (low, medium, and high, from left to right, respectively) and corresponding line profiles across the embedded feature of interest.

therefore used to describe their performance. As defined in equation 10, Detector Quantum Efficiency (DQE) describes the efficiency of the imaging system for translating the input SNR available in the x-ray fluence to the SNR in its output such as an image.

$$DQE(f) = \frac{SNR^2_{output}(f)}{SNR^2_{input}(f)} \qquad (10)$$

Although it is hard to interpret DQE in terms of the quality and utility of the output images, it provides an assessment of the image-forming process within an imaging system and, hence, is usually employed for the comparisons of different imaging systems. Ideal imagers, by definition, transfer all image information (e.g., SNR) to generated images and, hence, have DQE of 1.0 (or 100%). On the other hand, DQE of commercially available portal images is typically about 0.01 (1%). It is important to note

that this low DQE is not only attributable to the sensitivity or the geometric acceptance of the imaging detector but also to how efficiently the incident x-ray photons are converted to those that can be detected by the image sensors. Because of the high energy of photons and reduced attenuation in MV imaging, only 5% to 7% of the incident x-rays interact with the combined phosphor screen and metal plate of the conventional imagers.[25]

Camera-Based Imagers

Early experience with electronic imaging technologies originates from the use of camera-based systems. Camera-based fluoroscopic imaging systems were quickly integrated into thc realm of portal imaging because they incorporated other mature technologies such as the use of metal-phosphor for radiological film imaging as well as the developments in camera and optical recording systems. Another advantage of these systems was the high spatial and temporal resolution (video rate, e.g., 30 frames per second) achievable in the image acquisition.

Some commercial models utilized video camera tubes (scanning cathode ray tubes) and others implemented solid-state image sensors (charge-coupled devices or CCDs) forming the pixel elements of portal imagers.[84–87] Both sensors are sensitive to light radiation in the visible wavelength range and, therefore, high-energy radiation must be converted to visible light for detection. Therefore, camera-based systems are indirect radiation detectors designed with a metal plate (typically 1-mm- or 2-mm-thick copper, steel, or brass plate) acting as a converter medium and various thicknesses (typically 400 mg/cm^2) of scintillating layer (e.g., gadolinium oxysulfide doped with terbium Gd2O2S:Tb, or, simply, Gadox) as the phosphor screen.[88–90] In this ensemble, the metal plate converts the high-energy radiation to multiple Compton electrons, which are absorbed in the phosphor screen and converted into visible photons with typical gains of 1:10 000 for MV beams.

Selection of appropriate converter material and its design is crucial to the optimal use of these detectors because of a variety of factors contributing to the final image quality. Phosphors suitable for imaging applications require a high atomic number (Z) and density for increased photo-electric interaction cross-section as well as high quantum efficiency for conversion of high-energy x-rays into visible light photons that can finally be transferred and recorded by an optical camera. Furthermore, the structural design of the phosphor screen has also been shown to be a contributing factor to the final image quality.[91–92]

Customarily, the screens are constructed as a homogeneous layer of small crystalline elements and an optical photon created inside this homogeneous phosphor layer is highly diffused before it leaves the screen. This reduces the spatial resolution and also prevents the use

of thicker and more efficient scintillator materials that would improve the quantum efficiency. Different structural materials such as columnar CsI elements, typically 5 µm to 10 µm in width, are also designed to improve the optical gain without any degradation in the spatial resolution of the final image.[93,94] The needlelike crystalline structures serve the purpose of channeling light within each needle because of the difference in index of refraction between the crystal and the surrounding medium of air. They thus limit the diffusion of the optical photons into adjacent pixels similar to the process responsible for the transfer of optical signals via fiberoptic cables. The interplay between the spatial resolution and image signal generated from different designs of phosphor screens is illustrated in Figure 7-8.

In fluoroscopic portal imaging systems, the camera and associated electronics are often placed outside the limits of the radiation beam to prevent potential damage to these radiation-sensitive components. For this reason a mylar mirror placed at 45° angle between the central axis of the beam and the camera is integrated to enable the transfer of the optical light. The entire optical assembly is encased within a light-tight housing to prevent image degradation from ambient light. A typical design for the elements of these portal imagers is shown in Figure 7-9. Design requirements of camera-based portal imagers and their integration to the accelerator gantry often result in a bulky structure that presents functional problems for achieving various treatment geometries and also for the therapists working around the patient. Furthermore, the presence of multiple elements such as the mirror and lenses requires very accurate optical coupling to limit image deformations. Changes in the gantry rotation as well as the motion of the imager itself subject the imager to misalignment problems between its optical elements, potentially resulting in systematic errors in the assessment of the images for geometric verification purposes.

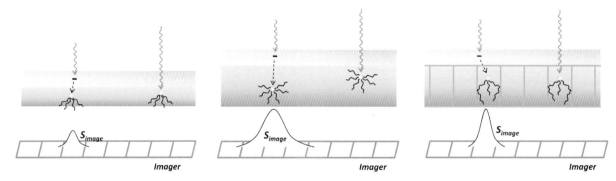

FIGURE 7-8. Interplay between the thickness of the phosphor screen and resulting spatial resolution is shown. Thin layer of phosphor (left) is necessary for achieving high spatial resolution but the thickness of the phosphor screen also regulates the conversion efficiency. A thicker screen (middle) achieves better signal efficiency but at the cost of reduced spatial resolution because of increased spread of the optical photons within the phosphor material. Structured crystals such as the needlelike design of Cesium Iodide (CsI) phosphor screen can be used to limit the spread of the photons and, therefore, can be constructed with larger thicknesses without significant degradation in spatial resolution.

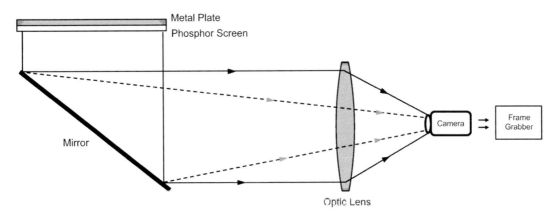

FIGURE 7-9. A schematic construction of the camera-based portal imagers incorporating metal plate and phosphor screen converter layer as well as mirror, lens, camera, and electronic read-out components. The optical acceptance of the camera is also demonstrated with the paths of the light beams (solid and dashed lines with arrows) with and without the presence of the large aperture lens. Figure is not drawn to scale.

The efficiency of the camera-based systems is documented in the literature.[95–97] Bissonnette et al. used Monte Carlo simulations to demonstrate the image quality at multiple levels of the acquisition through the metal-plate, phosphor, mirror, and camera components of a virtual camera-based portal imaging system.[98] Based on a theoretical design of a camera-based portal imager incorporating a copper conversion plate, 358 mg/cm^2 Gadox screen, a 45° mirror, large aperture lens, and the camera, their

study modeled the full imaging process starting from the conversion of x-rays to the detection of light quanta by the camera. In the process, the diffusion of light at the phosphor screen, lens, and camera as well as electronic noise was also included. The input x-ray fluence and corresponding virtual images generated at successive stages of the imaging chain (such as lens, camera, etc.) are shown in Figures 7-10 and 7-11, respectively. Loss of contrast and increased quantum mottle is evident in these

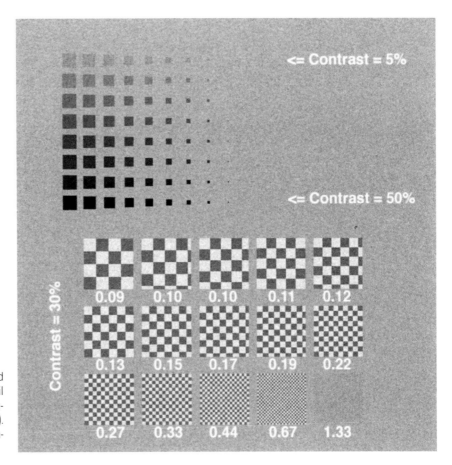

FIGURE 7-10. Image of the simulated x-ray fluence including contrast-detail (black squares) and varying spatial frequency patterns (checkerboard pattern). Reproduced with permission from Bissonnette et al.[98]

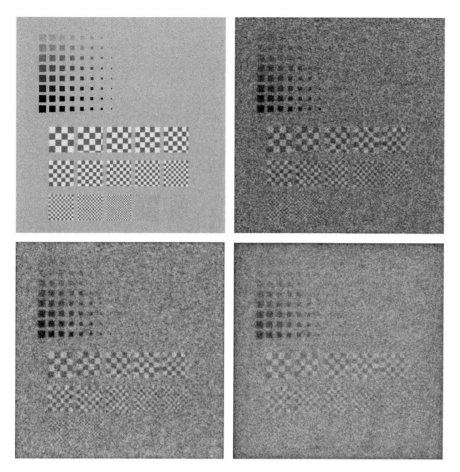

FIGURE 7-11. Monte Carlo simulation of images generated at different components of a camera-based portal imager. Input fluence used for these images was shown in Figure 7-10. Reproduced with permission from Bissonnette et al.[98]

images as light moves through the imaging chain. The theoretical DQE values achievable from this type of portal imagers are also extracted and shown in Figure 7-12.

One of the most prominent characteristics of these radiographic imagers is the light collecting size of their cameras. The typical size of CCD cameras used in these imagers is 2 cm^2 to 4 cm^2, which is much smaller than the typical aperture of the radiation beam being imaged. Although the phosphor screen can be made to cover the largest beam apertures possible with the accelerator, the spatial size of the available optical information is much larger than the size of the camera at the end of the optical imaging chain. This is the largest factor contributing to the low light collection efficiency of camera-based systems that restrict the collection of the light photons only to those emitted within the solid angle spanned by the size of the camera. Swindell[99] formulated an analytical description of the lens-coupling efficiency in camera-based megavoltage imaging devices. It can be shown[99,100] that the system DQE can be expressed as:

$$DQE = 1 + \frac{1}{\epsilon} \qquad (11)$$

where ϵ describes the total light collection efficiency and is defined as the ratio of mean number of detected light

quanta for every detected x-ray photon. In this formalism, the total light collection efficiency is divided in to three components ϵ_1, ϵ_2, and ϵ_3, the product of which is equal to the total efficiency, ϵ. The scintillation efficiency, ϵ_1, is the average number of light photons produced for every scintillation event generated by the x-ray in the phosphor

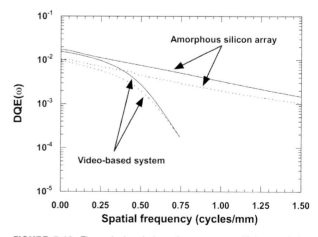

FIGURE 7-12. The calculated detective quantum efficiency of the camera-based and amorphous silicon portal imagers as a function of object spatial frequency from simulations of Bissonnette et al.[98] Reproduced with permission from Bissonnette et al.[98]

screen. In a typical phosphor screen, this efficiency is on the order of 10,000-20,000. The second component, ϵ_2, is the optical coupling efficiency and, as described earlier, it is purely a geometrical factor equal to the ratio of number of detectable photons at the camera to all photons produced at the phosphor. The coupling efficiency of lens optics is given by the following expression[99,101]:

$$\epsilon_2 = \frac{k \cdot (m+1)^2}{f^2 \cdot m^2} \tag{12}$$

where m is the lens magnification (ratio of the size of the image on the camera to the size on the converter screen), f is the focal ratio or relative aperture size of the lens (ratio of the focal length to the diameter size of the camera aperture), and k is a factor that incorporates the light emission distribution from the phosphor and geometric coverage of the camera.

Swindell argues that the optical coupling efficiency should be estimated with consideration of the fact that the phosphor is a self-luminous object and the photons are generated isotropically within its transparent medium. Therefore, coupling efficiency is equal to the solid angle spanned by the camera aperture, Ω, normalized by 4π:

$$\epsilon_2 = \Omega/4\pi. \tag{13}$$

Following equation 13, an appropriate selection for k in equation 12 would be $1/16n^2$ where n is the optical refractive index of the scintillating medium ($n \sim 1.6$). Consequently, a typical figure for overall coupling efficiency is on the order of 0.01% or, in other words, only one out of every 10 thousand light photons reaches the camera.

The last factor, ϵ_3, is the product of the efficiency attributable to other sources of light photon loss such as scattering and absorption in the phosphor screen and lens of the camera, which amount to about 30% and 90%, respectively. Other losses also occur in the camera because a fraction of the light sensor area is dedicated to nondetector functions, which reduce the quantum efficiency of the camera to about half (50%).

To address the low optical coupling efficiency of conventional mirror-camera systems, the focus has been directed to development of higher quantum efficiency phosphor screens as described previously or tapering the optical light to the physical dimensions of the camera. The latter was achieved by two distinct approaches: use of optic lenses and fiberoptic channeling. Large aperture lenses placed in front of the camera increase light collection efficiency by focusing the light that would otherwise be outside the geometric field of view of the camera, widening the effective solid angle covered by the camera and, therefore, increasing the light collection efficiency.

However, the addition of large area lenses introduces geometric distortions such as pin cushion or barrel distortions in addition to nonuniform spatial resolution with respect to the location of light falling onto the lens. Furthermore, the addition of another element in the imaging chain increases the sensitivity of the optical coupling to mechanical instabilities caused by the motion of the imager or mounted gantry.

The second approach to solving the low collection efficiency of the camera systems is the integration of fiberoptic cables to channel light directly from the phosphor screen to the camera.[102,103] In this design, a direct map of the camera pixels is replicated at the rear phosphor screen with individual fiberoptic cables accomplishing the mapping. Although the size of the camera is no longer the limiting factor with respect to the size of the typical radiation fields, the light collection efficiency in fiberoptic systems was governed by the acceptance angle for which full reflection of the light was achievable within the fiber, on the order of 2 degrees. This places another geometric limit on the collection efficiency because only those photons incident on the fiber surface by an angle smaller than the acceptance angle were fully transferred down the fibers onto the collecting surface of the camera. Other design details such as the length of the fibers and the optical properties of the glue used at each end of the cable are also contributing factors for the overall light collection efficiency of the fiberoptic systems. As a result, the overall efficiency of the fiberoptic systems is similar to an efficient camera system incorporating large-aperture lenses.[25]

Matrix Ionization Chamber Imagers

Use of liquid- or gas-filled chambers is a well-established technique for the detection of x-rays via the measurement of ionization current collected at chamber electrodes. Ionization chambers are ubiquitously used in today's diagnostic and therapeutic radiation applications for accurate radiation dosimetry. Their use as imaging devices was also explored in the 1980s and 1990s. The first such imager was designed as a matrix ion liquid chamber (for the pixilated design) in the form of a flat panel portal imager and developed at the Netherlands Cancer Institute by Merteens, van Herk, and colleagues.[104-107]

The matrix ion portal imager is formed by two bands of electrode strips constructed perpendicular to each other and separated by a 0.8-mm gap that is filled with a liquid (2,2,4-trimethylpentane) serving as the ionizing medium. Although the original prototype was developed with 32 copper strips, later commercial models increased the size of the imager to include 256 strips separated by 1.27 mm. The design of perpendicular bands of electrodes on each side of the liquid film actively forms a 256 × 256 matrix of individual ion chambers. The active area of the imager in this configuration was 325 mm × 325 mm. A schematic of the imager and associated electronics is shown in Figure 7-13. In addition to the detector components, the imager also incorporated a 1-mm-thick plastoferrite plate positioned upstream in the x-ray fluence to act as a converter layer for a generation of high-energy electrons and also as an absorber for low-energy scattered photons from the patient.

In this design, the front array of strips, called selection strips, are connected to a switchboard of high voltage source providing the collecting potential for each ionization pixel. Rear strips, called detection strips, are connected to a multichannel electrometer, which read out the ionization current generated by irradiation. Data acquisition is performed sequentially by scanning the imager row by row. In this mode, each selection strip is applied a high potential (300 V to 500 V), which activates all rows of ion chambers under the selected strip. Ionization current collected in all detection strips are then read out via the multiplexed electrodes. Therefore, a specific row of imager (i^{th}) is activated by the applied voltage and a specific column of imager (j^{th}) is activated by the reading of associated electrodes. This sequence registers a signal for the pixel positioned in (i,j) coordinates of the imager matrix. After a row is activated and read out, the high

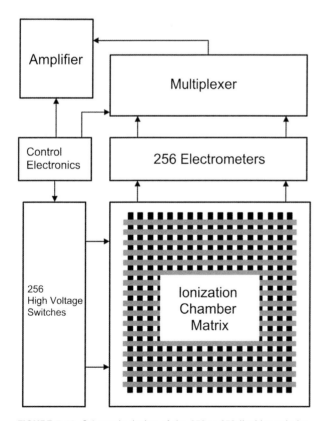

FIGURE 7-13. Schematic design of the 256 × 256 liquid matrix ion portal imaging system with associated electronics such as electrometers and pixel switching high-voltage source. Adapted with permission from Boyer et al.[25]

voltage switcher progresses to the strip in the next row until all rows are scanned this way. Typical current produced by each pixel of ion chamber is about 40 pA while exposed to a ^{60}Co beam with air kerma rate of 50 cGy/min at the position of the detector[104] (noise about 0.5%). Each detection strip is switched on for about 20 milliseconds. For 256 strips, the entire process takes about 5.5 seconds in order to create an image frame.[28]

Although matrix ion chambers are designed to exploit very high ion collection efficiencies, the read-out design of the existing imagers has been a limiting factor for their clinical efficiency. Because of the sequential scanning nature of the matrix ion imager, only a row of the imager is used for imaging purposes at a time while the rest of the imager receiving the radiation had to be ignored. Although total imaging time could be as little as a few seconds, the total utilization of x-ray quanta is considered to be poor with the scanning acquisition mode of these imagers. Another disadvantage of the scanning read out is that variations in the dose rate as the x-ray turned on reflect themselves as intensity variations across the image (in the direction of the high-voltage progression). For better-quality images, the image acquisition has to be delayed until the radiation beam is stabilized (about 1 second) which produces an additional loss of x-ray quanta not utilized for imaging. However, this undesirable consequence of the scanning mode is remedied in systems where the image acquisition is synchronized with the electron pulsing of the linear accelerator.

To increase quantum utilization of the imager, other read-out modes have also been investigated.[107] These modified modes, which included a scanning method with faster high-voltage switching (10 millisecond) and a low-resolution mode with only half of the strips turned on, resulted in a factor of 2 reduction in imaging time. However, these faster acquisition modes also were observed to affect the quantum mottle and image SNR in a negative way but are still considered useful especially for double-exposure images. More recent commercial systems such as the PortalVision Mark II (Varian Medical Systems, Palo Alto, CA) utilized a collecting potential of 500 V and 5 millisecond switching time to obtain an image frame in 1.25 second. To reduce image noise, frame averaging techniques were also used. In addition, the slow ion-recombination rate of the ionization liquid (2,2,4-trimethylpentane) was also observed to reduce image noise. With full recombination time of ~0.5 second, the concentration of ion pairs increases over a period of time.[28] Because of this effect, the signal measured by a collecting electrode is in fact largely attributable to the previous irradiation history of the pixels rather than the 5 millisecond to 20 millisecond high-voltage period. Although the recombination is still much shorter than the single-frame acquisition time of 1.25 second to 5 second, the presence of the extra signal (as much as three to five times more than that is acquired when the voltage is turned on) provides an averaging effect and reduces relative noise in the images.

Because of their compact size and the availability of a robotic arm mount enabling complete retraction of the PortalVision system, these imagers are successfully integrated into clinical operations. The robotic arm also provides the ability to set various source-to-detector distances, which introduced added flexibility for patient setup as well as image magnification. Compared with some optical imaging options, the matrix ion imagers also result in distortion-free images.

Active Matrix Flat Panel Imagers

Following technological advances on use of amorphous silicon arrays in liquid crystal displays as well as optical document scanners, active matrix flat panel imagers (AMFPI) were also developed for digital radiography applications.[108-111] Because of the superb imaging characteristics and convenience they provide in their integration with the day-to-day operations, these imagers have established themselves as the portal imaging device of choice in the majority of RT clinics today.

The fundamental construction of commercially available AMFPI devices is similar to that of other portal imaging devices discussed previously. A converter metal plate (typically 1.0 mm copper) encounters incident x-ray fluence for generation of high-energy electrons. These electrons (as well as nonattenuated primary x-ray photons) are then absorbed by a phosphor screen, which then emits visible light photons. In most MV imaging applications, a gadolinium oxysulphide (Gd_2O_2S) screen is used to generate scintillation photons. A pixilated image sensor panel is placed downstream of the phosphor screen to detect and accumulate raw imaging signal, which is,

to first order, proportional to the original x-ray fluence. Although direct detection image sensors are also being developed, these indirect imagers that work in combination with a phosphor screen are the only commercial active matrix portal imaging systems available as of this publication. Pixel switching/activating electronics, amplifiers, and analog-to-digital converters are, again, parts of the AMFPI devices that help create the final digital image. A typical design of indirect detection image sensor incorporating photodiodes is shown in Figure 7-14.

Despite the similarities with other portal imagers, the novel feature of the AMFPI devices comes from its imaging panel, which incorporates image sensor elements as well as pixel switching electronics as a thin detector layer. The basic image sensor element in (indirect detection) AMFPI is a hydrogenated amorphous silicon (aSi:H) photodiode located at each pixel of the imaging matrix. Hydrogenated amorphous silicon is a noncrystalline form of silicon that is deposited on a 1.0-mm glass substrate as thin film through a plasma-enhanced chemical vapor deposition (PEVCD) process. Operating at high pressures, an electric discharge ionizes the hydrogen (H_2) and silane gas (SiH_4) in the PEVCD plasma reactor to grow aSi:H film on a suitable substrate. The aSi film thickness is about 1.0 μm and its material is a semiconductor with sensitivity to light at energies beyond its band gap of 1.7 eV (photon wavelength of 730 nm). Typical spectral response of an aSi photosensor has a maximum quantum efficiency for detecting light photons at the end of the green light spectrum (550 nm to 600 nm), very close to the emission light wavelength from a common phosphor in imaging applications, gadolinium oxysulphide (Gd_2O_2S).

The electronic circuitry controlling the pixel switching and data read out are also embedded within a thin layer via similar vapor deposition and etching technologies. Thin field transistors (TFT) are used as fast-switching

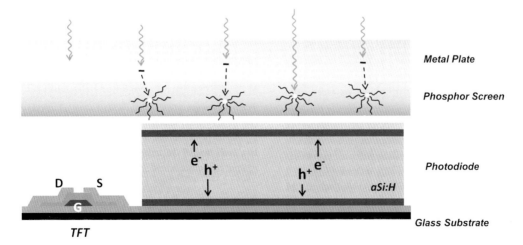

FIGURE 7-14. Schematic design of an hydrogenated amorphous silicon indirect detection photodiode detector with the thin field transistor pixel switch and converter layers. Generation of high-energy electrons, optical photons, and electron–hole pairs within the material of the photodiode are also depicted. Figure is not drawn to scale.

devices that are connected to each pixel sensor. A special kind of field effect transistors, TFTs feature three terminals (i.e., source, gain, and drain terminals). The source terminal is connected to the capacitive element of the photodiode image sensor. Thin field transistors in the same row are connected with a single gate line and they are controlled by the gate driver electronics positioned outside the image-sensitive area. Because of the potential difference between the source and drain terminals, TFTs are normally conducting but become nonconducting at a few volts of negative-gate bias. The on/off resistive ratio of TFTs is typically $1:10^6$ to 10^7 and such large differences are particularly important for imaging arrays to minimize leakage current from unaddressed pixels. During imaging, the TFTs are kept nonconducting so that no charge flows through the transistor terminals allowing the pixel capacitive element to accumulate charges because of interaction of photons within the sensor. When the gate potential is turned off through a row of TFTs, the TFTs become conducting, allowing accumulated charge to flow from source to drain, which are then collected through data lines and transferred to a series of amplifiers and digitizers. All pixels in the same column (e.g., j^{th}), are connected through the same data line and all pixels in the same row (e.g., i^{th}), are activated through a single gate line; therefore, the image signal from a particular pixel location (e.g., $[i,j]$), is decoded for the creation of an image frame. This sequential readout also re-initializes the pixels for subsequent data collection. A schematic design of the components of an active matrix aSi:H electronic portal imager is demonstrated in Figure 7-15.

Owing to the fast switching properties of the TFTs and sequential read out, an image frame acquisition can occur within a fraction of a second (typically five to 10 frames per second). Fast frame acquisition also makes AMFPI devices a suitable choice for fluoroscopic applications (continuous acquisition).

Specifications for a list of commercial electronic portal imagers incorporating aSi:H indirect detection technology are summarized in Table 7-1. Pictures of the commercial portal imaging devices listed in Table 7-1 are also shown in Figure 7-16. As a result of advances in photolithography techniques and minimization of electronic components, the fill factor (ratio of the size of the active image sensitive area to the entire surface of the imaging panel) in contemporary imagers reaches up to 84% for the aSi EPID (Varian Medical Systems, Palo Alto, CA) providing outstanding utilization of the incident x-ray fluence.

In addition to their implementation as portal imaging devices for megavoltage imaging, aSi imagers are also used for kV imaging applications because of their excellent image quality, fast image acquisition, and ease in their integration into clinical operations. Kilovoltage imaging panels are used to acquire 2D digital radiographs or multiple cone-beam images for reconstruction of a 3D image

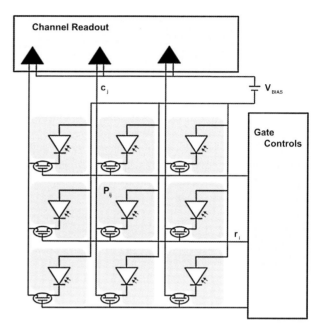

FIGURE 7-15. Schematic for the pixilated design of the aSi:H flat-panel PortalVision (Varian Medical Systems, Palo Alto, CA) imager with gate control and channel read-out electronics actively switching each pixel of the imager.

of the patient. Although the same amorphous silicon semiconductor material is used as photodiodes and TFTs are integrated as pixel switches, there are significant differences between the flat panel imagers used in kV and MV applications. Diagnostic quality spatial resolution is usually achieved with pixel dimensions smaller than those used in MV imagers. For example, the On-Board Imager (OBI; Varian Medical Systems, Palo Alto, CA) employs a 2048 × 1536 matrix of aSi sensors at a pixel pitch of 192 μm, half that of its similar MV imagers. Furthermore, the metal plate used as converter and absorber of scatter x-rays in MV imagers, would attenuate a large fraction of kV fluence and, therefore, is not included in the OBI. Because of increased scatter of photons within the kV range, a scatter grid is placed instead of the metal plate to achieve higher contrast in kV images. The OBI incorporates a 70% attenuating grid with a grid ratio of 10 to 1. Scintillator layer design can also show differences between MV and kV imagers. As discussed before, the efficiency of Gd_2O_2S:Tb screens are limited because larger thickness sizes degrade the spatial resolution. In the OBI, CsI:Tb screens are utilized to benefit from their larger thickness and columnar structure, which limit the spread of photons within the detector.

The spatial resolution and efficiency of AMFPI devices are in principle superior to camera-based and matrix liquid ion chamber portal imaging devices. Several studies[112-114] have explored the imaging characteristics of aSi flat panel imagers. A theoretical analysis of detector quantum efficiency of aSi arrays was performed by Bissonnette

TABLE 7–1 Design Specifications for Amorphous Silicon Active Matrix Flat Panel Imagers From Three Major Linear Accelerator Manufacturers

	Varian[a]		Elekta[b]	Siemens[c]	
Imager name	aS500	aS1000	iViewGT	Optivue 500	Optivue 1000
Panel dimensions, cm²	40.1 × 30.1	40.1 × 30.1	41.0 × 41.0	41.0 × 41.0	41.0 × 41.0
Focus detector distance, cm		105 to 180	160	115 to 160	
Metal plate			1 mm copper		
Phosphor screen			Gadolinium oxysulphide doped with terbium (Gd_2O_2S:Tb)		
Matrix resolution, pixels	512 × 384	1024 × 768	1024 × 1024	512 × 512	1024 × 1024
Pixel pitch, μm	784	392	400	800	400
Pixel bit depth	14	14	16	16	16
Image acquisition rate, fps	3	10	3	3.5	7

Note. fps = frames per second.
[a]Varian Medical Systems, Palo Alto, CA.
[b]Elekta AB, Stockholm, Sweden.
[c]Siemens Medical Solutions USA, Malvern, PA.

et al. and it was shown to be superior to that of camera-based systems (Figure 7-12).[98] In this study, investigators devised a virtual aSi flat panel imager with similar characteristics as Varian aS500 imagers and used Monte Carlo simulations to analyze input formation as well as input/output image quality comparisons. Similar to their simulation of camera-based EPIDs, the contrast-detail input x-ray fluence image depicted in Figure 7-10 was used and corresponding output images were generated after simulation of x-ray interaction through the imaging components. As shown in Figure 7-17, the replacement of optical imaging components (such as the lens, mirror, and camera) with aSi array improves image quality as a result of improvements in detection efficiency.

In a prototype aSi imager with pixel pitch of 0.75 mm a incorporating a 1.5-mm copper plate and 134 mg/cm² Gd_2O_2S:Tb phosphor screen, Munro and Bouius measured the detector quantum efficiency and observed that it does not vary significantly as a function of beam energy within therapeutic ranges and is approximately 1% at low spatial frequencies (< 0.3 lp/mm).[112] This DQE figure is still higher than those achievable with camera-based imager systems or scanning liquid ion matrix imagers. In addition, the MTF for the prototype system was measured

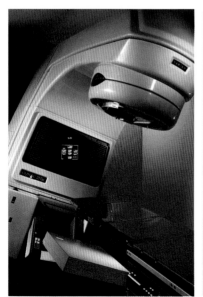
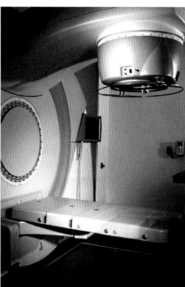
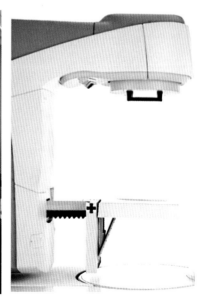

FIGURE 7-16. Pictures of the commercial amorphous silicon flat-panel imagers listed in Table 7-1. All displayed imagers can be retracted fully to their gantry housing by an electronic arm. Photos are courtesy of Varian Medical Systems, Elekta AB (publ) and Siemens Healthcare Inc. All rights reserved.

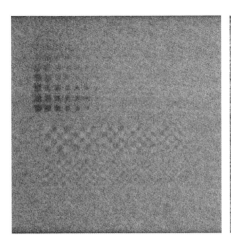
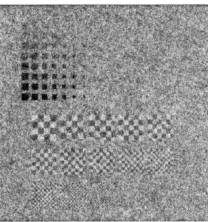

FIGURE 7-17. Comparisons of images obtained with camera-based and amorphous silicon portal imagers from simulations of Bissonnette et al.[98] Reproduced with permission from Bissonnette et al.[98]

with the narrow slit technique. Figure 7-18 shows the LSF for an 80-μm narrow slit measured for the aSi imager irradiated with 6 MV and 18 MV beams. The full width at half maximum for the LSFs is 0.77 mm and 0.85 mm for 6-MV and 18-MV beams, respectively. The tails of the LSF are larger for 18 MV suggesting that they are caused by Bremsstrahlung photons generated within the copper plate and phosphor screen. The MTF of the aSi imager system compared with the camera-based system is shown in upper panel of Figure 7-19. These curves are almost identical suggesting that the spatial resolution of aSi imagers is similar to what could be expected from a camera-based portal imager. Furthermore, limitations in spatial resolution of aSi panel are investigated by obtaining the MTF of the x-ray detector alone (metal plate and phosphor screen) with film instead of the aSi panel (Figure 7-19). A reduction in detector MTF when one is using aSi imagers could either be because of the optical spread in the imaging sensor or the limited pixel pitch

for the photosensors. Munro et al. filtered the detector MTF by using a virtual imager aperture of 0.75 mm.[112] This reflects a perfect imaging sensor with finite detective element resolution but no extra loss of spatial resolution. The actual MTF from the aSi imager is also overlaid in the same plot (lower panel of Figure 7-19) and a comparison with the filtered MTF shows that the finite size of the pixels in the aSi panel is the limiting factor governing the spatial resolution of these imagers rather than loss of spatial resolution within the image sensor.

The source of image noise in these systems is twofold: x-ray quantum noise and system noise caused by electronics and other components. Munro et al. evaluated the quantum noise by irradiating the imager while the copper plate was not in contact but was suspended 2 cm above the surface of the phosphor screen.[112] Quantum noise levels were measured to be negligible at nonzero spatial frequencies. This was confirmed by placing a 2-cm-thick lead block (2.5 cm² × 4 cm²) in contact with the phosphor screen. When irradiated, no image of the block was visible in the image.

These image quality studies suggest that the aSi imagers are very suitable choices for portal imaging applications. The linear response and other dose response characteristics of aSi imagers have also been studied extensively.[115–117] These studies have demonstrated that the imager response is highly linear with respect to expected x-ray fluence (as shown with different irradiation times at fixed air kerma strength or fixed integration time with varying air kerma strength). Linearity and long-term stability of the aSi imagers combined with accurate modeling of their response also allow these imagers to be used as dosimeters. Clinical protocols are being developed to utilize aSi imagers as in-vivo dosimeters for patient exit dose measurements as well as QA devices for their use in intensity-modulated RT (IMRT) fluence verification procedures.

Despite the success of existing amorphous silicon imagers, further developments in detector design as well as the read-out techniques still play an important role in

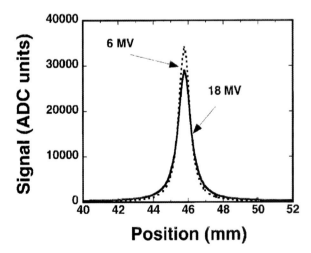

FIGURE 7-18. The line spread functions measured for the amorphous silicon imager irradiated with 6-MV and 18-MV beams by using an 80-μm narrow slit source. Reproduced with permission from Munro et al.[112]

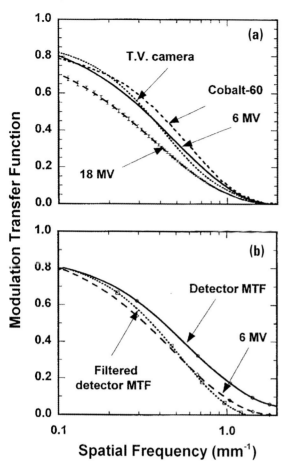

FIGURE 7-19. Modulation transfer function (MTF) of the hydrogenated amorphous silicon (aSi:H) imager irradiated with 6-MV and 18-MV (Co⁶⁰) beams by using an 80 μm (380 μm) narrow slit source is demonstrated in top panel. The flat panel imager response is also compared with a camera-based portal imaging system. In bottom panel, MTF of the aSi:H imager is compared with the MTF of the metal plate/phosphor screen detector (using a radiographic film, depicted as "Detector MTF"). The MTF of the detector is also filtered for the differences in the pixel sizes of the aSi:H imager and the film (depicted as "Filtered detector MTF" in bottom panel). Reproduced with permission from Munro et al.[112]

improving the quality of the images obtained with these imagers. The aSi image sensor was shown to withstand very large doses of radiation ($> 10^4$ Gy) with very small changes in its sensitivity (~1.3 %).[118,119] However, a challenge with the current technology of AMFPI panels is that the surrounding auxiliary electronic components such as gate drivers and amplifier circuits are prone to radiation damage and, thus, extra care must be taken to ensure that the radiation field is restricted to the active surface of the imager.

Another problem with images obtained with aSi AMFPI is the image artifact in the appearance of horizontal line patterns overlaying the anatomical image. These artifacts occur because of the pulse nature of radiation delivery with the linac. In AMFPI devices, rows of the imager pixels are read out in sequential mode and, therefore, this signal collection occurs in between two pulse trains of the linac when no x-ray fluence is generated. To avoid this, the imager read out can be synchronized with the radiation pulse signal received from the linac and frame acquisition could be paused between pulses. This synchronization leads to removal of the line artifacts and more uniform fluence across the image.

Direct Detection Flat Panel Imagers

Although indirect detection aSi imaging technology is the standard choice for today's electronic portal imaging solutions, an alternative method based on direct detection of x-rays is currently being researched by several investigators.[120-123] Because of the relatively low atomic number of silicon, the x-ray absorption within the bulk of the aSi image sensor is limited requiring the use of additional converters such as phosphor screens. Phosphor screens typically generate many optical photons (order of 10 000) for every incident x-ray quanta, which are emitted at wavelengths close to the optimum absorption spectrum of the silicon photodiodes. However, a disadvantage with the use of phosphor screens is that the presence of such translucent materials upstream of the image sensor spreads the spatial distribution of optical photons and, hence, degrades the spatial resolution in final images.

Conversely, directly converting semiconductor materials avoids the limitations caused by the two-step quantum process found in phosphor/sensor devices and uses photoconductor materials instead to provide the detection efficiency and spatial resolution necessary from such imaging devices. Having a relatively high atomic number, amorphous selenium (aSe) is considered to be an efficient x-ray detection material to be used for radiological imaging purposes. Amorphous selenium can also be constructed as a very thin layer (< 1 mm) to avoid a reduction of spatial resolution because of quanta with oblique incidence. An illustration of direct detection imaging devices incorporating aSe photoconductors and aSi TFT switches is shown in Figure 7-20. In such devices, high-energy electrons created in the metal converter plate interact with aSe and create electron–hole pairs within the bulk material of the image sensor. An external electric potential is required to collect the charge and store in the capacitive element of the pixels. Collected charge is then read out by the TFTs in a manner very similar to aSi AMFPI devices.

A commercial aSe imager originally designed for diagnostic imaging applications was investigated by Pang et al. for its use in megavoltage imaging.[123] Having an active aSe layer thickness of 500 μm, the matrix of 3072 by 2560 pixels (each with 139 $\mu m^2 \times$ 139 μm^2) was created by pixel electrodes keeping the photoconductor at a voltage bias of 1000 V. In this arrangement, they achieved a geometric fill factor of 86% (although it is argued that *effective*

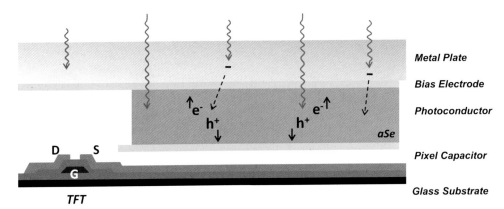

FIGURE 7-20. Schematic design of an amorphous selenium direct detection photodiode detector with the thin field transistor pixel switch. These detectors are directly sensitive to high-energy electrons and photons, therefore eliminating the need for an additional phosphor screen. Electron–hole pairs created in the material of photoconductor are collected via the pixel electrodes and generated signal is stored in pixel capacitors.

fill factor is closer to 100% because of the bulging shape of the electric field between two electrodes). As shown in the left panel of Figure 7-21, the MTF of the system was measured to be superior to that of an indirect detector (prototype aSi imager studied by Munro and Bouius[112]) especially at higher spatial frequencies. This result was partly attributable to the different pixel sizes of the two detectors (139 μm vs 750 μm) and, therefore, Pang et al.[123] provided a convolution of their measured MTF with different down-sampling functions to provide a more direct comparison. These simulations also confirmed a better MTF was achievable with aSe imagers. Similar comparative analysis for DQE demonstrated that the efficiency of their imager was high as 2% and, thus, comparable to the aSi imager. The DQE comparison from this study is also shown in Figure 7-21 (right panel).

Because of their primary use in diagnostic applications, the aSe imagers still require further optimization to prove as suitable alternatives to amorphous silicon-based indirect detectors for MV electronic portal imaging. Frame read-out times with aSe imagers are as large as 5 seconds, an order of magnitude higher than aSi panels, which leads to increased patient doses for MV imaging. The radiation hardness of the imaging panel as well as the accompanying electronics also needs to be improved.

Conclusions

Over the past two decades, there have been great advances in the development of electronic portal imaging solutions in the realm of MV RT. Although the improvement of image quality has always been a key issue, the trend of emerg-

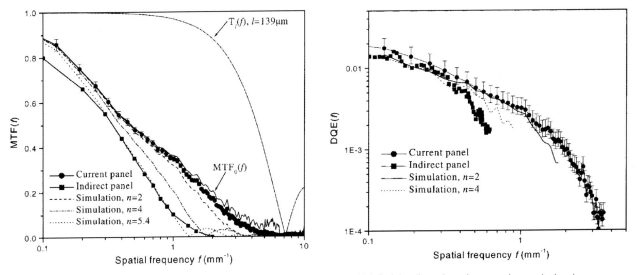

FIGURE 7-21. Modulation transfer function (left) and Detector Quantum Efficiency (right) of the direct detection amorphous selenium imager compared with the prototype indirect amouphous silicon imager of Munro and Bouius. Because of differences in the pixel sizes of the two imagers, the pixilated signal of the direct-detection imager is re-binned (n = 2,3) and its response with respect to a larger pixel size is simulated. Reproduced with permission from Pang et al.[123]

ing technologies has been toward devices that fit better into the daily operations and needs of RT clinics. The integration of compact and portable flat-panel imagers into conventional accelerator gantries enabled more convenient operation of these devices compared with their bulky predecessors. The availability of fast read-out electronics synchronized with the pulsing of the accelerator beam provided users with more imaging capacity without raising too much concern about imaging dose. The development of new operation modes, such as volumetric imaging and dosimetric applications, offered clinics much more utilization than the original function of these devices as portal imagers. All these factors contributed to the success of current electronic portal imagers and paved the way for the realization of IGRT in modern clinics.

Acknowledgements

I would like to thank Jong O. Kim, Ergun Ahunbay, and Chris Beltran for providing technical specifications for commercial EPIDs discussed in the text.

References

1. Mohan R, Barest G, Brewster LJ, et al. A comprehensive three-dimensional radiation treatment planning system. *Int J Radiat Oncol Biol Phys.* 1988;15(2):481–495.
2. Kuszyk BS, Ney DR, Fishman EK. The current state of the art in three dimensional oncologic imaging: an overview. *Int J Radiat Oncol Biol Phys.* 1995;33(5):1029–1039.
3. Armstrong J, McGibney C. The impact of three-dimensional radiation on the treatment of non-small cell lung cancer. *Radiother Oncol.* 2000;56(2):157–167.
4. Khoo VS, Dearnaley DP, Finnigan DJ, et al. Magnetic resonance imaging (MRI): considerations and applications in radiotherapy treatment planning. *Radiother Oncol.* 1997;42(1):1–15.
5. Pötter R, Heil B, Schneider L, et al. Sagittal and coronal planes from MRI for treatment planning in tumors of brain, head and neck: MRI assisted simulation. *Radiother Oncol.* 1992;23(2):127–130.
6. Grégoire V, Bol A, Geets X, et al. Is PET-based treatment planning the new standard in modern radiotherapy? The head and neck paradigm. *Semin Radiat Oncol.* 2006;16(4):232–238.
7. Heron DE, Smith RP, Andrade RS. Advances in image-guided radiation therapy—the role of PET-CT. *Med Dosim.* 2006;31(1):3–11.
8. Nestle U, Kremp S, Grosu A. Practical integration of [¹⁸F]-FDG-PET and PET-CT in the planning of radiotherapy for non-small cell lung cancer (NSCLC): the technical basis, ICRU-target volumes, problems, perspectives. *Radiother Oncol.* 2006;81(2):209–225.
9. Huang G, Medlam G, Lee J, et al. Error in the delivery of radiation therapy: results of a quality assurance review. *Int J Radiat Oncol Biol Phys.* 2005;61(5):1590–1595.
10. Rudat V, Flentje M, Oetzel D, et al. Influence of the positioning error on 3D conformal dose distributions during fractionated radiotherapy. *Radiother Oncol.* 1994;33(1):56–63.
11. Escó R, López P, Bellosta R, et al. Accidental over-irradiation syndrome. *Radiother Oncol.* 1993;28(2):177–178.
12. Ostrom LT, Rathbun P, Cumberlin R, et al. Lessons learned from investigations of therapy misadministration events. *Int J Radiat Oncol Biol Phys.* 1996;34(1):227–234.
13. Vatnitsky S, Ortiz Lopez P, Izewska J, et al. The radiation over-exposure of radiotherapy patients in Panama. *Radiother Oncol.* 2001;60(3):237–238.
14. Thomadsen BR. Principles in positioning cross-projecting lasers. *Med Phys.* 1981;8(3)375–377.
15. Byhardt RW, Cox JD, Hornburg A, et al. Weekly localization films and detection of field placement errors. *Int J Radiat Oncol Biol Phys.* 1978;4(9):881–887.
16. Dong L, Boyer AL. A portal image alignment and patient setup verification procedure using moments and correlation techniques. *Phys Med Biol.* 1996;41(4):697–723.
17. Herman MG, Abrams RA, Mayer RR. Clinical use of on-line portal imaging for daily patient treatment verification. *Int J Radiat Oncol Biol Phys.* 1994;28(4):1017–1023.
18. Sirois LM, Hristov DH, Fallone BG. Three-dimensional anatomy setup verification by correlation of orthogonal portal images and digitally reconstructed radiographs. *Med Phys.* 1999;26(1):2422–2428.
19. de Boer HC, van Sörnsen de Koste JR, Creutzberg CL, et al. Electronic portal image assisted reduction of systematic setup errors in head and neck irradiation. *Radiother Oncol.* 2001; 61(3):299–308.
20. Droege RT, Stefanakos TK. Portal film technique charts. *Int J Radiat Oncol Biol Phys.* 1985;11(11):2027–2031.
21. Haus AG, Dickerson RE, Huff KE, et al. Evaluation of a cassette-screen-film combination for radiation therapy portal localization imaging with improved contrast. *Med Phys.* 1997;24(10):1605–1608.
22. Munro P, Rawlinson JA, Fenster A. Therapy imaging: a signal-to-noise analysis of metal plate/film detectors. *Med Phys.* 1987;14(6):975–984.
23. Reinstein LE, Alquist L, Amols HI, et al. Quantitative evaluation of a portal film contrast enhancement technique. *Med Phys.* 1987;14(3):309–313.
24. Baily NA, Horn RA, Kampp TD. Fluoroscopic visualization of megavoltage therapeutic x ray beams. *Int J Radiat Oncol Biol Phys.* 1980;6(7):935–939.
25. Boyer AL, Antonuk L, Fenster A, et al. A review of electronic portal imaging devices (epids). *Med Phys.* 1992;19(1):1–16.
26. Munro P. Portal imaging technology: past, present, and future. *Semin Radiat Oncol.* 1995;5(2):115–133.
27. Herman MG, Kruse JJ, Hagness CR. Guide to clinical use of electronic portal imaging. *J Appl Clin Med Phys.* 2000;1(2):38–57.
28. Herman MG, Balter JM, Jaffray DA, et al. Clinical use of electronic portal imaging: report of AAPM radiation therapy committee task group 58. *Med Phys.* 2001;28(5):712–737.
29. Langmack KA. Portal imaging. *Br J Radiol.* 2001;74(885):789–804.
30. Antonuk LE. Electronic portal imaging devices: a review and historical perspective of contemporary technologies and research. *Phys Med Biol.* 2002;47(6):R31–R65.
31. Herman MG. Clinical use of electronic portal imaging. *Semin Radiat Oncol.* 2005;15(3):157–167.

32. Kirby MC, Glendinning AG. Developments in electronic portal imaging systems. *Br J Radiol.* 2006;79(1):S50–S65.

33. Stroom JC, de Boer HC, Huizenga H, et al. Inclusion of geometrical uncertainties in radiotherapy treatment planning by means of coverage probability. *Int J Radiat Oncol Biol Phys.* 1999;43(4):905–919.

34. Stroom JC, Heijmen BJM. Geometrical uncertainties, radiotherapy planning margins, and the ICRU-62 report. *Radiother Oncol.* 2002;64(1):75–83.

35. van Herk M. Errors and margins in radiotherapy. *Semin Radiat Oncol.* 2004;14(1):52–64.

36. Bel A, van Herk M, Lebesque JV. Target margins for random geometrical treatment uncertainties in conformal radiotherapy. *Med Phys.* 1996;23(9):1537–1545.

37. Stapleton S, Zavgorodni S, Popescu IA, et al. Implementation of random set-up errors in Monte Carlo calculated dynamic IMRT treatment plans. *Phys Med Biol.* 2005;50(3):429–439.

38. van Herk M, Witte M, van der Geer J, et al. Biologic and physical fractionation effects of random geometric errors. *Int J Radiat Oncol Biol Phys.* 2003;57(5):1460–1471.

39. Lebesque JV, Bel A, Bijhold J, et al. Detection of systematic patient setup errors by portal film analysis. *Radiother Oncol.* 1992;23(3):198.

40. Rosenthal SA, Galvin JM. Assessment of systematic error during radiotherapy. *Int J Radiat Oncol Biol Phys.* 1993;25(3):572.

41. Hoogeman MS, van Herk M, de Bois J, et al. Strategies to reduce the systematic error due to tumor and rectum motion in radiotherapy of prostate cancer. *Radiother Oncol.* 2005;74(2):177–185.

42. Wu Q, Lockman D, Wong J, et al. Effect of the first day correction on systematic setup error reduction. *Med Phys.* 2007;34(5):1789–1796.

43. Kirby MC. A multipurpose phantom for use with electronic portal imaging devices. *Phys Med Biol.* 1995;40(2):323–334.

44. Althof VG, Hoekstra CJ, te Loo HJ. Variation in prostate position relative to adjacent bony anatomy. *Int J Radiat Oncol Biol Phys.* 1996;34(3):709–715.

45. Bonin SR, Lanciano RM, Corn BW, et al. Bony landmarks are not an adequate substitute for lymphangiography in defining pelvic lymph node location for the treatment of cervical cancer with radiotherapy. *Int J Radiat Oncol Biol Phys.* 1996;34(1):167–172.

46. McNair HA, Hansen VN, Parker CC, et al. A comparison of the use of bony anatomy and internal markers for offline verification and an evaluation of the potential benefit of online and offline verification protocols for prostate radiotherapy. *Int J Radiat Oncol Biol Phys.* 2008;71(1):41–50.

47. Schallenkamp JM, Herman MG, Kruse JJ, et al. Prostate position relative to pelvic bony anatomy based on intraprostatic gold markers and electronic portal imaging. *Int J Radiat Oncol Biol Phys.* 2005;63(3):800–811.

48. Balter JM, Sandler HM, Lam K, et al. Measurement of prostate movement over the course of routine radiotherapy using implanted markers. *Int J Radiat Oncol Biol Phys.* 1995;31(1):113–118.

49. Kaatee RSJP, Olofsen MJJ, Verstraate MBJ, et al. Detection of organ movement in cervix cancer patients using a fluoroscopic electronic portal imaging device and radiopaque markers. *Int J Radiat Oncol Biol Phys.* 2002;54(2):576–583.

50. Bijhold J, Gilhuijs KG, van Herk M, et al. Radiation field edge detection in portal images. *Phys Med Biol.* 1991;36(12):1705–1710.

51. Lasserre P, Cutt B, Moffat J. Edge detection of the radiation field in double exposure portal images using a curve propagation algorithm. *J Appl Clin Med Phys.* 2008;9(4):2710.

52. Wang H, Fallone BG. A mathematical model of radiation field edge localization. *Med Phys.* 1995;22(7):1107–1110.

53. Kutcher G, Mageras G, Liebel S. Control, correction, and modeling of setup errors and organ motion. *Semin Radiat Oncol.* 1995;5(2):134–145.

54. Mageras GS, Kutcher GJ, Leibel SA, et al. A method of incorporating organ motion uncertainties into three-dimensional conformal treatment plans. *Int J Radiat Oncol Biol Phys.* 1996;35(2):333–342.

55. Stroom JC, Koper PC, Korevaar GA, et al. Internal organ motion in prostate cancer patients treated in prone and supine treatment position. *Radiother Oncol.* 1999;51(3):237–248.

56. Langen KM, Jones DT. Organ motion and its management. *Int J Radiat Oncol Biol Phys.* 2001;50(1):265–278.

57. Meijer GJ, Rasch C, Remeijer P, et al. Three-dimensional analysis of delineation errors, setup errors, and organ motion during radiotherapy of bladder cancer. *Int J Radiat Oncol Biol Phys.* 2003;55(5):1277–1287.

58. Keall PJ, Mageras GS, Balter JM, et al. The management of respiratory motion in radiation oncology report of AAPM task group 76. *Med Phys.* 2006;33(10):3874–3900.

59. Oelfke U, Tücking T, Nill S, et al. Linac-integrated kV cone beam CT: technical features and first applications. *Med Dosim.* 2006;31(1):62–70.

60. Morin O, Gillis A, Chen J, et al. Megavoltage cone-beam CT: system description and clinical applications. *Med Dosim.* 2006;31(1):51–61.

61. Gayou O, Miften M. Commissioning and clinical implementation of a mega-voltage cone beam CT system for treatment localization. *Med Phys.* 2007;34(8):3183–3192.

62. Chen J, Morin O, Aubin M, et al. Dose-guided radiation therapy with megavoltage cone-beam CT. *Br J Radiol.* 2006;79(1):S87–S98.

63. Morin O, Chen J, Aubin M, et al. Dose calculation using megavoltage cone-beam CT. *Int J Radiat Oncol Biol Phys.* 2007;67(4):1201–1210.

64. Yang Y, Schreibmann E, Li T, et al. Evaluation of on-board kV cone beam CT (CBCT)-based dose calculation. *Phys Med Biol.* 2007;52(3):685–705.

65. Kirby MC, Williams PC. The use of an electronic portal imaging device for exit dosimetry and quality control measurements. *Int J Radiat Oncol Biol Phys.* 1995;31(3):593–603.

66. Hansen VN, Evans PM, Swindell W. The application of transit dosimetry to precision radiotherapy. *Med Phys.* 1996;23(5):713–721.

67. Pasma KL, Kroonwijk M, Quint S, et al. Transit dosimetry with an electronic portal imaging device (EPID) for 115 prostate cancer patients. *Int J Radiat Oncol Biol Phys.* 1999;45(5):1297–1303.

68. Grein EE, Lee R, Luchka K. An investigation of a new amorphous silicon electronic portal imaging device for transit dosimetry. *Med Phys.* 2002;29(10):2262–2268.

69. Partridge M, Symonds-Tayler JR, Evans PM. IMRT verification with a camera-based electronic portal imaging system. *Phys Med Biol.* 2000;45(12):N183–N196.

70. Arnfield MR, Wu Q, Tong S, et al. Dosimetric validation for multileaf collimator-based intensity-modulated radiotherapy: a review. *Med Dosim.* 2001;26(2):179–188.

71. Warkentin B, Steciw S, Rathee S, et al. Dosimetric IMRT verification with a flat-panel EPID. *Med Phys.* 2003;30(12):3143–3155.

72. Luchka K, Chen D, Shalev S, et al. Assessing radiation and light field congruence with a video based electronic portal imaging device. *Med Phys.* 1996;23(7):1245–1252.

73. Prisciandaro JI, Herman MG, Kruse JJ. Utilizing an electronic portal imaging device to monitor light and radiation field congruence. *J Appl Clin Med Phys.* 2003;4(4):315–320.

74. Curtin-Savard A, Podgorsak EB. An electronic portal imaging device as a physics tool. *Med Dosim.* 1997;22(2):101–105.

75. Geyer P, Blank H, Evers C, et al. Filmless evaluation of the mechanical accuracy of the isocenter in stereotactic radiotherapy. *Strahlenther Onkol.* 2007;183(2):76–80.

76. Baker SJK, Budgell GJ, MacKay RI. Use of an amorphous silicon electronic portal imaging device for multileaf collimator quality control and calibration. *Phys Med Biol.* 2005;50(7):1377–1392.

77. Mohammadi M, Bezak E. Evaluation of MLC leaf positioning using a scanning liquid ionization chamber EPID. *Phys Med Biol.* 2007;52(1):N21–N33.

78. Clarke MF, Budgell GJ. Use of an amorphous silicon EPID for measuring MLC calibration at varying gantry angle. *Phys Med Biol.* 2008;53(2):473–485.

79. Motz JW, Danos M. Image information content and patient exposure. *Med Phys.* 1978;5(1):8–22.

80. Sandrik JM, Wagner RF. Absolute measures of physical image quality: measurement and application to radiographic magnification. *Med Phys.* 1982;9(4):540–549.

81. Droege RT. A megavoltage MTF measurement technique for metal screen-film detectors. *Med Phys.* 1979;6(4):272–279.

82. Sones RA, Barnes GT. A method to measure the MTF of digital x-ray systems. *Med Phys.* 1984;11(2):166–171.

83. Bradford CD, Peppler WW, Waidelich JM. Use of a slit camera for MTF measurements. *Med Phys.* 1999;26(11):2286–2294.

84. Althof VG, de Boer JC, Huizenga H, et al. Physical characteristics of a commercial electronic portal imaging device. *Med Phys.* 1996;23(11):1845–1855.

85. Johnson LS, Milliken BD, Hadley SW, et al. Initial clinical experience with a video-based patient positioning system. *Int J Radiat Oncol Biol Phys.* 1999;45(1):205–213.

86. Drake DG, Jaffray DA, Wong JW. Characterization of a fluoroscopic imaging system for kv and mv radiography. *Med Phys.* 2000;27(5):898–905.

87. de Boer JC, Heijmen BJ, Pasma KL, et al. Characterization of a high-elbow, fluoroscopic electronic portal imaging device for portal dosimetry. *Phys Med Biol.* 2000;45(1):197–216.

88. Munro P, Rawlinson JA, Fenster A. A digital fluoroscopic imaging device for radiotherapy localization. *Int J Radiat Oncol Biol Phys.* 1990;18(3):641–649.

89. Munro P, Rawlinson JA, Fenster A. Therapy imaging: a signal-to-noise analysis of a fluoroscopic imaging system for radiotherapy localization. *Med Phys.* 1990;17(5):763–772.

90. Wowk B, Radcliffe T, Leszczynski KW, et al. Optimization of metal/phosphor screens for on-line portal imaging. *Med Phys.* 1994;21(2):227–235.

91. Wowk B, Shalev S. Thick phosphor screens for on-line portal imaging. *Med Phys.* 1994;21(8):1269–1276.

92. Bissonnette JP, Cunningham IA, Munro P. Optimal phosphor thickness for portal imaging. *Med Phys.* 1997;24(6):803–814.

93. Rong XJ, Shaw CC, Liu X, et al. Comparison of an amorphous silicon/cesium iodide flat-panel digital chest radiography system with screen/film and computed radiography systems—a contrast-detail phantom study. *Med Phys.* 2001;28(11):2328–2335.

94. Zhao W, Ristic G, Rowlands JA. X-ray imaging performance of structured cesium iodide scintillators. *Med Phys.* 2004;31(9):2594–2605.

95. Bissonnette JP, Cunningham IA, Jaffray DA, et al. A quantum accounting and detective quantum efficiency analysis for video-based portal imaging. *Med Phys.* 1997;24(6):815–826.

96. Cremers F, Frenzel T, Kausch C, et al. Performance of electronic portal imaging devices (EPIDs) used in radiotherapy: image quality and dose measurements. *Med Phys.* 2004;31(5):985–996.

97. Samant SS, Gopal A. Study of a prototype high quantum efficiency thick scintillation crystal video-electronic portal imaging device. *Med Phys.* 2006;33(8):2783–2791.

98. Bissonnette J, Munro P, Cunningham IA. Monte Carlo simulation of the image formation process in portal imaging. *Med Phys.* 2003;30(12):3243–3250.

99. Swindell W. The lens coupling efficiency in megavoltage imaging. *Med Phys.* 1991;18(6):1152–1153.

100. Barrett HH, Swindell W. *Radiological Imaging - The Theory of Image Formation, Detection, and Processing.* New York, NY: Academic; 1981.

101. Nelson RS, Barbaric ZL, Gomes AS, et al. An evaluation of a fluorescent screen-isocon camera system for x-ray imaging in radiology. *Med Phys.* 1982;9(5):777–783.

102. Wong JW, Binns WR, Cheng AY, et al. On-line radiotherapy imaging with an array of fiber-optic image reducers. *Int J Radiat Oncol Biol Phys.* 1990;18(6):1477–1484.

103. Wong JW, Cheng AY, Binns WR, et al. Development of a second-generation fiber-optic on-line image verification system. *Int J Radiat Oncol Biol Phys.* 1993;26(2):311–320.

104. Meertens H, van Herk M, Weeda J. A liquid ionisation detector for digital radiography of therapeutic megavoltage photon beams. *Phys Med Biol.* 1985;30(4):313–321.

105. van Herk M, Meertens H. A matrix ionisation chamber imaging device for on-line patient setup verification during radiotherapy. *Radiother Oncol.* 1988;11(4):369–378.

106. Meertens H, van Herk M, Bijhold J, et al. First clinical experience with a newly developed electronic portal imaging device. *Int J Radiat Oncol Biol Phys.* 1990;18(5):1173–1181.

107. van Herk M, Bijhold J, Hoogervorst B, et al. Sampling methods for a matrix ionization chamber system. *Med Phys.* 1992;19(2):409–418.

108. Antonuk LE, Boudry J, Huang W, et al. Demonstration of megavoltage and diagnostic x-ray imaging with hydrogenated amorphous silicon arrays. *Med Phys.* 1992;19(6):1455–1466.

109. Antonuk LE, Yorkston J, Huang W, et al. A real-time, flat-panel, amorphous silicon, digital x-ray imager. *Radiographics.* 1995;15(4):993–1000.

110. Antonuk LE, Yorkston J, Huang W, et al. Megavoltage imaging with a large-area, flat-panel, amorphous silicon imager. *Int J Radiat Oncol Biol Phys.* 1996;36(3):661–672.

111. Granfors PR, Aufrichtig R. Performance of a 41x41-cm² amorphous silicon flat panel x-ray detector for radiographic imaging applications. *Med Phys.* 2000;27(6):1324–1331.

112. Munro P, Bouius DC. X-ray quantum limited portal imaging using amorphous silicon flat-panel arrays. *Med Phys.* 1998;25(5):689–702.

113. Antonuk LE, El-Mohri Y, Huang W, et al. Initial performance evaluation of an indirect-detection, active matrix flat-panel imager (AMFPI) prototype for megavoltage imaging. *Int J Radiat Oncol Biol Phys.* 1998;42(2):437–454.

114. Lachaine M, Fourkal E, Fallone BG. Investigation into the physical characteristics of active matrix flat panel imagers for radiotherapy. *Med Phys.* 2001;28(8):1689–1695.

115. Greer PB, Popescu CC. Dosimetric properties of an amorphous silicon electronic portal imaging device for verification of dynamic intensity modulated radiation therapy. *Med Phys.* 2003;30(7):1618–1627.

116. McDermott LN, Louwe RJW, Sonke JJ, et al. Dose-response and ghosting effects of an amorphous silicon electronic portal imaging device. *Med Phys.* 2004;31(2):285–295.

117. Winkler P, Hefner A, Georg D. Dose-response characteristics of an amorphous silicon EPID. *Med Phys.* 2005;32(10):3095–3105.

118. Antonuk L, Yorkston J, Huang W, et al. Radiation response characteristics of amorphous silicon arrays for megavoltage radiotherapy imaging. *IEEE Trans Nucl Sci.* 1992;39(4):1069–1073.

119. Boudry JM, Antonuk LE. Radiation damage of amorphous silicon, thin-film, field-effect transistors. *Med Phys.* 1996;23(5):743–754.

120. Papin PJ, Huang HK. A prototype amorphous selenium imaging plate system for digital radiography. *Med Phys.* 1987;14(3):322–329.

121. Mah D, Rowlands JA, Rawlinson JA. Sensitivity of amorphous selenium to x rays from 40 kVp to 18 MV: measurements and implications for portal imaging. *Med Phys.* 1998;25(4):444–456.

122. Falco T, Wang H, Fallone BG. Preliminary study of a metal/a-Se-based portal detector. *Med Phys.* 1998;25(6):814–823.

123. Pang G, Lee DL, Rowlands JA. Investigation of a direct conversion flat panel imager for portal imaging. *Med Phys.* 2001;28(10):2121–2128.

Chapter 8

INTEGRATED COMPUTED TOMOGRAPHY/LINAC SYSTEMS

C-M CHARLIE MA, PhD

Accurate patient setup, immobilization, and target localization before radiation treatment are important steps in image-guided radiation therapy (IGRT). These have become more critical as treatment margins are reduced and target doses are increased. Historically, patient positioning has been performed on the basis of skin marks and verified with portal films. These films are often of poor quality and verification is generally not performed in real time. Therefore, a safety margin is added to the clinical target volume (CTV) to form the planning target volume (PTV), accounting for the geometric uncertainties associated with patient positioning, target localization, and beam delivery. As a result, the prescription dose may be limited because of the overlap of the PTV with surrounding normal tissues. To increase the target dose for advanced radiotherapy (RT) approaches utilizing dose escalation or hypofractionation, it is necessary to reduce treatment margins to minimize the risk of damage to normal tissues. Different techniques have been investigated to improve the accuracy of patient setup and target localization including kilovoltage (kV), megavoltage (MV) x-ray computed tomography (CT), ultrasound imaging, magnetic resonance (MR) imaging, and kV or MV imaging with flat panel detectors. Among them, target localization with in-room CT techniques has played a significant role in the evaluation and clinical implementation of these on-line imaging modalities for IGRT.

Different CT systems have been developed for patient setup and target localization in RT. Currently available commercial kV CT systems used in the treatment room can be classified as either gantry-mounted or free-standing systems. A gantry-mounted CT system has its kV x-ray tube mounted on the treatment gantry of a clinical linear accelerator so that the tube and the detectors are fixed relative to the gantry and, thus, move with it during imaging. The major advantage of a gantry-mounted CT system is its ability to scan the patient in the treatment position. However, the currently available gantry-mounted cone-beam CT (CBCT) systems have much poorer image quality compared with a diagnostic CT scanner. A free-standing CT system, such as the CT-on-rails system, has its x-ray tube and detectors mounted in a conventional CT frame, which can move on "rails" when one is performing a CT scan. Such a system can be relocated in the treatment room depending on its configuration and applications. The principal advantage of a CT-on-rails system is its superior image quality as it is actually a diagnostic CT scanner. However, its major disadvantage is the requirement of the patient's relocation from the treatment position through a couch rotation to perform the CT scan. The use of CT-on-rails systems for IGRT has been reviewed by Ma and Paskalev.[1]

In this chapter, the current status of daily CT-guided RT with a focus on the hardware available commercially, the software tools for CT image processing, data analysis, and treatment guidance, and the applications of CT-on-rails for daily target localization and related clinical research in IGRT are discussed. Most clinical results reported here are based on the experiences at the Fox Chase Cancer Center (FCCC).

Commercially Available CT-on-Rails Systems

Commercial CT-on-rails systems consist of a conventional CT scanner installed in the treatment room such that it can be moved into a position for acquiring CT scans of the patient on the treatment couch. The scanner is mounted on rails along which it can move. In all systems, both the treatment couch and the CT scanner are mobile, and with known couch movement uncertainties a fixed geometrical relationship can be established between the CT coordinates and the treatment isocenter. Currently, two manufacturers provide CT-on-rails systems: Siemens AG (Erlangen, Germany) and GE Medical Systems (Waukesha, WI). It was estimated that in 2007 there were about 15 installations worldwide (13 by Siemens with five in the United States and two by GE with one in

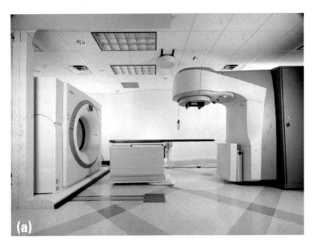 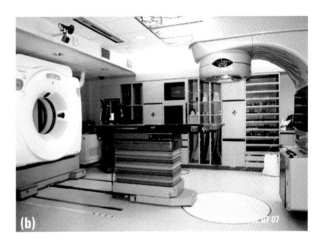

FIGURE 8-1. (a) The Siemens Primatom system that combines a Primus accelerator and a Somatom computed tomography (CT)-on-rails system (courtesy of Allen Li, PhD, Medical College of Wisconsin). **(b)** The GE-Varian Exact Targeting system that combines a Varian 21EX accelerator and a GE SmartGantry CT-on-rails system (courtesy of Lei Dong, PhD, M.D. Anderson Cancer Center, TX).

the United States), and several pending according to the manufacturers.

Siemens CT-on-Rails System

The Primatom system (Siemens AG, Erlangen, Germany) is a multifunctional hybrid configuration, consisting of a Siemens Primus linear accelerator and a modified Somatom diagnostic CT scanner that travels on two parallel rails in the treatment room (Figure 8-1a). The gantry is installed on a motor-driven carriage, which runs on rails on the floor (Figure 8-2a). The gantry is driven by a belt motor, located behind the gantry park position. The control signals and power outlet are connected to a ceiling-mounted tract to avoid collisions during operation. The accelerator gantry and the CT gantry can be positioned on opposite ends of the treatment couch. By rotating the couch 180° (or different angles depending on the configuration), the system allows a three-dimensional (3D) CT localization while the patient remains in an immobilized treatment position. The tabletop of the treatment couch is made of carbon fiber to eliminate any scanning artifacts.

The Primatom system has evolved significantly since its first installation in 2000 at Morristown Memorial Hospital, Morristown, NJ. Initially the system was equipped with a Balance Somatom scanner, which is a single-slice scanner with a minimum slice thickness of 1 mm and scan time of 1 second per rotation. The diameter of the CT gantry was 70 cm and the field of view (FOV) was 50 cm in diameter. More advanced CT scanners of the same family (Somatom) have been used in later versions of Primatom (e.g., 16-slice four-dimensional [4D] CT scanner). The gantry speed can vary between 1 mm and 100 mm per second and the gantry position accuracy is 0.5 mm.

Specially designed carbon fiber tabletops have been used to lower the position in the CT gantry. In the current version, the useable size of the FOV in the anterior–superior direction is 40 cm, which is sufficient for most applications including scans of extracranial stereotactic radiosurgery frames. The table column rotation is a standard feature for Primus treatment tables, so no further modifications are needed as far as the treatment couch is concerned. The Primus couch also has a digital readout, which is very useful when one is scanning large patients. The read out allows the user to "zero" the position of the tabletop right after the 180° rotation of the column.

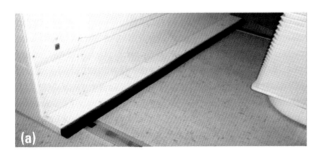 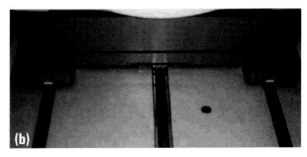

FIGURE 8-2. (a) The two rails and the collision interlock bar of the Siemens computed tomography (CT)-on-rails system and **(b)** the three rails of the GE CT-on-rails system.

The user can then move the top in all three directions to maximize the clearance in the CT gantry and to avoid potential collisions. After the scan is completed, the tabletop can be brought back to the "zero" position.

GE-Varian CT-on-Rails System

The GE-Varian (ExaCT Targeting) system combines a Varian Clinac 21EX linear accelerator (Varian Medical Systems, Palo Alto, CA) with a slightly modified Varian Exact couch with indexed immobilization, and a GE SmartGantry CT scanner (HiSpeed FX/I, GE Medical Systems, Waukesha, WI). Figure 8-1b shows the GE-Varian Exact Targeting system installed at the M.D. Anderson Cancer Center. The first GE CT-on rails system reported by Kuriyama and colleagues used the same CT scanner (SmartGantry, GE-Yokogawa Medical Systems, Tokyo, Japan) although they combined it with an EXL-15DP accelerator (Mitsubishi Electric Co, Tokyo, Japan) and a modified ram-type couch (MTC-22CS, Mitsubishi Electric Co, Tokyo, Japan).[2] The GE CT-on-rails system has three rails for the CT gantry (Figure 8-2b). The rail in the middle guides the gantry to move forward and backward linearly in the direction of scanning and the other two rails provide stability in leveling the system horizontally during scanning. A magnetic strip containing a linear scale is placed on the sidebars of the middle rail, along with a number of reference markers, which are spaced at fixed intervals, providing precise positional calibration along the rail. The gantry moves while reading the magnetic data and the reference markers to ensure accurate scanning. The CT gantry has an aperture diameter of 70 cm and the maximum gantry rotation speed is 1 second per rotation. The maximum table speed is 3.0 cm per second during helical scanning mode and 7.5 cm per second in scout scanning mode. The CT images are so calibrated that after a $180°$ couch rotation, a point at the isocenter position at the accelerator side can be mapped to the center of the acquired CT image at slice "0.0" location, thus creating a mirrored isocenter position in the CT image.

To provide a lower vertical limit for the treatment couch to scan a larger patient, the ExaCT couch top was slightly modified with a reduced width. The couch is in the left-right center position during CT scanning to avoid collision of the moving CT gantry with the treatment couch. There are other geometrical limits such as how far the CT gantry can move past the mirrored isocenter position in the CT side. For example, the CT gantry only allows 20 cm movement inferiorly past the isocenter for a head-in-first setup. This is usually not a problem because the treatment couch top (which supports the patient) can also move toward the CT gantry independently, increasing the CT imaging range in the superior–inferior direction. The CT unit is a single-slice helical CT scanner, and scanning usually takes less than 2 minutes. There have

been no recent installations of the GE-Varian ExaCT Targeting system with later CT models.

Clinical Implementation

The CT-on-rails systems that are being investigated for IGRT are based on established CT technologies. The performance criteria for these technologies have been established for diagnostic imaging and are readily adaptable for RT.

Room Configuration and Shielding

The installation of a kV imaging system will generally not impact the shielding requirement for clinical linear accelerator rooms because the shielding present in existing vaults far exceeds the requirements for kV imaging. The installation of a CT-on-rails system does, however, impact room design and functionality. For example, besides the railing and floor design considerations for a CT-on-rails system, the cost involved with larger room sizes and associated larger secondary barriers required for systems involving CT scanners complicates the introduction of such systems into existing RT rooms. On the other hand, although integrated cone-beam CT devices are more compact, one must consider the clearance of the imaging components as they move with respect to the patient as well as the treatment couch, whose isocentric rotation may become limited.

Safety Issues

Special safety procedures have been developed in the clinical implementation of CT-on-rails systems to prevent injuries to personnel and patients. Besides simple visual inspection, particular attention must be brought to those systems that use motorized or detachable mechanical components. Such components are usually equipped with collision detectors or manual interlocks that disable gantry, couch, and imager movement when triggered. For example, the Siemens sliding CT gantry has one collision safety bar on each side (Figure 8-2a) to stop the CT gantry movement if its base bar encounters an object. The procedure can only resume after the user manually clears the interlock. Users should perform routine checks to ensure that all collision detectors, switches, interlocks, and bypass systems are operational.

Geometric Accuracy

The acceptance criteria for CT-on-rails systems include the verification of the accuracy of motions from the following components: the CT gantry, the remote-controlled accelerator couch, the coincidence of the CT and linac isocenters, and the accuracy of the entire image-guidance procedure. First, the accuracy of automated couch motion and rotation, and the automatic positioning of the CT must be verified. The accuracy and precision of couch motions can be verified by using an acrylic ball bearing located at a known position within a visually opaque phantom.[2,3] Before image acquisition with the CT device, virtual simulation and planning is performed to generate a reference image with the ball bearing at the isocenter coordinates. The CT images can then be registered with respect to the reference CT scan to determine required table displacements to reposition the ball bearing at the accelerator isocenter by using the remote-controlled treatment couch. Subsequent CT imaging can confirm whether the automated couch displacements are performed accurately. The coincidence of the CT and linac isocenters can be verified by placing an acrylic ball bearing at the accelerator isocenter and rotating the couch by 180°; the ball bearing should then be at the CT isocenter. Stereotactic head or body frames can also be used for this purpose. The accuracy of the CT scanner position is assessed by imaging a crosswire phantom at selected positions, which are confirmed by the relative separation of the crosswires on the images.[2] Protocols have also been suggested to assess the mechanical accuracy of the entire patient alignment process, based on rigid phantoms.[4] Special attention should be paid to the table position (lateral, longitudinal, vertical, and isocentric rotation), as determined by read outs, imaging, and actual measurements.

Quality Assurance

The quality assurance (QA) program for an IGRT process based on CT-on-rails systems must evaluate the entire treatment process, including patient immobilization, setup, simulation imaging, treatment planning (including the production of reference images to guide corrections), verification imaging, image registration, patient position correction, and treatment. Tests that assess the entire process from beginning to end inspire confidence that the overall process is accurate and robust. In such as study, planning images of a phantom are acquired and transferred to the treatment planning system. A treatment plan is designed and reference images are produced. The phantom is then taken to the treatment unit and positioned for treatment. A verification image is acquired and registered to the reference image. Any necessary corrections to the position are made. Treatment is then delivered and measured by using an ion chamber and/or film. The dosimeter readings are compared with the expected values from the treatment plan. The frequency of such tests should be based upon an analysis of system stability during the initial operation of the CT-on-rails system. Also, the image-guidance procedures should be reviewed on a regular basis to ensure that the procedures are consistent with the initial design and to initiate appropriate changes if necessary. The review results and any new changes must be communicated among staff. The review of the guidance elements of a patient's treatment can be integrated into the institutional chart rounds and quality control programs to verify that the image-guidance procedure is operating correctly.

Clinical Applications

The first clinical application of a combined linear accelerator–CT scanner was reported for frameless, fractionated stereotactic treatments of brain and lung cancers at the National Defense Medical College, Saitama, Japan.[5-9] This system combined a conventional CT scanner with a sliding couch top to achieve the positional alignment of CT images with radiation treatment beams. A similar system with a movable couch top was later reported for paraspinal lesion and prostate cancer treatments at the Memorial Sloan-Kettering Cancer Center.[10,11]

The first CT-on-rails system that used a common couch approach was developed at the University of Yamanashi, Yamanashi, Japan.[2] Unlike previous in-room CT systems, the treatment couch was fixed and the CT scanning was accomplished by a movable gantry mounted on rails. The CT system was therefore called the "self-moving gantry CT" or the "CT-on-rails." Kuriyama and colleagues showed that this approach was practical; the positional accuracy of the common couch was 0.20 mm, 0.18 mm, and 0.39 mm in the lateral, longitudinal, and vertical directions, respectively.[2] The scan-position accuracy of the CT gantry was less than 0.4 mm in the lateral, longitudinal, and vertical directions.

Similar CT-on-rails systems have been since commercialized by major RT vendors. The initial clinical experience with the Siemens Primatom system was reported by Wong et al.[12] and Cheng et al.[13] The mechanical accuracy of the first GE-Varian ExaCT Targeting system was systematically investigated with a phantom by Court and Dong.[4] By analyzing different sources of uncertainties when one was using the system, it was found that the accuracy of the overall system was within 0.5 mm.

Although the installation of an independent diagnostic CT scanner in the treatment room is perceived to be costly and less efficient, it has a clear advantage in that it leverages all the development that has been invested in conventional CT technology over the past 20 years, leading to unquestioned image quality and clinical robustness. The geometry accuracy, in combination with excellent image quality, provides a reliable platform for the clinical evaluation of the rapidly developing in-room CT technology and its impact on different treatment sites.[1]

Many initial studies and clinical experiences with the CT-on-rails systems were focused on prostate cancer treatment. Because of its excellent image quality and its ability to image a patient's internal anatomy while the patient is in the immobilized treatment position, the CT-on-rails system was used to study the anatomical variation and soft-tissue target localization during the course of prostate treatment. Figure 8-3 shows the localization of the prostate by using the Siemens CT-on-rails system and the Volume Targeting (Siemens AG, Erlangen, Germany) prototype software. When one is using this software, the treatment planning contours and isocenter coordinates

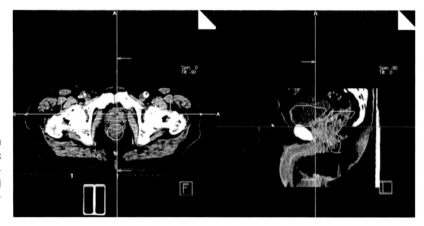

FIGURE 8-3. Localization of the prostate with the Siemens computed tomography on-rails system and Volume Targeting prototype software. The sagittal view shows that the proximal seminal vesicles are used as a landmark for longitudinal alignment.

are imported via DICOM RT. The contours are aligned with the anatomy in the pretreatment scan. The machine isocenter (before the shift) is obtained with radio-opaque markers. The sagittal view shows that the proximal seminal vesicles are used as a landmark for longitudinal alignment. Figure 8-4 shows the flowchart for the target localization procedure with the CT-on-rails system before a prostate IMRT treatment. Such a daily target alignment procedure adds an extra of ~5 minutes to the total duration for an IMRT prostate treatment time.

Extensive studies on the accuracy of prostate localization with CT-on-rails approaches were carried out by investigators from the M.D. Anderson Cancer Center and FCCC, where vast experiences with the ultrasound-based daily prostate localization technique were also accumulated. O'Daniel and coworkers showed that the systematic differences between CT-on-rails and ultrasound alignments were smaller than 1 mm, and the standard deviations (SDs) of the random differences were in the range of 3.6 mm to 4.5 mm.[14] Feigenberg et al. confirmed such low systematic differences but observed SDs of the random differences between 2.2 mm and 2.4 mm (Figure 8-5).[15] These studies demonstrated that CT-on-rails could be used as a gold standard to evaluate other alignment technologies. Their results also suggest that, contrary to the findings of Langen et al.[16] and Van den Heuvel et al.,[17] if performed by a well-trained user and with a proper technique, ultrasound-based prostate localization can be a reliable technique for prostate alignment.

The ability to acquire the 3D patient geometry before an RT treatment also allows for the evaluation of target coverage and critical structure sparing for dose escalation and hypofractionation studies. A randomized clinical trial was carried out at FCCC to compare 76 Gy in 38 fractions (Arm I: standard IMRT) to 70.2 Gy in 26 fractions (Arm II: hypofractioned IMRT). The PTV margins in arms I and II were 5 mm and 3 mm posteriorly, respectively, and 8 mm and 7 mm, respectively, in all other dimensions. The PTV dose to 95% of the volume (D95%) was at least the prescription dose, with a desired

dose gradient of 20% or less. For arm I, the rectal volume receiving 65 Gy (V65Gy) and V40Gy parameters were ≤ 17% and ≤ 35%. The bladder V65Gy and V40Gy parameters were ≤ 25% and ≤ 50%. For Arm II, the rectal V50Gy and V31Gy parameters were ≤ 17% and ≤ 35%. The bladder V50Gy and V31Gy parameters were ≤ 25% and ≤ 50%. The CT-on-rails system was used for target localization for both arms and a retrospective study was performed on the target coverage and rectal sparing based on 98 CT-on-rails scans immediately after the dose delivery for 15 patients. The results showed that 7.1% of the treatment fractions exhibited compromised target coverage; the minimal PTV dose was less than 65 Gy for these fractions assuming that the CT-on-rails scans represented the actual patient geometry during the treatment. Chen and coworkers demonstrated the benefits of an empty rectum during CT simulation; it is relatively easier to achieve the rectal dose criteria for a large rectal volume

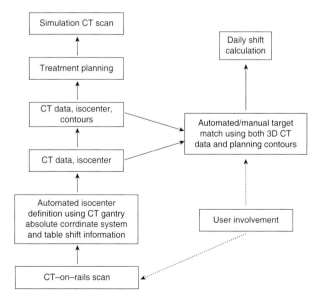

FIGURE 8-4. The workflow for the daily target alignment procedure using the CT-on-rails system.

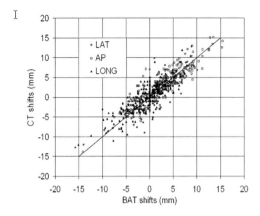

FIGURE 8-5. System-versus-system shifts for the B-mode Acquisition and Targeting ultrasound system (Nomos, Sewickley, PA) and the Primatom CT-on-Rails system (Siemens Medical Solutions, Concord, CA). Data for 218 alignments are presented. The solid line is the line of perfect agreement between the two systems. The correlation coefficients are 0.877 (anterior–posterior), 0.842 (lateral), and 0.831 (longitudinal).

during treatment planning but the actual doses received by the rectum can be worse for some patients when the rectal volume becomes smaller in subsequent treatments (Figure 8-6).[18]

The CT-on-rails system can also significantly improve the localization of the prostate bed in post-prostatectomy patients. For such patients, the prostate bed is a target that is not associated with a given anatomical shape and, thus, the target alignment is a very challenging task. A technique that employs CT-based ultrasound templates was developed and evaluated by Paskalev and colleagues at FCCC.[19] In this technique the user performs ultrasound localization of the prostate bed with the aid of a template ultrasound alignment. The template is made on the basis of a real-time CT alignment on the first day of the treatment. The distribution of the differences between the

template-assisted ultrasound alignments and control CT alignments are shown in Figure 8-7. These data were from the first 30 patients who underwent treatment to the prostate bed, after the evaluation study was completed. The results show that a clinical margin of 8 mm fully covers the target for all but three alignments (n = 183), clearly demonstrating the improvement in alignment accuracy with the template-assisted ultrasound technique.

In addition to soft-tissue target localization, the CT-on-rails system also plays an important role in the alignment of patients with brain tumors, because matching bone intensity of the skull is an easy task in terms of automated 3D image fusion. One of the most clinically important applications is the alignment of patients undergoing fractionated stereotactic radiosurgery (SRS), where the dose gradients outside the target are steep and the margins are small. In such cases, both precise CT-to-CT image fusion and correct transformation of the SRS coordinates defined by the SRS frame are required. Paskalev and others developed an integrated software system in conjunction with the SRS planning system for full 3D transformation between the SRS coordinate systems.[20] The software was tested by using CT-on-rails scans of patients undergoing single-fraction treatment with a frame fixed to the outer table of the skull. For these patients, the initial and recalculated SRS coordinates of any point should be identical and any discrepancies can be attributed to uncertainties of the method. Figure 8-8 shows a plot of the differences between initial and recalculated SRS coordinates. Robar and coworkers used small alignment contours to track the SRS coordinates of anatomically identical points (the centers of the contours) in both localization and simulation scans, and subsequently used these points for coordinate transformation.[21]

The stereotactic application of the CT-on-rails technique covers not only brain patients but also extracranial

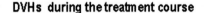

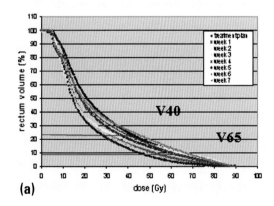

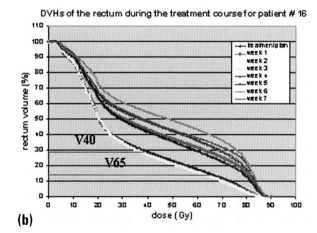

(a)   **(b)**

FIGURE 8-6. The rectal dose volume histogram (DVHs) based on the recomputed dose distributions using the computed tomography–on-rails scans immediately after an intensity-modulated radiation therapy (IMRT) treatment. The rectal DVHs for the original treatment plans are also shown. The original plan was generated on the basis of an empty rectum (a) and the original plan was generated on the basis of a large rectum (b).

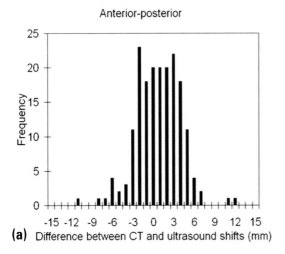

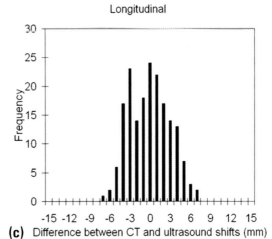

FIGURE 8-7. Histograms of the differences between ultrasound alignments performed with the aid of a computed tomography (CT)–based template, and those based on the control CT scans acquired on the same day. In almost all cases the clinical margin of 8 mm fully covers the target.

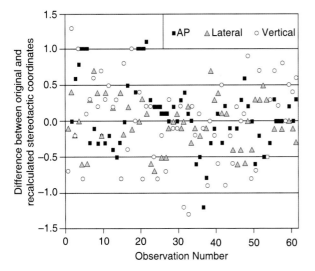

FIGURE 8-8. Testing results of an automated alignment method for stereotactic brain tumor patients. The stereotactic coordinates are recalculated on the basis of a pretreatment scan acquired with the Siemens computed tomography–on-rails system. All patients had the frame fixed to the outer table of the skull; therefore, the coordinates of any anatomical point should be identical in the two different scans. The differences are attributed to the uncertainties of the algorithm.

procedures. In these cases, the issues related to intrafraction target motion need to be addressed separately. For targets that move considerably during the treatment (such as lung tumors) the interfraction shifts are usually determined on the basis of an anatomical structure that is adjacent to the tumor but does not experience intrafraction motion. Such a structure may be the vertebra, for example. A procedure for treating paraspinal lesions using the CT-on-rails system was developed by Shiu and coworkers.[22] Wong and colleagues also reported a retrospective study to evaluate the target coverage for stereotactic lung RT in which the CT-on-rails system was used in the pretreatment setup.[12]

The CT-on-rails systems have also played an important role in the evaluation and clinical implementation of adaptive RT. A study was carried out on volume changes of head and neck tumors during the course of treatment by Barker and others.[23] Their results showed that in some cases the internal anatomy changed so significantly during the course of treatment that repeated simulation and planning were necessary. Such an adaptive procedure is already achievable with CT-on-rails because of its superior image quality. Ideally, the daily CT images and the actual treatment positions will be used to compute the daily delivered dose distributions for some sites where large deviations may occur to the target volume or the nearby critical structures. Deformable image registration will be performed automatically to map the daily delivered dose to the original planning CT to compute a cumulative delivered dose distribution. This up-to-date cumulative dose distribution will then be compared with the planned dose distribution on weekly basis to determine if an interventional treatment plan should be created for subsequent treatment fractions. This adaptive and image feedback-based treatment procedure is under development by many investigators.[24-30] Many technical challenges exist such as real-time target or structure delineation, treatment optimization, and dosimetry verification. The current infrastructure may also limit the daily use of CT images because of enormous storage and manpower requirements. Therefore, image-guided on-line adaptive radiotherapy has not been effectively used in routine clinical practice yet.

Clinical Considerations

Radiotherapy treatment setup is traditionally performed by therapists who manually position the patient based on skin marks and alignment lasers. Portal films or electronic portal imaging devices (EPIDs) have been used to facilitate target localization based on bony structures and/or implanted fiducial markers for conformal RT. Software tools were developed to improve image processing, data analysis, and structure recognition for EPID patient alignment. CT-on-rails systems can provide real-time 3D geometric information that requires effective and efficient software tools to perform either off-line or on-line image-guided and adaptive RT. Other important issues must also be considered in the clinical implementation of such advanced techniques including image acquisition, data analysis, structure recognition, margin determination, and decision-making in daily image-guided treatment procedures.

Image Acquisition

An important parameter in image acquisition is the volume of interest. Depending on the purpose of the image guidance process, either a full volume or a reduced volume may be selected. The slice spacing is crucial to the CT resolution in the superior–inferior direction and, therefore, should not be more than 3 mm for a target localization scan. In earlier CT-on-rails systems, the rate of image acquisition depends upon the frequency of intervention that is intended or possible. Clearly, correction of respiratory motion would not only require a high frame rate (> 5 frames per second) for imaging, but also would require a similarly fast mechanism for correcting the patient and beam coregistration. Newer Siemens and GE CT-on-rails systems are capable of 4D scans that are especially

useful for target localization in the thoracic regions. Other issues that need to be considered include the integration of various devices into the image-guidance procedure and the design of an appropriate image acquisition sequence for them. Typical systems being used clinically include breath-hold devices, gating systems, and tracking systems.

The frequency of imaging is another parameter for the image guidance: real-time, once or twice per treatment session, or weekly. The frequency may be determined on the basis of the capabilities of the imaging system and the goal of the image-guidance procedure. CT-on-rails systems have the highest image quality for high-precision target localization, which have been used to develop practical guidelines for IGRT. Daily on-line CT-based target localization has been performed at FCCC for stereotactic SRS and stereotactic body RT (SBRT) of lung cancer as well as prostate and post-prostatectomy RT. The CT-based target localization process typically adds an additional 5 minutes to the treatment procedure. Pre- and posttreatment CT scans have been acquired for special protocol patients to investigate proper margins for dose escalation and hypofractionation studies. Weekly image acquisition has been found to be adequate to monitor the geometrical changes of the treatment geometry for head and neck cancer patients, which, if determined to be significant, will require replanning, dosimetric verification, and approval of the new treatment plans.

Software Tools

Effective and efficient software tools are essential to the clinical implementation and the integration of in-room CT techniques with routine clinical treatments. The earlier CT-on-rails systems from both commercial vendors were not utilized in their fullest capacity because of the lack of software tools for CT-guided image registration. Hua and colleagues developed a semiautomatic image-alignment tool that only requires contouring of the extent of the prostate in five axial slices, instead of the whole prostate volume, for image registration.[10] Such limited manual contouring still takes time and the curve fitting may not work well when the curvature of the prostate is flat in the superior–inferior direction for the selected axial slices.

An in-house software image analysis tool was proposed by Court et al. and O'Daniel et al. for their GE CT-on-rails system that employed a gray-scale image-based automatic image-registration technique.[4,14] The algorithm took advantage of the well-calibrated CT numbers for prostate images and used the gray-scale information to directly compare with the image intensity in the same region of interest in the planning CT, allowing direct soft tissue registration for the prostate. The algorithm was shown to be reliable (less than 1% failure rate as tested in 120 CT images of seven prostate patients) and could tolerate some minor changes in the shape of the prostate caused by variable rectal and bladder filling.

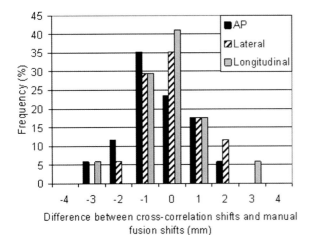

FIGURE 8-9. Distribution of the differences between daily shifts, automatically calculated by using a cross-correlation objective function and shifts derived through manual fusion for the same prostate cancer patients.

Paskalev and coworkers used an image correlation technique to developed a similar gray-scale–based image registration algorithm for their Siemens CT-on-rails system.[31] The algorithm was tested on 23 CT images from six different patients and was demonstrated to be effective and reliable. Figure 8-9 shows the distribution of the differences between the shifts, automatically calculated with this cross-correlation method and shifts derived through manual image fusion for the same patients. These investigators also showed that this method was very reliable when they were coregistering images with significant noise. Currently available CT-on-rails systems provide advanced software tools for image registration and are well-integrated with the treatment systems to improve the efficiency of the target localization procedure.

Determination of Treatment Margins

The application of advanced target localization techniques can significantly reduce, but not eliminate, geometric uncertainties. For example, it is hoped that if target localization uncertainties can be reduced with advanced imaging techniques, a smaller PTV may be used, leading to a possible reduction of normal tissue complications and/or the opportunity for dose escalation. One must consider many clinical issues in determining an appropriate PTV margin, such as the nature and magnitude of uncertainties because of patient positioning and organ motion (both random and systematic), as well as the desired goals of image-guided treatment modifications.

The PTV margin should be determined on the basis of clinical experience and the estimated impact of geometric uncertainties. It is difficult to simultaneously consider the impact of all factors that influence the selection of a margin. A common approach is to add a margin that is twice the SD of combined geometric uncertainties. Assuming a Gaussian distribution of uncertainties, two SDs will include 95% of all displacements. This approach

leads to population-based PTV margins that may not be optimal for many clinical situations. For example, it does not consider the importance of the dose gradients at the edge of the PTV and does not separate the effects of random and systematic uncertainties. Additionally, Gaussian distributions may not be appropriate for some uncertainties, such as those associated with respiratory motion, and for target localization uncertainties with few treatment fractions.

Alternative approaches have been proposed including margin recipes and margin calculators.[32–36] The former is a set of linear equations that describe the required margin in terms of the SDs of random and systematic uncertainties based on specific, clinically relevant criteria (e.g., 90% of patients receive 95% of the prescription dose). The strengths of margin recipes are the explicit separation of random and systematic uncertainties, the incorporation of dose gradients, and clinically meaningful criteria. However, they only consider the treatment target, not the nearby critical structures, and still assume the uncertainty distribution is Gaussian, thus, they will only work for a large number of treatment fractions. Margin calculators can use dose distributions, anatomical contours, and distributions of geometric uncertainty as input, simulate the effect of uncertainties, and return an appropriate margin to the treatment planner. Only the intentions of the planner need to be provided to the software (i.e., a PTV margin that will lead to 90% of patients receiving a minimum CTV dose of 95%). Such tools can use any evaluation parameters, including, but not limited to, the minimum or mean CTV dose, dose-volume specifications, and the tumor control probability. A margin calculation process can be considered as "inverse margin calculation," analogous to inverse treatment planning; it receives treatment criteria as input and returns an optimal margin as output.

It should be mentioned that all the methods described previously are population-based, meaning that individual patients are planned with the same general PTV margin, regardless of their individual geometric uncertainties. With the use of a CT-on-rails system, treatment verification and PTV definition can be used iteratively to produce patient-specific PTVs. This will be the ultimate form of adaptive RT. Recent studies have proposed to incorporate geometric uncertainties in the planning process and, therefore, reduce or eliminate the use of a PTV.[37–45] Before this approach is tested and accepted for clinical applications, the PTV remains an excellent concept for standardizing practice in routine RT.

Decision-Making in Daily Target Localization Procedures

For one to implement daily target localization procedures with CT-on-rails, an assessment must be made of the information available, the decisions to be made, and the individuals or disciplines that are responsible for these decisions. These procedures must be carried out with rigorous and documented strategies that are based on the daily image information, which will significantly impact the appropriate PTV margins to be used at various steps throughout the course of therapy and the efficiency of these image-guided procedures. Communication between the implementation team members and the routine operators is an important area of the utmost concern from a safety perspective. The implementation team should also review the strategies periodically and make adjustments if necessary.

Conclusions

This chapter has reviewed the CT-on-rails systems and their applications in IGRT. As described in detail, freestanding CT systems such as the CT-on-rails systems that use conventional diagnostic CT scanners provide the best image quality and appropriate geometric accuracy for patient setup and target localization for advanced treatment techniques involving high fractional doses and small treatment margins. These systems are playing an important role in the evaluation of other recently developed in-room CT techniques for image guidance and the results based on these systems will provide definitive answers to some important clinical questions concerning the effectiveness, efficiency, and cost of on-line 3D image guidance and its impact on cancer management.

In the past decade, the introduction of image guidance has provided new opportunities to further improve treatment accuracy and precision as well as new challenges for its efficient and effective implementation. The goal of IGRT is to match the clinical objective with the appropriate technology. Implementation of an advanced imaging technique requires rigorous characterization and validation of its performance, properly established quality assurance procedures, and adequate expertise for routine and specific clinical applications. Because of the inherent uncertainties of any image-guidance techniques, the truth is often not known and one should be aware of the residual error related to the implementation of the correction based on the imaging technique used.

References

1. Ma C-M, Paskalev K. In-room CT techniques for image-guided radiation therapy. *Med Dosim.* 2006;31(1):30–39.
2. Kuriyama K, Onishi H, Sano N, et al. A new irradiation unit constructed of self-moving gantry-CT and linac. *Int J Radiat Oncol Biol Phys.* 2003;55:428–435.
3. Sharpe MB, Moseley DJ, Haycocks T, et al. An integrated volumetric imaging and guidance system for targeting of soft-tissue structures in radiotherapy. *Int J Radiat Oncol Biol Phys.* 2003;57:S183.
4. Court LE, Dong L. Automatic registration of the prostate for computed-tomography-guided radiotherapy. *Med Phys.* 2003;30:2750–2757.
5. Uematsu M, Fukui T, Shioda A, et al. A dual computed tomography linear accelerator unit for stereotactic radiation therapy: a new approach without cranially fixated stereotactic frames. *Int J Radiat Oncol Biol Phys.* 1996;35:587–592.
6. Uematsu M, Shioda A, Tahara K, et al. Focal, high dose, and fractionated modified stereotactic radiation therapy for lung carcinoma patients: a preliminary experience. *Cancer.* 1998;82:1062–1070.
7. Uematsu M, Sonderegger M, Shioda A, et al. Daily positioning accuracy of frameless stereotactic radiation therapy with a fusion of computed tomography and linear accelerator (focal) unit: evaluation of z-axis with a z-marker. *Radiother Oncol.* 1999;50:337–339.
8. Uematsu M, Shioda A, Suda A, et al. Intrafractional tumor position stability during computed tomography (CT)-guided frameless stereotactic radiation therapy for lung or liver cancers with a fusion of CT and linear accelerator (FOCAL) unit. *Int J Radiat Oncol Biol Phys.* 2000;48:443–448.
9. Uematsu M, Shioda A, Suda A, et al. Computed tomography-guided frameless stereotactic radiotherapy for stage I non-small cell lung cancer: a 5-year experience. *Int J Radiat Oncol Biol Phys.* 2001;51:666–670.
10. Yenice KM, Lovelock DM, Hunt MA, et al. CT image-guided intensity-modulated therapy for paraspinal tumors using stereotactic immobilization. *Int J Radiat Oncol Biol Phys.* 2003;55:583–593.
11. Hua CH, Lovelock DM, Mageras GS, et al. Development of a semi-automatic alignment tool for accelerated localization of the prostate. *Int J Radiat Oncol Biol Phys.* 2003;54:811–824.
12. Wong JR, Grimm L, Uematsu M, et al. Treatment of lung tumor with stereotactic radiation therapy using the world's first PRIMATOM system: a case report. *Electromedia.* 2001;69:127–130.
13. Cheng C-W, Wong J, Grimm L, et al. Commissioning and clinical implementation of a sliding gantry CT scanner installed in an existing treatment room and early clinical experience for precise tumor localization. *Am J Clinical Oncol.* 2003;26:e28–e36.
14. O'Daniel JC, Dong L, Zhang L, et al. Dosimetric comparison of four target alignment methods for prostate cancer radiotherapy. *Int J Radiat Oncol Biol Phys.* 2006;66(3):883–891.
15. Feigenberg S, Paskalev K, McNeeley S, et al. Comparing computed tomography localization with daily ultrasound during image-guided radiation therapy for the treatment of prostate cancer: a prospective evaluation. *J Appl Clin Med Phys.* 2007;8(3):2268.
16. Langen KM, Pouliot J, Anezinos C, et al. Evaluation of ultrasound-based prostate localization for image guided radiation therapy. *Int J Radiat Oncol Biol Phys.* 2003;57(3):635–644.
17. Van den Heuvel F, Powell T, Seppi E, et al. Independent verification of ultrasound based image guided radiation treatment, using electronic portal imaging and implanted gold markers. *Med Phys.* 2003;30:2878–2887.
18. Chen L, Paskalev K, Zhu J, et al. Image guided radiation therapy for prostate IMRT: daily rectal dose variations during the treatment course. In: Bissonnette JP, ed. Proc. of the 15th

International Conference on the Use of Computer in Radiation Therapy (ICCR). Ontario, CA: Novel Digital Publishing; 2007; Volume I: 410–414.

19. Paskalev K, Feigenberg S, Jacob R, et al. Target localization for post-prostatectomy patients using CT and ultrasound image guidance, *J Appl Clin Med Phys.* 2005;6(4):40–49.

20. Paskalev K, Feigenberg S, Wang L, et al. A method for repositioning of stereotactic brain patients with the aid of real-time CT image guidance. *Phys Med Biol.* 2005;50:N201–N207.

21. Robar J, Clark B, Schella J, Kim C. Analysis of patient repositioning accuracy in precision radiation therapy using automated image fusion. *J Appl Clin Med Phys.* 2005;6(1):71–83.

22. Shiu AS, Chang EL, Ye JS, et al. Near simultaneous computed tomography image-guided stereotactic spinal radiotherapy: an emerging paradigm for achieving true stereotaxy. *Int J Radiat Oncol Biol Phys.* 2003;57:605–613.

23. Barker JL, Garden AS, Ang KK, et al. Quantification of volumetric and geometric changes occurring during fractionated radiotherapy for head-and-neck cancer using an integrated CT/linear accelerator system. *Int J Radiat Oncol Biol Phys.* 2004;59:960–970.

24. Liang J, Yan D. Reducing uncertainties in volumetric image based deformable organ registration. *Med Phys.* 2003;30:2116–2122.

25. Birkner M, Yan D, Alber M, et al. Adapting inverse planning to patient and organ geometrical variation: algorithm and implementation. *Med Phys.* 2003;30:2822–2831.

26. Brock KK, McShan DL, Ten Haken RK, et al. Inclusion of organ deformation in dose calculations. *Med Phys.* 2003;30:290–295.

27. Keller H, Ritter MA, Mackie TR. Optimal stochastic correction strategies for rigid-body target motion. *Int J Radiat Oncol Biol Phys.* 2003;55:261–270.

28. Lu W, Chen M-L, Olivera G, et al. Fast free-form deformable registration via calculus of variations. *Phys Med Biol.* 2004;49:3067–3087.

29. Ma C-M, Shan G, Hu W, et al. A dose-guided, volumetric target localization technique for prostate IGRT. *Int J Radiat Oncol Biol Phys.* 2009;75(3):S579.

30. Shan G, Chen L, Hu W, et al. Dosimetric evaluation of image guided radiation therapy for prostate cancer. *Med Phys.* 2009;36(6):2496.

31. Paskalev K, Ma C-M, Jacob R, et al. Daily target localization for prostate patients based on 3D image correlation. *Phys Med Biol.* 2004;49:931–939.

32. Bel A, van Herk M, Lebesque JV. Target margins for random geometrical treatment uncertainties in conformal radiotherapy. *Med Phys.* 1996;23:1537–1545.

33. McKenzie AL, van Herk M, Mijnheer B. The width of margins in radiotherapy treatment plans. *Phys Med Biol.* 2000;45:3331–3342.

34. Stroom JC, de Boer HCJ, Huizenga H, et al. Inclusion of geometrical uncertainties in radiotherapy treatment planning by means of coverage probability. *Int J Radiat Oncol Biol Phys.* 1999;43:905–919.

35. van Herk M, Remeijer P, Rasch C, et al. The probability of correct target dosage: dose-population histograms for deriving treatment margins in radiotherapy. *Int J Radiat Oncol Biol Phys.* 2000;47:1121–1135.

36. Craig T, Sharpe M, Haycocks T, et al. Comparison of correction protocols for image-guided radiation therapy. *Lecture Notes in Computer Science.* 2003;2879:264–270.

37. Niemierko A, Goitein M. Implementation of a model for estimating tumor control probability for an inhomogeneously irradiated tumor. *Radiother Oncol.* 1993;29:140–147.

38. Leong J. Implementation of random positioning error in computerised radiation treatment planning systems as a result of fractionation. *Phys Med Biol.* 1987;32:327–334.

39. Beckham WA, Keall PJ, Siebers JV. A fluence-convolution method to calculate radiation therapy dose distributions that incorporate random set-up error. *Phys Med Biol.* 2002;47:3465–3473.

40. Brock KK, McShan DL, Ten Haken RK, et al. Inclusion of organ deformation in dose calculations. *Med Phys.* 2003;30:290–295.

41. Craig T, Battista J, Van Dyk J. Limitations of a convolution method for modeling geometric uncertainties in radiation therapy. I. The effect of shift invariance. *Med Phys.* 2003;30:2001–2011.

42. Jaffray DA, Yan D, Wong JW. Managing geometric uncertainty in conformal intensity-modulated radiation therapy. *Semin Radiat Oncol.* 1999;9:4–19.

43. Keall PJ, Beckham WA, Booth JT, et al. A method to predict the effect of organ motion and set-up variations on treatment plans. *Australas Phys Eng Sci Med.* 1999;22:48–52.

44. Craig T, Battista J, Van Dyk J. Limitations of a convolution method for modeling geometric uncertainties in radiation therapy. II. The effect of a finite number of fractions. *Med Phys.* 2003;30:2012–2020.

45. Lujan AE, Larsen EW, Balter JM, et al. A method for incorporating organ motion due to breathing into 3D dose calculations. *Med Phys.* 2003;26:715–720.

Chapter 9

KILOVOLTAGE IMAGING SYSTEMS

MASAYORI ISHIKAWA, PhD, SRIJIT KAMATH, PhD, CHENG B. SAW, PhD,
ANIL SETHI, PhD, HIROKI SHIRATO, MD, WILLIAM Y. SONG, PhD

With the advent of modern radiotherapy (RT) treatment techniques, such as intensity-modulated RT (IMRT), stereotactic radiosurgery (SRS), and stereotactic body RT (SBRT), clinicians have become acutely aware of the necessity for image guidance. To satisfy this need, several manufacturers have incorporated kilovoltage (kV) x-ray imaging systems with their existing designs. The lower energy produced by these x-rays provides enhanced contrast particularly between soft tissue and bone. These imagers can provide image guidance through two distinct mechanisms. The first is through planar imaging in which standard x-ray images are compared with digitally reconstructed radiographs (DRRs) from the planning computed tomography (CT) scan. By aligning these images with image registration software, the patient position can be modified primarily on the basis of bony anatomy. In the cone beam CT (CBCT) mode, volumetric images are acquired while the patient is on the treatment table. Three-dimensional (3D) image registration is then performed that can be used to ensure alignment of soft tissue. The technologies associated with these approaches will be described in this chapter.

Accuray CyberKnife

The technology of the CyberKnife Robotic Radiosurgery System (Accuray Inc, Sunnyvale, CA) has been recently described by Saw et al.[1] on the implementation of the fiducial-based image registration and Ozhasoglu et al.[2] on the Synchrony, the respiratory tracking system. In addition, image registration techniques, which are essential components for this system, have been published by Saw et al.[3] These articles are contributions to the fourth special issue published in the journal *Medical Dosimetry* in the Image-Guided Radiation Therapy (IGRT) series. Much of the materials described here are included in these three articles.

The CyberKnife is a frameless robotic radiosurgery system consisting of a lightweight X-band 6-MV lin-

ear accelerator mounted onto a precisely controlled industrial robotic arm and an image-guidance system (Figure 9-1). Because the design of this delivery system is different from that of conventional medical linear accelerators, it is considered a specialized delivery system having its own acceptance testing and commissioning protocols, treatment planning system, and quality assurance program. The CyberKnife was introduced by the neurosurgeon, John R. Adler, at Stanford University in 1990.[4] Since its introduction, the CyberKnife has undergone several generations of modifications. The third generation is shown in Figure 9-1.

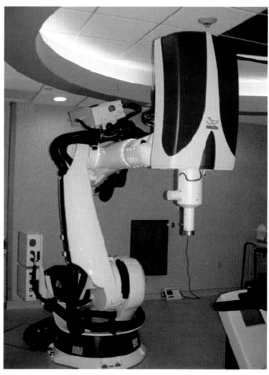

FIGURE 9-1. A third-generation CyberKnife robotic radiosurgery system. Reproduced with permission from Saw et al.[1]

The flexibility of the robotic arm allows the Cyber-Knife to position and/or reposition accurately the radiation source in the space around a patient. The earlier version of the robotic arm in the CyberKnife was from the Japanese Fanuc robot[5] and the later version, the German KUKA KR 240 robot.[6] The movement of the robotic arm is computerized and controlled by a six-axis robotic manipulator. This robotic arm movement offers significantly increased range of beam directions for aiming at the target compared with a gantry-mounted medical linear accelerator as shown in Figure 9-2. The system is also capable of performing noncoplanar and nonisocentric beam delivery and can be used to generate a highly conformal radiation dose distribution to irregularly shaped target volume with steep dose gradients, minimizing the radiation dose to surrounding normal tissues.

The 6-MV photon beam produced by the CyberKnife is highly focused and limited to circular beam sizes. It is collimated with a set of fixed tungsten collimators producing a beam of sizes 5 mm, 7.5 mm, 10 mm, 12.5 mm, 15 mm, 20 mm, 25 mm, 30 mm, 35 mm, 40 mm, 50 mm, and 60 mm in diameter at a distance of 80 cm source-axial distance (SAD) from the radiation source. The dose rate for the third-generation CyberKnife is 400 monitor units per minute (MU/min) but has been increased to 600 MU/min for the fourth-generation system, significantly reducing overall treatment times. The latest version of the CyberKnife is capable of producing a dose rate as high as 800 MU/min. Accuray has also announced the introduction of the IRIS, a dynamic variable-aperture collimator to replace the fixed collimators.[7] The IRIS has two offset banks of six prismatic tungsten segments to form 12 unique beam field sizes that are virtually identical to those created with the set of fixed collimators.

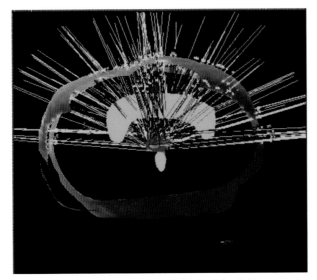

FIGURE 9-2. A number of nodes available on CyberKnife system for dose delivery. Reproduced with permission from Saw et al.[1]

The CyberKnife also has a target locating subsystem (TLS) to perform IGRT by localizing the target and subsequently tracking it. The TLS consists of two diagnostic x-ray sources—detection system pairs and software for image registration—mounted on the ceiling of the treatment vault. When the x-ray sources are energized, they will produce two real-time orthogonal radiographs (referred as live radiographs) captured on the two detection systems positioned on the left and right sides of the treatment couch. The image detection systems consist of 20 cm × 20 cm amorphous silicon detectors for the third-generation unit (41 cm × 41 cm for the fourth-generation unit but mounted in the floor) capable of generating high-resolution digital images. These images are processed automatically and image registration is performed to determine the target position.

Initially, the target must be brought within the geometrical treatment range of the CyberKnife. To comply with this requirement, a robotic treatment couch that has six degrees of freedom (DOF) or motions is used in the newer generation CyberKnife. The target position as determined from the live radiographs is then communicated through a real-time control loop to the robotic manipulator that adjusts and directs the radiation beam accordingly to within 1 mm spatial accuracy.

The CyberKnife can adapt to the changes in the patient position during the dose delivery period. Typically, 100 to 150 beams are used in a single fraction or treatment session. Each beam is defined by a node (x, y, z) position. At each node, the linear accelerator has 12 rotational positions defined by the solid angles (α, β, γ) for beam orientation. The radiation beam is turned off during robotic arm movement between nodes that are specified in the treatment plan. After the linear accelerator moves to the next node, live radiographs can be acquired to assess the target position again. If there is a change in the target position, the linear accelerator is adjusted accordingly to the required beam orientation for accurate conformal dose delivery. Although the target position can be evaluated after each nodal dose delivery, the evaluation is commonly done after irradiating through a few nodes to reduce treatment time. As presented, the machine essentially tracks the target position during treatment to perform adaptive radiosurgery or radiotherapy. An analysis of the accuracy of the CyberKnife system found that the machine has a clinically relevant accuracy of less than 1 mm. Hence, the CyberKnife precision is comparable with published localization errors in current frame-based irradiation systems.[8-9]

Patient Alignment and Target Localization

The CyberKnife robotic system offers no stereotactic frame-based option but relies on image guidance for patient alignment and target localization. Patient alignment and target localization are performed by taking orthogonal live radiographs and comparing them with a library of DRRs. This DRR library is generated from the CT image data set acquired for treatment planning with systematic variation of patient positions and orientations to simulate patient movements. A particular DRR that best matches the live radiographs is identified through an image registration methodology, such as the landmark-based technique using bony structures or fiducial markers. The use of this technique differentiates the CyberKnife as a frameless radiosurgery system. It should be noted that this landmark-based image registration methodology assumes the relationship between the landmarks and the tumor is fixed, which is not always valid, especially in those anatomical regions where the tumor is at distance from the bony structures. However, newer technologies such as the Xsight Spine Tracking System (Accuray Inc, Sunnyvale, CA) is capable of tracking the tumor based on the spinal processes that are less rigid by using deformable algorithms. The new target position is transmitted to the robotic arm manipulator so that the radiation beams will be redirected based on the updated target position. This process can be repeated between nodes and, thus, allows the treatment unit to track patient position changes during treatment.

An essential component of the CyberKnife is the use of image-guided technology for locating and tracking targets. The procedure referred to as image registration compares a live image data set to a reference image data set giving the current patient position relative to reference position defined at the time of CT scanning for planning purposes. There is a number of methodologies for performing image registration as described in a recent article published by Saw et al.[3] See Chapters 15D, 19E, 20F, 24D, and 24G for discussions on the application of the Cyber-Knife technology in a variety of tumor sites.

Motion-Gated Dose Delivery

The CyberKnife technology also addresses the issue of target motion when one is using the Synchrony Respiratory Tracking System (Accuray Inc, Sunnyvale, CA). The Synchrony system is used primarily to treat lung tumors, which are in motion because of breathing. The system uses a combination of surgically implanted internal fiducials and light-emitting optical fibers (external markers) mounted onto a vest worn by the patient. The external markers are adjusted on the vest so that they are located at the abdominal area to mimic the movement of the diaphragm and lung. Because the tumor is in continuous motion, the use of multiple live radiographs to track it would lead to a prohibitively high radiation dose to the patient. To overcome this issue, the CyberKnife system acquires live radiographs of the internal fiducials periodically and predicts their location at future times by using the motion of the external markers. The light from the external markers is tracked continuously with a charged

couple device (CCD) camera with the signals fed into the TLS. A computer algorithm is used to create a functional correlation model that represents the motion of the internal fiducials in correspondence to the external markers. Based on the motion of the external markers, the Synchrony system tracks the location of the internal fiducial markers and, hence, the tumor. The correlation model can be updated at any time if the breathing pattern changes during treatment. As such, there is no assumption made regarding the reproducibility of the patient breathing pattern. See Chapter 17B for an illustration of the use of the Synchrony Respiratory Tracking System in an early stage lung cancer patient.

BrainLAB Novalis - ExacTrac

The ExacTrac (BrainLAB, Feldkirchen, Germany) is an automated 6D patient positioning and verification system that uses infrared (IR) markers and stereoscopic x-ray image guidance (Figure 9-3a and b). The system is capable of delivering with submillimeter precision image-guided cranial and extracranial SRS treatments. The treatment unit is a 6-MV linear accelerator equipped with a micro-multileaf collimator (MLC; m3). The m3 is composed of two banks of 26 pairs of tungsten alloy (95% W, 3.4% Ni, and 1.6% Fe) leaves with variable leaf width.[10] The innermost 14 leaf pairs are 3-mm wide, followed by six pairs of 4.5-mm leaves and, finally, the outermost leaves are 5.5-mm thick. The leaves can create any field shape up to 9.8 $cm^2 \times 10\ cm^2$. In addition to the MLC leaves, the system is also capable of treatments involving circular cones of diameter ranging from 4 mm to 40 mm.

System Components

The BrainLAB image guidance system has two main components: an IR-based patient positioning and tracking system and a radiographic kV x-ray system.[11-13] The unique design features of the system are: (a) integrated with the treatment planning system (TPS); (b) capable of fully automated patient setup and position verification; and (c) able to provide continuous monitoring of patient position in real time via IR markers. These special features allow for a more efficient clinical workflow.

Briefly, the image-guided treatment begins with CT scanning of the patient with IR markers. The latter are automatically registered in the TPS and, hence, are spatially related to the treatment isocenter. In the treatment room, the patient is first automatically set up by using the IR markers with feedback from the TPS (Figure 9-4). Next, kV x-ray images are acquired to correct patient positioning and verify alignment with the treatment isocenter.

The IR system consists of a ceiling-mounted IR/video camera that sends a low-intensity signal to the IR reflecting spheres (markers) placed on the patient's surface.

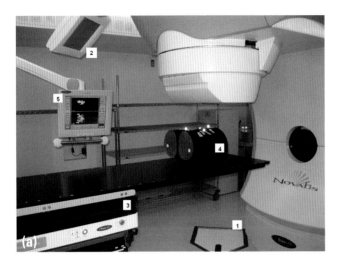
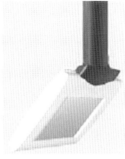
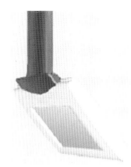
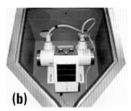
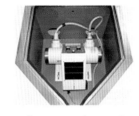

FIGURE 9-3. (a) BrainLAB Novalis linear accelerator equipped with the ExacTrac image-guidance system. Shown are floor-mounted x-ray tubes (1), flat panel detectors (2), robotics (3), phantom IR spheres (4), and touch screen (5) for software controls. Not shown is infrared/video camera. (b) Floor-mounted recessed x-ray tubes (cover removed) and amorphous-silicon flat panel detectors.

Generally, four to six spheres are used in a unique pattern. The IR signal from the camera is reflected back by the IR markers to yield position information. The IR system samples marker position at a frequency of 20 Hz with an accuracy better than 0.3 mm and is, thus, ideally suited as a real-time monitor of the patient position during treatment. The system also uses a couch-mounted robotics system to automatically move the treatment couch to the desired location based on IR markers match.

The external markers have to be placed in a stable location to achieve accurate setup. Sometimes, a reference "star" attached to the side rails of the treatment table may be used if the skin markers are prone to large respiratory motion. The reference star consists of four reflecting IR markers in a fixed position. With the reference star is attached to the couch for position verification, the couch's movement can be precisely determined. In addition to IR tracking, the built-in video camera can also be used for independent verification of patient position. A video image of the initial setup position of the patient is recorded and compared with images taken at subsequent fractions. All software functions can be operated either from a touch screen monitor inside the linac room or from a console computer located outside.[11]

The ExacTrac x-ray system uses an x-ray generator, two floor-mounted x-ray tubes (K&S Rontgenwerk, Bochum, Germany), and two ceiling-mounted amorphous silicon (aSi) flat-panel detectors (PerkinElmer Optoelectronics GmbH, Wiesbaden, Germany). The tubes are mounted in watertight wells recessed 43 cm in the floor on either side of the linac (Figure 9-3b).[11] The x-ray tubes emit orthogonal stereoscopic x-rays in the energy range of 40 kV to 150 kV in the exposure mode, and 40 kV to 125 kV in the fluoroscopic mode. The flat panel detectors consist of 512×512 pixels with an active area of 20 cm $\times$ 20 cm, which provides a field of view of 13 cm $\times$ 13 cm at the isocenter with an image pixel size of 0.4 mm $\times$ 0.4 mm (Figure 9-3b). The x-rays project in a $45°$ oblique direction, $42°$ tilted from the horizontal. The source-to-isocenter distance is 224 cm and the source-to-detector distance is 362 cm. The fixed source-detector geometry virtually eliminates any drifts in x-ray isocenter calibration. Two x-ray images are obtained after initial patient setup with the Exactrac system. These x-ray images are compared with DRRs obtained from the CT simulation scan.

The software allows various methods of matching images: automated fusion of x-rays with DRRs using bony anatomy, matching of implanted markers, or manual fusion. The fusion algorithm is based on a gradient search optimization employing six DOF (three linear and three angular) to obtain an acceptable match. First, the acquired planar x-rays are matched to the DRR images to obtain a 3D shift vector. In this first step, only linear shifts are considered (3D match). Subsequently, x-ray–DRR fusion is performed iteratively by using the full six DOF. For each step in the fusion process, a new set of DRRs is derived from the CT data corresponding to x-rays acquired in the new patient position. Both rotational and translational shifts (6D match) are applied to the CT data before generating DRRs to match with x-rays.[14] The fusion algorithm works best when sharp edges are visible in the image process. The system also offers an option for the

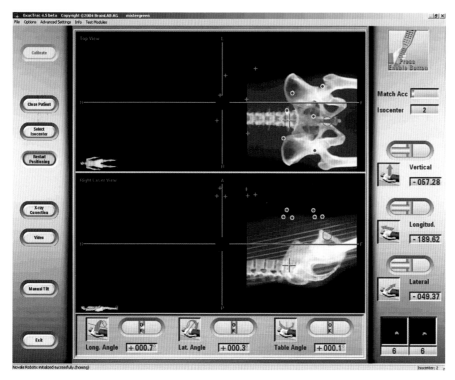

FIGURE 9-4. Computer screen showing workflow for automated patient setup using BrainLAB image guidance. Anterior and lateral digitally reconstructed radiographs generated by the planning system are shown along with target outline (large pink circle). The couch is robotically moved to align the current position of the infrared markers (small red circles) with the isocenter (blue crosses). The right panel shows required linear shifts and bottom panel angular shifts.

region of interest fusion by excluding potential sources of ambiguity from the match process, such as IR markers that are susceptible to breathing motion, patient immobilization devices, etc. The system also has an option for acquiring x-ray images (snap verification) during treatment delivery or between fields to detect any shifts in target position. This approach can be used to minimize intrafractional treatment errors. See Chapters 15E, 20E, and 21F for presentations on the use of the Novalis system in a variety of tumor sites.

Gated Delivery

The ExacTrac system is capable of image-guided positioning and gated treatments.[11] The purpose of gating is to irradiate the tumor volume when it is within a defined portion of the breathing cycle, thereby limiting the volume of normal tissue irradiated. Generally, the end-exhale phase is chosen for treatment as it is considered more stable and reproducible. A gating window corresponding to 20% to 30% of the breathing cycle may be selected for beam-on time. External IR markers placed on the patient surface and internal fiducial markers implanted in the target close to the isocenter are necessary to perform gated delivery. The infrared markers yield a respiratory signal for tracking and gating of the treatment beam. The x-ray system provides periodic confirmation of the patient position relative to the gating window throughout the duration of the gated delivery.

A high degree of correlation between external surface markers and internal fiducial markers is assumed in adaptive gating.[15] During the treatment process, the patient is set up on the couch with several IR markers attached to the abdomen to monitor breathing motion. The reference star is also used to monitor motion of IR markers and to precisely guide couch motion. Based on the time-dependent motion of the IR markers, the ExacTrac system displays the patient breathing curve. A gating reference level and beam-on window can be specified on this curve. Typically, kV x-ray images are acquired for target localization at the instant the breathing curve crosses the gating level. The implanted fiducials are identified in each x-ray image and are compared with the DRRs generated from the four-dimensional (4D) CT scans corresponding to that phase of breathing cycle. Further target confirmation may also be done at the edges of the gating window by acquiring additional x-ray images.

Elekta Synergy – X-Ray Volumetric Imaging

The X-ray Volumetric Imaging (XVI) system integrated with the Synergy linear accelerator (Elekta AB, Stockholm, Sweden) consists of a kV x-ray source (70 kVp to 150 kVp) and an aSi/cesium iodide (CsI) flat-panel detector placed opposite to each other and orthogonal to the MV treatment beam trajectory (Figure 9-5). When in use, the source and the detector panel can be extended out to a preset position (this must be done inside the room) while the therapist, from the control room, must manually trigger the kV beam generation by using the XVI software

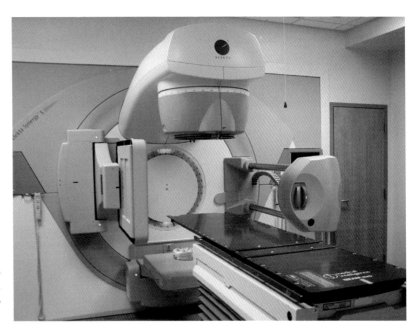

FIGURE 9-5. The commercial Elekta Synergy linear accelerator with the integrated X-ray Volumetric Imager (XVI) system. (Source: University of Florida, used with permission.)

and a foot-switch for image acquisition. Acquired projection images at each angle are stored in the XVI workstation, which controls the kV generator (not visible to the user) and the image acquisition synchronicity process, and from which the volumetric 3D CBCT images are reconstructed for clinical use.

Scanning Modes and Capabilities

The XVI is capable of imaging in either radiographic (2D), fluoroscopic (2D + time), or volumetric (3D) mode. Currently, a 4D (3D + time) imaging is not possible. In the radiographic mode, the XVI acquires one static planar kV image. This is achieved by acquiring a series of frames that are averaged to produce a single high-quality image. The acquired image(s), however, cannot be used for quantitative patient set-up at this time, because of the lack of physical or virtual cross-hairs in the images for reference. In the fluoroscopic mode, a sequence of planar images is acquired to visualize the motion of the tumor and/or its surrounding organs. During acquisition, the gantry can be held stationary or in rotation around the patient for different views as needed. Finally, in the volumetric mode, a set of planar images is acquired while the gantry rotates around the patient. For a full 360° rotation, approximately 650 planar images are acquired for volumetric reconstruction. Typically, the images are reconstructed in tandem with the acquisition process to facilitate a minimum wait time for image registration.

In the volumetric mode, there are three main types of acquisition: small (S), medium (M), and large (L) FOV, depending on the amount of axial FOV needed for adequate image registration. In the small FOV scan, the center of the detector panel is in line with the central axis

of the kV beam, whereas in the medium and large FOV scans, the center of the detector panel is shifted by 11.5 cm and 19.0 cm, respectively, to increase the geometrical limitation of FOV imposed by the physical setup.[16] The corresponding reconstructed FOVs can be up to 27.0 cm, 41.0 cm, and 50.0 cm in diameter for the three scans, respectively. In addition, at each scan mode, there is a matching cassette that defines the beam collimation along the gantry-target axis. Currently, there are three nominal length settings (2, 10, and 20 cm), which correspond to a longitudinal scan range from 3.5 cm up to 27.7 cm depending on the type of scan (i.e., S, M, or L). In addition to the collimator cassettes, there are two types of filtration cassettes available for beam filtration; namely, F0 and F1. F0 is simply an open or empty cassette and, therefore, does not change the filtration (i.e., beam quality) of the beam. The recently introduced F1 filter (also known as a bow-tie filter), however, can significantly change the x-ray beam spectrum and, therefore, cannot interchangeably be used with the F0 filter because the gain/range of the detector panel needs to be recalibrated. The main advantages of this hardware include the significant reduction of dose, decreased scatter for better image contrast, and the flattening of x-ray fluence variation across the field such that patient edge information is better preserved.[17-19] Investigations are ongoing at this time for optimal use of this technology.

Imaging Procedure for On-Line Guidance

Before any imaging procedure, the x-ray source should be adequately warmed up. This is done, typically, in the morning before the first treatment and at any time when the last scan was completed more than 4 hours ago. Also, it is important to not pull the imaging panel out for tube warm-ups to minimize the damage to the electronics.

Generally, the workflow of the XVI IGRT procedure is as follows. First, the patient is set up on the Elekta Precise Table with the laser-to-tattoo aligned as closely as possible. Second, a volumetric image of the patient is acquired and reconstructed on the XVI software. Third, the reconstructed image is registered with the planning CT image (see Figure 9-6). Fourth, a correction vector is calculated and translated to the treatment couch movement. Lastly, the couch corrections are made and the treatment begins. All of these steps are important and the quality assurance of each step is critical. However, the single most important step is in the registration of the CBCT to the planning CT. Unlike other steps, this step involves human judgment for final approval of the registration, which can directly affect the geometric accuracy of the treatment.

In the XVI software, there are currently three modes of registration and four modes of display available to aid in the registration and the evaluation of the image matching. The three modes of registration include (1) bone, (2) gray scale value, and (3) manual registrations. As their names suggest, the bone and gray scale value registrations are automatic procedures that focus mainly on the matching of the CT pixel values in the range of the bones or soft tissues, respectively. A clip box can be set to limit the registration to a local region of interest (typically includes the target volume). The manual registration is usually performed, if at all, after the previous automatic registrations.

The evaluation of the registration is aided by the four modes of display including (1) green-purple display, (2) cut, (3) localization-only, and (4) reference-only modes. The green-purple mode is shown in Figure 9-6. The planning CT image is shown in purple. This display mode gives a broad overview of the registration and, hence, is useful for gross and final registration evaluation. In the cut mode, the images are cut up in a checkerboard pattern of squares with the planning and CBCT images displayed in alternate squares. This mode is useful for making detailed comparisons of fine image structures and edge matching. The localization mode displays the CBCT image only and is typically useful when the contours in the planning CT are overlaid. Finally, the reference-only mode displays the planning CT image only and allows the therapists to familiarize themselves with the reference image before registration. Once the registration is finished and confirmed by a physician, the six-degree error vector (three translational, three rotational) is converted to the translational-only couch shifts in the room coordinates. This step is performed because the Elekta Precise Table cannot rotate in roll and pitch dimensions, and, hence, the necessity in conversion. See Chapters 16G, 18C, and 24J for presentations of patients treated with the Elekta system.

Mitsubishi Hokkaido RTRT

One of the most important problems to be solved in IGRT is the internal position of the tumor during the irradiation.[20–22] The real-time tumor-tracking radiotherapy

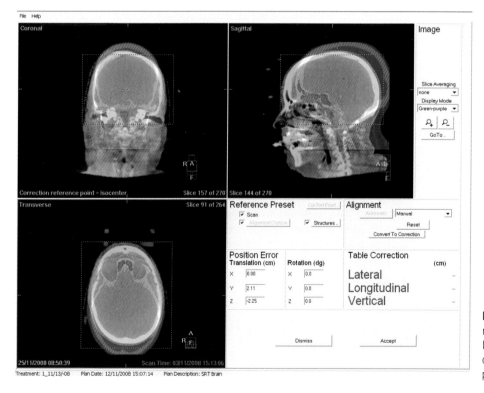

FIGURE 9-6. An example image registration on the X-ray Volumetric Imager (XVI) software of a stereotactic radiotherapy brain tumor patient.

(RTRT) system (Mitsubishi, Tokyo, Japan), which was first reported in 1999, can monitor the internal position of the tumor during treatment delivery with the aid of an internal (implanted) fiducial marker.[23,24] The location of a moving tumor can be detected every 0·033 seconds with an accuracy of ±1 mm, and the tumor is irradiated only when its location corresponds to the planned position with the aid of an internal fiducial marker near the tumor.[25,26]

A prototype RTRT system consisted of four sets of diagnostic x-ray television (TV) systems mounted in the treatment room (Figure 9-7). The second-generation RTRT system consists of two sets of diagnostic x-ray TV systems that can rotate in the treatment room and stop at the four positions. The x-ray images are fed to an image processor unit consisting of two image acquisition units, two image recognition units, and a central processor unit (CPU). The output of the RTRT system gates a dual-energy linear accelerator. The operating console and image display of the system (Figure 9-8) are placed adjacent to the console of the linac.

Each of the diagnostic x-ray TV units in the current RTRT system consists of a 1.5-MHU x-ray tube with a fixed collimator mounted under the floor, a 9-inch image intensifier mounted in the ceiling, and a high-voltage x-ray generator. The images from the intensifiers are digitized to 1024×1024 pixels, with 8 bits per pixel. The x-ray tubes are placed at right caudal, right cranial, left caudal, and left cranial position with respect to the patient couch at a distance of 280 cm from the isocenter. These positions correspond with the four corners of the floor. The image intensifiers are positioned opposite in the ceiling, i.e., at the left cranial, left caudal, right cranial, and right caudal position, at a distance of 180 cm from the isocenter. The beam axis of all four diagnostic x-ray units intersects the isocenter of the accelerator. In clinical use, only two positions of the four x-ray TV positions are ena-bled at a single time to avoid occlusion of the x-ray image by the gantry of the linac. In this way, tumor tracking is possible for all gantry angles.

The diagnostic x-ray units are pulsed in synchronization with the frame rate of the TV cameras. In addition, the x-ray units and the linac run in phase. The linac is gated in such a way that the treatment beam is never on at the same time as the diagnostic x-ray units are pulsed, i.e., pulses of the linac are dropped when an x-ray pulse is required. In this way, one avoids a rise in the background level of the fluoroscopic image, because of scattered therapeutic x-rays by the patient. This procedure is possible because the pulse rate of the linac is much higher than the highest pulse rate of the x-ray units. The image intensifiers are enabled only when the diagnostic x-ray tubes are pulsed. The gating of the linac is performed by means of a grid on the electron gun. The linac dose rate can thus be switched on and off instantaneously without powering down the rest of the linac.

Motion Tracking

The RTRT system has been used to reduce the uncertainty of interfractional and intrafractional motion of internal tumors, particularly those subjects with respiratory-induced motion. In preparation, a round gold marker with a diameter of 1.5 mm to 2.0 mm is inserted in or near the tumor.[15,27–30] The coordinates of the center of the tumor and the gold marker are then transferred from the CT to the RTRT system. Two sets of diagnostic fluoroscopes in the linac room detect the gold marker during RT and the central axis of the diagnostic radiographs is adjusted to cross at the isocenter of the linac where the tumor should be located during treatment.

The system is useful for precise setup of patients as usual IGRT with fiducial markers to reduce interfractional setup error.[31–35] Adding to it, real-time pattern recognition technology is used for automatic recognition of the

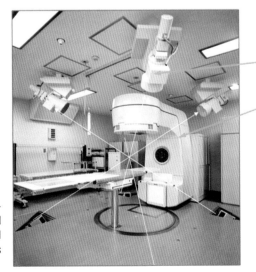
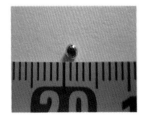

Treatment Room

Fluoroscopy

Linear accelerator

Gold Marker

FIGURE 9-7. Configuration of the real-time tumor-tracking system synchronized to a linear accelerator and an internal marker to be inserted near the patient's tumor.

projected figure of the gold marker in the fluoroscopic images during the delivery of the therapeutic beam. The 3D position of the marker is calculated from the two fluoroscopic images 30 times a second.[36] A linear accelerator is synchronized to irradiate the tumor only when the gold marker is located within the accepted volume as defined by the "allowed displacement" value from its planned position. Usually the "allowed displacement" is ±1.0 mm to 2.0 mm in the clinical practice. The period between recognition and actual irradiation is 0·05 seconds.

During treatment planning and daily setup in the treatment room, the trajectory of the internal fiducial marker was recorded for 1 to 2 minutes at the rate of 30 times per second by the RTRT system. To maximize gating efficiency, the patient's position on the treatment couch was adjusted by using the 4D setup system with fine on-line remote control of the treatment couch.[37] The trajectory of the marker detected in the 4D setup system was well visualized and used for daily setup. Various degrees of interfractional and intrafractional changes in the absolute amplitude and speed of the internal marker were detected. Readjustments were necessary during each treatment session, prompted by baseline shifting of the tumor position. The 4D setup system was shown to be useful for reducing the uncertainty of tumor motion and for increasing the efficiency of gated irradiation. Chapter 19D provides a discussion of a patient with a liver tumor treated with the RTRT system.

The benefit of the RTRT system to reduce the uncertainty in set-up and organ motion has been shown in various organs in the actual treatment.[38-44] However, the definitive role of the RTRT system to improve the clinical outcome of radiotherapy has not been established in clinical trials. However, several studies based on the trajectory data detected by the RTRT system have shown that predictive model of respiration may be useful to reduce the requirement for fluoroscopic monitoring during irradiation.[39-52]

Varian Trilogy – On-Board Imager

Varian provides a fully integrated CBCT system that is currently available on the market in the On-Board Imager (OBI) integrated with the Trilogy linear accelerator (Varian Medical Systems, Palo Alto, CA; Figure 9-9). The system consists of a kV x-ray source (KVS) and an aSi flat-panel detector (KVD), with an active area of 39.7 cm × 29.8 cm, that are attached to the fully motorized robotic arms (ExactArms) mounted in an orthogonal plane to the MV treatment beam trajectory.

Scanning Modes and Capabilities

The OBI is capable of imaging in either radiographic (2D), fluoroscopic (2D + time), or volumetric (3D) mode. Currently, a 4D (3D + time) imaging is not possible, although this is an active area of research at this time.[53-59] In the radiographic mode, the OBI acquires a static planar kV image at any given gantry angle (usually anterior and lateral). The acquired image(s) are readily available for quantitative patient setup by visually matching the planar images to the planning DRRs. This is done in a 2D2D Match software environment, where the match can be automated or performed manually (Figure 9-10a). Once

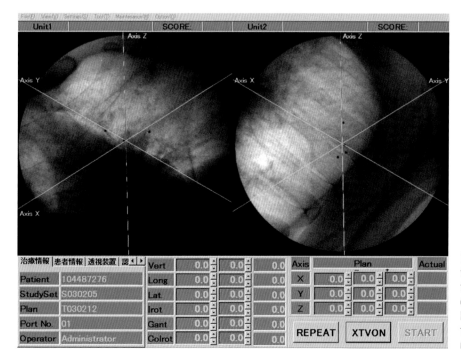

FIGURE 9-8. Display on the monitor of the second-generation real-time tumor-tracking system in a patient with lung cancer. Four markers are inserted through bronchial tree around a tumor and one of the markers is used for the real-time tumor tracking and gated radiotherapy.

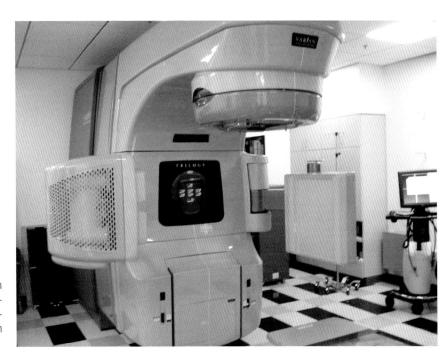

FIGURE 9-9. The commercial Varian Trilogy linear accelerator with the integrated On-Board Imager system. (Source: University of California, San Diego, used with permission.)

the desired match is reached, the couch shift parameters are downloaded to the treatment console and the couch is moved remotely.

In the fluoroscopic mode, a sequence of planar images is acquired in a specified time (set in minutes) to visualize the internal motions of the patient anatomy just before treatment to verify the consistency of target motion range with respect to the simulation and planning studies. During acquisition, the gantry can be held stationary or rotated around the patient for different views as needed. Finally, in the volumetric mode, a set of low-dose planar images is acquired while the gantry rotates around the patient. Typically, 200° and 360° rotations are used in conjunction with a head and body scanning modes, respectively. On average, approximately 360 and 670 planar images, respectively, are acquired for volumetric reconstruction (Figure 9-10b). Typically, the images are reconstructed in tandem with the acquisition process to facilitate a minimum wait time for image registration.

In the volumetric mode, there are two main types of acquisition available: full-fan and half-fan. In the full-fan mode, the reconstructed FOV is a circle of up to 24-cm diameter with a 15-cm length in volume. This mode is used for visualizing relatively small anatomic sites such as the brain and the head and neck. In the half-fan mode, the KVD is shifted in an orthogonal direction to the kV beam axis by 14.8 cm to increase the scanning area[16] such that the resulting FOV is a circle of 45-cm diameter with a 14-cm length in volume (the FOV can be set up to 50 cm). As one can imagine, this mode is used for visualizing larger sites such as the pelvis, chest, and abdomen. In

both modes, the beam collimation is accomplished automatically with a set of X and Y dynamic jaws mounted on the KVS unit.

To account for the variation in the beam path length, and the resulting differential attenuation (and fluence) along the beam trajectory in an axial plane,[17] the bow-tie filters are inserted in front of the kV source. The full and half bow-tie filters are used with the full-fan and half-fan modes, respectively. With these option settings, there are currently four possible scanning techniques available: full-fan mode with and without the full bow-tie filter, and half-fan mode with and without the half bow-tie filter. In addition, one can set a low-dose mode in which the same scans can be performed with a significant reduction in the total mAs used. This mode, however, also significantly degrades the image quality and, hence, is not recommended for clinical use.[60]

A scanning technique that is currently in the research phase of its development is the use of limited scan angles to reconstruct an orthogonal set of images to the x-ray source for use with patient registration, also known as digital tomosynthesis (DTS).[61-65] This technique is promising in that it provides a high-resolution images (i.e., in the viewing plane) for target registration and at same time requires significantly fewer projections for image reconstruction (e.g., < 45° scan rotation). This results in a marked reduction in scan time and the dose delivered for imaging (e.g., 0.5 cGy to 1 cGy for a 45° scan).[65] A downside to this technique is a reduction in the resolution of the slice thickness because of the narrow angle scan.[61,62] It is expected that DTS will be the scanning protocol of choice for at least some clinical sites.

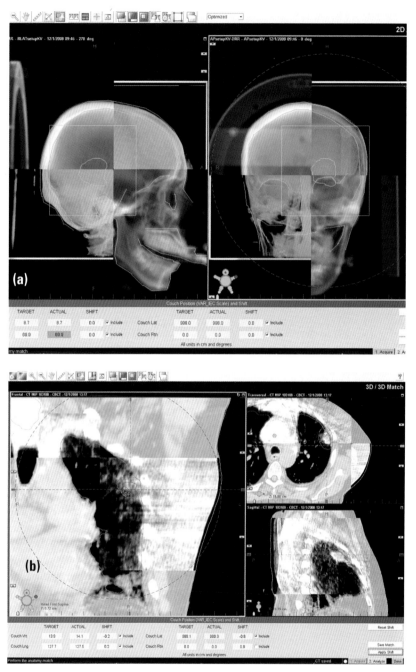

FIGURE 9-10. (a) A 2D2D Match software environment for registering kilovoltage (kV) x-ray setup images to its corresponding digitally reconstructed radiographs. An example shown here is for a stereotactic brain tumor patient. (b) A 3D3D Match software environment for registering volumetric cone beam computed tomography images to its corresponding planning computed tomography images. An example shown here is for a hypofractionated lung cancer patient.

Imaging Procedure for On-Line Guidance

Generally, the workflow of OBI-based IGRT procedure is similar to the Elekta XVI system. One notable exception is the optional use of kV planar radiographs because the virtual cross-hairs (i.e., graticules) are readily available for setup use in the 2D2D Match environment. In the 3D3D Match environment (software for volumetric mode), the registration is performed in one of two methods:

(1) automated gray scale value matching, or (2) manual matching. In the automated matching, a clip box cannot be set for a local registration and, hence, only a global matching is possible. Therefore, in general, the automated matching is performed first (to match the images globally) followed by the manual matching of detailed anatomy. Similar to XVI, there are a variety of standard registration evaluation tools available to aid in the manual matching of

the CT images. Once the registration is finished and confirmed by a physician or physicist, the four-degree-error vector (three translational, one rotational) is converted to the translational-only couch shifts in the room coordinates. The correction parameters are then downloaded to the Varian treatment console and the couch position is adjusted remotely from the control room. Presentations on the use of the Varian Trilogy system in different tumor sites are provided in Chapters 17D, 19C, 20H, 21I, 22E, and 23A.

References

1. Saw CB, Chen H, Wagner Jr H. Implementation of fiducial-based image registration in the CyberKnife robotic system. *Med Dosim.* 2008;33:156–160.
2. Ozhasoglu C, Saw CB, Chen H, et al. Synchrony – CyberKnife respiratory compensation technology. *Med Dosim.* 2008;33:117–123.
3. Saw CB, Chen H, Beatty RE, et al. Multimodality image fusion and planning and dose delivery for radiation therapy. *Med Dosim.* 2008;38:148–154.
4. Adler JR, Chang SD, Murphy MJ, et al. The CyberKnife: a frameless robotic system for radiosurgery. *Stereotactic Funct Neurosurg.* 1997;60:124–128.
5. Fanuc Robotics [Web site]. Available at: http://www.fanucrobotics.com. Accessed February 5, 2009.
6. Kuka Roboter GmbH [Web site]. Available at: http://www.kuka.com/en. Accessed February 5, 2009.
7. Accuray Inc [Web site]. Available at: http://www.accuray.com/Content.aspx?id=674. Accessed February 5, 2009.
8. Murphy MJ, Cox RS. The accuracy of dose localization for an imaged-guided frameless radiosurgery system. *Med Phys.* 1996;23:2043–2049.
9. Murphy MJ. Fiducial-based targeting accuracy for external beam radiotherapy. *Med Phys.* 2002;29:334–344.
10. Cosgrove VP, Jahn U, Pfaender M, et al. Commissioning of a micro multi-leaf collimator and planning system for stereotactic radiosurgery. *Radiother Oncol.* 1999;50:325–336.
11. *Clinical Users Guide Revision 1.0, Novalis Body/ExacTrac Version 5.0.* Heimstettan, Germany: BrainLAB AG;2009.
12. Verellen D, Soete G, Linthout N, et al. Quality assurance of a system for improved target localization and patient setup that combines real-time infrared tracking and stereoscopic x-ray imaging. *Radiother Oncol.* 2003;67:129–141.
13. Lutz W, Winston KR, Maleki N. A system for stereotactic radiosurgery with a linear accelerator. *Int J Radiat Oncol Biol Phys.* 1988;14:373–381.
14. Murphy MJ. An automatic six-degree-of-freedom image registration algorithm for image-guided frameless stereotaxic radiosurgery. *Med Phys.* 1997;24(6):857–866.
15. Shirato H, Harada T, Harabayashi T, et al. Feasibility of insertion/implantation of 2.0mm diameter gold internal fiducial markers for precise setup and real time tumor tracking in radiotherapy. *Int J Radiat Oncol Biol Phys.* 2003;56:240–247.
16. Cho P, Johnson RH, Griffin TW. Cone-beam CT for radiotherapy applications. *Phys Med Biol.* 1995;40:1863–1883.

17. Graham SA, Moseley DJ, Siewerdsen JH, Jaffray DA. Compensators for dose and scatter management in cone-beam computed tomography. *Med Phys.* 2007;34:2691–2703.
18. Ozawa S, Peng J, Song WY, et al. Comprehensive evaluation of the bow tie filter in the Elekta XVI CBCT system [abstract]. *Med Phys.* 2008;35;2769.
19. Mail N, Moseley DJ, Siewerdsen JH, Jaffray DA. The influence of bowtie filtration on cone-beam CT image quality. *Med Phys.* 2009;36:22–32.
20. Shimizu S, Shirato H, Xo B, et al. Three-dimensional movement of a liver tumor detected by high-speed magnetic resonance imaging. *Radiother Oncol.* 1999;50(3):367–370.
21. Shimizu S, Shirato H, Kagei K, et al. Impact of respiratory movement on the computed tomographic images of small lung tumors in three-dimensional (3D) radiotherapy. *Int J Radiat Oncol Biol Phys.* 2000;46(5):1127–1133.
22. Shimizu S, Shirato H, Aoyama H, et al. High-speed magnetic resonance imaging for four-dimensional treatment planning of conformal radiotherapy of moving body tumors. *Int J Radiat Oncol Biol Phys.* 2000;48(2):471–474.
23. Shirato H, Shimizu S, Shimizu T, et al. Real-time tumor-tracking radiotherapy. *Lancet.* 1999;353(9161):1331–1332.
24. Jiang SB. Technical aspects of image-guided respiration-gated radiation therapy. *Med Dosim.* 2006;31(2):141–151.
25. Shirato H, Shimizu S, Kitamura K, et al. Four-dimensional treatment planning and fluoroscopic real-time tumor tracking radiotherapy for moving tumor. *Int J Radiat Oncol Biol Phys.* 2000;48(2):435–442.
26. Shirato H, Shimizu S, Kunieda T, et al. Physical aspects of a real-time tumor-tracking system for gated radiotherapy. *Int J Radiat Oncol Biol Phys.* 2000;48(4):1187–1195.
27. Shimizu S, Shirato H, Kitamura K, et al. Use of an implanted marker and real-time tracking of the marker for the positioning of prostate and bladder cancers. *Int J Radiat Oncol Biol Phys.* 2000;48(5):1591–1597.
28. Harada T, Shirato H, Obura S, et al. Real-time tumor-tracking radiation therapy for lung carcinoma by the aid of insertion of a gold marker using bronchofiberscopy. *Cancer.* 2002;95(8):1720–1727.
29. Imura M, Yamazaki K, Shirato H, et al. Insertion and fixation of fiducial markers for setup and tracking of lung tumors in radiotherapy. *Int J Radiat Oncol Biol Phys.* 2005;63(5):1442–1447.
30. Imura M, Yamazaki K, Kubota KC, et al. Histopathologic consideration of fiducial gold markers inserted for real-time tumor-tracking radiotherapy against lung cancer. *Int J Radiat Oncol Biol Phys.* 2007;70(2):382–384.
31. Shirato H, Oita M, Fujita K, et al. Three-dimensional conformal setup (3D-CSU) of patients using the coordinate system provided by three internal fiducial markers and two orthogonal diagnostic x-ray systems in the treatment room. *Int J Radiat Oncol Biol Phys.* 2004;60(2):607–612.
32. Oita S, Ohmori K, Obinata K, et al. Uncertainty in treatment of head-and-neck tumors by use of intraoral mouthpiece and embedded fiducials. *Int J Radiat Oncol Biol Phys.* 2006;64(5):1581–1588.
33. Onimaru R, Shirato H, Aoyama H, et al. Calculation of rotational setup error using the real-time tracking radiation therapy (RTRT) system and its application to the treatment of spinal schwannoma. *Int J Radiat Oncol Biol Phys.* 2002;54(3):939–947.

34. Kitamura K, Shirato H, Shimizu S, et al. Registration accuracy and possible migration of internal fiducial gold marker implanted in prostate and liver treated with real-time tumor-tracking radiation therapy (RTRT). *Radiother Oncol.* 2002; 62(3):275–281.

35. Yamamoto R, Yonesaka a, Nishioka S, et al. High dose three-dimensional conformal boost (3DCB) using an orthogonal diagnostic x-ray set-up for patients with gynecological malignancy: a new application of real-time tumor-tracking system. *Radiother Oncol.* 2004;73(2):219–222.

36. Shimizu S, Shirato H, Ogura S, et al. Detection of lung tumor movement in real-time tumor-tracking radiotherapy. *Int J Radiat Oncol Biol Phys.* 2001;51(2):304–310.

37. Shirato H, Suzuki K, Sharp GC, et al. Speed and amplitude of lung tumor motion precisely detected in four-dimensional set-up and in real-time tumor-tracking radiotherapy. *Int J Radiat Oncol Biol Phys.* 2006;64(4):1229–1236.

38. Shirato H, Shimizu S, Kitamura K, Onimaru R. Organ motion in image-guided radiotherapy: lessons from real-time tumor-tracking radiotherapy. *Int J Clin Oncol.* 2007;12(1):8–16.

39. Kitamura Y, Shirato H, Seppenwoolde Y, et al. Three-dimensional intrafractional movement of prostate measured during real-time tumor-tracking radiotherapy in supine and prone treatment positions. *Int J Radiat Oncol Biol Phys.* 2002;53(5):1117–1123.

40. Kitamura K, Shirato H, Seppenwoolde Y, et al. Tumor location, cirrhosis, and surgical history contribute to tumor movement in the liver, as measured during stereotactic irradiation using a real-time tumor-tracking radiotherapy system. *Int J Radiat Oncol Biol Phys.* 2003;56(1):221–228.

41. Ahn YC, Shimizu S, Shirato H, et al. Application of real-time tumor-tracking and gated radiotherapy system for unresectable pancreatic cancer. *Yonsei Med J.* 2004;45(4):584–590.

42. Hashimoto K, Shirato H, Katoh M, et al. Real-time monitoring of a digestive tract marker to reduce adverse effects of moving organs at risk (OAR) in radiotherapy for thoracic and abdominal tumors. *Int J Radiat Oncol Biol Phys.* 2005;61(5):1559–1564.

43. Kitamura K, Shirato H, Shinohara N, et al. Reduction in acute morbidity using hypofractionated intensity-modulated radiation therapy assisted with a fluoroscopic real-time tumor-tracking system for prostate cancer: preliminary results of a phase I/II study. *Cancer J.* 2003;9(4):268–276.

44. Taguchi H, Sakuhara Y, Hige S, et al. Intercepting radiotherapy using a real-time tumor-tracking radiotherapy system for highly selected patients with hepatocellular carcinoma unresectable with other modalities. *Int J Radiat Oncol Biol Phys.* 2007;69(2):376–380.

45. Seppenwoolde Y, Shirato H, Kitamura Y, et al. Precise and real-time measurement of 3D tumor motion in lung due to breathing and heartbeat, measured during radiotherapy. *Int J Radiat Oncol Biol Phys.* 2002;53(4):822–834.

46. Shirato H, Seppenwoolde Y, Kitamura K, et al. Intrafractional tumor motion: lung and liver. *Semin Radiat Oncol.* 2004;14(1): 10–18.

47. Onimaru R, Shirato H, Fujino M, et al. The effect of tumor location and respiratory function on tumor movement estimated by Real-time Tracking RadioTherapy (RTRT) system. *Int J Radiat Oncol Biol Phys.* 2005;63(1):164–169.

48. Sharp GC, Jiang SB, Shimizu S, et al. Prediction of respiratory tumor motion for real-time image-guided radiotherapy. *Phys Med Biol.* 2004;49(3):425–440.

49. Berbeco R, Nishioka S, Shirato H, et al. Residual motion of lung tumors in gated radiotherapy with external respiratory surrogates. *Phys Med Biol.* 2005;50(16):3655–3667.

50. Berbeco RI, Nishioka S, Shirato H, Jiang SB. Residual motion of lung tumors in end-of-inhale respiratory gated radiotherapy based on external surrogates. *Med Phys.* 2006;33(11):4149–4156.

51. Kanoulas E, Aslam JA, Sharp GC, et al. Derivation of the tumor position from external respiratory surrogates with periodical updating of the internal/external correlation. *Phys Med Biol.* 2007;52(17):5443–5456.

52. Ren Q, Nishioka S, Shirato H, Berbeco RI. Adaptive prediction of respiratory motion for motion compensation radiotherapy. *Phys Med Biol.* 2007;52(22):6651–6661.

53. Sonke JJ, Zijp L, Remeijer P, van Herk M. Respiratory correlated cone beam CT. *Med Phys.* 2005;32:1176–1186.

54. Dietrich L, Jetter S, Tucking T, et al. Linac-integrated 4D cone-beam CT: first experimental results. *Phys Med Biol.* 2006;51: 2939–2952.

55. Purdie TG, Moseley DJ, Bissonnette JP, et al. Respiration correlated cone-beam computed tomography and 4DCT for evaluating target motion in Stereotactic Lung Radiation Therapy. *Acta Oncol.* 2006;45:915–922.

56. Li T, Xing L, Munro P, et al. Four-dimensional cone-beam computed tomography using an on-board imager. *Med Phys.* 2006;33:3825–3833.

57. Li T, Xing L. Optimizing 4D cone-beam CT acquisition protocol for external beam radiotherapy. *Int J Radiat Oncol Biol Phys.* 2007;67:1211–1219.

58. Sonke JJ, Lebesque J, van Herk M. Variability of four-dimensional computed tomography patient models. *Int J Radiat Oncol Biol Phys.* 2008;70:590–598.

59. Thompson BP, Hugo GD. Quality and accuracy of cone beam computed tomography gated by active breathing control. *Med Phys.* 2008;35:5595–5608.

60. Yoo S, Kim GY, Hammoud R, et al. A quality assurance program for the on-board imager. *Med Phys.* 2006;33:4431–4447.

61. Dobbins J, Godfrey D. Digital x-ray tomosynthesis: current state of the art and clinical potential. *Phys Med Biol.* 2003;48: R65–R106.

62. Godfrey D, McAdams H, Dobbins J. Optimization of the matrix inversion tomosynthesis (MITS) impulse response and modulation transfer function characteristics for chest imaging. *Med Phys.* 2006;33:655–667.

63. Godfrey D, Yin F, Oldham M, et al. Digital tomosynthesis with an on-board kilovoltage imaging device. *Int J Radiat Oncol Biol Phys.* 2006;65:8–15.

64. Wu Q, Godfrey D, Wang Z, et al. On-board patient positioning for head and neck IMRT – Comparing digital tomosynthesis to kV radiograph and cone-beam CT. *Int J Radiat Oncol Biol Phys.* 2007;69:598–606.

65. Yoo S, Wu Q, Godfrey D, et al. Clinical evaluation of positioning verification using digital tomosynthesis and bony anatomy and soft tissues for prostate image-guided radiotherapy. *Int J Radiat Oncol Biol Phys.* 2009;73:296–305.

Chapter 10

MEGAVOLTAGE IMAGING SYSTEMS

THOMAS R. MACKIE, PhD, OLIVIER MORIN, PhD,
GUSTAVO H. OLIVERA, PhD, JEAN POULIOT, PhD

Portal imaging that uses the beam directly from the radiotherapy (RT) treatment unit has been the mainstay of image guidance in the latter half of the 20th century. Up until the 1990s, portal images were obtained by using screen-film systems. Physicians would compare portal and simulation films side-by-side on a light box and indicate positioning changes on these films with colored pencils. With the advent of electronic portal imaging devices (EPIDs), physicians obtained the ability to review images digitally, allowing them to potentially make adjustments with the patient on the treatment table. A further evolution in portal imaging was the creation of volumetric images with EPIDs. Through the use of megavoltage (MV) cone beam computed tomography (CBCT), a three-dimensional (3D) analysis of patient positioning and organ motion could be performed. Megavoltage CBCT has a number of distinct advantages including use of the same beam that is treating the patient, as well as no additional hardware requirements. Beyond MV CBCT, MV computed tomography (CT) has also been utilized within the novel design of the Tomotherapy unit (Tomotherapy Inc, Madison, WI). Each of these technologies will be discussed in this chapter.

Siemens Oncor

The only MV CBCT system currently available (MVision, Siemens AG, Erlangen, Germany) is the most recent addition to the family of in-room 3D systems designed for image-guided RT (IGRT). The use of MV photons for imaging is a departure from conventional preferences of using kilovoltage (kV) photons, which have resulted in superior image quality for diagnostic purposes. Some of the advantages and disadvantages of using MV systems will be discussed.

Megavoltage CBCT consists of a 3D image of the patient anatomy acquired with the linear accelerator. Similar to a conventional kV CT, MV CBCT images can be displayed in axial, sagittal, and coronal planes of the patient anatomy. Both kV CT and MV CBCT images

share the concept of computerized tomography reconstruction where the volumetric element (voxel) intensities represent the attenuation coefficient of the patient body to the x-ray source used for imaging.[1] The design and mode of acquisition of CT and MV CBCT, however, have key differences with regard to the radiation field geometry, the x-ray source energy, the image acquisition, and the reconstruction algorithm used. In the case of CT, narrow slices are imaged as the x-ray source rotates around the patient. The patient table, therefore, has to be translated to capture a complete volume. For MV CBCT, an open two-dimensional (2D) cone beam of radiation penetrates the patient before reaching a 2D detector; thus, no couch movement is required during acquisition.

Historical Perspective

The first utilization of a linear accelerator for 3D imaging was performed nearly 30 years ago soon after the invention of CT.[2] A similar imaging system was also investigated for patient setup and verification.[3] These early prototypes used fan-beam geometry to collect the anatomical information. As EPID technology advanced, cone-beam reconstruction systems became increasingly feasible.[4–10] Since 2001, the University of California San Francisco (UCSF) has worked in collaboration with Siemens Oncology Care Systems on the first clinical implementation of a MV CBCT system. Over the past 8 years, a number of publications have covered the work done to introduce MV CBCT imaging to the clinic.

In early 2002, a proof of feasibility was demonstrated with a low-exposure MV CBCT acquisition and sufficient image quality for 3D registration with the reference CT.[11] The first MV CBCT system approved by the US Food and Drug Administration (FDA) was described in 2005.[12] An overview of the possible IGRT clinical applications with this system is also available.[13]

Following these initial publications, the dose delivered to patients from MV CBCT imaging was thoroughly reviewed and discussed by two independent groups.[14–16] Two methods to include the patient dose in the treatment

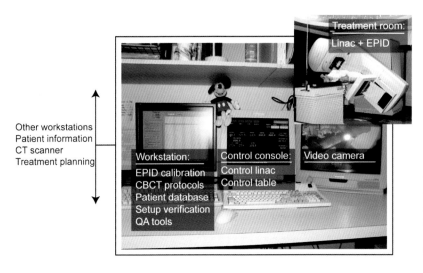

FIGURE 10-1. Major system components for the megavoltage (MV) cone beam computed tomography (CBCT) imaging system. Nearly all the calibrations and clinical tasks related to MV CBCT are performed with the computer workstation. *Note.* EPID = electronic portal imaging device; QA = quality assurance.

plan were described for cases where routine high-quality images are needed. The image quality obtained from a limited set of image acquisition protocols available in the first generation of the MV CBCT system has also been evaluated.[16] A set of recommendations on how to optimize image quality with the system for given clinical applications and body sites was published.[17] Finally, implementations of quality assurance programs for the MV CBCT system have been discussed.[18,19]

System Components, Design, and Workflow

The MV CBCT imaging system presented in Figure 10-1 consists of a 6-MV x-ray beam produced by a conventional linear accelerator (Oncor, Siemens AG, Erlangen, Germany) equipped with an amorphous-silicon EPID (AG9-ES, PerkinElmer Optoelectronics, Waltham, MA) flat panel detector. More specific technical details on the system components are available in the literature.[13] The system is controlled by a computer workstation (Syngo Coherence RTT, Siemens AG, Erlangen, Germany) that is responsible for all tasks related to portal or MV CBCT imaging, including calibration of the system, quality assurance, image acquisition, and image registration (2D or 3D) for patient alignment. Some system parameters in this first generation of the MV CBCT system (acquisition starting position, arc range, source detector distance, etc.) are fixed, whereas others (total exposure, patient orientation, craniocaudal imaging length, and several reconstruction parameters) can be modified. Future generations of the system will likely allow more flexibility.

The MV CBCT acquisition field is transferred from the workstation to the control console of the linear accelerator and the system components (gantry, jaws, and detector) are placed to start the acquisition. The patient reference information (CT, anatomical contours, and treatment isocenter) is automatically loaded in a 3D registration application at the workstation upon transfer of the MV CBCT field to the control console. The gantry then rotates in a continuous 200° arc (270° to 110°) while acquiring one low-dose portal image per degree. While the gantry rotates without interruption, the radiation output follows a beam-on and beam-off sequence. The 200 projection images acquired are then used for MV CBCT reconstruction, which is completed approximately 2 minutes after the start of the acquisition. Immediately after the reconstruction, the MV CBCT is aligned to the reference CT in the 3D registration application. The image alignment starts with an automatic registration, based on a maximization of mutual information algorithm, which utilizes all information in both 3D images (CT and MV CBCT) to maximize the alignment of similar structures. Manual adjustment of the registration is possible and often needed because the automatic algorithm tries to match all anatomical structures including air cavities, movable bony structures, and all structures outside the target volume.

A systematic method has been developed to facilitate the registration of MV CBCT with CT. First, the slice thickness of MV CBCT is adjusted to 3 mm, which is generally the same slice thickness utilized for CT. The window level of both 3D images is adjusted such that identical bony structures have the same visual texture. The colormaps of MV CBCT and CT are respectively set to gray-scale and inverse gray-scale 16-bit. The blending tool is set to 30% opacity for CT and 70% opacity for MV CBCT. Manual alignment is performed on specific bony features near the target area. Finally, the blending tool is moved back and forth (0% to 100%) between CT and MV CBCT to ensure acceptable image registration. Other planes crossing the target volume are also quickly analyzed. The user can then accept the registration, read the patient shift needed for 3D alignment, and remotely adjust the patient couch.

Physical Performance

Recent publications have set the expectations and limitations of the initial MV CBCT system for clinical applications[13,16,17] (see Chapter 20G). The MV CBCT system is capable of measuring setup errors of fiducials in an anthropomorphic head phantom with submillimeter accuracy and reproducibility. Routine quality assurance on the system has also demonstrated that the calibrated MV CBCT imaging isocenter remained within 1 mm to the machine treatment isocenter over a period of 1 year. As for the field-of-view, anatomical information situated in a 27 cm^3 × 27 cm^3 × 27 cm^3 volume centered at isocenter is reconstructed in the MV CBCT image. The new generation of MV CBCT system with a half-beam acquisition mode should increase the reconstruction size in the axial plane by up to 40 cm.[20]

One practical feature of MV CBCT is the capability to change the craniocaudal imaging length by independently moving the upper jaws. One can, therefore, for example, exclude the patient eyes from the radiation field during a head and neck MV CBCT acquisition while still capturing the anatomy needed to evaluate patient positioning. For a typical MV CBCT (anterior arc), the dose delivered to the patient forms a small anterior–posterior gradient ranging from 1.2 cGy to 0.6 cGy per MV CBCT unit of exposure. It has been demonstrated that MV CBCT monitor units (MUs) have a strong impact on image quality. Although three MUs is sufficient for fiducial alignment, nine MUs or more will provide some soft-tissue structures. The decision on the number of MUs should be based on the overall objective of the IGRT procedure.

Figure 10-2 shows side-by-side views of conventional CT and MV CBCT for typical pelvis (right) and head-and-neck (left) patients. Soft tissue structures such as the trapezius, the obturator internus, the gluteus maximus, and the prostate gland are easily identified on both the CT and MV CBCT images of Figure 10-2. Megavoltage CBCTs with exposure as low as two MUs and 10-cm imaging length in the craniocaudal direction have been used in the clinic for simpler setup cases such as prostate patients with implanted gold seeds. The total MV CBCT dose comprises a small percentage of the total prescription dose (< 4%). Strategies of including the MV CBCT dose in the treatment plan have been presented for the case where routine high MU MV CBCT acquisitions are required.[14,15]

Imaging High-Density Materials

The presence of high atomic number (Z) materials such as metallic implants complicate the use of conventional CT images for treatment planning because of severe imaging artifacts that may affect both contouring and dose calculation. Several postprocessing algorithms have been developed to reduce the image degradation.[21] However, the level of artifact reduction is still only adequate on images affected by small metal objects, such as gold seeds, and cannot resolve artifacts that accompany the use of larger metallic structures such as femoral and spinal implants, dental fillings, and arterial stents. In contrast, the image quality of MV CBCT is nearly unaffected (see Figures 10-2 and 10-3) by high-Z materials because of the predominance of Compton interactions in the MV x-ray energy range. In fact, MV CBCT CT numbers scale linearly with electron density. For these reasons, MV CBCT images have been used for prostate delineation in presence of bilateral hip prostheses.[22] Megavoltage imaging has also been used in patients undergoing brachytherapy to facilitate the digitization of catheters in presence of metallic implants.[23]

The presence of metal artifacts in CT makes it difficult to use the image quantitatively for dose calculation. Not only do the image artifacts produce errors in the measured tissue electron density, but the superposition convolution algorithm use for dose calculation does not perform well in such circumstances.[24] For these cases, the treated volume is usually assumed to be water-equivalent in the treatment plan calculations. Treating the volume as water and ignoring the presence of metal may cause severe deviations between the planned dose distribution and the real dose delivered. Increasingly, MV CBCT is

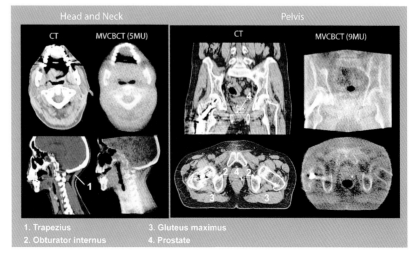

FIGURE 10-2. Typical images for head and neck (5 monitor unit [MU]) cancer and prostate (9 MU) cancer patients compared with conventional computed tomography (CT). The image quality of megavoltage (MV) cone beam CT (CBCT) is sufficient to perform three-dimensional alignment based on bony anatomy and soft tissue. Several muscles and the prostate can be identified on both CT and MV CBCT images. Both CT and MV CBCT images are displayed with 3-mm slice thickness but with different window levels.

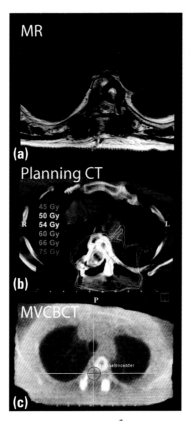

FIGURE 10-3. Magnetic resonance (MR), computed tomography (CT), and megavoltage (MV) cone beam CT (CBCT) images of a 62-year-old woman treated with radiation for a paraspinous tumor in presence of metallic hardware. (a). Postoperative axial pure T2 MR with metallic artifact. (b). Intensity-modulated radiation therapy plan calculated on CT with the 45 Gy isodose line surrounding the spinal cord. (c). MV CBCT image (8 monitor units) used for daily alignment showing nearly no degradation in image quality in the presence of a metallic structure.

also being proposed as an alternative for measuring the true tissue electron density. Optimal dose simulation could be obtained with a Monte Carlo calculation engine that better reproduces the physical interactions of high-energy x-ray in metal. Megavoltage CBCT and Monte Carlo are being used to evaluate the dosimetric implications of having x-ray beam entering through metallic structures before reaching the target volumes of different treatment plans.

Future Directions

Megavoltage CBCT has improved tremendously in a short time and the system advantages for patient set-up accuracy now largely outweigh initially perceived weaknesses in image quality and patient dose. New developments with use of an optimized MV beam line for imaging and more sensitive detectors have demonstrated that significant improvements can be made in image quality for the next generation MV CBCT systems.[25] With use of this new MV CBCT imaging beam line, soft-tissue structures in the head and neck region can be resolved with

a dose of only 1 cGy. The new 3D anatomical information of the patient over their course of treatment can be used to tailor the treatment plan for future fractions to account for individual variations. In addition, software tools and image corrections are being developed to apply the original plan to MV CBCT images. The deposited dose on treatment day will be obtained within minutes and, compared with the planned dose distributions either within specific volumes or as an overall distribution, will provide an accurate estimate of the dosimetric impact of observed anatomical changes. Dosimetric considerations could also be used to determine the most effective time for patient replanning. Additionally, tumor response and radiation side effects can be understood based on actual absorbed dose during treatment. With these new developments, MV CBCT could become a crucial component in personalized treatment strategies and adaptations.

TomoTherapy Hi-Art

Tomotherapy is CT-guided intensity-modulated rotational therapy (Figure 10-4). A fan beam is modulated by a binary multileaf collimator (MLC), whereby the leaves rapidly cross the width of the fan beam to open and closed positions during arc segments of the rotational delivery.[26] Each leaf transit, from a closed to open and back to a closed position, defines a "beamlet." The highest intensities through a beamlet are delivered by opening a leaf at the beginning of the angular segment and closing it at the end. Conversely, a small intensity is delivered by opening a leaf just before the midpoint of the arc segment and closing it just after the midpoint. Other than zero intensity with a leaf closed during the whole angular segment, about 100 intensity levels spanning a range from 5% open to 95% open can be delivered. Helical tomotherapy is tomotherapy delivered with the gantry and couch in simultaneous motion in a fashion similar to a helical CT scanner.[27–30]

Like all general purpose diagnostic CT scanners, the Hi-Art Helical TomoTherapy system uses a CT-like ring gantry. The stability that can be achieved with a ring gantry platform is unrivalled to prevent reconstruction artifacts for the integrated CT scanner. The Hi-Art ring gantry maintains its isocenter to tens of microns compared with a millimeter diameter on the best C-arm linac gantries. The x-ray source for imaging is the treatment linac with the beam lowered in energy to about 3 MV (with a mean energy less than 1 MV). Using the same beam line for therapy and imaging ensures that what is imaged is what is being treated. The image enables lung, fat, muscle, and bone to be clearly distinguished.[31] The kidney, lens of the eye, prostate capsule, and bowel are rendered visible with a dose to the patient of about 1 cGy to 2 cGy, which is sufficiently low for daily use. As described previously, when metal is in the treatment field, an MV CT image

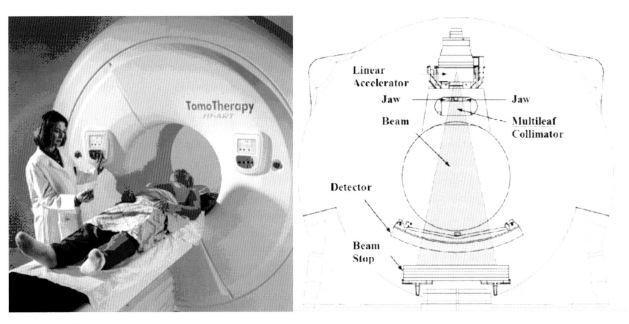

FIGURE 10-4. The left panel is a photograph of a TomoTherapy Hi-Art unit and the right panel shows the integrated beam line for imaging and treatment delivery.

is preferable to that of a kV CT image because fewer streak artifacts are produced.[32] More than 95% of treatments on the Hi-Art Helical TomoTherapy unit use daily CT guidance.

The TomoTherapy Hi-Art unit has an integrated design. Optimized planning, delivery quality assurance, CT-guided delivery, record and verify, and image archiving are all integrated around a central database server. The treatment unit, the planning console, the operator console, and a computer cluster are directly attached to the database. Diagnostic CT scans are sent into this database. The MV CT scan from the unit may be used for the purposes of planning. The physician follows processes identical to 3D RT planning in terms of outlining target volumes and regions at risk. The contouring may be done on the planning console or obtained from a CT-simulator or another planning station.

The process of optimized planning is similar to intensity-modulated RT (IMRT). Dose constraints are given to both the target volumes and the regions at risk. The constraints may be changed through the iterative phase in planning without starting over. Because there are so many beam directions, the probability of doses similar to the prescription appearing in normal tissue a long way away, as is common in more conventional IMRT, is reduced for helical tomotherapy.

Image Registration

The operator console controls the CT scanning parameters. The setup of the patient is adjusted by using registration of the daily MV CT onto the planning CT images. To start, a patient is selected from a hierarchical

menu of patients, diseases, and plans. On the operator console, an image panel displays a sagittal view of the patient on which the CT scan range is selected. The CT images are reconstructed and displayed during acquisition. At the end of the CT acquisition, the registration begins. There are several methods for autoregistration of the image sets such as using bony alignment or the whole image set. The registration results can be checked in three orthogonal directions (axial, sagittal, and coronal). Tools to assist in the evaluation include a checkerboard pattern with alternating planning CT and daily image CT sets displayed, display of regions of interest, isodose lines, and dose colorwashes. Because of local shifts or deformation, manual registration is often necessary. The adjustments can be made in the three translation directions and in the rotational dimensions of roll, pitch, and yaw. When the registration is deemed satisfactory, the couch automatically moves longitudinally and vertically. Lateral adjustments are made by using a motor to move the tabletop. A roll rotational adjustment is accounted for automatically by changing the angular indexing of the gantry. Pitch and yaw adjustments must be made manually. The treatment delivery begins following the setup adjustment. As the treatment is one continuously delivered helical field, there is only one treatment initialization.

Computed tomography image guidance is performed daily for the vast majority of tomotherapy patients (see Chapters 16F, 17C, 18B, and 20I). This is made practical by the tight integration of imaging and delivery, as well as the low CT dose. Figure 10-5 is an example of an MV CT and planning CT registration before treatment of a patient with prostate cancer. The goal is soft tissue alignment.

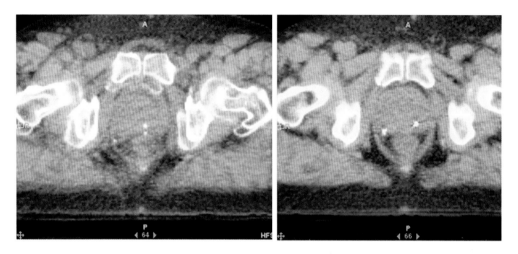

FIGURE 10-5. Illustration of registration of a megavoltage (MV) computed tomography (CT; yellow-scale image) with a planning CT (gray-scale image). The left is before registration and the right is after registration. Notice that the bones do not line up perfectly because the goal is to line up the soft tissue, such as the prostate and rectal wall, as best as possible.

In the particular case of the prostate, differential filling of the rectum and bladder can alter the prostate position significantly. The need for daily CT guidance for prostate radiotherapy was never much in doubt.[33] What was surprising to many was the setup variability for patients with head and neck cancer. Researchers at M.D. Anderson Orlando retrospectively asked what would have been the setup accuracy if they had not done daily CT setup guidance and instead did other schedules such as weekly or every-second-day image acquisition.[34] Daily CT image sets were used as the basis for the comparisons. They observed that weekly set-up adjustment would have resulted in more than 5 mm error about 30% of the time.

Adaptive Radiotherapy

Adaptive radiotherapy is a set of procedures that collectively ensures quality assurance of the whole course of radiotherapy. The actual dose delivered is computed on the daily CT image after the registration of the patient is taken into account.[35] The dose distribution is compared to the desired dose distribution. If the dose was too low to the target volume, the dose can be reoptimized so that on subsequent fractions the dose can be increased (Figure 10-6). A typical workflow might be to accumulate the dose for several weeks, evaluate, and then adjust the treatment for the subsequent week. A single adaptive correction between the halfway point and two thirds of the fractions delivered may be sufficient to ensure the course is being delivered correctly.

To date, there are approximately 300 Hi-Art systems worldwide, treating patients in both academic and community hospital settings. Some of these centers are operating under strict research protocols so that the efficacy and efficiency of the units can be carefully documented. Other centers are treating a large number of image-guided IMRT patients (more than 40 per day) for a variety of cancer sites.

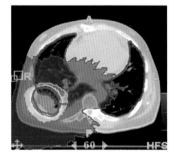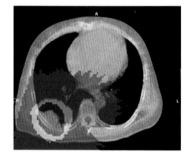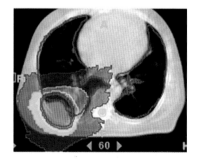

FIGURE 10-6. Example of replanning in a patient with lung cancer following dramatic changes in lung anatomy. On the left is the original plan shown on the planning computed tomography (CT) image showing good sparing of the spinal cord. In the center megavoltage (MV) CT image, fluid has drained from the normal lung significantly shifting the tumor. The patient shift enables the lung to be treated but the dose to the cord is unacceptably high. A replan on the right shown on the MV CT image restores the cord sparing for the remainder of the treatments.

References

1. Kak AC, Slaney M. Principles of computerized tomographic imaging. Piscataway, NJ: IEEE Service Center; 1988.

2. Swindell W, Simpson RG, Oleson JR, et al. Computed tomography with a linear accelerator with radiotherapy applications. *Med Phys.* 1983;10:416–420.

3. Nakagawa K, Akanuma KA, Aoki Y, et al. A quantitative patient set-up and verification system using megavoltage CT scanning. *Int J Radiat Oncol Biol Phys.* 1991;21:228.

4. Sillanpa J, Chang J, Mageras G, et al. Developments in megavoltage cone beam CT with an amorphous silicon EPID: reduction of exposure and synchronization with respiratory gating. *Med Phys.* 2005;32:819–829.

5. Sidhu K, Ford EC, Spirou S, et al. Optimization of conformal thoracic radiotherapy using cone-beam CT imaging for treatment verification. *Int J Radiat. Oncol Biol Phys.* 2003;55:757–767.

6. Seppi EJ, Munro P, Johnsen SW, et al. Megavoltage cone-beam computed tomography using a high-efficiency image receptor. *Int J Radiat Oncol Biol Phys.* 2003;55:793–803.

7. Ford EC, Chang J, Mueller K, et al. Cone-beam CT with megavoltage beams and an amorphous silicon electronic portal imaging device: potential for verification of radiotherapy of lung cancer. *Med Phys.* 2002;29:2913–2924.

8. Spies L, Ebert M, Groh BA, et al. Correction of scatter in megavoltage cone-beam CT. *Phys Med Biol.* 2001;46:821–833.

9. Mosleh-Shirazi MA, Evans PM, Swindell W, et al. A cone-beam megavoltage CT scanner for treatment verification in conformal radiotherapy. *Radiother Oncol.* 1998;48:319–328.

10. Midgley S, Millar RM, Dudson J. A feasibility study for megavoltage cone beam CT using a commercial EPID. *Phys Med Biol.* 1998;43:155–169.

11. Pouliot J, Aubin M, Verhey L, et al. Low dose megavoltage cone beam CT reconstruction for patient alignment [abstract]. Presented at: 7th International Workshop on Electronic Portal Imaging; Vancouver, BC, Canada; June 27, 2002.

12. Pouliot J, Bani-Hashemi A, Chen J, et al. Low-dose megavoltage cone-beam CT for radiation therapy. *Int J Radiat Oncol Biol Phys.* 2005;61:552–560.

13. Morin O, Gillis A, Chen J, et al. Megavoltage cone-beam CT: system description and clinical applications. *Med Dosim.* 2006;31:51–61.

14. Morin O, Gillis A, Descovich M, et al. Patient dose considerations for routine megavoltage cone-beam CT imaging. *Med Phys.* 2007;35:1819–1827.

15. Miften M, Gayou O, Reitz B, et al. IMRT planning and delivery incorporating daily dose from mega-voltage cone-beam computed tomography imaging. *Med Phys.* 2007;34:3760–3767.

16. Gayou O, Parda DS, Johnson M, Miften M. Patient dose and image quality from mega-voltage cone beam computed tomography imaging. *Med Phys.* 2007;34:499–506.

17. Morin O, Aubry JF, Aubin M, et al. Physical performance and image optimization of megavoltage cone-beam CT. *Med Phys.* 2009;36:1421–1432.

18. Morin O, Aubin M, Aubry JF, et al. Quality assurance of megavoltage cone-beam CT [abstract]. *Med Phys.* 2007;34:2634.

19. Gayou O, Miften M. Commissioning and clinical implementation of a mega-voltage cone beam CT system for treatment localization. *Med Phys.* 2007;34:3183–3192.

20. Smitsmans MHP, De Bois J, Sonke JJ, et al. Automatic prostate localization on cone-beam CT scans for high precision image-guided radiotherapy. *Int J Radiat Oncol Biol Phys.* 2005;63:975–984.

21. Mahnken AH, Raupach R, Wildberger JE, et al. A new algorithm for metal artifact reduction in computed tomography: in vitro and in vivo evaluation after total hip replacement. *Invest Radiol.* 2003;38:769–775.

22. Aubin M, Morin O, Chen J, et al. The use of megavoltage cone-beam CT to complement CT for target definition in pelvic radiotherapy in presence of hip replacement. *Br J Radiol.* 2006;79:918–921.

23. Descovich M, Morin O, Aubry JF, et al. Megavoltage cone-beam CT to complement CT-based treatment planning for HDR brachytherapy. *Brachytherapy.* 2006;5:85–86.

24. Huang CY, Chu TC, Lin SY, et al. Accuracy of the convolution/superposition dose calculation algorithm at the condition of electron disequilibrium. *Applied Radiation Isotopes.* 2002;57:825–830.

25. Faddegon BA, Wu V, Pouliot J, et al. Low dose megavoltage cone beam computed tomography with an unflattened 4 MV beam from a carbon target. *Med Phys.* 2008;35:5777–5786.

26. Swerdloff S, Mackie TR, Holmes TW. Method and apparatus for radiation therapy, US patent 5,317,616. 3/19/1992.

27. Mackie TR, Holmes T, Swerdloff S, et al. Tomotherapy: a new concept for the delivery of dynamic conformal radiotherapy. *Med Phys.* 1993;20:1709–1719.

28. Mackie TR, Holmes TW, Reckwerdt PJ, Yang J. Tomotherapy: optimized planning and delivery for radiation therapy. *Int J Imaging Sys Tech.* 1995;6:43–55.

29. Mackie TR, Kapatoes J, Ruchala K, et al. Image guidance for precise conformal radiotherapy. *Int J Radiat Oncol Biol Phys.* 2003;56:89–105.

30. Olivera GH, Shepard DM, Ruchala KJ, et al. Tomotherapy. In: *Modern Technology of Radiation Oncology.* Van Dyk J, ed. Madison, WI: Medical Physics Publishing; 1999: 521–587.

31. Ruchala KJ, Olivera GH, Schloesser EA, et al. Calibration of a tomotherapeutic MVCT system. *Phys Med Biol.* 2000;45: 27–36.

32. Holly R, Myrehaug S, Kamran A, et al. High-dose-rate prostate brachytherapy in a patient with bilateral hip prostheses planned using megavoltage computed tomography images acquired with a helical tomotherapy unit. *Brachytherapy.* 2009;8:70–73.

33. Kupelian PA, Langen KM, Willoughby TR, et al. Daily variations in the position of the prostate bed in patients with prostate cancer receiving postoperative external beam radiation therapy. *Int J Radiat Oncol Biol Phys.* 2006;66:593–596.

34. Zeidan OA, Langen KM, Meeks SL, et al. Evaluation of image-guidance protocols in the treatment of head and neck cancers. *Int J Radiat Oncol Biol Phys.* 2007;67:670–677.

35. Kapatoes JM, Olivera GH, Balog JP, et al. On the accuracy and effectiveness of dose reconstruction for tomotherapy. *Phys Med Biol.* 2001;46:943–966.

Chapter 11

Respiratory Management Technologies

Laura I. Cerviño, PhD, Steve B. Jiang, PhD

Improvements in staging, imaging, and precision radiotherapy (RT) delivery by means of three-dimensional (3D) conformal or intensity-modulated RT (IMRT) allow a more conformal dose to be delivered to the target, thereby reducing the dose to the nearby organs at risk (OARs). The net result is an improvement in the therapeutic gain.[1] In certain disease sites, however, there is a concern related to the potential increased risk of geometrical misses because of respiratory-induced motion. For tumors in the thorax and abdomen, the magnitude of such motion can be significant (~2 cm to 3 cm), depending on location and patient-specific characteristics.[2] However, even motion of pelvic tumors has been observed.[3–5]

Motion poses a number of special problems, including geometrical uncertainty[6,7] (moving targets may appear with distorted shapes and in wrong locations on treatment planning scans), and increased irradiation of normal tissues (large margins are often used to ensure that the tumor is not missed).[8–10] These sources of uncertainty may compromise the efficacy of conformal RT in the management of these lesions, especially when the treatment is delivered using a hypofractionated schedule. One consequence of respiration is that the treatment volume has to be increased, thus unnecessarily irradiating a larger normal tissue volume to higher doses. Breathing compensation strategies have been and are under investigation. Recommendations of the use of different imaging and treatment techniques for motion management has been provided in the American Association of Physicists in Medicine (AAPM) Task Group Report 76.[11]

An important goal of image-guided RT (IGRT) is to allow the use of reduced treatment field margins, thereby minimizing the dose delivered to normal tissues while ensuring that the target receives the full prescription dose. Image guidance provides useful information about tumor motion caused by respiration. Its clinical introduction is drastically changing imaging, treatment planning, and delivery. Additionally, new technologies are constantly being developed and investigated.[12] In this chapter,

techniques and technologies available to manage tumor motion during treatment are described. First of all, disease sites affected by respiration are reviewed. An overview of current techniques used in motion management is then provided, focusing on image-guided procedures.

Disease Sites Affected by Respiratory Motion

The lungs are the most relevant organ affected by respiratory motion. However, it is not the only site, for other anatomic sites are also affected by respiratory motion, including the breast, liver, pancreas, kidneys, and even the prostate. A brief summary of organ motion studies classified by disease site is given in Table 11-1. Tumor motion reported by these studies has been assessed with a variety of imaging modalities, including ultrasound, fluoroscopy, four-dimensional (4D) computed tomography (CT), and 4D magnetic resonance (MR) imaging.

Lung

Most studies of tumor motion with respiration, and most of the effort in developing new techniques for motion management in RT have focused on lung. Lung tumor motion depends on tumor location and other patient factors. It has been observed that tumors can move up to 2 cm to 3 cm during normal respiration, and even more during deep inspiration. Because of the complicated motion of lung tumors, only cranial–caudal motion has been shown in Table 11-1. The most comprehensive study to date on lung tumor motion has been performed by Seppenwoolde et al., who measured tumor motion in three directions (cranial–caudal, anterior–posterior, lateral), for different locations in the lung (upper lobe, lower lobe, middle lobe), making the additional distinction of whether tumor was or was not attached to any anatomical structure.[13] Image-guided RT techniques are used for either tracking the tumor or treating only when the tumor is in a given position (in the beam path).

TABLE 11–1 Organ Motion for Patients in the Supine Position

Site	Study	n	Motion, mm	
			Normal Breathing	Deep Breathing
Lung (motion in cranial–caudal direction)	Seppenwoolde et al.[13] (Upper/lower lobes)	20	2±2 / 12±6	–
	Ekberg et al.[18]	20	3.9 (0–12)	–
	Plathow et al.[19] (upper/middle/lower)	20	4.3±2.4 / 7.2±1.8 / 9.5±4.9	4±2 / 17±12 / 24±17
Liver	Weiss et al.[20]	12	11±3	–
	Harauz et al.[21]	51	14	–
	Suramo et al.[22]	50	25 (10–40)	55 (30–80)
	Davies et al.[23]	8	10±8 (5–17)	37±8 (21–57)
	Balter et al.[24]	9	17	–
Kidneys	Suramo et al.[22]	100	19 (10–40)	41 (20–70)
	Davies et al.[23]	8	11±4 (5–16)	–
	Balter et al.[24]	18	18	–
Pancreas	Suramo et al.[22]	50	20 (10–30)	43 (20–80)
	Bryan et al.[25]	36	18	–
	Bhasin et al.[15]	22	–	1–34
Diaphragm	Wade[26]	10	17±3	99±16
	Weiss et al.[20]	25	13±5	–
	Davies et al.[23]	9	12±7 (7–28)	43±10 (25–57)
	Korin et al.[27]	15	13	39
	Hanley et al.[28]	5	26.4 (18.8–38.2)	–

The displacement is provided in millimeters. Mean values and standard deviations (if available) are listed. Ranges of motion (if available) are listed in parentheses. Here, *n* indicates the number of participants in the study, except for kidneys, where it is the number of kidneys.

Liver

Liver RT has traditionally had a limited role in the treatment of liver cancers, mainly because of the low whole-liver radiation tolerance and tumor motion.[14] However, with the advancements of 3D conformal RT, IMRT, and IGRT, treatment can be applied. As can be seen in Table 11-1, respiratory motion in the liver has a larger effect than that observed previously in lung tumor motion. It is, therefore, an organ that will benefit greatly from IGRT, and is, with breast and lung, one of the tumor sites where IGRT techniques for tumor management have current use.

Breast

The breast moves mainly in anterior–posterior direction, although motion during regular breathing is of only 2 mm to 4 mm. Because this motion is relatively small, motion management techniques for breast treatment do not normally have the purpose of immobilizing the tumor, but of sparing healthy tissues. Treatment at deep-inspiration breath hold has the advantage of increasing the distance between the heart and chest wall.

Pancreas

Pancreas, as an upper-abdominal organ, suffers both from respiratory motion as well as from gastrointestinal motion. Respiratory motion occurs because of the contraction of the diaphragm, as for other abdominal organs. It has been observed that different portions of the pancreas have different motion modes and amplitude.[15] As with the liver, its motion may be larger than the motion observed in the lung.

Kidneys

It has been observed that kidneys may exhibit large motion because of respiration. Kidney motion has been evaluated with radiographs, ultrasound, CT, and MR. A summary of kidney motion is shown in Table 11-1.

Prostate

Although the prostate is not treated with respiratory motion management techniques, respiratory motion of the diaphragm has been linked to intrafraction prostate motion.[4,16,17]

Motion Management Techniques

Motion management techniques discussed in this chapter refer, in general, to treatment techniques applied once the plan has been prepared and the patient has been properly set up for treatment. This being said, some of the techniques presented here are also used during imaging and simulation. An important point to make is that respiration patterns can vary from day to day. Moreover, tumor deformation or regression may occur. It is therefore important to confirm on a daily basis that respiratory motion is compatible with the treatment plan. This could be done, for example, by imaging the patient with fluoroscopy or cone beam CT (CBCT) and setting up the patient so that the motion range of the day coincides with the planned motion range.

Two major classes of techniques have been developed to manage respiratory tumor motion during treatment. In one class, the tumor is allowed to move freely relative to the treatment beam and the goal is to integrate the motion effect into the treatment plan (geometrically or dosimetrically). These techniques include (1) patient population–based internal margin, (2) patient-specific internal margin, (3) internal target volume (ITV) method, and (4) IMRT optimization using motion probability density function (PDF).[12,29] In the second class of techniques, the goal is to "freeze" the tumor motion relative to the treatment beams, which includes two approaches: (1) to allow free tumor motion but adjust the treatment equipment to maintain a constant target position in the beam's eye view when the beam is on, through *respiratory gating, beam tracking,* or *couch-based motion compensation*[12] and (2) to control the tumor motion, using techniques such as *breath hold, forced shallow breathing,* or *abdominal compression*. The reader should be aware that not all of these techniques are unique to IGRT. Non-IGRT techniques will be briefly discussed; however, special attention will be paid to IGRT techniques.

Motion Encompassing Methods

The methods described in this section consist of developing a treatment plan by adding margins to the target volume that encompass tumor motion. A major drawback of these approaches is that tumor motion is measured at the time of simulation, and this motion can vary greatly from simulation to treatment time as well as between different treatment days. Therefore, it is important to use some image guidance technique to monitor tumor motion during treatment or to ensure a regular and stable breathing pattern by using breath-coaching techniques.

Population-Based Margins

Motion management is, at many institutions, accounted for by the use of margins encompassing tumor motion. Definition of relevant terminology is included in the International Commission on Radiation Units and Measurements (ICRU) Report 50.[30] The gross tumor volume (GTV) includes the demonstrable tumor as visualized on the planning scan. The clinical target volume (CTV) is generated by including areas of potential tumor involve-

ment. Lastly, the planning target volume (PTV) is defined as the CTV with the addition of a margin to account for geometrical variations such as patient movement, setup errors, and organ motion.

Adding population-based margins has been the standard clinical practice for many years. However, population-based margins used to expand the CTV into the PTV are only valid for the "average" patient. In patients where target motion is larger than the population average, the target will be underdosed. On the other hand, in patients where the target motion is smaller than the population average, the surrounding healthy tissues will be overdosed. Because, in general, margins are larger than tumor motion, this method to encompass tumor motion often leads to unnecessary normal tissue irradiation.

Patient-Specific Margins

A primary goal of IGRT is to safely adjust margins in order to not overdose healthy tissue and/or to not underdose the target. If information on tumor motion in the patient is available, these margins can be designed on a patient-by-patient basis. Tumor motion can be measured with fluoroscopy or a 4D CT scan, and a patient-specific internal margin, which is often asymmetric, can be designed according to these measurements.

Internal Target Volume

The ICRU Report 62 defines the ITV as the volume that encompasses the CTV and an internal margin (IM).[31] The IM is added to compensate for expected physiologic movements and variations in size, shape, and position of the CTV during therapy in relation to an internal reference point. The ITV is generally asymmetric with respect to the CTV. Because the ITV includes motion, it cannot be detected with a single static image of the patient, and it must be determined with imaging techniques that show the entire range of tumor motion. Such techniques include fluoroscopy, slow CT scans, 4D CT or respiration-correlated CT scans, 4D MR, and combined inhale and exhale breath-hold CT scans.[32] When CT scans are used to obtain the ITV, normally a maximum intensity projection (MIP) is used to obtain the tumor-motion–encompassing volume.[33]

In addition to the ITV, a setup margin (SM) needs to be added around the ITV to account for uncertainties in patient positioning and therapeutic beam alignment during treatment planning and all the treatment sessions. The ITV with the addition of the SM forms the PTV.

Motion PDF-Based Optimization

One way to account for real patient-specific tumor motion in IMRT is to include the motion into plan optimization. As mentioned earlier, motion of the tumor can be determined via 4D CT. A PDF of the tumor motion can then be derived from it by quantifying tumor and OAR positions in the different instances of the CT scan. This PDF is convolved with the pencil beam kernel during inverse optimization.[29,34] Based on the probability of tumor or an OAR being within a particular voxel, the dose to a particular voxel is adjusted lower relative to the prescription dose. This lower dose is compensated for by irradiating regions that are always occupied by tumor with a higher dose.

Respiratory Gating

Respiratory gating is a motion management technique that consists of delivering radiation only during the portion of the breathing cycle when the tumor is in the path of the beam.[35-40] Respiratory gating relies on the existence and knowledge of a breathing signal and the feasibility to trigger the beam during the desired portion (phase or amplitude) of the given breathing signal. Commonly used in the treatment of lung tumors, it is being used also for treatment of tumors in other organs such as liver.[41]

4D CT Imaging

Regular free-breathing CT scans do not properly reflect tumor motion. Depending on the tumor and scanning speeds, a variety of artifacts may appear in the free-breathing CT image.[42,43] One way to mitigate motion artifacts is through a gated CT, which consists of imaging only at a specified breathing phase.[44,45] Treatment should be delivered accordingly to the phase selected for imaging. A more powerful technique is 4D imaging, which is currently the most widely used method for planning of gated treatments. Longer scans at each couch position are obtained, and the acquisition time is synchronized with a breathing signal. Upon completion of the acquisition of the 4D CT, a series of CT scans is reconstructed at different phases of the breathing cycle. Normally 10 to 20 phases are used. A reduced number of phases is selected from the scan for gated treatment, and normally the MIP is used for lung cancer to combine them and define the gated ITV. Because only a few breathing phases are considered, the gated ITV is smaller than the one derived from motion-encompassing methods. Use of 4D CT is based on the assumption that the patient produces a regular and reproducible breathing signal. Because breathing is not always regular, and because of the mechanical limitations of CT scanners, artifacts may appear in the image. Verbal coaching techniques have been used to help patients achieve a regular and reproducible breathing signal in order to have an artifact-free image. Visual and audio coaching techniques have also been studied[46-52] (see Chapter 17E).

Respiration Monitoring

As previously mentioned, gating relies on the existence and knowledge of a breathing signal. Because tumor motion itself is not usually available, other surrogates have to be used to derive the breathing signal. Gating systems can be categorized depending on the surrogates they use: internal and external gating.[37] Internal gating consists of using internal surrogates such as implanted fiducial markers in or near the tumor to generate the gating signal, whereas external gating uses surrogates such as infrared markers placed on the abdomen or chest, surface motion derived from surface imaging cameras, air flow during breathing, etc.

Currently, the only internal gating system clinically available is the real-time tumor-tracking radiation therapy (RTRT) system developed jointly by Mitsubishi Electronics Co. (Tokyo, Japan) and Hokkaido University.[40,53] Gold seeds are implanted in or near the tumor, and their position is automatically tracked in three dimensions with the aid of a stereotactic kilovoltage x-ray imaging system. The imaging system acquires simultaneous orthogonal fluoroscopic images acquired at a rate of 30 Hz. When fiducials are within a small range of their target position (defined at simulation), the treatment beam is turned on.

External gating consists of deriving tumor position from external breathing signals. Breathing can be externally monitored in a variety of ways, which has led to the development of different systems. Early methods explored in the mid-1990s by Kubo and colleagues for gating included the use of thermistors, thermocouples, strain gauge methods, and a pneumotachograph.[54] These investigators have also developed a gated RT system that tracks infrared reflective markers on the patient abdomen by using a video camera, developed jointly with Varian Medical Systems Inc. (Palo Alto, CA).[39] This system was later commercialized by Varian and called the Real-Time Position Management (RPM) system (Figure 11-1). The RPM system has been extensively implemented and investigated clinically at a number of centers. Similar systems have been implemented, such as the ExacTrac Gating/Novalis Gating (BrainLab, Feldkirchen, Germany), which, in addition to the external markers, incorporates x-ray imaging capabilities for determining the internal anatomy position and for verifying the internal anatomy during treatment.

In external gating that uses surface motion, both chest motion and abdominal motion have been used as surrogates, the latter being the preferred method because of its higher amplitude. Siemens AG (Erlangen, Germany) has a linear accelerator gating interface that receives the respiratory signal from a belt around the patient with a pressure cell that senses changes as the patient breathes. More recently, 3D surface imaging video cameras have been used to obtain, track, and monitor images from the patient's surface. A commercially available 3D camera system is available from VisionRT Ltd (London, UK; Figure 11-2).[55]

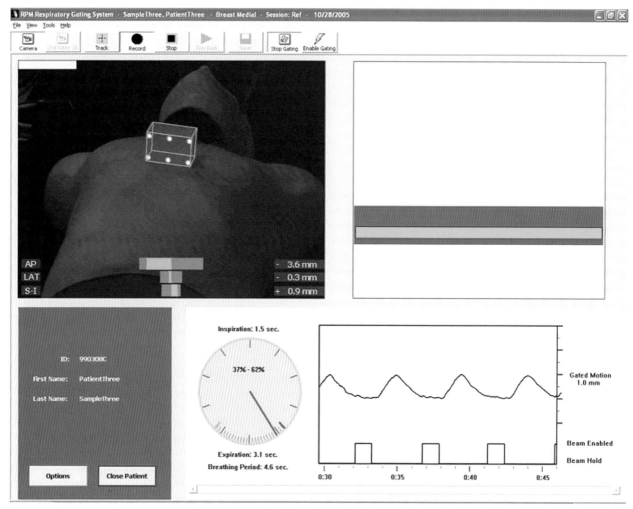

FIGURE 11-1. The Real-Time Position Management (RPM) system (Varian Medical Systems, Palo Alto, CA). A box with reflective markers is placed on the patient and is tracked by camera, providing the breathing signal for treatment gating.

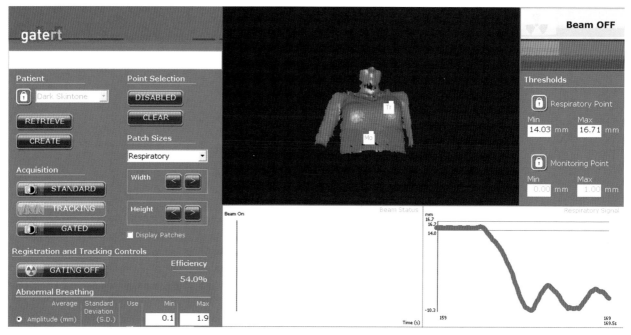

FIGURE 11-2. Surface image provided by AlignRT (VisionRT, London, UK). Surface points have been chosen to extract the respiratory signal.

Gating Window

The gating window is defined as the range of the surrogate signal when the radiation beam is turned on. Two important factors in respiratory gating are the linear accelerator duty cycle and the residual motion of the tumor during the gating window. The duty cycle is the ratio of the beam-on time to the total treatment time. While in a non-gated treatment the duty cycle is 100%, a typical range in gated treatments is 30% to 50%.[37] The objective in gating is to maximize the duty cycle and to minimize the residual motion of the tumor in the gating window. These goals are achieved best at end-of-inhale (EOI) and end-of-exhale (EOE). It has been shown that gating at EOE and EOI are equivalent in lung dose and toxicity, and, with proper coaching, in terms of duty cycle.[56,57] The PTV margins should be added in accordance to the residual motion during the beam-on time.

Breath Coaching

The main disadvantage of external gating is that it assumes a good and constant relationship between the surrogate and the tumor motion. This relationship, however, may change over time, both inter- and intrafractionally.[58] At the same time, it is important to maintain a reproducible breathing pattern in order to provide adequate treatment in an efficient way. Treatment efficiency in terms of duty cycle can be improved with the cooperation of the patient and with visual and audio respiratory coaching (Figure 11-3).[46,47,49–51] Audio coaching alone improves the periodicity of the patient's breathing pattern, but not amplitude or baseline drift.[47,50]

Tumor Tracking

Beam tracking techniques follow the target dynamically with the radiation beam.[59] In the previous section, the RTRT system was discussed that tracks in real-time gold markers implanted within the tumor. This system, however, is used for gating, and no beam tracking is performed. In this section, three techniques that provide beam tracking will be discussed: repositioning of the linear accelerator, adjustment of the collimating aperture, and electromagnetic steering of a charged particle beam.

Beam tracking was first implemented in a robotic radiosurgery system.[60–64] The Synchrony Respiratory Tracking system integrated with the CyberKnife robotic linear accelerator (Accuray Inc, Sunnyvale, CA) is the only robotic linear accelerator currently used clinically. Prior to treatment, the 3D position of the tumor is determined by automatically detecting implanted gold markers via orthogonal x-ray images, at the same time as the signal from an external surrogate on the patient's surface is recorded. A model that relates the external and internal motions is generated based on the x-ray images and the recorded signal. During treatment, tumor position is continuously predicted from the external surrogate and the model is modified. The model is updated for every new radiation beam by acquiring new x-ray images.

In linac-based RT, tumor motion can be compensated for by using a dynamic multileaf collimator (MLC).[50,65–75] The dynamic MLC continuously aligns or reshapes the treatment aperture to compensate for tumor motion. Theoretical and empirical investigations have shown the great potential of this technique; however, it has not been clinically implemented to date.

Other ideas have been proposed for heavy ion therapy, such as magnetic deflection of the pencil beam for lateral compensation and energy modulation for longitudinal compensation.[76,77]

Other Respiration Monitoring Strategies

Besides the techniques used for gating, new respiration monitoring strategies are being investigated for tumor tracking. One technique is fluoroscopic tracking of radioopaque fiducial markers implanted inside or near the tumor.[78,79] The accuracy of this technology is better than 1.5 mm for tracking moving targets, which is much higher than the external surrogates approach.[40] Another implementation of marker tracking is based on nonionizing electromagnetic fields, using small wireless transponders implanted in tissue.[80] A commercial system with electromagnetic transponders is the 4D Localization System of Calypso Medical Technologies (Seattle, WA). However, no matter how marker tracking is realized, as long as the percutaneous marker implantation is involved, the clinical implementation of this technology in lung cancer is limited because of the risk of pneumothorax.[81,82]

Tracking of lung tumor can also be achieved without implanted fiducial markers with fluoroscopic and with electronic portal imaging device (EPID) images (Figure 11-4). Template matching techniques, optical flow, active shape model, and principal component analysis

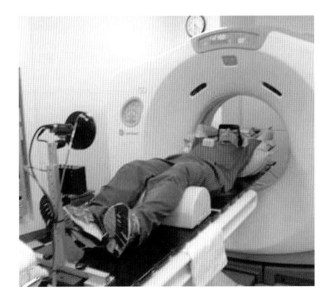

FIGURE 11-3. Visual coaching is provided to patients through video goggles.

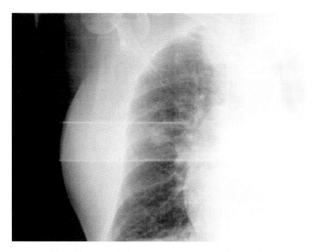

FIGURE 11-4. Fluoroscopic image where tumor and internal structures can be seen.

combined with artificial neural network have achieved promising results when the tumor has reasonably high contrast and clear boundary in the images.[83–86]

Couch Motion Compensation

Couch motion compensation is a technique that involves adjustments of the treatment couch opposite to tumor motion.[87] It uses a robotically controlled couch coupled with a target-tracking system. The motion is opposite to tumor motion as the patient breathes, therefore keeping the target at a fixed position in space. Although this technique is not commercially available, D'Souza and colleagues have proved its feasibility.[87,88] Nonetheless, there are several concerns associated with this technique. Couch motion may compensate for intrafractional motion; however, it will not compensate for tumor deformation. In addition, the patient may react to couch motion and may resist or try to compensate for it. To minimize this, good immobilization and patient coaching should be used. However, the main difficulty comes in implementing fast couch motion and associated position verification uncertainties. Mean tumor position, however, can be compensated for because of its slow-motion nature.[89,90]

Breath-Hold Techniques

Breath-hold techniques consist of freezing the tumor position by a voluntary or forced breath hold while the radiation beam is on. Used mainly for lung and breast radiation treatments, it has also evolved for the treatment of tumors in other organs such as liver and kidneys.[22,28,91–102] Each breath-hold technique presents different advantages, with tumor immobilization being common to all of them. A key issue in breath-hold treatment is that the treatment plan should always be designed according to the technique. Therefore, if treatment is going to be delivered at a

specified point in the breathing cycle, the plan and simulation should be performed at the same point. The aim is to achieve the same breath-hold position between fields during a single treatment fraction as well as between fractions. Therefore, reproducibility of the breath hold needs to be guaranteed.

One of the main problems of breath holding is patient compliance. As the duration of a treatment beam is generally 15 to 30 seconds, many patients are able to have the beam dose delivered within one breath hold. Some patients, such as breast cancer patients, will usually comply well with treatment; however, lung cancer patients may have a more difficult time holding their breath because of their compromised pulmonary status. Patient cooperation and patient comfort, thus, need to be considered when one is selecting this technique.

Most breath-hold methods use some means of monitoring during each breath hold. These methods range from spirometry to more sophisticated surface motion tracking and provide feedback to the patient for reproducibility. In addition, verbal coaching as well as visual coaching can be provided to the patient to improve reproducibility.

Respiration Monitoring

The most commonly used device to monitor breath hold is a spirometer.[28,92,93] These devices measure the time-integrated air flow, and, thus, provide the lung volume from a baseline (e.g., EOE). An occlusion valve can be added to the spirometer, forcing the breath-hold when desired, and leading to forced breath hold. This idea led to the development of what is known as the Active Breathing Control (ABC) system (Elekta AB, Stockholm, Sweden). The ABC system has been used in the treatment of diverse tumor sites at breath hold, such as lung, liver, breast, and Hodgkin's disease.[91,95,97,98,100,103]

Voluntary breath hold can be monitored with RPM. Predominantly used for lung gating treatments, it has also been used in breath-hold treatment of upper abdomen and breast.[101,102] More recently, magnetic sensors and optical tracking systems have been proposed for monitoring breath hold.[52,104] As in respiratory gating, a key issue is the accuracy of externally placed breath-hold monitors in predicting internal positions of the tumor and nearby organs. The external-to-internal correlation may change, not only by alterations in the breathing pattern, but also by changes in the internal anatomy, such as abdominal contents, ascites, and tumor growth or shrinkage with treatment. Thus, the external-to-internal constancy requires verification at simulation and throughout the treatment course.

Deep Inspiration Breath Hold

Deep inspiration breath hold (DIBH) is a maneuver that consists of a free-breathing interval followed by a breath hold at approximately 100% vital capacity during a prescribed period. Mainly explored for lung cancer and breast cancer treatments, DIBH has two main goals: (1) to increase the distance between the breast and the heart; this results in increased normal tissue sparing and reduces the risk of pneumonitis[96]; and (2) breath hold that immobilizes the tumor.[28,96]

Voluntary Breath Hold

Voluntary breath hold, or self-held breath hold, can be achieved with or without respiratory monitoring. The patient voluntarily holds his or her breath at a specified point in the breathing cycle, and the beam is turned on during breath hold. The duty cycle is larger than free-breathing respiratory gated techniques because delivery of radiation is continuous during the breath hold. It has been observed that maximum reproducibility is achieved at deep inhale or deep exhale.

Forced Breath-Hold

Assisting devices can be used for improving reproducibility of the breath hold. The ABC system was first developed at William Beaumont Hospital and is currently widely used in deep-inspiration breath-hold treatment, although it can suspend breathing at any predetermined position. The patient is verbally coached to help achieve steady breathing. Treatments at moderate DIBH, which consists of holding the breath at approximately 75% of the vital capacity, have been shown to achieve good reproducibility of internal organ position when one is using ABC, while being more comfortable for the patient.[100,105]

Shallow Breathing and Immobilization

One of the easiest ways to minimize respiratory-induced organ motion in the upper abdomen and thoracic area is to use abdominal compression, which is occasionally used in extracranial stereotactic radiosurgery (SRS) or stereotactic body radiotherapy (SBRT).[106,107] The use of SBRT with immobilization was first applied to treatments of lung, liver, and some extrahepatic lesions[108,109] The standard technique utilizes a stereotactic body frame with a vacuum pillow for body immobilization, with an attached plate that applies compression to the abdomen, therefore reducing diaphragmatic excursions, while still permitting limited normal respiration. There are currently only a few commercial systems, such as the Stereotactic Body Frame (Elekta AB, Stockholm, Sweden), and some institutions have designed their own systems.[108,110]

The body frame is used for defining and fixing a coordinate system for stereotactic treatment, while abdominal compression is used to manage tumor motion. The abdominal plate is attached to the body frame by a rigid arc and a scaled screw is used to achieve reproducible pressure. Abdominal compression is used when tumor motion exceeds clinical goals. Usually, the maximum

pressure that the patient can tolerate for the duration of the treatment is used. During the CT scan, the range of tumor motion attributable to pulmonary and cardiac motion is determined fluoroscopically. Negoro and coworkers observed tumor motion in 18 lung cancer patients (20 lesions) and applied abdominal compression (or diaphragm control) to 10 of them. The tumor motion range was larger than 5 mm.[111] Tumor motion was reduced from a mean of 12.3 mm during free respiration to 7.0 mm with compression. Of note, there was one patient whose tumor motion increased when compression was applied, probably because of an effort to overcome compression. Therefore, after abdominal compression is applied, motion needs to be fluoroscopically evaluated and the pressure should be adjusted as needed.

Because of the high doses delivered in the few fractions in SBRT approaches, precision is very important. Approaches that aid in the accurate treatment delivery include whole-body immobilization and image-based assessment of patient and target position immediately prior to the delivery of radiation. Two major factors have to be considered for image-guidance of SBRT. First, patient setups for body treatments are rarely as reliable and accurate as setups for intracranial treatment. Second, target motion (either intrafraction or interfraction) frequently occurs. To assess the accuracy of patient positioning, usually verification portal images are obtained prior to each treatment.[110,112] However, other approaches are available and under investigation, such as kilovoltage (kV) CT, megavoltage (MV) CT, on-board CBCT, and ultrasound guidance.[113] Measurements of diaphragm motion under fluoroscopy on different days can also be made to verify reproducibility.[11]

Conclusions

It is well known that respiratory motion poses a challenge for the radiotherapeutic treatment of some tumor sites, such as those of the lung, liver, and pancreas. However, some organs are more affected than others by respiratory motion, and the effect is also patient-specific. Recently, tumor motion has begun to be a focus of research and technology development in RT. Image-guided RT, in its different varieties, has brought about the possibility of obtaining tumor motion information and to improve therapy yielding a more conformal dose to a moving tumor. Fluoroscopy, CT, 4DCT, MR, surface imaging, and the use of electromagnetic transponders are some of the currently available modalities to obtain tumor motion information.

Although tumor is in general hard to track and distinguish in images during treatment, some surrogates may be easier to visualize. Ionizing imaging techniques such as fluoroscopy provide internal organ motion information, and surface imaging provides external surface information. However, when one is using surrogates to derive tumor motion, a good and consistent correlation with tumor motion needs to be proved. This correlation can be improved with proper patient breathing coaching. Although great advances in IGRT have been made to manage tumor motion, much remains to be done to optimize treatment.

References

1. Fang LC, Komaki R, Allen P, et al. Comparison of outcomes for patients with medically inoperable stage I non-small-cell lung cancer treated with two-dimensional vs. three-dimensional radiotherapy. *Int J Radiat Oncol Biol Phys.* 2006;66:108–116.

2. Keall PJ, Mageras GS, Balter JM, et al. The management of respiratory motion in radiation oncology report of AAPM Task Group 76. *Med Phys.* 2006;33:3874–3900.

3. Kitamura K, Shirato H, Seppenwoolde Y, et al. Three-dimensional intrafractional movement of prostate measured during real-time tumor-tracking radiotherapy in supine and prone treatment positions. *Int J Radiat Oncol Biol Phys.* 2002;53:1117–1123.

4. Malone S, Crook JM, Kendal WS, et al. Respiratory-induced prostate motion: quantification and characterization. *Int J Radiat Oncol Biol Phys.* 2000;48:105–109.

5. Weiss E, Vorwerk H, Richter S, et al. Interfractional and intrafractional accuracy during radiotherapy of gynecologic carcinomas: a comprehensive evaluation using the ExacTrac system. *Int J Radiat Oncol Biol Phys.* 2003;56:69–79.

6. Chen GTY, Kung JH, Beaudette KP. Artifacts in computed tomography scanning of moving objects. *Sem Radiat Oncol.* 2004;14:19–26.

7. Yamamoto T, Langner U, Loo Jr BW, et al. Retrospective analysis of artifacts in four-dimensional CT images of 50 abdominal and thoracic radiotherapy patients. *Int J Radiat Oncol Biol Phys.* 2008;72:1250–1258.

8. Prescribing, recording, and reporting photon beam therapy. ICRU Report 62. Bethesda, MD: International Commission on Radiation Unit and Measurements (ICRU); 1999.

9. Ramsey CR, Scaperoth D, Arwood D, et al. Clinical efficacy of respiratory gated conformal radiation therapy. *Med Dosim.* 1999;24:115–119.

10. Langen KM, Jones DTL. Organ motion and its management. *Int J Radiat Oncol Biol Phys.* 2001;50:265–278.

11. Keall PJ, Mageras GS, Balter JM, et al. The management of respiratory motion in radiation oncology report of AAPM Task Group 76. *Med Phys.* 2006;33:3874–3900.

12. Jiang SB. Radiotherapy of mobile tumors. *Semin Radiat Oncol.* 2006;16:239–248.

13. Seppenwoolde Y, Shirato H, Kitamura K, et al. Precise and real-time measurement of 3D tumor motion in lung due to breathing and heartbeat, measured during radiotherapy. *Int J Radiat Oncol Biol Phys.* 2002;53:822–834.

14. Ingold J, Reed G, Kaplan H, et al. Radiation hepatitis. *Am J Roentgenol.* 1965;93:200–208.

15. Bhasin DK, Rana SS, Jahagirdar S, et al. Does the pancreas move with respiration? *J Gastroenterol Hepatol.* 2006;21:1424–1427.

16. Souchon R, Rouvière O, Gelet A, et al. Visualisation of HIFU lesions using elastography of the human prostate in vivo: preliminary results. *Ultrasound Med Biol.* 2003;29:1007–1015.

17. Dawson LA, Litzenberg DW, Brock KK, et al. A comparison of ventilatory prostate movement in four treatment positions. *Int J Radiat Oncol Biol Phys.* 2000;48:319–323.

18. Ekberg L, Holmberg O, Wittgren L, et al. What margins should be added to the clinical target volume in radiotherapy treatment planning for lung cancer? *Radiother Oncol.* 1998;48:71–77.

19. Plathow C, Ley S, Fink C, et al. Analysis of intrathoracic tumor mobility during whole breathing cycle by dynamic MRI. *Int J Radiat Oncol Biol Phys.* 2004;59:952–959.

20. Weiss PH, Baker JM, Potchen EJ. Assessment of hepatic respiratory excursion. *J Nucl Med.* 1972;13:758–759.

21. Harauz G, Bronskill MJ. Comparison of the liver's respiratory motion in the supine and upright positions: concise communication. *J Nucl Med.* 1979;20:733–735.

22. Suramo I, Päivänsalo M, Myllylä V. Cranio-caudal movements of the liver, pancreas and kidneys in respiration. *Acta Radiol Diagn.* 1984;25:129–131.

23. Davies SC, Hill AL, Holmes RB, et al. Ultrasound quantitation of respiratory organ motion in the upper abdomen. *Br J Radiol.* 1994;67:1096–1102.

24. Balter JM, Ten Haken RK, Lawrence TS, et al. Uncertainties in CT-based radiation therapy treatment planning associated with patient breathing. *Int J Radiat Oncol Biol Phys.* 1996;36:167–174.

25. Bryan PJ, Custar S, Haaga JR, et al. Respiratory movement of the pancreas: an ultrasonic study. *J Ultrasound Med.* 1984;3:317–320.

26. Wade OL. Movements of the thoracic cage and diaphragm in respiration. *J Physiol.* 1954;124:193–212.

27. Korin HW, Ehman RL, Riederer SJ, et al. Respiratory kinematics of the upper abdominal organs: a quantitative study. *Magn Reson Med.* 1992;23:172–178.

28. Hanley J, Debois MM, Mah D, et al. Deep inspiration breath-hold technique for lung tumors: the potential value of target immobilization and reduced lung density in dose escalation. *Int J Radiat Oncol Biol Phys.* 1999;45:603–611.

29. Trofimov A, Rietzel E, Lu HM, et al. Temporo-spatial IMRT optimization: concepts, implementation and initial results. *Phys Med Biol.* 2005;50:2779–2798.

30. Prescribing, recording and reporting photon beam therapy. ICRU Report 50. Bethesda, MD: International Commission on Radiation Units and Measurements; 1993.

31. Prescribing, recording, and reporting photon beam therapy (supplement to ICRU Report 50). ICRU Report 62. Bethesda, MD: International Commission on Radiation Units and Measurements; 1999.

32. Liu HH, Balter P, Tutt T, et al. Assessing respiration-induced tumor motion and internal target volume using four-dimensional computed tomography for radiotherapy of lung cancer. *Int J Radiat Oncol Biol Phys.* 2007;68:531–540.

33. Underberg RW, Lagerwaard FJ, Slotman BJ, et al. Use of maximum intensity projections (MIP) for target volume generation in 4DCT scans for lung cancer. *Int J Radiat Oncol Biol Phys.* 2005;63:253–260.

34. Unkelbach J, Oelfke U. Inclusion of organ movements in IMRT treatment planning via inverse planning based on probability distributions. *Phys Med Biol.* 2004;49:4005–4029.

35. Ohara K, Okumura T, Akisada M, et al. Irradiation synchronized with respiration gate. *Int J Radiat Oncol Biol Phys.* 1989;17:853–857.

36. Inada T, Tsuji H, Hayakawa Y, et al. Proton irradiation synchronized with respiratory cycle [in Japanese]. *Nippon Igaku Hoshasen Gakkai Zasshi.* 1992;52:1161–1167.

37. Jiang SB. Technical aspects of image-guided respiration-gated radiation therapy. *Med Dosim.* 2006;31:141–151.

38. Kubo HD, Wang L. Compatibility of Varian 2100C gated operations with enhanced dynamic wedge and IMRT dose delivery. *Med Phys.* 2000;27:1732–1738.

39. Kubo HD, Len PM, Minohara S, et al. Breathing-synchronized radiotherapy program at the University of California Davis Cancer Center. *Med Phys.* 2000;27:346–353.

40. Shirato H, Shimizu S, Kunieda T, et al. Physical aspects of a real-time tumor-tracking system for gated radiotherapy. *Int J Radiat Oncol Biol Phys.* 2000;48:1187–1195.

41. Wagman R, Yorke E, Ford E, et al. Respiratory gating for liver tumors: use in dose escalation. *Int J Radiat Oncol Biol Phys.* 2003;55:659–668.

42. Chen GT, Kung JH, Beaudette KP. Artifacts in computed tomography scanning of moving objects. *Semin Radiat Oncol.* 2004;14:19–26.

43. Lewis JH, Jiang SB. A theoretical model for respiratory motion artifacts in free-breathing CT scans. *Phys Med Biol.* 2009;54:745–755.

44. Shen S, Duan J, Fiveash JB, et al. Validation of target volume and position in respiratory gated CT planning and treatment. *Med Phys.* 2003;30:3196–3205.

45. D'Souza WD, Kwok Y, Deyoung C, et al. Gated CT imaging using a free-breathing respiration signal from flow-volume spirometry. *Med Phys.* 2005;32:3641–3649.

46. Mageras GS, Yorke E, Rosenzweig K, et al. Fluoroscopic evaluation of diaphragmatic motion reduction with a respiratory gated radiotherapy system. *J Appl Clin Med Phys.* 2001;2:191–200.

47. Kini VR, Vedam SS, Keall PJ, et al. Patient training in respiratory-gated radiotherapy. *Med Dosim.* 2003;28:7–11.

48. Nelson C, Starkschall G, Balter P, et al. Respiration-correlated treatment delivery using feedback-guided breath hold: a technical study. *Med Phys.* 2005;32:175–181.

49. George R, Chung TD, Vedam SS, et al. Audio-visual biofeedback for respiratory-gated radiotherapy: impact of audio instruction and audio-visual biofeedback on respiratory-gated radiotherapy. *Int J Radiat Oncol Biol Phys.* 2006;65:924–933.

50. Neicu T, Berbeco R, Wolfgang J, et al. Synchronized moving aperture radiation therapy (SMART): improvement of breathing pattern reproducibility using respiratory coaching. *Phys Med Biol.* 2006;51:617–636.

51. Baroni G, Riboldi M, Spadea MF, et al. Integration of enhanced optical tracking techniques and imaging in IGRT. *J Radiat Res.* 2007;48:A61–A74.

52. Cerviño LI, Gupta S, Rose MA, et al. Using surface imaging and visual coaching to improve reproducibility and stability of deep-inspiration breath hold for left breast cancer radiotherapy. *Phys Med Biol.* 2009;54(22):6853–6865.

53. Shirato H, Shimizu S, Shimizu T, et al. Real-time tumour-tracking radiotherapy. *Lancet.* 1999;353:1331–1332.

54. Kubo HD, Hill BC. Respiration gated radiotherapy treatment: a technical study. *Phys Med Biol.* 1996;41:83–91.

55. Bert C, Metheany KG, Doppke K, et al. A phantom evaluation of a stereo-vision surface imaging system for radiotherapy patient setup. *Med Phys.* 2005;32:2753–2762.

56. Berbeco RI, Nishioka S, Shirato H, et al. Residual motion of lung tumors in end-of-inhale respiratory gated radiotherapy based on external surrogates. *Med Phys.* 2006;33:4149–4156.

57. Wu J, Li H, Shekhar R, et al. An evaluation of planning techniques for stereotactic body radiation therapy in lung tumors. *Radiother Oncol.* 2008;87:35–43.

58. Seppenwoolde Y, Berbeco RI, Nishioka S, et al. Accuracy of tumor motion compensation algorithm from a robotic respiratory tracking system: a simulation study. *Med Phys.* 2007;34:2774–2784.

59. Murphy MJ. Tracking moving organs in real time. *Semin Radiat Oncol.* 2004;14:91–100.

60. Adler JR Jr, Murphy MJ, Chang SD, et al. Image-guided robotic radiosurgery. *Neurosurgery.* 1999;44:1299–1306; discussion 1306–1297.

61. Schweikard A, Glosser G, Bodduluri M, et al. Robotic motion compensation for respiratory movement during radiosurgery. *Comput Aided Surg.* 2000;5:263–277.

62. Ozhasoglu C, Murphy MJ, Glosser G, et al. Real-time tracking of the tumor volume in precision radiotherapy and body radiosurgery - a novel approach to compensate for respiratory motion. In: Lemke HU, Vannier MW, Inamura K, et al., eds. *Proc. 14th Int. Conf. on Computer Assisted Radiology and Surgery (CARS 2000)*; San Francisco, CA; 2000: 691–696.

63. Murphy MJ, Chang SD, Gibbs IC, et al. Patterns of patient movement during frameless image-guided radiosurgery. *Int J Radiat Oncol Biol Phys.* 2003;55:1400–1408.

64. Murphy MJ. Fiducial-based targeting accuracy for external-beam radiotherapy. *Med Phys.* 2002;29:334–344.

65. Keall PJ, Kini VR, Vedam SS, et al. Motion adaptive x-ray therapy: a feasibility study. *Phys Med Biol.* 2001;46:1–10.

66. Neicu T, Shirato H, Seppenwoolde Y, et al. Synchronized moving aperture radiation therapy (SMART): average tumour trajectory for lung patients. *Phys Med Biol.* 2003;48:587–598.

67. Suh Y, Yi B, Ahn S, et al. Aperture maneuver with compelled breath (AMC) for moving tumors: a feasibility study with a moving phantom. *Med Phys.* 2004;31:760–766.

68. Papiez L. The leaf sweep algorithm for an immobile and moving target as an optimal control problem in radiotherapy delivery. *Math Comput Modelling.* 2003;37:735–745.

69. Rangaraj D, Papiez L. Synchronized delivery of DMLC intensity modulated radiation therapy for stationary and moving targets. *Med Phys.* 2005;32:1802–1817.

70. Papiez L, Rangaraj D. DMLC leaf-pair optimal control for mobile, deforming target. *Med Phys.* 2005;32:275–285.

71. Keall PJ, Joshi S, Vedam SS, et al. Four-dimensional radiotherapy planning for DMLC-based respiratory motion tracking. *Med Phys.* 2005;32:942–951.

72. Wijesooriya K, Bartee C, Siebers JV, et al. Determination of maximum leaf velocity and acceleration of a dynamic multileaf collimator: implications for 4D radiotherapy. *Med Phys.* 2005;32:932–941.

73. Webb S. The effect on IMRT conformality of elastic tissue movement and a practical suggestion for movement compensation via the modified dynamic multileaf collimator (dMLC) technique. *Phys Med Biol.* 2005;50:1163–1190.

74. Webb S. Limitations of a simple technique for movement compensation via movement-modified fluence profiles. *Phys Med Biol.* 2005;50:N155–N161.

75. Sawant A, Venkat R, Srivastava V, et al. Management of three-dimensional intrafraction motion through real-time DMLC tracking. *Med Phys.* 2008;35:2050–2061.

76. Grozinger SO, Rietzel E, Li Q, et al. Simulations to design an online motion compensation system for scanned particle beams. *Phys Med Biol.* 2006;51:3517–3531.

77. Bert C, Saito N, Schmidt A, et al. Target motion tracking with a scanned particle beam. *Med Phys.* 2007;34:4768–4771.

78. Shirato H, Harada T, Harabayashi T, et al. Feasibility of insertion/implantation of 2.0-mm-diameter gold internal fiducial markers for precise setup and real-time tumor tracking in radiotherapy. *Int J Radiat Oncol Biol Phys.* 2003;56:240–247.

79. Tang X, Sharp GC, Jiang SB. Fluoroscopic tracking of multiple implanted fiducial markers using multiple object tracking. *Phys Med Biol.* 2007;52:4081–4098.

80. Balter JM, Wright JN, Newell LJ, et al. Accuracy of a wireless localization system for radiotherapy. *Int J Radiat Oncol Biol Phys.* 2005;61:933–937.

81. Arslan S, Yilmaz A, Bayramgurler B, et al. CT-guided transthoracic fine needle aspiration of pulmonary lesions: accuracy and complications in 294 patients. *Med Sci Monit.* 2002;8:CR493–CR497.

82. Geraghty PR, Kee ST, McFarlane G, et al. CT-guided transthoracic needle aspiration biopsy of pulmonary nodules: needle size and pneumothorax rate. *Radiology.* 2003;229:475–481.

83. Cui Y, Dy JG, Sharp GC, et al. Multiple template-based fluoroscopic tracking of lung tumor mass without implanted fiducial markers. *Phys Med Biol.* 2007;52:6229–6242.

84. Xu Q, Hamilton RJ, Schowengerdt RA, et al. A deformable lung tumor tracking method in fluoroscopic video using active shape models: a feasibility study. *Phys Med Biol.* 2007;52:5277–5293.

85. Xu Q, Hamilton RJ, Schowengerdt RA, et al. Lung tumor tracking in fluoroscopic video based on optical flow. *Med Phys.* 2008;35:5351–5359.

86. Lin T, Cerviño LI, Tang X, et al. Fluoroscopic tumor tracking for image-guided lung cancer radiotherapy. *Phys Med Biol.* 2009;54:981–992.

87. D'Souza WD, Naqvi SA, Yu CX. Real-time intra-fraction-motion tracking using the treatment couch: a feasibility study. *Phys Med Biol.* 2005;50:4021–4033.

88. D'Souza WD, McAvoy TJ. An analysis of the treatment couch and control system dynamics for respiration-induced motion compensation. *Med Phys.* 2006;33:4701–4709.

89. Wilbert J, Meyer J, Baier K, et al. Tumor tracking and motion compensation with an adaptive tumor tracking system (ATTS): system description and prototype testing. *Med Phys.* 2008;35:3911–3921.

90. Trofimov A, Vrancic C, Chan TCY, et al. Tumor trailing strategy for intensity-modulated radiation therapy of moving targets. *Med Phys.* 2008;35:1718–1733.

91. Wong JW, Sharpe MB, Jaffray DA, et al. The use of active breathing control (ABC) to reduce margin for breathing motion. *Int J Radiat Oncol Biol Phys.* 1999;44:911–919.

92. Rosenzweig KE, Hanley J, Mah D, et al. The deep inspiration breath-hold technique in the treatment of inoperable non-small-cell lung cancer. *Int J Radiat Oncol Biol Phys.* 2000;48:81–87.

93. Mah D, Hanley J, Rosenzweig KE, et al. Technical aspects of the deep inspiration breath-hold technique in the treatment of thoracic cancer. *Int J Radiat Oncol Biol Phys.* 2000;48:1175–1185.

94. Schwartz LH, Richaud J, Buffat L, et al. Kidney mobility during respiration. *Radiother Oncol.* 1994;32:84–86.

95. Stromberg JS, Sharpe MB, Kim LH, et al. Active breathing control (ABC) for Hodgkin's disease: reduction in normal tissue irradiation with deep inspiration and implications for treatment. *Int J Radiat Oncol Biol Phys.* 2000;48:797–806.

96. Barnes EA, Murray BR, Robinson DM, et al. Dosimetric evaluation of lung tumor immobilization using breath hold at deep inspiration. *Int J Radiat Oncol Biol Phys.* 2001;50:1091–1098.

97. Dawson LA, Brock KK, Kazanjian S, et al. The reproducibility of organ position using active breathing control (ABC) during liver radiotherapy. *Int J Radiat Oncol Biol Phys.* 2001;51:1410–1421.

98. Sixel KE, Aznar MC, Ung YC. Deep inspiration breath hold to reduce irradiated heart volume in breast cancer patients. *Int J Radiat Oncol Biol Phys.* 2001;49:199–204.

99. Kim DJ, Murray BR, Halperin R, et al. Held-breath self-gating technique for radiotherapy of non-small-cell lung cancer: a feasibility study. *Int J Radiat Oncol Biol Phys.* 2001;49:43–49.

100. Remouchamps VM, Letts N, Vicini FA, et al. Initial clinical experience with moderate deep-inspiration breath hold using an active breathing control device in the treatment of patients with left-sided breast cancer using external beam radiation therapy. *Int J Radiat Oncol Biol Phys.* 2003;56:704–715.

101. Berson AM, Emery R, Rodriguez L, et al. Clinical experience using respiratory gated radiation therapy: comparison of free-breathing and breath-hold techniques. *Int J Radiat Oncol Biol Phys.* 2004;60:419–426.

102. Pedersen AN, Korreman S, Nystrom H, et al. Breathing adapted radiotherapy of breast cancer: reduction of cardiac and pulmonary doses using voluntary inspiration breath-hold. *Radiother Oncol.* 2004;72:53–60.

103. Remouchamps VM, Letts N, Yan D, et al. Three-dimensional evaluation of intra- and interfraction immobilization of lung and chest wall using active breathing control: a reproducibility study with breast cancer patients. *Int J Radiat Oncol Biol Phys.* 2003;57:968–978.

104. Remouchamps VM, Huyskens DP, Mertens I, et al. The use of magnetic sensors to monitor moderate deep inspiration breath hold during breast irradiation with dynamic MLC compensators. *Radiother Oncol.* 2007;82:341–348.

105. Remouchamps VM, Vicini FA, Sharpe MB, et al. Significant reductions in heart and lung doses using deep inspiration breath hold with active breathing control and intensity-modulated radiation therapy for patients treated with locoregional breast irradiation. *Int J Radiat Oncol Biol Phys.* 2003;55:392–406.

106. Potters L, Steinberg M, Rose C, et al. American Society for Therapeutic Radiology and Oncology* and American College of Radiology Practice Guideline for the Performance of Stereotactic Body Radiation Therapy. *Int J Radiat Oncol Biol Phys.* 2004;60:1026–1032.

107. Murray B, Forster K, Timmerman R. Frame-based immobilization and targeting for stereotactic body radiation therapy. *Med Dosim.* 2007;32:86–91.

108. Lax I, Blomgren H, Naslund I, et al. Stereotactic radiotherapy of malignancies in the abdomen. Methodological aspects. *Acta Oncol.* 1994;33:677–683.

109. Blomgren H, Lax I, Naslund I, et al. Stereotactic high dose fraction radiation therapy of extracranial tumors using an accelerator. Clinical experience of the first thirty-one patients. *Acta Oncol.* 1995;34:861–870.

110. Lee S-W, Choi EK, Park HJ, et al. Stereotactic body frame based fractionated radiosurgery on consecutive days for primary or metastatic tumors in the lung. *Lung Cancer.* 2003;40:309–315.

111. Negoro Y, Nagata Y, Aoki T, et al. The effectiveness of an immobilization device in conformal radiotherapy for lung tumor: reduction of respiratory tumor movement and evaluation of the daily setup accuracy. *Int J Radiat Oncol Biol Phys.* 2001;50:889–898.

112. Wulf J, Hädinger U, Oppitz U, et al. Stereotactic radiotherapy of extracranial targets: CT-simulation and accuracy of treatment in the stereotactic body frame. *Radiother Oncol.* 2000;57:225–236.

113. Fuss M, Boda-Heggemann J, Papanikolau N, et al. Image-guidance for stereotactic body radiation therapy. *Med Dosim.* 2007;32:102–110.

Chapter 12

ELECTROMAGNETIC TRACKING

DALE W. LITZENBERG, PhD

The systems used for target volume localization guidance described throughout this textbook are based on two-dimensional (2D) or three-dimensional (3D) image acquisition technologies. Electromagnetic localization and tracking systems are unique in several respects. They do not use ionizing radiation or generate 2D or 3D anatomical images. Moreover, tracking data are generated continuously (currently at a rate of 10 Hz) and require little to no postprocessing or interpretation.

Interestingly, the precursor technologies that led to electromagnetic tracking for radiation therapy (RT) were developed in the early 1960s. The ability to determine the orientation and origin of a magnetic dipole field[1] helped spur the development of technologies to find the location of trapped miners,[2] provide surface navigation for ships,[3] enable subsurface navigation for tunneling devices,[4] and produce helmet-mounted sights for fighter aircraft.[5] One of the first companies to commercialize the related technology was Polhemus Associates, which was founded in 1964. The company developed a system ubiquitously called "The Polhemus" in the virtual reality and entertainment industries, for capturing and simulating the motion of people and objects.

Early efforts to introduce electromagnetic guidance into medical devices involved the localization and guidance of catheters during magnetocardiographic procedures.[6] By the mid- to late-1990s, electromagnetic guidance systems were available for use during surgery with results of multiinstitutional trials being reported.[7] Systems with multiple sensors have also been used to study the properties of ligaments and ligament reconstruction methods in articulating joints, particularly in the elbow and knee.[8–10] Similarly, a Polhemus System with two sensors was implemented as a 3D digitizer for cranial neurosurgical planning.[11] However, before the discussion of applications in RT, the theory of electromagnetic tracking will be discussed briefly.

Electromagnetic Localization and Tracking Theory

In this section the basic theory of electromagnetic tracking will be discussed, though further details may be found elsewhere.[5,12] The essential components of an electromagnetic localization and tracking system consist of a magnetic dipole source and a set of sensors, and their associated electronics, for measuring the magnetic flux field produced by the dipole at many different locations. In its simplest form, the source is formed by a single loop of wire carrying an oscillating current, which forms an oscillating magnetic dipole field. A magnetic dipole field is cylindrically symmetric about the axis of the wire loop and resembles concentric toroids or doughnuts. The shape of the dipole field is fixed and depends only on the geometry of the loops of wire in the source, as shown in Figure 12-1. In a practical source, many loops of wire are wound about a small iron cylinder. For a fixed-source geometry, the strength and direction of the magnetic field at any point away from the dipole source is determined by the amount and direction of the current.

The sensor also consists of a loop of wire. When the magnetic flux through the sensor loop changes, a current is induced in the sensor loop (Faraday's Law) that is proportional to the rate of change of the magnetic flux at that location. The direction of the change in the magnetic field can be determined from the direction of the induced current (Lenz's Law). Consequently, many sensors placed in a known configuration may be used to measure the magnetic field flux and strength at several locations, and the data used to fit the origin and orientation of the magnetic dipole that would produce such measurements.

In commercial systems, the components are more complex than these simple descriptions. In practice, the current in the source will vary with a specified frequency to produce the changing magnetic flux needed for detection by the sensors. This may be accomplished by using

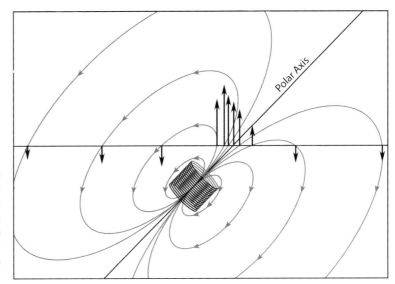

FIGURE 12-1. Illustration of the shape of the dipole magnetic field created by a coil of wire carrying a current. The horizontal line represents the plane of a two-dimensional array containing sensor coils. The coils measure the changing magnetic flux normal to their cross-sectional area. The vertical arrows represent the component of the dipole field that is normal to the coils.

wired sources connected to a sinusoidally varying voltage source. Alternatively, wireless sources may be used where the wire loop used to generate the magnetic dipole field is connected to a capacitor. Such a wireless source has a resonant frequency determined by the geometry of the loop and the size of the capacitor. As illustrated in Figure 12-2, the source is then excited by an externally applied resonant radiofrequency signal, which is typically produced by excitation coils housed near the sensors. When the external signal is removed, the charge induced on the capacitor is discharged through the wire loop at the resonant frequency and the oscillating magnetic dipole produced by this de-excitation signal is detected by the sensors. In either case, the ability to drive or tune each source at a different frequency allows several different sources to be uniquely identified and tracked in quick sequential order by the same set of sensors.

The intended application places stringent constraints on the design of the source. For real-time target tracking of an internal device, the sources must be as small as possible so they can be implanted in a minimally invasive procedure, such as through a biopsy needle. Likewise, in surgical applications, they must be deliverable through small catheter lumens and possibly attachable to remotely guided surgical instruments without impeding their mobility or function. In either case, the source must also be protected in a bio-inert casing.

Sensor configurations will also vary depending on the application. In surgical applications a limited number of sensors may be used, each of which may measure the three vector components of the magnetic field at each location. In other implementations, a 2D array of single-axis (coil) sensors may sample the magnetic flux through sensors arrayed in a 2D plane, through the 3D magnetic dipole

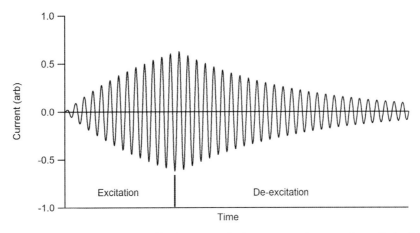

FIGURE 12-2. Schematic illustration of the current excited in the transponder in response to the externally applied radiofrequency signal. The amplitude of the current decays while oscillating at its resonant frequency, producing the detected dipole magnetic field. This figure illustrates the response of the 400-kHz transponder over about a 100 μs timescale. This process is typically repeated many times to increase the signal-to-noise ratio.

field of each source. Because the strength of the magnetic dipole field decreases as r^{-3} on the dipole axis, the sensors have very limited range and are typically placed as close as possible to the sources to provide a sufficient signal-to-noise ratio.

Electromagnetic tracking systems are also susceptible to the proximity of conducting metal objects, especially alloys containing iron and nickel, which have high magnetic permeability.[5,13] These objects distort and reflect the dipole source fields leading to errors in determining position and orientation, as well as reducing the signal-to-noise ratio. However, the distortions caused by the presence of these objects in known orientations, such as the treatment machine gantry, may be compensated for in the processing of the detected signals.[5] In wired systems for guiding instrumentation, positional deviations of up to 2 mm are typical, though in the most extreme circumstances have been reported to be almost 10 mm.[13,14] Consequently, patients who have metallic implants, such as artificial hips and metallic or conductive implants in the tracking region, should be excluded from electromagnetic tracking procedures. Likewise, patients should remove all metallic and conducting objects such as watches, belts, and electronic devices, before undergoing electromagnetically guided procedures. As will be discussed subsequently, this also precludes the use of conducting carbon-fiber treatment tables, which will produce a mirror image of the dipole source, confounding localization and leading to potential errors in determining position and orientation. Additional precautions must be taken if electronic devices that could be affected by radiofrequency (RF) electromagnetic emissions are present. These include digital flat-panel imaging devices, which may show image artifacts, as well as pacemakers and defibrillators.

Radiation Therapy Applications - Wired Systems

One of the earliest applications of electromagnetic tracking in RT was for the nonradiographic localization of interstitial abdominal implants for intraoperative high-dose-rate (HDR).[15] In this application a then–commercially available 3SPACE-FASTRAK system (Polhemus Inc, Colchester, VT) was configured to fit in the lumen of a catheter. The system was then used to measure the spatial path of all catheters by inserting the wired sensor sequentially into each catheter. This information was then used by the planning system to accurately determine and calculate dwell positions and times. The stated accuracy of the system was a root mean square (RMS) of 0.8 mm, but measurements in the operating environment found the RMS accuracy to be 0.38 mm in the absence of metallic surgical retractors and 0.70 mm in the presence of three retractors, with maximum absolute errors of 2.1 mm or less.

In 1995, Lennernäs and Nilsson reported a system that could track permanent magnets composed of neodymium-iron and boron by using an array of magnetic Hall effect sensors.[16,17] The permanent magnets ranged in size from a 3 mm³ by 3 mm³ by 1 mm³ rectangular, to circular with a diameter of 9.5-mm by 3-mm thick. The system was capable of submillimeter resolution measurements at 100 Hz, but had a very limited range of less than 13 mm for even the largest magnet. The intention was to either temporarily implant the permanent magnets, which would be removed after RT, or insert them through an implanted catheter. This effort led to the founding of the company Micropos Medical AB (Gothenburg, Sweden) in 2003.[18] Subsequently, the permanent magnet was replaced by an active wired magnetic dipole antenna placed at the tip of a catheter that operates at 10 Hz. Initial studies in patients resulted in an absolute positional accuracy of 2.7 mm +/- 1.2 mm. At the time of writing, the Micropos RayPilot system was still under development for commercial use.

In 2000, the Paul Scherrer Institute reported on an electromagnetic tracking system they had developed for real-time (50 Hz) target volume tracking during proton therapy with continuous spot scanning delivery.[19] This system consisted of an external magnetic field generator, a wired implantable sensor, and the associated signal processing electronics. When compared with an optical tracking device with 30 μm accuracy, the RMS spatial accuracy was reported to be 1 mm to 2 mm, whereas the RMS angular accuracy of determining the orientation of the dipole was 0.5° to 1°. The system's ability to track and gate was tested in a moving phantom and qualitatively shown to very nearly restore the dose distribution to the planned static distribution when a 3-mm gating window was implemented. The technology for this system was developed by a spin-off company from the Paul Scherrer Institute called Mednetix AG, which was acquired by Northern Digital Inc (Waterloo, ON, Canada). Further development efforts have focused on a wired electromagnetic tracking system for guidance of medical instruments, which is commercially available in the Aurora system.[20] A similar system is manufactured by Medtronic (Minneapolis, MN) called the StealthStation Treon-EM.[13] A system that used DC magnetic fields is also available from Ascension Technology Corporation (Milton, VT) called the microBird.

Radiation Therapy Applications— Wireless Electromagnetic Tracking

The first, and, to date, only, commercially available electromagnetic tracking system designed for use in RT was developed by Calypso Medical Technologies Inc (Seattle, WA). This system has been described extensively in many scientific publications[12,21,22] and its physical components will only be described briefly here. As illustrated

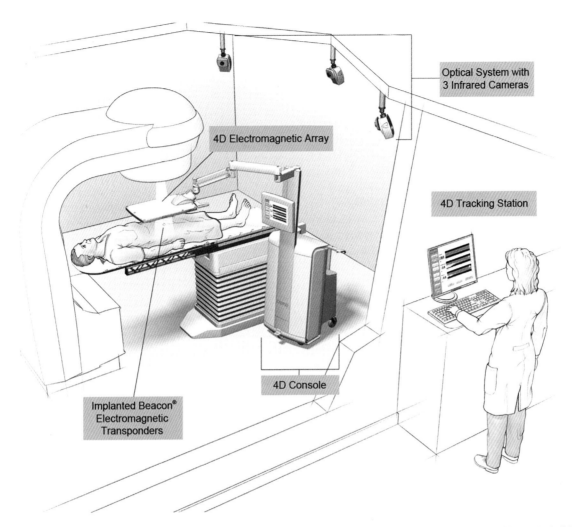

FIGURE 12-3. Components of the Calypso System include the implanted transponders, the four-dimensional (4D) console with attached 4D Electromagnetic Array, ceiling-mounted infrared cameras, and the 4D Tracking Station. Figure used with permission from Calypso Medical Technologies, Seattle WA.

in Figure 12-3, the Calypso System consists of implantable wireless transponders, an in-room four-dimensional (4D) console with 4D electromagnetic array, and an optical system with infrared cameras, along with a tracking station, which is located in the therapy control room.

The in-room console contains the signal processing unit and supports a moveable flat panel that houses the excitation and receiver coil arrays. The array is placed over the patient and tracks the relative geometry of the implanted transponders in relation to the panel. The position of the array relative to the treatment machine and isocenter is determined by three infrared cameras that are mounted to the ceiling and calibrated to the room geometry. The positions are used to determine the location of the planned treatment isocenter. The offset of the isocenter from the machine isocenter is displayed on the screen of the in-room console, as well as on the Tracking Station in the therapy control room. The real-time tracking data displayed on the Tracking Station are monitored

throughout treatment delivery. The Tracking Station also supports administrative activities including data storage report generation and the creation of localization plans for each patient. These plans consist of patient identification information; treatment and data description information such as patient position, coordinate system conventions, and motion tolerances; and the coordinates of the plan isocenter and of the three implanted transponders.

Implantation and Stability of Transponders

The use of this technology requires that transponders are implanted into the patient. Before proceeding with implantation, however, consideration should be given to the eligibility of the patient and the imaging modality that will be used for simulation. For a prostate cancer patient, it should be verified that the patient does not have metallic implants in the pelvic region such as an artificial hip, metallic rod in the upper leg, and supporting structures in the lower spine, as these are a contraindication for the use of electromagnetic tracking. Additionally, compatibility with surgical clips for post-prostatectomy patients has not been evaluated. Consideration should also be given to the patient's size. In larger patients, for whom the treatment isocenter will be greater than 19 cm from the array when the patient is supine, tracking during therapeutic delivery will not be possible. The patient could be treated prone[23,24] to reduce the distance to within the operational range and utilize the real-time tracking capabilities, or the technology can be limited to localization before, or as needed, during treatment. If the patient is eligible for implantation, but magnetic resonance (MR) imaging will be used for simulation, the MR should be obtained before implanting the transponders. Patients with implanted transponders may safely be imaged with MR; however, each transponder produces an artifact approximately 1.5 cm to 2 cm in diameter where no anatomical information is present in 1.5-Tesla (T) MR scanners.[25] In 3-T systems, these void artifacts may be as large as 4 cm. This dark area in the image is caused by an increase in the Larmor frequency caused by the presence of the ferrous core of the transponder, resulting in a loss of signal from the affected region.[25]

Prostate cancer patients typically have three transponders implanted transrectally through a 14-gauge needle under ultrasound guidance into the apex and left- and right-midbase of the prostate. Because the anterior rectal wall is the closest critical structure, some institutions aim to have the transponders placed in the posterior portion of the prostate. This provides the most accurate localization of the interface between the prostate and rectum in the event of local anatomical deformations. For post-prostatectomy patients, two Beacon transponders are placed between the bladder and rectal wall, one on the right side and one on the left side and the remaining transponder is placed on the right side of the anastomosis site. For both intact prostate and post-prostatectomy patients it is recommended that transponders be placed a minimum of 1 cm apart in a triangular configuration. The implantation procedure typically takes about 10 minutes and is performed under local anesthesia. The procedure may lead to some temporary swelling of the gland. Consequently, it is recommended that the planning computed tomography (CT) study be performed at least 4 to 7 days after implantation to allow swelling to resolve.[26]

The relative positional stability of the transponders after implantation has also been studied and found to be similar to that of implanted fiducials, with standard deviations about the expected intratransponder distances of about 0.1 cm.[26-28] Although migration of fiducials and transponders has been observed, it is rare.[27-32] These events are typically associated with isolated incidences of poor implantation technique that result in a fiducial being implanted completely or partially outside the prostatic capsule or within the urethra.

Simulation and Treatment Planning

Good simulation practice requires that the planning CT scan be performed with the same positioning and immobilization as well as bladder and bowel preparation conditions that will be used during therapy. Advanced localization technology should not be relied upon to overcome poor simulation technique. It is common for institutions to require a full bladder and empty rectum during the time of simulation and treatment to minimize daily variation in position and motion. In particular, if significant rectal filling (fecal or gas) is observed on the initial planning CT, it is a strong indication of prostate deformation and rotation about its typical configuration. In this case, the condition should be relieved and the planning CT repeated.

Patients are typically treated in the supine position because of the reduced intrafraction breathing motion observed compared with that seen when patients are in the prone position.[33-37] Computed tomography slices through the gland should be obtained with about 0.1-cm thickness to allow the centers of the transponders to be found with reasonable accuracy during planning. To verify the patient's eligibility for use of the technology, the distance from the most anterior aspect of the patient, when supine, to the farthest transponder should be determined and confirmed to be within the range allowed by the system. Because of the sensitivity of the system, the transponders must be within 19 cm to allow real-time tracking and 25 cm for pretreatment verification only. If the limits are exceeded and prone positioning will be used, simulation should be performed accordingly. As described earlier, the absence of metallic implants, such as artificial hips, should also be verified.

Once the physical requirements of eligibility are satisfied, the isocenter location is set and the treatment plan is created. The choice of isocenter position requires special consideration. If the isocenter is close to the centroid of the transponders, local anatomical deformations will have little impact on their relative orientation. However, as the distance increases, the uncertainty in the relative orientation will increase. Consequently, it is recommended that the isocenter be chosen near the geometrical centroid of the transponder locations. The spatial positions of the three transponders are then found from the planning CT, along with the coordinates of the plan's isocenter. These are entered into the Calypso System when the patient's localization plan is created.

Localization

Because of the sensitivity of electromagnetic tracking to the proximity of metallic objects, some preparations and precautions are required before beginning treatment. A nonconducting table overlay is used to increase the distance from the array to the conducting components of the treatment table, which commonly contains metals or carbon fiber. Alternatively, nonconducting replacement table tops may be obtained. Patients must also remove conducting objects as per standard practice during RT.

During a typical treatment fraction, patients are initially set up according to skin tattoos placed during simulation. As usual, particular care should be taken to make sure the patient is level and not rotated. The array of the Calypso System is then placed above the patient and localization begins. During initial localization, longer signal integration is used, resulting in increased accuracy and the ability to localize transponders at greater distances (up to 25 cm). Each of the transponders is uniquely identified by its resonant frequency and their positions are determined. This information allows many safety and quality assurance (QA) checks to then be conducted. Because the transponder implant configuration of each patient varies to a degree that may be measured accurately, this information may be used to verify that the correct patient has been selected within the Calypso System. The allowable deviation by which the measured and expected relative orientation of the transponders varies may be configured by the user and is typically set to 0.2 cm deviation in an unspecified least-squares fit metric. If this threshold is exceeded, it is an indication that the wrong patient may have been selected for localization, that one or more of the transponders may have migrated, or that significant local deformation has occurred.

The presence of three transponders also allows rotations of the prostate to be calculated (Euler angle convention of roll, pitch, and yaw). These angles are compared against a user configurable tolerance, which is typically set at 10°. If any of these angles exceeds the tolerance, a dialog is displayed giving the largest rotation. These events are fairly uncommon and the policy for the action taken will vary by institution. These rotational events may be transient events, caused by changes in the bladder or rectal volumes that resolve themselves, or can be resolved by simply sitting the patient up to allow the bowels to adjust to a more normal position, and then performing the setup and localization again. However, repeated incidents of rotational misalignment may also indicate a systematic deviation from anatomical positioning during the treatment planning simulation. In these cases, the planning CT should be examined for excessive rectal filling, which was likely alleviated during subsequent daily treatments, possibly indicating the need for a new planning CT.

One of two methods for determining the offsets from isocenter is used, depending on the distance of isocenter from the centroid of the transponders, the distances between transponders, and other plan geometry attributes. As previously discussed, placing the isocenter near the centroid of the transponders minimizes the impact of deformations on the relative geometry of the transponders and isocenter. In this case, the additional translations of the planning isocenter caused by

any rotation of the prostate may be accurately included in the reported translations necessary to move the planning isocenter back to the treatment machine isocenter. However, if the isocenter is placed a significant distance away from the geometric center of the transponders, this rigid body relationship is less reliable. In this case, the deviation of the centroid of the transponders from their planned position is reported, without including translations attributable to prostate rotation that might impact the isocenter. In the first method, the distance allowed between the isocenter and the centroid of the transponders is roughly the radius of the circle that could be transcribed within the triangle formed by the transponders. To include rotations in the translational correction of isocenter, it is also necessary that rotations can be determined accurately from the transponder geometry. As previously mentioned, they should be implanted in a triangular configuration with separations of at least 1 cm. However, if two transponders are very close together compared with the distance to the third, then the transponders effectively become colinear and the accuracy of determining rotations decreases. In this situation, positional deviations are reported based on the centroid of the transponders.

The localization method that will be used is determined before the first treatment, when the isocenter and transponder coordinates are entered into the system and do not require any input or decisions from the therapists during treatments. The therapist simply places the array over the patient in the appropriate position, with guidance from the system, and moves the treatment couch to place the target volume at isocenter, such that the system reports a deviation of typically +/− 0.05 cm or less. Once localization is complete, the therapist places the system into tracking mode and it is ready to begin treatment.

Real-Time Tracking and Treatment Delivery
When placed in tracking mode, the system uses a shorter signal integration time resulting in a reduced tracking range of 19 cm. This tracking range dictates the patient screening criteria described previously. Signal processing by the electromagnetic system is also employed to remove the impact of the presence of the metallic gantry at variable positions. Deviations from the planned position, as described previously, are reported at 10 Hz in current commercial systems (25 Hz in research systems) and displayed on the in-room console and the Tracking Station in the treatment control room, as illustrated in Figure 12-3. In the initial implementation of the technology, visual and audio queues are given when the displayed motion data exceed the tolerance set for any given direction.

Several types of motion are commonly observed including slow constant drifts in one or more directions, sudden transient motions that resolve within 20 to 30 seconds, sudden offsets to a different stable position,

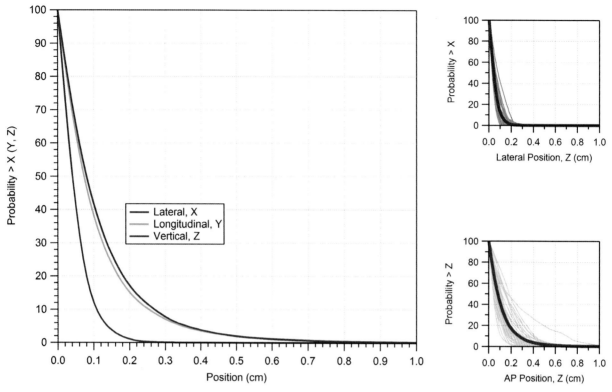

FIGURE 12-4. The probability of a displacement greater than some value in any single direction for a population of patients. The insets show the variability by patient over the course of treatment in the lateral and anterior–posterior (AP) directions. Note that the superior–inferior (SI) variations are very similar to those shown for the AP direction.

and periodic motion about isocenter. There may also be combinations of these motions.[38,39] As described by Langen et al., the magnitude of the vector displacement from isocenter was greater than 3 mm roughly 14% of the time and greater than 5 mm about 3% of the time.[38] However, the variation among patients is large, with the displacements of greater than 3 mm and 5 mm, occurring 36% and 11% of the time , respectively, in a single patient over all fractions. For an individual fraction of any given patient, the deviation may exceed 3– 5 mm 98% of the time. The probability of a displacement greater than some value in any single direction, for the same cohort of patients, is shown in Figure 12-4. The insets show the variability by patient over the course of treatment. Below 2 mm to 3 mm (on average across this cohort) it can be seen that the frequency of displacements beyond these tolerances rises rapidly; for several individual patients, prostate motion well beyond these limits is likely. Consequently, setting displacement tolerances below 3 mm will result in a sharp increase of corrective action at the treatment unit. However the increase in intervention is generally warranted by the fact that the tighter tolerance may reflect tighter, more conformal treatment.

Procedures vary among institutions on the action that should be taken when the positional deviation exceeds

the tolerance level and the nature of the deviation.[39–43] Although the dosimetric impact of very short excursions will vary depending on the margins used and other plan attributes, therapists generally feel compelled to turn the beam off manually unless it is obvious that the deviation will resolve itself within a few seconds, which is often the case. Malinowski and colleagues reported that 59% of excursions greater than 0.3 cm, and 45% of those greater than 1.0 cm resolve within 5 seconds, without any intervention.[41] The most important deviations to correct are the slow drifts, primarily caused by steady bladder and rectal filling over the course of a fraction. Although the initial implementation of the technology required the therapist to enter the room to make a correction using the treatment couch, integration with the treatment control system has allowed the couch moves to be made remotely in a semiautomated manner. This greatly increases the accuracy and speed of corrections. In the case where therapists have to enter the room to make corrections, Malinowski et al. recommended manually gating the beam for 11 to 21 seconds, for 3 mm to 5 mm tolerances, before entering the room to make corrections.[41] Further integration will allow real-time correction.

An institution's policy and procedure for corrective action should be developed in close consideration with the simulation imaging technology used and the treatment planning techniques and objectives. It has been shown that increased levels of corrective action may allow the use of smaller clinical target volume (CTV) to planning target volume (PTV) margins.[40] However, as electromagnetic guidance becomes more integrated with the treatment delivery process, the limiting factor on margin reduction will become the uncertainty in our ability to accurately define the target volume. Although gross tumor volume (GTV) determined from CT may be larger than those defined from MR simulations,[44] they may be systematically shifted in some cases.[45] In addition, daily prostate deformations of several millimeters will also limit the ability to conform dose to the target volume.[46,47]

Clinical Impact

The clinical impact of systematic errors while contouring prostate volumes was clearly demonstrated by de Crevoisier and coworkers in 2005.[48] In this study, the biochemical relapse-free survival of 127 prostate cancer patients was investigated based on rectal distention at the time of the planning CT. Patients with distended rectums at the time of simulation demonstrated a systematic displacement of the contoured prostate volumes relative to the undistended position, which was presumably more common during subsequent treatment fractions. Patients whose rectal distention was less than the median value had a 5-year biochemical control rate of 92%, whereas for patients with greater than the median distention, the control rate was only 63%.

The clinical significance of image-guided prostate localization was demonstrated by Kupelian et al. in 2008.[49] In this retrospective study, daily pretreatment localization was performed using ultrasound guidance in 488 patients. It was found that the degree of rectal distention did not have a statistically significant impact on 5-year biochemical survival when daily pretreatment image guidance was implemented. The study concluded that daily image guidance could eliminate systematic errors during simulation and treatment planning that could adversely impact outcomes. Although ultrasound guidance has fallen out of favor in the intervening years, with preference to more accurate implanted marker and electromagnetic techniques,[50,51] the study still clearly demonstrates the advantage of image guidance.

At the time of writing, the additional clinical significance of electromagnetic tracking is just beginning to be reported. Because the technology has only been commercially available for a few years, no long-term survival data are available yet. However, the impact on quality of life and toxicity, attributable to the further reduction of the CTV-to-PTV margin, is starting to become available.[52–54] A clinical trial has been completed that enrolled prostate cancer patients who were treated with IMRT planned

with a 3-mm PTV margin to a median dose of 81 Gy. All fractions employed electromagnetic guidance with a 2-mm action threshold. The Expanded Prostate Cancer Index Composite (EPIC) questionnaire was completed by patients before and after treatment. In an initial cohort of 20 patients, bowel and rectal scores improved by more than 12% compared with a non–image-guided four-field 3D conformal treatment technique planned to a median dose of 75.6 Gy.[55,56]

In another study, toxicity was evaluated between prostate patients without image guidance and 10 mm PTV margins and patients with daily guidance based on implanted fiducials while using 2 mm to 3 mm PTV margins. Grade 2 rectal toxicity was reduced from 80% to 13% in the image-guided group, and grade 2 bladder toxicity was reduced from 60% to 13%. These reductions in toxicity were attributed to the use of smaller PTV margins, allowed by image guidance, which resulted in reduced dose to the organs at risk.

Although the use of smaller PTV margins to reduce toxicity is quite alluring, one must proceed with great caution. In a study by Engels et al., the outcomes of prostate cancer patients treated with daily bony alignment with 6-mm left–right PTV margins and 10-mm margins in all other directions, were compared with patients who were aligned daily with gold markers and had asymmetrical PTV margins of 3 mm to 5 mm. Unexpectedly, the patients with daily setup with implanted gold markers had significantly worse freedom from biochemical failure after 5 years compared with those who had bony setup—58% versus 91% ($P = .02$).[57,58] The authors concluded by cautioning that margins must be determined on the basis of the residual error for the guidance technique used and the available data on organ motion, which include deformations and rotations. Consequently, real-time electromagnetic tracking shows great promise for enabling tighter margins but other institutional factors must also be considered.

Lung

Because of the large amplitude of intrafraction motion in the lung, and the high prevalence rate of lung cancer, there is great interest in the application of electromagnetic tracking to this site. To date, transponders have been implanted in canines[59–61] and in two humans.[62] Published results from an implantation study in canines showed low stability and retention of the transponders at the implantation site.[59] The transponders were placed bronchoscopically into small airways under fluoroscopic guidance. At 60 days postimplantation only six transponders remained in place. In the two humans, one had three transponders implanted and the other had two, both implanted bronchoscopically. The patient with two implants lost one transponder, which was recovered after being expelled by coughing. To address the low retention rate, a five-legged anchoring device was developed. In a subsequent study, 54 anchored transponders were implanted in nine canines with 100% stability and retention at 60 days.[61] Excision of the lobes containing the transponders and examination of the implantation sites showed that the anchors were well-tolerated. Little to no inflammation was found around 16 of 18 sites, wheras severe inflammation was seen at one of 18 sites.[60] Based on these results, it is anticipated that a clinical study will begin in 2010.

Spine

At the M.D. Anderson Cancer Center in Orlando, Florida, at least four spine patients were implanted with transponders to assess the implantation technique, transponder stability, and the ability to track during clinical use.[62] The transponders were implanted transcutaneously into the paraspinal muscles near the vertebra to be treated. All transponders were reported to be stable as verified with repeat CT studies and daily kV x-rays. While tracking was possible, the patients were treated in the supine position, which placed the transponders near the 25-cm limit of operation in three of the four patients. No side effects of the implantation were reported.

Breast

The Swedish Medical Center (Seattle, WA) has initiated a partial breast irradiation study using implanted gold markers and transponders for guidance of external beam radiation. Modifications to the Calypso System workflow were made to the Calypso System to allow couch rotations of +/– 90°.[63] Three transponders and gold markers were implanted percutaneously under ultrasound guidance into perilumpectomy tissue in six patients. In four patients who required MR follow-up imaging, transponders and gold markers were afterloaded in two interstitial catheters. Setup corrections were determined radiographically from the gold markers. Residual shifts after correction based on gold markers were made using the Calypso System and found to agree within 1.5 mm. Real-time electromagnetic tracking demonstrated intrafraction motion with an average deviation of 1.9 mm and a range of 0.5 mm to 7.1 mm.

Pancreas

The University of Pennsylvania's Abramson Cancer Center has laparoscopically implanted transponders in pancreatic cancer patients.[64] No complications or transponder migrations have been observed. Preliminary range-of-motion results showed the greatest intrafraction motion in the superior–inferior direction with a mean value of 6.3 mm and a range of 25 mm. With some respiratory training, deviations were reduced to a mean of 3.3 mm and a range of 10 mm.

Prostate Prone Position

Because of the availability of electromagnetic tracking, a renewed interest has been explored by some groups in treating prostate patients in the prone position.[23,24] This position offers the possibility of increasing the separation between the prostate and the anterior rectal wall in some patients as reported by Zelefsky and colleagues.[65] Although the prone position fell out of favor because of interfraction setup uncertainties and large respiratory motion, electromagnetic tracking offers the possibility of reducing these uncertainties and taking advantage of the potentially increased separation between the prostate and rectum. Figure 12-5 shows the motion of a patient treated in the prone position. Motion patterns for prone patients are largely similar to those of supine patients with the additional superposition of respiratory motion, which itself may have a peak-to-peak amplitude of many millimeters.[33]

Shah et al. evaluated 200 fractions of prone motion data from 20 patients. After treating the patients in the supine position, they were placed in the prone position and the prostate motion was tracked for 10 minutes.[23] They found that, averaged over all fractions, deviations beyond 3 mm and 5 mm occurred 28.7% and 4.2% of the

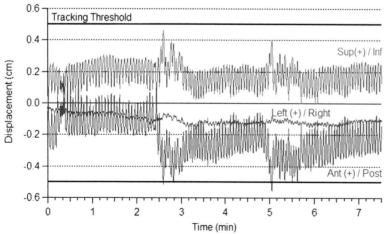

FIGURE 12-5. Sample motion data for a patient treated in the prone position.

time while prone, compared with 13.6% and 3.3% of the time while supine, respectively. Consequently, electromagnetic tracking enables accurate targeting in the prone positioning, with modest impact on workflow, compared with supine positioning. As with supine patients, determining how to address any motion with intervention and appropriate treatment planning margins is important.

Prostate Bed

Investigators at the University of Miami conducted a study comparing the relative geometrical stability of three implanted transponders between intact prostate and the prostate bed.[66] In the prostate bed, transponders were implanted between the bladder and rectal wall near the right and left sides of the trigone, and the third transponder was placed near the anastomosis site of the urethra. Variations in the distances and the angles between the transponders were evaluated. The distances between transponders varied on average by 1.1 mm +/-1.0 mm and 1.7 mm +/- 1.3 mm, for intact prostate and prostate bed, respectively. The maximum deviations were 4.8 mm and 6.4 mm, respectively. No migration or deleterious side effects were reported.

Head and Neck Tracking

In preparation for possible trials to study real-time tracking in the head and neck region, the Swedish Cancer Institute has conducted tests in phantoms. The primary concern of this study was the magnitude of the backscatter from the transponders. A custom mouthpiece was imbedded with three transponders and fit to a dental phantom in which 16 of 28 teeth contained amalgam. The transponders were not found to cause any measurable backscatter. However, the impact of the metallic amalgam on the spatial accuracy of electromagnetic tracking was not reported.[67]

Future Technology Integration

Electromagnetic tracking has only been commercially available since 2006; therefore, its development and integration into the treatment delivery process is still in its infancy. Because the system provides real-time numeric data in a digital format, which requires no human interpretation or further processing, its integration with the treatment delivery system is conceptually straightforward. Indeed, subsequent software integrations have already allowed the measured deviations to be transferred to the computer-controlled delivery system to make couch shifts remotely from the treatment control room. This commercially available option eliminates the time associated with entering the room, manually making corrections, and leaving the treatment room to resume treatment. Consequently, corrections can be made more frequently and accurately while reducing overall treatment time.

Using the system to gate the treatment beam is also an obvious and simple form of integration. Because the system measures the deviation, and the tolerance level is configurable by the user and known before treatment, it is a very simple task to generate a logic signal to gate off the treatment beam when the threshold deviation is exceeded. Additionally, major manufacturers of treatment delivery systems already have an interface in place to accept a logic signal for beam gating. Smith et al. have described the integrated behavior of such a system.[68] Experiments were conducted with a moving phantom to determine the latency for turning the beam on and off when the deviation crossed the threshold level. The mean time to turn the beam off when the threshold was exceeded was 65 milliseconds +/- 13 milliseconds, while the time to turn the beam back on was 75 milliseconds +/-13 milliseconds. Dosimetric tests were conducted in phantoms using a 3D motion stage capable of reproducing measured physiologic motions. A 3D conformal lung plan using four 6-MV beams, delivering 200 cGy, was chosen for the tests. Film measurements were made in the moving phantom with and without gating and compared with measurements made in a static phantom. Without gating, 32% of points within the beam were more than +/- 10 cGy from the desired dose, compared to 3% with gating. Similarly, deviations of +/- 20 cGy occurred over 9% of the field without gating and 0% with gating.

Although these beam gating and remote correction capabilities save time and improve treatment accuracy, they still require the beam to be turned off while positional corrections are applied to the patient. Sawant et al. at Stanford University have demonstrated an integrated system wherein the real-time tracking data are used to dynamically move the beam, rather than the patient, using the multileaf collimator (MLC) leaves.[43,69] Such a system, when commercially available, would likely incorporate target volume tracking during intensity-modulated RT (IMRT) delivery, beam gating, and possibly remote couch corrections all in one package. The prototype system has demonstrated better than 2 mm accuracy for tracking lung motion trajectories and better than 1 mm accuracy for prostate motion trajectories, with a system latency of 220 milliseconds.[69] Dosimetric measurements of single beams in moving phantoms were made to evaluate the effectiveness of reducing dosimetric deviations when beam gating and tracking were used, with both step-and-shoot and dynamic IMRT delivery. Without gating or tracking, deviations greater than +/- 3 cGy were observed over 10.86% and 13.06% of the field for static MLC (SMLC) and dynamic MLC (DMLC), respectively. With beam gating implemented, the deviations were 10.91% and 3.30% for SMLC and DMLC, respectively, whereas MLC tracking resulted in dosimetric deviations of 7.53% and 7.20% for SMLC and DMLC, respectively. As expected, dramatic improvements in delivery time were observed with tracking compared with beam gating. Compared with gating, tracking reduced the delivery times for SMLC and DMLC delivery of IMRT fields by a factor of 2.8 and 4.4, respectively, when a +/– 2 mm gating window was used.

Because of the complementary nature of electromagnetic and kilovoltage x-ray imaging, it is natural to consider using them both during a treatment fraction. Rau et al. have reported on a system that simultaneously employs both technologies.[70] To achieve this, the systems must be synchronized such that x-ray imaging occurs between electromagnetic localization cycles to avoid line artifacts in the x-ray images. In such a system, large motions detected by electromagnetic tracking might be used to trigger a cone beam CT (CBCT) volumetric image acquisition to study motion and deformations in anatomy, especially away from the implanted transponders where rigid body assumptions lose their validity. Additionally, the ability to precisely track a known internal fiducial would allow much better motion correction during the reconstruction of the CBCT image. In the reconstruction of 4D CBCT, phase or amplitude sorting is typically used to reduce motion artifacts. However, these techniques typically assume a periodic respiratory motion with a fixed baseline position, amplitude, and frequency. Because all these parameters may vary from breath to breath in real patients, the extent to which motion artifacts can be reduced is limited by the variability of these parameters. However, using real-time tracking data based on absolute position would allow more accurate sorting of image projections for 4D CT reconstruction, further reducing motion artifacts as demonstrated by Rau et al.[70]

Quality Assurance

To realize the potential benefits of electromagnetic tracking, a comprehensive QA program must be implemented and integrated with standard treatment machine QA, including daily, monthly, and annual tests. Many daily and monthly calibration and QA tasks are suggested and semiautomated by the manufacturer, and additional tests should be implemented as a part of institutional policy.[71] Daily QA tests are typically performed as part of the morning warm-up procedure and by necessity must be relatively simple and quick to perform. This typically entails placing a standard phantom at isocenter with transponders embedded at known positions and verifying that each transponder may be uniquely identified and localized at a known location (relative to isocenter) with acceptable accuracy.

Other QA is performed on at least a monthly basis. This includes calibration of the three ceiling-mounted infrared cameras that track the detector array to establish the position of isocenter and map optical distortions in the system. Additionally, the calibrated position of isocenter should also be independently verified radiographically. Known

shifts of an electromagnetic QA phantom should also be verified by the tracking system at least monthly. In addition, because of the susceptibility of electromagnetic systems to metallic objects, the stability of a phantom in known positions should be verified while the gantry is rotated about the QA phantom. One a yearly basis, a thorough end-to-end test should be performed. A QA phantom should be used to follow standard patient procedures from simulation through real-time tracking of known motions and positions, including all data transfer procedures.

As the technology becomes more integrated with treatment delivery, QA procedures must be implemented to ensure the interface components and dependent capabilities function as expected. At a minimum this will include timely beam gating at user-configurable tolerance settings, accurate transfer and execution of treatment couch shifts, and stringent MLC tracking tests including known dynamic motions and accurate positional testing. The implementation of MLC tracking will also make routine maintenance of multileaf collimators much more important to ensure they meet the required performance characteristics.

Complementary and Competing Technologies

Electromagnetic tracking reports the position of implanted transponders. This requires that the geometrical relationship between the transponders and the target volume shape be well known and largely requires the assumption of a rigid body relationship between them. Technologies such as CBCT provide full geometrical information of the relevant anatomy but can not provide real-time data. Consequently, these technologies are complementary and both will be required to provide the highest degree of conformal treatment delivery, especially as new sites are studied that exhibit large motions and deformations.

This chapter has almost exclusively discussed studies performed with the electromagnetic tracking system available from Calypso Medical Technologies Inc, largely because it is the only commercially available wireless electromagnetic system available at the time of writing. Other real-time tracking systems are under development for commercial use. These include the Micropos RayPilot (Gothenburg, Sweden), as previously mentioned, which uses a single wired antenna that is temporarily inserted for each treatment fraction through a urethral catheter, and the Navotek (Yokneam, Israel) RealEye, which uses collimated scintillators to track an implantable microcoil containing approximately 50 μCi of ^{192}Ir.[72–76] Both systems had been demonstrated and studied in patients, but were not yet available commercially at the time of this writing.

Conclusions

This chapter has reviewed the development, principles, implementation, and preliminary clinical use of electromagnetic tracking. The use of this technology for guidance of external beam radiation therapy is still in its infancy and continues to evolve quickly. As this technology becomes more widely available in the coming years, the uncertainties in dosimetric delivery of treatment plans because of inter- and intrafraction positioning errors will be greatly reduced. While these remaining uncertainties will always have to be considered, uncertainties in delineating the CTV, containing microscopic disease, will become much more important. As always, the reduction of CTV-to-PTV margins must be approached with caution.[58] This, in turn, will emphasize the importance of complementary anatomical imaging techniques for defining the GTV in a consistent manner. As image-guided and real-time treatment guidance technologies improve, dose delivery will become ever more conformal leading to the reduction of toxicities, and potentially allowing dose escalation in some sites.

References

1. Kalmus HP. A new guiding and tracking system. *IRE Trans Aerosp Navig Electron.* 1962;9:7–10.

2. Olsen RG, Farstad AJ. Electromagnetic direction finding experiments for location of trapped miners. *IEEE Trans Geosci Electron.* 1973;GE–11:178–185.

3. Barta G, Olsen R. A short-range VLF navigation system for rivers and harbors. *IEEE Antenna Propagation Soc International Symp.* 1977:124–127.

4. Coyne J, Elia F, Southworth H Jr, inventors; Location detection and guidance systems for burrowing devices. US Patent 3529682. September 22, 1970.

5. Raab F, Blood E, Steiner T, Jones H. Magnetic position and orientation tracking system. *IEEE Transactions Aerospace Electronic Systems.* 1979;15:709–718.

6. Fenici RR, Covino M, Cellerino C, et al. Magnetocardiographically-guided catheter ablation. *J Interv Cardiol.* 1995;8:825–836.

7. Fried MP, Kleefield J, Gopal H, et al. Image-guided endoscopic surgery: results of accuracy and performance in a multicenter clinical study using an electromagnetic tracking system. *Laryngoscope.* 1997;107:594–601.

8. Bottlang M, Madey SM, Steyers CM, et al. Assessment of elbow joint kinematics in passive motion by electromagnetic motion tracking. *J Orthop Res.* 2000;18:195–202.

9. Hagemeister N, Long R, Yahia L, et al. Quantitative comparison of three different types of anterior cruciate ligament reconstruction methods: laxity and 3-D kinematic measurements. *Biomed Mater Eng.* 2002;12:47–57.

10. Kundra RK, Moorehead JD, Barton-Hanson N, Montgomery SC. Magnetic tracking: a novel method of assessing anterior cruciate ligament deficiency. *Ann R Coll Surg Engl.* 2006;88:16–17.

11. Tan KK, Grzeszczuk R, Levin DN, et al. A frameless stereotactic approach to neurosurgical planning based on retrospective patient-image registration. *J Neurosurg.* 1993;79:296–303.

12. Balter JM, Wright JN, Newell LJ, et al. Accuracy of a wireless localization system for radiotherapy. *Int J Radiat Oncol Biol Phys.* 2005;61:933–937.

13. Schicho K, Figl M, Donat M, et al. Stability of miniature electromagnetic tracking systems. *Phys Med Biol.* 2005;50:2089–2098.

14. Hummel J, Figl M, Birkfellner W, et al. Evaluation of a new electromagnetic tracking system using a standardized assessment protocol. *Phys Med Biol.* 2006;51:N205–N210.

15. Watanabe Y, Anderson LL. A system for nonradiographic source localization and real-time planning of intraoperative high dose rate brachytherapy. *Med Phys.* 1997;24:2014–2023.

16. Lennernas B, Edgren M, Nilsson S. Patient positioning using artificial intelligence neural networks, trained magnetic field sensors and magnetic implants. *Acta Oncol.* 1999;38:1109–1112.

17. Lennernas B, Nilsson S. A new patient positioning system using magnetic implants and magnetic field sensors. *Radiother Oncol.* 1995;37:249–250.

18. Kindblom J, Ekelund-Olvenmark AM, Syren H, et al. High precision transponder localization using a novel electromagnetic positioning system in patients with localized prostate cancer. *Radiother Oncol.* 2009;90:307–311.

19. Seiler PG, Blattmann H, Kirsch S, et al. A novel tracking technique for the continuous precise measurement of tumour positions in conformal radiotherapy. *Phys Med Biol.* 2000;45:N103–N110.

20. Yaniv Z, Wilson E, Lindisch D, et al. Electromagnetic tracking in the clinical environment. *Med Phys.* 2009;36:876–892.

21. Willoughby TR, Kupelian PA, Pouliot J, et al. Target localization and real-time tracking using the Calypso 4D localization system in patients with localized prostate cancer. *Int J Radiat Oncol Biol Phys.* 2006;65:528–534.

22. Balter JM, Wright N, Dimmer S, et al. Demonstration of accurate localization and continuous tracking of implantable wireless electromagnetic transponders. *Int J Radiat Oncol Biol Phys.* 2003;57:S264–S265.

23. Shah AP, Meeks SL, Willoughby TR, et al. Evaluating intrafraction motion of the prostate in the prone and supine positions using electromagnetic tracking. *Int J Radiat Oncol Biol Phys.* 2009;75:S597–S597.

24. Bittner N, Butler WM, Reed JL, et al. Electromagnetic tracking of intrafraction prostate displacement in patients externally immobilized in the prone position. *Int J Radiat Oncol Biol Phys.* 2010;77(2)490–495.

25. Zhu X, Bourland JD, Yuan Y, et al. Tradeoffs of integrating real-time tracking into IGRT for prostate cancer treatment. *Phys Med Biol.* 2009;54:N393–N401.

26. Litzenberg DW, Willoughby TR, Balter JM, et al. Positional stability of electromagnetic transponders used for prostate localization and continuous, real-time tracking. *Int J Radiat Oncol Biol Phys.* 2007;68:1199–1206.

27. Pouliot J, Shinohara K, et al. Positional stability and implant experience of AC magnetic beacon transponders used to localize patients for external beam radiation therapy. *Med Phys.* 2004;31:1847.

28. Willoughby TR, Kupelian PA, Pouliot J, et al. Implant experience and positional stability of AC magnetic beacon(TM) transponders used to localize patients for external beam radiation therapy of the prostate. *Int J Radiat Oncol Biol Phys.* 2004;60:S267–S268.

29. Kitamura K, Shirato H, Shimizu S, et al. Registration accuracy and possible migration of internal fiducial gold marker implanted in prostate and liver treated with real-time tumor-tracking radiation therapy (RTRT). *Radiother Oncol.* 2002;62:275–281.

30. Kupelian PA, Willoughby TR, Meeks SL, et al. Intraprostatic fiducials for localization of the prostate gland: monitoring intermarker distances during radiation therapy to test for marker stability. *Int J Radiat Oncol Biol Phys.* 2005;62:1291–1296.

31. Poggi MM, Gant DA, Sewchand W, Warlick WB. Marker seed migration in prostate localization. *Int J Radiat Oncol Biol Phys.* 2003;56:1248–1251.

32. Pouliot J, Aubin M, Langen KM, et al. (Non)-migration of radiopaque markers used for on-line localization of the prostate with an electronic portal imaging device. *Int J Radiat Oncol Biol Phys.* 2003;56:862–866.

33. Dawson LA, Litzenberg DW, Brock KK, et al. A comparison of ventilatory prostate movement in four treatment positions. *Int J Radiat Oncol Biol Phys.* 2000;48:319–323.

34. Huang E, Dong L, Chandra A, et al. Intrafraction prostate motion during IMRT for prostate cancer. *Int J Radiat Oncol Biol Phys.* 2002;53:261–268.

35. Mah D, Freedman G, Milestone B, et al. Measurement of intrafractional prostate motion using magnetic resonance imaging. 2002;54:568.

36. Malone S, Crook JM, Kendal WS, Szanto J. Respiratory-induced prostate motion: quantification and characterization. *Int J Radiat Oncol Biol Phys.* 2000;48:105–109.

37. Nederveen AJ, Van Der Heide UA, Dehnad H, et al. Measurements and clinical consequences of prostate motion during a radiotherapy fraction. *Int J Radiat Oncol Biol Phys.* 2002;53:206–214.

38. Langen KM, Willoughby TR, Meeks SL, et al. Observations on real-time prostate gland motion using electromagnetic tracking. *Int J Radiat Oncol Biol Phys.* 2008;71:1084–1090.

39. Kupelian P, Willoughby T, Mahadevan A, et al. Multi-institutional clinical experience with the Calypso System in localization and continuous, real-time monitoring of the prostate gland during external radiotherapy. *Int J Radiat Oncol Biol Phys.* 2007;67:1088–1098.

40. Litzenberg DW, Balter JM, Hadley SW, et al. Influence of intrafraction motion on margins for prostate radiotherapy. *Int J Radiat Oncol Biol Phys.* 2006;65:548–553.

41. Malinowski KT, Noel C, Roy M, et al. Efficient use of continuous, real-time prostate localization. *Phys Med Biol.* 2008;53:4959–4970.

42. Santanam L, Malinowski K, Hubenshmidt J, et al. Fiducial-based translational localization accuracy of electromagnetic tracking system and on-board kilovoltage imaging system. *Int J Radiat Oncol Biol Phys.* 2008;70:892–899.

43. Smith RL, Sawant A, Santanam L, et al. Integration of real-time internal electromagnetic position monitoring coupled with dynamic multileaf collimator tracking: an intensity-modulated radiation therapy feasibility study. *Int J Radiat Oncol Biol Phys.* 2009;74:868–875.

44. Rasch C, Steenbakkers R, Van Herk M. Target definition in prostate, head, and neck. *Semin Radiat Oncol.* 2005;15:136–145.

45. Gao Z, Wilkins D, Eapen L, et al. A study of prostate delineation referenced against a gold standard created from the visible human data. *Radiother Oncol.* 2007;85:239–246.

46. Deurloo KEI, Steenbakkers RJHM, Zijp LJ, et al. Quantification of shape variation of prostate and seminal vesicles during external beam radiotherapy. *Int J Radiat Oncol Biol Phys.* 2005;61:228–238.

47. Nichol AM, Brock KK, Lockwood GA, et al. A magnetic resonance imaging study of prostate deformation relative to implanted gold fiducial markers. *Int J Radiat Oncol Biol Phys.* 2007;67:48–56.

48. De Crevoisier R, Tucker SL, Dong L, et al. Increased risk of biochemical and local failure in patients with distended rectum on the planning CT for prostate cancer radiotherapy. *Int J Radiat Oncol Biol Phys.* 2005;62:965–973.

49. Kupelian PA, Willoughby TR, Reddy CA, et al. Impact of image guidance on outcomes after external beam radiotherapy for localized prostate cancer. *Int J Radiat Oncol Biol Phys.* 2008;70:1146–1150.

50. Johnston H, Hilts M, Beckham W, Berthelet E. 3D ultrasound for prostate localization in radiation therapy: a comparison with implanted fiducial markers. *Med Phys.* 2008;35:2403–2413.

51. Fuller CD, Thomas CR, Schwartz S, et al. Method comparison of ultrasound and kilovoltage x-ray fiducial marker imaging for prostate radiotherapy targeting. *Phys Med Biol.* 2006;51:4981–4993.

52. Khan DC, Tropper S, Liu P, Mantz CA. Patient-reported reduction in acute GU and GI side effects for prostate cancer patients treated with 81 Gy IMRT using reduced PTV margins and electromagnetic tracking. *Int J Radiat Oncol Biol Phys.* 2009;75:S113–S114.

53. Tropper SE, Khan D, Mantz CA. Efficiency and clinical workflow of delivering IMRT to the prostate within 2 mm tolerances. *Int J Radiat Oncol Biol Phys.* 2009;75:S580–S580.

54. Chung HT, Xia P, Chan LW, et al. Does image-guided radiotherapy improve toxicity profile in whole pelvic-treated high-risk prostate cancer? Comparison between IG-IMRT and IMRT. *Int J Radiat Oncol Biol Phys.* 2009;73:53–60.

55. Shipley WU, Thames HD, Sandler HM, et al. Radiation therapy for clinically localized prostate cancer: a multi-institutional pooled analysis. *JAMA.* 1999;281:1598–1604.

56. Sanda MG, Dunn RL, Michalski J, et al. Quality of life and satisfaction with outcome among prostate-cancer survivors. *N Engl J Med.* 2008;358:1250–1261.

57. Soete G, Verellen D, Michielsen D, et al. Image-guided conformation arc therapy for prostate cancer: early side effects. *Int J Radiat Oncol Biol Phys.* 2006;66:S141–S144.

58. Engels B, Soete G, Verellen D, Storme G. Conformal arc radiotherapy for prostate cancer: increased biochemical failure in patients with distended rectum on the planning computed tomogram despite image guidance by implanted markers. *Int J Radiat Oncol Biol Phys.* 2009;74:388–391.

59. Mayse ML, Parikh PJ, Lechleiter KM, et al. Bronchoscopic implantation of a novel wireless electromagnetic transponder in the canine lung: a feasibility study. *Int J Radiat Oncol Biol Phys.* 2008;72:93–98.

60. Mayse ML, Peauroi JR, Parikh PJ, et al. Long-term interaction and tissue response of a bronchoscopically implanted, anchored electromagnetic transponder in the canine lung. *Int J Radiat Oncol Biol Phys.* 2009;75:S37.

61. Mayse ML, Smith RL, Park M, et al. Development of a non-migrating electromagnetic transponder system for lung tumor tracking. *Int J Radiat Oncol Biol Phys.* 2008;72:S430–S430.

62. Willoughby TR, Shah AP, Forbes AR, et al. Clinical use of electromagnetic guidance for lung and spine radiation therapy. *Int J Radiat Oncol Biol Phys.* 2008;72:S642–S643.

63. Eulau S, Zeller T, Afghan MKN. Adaptation of the Calypso 4D localization system to accommodate complex treatment geometry. *Int J Radiat Oncol Biol Phys.* 2009;75:S598–S598.

64. Metz JM, Kassaee A, Ingram M, et al. First report of real-time tumor tracking in the treatment of pancreatic cancer using the Calypso system. *Int J Radiat Oncol Biol Phys.* 2009;75: S54–S55.

65. Zelefsky MJ, Happersett L, Leibel SA, et al. The effect of treatment positioning on normal tissue dose in patients with prostate cancer treated with three-dimensional radiotherapy. *Int J Radiat Oncol Biol Phys.* 1997;37:13–19.

66. Wang K, Wu X, Bossart E, et al. The uncertainties in target localization for prostate and prostate-bed radiotherapy with Calypso 4D. *Int J Radiat Oncol Biol Phys.* 2009;75:S594–S594.

67. Ye J, Werner B, Mate T, Zeller T. Assessment of dental amalgam backscatter with a beacon transponder embedded mouthpiece for real-time tracking during head and neck IMRT. *Med Phys.* 2006;33:2073–2073.

68. Smith RL, Lechleiter K, Malinowski K, et al. Evaluation of linear accelerator gating with real-time electromagnetic tracking. *Int J Radiat Oncol Biol Phys.* 2009;74:920–927.

69. Sawant A, Smith RL, Venkat RB, et al. Toward submillimeter accuracy in the management of intrafraction motion: the integration of real-time internal position monitoring and multileaf collimator target tracking. *Int J Radiat Oncol Biol Phys.* 2009;74:575–582.

70. Rau AW, Nill S, Eidens RS, Oelfke U. Synchronized tumour tracking with electromagnetic transponders and kV x-ray imaging: evaluation based on a thorax phantom. *Phys Med Biol.* 2008;53:3789–3805.

71. Santanam L, Noel C, Willoughby TR, et al. Quality assurance for clinical implementation of an electromagnetic tracking system. *Med Phys.* 2009;36:3477–3486.

72. Alezra D, Schifter D, Shchory T, et al. Robustness of a gantry-mounted radioactive tracking system in a clinical radiation therapy environment. *Med Phys.* 2009;36:2490–2490.

73. Alezra D, Shchory T, Lifshitz I, et al. Localization accuracy of a gantry-mounted radioactive tracking system in the clinical radiation therapy environment. *Med Phys.* 2009;36:2486–2486.

74. Neustadter D, Corn B, Shchory T, et al. Analysis of dose to patient, spouse/caretaker, and staff, from an implanted trackable radioactive fiducial for use in the radiation treatment of prostate cancer. *Med Phys.* 2008;35:2921–2921.

75. Neustadter D, Tune M, Zaretsky A, et al. Stability and visibility of a novel non-migrating radiographic/radioactive fiducial marker: implications for external beam treatment of prostate cancer. *Med Phys.* 2008;35:2719–2719.

76. Shchory T, Schifter D, Lichtman R, et al. Static and dynamic tracking accuracy of a novel radioactive tracking technology for target localization and real time tracking in radiation therapy. *Med Phys.* 2008;35:2719–2719.

Chapter 13

Emerging In-Room Imaging Technologies

James Bowsher, PhD, James F. Dempsey, PhD, Jan J.W. Lagendijk, PhD,
Masatoshi Mitsuya, PhD, Bas W. Raaymakers, PhD, Richard H. Stark, MS,
Yoshihiro Takai, MD, PhD, Fang-Fang Yin, PhD

Currently, the technologies associated with image-based planning have been considered separate and distinct from image-guided treatment devices. Single-photon emission computed tomography (SPECT), positron emission tomography (PET), and magnetic resonance (MR) imaging scanners often reside in radiology departments and are primarily used during the planning stages of treatment. Recently, there has been an interest in combining these modalities with radiotherapy (RT) treatment devices to provide enhanced image guidance. Moreover, the currently available image-guided technologies, which are primarily x-ray based, are also undergoing significant changes. By incorporating continuous imaging during treatment, the tumor may be tracked such that treatment can be modified in near-real time. The technologies associated with these emerging systems are the subject of this chapter.

Magnetic Resonance Onboard Imaging

The functionality of MR integrated with a RT device offers superb soft-tissue contrast imaging directly on the treatment table. The value of MR for target definition has already been shown extensively for treatment planning purposes. Not only does it provide improved target localization, but it also provides better tumor characterization by means of functional imaging.[1-3] Furthermore, because of the dynamic capability of MR, a full inventory of motion, deformation, and response can be assessed to minimize the margins required for geometrical uncertainties in the tumor position.

Given the advantages of MR for target definition, MR for treatment guidance is the logical next step.[4] For treatment guidance, MR can visualize the tumor without the need of surrogates, and can also visualize the surrounding organs at risk (OARs). This can be done not only prior to each fraction but also continuously *during* treatment delivery so that intrafraction motion (e.g., breathing-related motion) can be tracked and corrected. Integrated MR RT systems are currently under construction and rapidly approaching clinical introduction. This section will present a brief overview of these designs.

Challenges for Integrating MR Functionality With a Radiotherapy Device

Integrating MR with a RT device is not straightforward. The main hardware-related concerns for integration are magnetic interference, radiofrequency (RF) interference, and dose delivery while a patient is inside a MR system.

Magnetic interference has two effects. The strong, permanent magnetic field of the MR may hamper the operation of the RT device; at the same time, magnetization of moving components within that device may reduce the field homogeneity and, thus, MR image quality. Furthermore the stray magnetic field may also affect accelerators in neighboring treatment rooms.[5]

Radiofrequency interference is a problem that affects MR acquisition. Normally an MR is installed in a Faraday cage to shield the outer world from the high-power RF emission of the MR, while it also protects the MR from outside RF noise. Installation of a RT device inside this Faraday cage cannot be done without measures to prevent RF noise from the device itself.

The last issue is beam delivery to a patient inside an MR system. The choice for a closed-bore MR implies beam attenuation and scatter induction whereas the choice for an open system implies a lower magnetic field strength, resulting in a lower signal-to-noise in the MR images and deteriorated gradient performance. Additionally the presence of a magnetic field will affect the dose distribution. Although the primary photon beam will not be affected, the secondary electrons experience a Lorentzian force that will alter the dose distribution as will be discussed later in this chapter.

Hybrid Designs

Currently, five designs for RT devices with integrated MR functionality have been proposed in the literature. Ordered by publication date these are:

1. The MR accelerator from UMC Utrecht, the Netherlands. This unit consists of a 1.5-Tesla (T) MR scanner with a 6-megavoltage (MV) linear accelerator.[6] It is the only closed-bore MR solution. A prototype is operational and will be discussed in more detail later in this chapter.
2. The Renaissance from ViewRay (Oakwood Village, OH). This system is comprised of an open 0.3-T MR scanner. By using three ^{60}Co irradiation sources that rotate in the mid-plane of the MR, the RF interference is likely to be less severe.[7] This system is currently under construction and will be described in more detail later in this chapter.
3. A design presented by Kron and coworkers.[8] An open, resistive 0.25-T MR with a single ^{60}Co source for helical radiation delivery. No implementation details are known.
4. The linac-MR system at the Edmonton Cross Cancer Institute, Canada.[9] This systems consists of an open, small-bore 0.2-T MR combined with a 6-MV accelerator. The accelerator and MR are rigidly connected and passive magnetic shielding is used to shield the accelerator. The rigid connection ensures that the magnetic impact of the shielding can be compensated. A separate Faraday cage around the

accelerator is used to prevent RF interference. The beam is perpendicular to the magnetic field. The entire system, including the MR, has to rotate around the patient to irradiate from different directions.

This 28-cm small-bore, nonrotating system has been operational since December 2008 and simultaneous 6-MV irradiation and MR imaging has been shown on phantoms.[10] Fallone and coworkers also reported on the development of an open human-sized MR of 0.5 T or 1.0 T with a 6-MV accelerator, again rigidly connected and now with the beam direction parallel to the magnetic field to minimize the impact of the magnetic field on the dose distribution.[11]

5. A preliminary proposal by Varian and Stanford University of an open MR with a linear accelerator positioned in line with the primary magnetic field. The latter is to minimize the impact of the magnetic field on the dose distribution, similar to the previous design.[12] No implementation details are known.

1.5-T MR and a 6-MV Accelerator at the UMC Utrecht

The earliest design of a hybrid system is a modified closed-bore 1.5-T Achieva MR scanner (Philips Medical Systems, Andover, MA) with an Elekta (Elekta AB, Stockholm, Sweden) 6-MV accelerator. A schematic of the design is shown in Figure 13-1.[6,13] The high field strength and diagnostic gradient coil performance are required for high spatial and temporal resolution imaging. In this system, both the magnet and the gradient coil are adapted.[14] The result is a circumferential beam portal in the midplane of the MR where the mass is minimized and absorption is completely homogeneous. In the prototype system, the total mass in the beam's-eye-view is the equivalent of approximately 10 cm of aluminium. In the next generation,

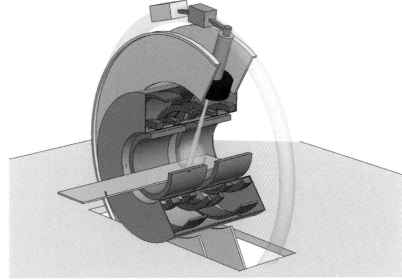

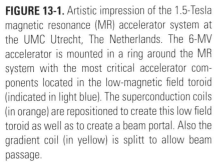

FIGURE 13-1. Artistic impression of the 1.5-Tesla magnetic resonance (MR) accelerator system at the UMC Utrecht, The Netherlands. The 6-MV accelerator is mounted in a ring around the MR system with the most critical accelerator components located in the low-magnetic field toroid (indicated in light blue). The superconduction coils (in orange) are repositioned to create this low field toroid as well as to create a beam portal. Also the gradient coil (in yellow) is splitt to allow beam passage.

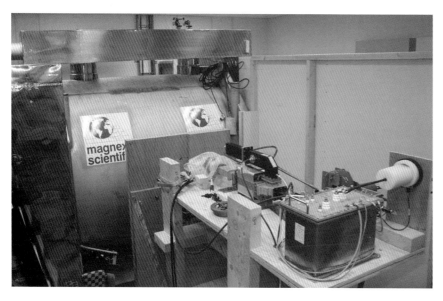

FIGURE 13-2. Photograph of the prototype magnetic resonance accelerator at the UMC Utrecht, The Netherlands. The accelerator is positioned on the wooden stand, and the magnet is shown behind it. Also, the copper radiofrequency cage at the service side of the magnet is shown.

this thickness is planned to be decreased to 5 cm. The magnetic interference between the MR and accelerator is overcome by adapting the active shielding of the magnet in such a way that a low magnetic field toroid (Figure 13-1) is created around the MR in which the most critical accelerator components can be placed (i.e., the gun section).[14] The RF interference is solved by building two Faraday cages, one at either end of the MR. In this way, the accelerator and its peripheral systems are in the same room as the MR but RF-wise separated from the MR.

Since March 2009 a prototype of this system has been functional (Figure 13-2).[15] It has been demonstrated that simultaneous radiation delivery and MR imaging is possible while maintaining the diagnostic 1.5-T MR image quality. Because the MR electronics and peripherals are from a standard Philips Achieva system, any diagnostic sequence can be run on this hybrid unit.

An appealing feature of a RT system with integrated MR functionality is the possibility of three-dimensional (3D) dosimetry using Fricke or polymer gels.[16] These phantoms have dose-dependent MR properties and can be read simultaneously with dose delivery, potentially facilitating 4D dose quantification. Even more appealing is the possibility of beam visualization directly in the patient. Researchers are investigating if, for very specific MR sequences, the secondary electrons released by the photon beam can alter the MR images.

ViewRay

ViewRay is developing an MR-guided RT system that can continuously image the patient during therapy and, when the tumor deviates from the intended position, shut off the beam in a fraction of a second. Additionally, when the tumor is on target, the real-time imaging will capture the dose delivered to the patient. This system will utilize

cutting-edge MR technology for real-time imaging, a sophisticated multileaf collimator (MLC), and beam delivery system (Figure 13-3). This comprehensive system will include treatment planning and accompanying software along with rapid computerized processing of data. The ViewRay system incorporates three high-intensity cobalt sources and three double-focused MLCs. The net result is high dose rate capability and sharpened penumbra equivalent to typical linacs employing MLC. Surface doses are reduced by the presence of a 0.35-T magnetic field and intensity-modulated radiation therapy (IMRT) dose distributions are comparable to 6-MV linacs.

Preliminary features of the ViewRay system include:

- Superconducting open 0.35-T MR with 50-cm field of view (FOV) and 70-cm bore
- Pilot volumetric scans in 15 seconds or less (3-mm voxel)
- Planning volumetric scans in 1 to 2 minutes (1.5-mm voxel)
- Anatomy-based gating at four frames per second
- 3 KCi × 15 KCi sources with at dose rate of 600 cGy/min at 1 meter and double-focused MLC
- Field sizes up to 30 cm × 30 cm for IMRT and/or conformal RT
- Fast Monte Carlo and pencil beam calculation algorithms
- Real-time deformable image registration
- Fast optimization, dose prediction, and adaptive planning capability

The choice of a ^{60}Co source and 0.35-T MR system was made to reduce the interaction between the RT device and MR imaging while achieving all clinical goals. Low magnetic susceptibility at 0.35 T results in very high spatial integrity compared with higher field-strength magnets and a larger electron radius of gyration at 0.35 T

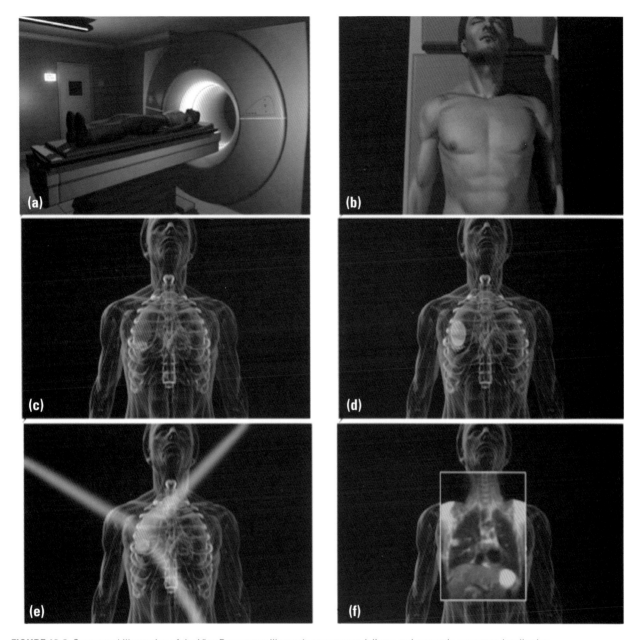

FIGURE 13-3. Conceptual illustration of the ViewRay system illustrating treatment delivery and magnetic resonance localization.

practically eliminates the electron return effect that may cause up to 40% hot spots at 6 MV and 1.5 T.

Onboard SPECT Imaging

Onboard SPECT external-beam treatment machines have been proposed for RT target localization.[17,18] SPECT imaging utilizes radiotracers that are injected into the patient that consist of a biologically active molecule that incorporates or is attached to an x-ray– or gamma-ray–emitting radionuclide. Biological properties imaged by SPECT radiotracers include cell proliferation[19]; apoptosis[20,21]; angiogenesis[19]; COX-2 expression[19]; epidermal growth factor

receptor (EGFR)[19,22]; hypoxia[19,23]; glucose metabolism[19,24]; amino acid transport[25]; and multidrug resistance[26]. Such radiotracers are in various stages of development. For example, Phase 2 clinical trials have been undertaken with radiotracers for hypoxia and glucose metabolism.[27] Other SPECT radiotracers—^{99m}Tc-Prostascint, ^{99m}Tc-CEA, and ^{99m}Tc-Depreotide—are already approved, respectively, for imaging prostate, colon, and lung cancers.[27]

The photon energy of the emission depends on the radionuclide. The most widely employed SPECT radionuclide is ^{99m}Tc, which emits photons at approximately 140 keV. Other radionuclides utilized for SPECT imaging include ^{123}I, ^{111}In, ^{201}Tl, and ^{67}Ga. The half-lives of these radionuclides range from 6 to 78 hours. To utilize these photons, the SPECT imaging hardware includes a scintillator and a collimator covering the scintillator. The collimator, which is typically an array of long narrow holes formed from lead, defines the direction of photons that reach the scintillator. The line along which a given photon was emitted can then be established by that direction combined with the location on the scintillator at which the photon is detected. By detecting many individual (single) photons, the SPECT hardware can thereby measure a set of line integrals through the radiotracer distribution. From a properly chosen set of line integrals, an image of the radiotracer distribution can be reconstructed.

Computer Simulations

As an initial step toward developing onboard SPECT, researchers have recently conducted a computer-simulation study into its potential localization accuracy.[18] The experimental design is illustrated in Figure 13-4. Starting with the NURBS-based cardiac–torso phantom[28] as a base, three phantom radiotracer distributions were simulated, one for each of three tumor diameters: 10.8 mm, 14.4 mm, and 21.6 mm. Tumor-to-background uptake ratios were six to one (left side of phantom) and three to one (right side of phantom). Tumors in the lung were blurred to simulate lung motion. A 180° trajectory was computer-simulated for a full-size SPECT gamma camera orbiting about the sides and anterior portions of the phantom. The modeled detector radius of rotation was the same at all detector angles, and was somewhat large relative to the phantom, to prevent collision with the modeled RT treatment couch.

Shown in Figure 13-5 are sample SPECT images reconstructed from simulated 4-, 8-, and 20-minute SPECT acquisitions. The Figure 13-5 results are anecdotal

in that only a single noisy reconstructed image is shown for each combination of scan time and tumor diameter. With six-to-one uptake ratio (left side of phantom), some 14.4-mm-diameter tumors are visible in a 4-minute scan, and most 21.6-mm-diameter tumors are visible. Quantitative results—computed across ensembles of reconstructed images—are given in Figure 13-6. For anterior locations, localization accuracy is around 2 mm or 3 mm for 14.4-mm-diameter tumors and a 4-minute scan.

This study touches on several factors that are likely to be key both in the development of onboard SPECT and in its clinical use.[18] Radiotracer uptake ratio is important. Figure 13-2 illustrates that tumors with six-to-one uptake ratio are much more visible than those with three-to-one uptake ratio, and Figure 13-6 shows that tumors with six-to-one uptake ratio are more accurately and precisely localized. It follows that research into improved SPECT radiotracers could substantially advance onboard SPECT. Regarding clinical practice, these results suggest that uptake ratios observed during planning SPECT scans may be useful as predictors of the localization accuracy of onboard SPECT for that specific patient.[18]

Detector proximity to target is also important. The least visible tumors are posterior tumors—i.e., those tumors that are on average the farthest from the detector. This effect—poorer image quality at greater average distances from the detector—arises because SPECT spatial resolution worsens with distance from the collimator, and because the amount of tissue traversed also tends to increase with distance from the collimator, thus increasing attenuation of the outgoing photons and thereby increasing noise. The study[18] is conservative in maintaining a fixed and somewhat loose detector radius of rotation for the detector. Improved spatial resolution—and, therefore, presumably improved localization—could be obtained by

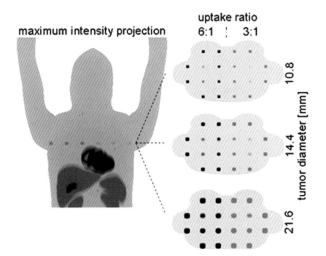

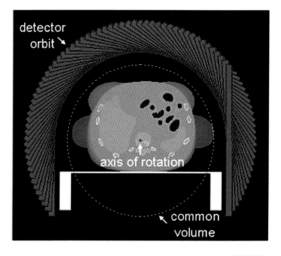

FIGURE 13-4. Design for the computer-simulation study of target localization using onboard single photon emission computed tomography (SPECT). Left: Phantom, with additional tumors positioned periodically. Right: Transverse section through computer-simulated phantom, radiotherapy patient table, and 180° trajectory of a full-size SPECT gamma camera.

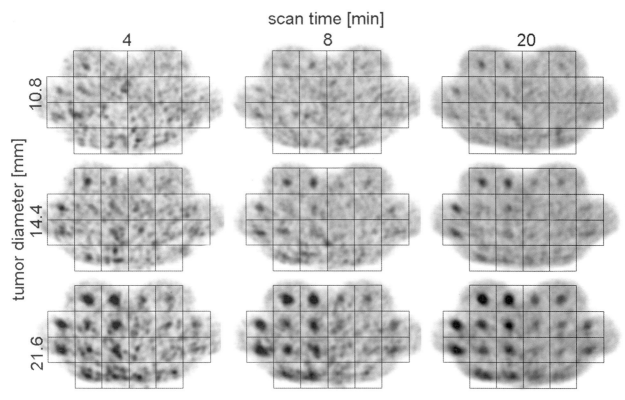

FIGURE 13-5. Sample single photon emission computed tomography (SPECT) images reconstructed from simulated 4-, 8-, and 20-minute SPECT acquisitions.

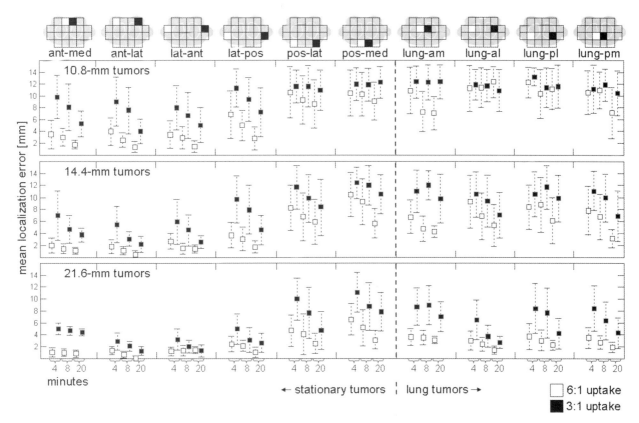

FIGURE 13-6. Localization results computed from ensembles of reconstructed images.

varying the detector radius of rotation so as to minimize detector-to-patient distance at each detector angle.[18]

During onboard target localization, the approximate location of the tumor target is known. However, onboard SPECT need only image in the vicinity of this target location. Imaging of the entire patient is not required. Of the various tumor locations considered in Figure 13-6, the anterior–medial (ant–med), anterior–lateral (ant–lat), and lateral–anterior (lat–ant) locations best indicate the potential task performance of on-board SPECT, at least for imaging more superficial tumors, because these are the locations best imaged by the detector trajectory used in this study. This trajectory might be utilized for a patient with a tumor target in the ant–med, ant–lat, or lat–ant locations. For a patient with tumor target in a posterior superficial region, a different detector trajectory would presumably be utilized, such that localization in the posterior region more nearly matches that seen in Figure 13-6 for anterior regions.

Figure 13-4 shows that spatial constraints imposed by the patient bed—typically a heavier, more rigid bed than those utilized for diagnostic imaging—may hamper imaging of posterior regions. This illustrates that development of onboard SPECT involves unique challenges. The task of onboard SPECT—to localize a target whose approximate location is already known—is also distinct, and there is opportunity and potential for onboard SPECT systems developed and optimized to that distinct task.[18]

There is room for considerable development beyond the SPECT system considered in the initial exploratory study.[18] The full-size gamma camera previously simulated may be cumbersome and unnecessarily expensive.[18] A smaller gamma camera may be well suited to imaging a limited region about the approximately known tumor target location, potentially lowering cost while improving maneuverability, including closer approach to the target region, thus enhancing spatial resolution. There is also considerable potential for improving imaging of specific regions, superficial and interior, through use of pinhole[29] and converging-beam[30] collimation.

Dual kV X-Ray Onboard Imager for Tumor Tracking

Researchers at the Tohoku University Graduate School of Medicine in Japan have developed an accelerator-mounted dual fluoroscopy system using two amorphous silicon flat-panel detectors (dual fluoroscopy with flat panel system: DFFP system) to image and track the motion of a gold marker implanted in the tumor.[31,32]

This DFFP system comprises two conventional diagnostic x-ray tubes that have been mounted directly onto the gantry of the accelerator (Clinac 23EX, Varian Medical Systems, Palo Alto, CA) and two sets of amorphous silicon (aSi) flat-panel x-ray sensors (PaxScan 2520, Varian Medical Systems, Palo Alto, CA) that are mounted opposite the x-ray tubes (Figure 13-7). The focal spots of the tubes are located ±45 degrees to the accelerator target, and two sets of aSi flat panel are located at a gantry position of ±135 degrees on retractable arms that extend from the lower part of the accelerator gantry. The flat panel imager is operated at a frame time of 33 milliseconds, and the images obtained are outputted as digital video signals. These 16-bit video signals are sent to a frame-grabber on a standard personal computer, and are visualized on the video graphic array monitor. The orthogonal images demonstrate the

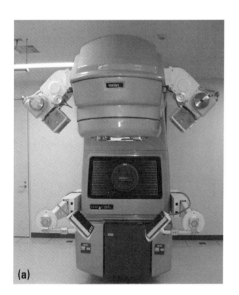
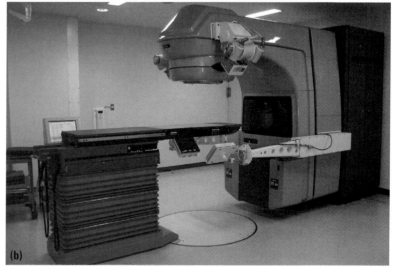

FIGURE 13-7. The front (a) and side (b) views of an accelerator-mounted dual fluoroscopy system using two amorphous silicon flat-panel detectors (dual fluoroscopy with flat panel system).

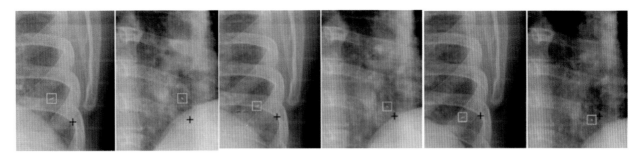

End-exhale $\longrightarrow$ End-inhale

FIGURE 13-8. Orthogonal pair images showing the gold seed motion with respiration, from end of normal exhalation to end of normal inhalation. The rectangles mark the region encompassing the implanted gold seed, which is analyzed in real time for tracking.

location of the markers (Figure 13-8). Under computer control, the 3D coordinates of the center position of a rod-shaped gold marker as small as 0.8 mm in diameter and 2 mm to 3 mm in length in prostate or lung tumor can be calculated and expressed as digital figures with 0.1 mm increment. As a conceptual demonstration, the dynamic MLC may be used to track the marker position throughout the range of motion.

Studies have reported on the utility of this system for positioning patients who are receiving IMRT for prostate cancer and stereotactic body radiotherapy for early-stage non-small cell lung cancer.[33,34] These studies have demonstrated that the daily use of the DFFP system was able to considerably reduce motion uncertainty and is feasible to improve the accuracy of stereotactic irradiation, IMRT, and conventional radiotherapy.

References

1. Haie-Meder C, Pötter R, Van Limbergen E, et al. Gynaecological (GYN) GEC-ESTRO Working Group. Recommendations from Gynaecological (GYN) GEC-ESTRO Working Group (I): concepts and terms in 3D image based 3D treatment planning in cervix cancer brachytherapy with emphasis on MRI assessment of GTV and CTV. *Radiother Oncol.* 2005;74(3): 235–245.
2. Villeirs GM, De Meerleer GO. Magnetic resonance imaging (MRI) anatomy of the prostate and application of MRI in radiotherapy planning. *Eur J Radiol.* 2007;63(3):361–368.
3. Narayana A, Chang J, Thakur S, et al. Use of MR spectroscopy and functional imaging in the treatment planning of gliomas. *Br J Radiol.* 2007;80(953):347–354.
4. Lagendijk JJW, Raaymakers BW, Raaijmakers AJE, et al. MRI/linac integration. *Radiother Oncol.* 2008;86(1):25–29.
5. Kok JGM, Raaymakers BW, Lagendijk JJW, et al. Installation of the 1.5 T MRI accelerator next to clinical accelerators: impact of the fringe field. *Phys Med Biol.* 2009;54(18):N409–N415.
6. Lagendijk JJW, Raaymakers BW, Van der Heide UA, et al. MRI guided radiotherapy: MRI as position verification system for IMRT. *Radiother Oncol.* 2002;64(S1):S75–S76.

7. Dempsey J, Dionne B, Fitzsimmons J, et al. A real-time MRI guided external beam radiotherapy delivery system. *Med Phys.* 2006;33(6):2254.
8. Kron T, Eyles D, Schreiner JL, Battista J. Magnetic resonance imaging for adaptive cobalt tomotherapy: a proposal. *Med Phys.* 2006;31(4):242–254.
9. Fallone BG, Carlone M, Murray B, et al. Development of a linac-MRI system for real-time ART. *Med Phys.* 2007;34(6):2547.
10. Fallone BG, Murray B, Rathee S, et al. First MR images obtained during megavoltage photon irradiation from a prototype integrated linac-MR system. *Med Phys.* 2008;36(6):2084–2088.
11. Fallone BG. Real-time MR-guided radiotherapy: integration of a low-field MR system. *Med Phys.* 2009;36(6).2774–2775.
12. Green M. Magnetic field effects on radiation dose distribution. *Med Phys.* 2009;36(6):2774.
13. Raaymakers BW, Lagendijk JJW, Van der Heide UA, et al. Integrating a MRI scanner with a radiotherapy accelerator: a new concept of precise on line radiotherapy guidance and treatment monitoring. *Proceedings of the XIVth International Conference on the Use of Computers in Radiation Therapy (ICCR).* Seoul, Korea: Jeong Publishing; 2004: 89–92.
14. Overweg J, Raaymakers BW, Lagendijk JJW, Brown K. System for MRI guided radiotherapy. In: *Proceedings ISMRM 2009.* Abstr. 593. International Society for Magnetic Resonance in Medicine, April 18-24, 2009. Published by society, Berkeley, CA.
15. Raaymakers BW, Lagendijk JJW, Overweg J, et al. Integrating a 1.5 T MRI scanner with a 6 MV accelerator: proof of concept. *Phys Med Biol.* 2009;54(12):N229–N237.
16. Vergote K, De Deene Y, Claus F, et al. Application of monomer/polymer gel dosimetry to study the effects of tissue inhomogeneities on intensity-modulated radiation therapy (IMRT) dose distributions. *Radiother Oncol.* 2003;67(1):119–128.
17. Bowsher J, Yin FF, Greer, K, et al. Preliminary investigations into combined CT/SPECT imaging onboard therapy machines. *Med Phys.* 2006;33(6):2221.
18. Roper JR, Bowsher JE, Yin FF. On-board SPECT for localizing functional targets: a simulation study. *Med Phys.* 2009;36(5): 1727–1735.
19. Yang DJ, Azhdarinia A, Kim EE. Tumor specific imaging using Tc-99m and Ga-68 labeled radiopharmaceuticals. *Curr Med Imag Rev.* 2005;1:25–34.

20. Boersma HH, Kietselaer BL, Stolk LM, et al. Past, present, and future of annexin A5: from protein discovery to clinical applications. *J Nucl Med.* 2005;46(12):2035–2050.
21. Blankenberg FG. In vivo detection of apoptosis. *J Nucl Med.* 2008;49:81s–95s.
22. Cai W, Niu G, Chen X. Multimodality imaging of the HER-kinase axis in cancer. *Eur J Nucl Med Mol Imag.* 2008;35(1):186–208.
23. Chapman JD, Zanzonico P, Ling CC. On measuring hypoxia in individual tumors with radiolabeled agents - Invited commentary. *J Nucl Med.* 2001;42(11):1653–1655.
24. Xiong QF, Chen Y. Review: Deoxyglucose compounds labeled with isotopes different from 18-fuoride: is there a future in clinical practice? *Cancer Biother Radiopharm.* 2008;23(3):376–381.
25. Plathow C, Weber WA. Tumor cell metabolism imaging. *J Nucl Med.* 2008;49:43s–63s.
26. Sharma V, Prior JL, Belinsky MG, et al. Characterization of a Ga-67/Ga-68 radiopharmaceutical for SPECT and PET of MDR1 P-glycoprotein transport activity in vivo: validation in multidrug-resistant tumors and at the blood-brain barrier. *J Nucl Med.* 2005;46(2):354–364.
27. Imam SK. Molecular nuclear imaging: the radiopharmaceuticals (review). *Cancer Biother Radiopharm.* 2005;20(2):163–172.
28. Segars WP, Tsui BM. Study of the efficacy of respiratory gating in myocardial SPECT using the new 4D NCAT Phantom. *IEEE Trans Nucl Imaging.* 2002;49(3):675–679.
29. Bobkov KV, Bowsher JE, Greer KL, et al. Phantom assessment of new acquisition geometries for breast pinhole SPECT imaging. *IEEE Trans Nuclear Science.* 2006;53(3):1162–1167.
30. Ter-Antonyan R, Jaszczak RJ, Bowsher JE, et al. Quantitative evaluation of half-cone-beam scan paths in triple-camera brain SPECT. *IEEE Trans Nucl Sci.* 2008;55(5):2518–2526.
31. Takai Y, Mitsuya M, Nemoto K, et al. Development of a new linear accelerator with dual x-ray fluoroscopy using amorphous silicon flat panel x-ray sensors to detect a gold seed in tumor at real treatment position. *Int J Radiat Oncol Biol Phys.* 2001;51:381.
32. Takai Y, Mitsuya M, Nemoto K, et al. Development of a real-time tumor tracking system with DMLC with dual x-ray fluoroscopy and amorphous silicon flat panel on the gantry of linear accelerator. *Int J Radiat Oncol Biol Phys.* 2002;54:193–194.
33. Britton KR, Takai Y, Mitsuya M, et al. Evaluation of inter- and intrafraction organ motion during intensity modulated radiation therapy (IMRT) for localized prostate cancer measured by a newly developed on-board image-guided system. *Radiat Med.* 2005;23:14–24.
34. Koto M, Takai Y, Ogawa Y, et al. A phase II study on stereotactic body radiotherapy for stage I non-small cell lung cancer. *Radiother Oncol.* 2007;85:429–434.

Chapter 14

Quality Assurance in the Image-Guided Era

Erica Kinsey, PhD, Daniel J. Scanderbeg, PhD,
Jia-Zhu Wang, PhD, Trent Ning, PhD, Todd Pawlicki, PhD

An important goal of a quality assurance (QA) program is to instill confidence that patients are receiving their prescribed treatments accurately. The goal should not be simply getting through some mandatory tests as quickly and painlessly as possible. Unfortunately, many catastrophic events are produced by failures happening at a moment that cannot be predicted or caught by routine quality control (QC) procedures.[1] As there are built-in interlocks in treatment devices, most failures occur in human processes rather than in equipment.[1] Finding the proper balance between effort spent on specific QC procedures and effort spent on an overall quality management program is a major challenge at most institutions.

The words "assurance" and "control" can have multiple definitions. For example, "assurance" can mean confidence of mind, the state of being certain, or something that inspires confidence. The word "control" can mean to check, test, or verify; the act of guiding; or to exercise restraint over. In this chapter, quality assurance (QA) is defined as all the actions necessary to provide confidence in patient treatments, whereas QC is defined as the procedures that are the operational techniques used to fulfill the requirements for quality. Quality management is a formalized system that documents the structure, responsibilities, and procedures required to achieve optimal quality.

In 2007, the American Society for Therapeutic Radiology and Oncology (ASTRO), and the American Association of Physicists in Medicine (AAPM) jointly sponsored a symposium on QA for advanced technologies. The conference proceedings were presented in a supplement issue of the *International Journal of Radiation Oncology, Biology and Physics* (Volume 71). The issues relevant to image-guided radiation therapy (IGRT) QA will be discussed here. A major difficulty in discussing IGRT QA is that for newer advanced technologies, guidance on QA may be quickly outdated because of rapid development and implementation of devices and techniques.[2] Moreo-

ver, there is a large diversity of treatment devices on the market. For this reason, one of the symposium findings was that it will be extremely difficult to continue development of specific QA guidelines for each treatment device and process. Scientific bodies such as the AAPM should instead focus on overall process QA, which each institution can adapt to its individual environment.

The use of image-guided technologies can be considered a type of QA for patient setup and treatment. However, some may neglect the need for ensuring quality and proper operation of the IGRT equipment itself. As IGRT is increasingly automated, one needs to include an increasing amount of QC to independently verify computer actions. Quality assurance becomes more complicated and time-consuming as technology and processes become increasingly complex. Complicated QA practices can lead to QC not being performed at all, which introduces risk into clinical practice.

In terms of equipment and resources, comprehensive QA protocols for IGRT can be costly and time-consuming. Furthermore, they can still fail to safeguard patients because potential process errors are not necessarily included in traditional QA. Institutions may not realize that the increasing QA demands accompanying advanced technology require increased staffing. Additionally, traditional guidelines focus on specific devices rather than overall processes. The overall recommendations of the QA Symposium are to focus on process-centered quality management that is based on error prevention and analysis techniques, including adapting modern QA and quality management methods used in many other industries.[2,3] For example, failure mode and effects analysis (FMEA) is a newly recommended method to evaluate QA needs, and will be the subject of the upcoming AAPM Task Group (TG)-100 report.[4]

Potential errors of primary importance in IGRT include patient imaging, image registration, delineation between systematic and random motion, plan adaptation, and treatment dose calculation.[5] Some of these issues are difficult to test and verify. Many institutions rely on phantom studies to test their IGRT methods, but creating a phantom that is as deformable and seemingly random as a human patient is nearly impossible. Aspects of IGRT that are not fully automated introduce interuser variability. This variability is not as much of an issue in conventional radiotherapy (RT), but can be detrimental in IGRT where precision and accuracy are assumed to be high, and margins for error (i.e., planning margins) have been reduced.

Although this chapter is not intended to be an exhaustive report or a checklist, it is a compilation of current practices and recommendations, and will provide a starting point for the development of a comprehensive IGRT QA program. The overall goal of this chapter is to address QA issues for several major aspects of IGRT.

Conventional Linac IGRT

Conventional linear accelerator-based IGRT consists of imaging in the treatment room during a course of radiotherapy. Planar (two-dimensional [2D]) and volumetric (three-dimensional [3D]) imaging are used for repositioning the patient immediately prior to treatment. Volumetric imaging has the additional ability to utilize soft-tissue anatomic information for patient setup and may eventually allow adaptation of the daily treatment based on soft-tissue changes during the course of RT. This section will discuss the QA features of these techniques and systems. We also describe the QA of moving tumors even though this is still a developing modality. As the technology matures, QA and QC recommendations for moving tumors will undoubtedly be updated.

Modern kilovoltage (kV) imaging systems attached to linear accelerators make image guidance easier and provide added functionality. Image guidance, however, has been a part of radiotherapy treatments for many years (e.g., weekly port films). Megavoltage (MV) planar imaging is part of the image guidance paradigm and was initially implemented as a technique to increase efficiency by eliminating the use of radiographic film. Electronic portal imaging devices' (EPIDs') operational and QA issues are discussed in the AAPM TG-58 report.[6] In terms of QA, these systems should be checked for safety, mechanical stability, image quality, and quantitative reporting of patient shifts detected by the EPID device. All of these qualities are also important for current linac-based image-guided technologies.

The kV source and flat panel imager mounted to the linear accelerator gantry has changed linear accelerator QA requirements considerably. Geometric errors can occur in this imaging chain for both 2D projection imaging and 3D cone-beam computed tomography (CBCT). This is generally because of the sagging of the linac head and the flexing of the robotic arms that mount the kV

x-ray tube and flat-panel detector. Geometric parameters are usually established during commissioning and incorporated into correction software to be used as baseline values. Quality assurance of the coincidence between the treatment isocenter and imaging isocenter of orthogonally mounted systems is of paramount importance. It should be noted that different technologies have different strengths or weaknesses related to QA. For example, tomotherapy systems do not have an issue with imaging–treatment isocenter coincidence because their treatment beams and imaging beams utilize the same axis.

Quality assurance approaches have been proposed for systems that use a kV source and imager attached orthogonally to the treatment beam on the linear accelerator gantry. Some tests are typically performed before the clinical implementation of the imaging system whereas others are used to monitor the system's performance. These have been discussed in regard to MV imaging systems using phantom-based tests to establish the geometric accuracy and precision.[7] For kV imaging systems, QA procedures have been presented for both Elekta linacs (Elekta AB, Stockholm, Sweden) and Varian linacs (Varian Medical Systems Inc, Palo Alto, CA).[8,9] The common elements of a QA program for these orthogonally mounted kV systems include: (1) safety and functionality, (2) geometric accuracy (agreement of MV and kV beam isocenters), (3) image quality, (4) registration and correction accuracy, and (5) dose to patient and dosimetric stability. Safety and functionality tests evaluate these features and clinical operation of the entire system during the tube warm-up. Geometry QA verifies the geometric accuracy and stability of the kV system hardware and software. Quality assurance of the image requires one to regularly check spatial resolution and contrast sensitivity of the radiographic images.

Image QA for CBCT includes tests for Hounsfield unit (HU) linearity, HU uniformity, spatial linearity, and scan slice geometry. Image noise and spatial and contrast resolution can be assessed with standard computed tomography (CT) phantoms. Dose to the patient depends on the machine settings and patient geometry, and can be determined both by calculations and measurements. A QC procedure verifying agreement of the MV and kV isocenters using a simple phantom should be performed daily by a therapist and verified by a physicist. Alignment systems are generally accurate to within 1 mm to 2 mm and 1 degree. In a robust QA program, items (1), (2), and (3) should be performed monthly and items (4) and (5) should be performed at least annually. One can evaluate the frequency of all checks based on the system performance during the course of the first year of operation. For the interested reader, Balter and Antonuk have provided a general discussion of QA for these systems.[10] Bissonnette and colleagues have provided specific guidelines and tolerance levels for geometric accuracy of CBCT systems.[11]

Quality assurance issues for linac-based motion-adaptive radiation therapy involves challenges attributable to the added temporal dimension.[12] The main problem with gated treatments is the correlation of the internal tumor motion with the external marker system (e.g., reflecting block, pressure device, etc.). For breath-hold approaches, the patient is required to hold his or her breath at the same position within the same fraction and possibly between fractions as well. Minimizing errors for both of these approaches requires patient training appropriate to the particular approach. Patient training and coaching are essential components of a patient-specific QA program.[13] As a matter of safety, proper hygienic techniques should be followed for any parts of these systems that come in contact with the patient. Either for gating or breath hold, the instantaneous tumor position can be verified prior to treatment using fluoroscopy afforded by the kV imaging systems mounted on the linear accelerator. The average tumor position can be verified by using CBCT, for example. Definitive recommendations on this topic are provided by AAPM TG-76.[14] Interested readers are advised to follow the peer-reviewed literature as this is a treatment technique that will mature over time.

Tomotherapy

Helical Tomotherapy (Tomotherapy Inc, Madison, WI) delivers IGRT and IMRT using the combined features of a linear accelerator and a helical CT scanner. The 40-cm wide, by 1.0 cm, 2.5 cm, or 5.0 cm in length jaws are equipped with 64 binary multileaf collimator (MLC) leaves. Intensity modulation is accomplished by varying the fraction of time for which different leaves are open, while the gantry rotates at a constant velocity and the couch continuously translates the patient through the bore of the Tomotherapy machine. Analogous to the QA program of AAPM TG-40 for the conventional linac, mechanical and dosimetry checks need to be performed on a daily, monthly, and yearly schedule. Quality assurance on the dynamic and synchrony features unique to Tomotherapy also need to be implemented.

In Tomotherapy, there is a stationary laser system defining a virtual isocenter used for patient setup, which is offset 70 cm longitudinally from the machine isocenter. A second moveable laser system is used to align with fiducial markers on the patient. Therefore, the accuracy of the virtual isocenter, the machine isocenter, and couch translation between them are essential for correct patient setup and QA verification needs to be performed on a daily basis.

Tomotherapy has an inherent image-guidance system for patient setup, using the actual treatment beam as the x-ray source for image acquisition. An MV CT scan is obtained of the patient in the setup position before delivery of each treatment fraction. Fusion of the MV CT with

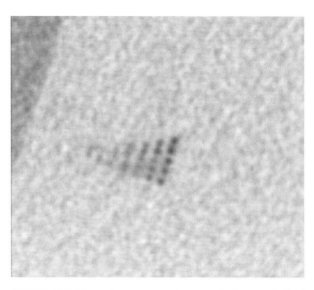

FIGURE 14-1. Megavoltage computed tomography images obtained of a diagnostic computed tomography phantom. This quality assurance phantom has eight sets of holes (five in each) with circular diameters ranging from 0.4 mm to 1.75 mm.

the planning CT allows for adjustment of the daily treatment position. Because the same x-ray source is used for the daily MV CT and treatment, registration of the daily image with the treatment isocenter is straightforward. However, QC on the performance and spatial resolution of the MV CT images needs to be performed because it plays an important role in IGRT. For this purpose, a CT phantom with holes of different diameters can be used, as shown in Figure 14-1.[15,16]

Tomotherapy requires synchrony of gantry rotation, couch translation, linear accelerator pulsing, and opening and closing of the binary MLC leaves used to modulate the radiation beam. The accuracy of this highly dynamic treatment process depends on the correct performance of the radiation source, MLC, gantry, and couch table. The dose delivered to the patient depends on the static beam dosimetry, system geometry, system dynamics, and system synchrony. Systematic QA of the system dynamics and synchrony has been suggested, which includes jaw width constancy, actual fraction of time leaves are open, couch drive distance, speed and uniformity, linear accelerator pulsing and gantry synchrony, leaf opening and gantry synchrony, and couch drive and gantry synchrony.[15,17]

For QA checks of the synchrony of leaf opening and gantry angle, Fenwick and colleagues developed a test using a pair of star patterns, using two S-Omat V films (Eastman Kodak, Rochester, NY) placed on the couch, sandwiched by solid water.[17] Accuracy of the couch translation and gantry synchrony is assessed with a Kodak EDR-2 film taped onto the couch. With the jaw opening set to 40 cm by 1 cm, the couch moves into the gantry at 1 cm per gantry rotation and the leaf opens every five gantry rotations centered at 0 gantry angle. The film results in three peaks of the irradiated segments 5 cm apart along the direction of couch drive.

CyberKnife

CyberKnife (Accuray Inc, Sunnyvale, CA) is a robotic radiosurgery system with a compact 6-MV linear accelerator mounted on a robotic arm with six degrees of freedom. Radiation is delivered at a discrete set of positions, known as the nodes, distributed on the surface of a semisphere centered on the treatment site, and the source-to-skin distance (SSD) can vary from 65 cm to 100 cm (Figure 14-2). The radiation beam is modulated with a circular collimator of diameter ranging from 5 mm to 60 mm at 80 cm SSD. This system uses frameless patient positioning for radiosurgery, and radiation is delivered as the robotic arm moves around the patient.

Patient setup on the CyberKnife system is guided by an orthogonal kV source–flat-panel image pair in the room coordinate system before treatment. Two x-ray cameras are mounted on the ceiling and two image detectors are mounted on the floor at either side of the treatment table. Patient position is monitored during the treatment for every few nodes and compared with digitally reconstructed radiographs (DRRs). The robot position is adjusted accordingly to correct for patient movement. Two important aspects distinguish the CyberKnife system from conventional external beam IGRT systems: (1) automated motion correction and (2) planning, imaging, and delivery combined with robotics.

Analogous to the QA program of AAPM TG-40 for a conventional linac system, mechanical and dosimetry checks of the CyberKnife need to be performed on a daily, monthly, and annual basis. Because of the unique robotic-based feature of CyberKnife, some specific procedures need to be added.[18–20] One such procedure is a daily check of the robot perch position through an internal laser from the robot to verify that the laser is aligning correctly. Another daily QA test needs to verify the coincidence of the treatment beam with the imaging center.

On a monthly basis, an end-to-end test should be performed to measure the total robotic targeting accuracy of the system, including localization, mechanical targeting, and planning errors. This is done by using an anthropomorphic head phantom or a ball-cube phantom (Figure 14-3) containing a film cassette to hold orthogonal pieces of GafChromic film (International Specialty Products, Wayne, NJ). After delivery, the orthogonal films are scanned and analyzed, and the delivered dose is compared with the planned distribution. This test also checks the geometric, mechanical, and radiation targeting accuracy. Such an analysis may also be repeated for each tracking technique, such as skull tracking, fiducial tracking, spine tracking, and synchrony-based tracking. The existing QA approaches and guidelines are being evaluated and the AAPM TG-135 is formalizing QA guidelines for robotic radiosurgery.

Ultrasound IGRT

Ultrasound target localization offers multiple benefits to patients and departments through its relatively inexpensive nature, fast real-time feedback, and lack of additional radiation dose to patients. Tome and Orton provide an overall review of ultrasound including a description of potential pitfalls as well as tests and references to minimize problems.[21]

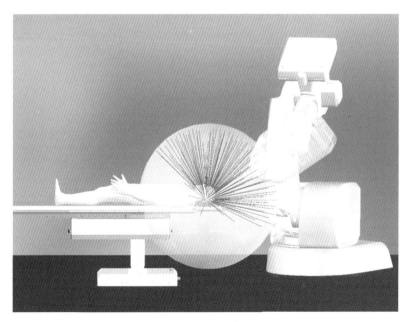

FIGURE 14-2. Illustration of the CyberKnife system (Accuray Inc, Sunnyvale, CA). The robotic arm has six degrees of freedom and the nodes are distributed on a spherical surface. Image used with permission from Accuray Incorporated.

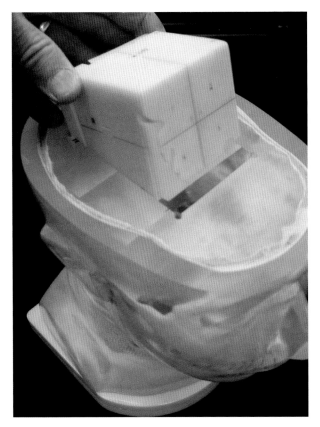

FIGURE 14-3. Head phantom used for quality assurance. The cube that is inserted into the phantom holds GafChromic film (International Speciality Products, Wayne, NJ) in an orthogonal arrangement for end-to-end tests. Image used with permission from Accuray Incorporated.

The first issue to address with ultrasound IGRT is the accuracy of target localization with well-defined boundaries. To perform this test, a test phantom can be utilized to verify target position agreement between the ultrasound measurement and the predicted target location from the treatment planning system.[22,23] A standard commercially available phantom can be used for this test; however, an article by Drever and Hilts describes a custom-made phantom that can also be used for daily QA.[24]

A second test should be to verify the accuracy of the system by using an unknown target. This means that the localization accuracy should be tested with target motion of a varying, unknown degree.[22,23] Patient target volumes can move erratically and unpredictably, so localization should be tested under similar conditions.

Ultrasound operation requires specialized training and skills, which are not as routinely used in RT. Therefore, there can be a high degree of user variability according to the experience or training level of the operator. A test of interuser variability may also be useful to quantify the extent of this potential problem. Ideally, users would be interchangeable with zero influence on the daily localization, but, in reality, there is always a discrepancy in training and experience. It should be noted that this issue of variability attributable to user experience is not specific to ultrasound images but also occurs in planar and volumetric radiographic images. This operator discrepancy leads to an additional margin needed on top of the usual setup error. A baseline test of the interuser variability will help establish reasonable target margins. A more thorough description of the test is found in another article written by Orton and Tome.[25]

Surface Imaging

Real-time 3D surface mapping techniques are available for patient setup and surveillance (for example: VisionRT, London, UK; and C-RAD, Uppsala, Sweden). An advantage of these systems, similar to ultrasound systems, is that they add no additional radiation dose to the patient as part of the imaging procedure. Because these are relatively new products, available literature is limited, especially in the area of QA. The majority of publications are feasibility-type studies and error analysis, proving the utility of the devices in clinical operations.[26-29]

An important QA issue related to these devices is camera stability.[30,31] Ideally, the cameras are mounted in a secure position to minimize the potential for movement; however, unexpected motion can occur. To test for this, a target image (e.g., calibration template) can be set at the treatment machine isocenter (Figure 14-4). An image is acquired and automatically compared with the system calibration file. Then, the system either passes or fails, in which case the system would need to be recalibrated. A daily calibration test along with a monthly system recalibration is recommended when one is beginning to use these systems.

One potential for error with these systems is related to the reference images. Ideally, one would take a reference image at the time of simulation and use this for treatment setup to ensure reproducible patient positioning between the time of simulation and treatment. This requires a camera system in the simulator room. This is not a major problem except for the positioning of the camera system. The camera system must be positioned like that of treatment room setup and the isocenter of each room must match. If not, then a transformation of coordinate systems must be made between the simulation reference image and the treatment images.[31] In place of reference images in the simulation room are reference images created from the patient CT scans, which serve the same purpose. This approach is equally accurate for regions of the body that are not prone to motion artifacts during simulation.

4DCT and Respiratory Gating

The issue of respiratory management is a major challenge in radiation oncology today. Motion caused by

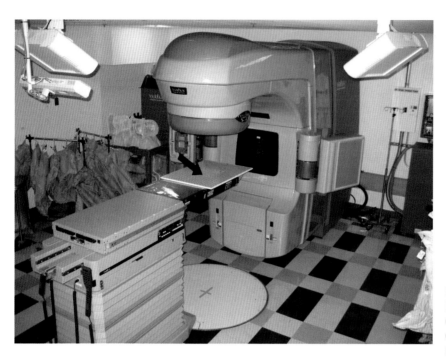

FIGURE 14-4. VisionRT system (Vision RT Ltd, London, UK) calibration verification. The calibration template, placed on the linac couch (arrow), is set up to image and compare with the system calibration file.

respiration definitely affects tumors in the thorax and abdomen and possibly beyond these regions. The importance of respiratory management is reflected in the formation of an AAPM Task Group dedicated solely to this issue. The AAPM TG-76 report, which includes QA recommendations for motion management, has been published in *Medical Physics*.[14] Additionally, in a special issue of the *International Journal of Radiation Oncology, Biology and Physics* dedicated to IGRT, Jiang and colleagues discuss fundamental challenges for three techniques of respiratory management: respiratory gating, breath hold, and 4DCT.[12] Four-dimensional CT has three major sources of potential error: (1) irregular patient respiration, (2) CT image reconstruction algorithms, and (3) re-sorting of reconstructed CT images with respiratory signal.[12]

One of the key components of gated treatments is the correlation between the external monitor to the internal target motion. Irregular breathing of the patient can lead to irregular motion of the tumor/organs, image artifacts during the scan, and improper sorting or binning of the images. Therefore, reproducible respiration from the patient is the key to the best treatment and, hence, breath coaching is necessary. Breath coaching helps ensure a more reproducible breathing cycle between simulation and treatment. Coaching is useful for improved reproducibility even with a breath-hold technique as it helps with inspiration and exhalation limits.

Reconstruction algorithms come in two forms with either a prospective-based reconstruction with a fixed-interval or a respiratory signal–based reconstruction. In both cases, the reconstruction can be sensitive to

temporal parameters. Computed tomography image re-sorting falls in one of two categories, namely, phase-based or amplitude-based. Phase-based sorting matches the recorded respiratory signal with the CT images taken and estimates the phase, re-sorting the images accordingly. Amplitude-based sorting re-sorts the images according to amplitude and does not consider any phase information from the breathing trace.

Reconstruction algorithms and re-sorting of the CT images can be checked by using a respiratory motion phantom.[12] There are several respiratory motion phantoms on the market that can be used to characterize the system from simulation through treatment. The phantom can be used for 4DCT simulation, planned as if it were a patient, and finally used to check delivered dose with film and/or an ion chamber. Additionally, some of the phantoms can be programmed with the same respiratory cycle as the patient such that the patient's treatment plan can be delivered to the phantom. This ensures each patient's treatment plan is being accurately delivered with his or her own respiratory cycle. However, as a matter of clinical implementation, it is best to ensure that the patient breathes reproducibly by using some type of breath coaching for patients that are receptive to the coaching process.[13]

Respiratory management through 4DCT allows the reduction of treatment margins, normal tissue exposure, and potentially allows for dose escalation. A major quality issue to address (besides equipment functionality) with regard to 4DCT is reproducing the patient's breathing pattern between simulation, treatment, and each subsequent fraction delivered. If a patient is breathing irregularly, then there is no guarantee that the tumor and organ motion is the same as that represented in the 4DCT scan.

Image Registration, Fusion, and Segmentation

Image registration (alignment), fusion (superposition), and segmentation (automatic contouring) have become an integral part of RT planning and treatment, especially within the realm of IGRT. Image registration is used for treatment planning, to check delivery setup, and to adapt treatment based on actual dose delivered.[32] New methods and software are continually being developed, and the field is quickly becoming increasingly sophisticated. These technologies are helping advance IGRT capabilities, and, with many institutions eager to implement new technology as it comes online, care needs to be taken to address the safety and reliability of such systems.

One type of QA is manual inspection of the results. Image registration, fusion, and segmentation have a built-in QA, albeit rudimentary, because it is difficult to get an optimal result if there is a major problem somewhere in the process (i.e., trying to register images from two separate patients, for example). Many institutions rely heavily on this built-in safety net and might be careless with the process. There are still many errors that can produce apparently reasonable but incorrect results (e.g., fusing a positron emission tomography [PET] scan from one patient onto a CT from a similar patient). In addition, extra care needs to be taken when deformable algorithms are used.[33] There are numerous papers assessing the validity of such systems, but most are for in-house algorithms or for one specific clinical setup, thus resulting in a lack of general QA guidance regarding image registration, fusion, and segmentation. This section will give an overview of the potential pitfalls, along with advice from literature as a starting point for developing QA programs for image registration, fusion, and segmentation.

Potential dangers and pitfalls during image registration, fusion, and segmentation include accuracy and specificity issues, orientation, chirality, spatial distortion, spatial resolution, partial volume effect (PVE), and the use of rigid body models on a nonrigid body. Accuracy and specificity issues include errors such as registering images from two different patients. This type of problem should be relatively easy to catch if it is a CT–CT or CT–magnetic resonance (MR) registration, but would be less obvious for a CT–PET registration. Orientation issues include problems of registering to the wrong anatomic location, such as trying to register a small spinal portal image to an incorrect section of vertebrae. The ability to detect this type of error depends on the anatomical location. An example of a chirality issue would be registering to a mirror image. This type of error would most likely be caused by a data transmission or data export or import problem and the ability to detect it depends on anatomic location (an abdomen would be easier to differentiate than a head) and image type (CT and MR would be easier to differentiate than PET). Spatial distortion becomes an issue if one of the image sets is from MR.[34,35] Spatial resolution is an issue for PET and single photon emission CT (SPECT) images.[35] In addition, CT, MR, and PET images are all prone to PVE from the voxelization process, which can influence the perceived size of objects.[36] Finally, aside from the head and extremities, one cannot assume rigid movement, and using rigid body registration models on a nonrigid body would introduce errors.[34,37]

The AAPM has formed TG-132 to focus on image registration, which will include QA issues.[37] Until their suggestions are published, it is at the discretion of individual institutions to determine the level and type of QA needed. Mutic and colleagues proposed image registration QA tests to be used during annual QA or whenever software or scanners are upgraded.[35] These tests utilized a modified commercial phantom (RSVP Phantom, The Phantom Laboratory, Salem, NY) to verify CT-CT, CT-MR, and CT–PET registration. The phantom was filled with contrast material compatible with each imaging modality, scans were performed, and the images were registered to a reference CT scan. The registrations were verified by using both contrast objects within the phantom and fiducials placed on the exterior of the phantom. These investigators emphasized the importance of periodic QA checks of the entire image fusion process.

Dalah and colleagues used a commercial body phantom (NEMA IEC Body Phantom, Data Spectrum Corp, Hillsborough, NC) specifically for testing commercial image registration software packages.[36] They proposed several tests to check the performance and reliability of ProSoma (Pi Medical, Athens, Greece) with the intention that the tests could be translated to any system that is used for CT-CT, CT-MR, or CT–PET registration. The phantom was filled with contrast material that was compatible to each imaging modality, and scans were performed. The scans were registered by using the three types of ProSoma registration (manual, semiautomatic, and automatic), and the registrations were verified by using both contrast objects within the phantom and fiducials placed on the exterior of the phantom. Kashani and colleagues proposed a way to test deformable registration with a modified deformable phantom.[33] Numerous small markers were added to a deformable phantom, and CT scans were acquired at various levels of deformation. The locations of all of the markers were identified, and they were digitally removed from the images before registration. Multiple in-house deformable registration algorithms were applied, and the resulting transforms were applied to the marker positions to enable comparison with the reference marker locations.

Although image registration, fusion, and segmentation have an inherent level of human review QA (at least as long as it is not a completely automated process) that should catch most process errors, more QA is needed to protect against errors that are less-detectable by human review, such as chirality in a brain scan. Image registration should always be validated before any clinical decisions are made based on the results.[32] Even if the registration is checked by visual inspection of anatomical landmarks, precision depends greatly on the user, the respective slice thicknesses, and resolutions.[33] Some guidance can be found in literature, but general guidelines are lacking. Many QA methods presented in literature are only applicable to in-house systems, or specific machine equipment and/or software setups. To date, very little has been published on QA for automatic image segmentation, other than the fact that extreme care needs to be taken when imaging artifacts exist.[38]

Image-Guided Brachytherapy

In recent years, treatment planning for both high-dose-rate (HDR) and low-dose-rate (LDR) brachytherapy has evolved from using orthogonal x-ray films to using volumetric imaging such as CT, MR, or ultrasound. Trans Rectal UltraSonography (TRUS) has been used in permanent prostate seed implants since the 1980s.[39] Image-guided brachytherapy has been utilized in prostate brachytherapy (permanent seed or HDR implantation), partial breast irradiation, gynecological and endobronchial brachytherapy, etc. Quality control procedures are essential to reduce the chance for errors and minimize uncertainties.

Patient identity is one issue that needs to be addressed during QA for image-guided brachytherapy. When x-ray film is used in brachytherapy, the date of acquisition and patient identification should be unambiguously marked on the film.[39] With digital equipment, the operator needs to verify the information in the computer for each patient and update it if necessary. The verification is more important if the same procedures are scheduled side by side in the same location. For example, multiple prostate seed implants are scheduled in the same operating room. If the image of implanted seeds was taken with a digital x-ray unit and the patient information in the unit was not updated, the new image would be stored with an incorrect patient name.

Source and/or applicator localization is another issue to be addressed to ensure quality. Although computer-reconstructed 3D images provide more anatomical information along with the correlation between the anatomy and applicator(s), the longitudinal resolution is limited by the slice thicknesses of the images. Small slice thicknesses provide better resolution and therefore may help to identify markers and other structures. However, for prostate seed implants, because of the length of seeds (4.5 mm), small slice thicknesses might not help identify seeds in postimplant CT scans used for postimplant dosimetry evaluation.

Anatomic and dosimetric concerns are another important part of QA. Because the dose rate of a brachytherapy source decreases rapidly with increasing distance from the source, a small change in target contour could increase or decrease treatment time significantly. Accurate target contouring and source localization are necessary for optimal dose coverage. Therefore, QA is needed for both the planning computer and the imaging device to reduce errors in target and critical organ contouring.

In addition to these specific issues, imaging devices for brachytherapy also need to be included in the QA process. Prostate brachytherapy uses a grid template as a guide for needle insertion under ultrasound guidance. The position of the template relative to the ultrasound probe should be calibrated by viewing the ultrasound image with an overlapping image of the grid. The coordinates of the template, and that of the ultrasound images of the needles, should be in agreement within acceptable tolerance (~2 mm). The calibration should be performed initially and periodically afterward, or whenever the positioning of the template is in question. Additionally, because the needle's ultrasound image is model dependent because of the manufacturing process used to enhance echogenicity, the templates should be recalibrated if different needles are used.[39]

For CT or MR imaging, the applicator should be CT/MR compatible. Artifacts introduced by metal markers or other objects should be evaluated carefully. As a part of treatment QA, orthogonal planar x-ray images or scout images from the CT-simulator can be used to verify the positions of the applicator and markers. The images combined with a source-position-check function of the HDR unit provide a good reference-position check immediately before treatment. Also, image fusion provides an efficient tool for contouring if the target is not visible on both image modes. The registration of image sets from different modes has to be done using the other structures that are visible in both image sets. Consequences of the registration uncertainty on the treatment plan should be evaluated as previously discussed in this chapter.

Additional sources of uncertainty in image-guided brachytherapy include image accuracy, applicator reconstruction (e.g., digitizing of catheters), and target and region of interest contouring. Image uncertainty can be minimized with an appropriate QA procedure conducted by a qualified medical physicist with a well-designed phantom. For reconstruction, a thorough understanding of the physical aspects of the applicator can help limit the uncertainty to within acceptable tolerance (~2 mm). Contouring uncertainty is minimized by a planner with a good knowledge of human anatomy and an appropriate peer-review program in place.

Most currently available brachytherapy QA recommendations are relatively fixed protocols of specific tests, end points, tolerances, and frequencies. The protocols reflect practice patterns that predate the image-based planning era. More process-focused guidance is needed for all clinical applications using image-based planning, image-guidance, non-CT imaging modalities, and image processing and registration techniques.[40]

Phantoms for IGRT

Phantoms are a necessary component of IGRT QC procedures. There are many phantoms that have been developed for IMRT QC and a similar effort is being put forth for IGRT QC. Some phantoms appropriate for IGRT QC have been presented throughout this chapter. In this section, a brief discussion of three recently introduced QC phantoms is presented, primarily used for linac-based IGRT.

A need exists for 4D QC devices that can analyze intrafraction motion as it relates to dose delivery and respiratory gating, including IMRT treatments. A 4D phantom prototype device has been built that utilizes a well-known IMRT QC phantom (MapCheck, Sun Nuclear Corporation, Melbourne, FL). This system can mimic breathing motion as entered by the user and preview that motion in real time as well as drive a motorized device that has a mounted planar IMRT QC measurement device.[41] This type of tool can be used for dose delivery verification under conditions of intrafraction motion.

Another phantom has been developed for QC of linear accelerators capable of CBCT image guidance and IMRT. This phantom is to be used in an integral test to quantify in real time both the performance of the image guidance and the dose delivery systems in terms of dose localization.[42] The prototype QC phantom consisted of an existing cylindrical imaging phantom (CatPhan 500, Phantom Laboratories, Salem, NY) combined with an array of 11 radiation diodes mounted on a 10-cm-diameter disk, oriented perpendicular to the phantom axis. For single-beam geometry, errors in phantom placement as small as 0.5 mm could be accurately detected. In the clinical setting, MLC systematic errors of 1 mm on a single MLC bank introduced in the IMRT plan were detectable with the QC phantom.

The last phantom discussed provides a method to determine CBCT to MV isocenter alignment using another commercially available phantom (QUASAR Penta-Guide phantom, Modus Medical Devices Inc, London, Ontario, Canada).[43] This system will allow measurement of image sharpness from the edge response function of a spherical air cavity within the Penta-Guide phantom.

These newly-developed QC tools have the potential to streamline this QC process and improve the level of performance of IGRT. There are many more phantoms on the market for IGRT (and IMRT) QC and many more will surely be introduced in the future.

Conclusions

Image-guided RT has introduced the potential to realize a higher level of precision and accuracy in RT, but along with the increased performance comes an increased responsibility to verify treatment delivery. Quality assurance programs for IGRT are not easy to implement. Rapid development of new IGRT techniques and devices is quickly making traditional QA guidelines outdated. Because of the diversity of IGRT, it is extremely difficult to develop industry-wide specific QA guidelines, forcing a conversion to process-centered quality management guidelines, which each institution can tailor to its individual needs. Commissioning and clinical implementation is a good time to develop a QA plan and to set baseline values for performance. Ideally, some portion of this should be done in a clinical setting with clinical images and end-to-end tests. A key component of any IGRT QA program is using the right tools for the job, along with appropriately trained staff. An optimal QA program is always a balance between available resources, manpower, and time to perform the work.

References

1. Thomadsen B. Critique of traditional quality assurance paradigm. *Int J Radiat Oncol Biol Phys.* 2008;71(1 Suppl):S166–S169.
2. Williamson JF, Dunscombe PB, Sharpe MB, et al. Quality assurance needs for modern image-based radiotherapy: recommendations from 2007 interorganizational symposium on "Quality assurance of radiation therapy: Challenges of advanced technology." *Int J Radiat Oncol Biol Phys.* 2008;71(1 Suppl):S2–S12.
3. Hendee WR. Safety and accountability in healthcare from past to present. *Int J Radiat Oncol Biol Phys.* 2008;71(1 Suppl):S157–S161.
4. Huq MS, Fraass BA, Dunscombe PB, et al. A method for evaluating quality assurance needs in radiation therapy. *Int J Radiat Oncol Biol Phys.* 2008;71(1 Suppl):S170–S173.
5. Yan D. Developing quality assurance processes for image-guided adaptive radiation therapy. *Int J Radiat Oncol Biol Phys.* 2008;71(1 Suppl):S28–S32.
6. Herman MG, Balter JM, Jaffray DA, et al. Clinical use of electronic portal imaging: report of AAPM Radiation Therapy Committee Task Group 58. *Med Phys.* 2001;28(5):712–737.
7. Langen KM, Meeks SL, Pouliot J. Quality assurance of onboard megavoltage computed tomography imaging and target localization systems for on- and off-line image-guided radiotherapy. *Int J Radiat Oncol Biol Phys.* 2008;71(1 Suppl):S62–S65.
8. Lehmann J, Perks J, Semon S, et al. Commissioning experience with cone-beam computed tomography for image-guided radiation therapy. *J Appl Clin Med Phys.* 2007;8(3):2354.

9. Yoo S, Kim GY, Hammoud R, et al. A quality assurance program for the on-board imagers. *Med Phys.* 2006;33(11):4431–4447.

10. Balter JM, Antonuk LE. Quality assurance for kilo- and megavoltage in-room imaging and localization for off- and online setup error correction. *Int J Radiat Oncol Biol Phys.* 2008;71 (1 Suppl):S48–S52.

11. Bissonnette JP, Moseley D, White E, et al. Quality assurance for the geometric accuracy of cone-beam CT guidance in radiation therapy. *Int J Radiat Oncol Biol Phys.* 2008;71(1 Suppl):S57–S61.

12. Jiang SB, Wolfgang J, Mageras GS. Quality assurance challenges for motion-adaptive radiation therapy: gating, breath holding, and four-dimensional computed tomography. *Int J Radiat Oncol Biol Phys.* 2008;71(1 Suppl):S103–S107.

13. Neicu T, Berbeco R, Wolfgang J, Jiang SB. Synchronized moving aperture radiation therapy (SMART): improvement of breathing pattern reproducibility using respiratory coaching. *Phys Med Biol.* 2006;51(3):617–636.

14. Keall PJ, Mageras GS, Balter JM, et al. The management of respiratory motion in radiation oncology report of AAPM Task Group 76. *Med Phys.* 2006;33(10):874–900.

15. Balog J, Holmes T, Vaden R. A helical tomotherapy dynamic quality assurance. *Med Phys* 2006;33(10):3939–3950.

16. Meeks SL, Harmon JF Jr, Langen KM, et al. Performance characterization of megavoltage computed tomography imaging on a helical tomotherapy unit. *Med Phys* 2005;32(8):2673–2681.

17. Fenwick JD, Tomé WA, Jaradat HA, et al. Quality assurance of a helical tomotherapy machine. *Phys Med Biol.* 2004;49(13): 2933–2953.

18. Chang SD, Main W, Martin DP, et al. An analysis of the accuracy of the CyberKnife: a robotic frameless stereotactic radiosurgical system. *Neurosurgery* 2003;52:140–146

19. Dieterich S,. Pawlicki T. Cyberknife image-guided delivery and quality assurance. *Int J Radiat Oncol Biol Phys.* 2008;71 (1 Suppl):S126–S130.

20. Yu C, Main W, Taylor D, et al. An anthropomorphic phantom study of the accuracy of Cyberknife spinal radiosurgery. *Neurosurgery.* 2004;55:1138–1149.

21. Tome WA, Orton NP. Quality assurance of ultrasound imaging systems for target localization and online setup corrections. *Int J Radiat Oncol Biol Phys.* 2008;71(1 Suppl):S53–S56.

22. Tome WA, Meeks S, Orton NP, et al. Patient positioning in radiotherapy using optical guided 3-D ultrasound techniques. In: Schlegel W, Bortfeld T, Grosu A, eds. *New Technologies in Radiation Oncology.* Berlin, Germany: Springer; 2006: 151–163.

23. Tome WA, Meeks SL, Orton NP, et al. Commissioning and quality assurance of an optically guided three-dimensional ultrasound target localization system for radiotherapy. *Med Phys.* 2002;29:1781–1788.

24. Drever LA, Hilts M. Daily quality assurance phantom for ultrasound image guided radiation therapy. *J Appl Clin Med Phys.* 2007;8:2467.

25. Orton NP, Tome WA. The impact of daily shifts on prostate IMRT dose distributions. *Med Phys.* 2004;31:2845–2848.

26. Bert C, Metheany KG, Doppke K, Chen GT. A phantom evaluation of a stereo-vision surface imaging system for radiotherapy patient setup. *Med Phys.* 2005;32:2753–2762.

27. Bert C, Metheany KG, Doppke KP, et al. Clinical experience with a 3D surface patient setup system for alignment of partial-breast irradiation patients. *Int J Radiat Oncol Biol Phys.* 2006; 64:1265–1274.

28. Gierga DP, Riboldi M, Turcotte JC, et al. Comparison of target registration errors for multiple image-guided techniques in accelerated partial breast irradiation. *Int J Radiat Oncol Biol Phys.* 2008;70:1239–1246.

29. Schoffel PJ, Harms W, Sroka-Perez G, et al. Accuracy of a commercial optical 3D surface imaging system for realignment of patients for radiotherapy of the thorax. *Phys Med Biol.* 2007;52:3949–3963.

30. Johnson LS, Milliken BD, Hadley SW, et al. Initial clinical experience with a video-based patient positioning system. *Int J Radiat Oncol Biol Phys.* 1999;45:205–213.

31. Milliken BD, Rubin SJ, Hamilton RJ, et al. Performance of a video-image-subtraction-based patient positioning system. *Int J Radiat Oncol Biol Phys.* 1997;38:855–866.

32. Kessler ML. Image registration and data fusion in radiation therapy. *Br J Radiol.* 2006;79(Spec no. 1):S99–S108.

33. Kashani R, Hub M, Kessler ML, Balter JM. Technical note: a physical phantom for assessment of accuracy of deformable alignment algorithms. *Med Phys.* 2007;34:2785–2788.

34. Balter JM, Kessler ML. Imaging and alignment for image-guided radiation therapy. *J Clin Oncol.* 2007;25:931–937.

35. Mutic S, Dempsey JF, Bosch WR, et al. Multimodality image registration quality assurance for conformal three-dimensional treatment planning. *Int J Radiat Oncol Biol Phys.* 2001;51:255–260.

36. Dalah EZ, Nisbet A, Reise S, Bradley D. Evaluating commercial image registration packages for radiotherapy treatment planning. *Appl Radiat Isot.* 2008;66:1948–1953.

37. Sharpe M, Brock KK. Quality assurance of serial 3D image registration, fusion, and segmentation. *Int J Radiat Oncol Biol Phys.* 2008;71:S33–S37.

38. Wijesooriya K, Weiss E, Dill V, et al. Quantifying the accuracy of automated structure segmentation in 4D CT images using a deformable image registration algorithm. *Med Phys.* 2008;35:1251–1260.

39. Cormack RA. Quality assurance issues for computed tomography-, ultrasound-, and magnetic resonance imaging-guided brachytherapy. *Int J Radiat Oncol Biol Phys.* 2008;71(1 Suppl): S136–S141.

40. Williamson JF. Current brachytherapy quality assurance guidance: does it meet the challenges of emerging image-guided technologies? *Int J Radiat Oncol Biol Phys.* 2008;71(1 Suppl):S18–S22.

41. Nelms BE, Ehler E, Bragg H, Tomé WA. Quality assurance device for four-dimensional IMRT or SBRT and respiratory gating using patient-specific intrafraction motion kernels. *J Appl Clin Med Phys.* 2007;8:2683.

42. Letourneau D, Keller H, Sharpe MB, Jaffray DA. Integral test phantom for dosimetric quality assurance of image guided and intensity modulated stereotactic radiotherapy. *Med Phys.* 2007;34:1842–1849.

43. Sykes JR, Lindsay R, Dean CJ, et al. Measurement of cone beam CT coincidence with megavoltage isocentre and image sharpness using the QUASARtrade mark Penta-Guide phantom. *Phys Med Biol.* 2008;53:5275–5293.

Central Nervous System Tumors: Overview

Ashwatha Narayana, MD, Jenghwa Chang, PhD

Radiation therapy (RT) plays an important role in the management of intracranial tumors. Although significant improvement in survival has been achieved in pediatric brain tumors such as medulloblastoma, local control remains a problem in many tumors, notably gliomas. The pattern of recurrence in most brain tumors including gliomas is predominantly local.[1] The inability to deliver adequate radiation dose to the precise target volume often remains the cause for local failure. This is particularly frustrating because distant metastasis is not an issue in primary intracranial tumors and leptomeningeal dissemination happens rarely in these tumors. The difficulty in identifying the region of high-grade tumor as well as areas of tumor extension within the area of radiological abnormality contributes significantly to the risk of local recurrence.[1] Because gliomas are the most common primary intracranial tumors, they will be used as the model for discussion throughout the section, although frequent references to other tumors such as metastases and meningiomas will be made frequently.

Randomized clinical trials have clearly established the benefit of RT in high-grade gliomas using conventional doses.[1] An improvement in both local control and survival has been clearly shown when the radiation dose has been escalated from 40 Gy to 60 Gy.[2] Despite a lack of consistent evidence for a strong dose–response curve beyond 60 Gy when one is using radiation to treat gliomas, there is interest in employing higher doses, because of the benefit seen in other locations.[3,4] However, dose escalation carries with it an increased incidence of side effects.[5] It can be postulated that the use of such high doses may be of greatest clinical value only if all the active disease receives a certain dose and if normal tissue is spared as much as possible. A possible approach would be to use intensity-modulated RT (IMRT) to spare the critical structures. Its ability to improve tumor coverage while decreasing the dose to critical structures has been demonstrated in several studies for skull base tumors, meningiomas, and in head and neck sites.[6–8] The preliminary data with IMRT in high-grade gliomas has indicated that it is unlikely that

its use with conventional doses and volume definition would improve the local control.[9] However, it did result in decreased acute and late toxicities. No increased acute or late toxicities were noted in another prospective phase I dose escalation trial for glioblastoma done at Wake Forest University.[10]

The limiting factor for dose escalation in brain tumors is the increased risk of radiation-induced brain injury. The risk of radiation-induced brain injury increases with total dose, dose per fraction, and volume of radiation.[11] The dose and volume constraints for anatomically critical structures such as brain stem and optical structures have been well studied and documented. However, little is known about the limiting dose for functionally critical structures such as the motor cortex, Broca's area, Wernicke's area, and visual cortex because of the lack of imaging tools to identify those structures. Cognitive impairment attributable to late delayed effects of radiation damages to functionally critical structures ranges from mild apathy to incapacitating dementia and is clearly observed in patients undergoing whole-brain RT, hypofractionated RT, and concurrent neurotoxic chemotherapy.[12] Treatment of cognitive sequelae of cranial irradiation is still limited at this time.[11,12]

Magnetic resonance (MR) imaging remains the modality of choice for defining the tumor extent in intracranial tumors, treatment planning, and image-guided therapies because of its multiplanar capability, anatomic detail, and superior resolution.[13] Its ability to characterize tissue has allowed improved assessment of fatty, hemorrhagic, cystic, necrotic, and vascular components as well as mass effect and location. The approach to defining target volumes for RT in patients with gliomas at the present time is to deliver a certain dose to the contrast-enhancing area, as determined from a contrast-enhanced T1-weighted MR or fluid-attenuated-inversion-recovery (FLAIR) images plus a margin of 2 cm to 3 cm.[14,15] The size of this margin is generally chosen because serial biopsies of patients undergoing craniotomy for malignant gliomas have revealed tumor cells up to 3 cm distance from the contrast-enhancing margin in a majority of the patients. However, lacking with conventional MR is an assessment of physiological and functional information about the tumor. The contrast-enhancing lesion on T1-weighted MR images only reflects areas with a breakdown of the blood–brain barrier. This has been shown to be not always a reliable indicator of high-grade tumor because of the presence of both nonenhancing high-grade tumor and contrast-enhancing necrosis.[16] Similarly, T2- or FLAIR-defined volume either overestimates or underestimates the low-grade tumor in a majority of patients.[17] As a result, new diagnostic tools are being explored that would assist the treating radiation oncologist in better defining the volumes to which dose should be delivered.

The volume of radiation can be optimized with better target delineation by using newer imaging techniques, including MR spectroscopy (MRS), perfusion imaging, positron emission tomography (PET), and more accurate patient setup using image-guided RT (IGRT) to reduce the planning target volume (PTV) and clinical target volume (CTV) margins. The therapeutic ratio can further be improved if dose to critical structures can be minimized by using functional imaging studies. Because there are not enough clinical data at present to suggest the limiting dose, efforts should be made to correlate the dose to and the complication of the functionally critical regions. The following section details the new imaging modalities and the advances made in incorporating them in IGRT treatment planning of brain tumors.

Image-Guided Target Delineation

Magnetic Resonance Spectroscopic Imaging

Magnetic resonance spectroscopic imaging is a powerful diagnostic tool that can obtain proton (1H) spectra from selected regions within the brain.[18,19] Magnetic resonance spectroscopy can provide information about tumor activity based upon the levels of cellular metabolites, including choline-containing compounds (Cho), total creatine (Cr), N-acetylaspartate (NAA), and lactate/lipid. Each of these metabolites acts as a biochemical marker: Cho is a membrane component that is increased in viable tumor; Cr is a marker of cellular bioenergetic process; NAA is a neuronal marker that is decreased in tumors because of neuronal loss; and lactate is an end product of anaerobic metabolism. Clinical studies have shown that the degree of changes in metabolite levels may help differentiate normal brain from tumor in patients with suspected glioma.[6,20] It has been noted that gliomas exhibit a markedly high resonance in the spectral region of Cho and/or a low Cr and NAA resonance, implying increases in the Cho-to-Cr and/or Cho-to-NAA ratios. In addition, it has also been shown that the degree of elevation in Cho-to-Cr level correlates with an elevation in tumor cell density and/or the tumor grade.[21,22] The ability of MRS imaging to

demonstrate areas of high-grade tumor within low-grade gliomas has also been noted.[21]

In several studies, MRS was found to be a better tool than conventional MR alone in both defining the true extent of the tumor and in defining the grade of the tumor. In a pilot study, conventional MR failed to detect the tumor adequately in 50% of the patients that were noted in the MRS imaging.[21] Similarly, the postcontrast T1 sequences overestimated the gross tumor volume (GTV) defined by a Cho-to-Cr ratio of greater than 3 by 40%. In addition, the T2-based imaging overestimated the CTV defined by a Cho-to-Cr ratio of greater than 1 by 30% in half the patients indicating overtreatment of normal brain tissue. At the University of California San Francisco (UCSF), both Cho-to-Cr and Cho-to-NAA ratios have been used and categorization has been done based on abnormality index.[23] These investigators demonstrated metabolically active tumor outside MR-defined volumes in a nonuniform manner in both low-grade and high-grade tumors. See Chapter 15B for a description of the use of MRS-guided target delineation in a patient with recurrent glioblastoma multiforme.

Although MRS is a powerful tool, it has its limitations. Poor-quality spectroscopy because of the presence of clips, radioactive seeds, clotted blood, and skull bone within the measured volume may make it very difficult to interpret the findings.[1] Decreasing the size of the individual voxels improves the spatial resolution of MRS imaging data but can increase the scan time and/or decrease the signal-to-noise ratio (quality of the spectroscopy). Use of 3 Tesla (3T) MR and defining the volume of interest tightly around the FLAIR abnormality while avoiding the ventricles and bone may improve the target definition.

Perfusion/Diffusion Imaging

Relative cerebral blood volume (rCBV) and vascular permeability measurements from dynamic susceptibility contrast and dynamic contrast-enhanced perfusion MR have been shown to be closely correlated with histological measurements of microvascular density in gliomas.[24] Dynamic susceptibility contrast perfusion MR images are acquired with a gradient-echo echo-planar imaging (EPI) sequence during the first pass of a standard dose intravenous contrast administration. Application of pharmacokinetic models with an artery input function will allow estimation of vascular permeability in the region of interest. Relative CBV measurements have provided physiologic information about neovascularity and angiogenesis of the entire brain and have been shown to correlate well with the grade of the glioma.[25–27] It has also been shown that rCBV measurements are superior to conventional contrast-enhanced MR in predicting tumor biology and may even be superior to pathologic assessment in predicting patient clinical outcome, given the accepted limitations of pathologic assessment either from stereotactic biopsy or even from surgical resection.[27] In a large retrospective trial of 189 glioma patients, those with an rCBV of greater than 1.75 were found to have a shorter time to progression compared with those with an rCBV of less than or equal to 1.75.[28]

Changes in rCBV during the course of RT may be predictive of overall outcome in gliomas. Data from University of Michigan have indicated that patients with fractional tumor volume with high rCBV before RT had poor outcomes.[29] More interestingly, changes in rCBV in the first 3 weeks of RT were predictive of overall survival. Those patients who showed a continued reduction in the fractional volume of high rCBV from beginning of therapy to 1 week and then 3 weeks into RT had the best survival. Such data suggest that selective dose escalation to areas of high rCBV may have an impact on survival in gliomas.

Diffusion tensor imaging (DTI) and diffusion weighted imaging (DWI) have also demonstrated potentials for identifying tumor boundary and predicting treatment responses. Diffusion metrics are clearly altered within the vasogenic edema surrounding both high-grade gliomas and metastatic tumors,[30] and enable the differentiation of solitary intraaxial metastatic brain tumors and meningiomas from gliomas.[31,32] The functional diffusion maps have also been found to predict patient response as early as 3 weeks from the start of treatment.[33]

A major limitation of cerebral blood volume measurement and perfusion/diffusion imaging in brain tumors is the degree of inhomogeneity across the tumor as well as the intrinsic background perfusion in gray and white matter of the brain, respectively.[34] However, a combined parametric image of rCBV and perfusion imaging may be able to better define the tumor for RT target definition.

Positron Emission Tomography

Positron emission tomography imaging has emerged as valuable diagnostic tool to detect the metabolic rate and cellular proliferation in the field of oncology. In brain tumors, the most commonly used agent, ^{18}F-fluorodeoxyglucose (^{18}F-FDG) is not efficient because of the high glucose metabolism of the gray matter of the brain for the purpose of target delineation. However, newer tracers including ^{11}C-methionine (MET), ^{18}F-fluorothymidine (FLT), and ^{18}F-fluoro L-DOPA have shown the ability to provide the delineation between the tumor and the surrounding normal brain using PET imaging. Two studies have shown the accuracy of MET–PET in relation to stereotactic biopsy in gliomas. In one, seven out of 10 patients with increased MET–PET uptake corresponded with histopathological diagnosis of glioma following planned stereotactic biopsy.[35] In another series of 30 patients using a SUV threshold of 1.3, a sensitivity of 87% and a specificity of 89% were found with MET–PET.[36] In both, false-negative results were found mainly in the solid and not the necrotic region of the tumor. FLT–PET has

shown the ability to provide an early imaging biomarker response to therapy in recurrent glioma.[37] A 25% or more reduction in FLT uptake following Bevacizumab therapy in recurrent glioma correlated best with improved overall survival. In addition, changes in uptake within 1 to 2 weeks of therapy stood out as an independent predictor of survival.

Such data make a compelling argument for including PET imaging in RT treatment planning. In a prospective trial using MET–PET, those patients who underwent treatment planning using PET information had an improved survival compared with those where planning was done using CT–MRI alone (9 vs 5 months) in recurrent high-grade glioma.[38] Similarly, the role of MET–PET in defining the target in RT treatment planning in low-grade glioma has been studied.[39] The tumor area was clearly discernible on the baseline PET in 12 of 14 patients. In RT planning, MET–PET was helpful in outlining the gross tumor volume in three of 11 cases (27%), whereas PET findings either coincided with MR (46%) or were less distinctive (27%) in other cases. In quantitative evaluation, patients with a low tumor standardized uptake value (SUV) had significantly better prognosis than those with a high SUV. At the University of Michigan, researchers examined the potential utility of PET to identify the target volume at the highest risk of local failure.[4] They assessed whether the area of increased MET–PET activity was fully encompassed within the high-dose region and compared the patterns of failure for those with versus those without adequate high-dose coverage of the PET GTV in 19 patients with glioma. Among the 14 patients with adequately covered PET GTV, only two had noncentral failures. In another study using ^{18}F L-DOPA for treatment planning, the PTV had to be enlarged by greater than 20% in 25 patients where initial planning was done using CT–MR alone.[40] These studies indicate that a strategy of incorporating PET into RT treatment planning is practical especially for identifying areas for conformal boost therapy.

The main limitation of ^{11}C-MET–PET is the short half-life of the agent, which is approximately 20 minutes. However, FLT, which has a much longer half-life, can offset this problem. But the issue of spatial resolution with PET imaging as well as using clear cutoff values for SUV definition for RT treatment planning still needs to be clarified.

Functional Imaging

Functional MR (fMR) is gaining potential in clinical application recently as it can image the eloquent cortices that are difficult to identify on anatomical MR. Based on the blood oxygen level–dependent (BOLD) mechanism during brain function activation,[41,42] fMR uses paramagnetic deoxyhemoglobin in venous blood as a naturally occurring contrast agent for MR. BOLD fMR usually uses a gradient-echo EPI sequence to define the locations of functionally eloquent cortices. During fMR scans, patients are asked to perform certain tasks (e.g., motor paradigm, language paradigm, etc.) repeatedly to activate the eloquent cortex (e.g., the motor cortex, Broca's area, Wernicke's area, and the visual cortex) that is being studied. Mapping of such critical areas along with tracking of the corticospinal tract using diffusion MR tractography has helped in surgical resection of deep-seated brain tumors including craniopharyngioma and skull base meningioma.[43]

Activation maps from fMR have been retrospectively integrated into treatment planning to guide stereotactic radiosurgery (SRS)[44,45] (see Chapter 15C) and fractionated glioma IMRT[46] planning. The integration of cortical activation information into SRS treatment planning has provided an alternative to prevent or minimize radiation damage to the eloquent cortex. In a pilot study, three brain metastases patients were studied using this method with motor and/or visual paradigms.[44] The activation maps were subsequently transferred to a treatment planning workstation for SRS planning based on both functional and structural information. With a peripheral prescription dose of 16 Gy, the mean doses with and without fMR information to the eloquent cortices were 1.6 Gy and 2.4 Gy respectively, indicating a 32% dose reduction. In another pilot trial, the feasibility of incorporating fMR information for IMRT treatment planning of brain tumors was demonstrated in three glioma patients.[46] The fMR was acquired using a bilateral finger-tapping paradigm with a gradient-echo EPI sequence. The fMR data were processed using the Analysis of Functional Neuroimaging (AFNI) software package (NIMH, Bethesda, MD) for determining activation volumes, and the volumes were fused with the simulation computed tomography (CT) scans. The activated pixels in left and right primary motor cortexes (PMCs) were contoured as critical structures for IMRT planning. The mean dose to the contralateral PMC was reduced by 66%, 73%, and 69%, respectively, in these three patients indicating that IMRT optimization can reduce the dose to the PMC regions without compromising the PTV coverage or the sparing of other critical organs.

The limitations in fMR acquisition include the difficulty in obtaining cooperative patients, lack of reproducibility, and the difficulty of performing the defined paradigms on a consistent basis. The negative consequences of incorporating fMR information include a possible higher integral dose, higher dose to critical organs, and slightly increased hot spots.[46] However, these issues may be alleviated during planning by adding an avoidance structure consisting of brain tissue outside the PTV into the optimization.

Image Registration and Treatment Planning

All image registration methods require common anatomical information in different image sets and demand extensive computing power. Coregistered CT and MR scans using mutual information have been widely used for brain RT, resulting in more accurate target definition and better normal tissue sparing. However, the requirement for common anatomical features poses serious problems for incorporating information from functional imaging such as PET, MRS, or fMR into the treatment planning system. Most external markers or anatomical landmarks cannot be easily identified on functional imaging. Incomplete anatomical information in functional images also hinders the accuracy of surface matching or intensity matching with anatomical CT or MR images.

One successful approach for registering a functional image set with an anatomical image data set uses a reference anatomical image set acquired at the same scanning position as the functional image set. The reference scan can be registered with the simulation CT scan by using the conventional registration methods (e.g., mutual information). The transformation matrix between the reference scan and the simulation CT can then be directly applied to the functional scan because the reference scan and the functional scan are intrinsically registered. For example, CT has been successfully used as the reference in a PET–CT unit to transfer PET information to other imaging modalities.[47]

A similar approach has been adopted for registering MRS with treatment planning CT using reference MR images acquired in the same scanning position. Graves et al.[48] used an automatic registration scheme for incorporating the Cho-to-NAA index into glioma treatment planning. In this approach, multiple MR scans were acquired for each patient and were automatically aligned to the spoiled gradient recalled (SPGR) MR images acquired immediately before the MRS data. The SPGR MR images were then registered to the simulation CT images. Chang et al.,[22] on the other hand, developed a registration protocol that successfully overlaid the Cho-to-Cr ratio on top of the FLAIR MR in DICOM format and imported the registered images set into the treatment planning system for glioma IMRT. In the 12 cases reported in that study, the average positional difference was 0.29 mm with a standard deviation of 0.07 mm. Similar registration can also be used to incorporate fMR into the treatment planning process.[46]

Figure 15-1 illustrates the overlay of an MRS image set on top of a FLAIR image of a right frontal glioma using the coregistration method developed by Chang et al.[22] The FLAIR MR (Figure 15-1a) and MRS image (Figure 15-1b) were acquired at the same imaging position. Text files containing the interpolated Cho-to-Cr ratios for each MRS imaging voxel were generated using the GE FuncTool software (GE Medical Systems, Waukesha, WI). A new set of MRS images was then generated using the Cho-to-Cr grades to replace the image intensity of voxels inside the MRS acquisition box on the FLAIR images (Figure 15-1c),

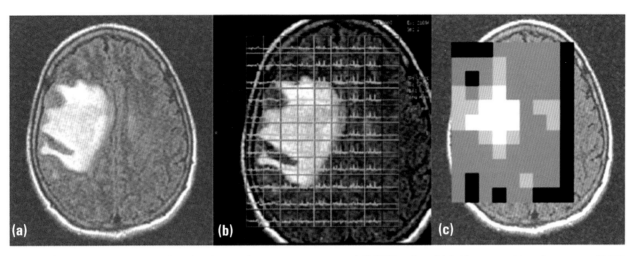

FIGURE 15-1. Illustration of the coregistration of magnetic resonance spectroscopic (MRS) imaging with fluid-attenuated inversion recovery (FLAIR) magnetic resonance (MR) imaging. **(a)** FLAIR image, **(b)** MRS image, **(c)** coregistered image. Reproduced with permission from Narayana A et al.[21]

with higher image intensity indicating higher Cho-to-Cr ratio, and more aggressive tumors. The resulting images can then be imported into the treatment planning system and fused with simulation CT for treatment planning purposes.

Once the treatment target and critical normal organs are delineated from anatomic and functional imaging, treatment planning can be performed. Because more critical organs may be identified from functional imaging, beam placement becomes critical to satisfy multiple planning constraints. In addition, if IMRT is used, the inverse planning may take longer as it will require more time to find the optimal beam modulation to satisfy the additional constraints.

Treatment planning may be further complicated if IGRT is used to set up the patient. Depending on the IGRT techniques, additional information needs to be generated by the treatment planning system for IGRT setup. This information may include the planning CT itself, digitally reconstructed radiographs (DRRs), or the relative position of implanted or external fiducial markers to the treatment isocenter. Most modern treatment planning systems have DICOM–RT export capability, allowing the export of the planning CT and/or DRR with contours of the planning target volume and critical organs. Export of fiducial marker positions is not standardized yet and usually requires vendor-specific software to transfer data from the treatment planning system to the monitoring device.

Image-Guided Treatment Delivery

Radiation therapy of primary and secondary brain tumors usually involves whole brain irradiation, partial brain RT, single-fraction SRS, and fractionated stereotactic RT (SRT). Generous margins (5 mm or higher) are generally adopted for conventional RT setup and

immobilization using thermoplastic masks. For SRS and SRT, specialized immobilization and setup devices, i.e., frame-based systems, are used to meet the more stringent criterion for treatment accuracy. Image-guided RT has recently gained popularity for conventional brain RT as well as brain SRS or SRT because of its superior treatment accuracy, or comparable treatment accuracy but with improved patient comfort. Unlike the mask- or frame-based system that is both an immobilization and a setup device, an IGRT system uses an imaging device for setup and a separate immobilization device for patient restriction.

Immobilization Devices

Both a thermoplastic mask and frame can be used in IGRT as an immobilization device. The thermoplastic mask has traditionally been used for setup and immobilization of brain and head/neck patients and the setup accuracy is on the order of 5 mm. Invasive frames (e.g., Brown-Roberts-Wells (BRW) frame[49,50]) have been used for SRS because of their very high (submillimeter) setup accuracy and excellent immobilization capability; however, these cause significant discomfort to the patient. Relocatable frames (e.g., Gill-Thomas-Cosman (GTC) frame[51,52]) cause less discomfort but have decreased accuracy (1 mm to 2 mm) and are less sturdy. Combining a good imaging device with an appropriate immobilization device, IGRT can potentially achieve accuracy closer to SRS but is less invasive.

Setup Imaging Devices

Various IGRT technologies have been developed for improving the setup accuracy of conventional brain RT. For example, stereotactic two-dimensional (2D) x-ray projection images such as On-Board Imaging (Varian Medical Systems, Palo Alto, CA) or the Novalis system (BrainLab, Feldkirchen, Germany) have been used with conventional

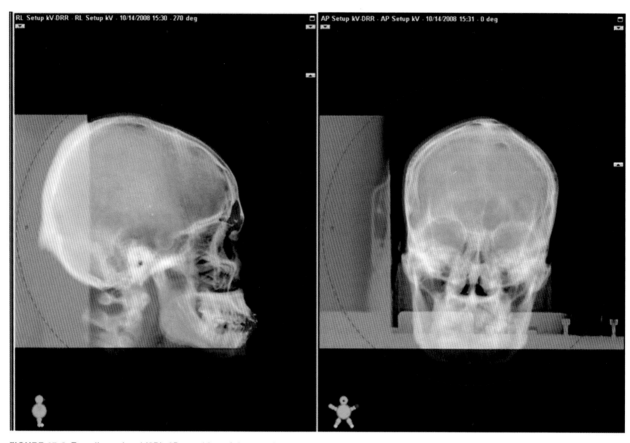

FIGURE 15-2. Two-dimensional (2D)–2D matching of the anterior–posterior and lateral kV images of a head; match verification using color blend. (Image courtesy of Varian Medical Systems of Palo Alto, CA. Copyright 2010, Varian Medical Systems. All rights reserved.)

thermoplastic masks for partial brain setup. For this IGRT technique, therapists visually compare the skull and other bony anatomies on the 2D projection images acquired during the treatment with that on the DRR generated from treatment planning, and adjust patient positions accordingly. Most of the adjustments are translational shifts although a rotational correction is possible (but less reliable). Figure 15-2 illustrates a 2D–2D matching example that uses the anterior–posterior and lateral kilovoltage (kV) head images to set up a patient using color blend match verification. Image-guided RT using 2D–2D matching can usually reduce the PTV margin to 3 mm.[53,54] This accuracy is superior to the 5-mm PTV margin that is usually adopted for conventional setup using the thermoplastic mask, and is comparable to the 3-mm PTV margin used for GTC frame for SRT.

More advanced 2D–2D, for example, CyberKnife (Accuray Inc, Sunnyvale, CA) or 3D–3D cone beam CT (CBCT) and Tomotherapy (Tomotherapy Inc, Madison, WI) or fiducial-based (e.g., infrared or implanted markers) IGRT systems have also been developed to compete with the frame-based system for SRS.

Real-time infrared tracking systems[55] have been used for frameless SRS/SRT for patient setup and monitoring

since 1995.[56,57] This approach uses multiple infrared emitters attached to a bite block, which was tracked by a stereo camera system mounted to the ceiling of the treatment room. Figure 15-3 shows the infrared bite plate used for a frameless SRS system and illustrates the attachment of the plate to a patient. The infrared light-emitting diodes on the bite block are tracked by a camera and the deviation of the patient from the isocenter position is calculated and displayed in real time. This technology can track the patient's position in six degrees (three translations and three rotations) of freedom after complex moves including table rotations and translations, and during treatment delivery.[57]

The CyberKnife system,[58] on the other hand, uses a pair of diagnostic x-ray fluoroscopes to image the patient periodically during treatment delivery. The system automatically registers the anatomy (skull) or implanted fiducial markers on the acquired radiographs with that on the DRRs derived from the treatment planning CT study (see Chapter 15D). The six-degree-of-freedom corrections are then calculated and used to align the beam of a 6-MV linac mounted on a robotic arm with the treatment target in real-time. Like the infrared tracking systems, stereoscopic x-ray imaging can be used for both patient setup

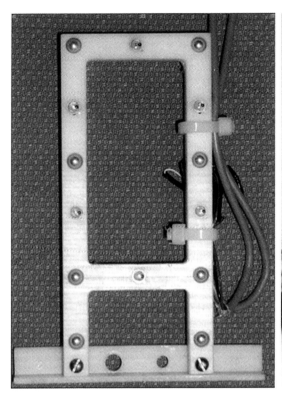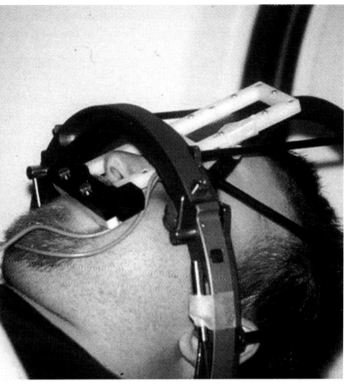

FIGURE 15-3. The infrared bite plate used for frameless SRS (left). The combination bite plate has aluminum fiducial markers for localization in the computed tomography (CT) scan and infrared light-emitting diodes for optical tracking in the treatment vault. Attachment of the plate to a patient (right). An invasive frame was also attached to the patient for comparison purposes. Reproduced with permission from Meeks SL et al.[57]

and monitoring. Similar stereoscopic x-ray imaging has been used to guide conventional linac-based irradiation. For example, the Novalis system[59] is equipped with both stereotactic x-ray imaging device and real-time infrared tracking; both can be used for IGRT setup and monitoring (see Chapter 15E).

Onboard MVCT[60] and kV/MV CBCT[61–64] systems use 3D–3D registration of the patient anatomies in the treatment and simulation positions for patient setup. This IGRT strategy provides the most accurate information for patient setup as the treatment targets are directly imaged and compared with the simulation CT in 3D. Studies have shown that CBCT of the brain does not present any significant geometric distortions and can be accurately coregistered with simulation CT scan.[65] Figure 15-4 illustrates one slice of the simulation CT and CBCT scan of a patient undergoing brain RT after coregistration. Coregistration of simulation CT and CBCT scans allows transfer and display of the isodose line from the treatment plan on the CBCT images so that dosimetric coverage can be evaluated in the treatment position. Although the CT number of CBCT is not sufficiently accurate for heterogeneity corrections, simulation and treatment planning using the CBCT scan has been proposed for SRS that does not require such correction.[65]

Apparatus Accuracy

A metric for evaluating the accuracy of a setup device is the "apparatus accuracy," the ability of a setup device to position a selected point at the center of the radiation beam. The apparatus accuracy is ~0.5 mm for the invasive frame[66] and ~1 mm for the relocatable GTC frame.[51,52] The 1-mm apparatus accuracy is easily achievable for most IGRT technologies, including kV CBCT, MV CBCT, MVCT, and fiducial marker tracking. However, it is questionable whether an IGRT system can achieve similar (0.5 mm) apparatus accuracy as the invasive frame system because image-guided setup relies on 2D–3D image fusion and a consistent study of image fusion for SRS remains to be published in clinical situations.[67]

The most important factor for determining the image coregistration accuracy is the slice thickness of simulation CT.[68] Because of the finite resolution and slice thickness, the position of an object shown on a brain CT–MR image can only be accurate within a half-pixel size or slice thickness. Because the slice thickness (e.g., 1 mm to 2 mm) is generally larger than the in-plane resolution (e.g., 0.7 mm), the localization accuracy is usually on the order of a half-slice thickness. Murphy and colleagues reported that the positional accuracy of the skull for frameless SRS using the stereotatic x-ray fluoroscopes of the CyberKnife

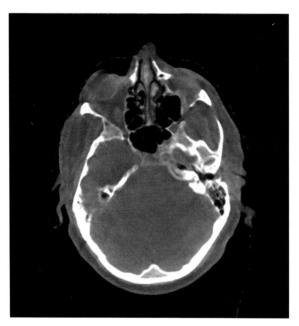 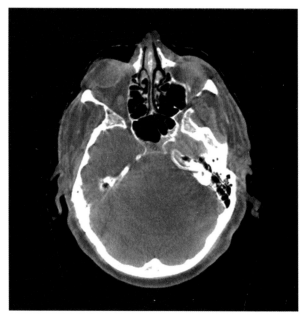

FIGURE 15-4. One slice of the coregistered (left) simulation computed tomography (CT) scan and (right) cone-beam CT scan of a patient undergoing brain radiotherapy.

system improved by a factor of 2 (mean radial error from 1.2 mm to 0.6 mm) when the CT slice thickness was reduced from 3.0 mm to 1.5 mm.[68] Similar amplification of localization error appears for optic-guided systems.[57] Because the most commonly used CT slice thickness is 1 mm to 2 mm for brain scan, the matching accuracy is expected to be greater than 0.5 mm unless a very thin CT slice (e.g., 0.625 mm) is used.

The uncertainty of the radiation isocenter is another source of apparatus error because the setup apparatus needs to be calibrated against the radiation isocenter before patient setup. For a conventional linac system, the calibration usually relies on the intersection of lasers, which has an uncertainly of ~0.5 mm. For the CyberKnife system, the linac on the robotic arm moves freely and has a pointing accuracy of ~0.7 mm.[69] Considering all these factors, it is very challenging for current IGRT systems to achieve accuracy significantly better than 1 mm until more precise systems are developed.

System Accuracy

System accuracy is the uncertainty of the whole setup and treatment process, including the uncertainty of the apparatus. For linac-based SRS, system accuracy can be estimated through an evaluation of the overall accuracy of planning, setup, and treatment process, as established by Lutz et al.[66] and Yeung et al.[70] The American Association of Physicists in Medicine (AAPM) Task Group 42 reports the overall achievable SRS treatment accuracy of 2.4 mm and 3.7 mm (one standard deviation of position uncertainty) using a stereotactic frame for target localization with CT images of 1 mm and 3 mm CT slice thick-

nesses, respectively.[71] Because the only difference between an IGRT system and a frame-based system is the setup apparatus, the system accuracy of an IGRT system should be slightly inferior to the frame-based system because of the slightly inferior apparatus accuracy.

However, this difference in system accuracy might not be clinically significant as the system accuracy is usually measured using a head (e.g., Rando head) phantom that does not account for some uncertainties from real patient setup. Figure 15-5 shows the overlay of a coregistered CBCT scan (amber) on CT scan (blue) for a framed-based SRS patient. Although the registration of skull anatomies of these two scans were reasonably good, the fiducial rods did not align as well (yellow arrows), indicating positional shift between the skull and CT localizer. Maciunas et al. studied the accuracy of stereotactic frames and concluded that, in addition to imaging uncertainty, clinically encountered levels of weight-bearing by stereotactic frames may have a pronounced effect on their mechanical accuracy.[72] Because the weight-bearing effect is not easy to detect with the current quality assurance procedure for frame-based SRS, a volumetric CBCT scan has been recommended even for invasive frame-based SRS.[73] The setup accuracy of IGRT, however, is not affected by this weight-bearing effect.

Intrafractional Motion

Once the patients are properly set up using image guidance, treatment delivery is essentially the same as conventional brain RT except that intrafractional motion needs to be monitored and corrected. If a monitoring device is not used, an additional margin should be used for the

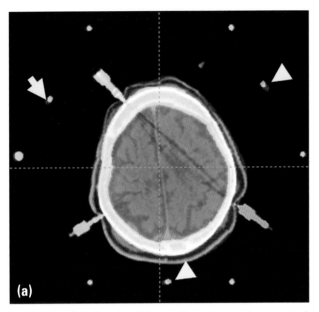 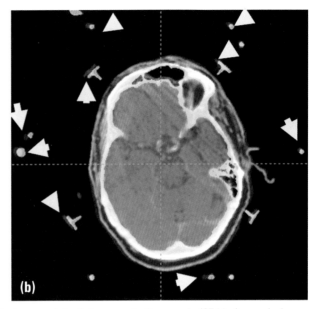

FIGURE 15-5. Coregistration of the cone-beam computed tomography (amber) scan and simulation computed tomography (CT; blue) scan of a frame-based stereotactic radiosurgery patient for **(a)** a slice close to isocenter and **(b)** a slice close to the Brown-Roberts-Wells frame. Yellow arrows point to the locations of the CT localizer that are significantly different on these two scans.

PTV expansion to account for intrafractional motion. However, this may defeat the purpose of image-guided setup, which is to achieve better setup accuracy than the mask-based system or similar setup accuracy as the frame-based system but with improved patient comfort and clinical flexibility.

Patient motion during the treatment is undesirable for fractionated treatment and is definitely unacceptable for SRS if it is greater than 1 mm. Significant motion during setup CT–CBCT scan also creates artifacts that adversely affect image-guided setup accuracy. Currently, the thermoplastic mask is the most commonly used immobilization device for IGRT because it is less rigid

and therefore more comfortable for the patients. Murphy et al.[74] studied the intrafractional motion for frameless SRS patients restrained using an AquaPlast mask (AquaPlast Corp, Wyckoff, NJ). Figure 15-6 shows a record of the position (in cm) over time of a cranial treatment site in this study. Significant intrafractional motions were observed in all three directions as the time of treatment increased. Overall, more than half the cases showed a systematic position shift in one or more directions that was at least 2.4 mm, indicating that it was inaccurate to assume that the patient maintained a consistent average position during the SRS treatment that lasted 30 to 45 minutes.[74]

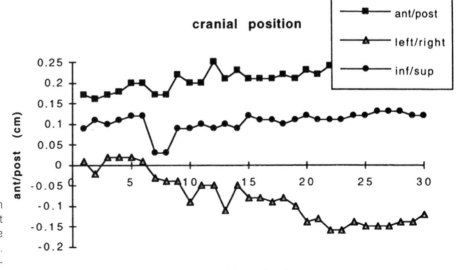

FIGURE 15-6. A record of the position (in cm) over time of a cranial treatment site. The position checks were made at approximately 1.5-minute intervals. Reproduced with permission from Murphy MJ et al.[74]

Based on these data, the intrafractional motion needs to be monitored and corrected. Most imaging devices used by IGRT systems for patient setup can also be used for tracking intrafractional motion. For example, real-time tracking can be performed using infrared systems[55,56] and stereotactic diagnostic x-ray fluoroscopes.[58,59] Monitoring intrafractional motion using an onboard kV or MV imager is also possible but not ideal because the motion can only be monitored in one direction. However, research studies are being pursued to interlace the MV beam and kV beam pulses so that both kV and MV imagers can be used during the treatment. A CT–CBCT–based IGRT system cannot be used to monitor the intrafractional motion because of the relative longer time required to perform the scan, and will rely on other add-on devices for this purpose.

Conclusions

The variations in tumor cell distribution and the tumor grade makes it difficult to define an effective, yet safe, margin for therapy using conventional CT–MR imaging alone in brain tumors. The assumption of a uniform margin will either encompass too much uninvolved brain or leave areas of tumor infiltration outside the treatment volume, both of which are unacceptable. New treatment algorithms incorporating spectroscopy, PET, and perfusion imaging for the management of brain tumors are being developed and need to be validated in the future. In addition, information from fMR will help establish the limiting doses for functionally critical structures. Because the goal of imaging-defined volume is tailored to tumor extension rather than uniformity, it is hoped that such an approach would improve both the quality of survival and local control. Furthermore, these imaging modalities can be utilized to triage patients who are more likely to benefit from adjuvant chemotherapy following surgery and radiation therapy. They can also be used as a prognostic biomarker for response to radiation therapy. Such an approach will help to customize the care of an individual patient and may aid in identifying patients who may benefit from further targeted treatment intensification.

Image-guided RT has replaced the mask-based system in many clinics for fractionated radiotherapy of brain tumors because of its higher accuracy and ability to monitor intrafractional motion. However, the advantages of image-guided SRS over the frame-based SRS are still being debated. Because frame-based SRS already has achieved excellent setup accuracy and local control, the major improvements of IGRT over the frame-based approach are primarily patient comfort and increased flexibility. Image-guided RT is generally more flexible but demands multiple imaging or computation devices, involves complex networking, and requires monitoring of intrafractional movement. In contrast, the invasive frame system is simple, reliable, and efficient. Therefore, the frame-based approach will remain a viable option for intracranial SRS in the near future even though image-guided frameless SRS has gained significant popularity in the past few years.

References

1. Narayana A, Leibel SA. "Primary and Metastatic Brain Tumors in Adults." *Textbook of Radiation Oncology.* Leibel SA, Phillips TL, eds. Philadelphia, PA: Saunders; 2002.
2. Bleehen NM, Stenning SP. A Medical Research Council trial of two radiotherapy doses in the treatment of grades 3 and 4 astrocytoma. The Medical Research Council Brain Tumour Working Party. *Br J Cancer.* 1991;64:769–774.
3. Nelson DF, Diener-West M, Horton J, et al. Combined modality approach to treatment of malignant gliomas—re-evaluation of RTOG 7401/ECOG 1374 with long-term follow-up: a joint study of the Radiation Therapy Oncology Group and the Eastern Cooperative Oncology Group. *NCI Monogr.* 1988;6:279–284.
4. Lee SW, Fraass BA, Marsh LH, et al. Patterns of failure following high-dose 3-D conformal radiotherapy for high-grade astrocytomas: a quantitative dosimetric study. *Int J Radiat Oncol Biol Phys.* 1999;43:79–88.
5. Roman DD, Sperduto PW. Neuropsychological effects of cranial radiation: current knowledge and future directions. *Int J Radiat Oncol Biol Phys.* 1995;31:983–998.
6. Pirzkall A, McKnight TR, Graves EE, et al. MR-spectroscopy guided target delineation for high-grade gliomas. *Int J Radiat Oncol Biol Phys.* 2001;50:915–928.
7. Hunt MA, Zelefsky MJ, Wolden S, et al. Treatment planning and delivery of intensity-modulated radiation therapy for primary nasopharynx cancer. *Int J Radiat Oncol Biol Phys.* 2001;49:623–632.
8. Huang E, Teh BS, Strother DR, et al. Intensity-modulated radiation therapy for pediatric medulloblastoma: early report on the reduction of ototoxicity. *Int J Radiat Oncol Biol Phys.* 2002;52:599–605.
9. Narayana A, Yamada J, Berry S, et al. Intensity-modulated radiotherapy in high-grade gliomas: clinical and dosimetric results. *Int J Radiat Oncol Biol Phys.* 2006;64:892–897.
10. Shaw EG, Stieber V, Tatter S, et al. A phase I dose escalating study of intensity modulated radiation therapy (IMRT) for the treatment of glioblastoma multiforme (GBM). *Int J Radiat Oncol Biol Phys.* 2002;54(2 suppl):206–207.
11. Butler JM, Rapp SR, Shaw EG. Managing the cognitive effects of brain tumor radiation therapy. *Curr Treat Options Oncol.* 2006;7:517–523.
12. Laack NN, Brown PD. Cognitive sequelae of brain radiation in adults. *Sem Oncol.* 2004;31:702–713.
13. Henson JW, Gaviani P, Gonzalez RG. MRI in treatment of adult gliomas. *Lancet Oncol.* 2005;6:167–175.
14. Thornton AF Jr, Sandler HM, Ten Haken RK, et al. The clinical utility of magnetic resonance imaging in 3-dimensional treatment planning of brain neoplasms. *Int J Radiat Oncol Biol Phys.* 1992;24:767–775.
15. Wallner KE. Radiation treatment planning for malignant astrocytomas. *Sem Radiat Oncol.* 1991;1:17–22.

16. Byrne TN. Imaging of gliomas. *Semin Oncol.* 1994;21:162–171.

17. Earnest FT, Kelly PJ, Scheithauer BW, et al. Cerebral astrocytomas: histopathologic correlation of MR and CT contrast enhancement with stereotactic biopsy. *Radiology.* 1988;166:823–827.

18. Moonen CT, von Kienlin M, van Zijl PC, et al. Comparison of single-shot localization methods (STEAM and PRESS) for in vivo proton NMR spectroscopy. *NMR Biomed.* 1989;2:201–208.

19. Duijn JH, Matson GB, Maudsley AA, et al. 3D phase encoding 1H spectroscopic imaging of human brain. *Magn Reson Imaging.* 1992;10:315–319.

20. De Stefano N, Caramanos Z, Preul MC, et al. In vivo differentiation of astrocytic brain tumors and isolated demyelinating lesions of the type seen in multiple sclerosis using 1H magnetic resonance spectroscopic imaging. *Ann Neurol.* 1998;44:273–278.

21. Narayana A, Chang J, Thakur S, et al. Use of MR spectroscopy and functional imaging in the treatment planning of gliomas. *Br J Radiol.* 2007;80:347–354.

22. Chang J, Thakur S, Perera G, et al. Image-fusion of MR spectroscopic images for treatment planning of gliomas. *Med Phys.* 2006;33:32–40.

23. Pirzkall A, Nelson SJ, McKnight TR, et al. Metabolic imaging of low-grade gliomas with three-dimensional magnetic resonance spectroscopy. *Int J Radiat Oncol Biol Phys.* 2002;53:1254–1264.

24. Cha S, Knopp EA, Johnson G, et al. Intracranial mass lesions: dynamic contrast-enhanced susceptibility-weighted echo-planar perfusion MR imaging. *Radiology.* 2002;223:11–29.

25. Lev MH, Ozsunar Y, Henson JW, et al. Glial tumor grading and outcome prediction using dynamic spin-echo MR susceptibility mapping compared with conventional contrast-enhanced MR: confounding effect of elevated rCBV of oligodendrogliomas. *AJNR Am J Neuroradiol.* 2004;25:214–221.

26. Shin JH, Lee HK, Kwun BD, et al. Using relative cerebral blood flow and volume to evaluate the histopathologic grade of cerebral gliomas: preliminary results. *Am J Roentgenol.* 2002;179:783–789.

27. Knopp EA, Cha S, Johnson G, et al. Glial neoplasms: dynamic contrast-enhanced T2*-weighted MR imaging. *Radiology.* 1999;211:791–798.

28. Law M, Young RJ, Babb JS, et al. Gliomas: predicting time to progression or survival with cerebral blood volume measurements at dynamic susceptibility-weighted contrast-enhanced perfusion MR imaging. *Radiology.* 2008;247:490–498.

29. Cao Y, Nagesh V, Hamstra D, et al. The extent and severity of vascular leakage as evidence of tumor aggressiveness in high-grade gliomas. *Cancer Res.* 2006;66:8912–8917.

30. Lu S, Ahn D, Johnson G, et al. Peritumoral diffusion tensor imaging of high-grade gliomas and metastatic brain tumors. *AJNR Am J Neuroradiol.* 2003;24:937–941.

31. Lu S, Ahn D, Johnson G, et al. Diffusion-tensor MR imaging of intracranial neoplasia and associated peritumoral edema: introduction of the tumor infiltration index. *Radiology.* 2004;232:221–228.

32. Provenzale JM, McGraw P, Mhatre P, et al. Peritumoral brain regions in gliomas and meningiomas: investigation with isotropic diffusion-weighted MR imaging and diffusion-tensor MR imaging. *Radiology.* 2004;232:451–460.

33. Moffat BA, Chenevert TL, Lawrence TS, et al. Functional diffusion map: a noninvasive MRI biomarker for early stratification of clinical brain tumor response. *Proc Natl Acad Sci U S A.* 2005;102:5524–5529.

34. Tsien CI, Cao Y, Lawrence TS. Functional and metabolic magnetic resonance imaging and positron emission tomography for tumor volume definition in high-grade gliomas. *Sem Radiat Oncol.* 2009;19:155–162.

35. Mosskin M, Ericson K, Hindmarsh T, et al. Positron emission tomography compared with magnetic resonance imaging and computed tomography in supratentorial gliomas using multiple stereotactic biopsies as reference. *Acta Radiol.* 1989;30:225–232.

36. Kracht LW Miletic H, Busch S, et al. Delineation of brain tumor extent with [11C]L-methionine positron emission tomography: local comparison with stereotactic histopathology. *Clin Cancer Res.* 2004;10:7163–7170.

37. Chen W, Delaloye S, Silverman DHS, et al. Predicting treatment response of malignant gliomas to bevacizumab and irinotecan by imaging proliferation with [18F] fluorothymidine positron emission tomography: a pilot study. *J Clin Oncol.* 2007;25:4714–4721.

38. Grosu A-L, Weber WA, Riedel E, et al. L-(methyl-11C) methionine positron emission tomography for target delineation in resected high-grade gliomas before radiotherapy. *Int J Radiat Oncol Biol Phys.* 2005;63:64–74.

39. Nuutinen J, Sonninen P, Lehikoinen P, et al. Radiotherapy treatment planning and long-term follow-up with [11C]methionine PET in patients with low-grade astrocytoma. *Int J Radiat Oncol Biol Phys.* 2000;48:43–52.

40. Alheit H, Oehme L, Winkler C, et al. Radiation treatment planning in brain tumours: potential impact of 3-O-methyl-6-[(18)F]fluoro-L-DOPA and PET. *Nuklearmedizin.* 2008;47:200–204.

41. Ogawa S, Lee TM, Kay AR, et al. Brain magnetic resonance imaging with contrast dependent on blood oxygenation. *Proc Natl Acad Sci U S A.* 1990;87:9868–9872.

42. Norris DG. Principles of magnetic resonance assessment of brain function. *J Magn Reson Imaging.* 2006;23:794–807.

43. Holodny AI, Schwartz TH, Ollenschleger M, et al. Tumor involvement of the corticospinal tract: diffusion magnetic resonance tractography with intraoperative correlation. *J Neurosurg.* 2001;95:1082–1082.

44. Liu WC, Narra SM, Kalnin V, et al. Functional magnetic resonance imaging aided radiation treatment planning. *Med Phys.* 2000;27:1563–1572.

45. Aoyama H, Kamada K, Shirato H, et al. Integration of functional brain information into stereotactic irradiation treatment planning using magnetoencephalopathy and magnetic resonance axonography. *Int J Radiat Oncol Biol Phys.* 2004;58:1177–1183.

46. Chang J, Kowalski A, Hou B, et al. Feasibility study of intensity-modulated radiotherapy (IMRT) treatment planning using brain functional MRI. *Med Dosim.* 2008;33:42–47.

47. Beyer T, Townsend DW, Brun T, et al. A combined PET/CT scanner for clinical oncology. *J Nucl Med.* 2000;41:1369–1379.

48. Graves EE, Pirzkall A, Nelson SJ, et al. Registration of magnetic resonance spectroscopic imaging to computed tomography for radiotherapy treatment planning. *Med Phys.* 2001;28:2489–2496.

49. Brown RA, Roberts T, Osborn AG. Simplified CT-guided stereotaxic biopsy. *Am J Neuroradiology.* 1981;2:181–184.
50. Brown RA, Roberts TS, Osborn AG. Stereotaxic frame and computer software for CT-directed neurosurgical localization. *Investig Radiology.* 1980;15:308–312.
51. Gill SS, Thomas DGT, Warrington AP, et al. Relocatable frame for stereotactic external beam radiotherapy. *Int J Radiat Oncol Biol Phys.* 1991;20:599–603.
52. Kooy HM, Dunbar SF, Tarbell NJ, et al. Adaptation and verification of the relocatable Gill-Thomas-Cosman frame in stereotactic radiotherapy. *Int J Radiat Oncol Biol Phys.* 1994;30:685–691.
53. Kuo L, Mechalakos J, Hunt M, et al. Setup accuracy of a thermoplastic mask system using two-dimensional (2D) on-board imager (OBI) for fractionated stereotactic radiotherapy (FSRT). *Med Phys.* 2008;35(6):2825.
54. Chang J, O'Meara W, Mechalakos J, et al. A feasibility study of image-guided non-invasive single-fraction stereotactic radiosurgery using the 2D2D match of an on-board imaging system. *Med Phys.* 2007;34:2375.
55. Meeks SL, Tome WA, Willoughby TR, et al. Optically guided patient positioning techniques. *Semin Radiat Oncol.* 2005;15:192–201.
56. Bova FJ, Buatti JM, Friedman WA, et al. The University of Florida frameless high-precision stereotactic radiotherapy system. *Int J Radiat Oncol Biol Phys.* 1997;38:875–882.
57. Meeks SL, Bova FJ, Wagner TH, et al. Image localization for frameless stereotactic radiotherapy. *Int J Radiat Oncol Biol Phys.* 2000;46:1291–1299.
58. Adler JR Jr, Murphy MJ, Chang SD, et al. Image-guided robotic radiosurgery. *Neurosurgery.* 1999;44:1299–1307.
59. Verellen D, Soete G, Linthout N, et al. Quality assurance of a system for improved target localization and patient set-up that combines real-time infrared tracking and stereoscopic x-ray imaging. *Radioter Oncol.* 2003;67:129–141.
60. Mackie TR, Kapatoes J, Ruchali K, et al. Image guidance for precise conformal radiotherapy. *Int J Radiat Oncol Biol Phys.* 2003;56:89–105.
61. Jaffray DA, Siewerdsen JH, Wong JW, et al. Flat-panel cone-beam computed tomography for image-guided radiation therapy. *Int J Radiat Oncol Biol Phys.* 2002;53:1337–1349.
62. Sillanpaa J, Chang J, Mageras G, et al. Developments in megavoltage cone beam CT with an amorphous silicon EPID: reduction of exposure and synchronization with respiratory gating. *Med Phys.* 2005;32:819–829.
63. Pouliot J, Chen J, Aubin M, et al. Low-dose megavoltage cone-beam CT for radiation therapy. *Int J Radiat Oncol Biol Phys.* 2005;61:552–560.
64. Yoo S, Kim GY, Hammoud R, et al. A quality assurance program for the on-board imager. *Med Phys.* 2006;33:4431–4447.
65. Chang J, Yenice KM, Narayana A, et al. Accuracy and feasibility of cone-beam computed tomography for stereotactic radiosurgery setup. *Med Phys.* 2007;34:2077–2084.
66. Lutz W, Winston KR, Maleki N. A system for stereotactic radiosurgery with a linear accelerator. *Int J Radiat Oncol Biol Phys.* 1988;14:373–381.
67. Lightstone AW, Benedict SH, Bova FJ, et al. Intracranial stereotactic positioning systems: report of the American Association of Physicists in Medicine Radiation Therapy Committee Task Group No. 68. *Med Phys.* 2005;32:2380–2398.
68. Murphy MJ. The importance of computed tomography slice thickness in radiographic patient positioning for radiosurgery. *Med Phys.* 1999;26:171–175.
69. Murphy MJ, Chang S, Gibbs I, et al. Image-guided radiosurgery in the treatment of spinal metastases. *Neurosurgical Focus [electronic resource].* 2001;11.
70. Yeung D, Palta J, Fontanesi J, et al. Systematic analysis of errors in target localization and treatment delivery in stereotactic radiosurgery (SRS). *Int J Radiat Oncol Biol Phys.* 1994;28:493–498.
71. Schell MC, Bova FJ, Larson DA, et al. AAPM Report No. 54: Stereotactic Radiosurgery. Woodbury, NY: American Institute of Physics; 1995.
72. Maciunas RJ, Galloway RL Jr., Latimer JW, et al. The application accuracy of stereotactic frames. *Neurosurgery.* 1994;35:682–695.
73. Chang J, O'Meara W, Yamada Y, et al. Analysis of setup accuracy for invasive frame-based stereotactic radiosurgery (SRS) patients using cone beam computed tomography (CBCT). *Med Phys.* 2007;34:2418–2419.
74. Murphy MJ, Chang SD, Gibbs IC, et al. Patterns of patient movement during frameless image-guided radiosurgery. *Int J Radiat Oncol Biol Phys.* 2003;55(5):1400–1408.

^{68}Ga-DOTATOC-PET–Guided Target Delineation in a Patient with an Intracranial Meningioma

Case Study

Stefanie Milker-Zabel, MD, Angelika Zabel du Bois, MD

Patient History

A 40-year-old woman presented with a right sphenoid wing meningioma and was treated with a complete neurosurgical resection. One year later, she developed moderate right-sided exophthalmus, ptosis, and swelling of the temple. No reduction in visual acuity or visual field deficits was noted. Workup, including computed tomography (CT) and magnetic resonance (MR) imaging of the brain, demonstrated a lesion of the lateral right orbital bone (Figure 15A-1). Although it was an unusual finding, this intraosseous lesion was felt to be consistent with a recurrence of her prior meningioma.

Because of the tumor's location, surgical resection was not recommended. We thus elected to treat the patient by using intensity-modulated radiotherapy (IMRT) with curative intent. We used ^{68}Ga-DOTATOC-PET to guide target delineation in this patient.

Simulation

The patient was simulated in the supine position and immobilized with a customized wrap-around head mask fixation (Scotch Cast, 3M Corp, St Paul, MN) attached to a stereotactic frame. This frame consisted of four triangular plates containing metal wire for CT or gadolinium-filled pipes for MR imaging. The center of the frame represents the origin of the stereotactic coordinate system. This immobilization device is associated with a setup accuracy of better than 2 mm, particularly in tumors of the base of skull. A planning CT scan was performed with the patient immobilized in the treatment position on our department CT simulator (Somatom Sensation 64, Siemens AG, Erlangen, Germany) with 3-mm slices. Contrast was administered before the CT simulation.

Imaging and Target Delineation

Following the CT simulation, the patient underwent a contrast-enhanced 1.5 T MR scan of the brain (Symphonie, Siemens AG, Erlangen, Germany) performed under stereotactic guidance with the stereotactic localization system described previously. The following MR sequences were obtained: T1-weighted axial and coronal images with and without contrast, T2-weighted fat saturation (FAT-SAT) axial and coronal images, T2-weighted turbo-spin echo axial images, and T1-weighted FATSAT axial images.

To improve target delineation, the patient also underwent a ^{68}Ga-DOTATOC-positron-emission tomography (^{68}Ga-DOTATOC-PET) PET scan (Figure 15A-2). DOTATOC is the somatostatin analog DOTA (o)-D-Phe (1)-Tyr (3)-Octreotide developed based on modifications of octreotide, which is commercially available for somatostatin receptor scintigraphy.[1] Labelled with the positron-emitting radionuclide ^{68}Ga, ^{68}Ga-DOTATOC is an attractive PET tracer in patients with intracranial meningiomas, because of their high expression of the somatostatin-receptor subtype 2 (SSTR2). In contrast to ^{18}F-fluorodeoxyglucose, ^{68}Ga-DOTATOC has been shown to exhibit a very high meningioma-to-background ratio.[2] Furthermore, ^{68}Ga-DOTATOC has been shown to provide additional information regarding the extension

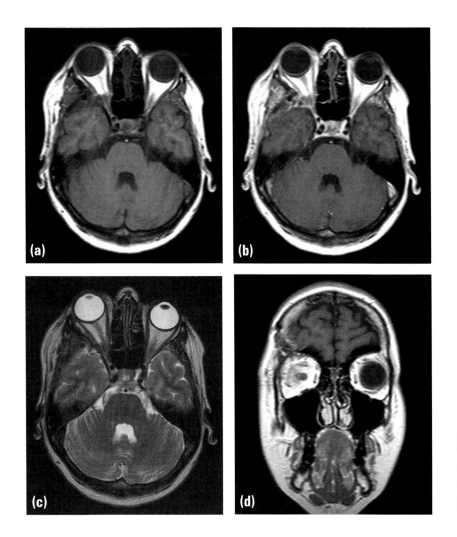

FIGURE 15A-1. Representative axial T1-weighted **(a)**, axial contrast-enhanced T1-weighted **(b)**, axial T2-weighted **(c)**, and coronal contrast-enhanced T1-weighted **(d)** magnetic resonance scans of the recurrent intraosseous meningioma located within the right orbital bone.

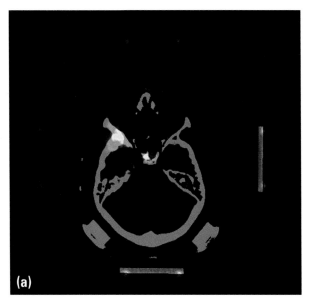
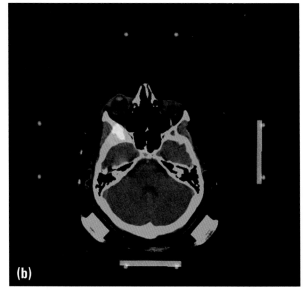

FIGURE 15A-2. Representative positron emission tomography (PET) **(a)** and PET–computed tomography **(b)** scan for treatment planning of the recurrent intraosseous meningioma. The pituitary gland also shows a high tracer uptake in the ⁶⁸Ga-DOTATOC PET image.

of meningiomas located at the skull base next to osseous structures.[2]

Dynamic PET scans were acquired over 60 minutes after intravenous injection of 155 MBq ^{68}Ga-DOTATOC. The PET studies were performed with an ECAT EXACT HR+ whole-body PET system (Siemens/CTI, Knoxville, TN) covering 155 mm in the axial field of view (63 transversal slices; 2.4 mm slice thickness). Data acquisition was performed in the three-dimensional (3D) mode without interslice tungsten septa. The matrix size was 128 × 128 pixels. Images were corrected for scatter and attenuation. Iterative image reconstruction used the ordered subsets–expectation maximization algorithm.

Treatment planning was performed on a 3D CT data cube generated from continuous 3-mm CT images. The MR data set was stereotactically fused to the CT. The PET images were imported into the 3D RT planning system, VOXELPLAN, developed at the German Cancer Research Center, Heidelberg.[3] Contours of the volumes of interest were performed by using the manual segmentation module, TOMAS, which is part of the planning system.

The clinical target volume (CTV) and organs at risk including the eyes, optic nerves, chiasm, and brain stem were delineated on each slice of the 3D data cube after image fusion. The CTV consisted of the contrast-enhanced lesion on T1-weighted MR, modified to include hyperostotic changes evident on CT. The planning target volume (PTV) was defined as macroscopic tumor visible on CT and T1-MR contrast-enhanced scans with a safety margin of 1 mm to 2 mm to the normal brain tissue, 5 mm to 10 mm to adjacent osseous structures optimized by the information from the PET scan. ^{68}Ga-DOTATEC showed very high meningioma-to-background ratios and, therefore, we confirmed the diagnosis of a rare intraosseous meningioma. Furthermore, we achieved additional information for target delineation concerning the extension of the meningioma. The CTV and surrounding critical normal tissues were defined on the image modality with best visualization and then transferred onto the CT cube for dose calculation by using the stereotactic localization technique within VOXELPLAN. The resulting PTV in this patient was 27.9 cc.

Treatment Planning

The IMRT treatment planning was performed with the inverse planning system KONRAD, developed at our institution. A total dose of 55.8 Gy was prescribed in a daily fractionation of 1.8 Gy delivered five times a week. Three-dimensional dose distributions were calculated by the module VIRTUOS within VOXELPLAN. Nine coplanar 6-MV beams with 69 sub-segments were defined because of the complexity of the target volume. The PTV was covered by the 95% isodose. Representative images illustrating the dose distribution for the optimized treatment plan are shown in Figure 15A-3. Mean doses of the right and left eyes were 18.3 Gy and 9.7 Gy, respectively (Figure 15A-4). Mean doses of the right and left lenses were 10.9 Gy and 4.0 Gy, respectively. Mean and maximum

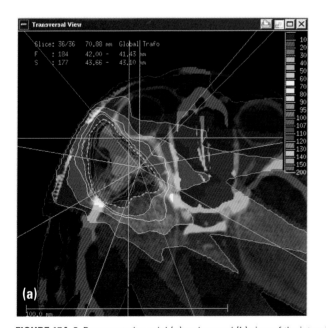
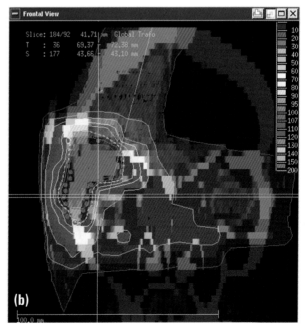

FIGURE 15A-3. Representative axial (a) and coronal (b) view of the intensity-modulated treatment plan with dose distribution used in this patient. The isodose lines are 100%, 95%, 90%, 80%, 70%, 50%, 30%, and 10%, respectively.

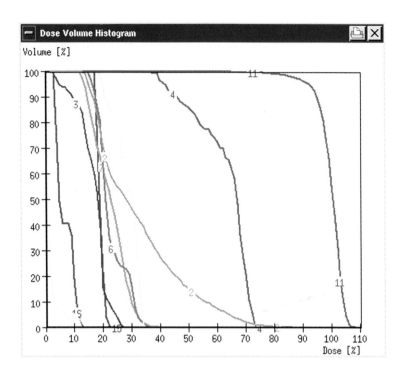

FIGURE 15A-4. Dose-volume-histogram (DVH) of the optimized intensity-modulated treatment plan: 2=right eye; 3=left eye; 4=right optic nerve; 5=left optic nerve; 6=chiasm; 7=brain stem; 8=spinal cord; 11=planning target volume; 15=right lens.

doses of the right optic nerve were 25.3 Gy and 41.6 Gy, of the left optic nerve were 16.3 Gy and 19.4 Gy, and for the chiasm were 12.9 Gy and 20.4 Gy, respectively. The IMRT treatments were delivered on a Mevatron linear accelerator (Siemens AG, Erlangen, Germany).

Clinical Outcome

The patient tolerated the treatment well without any significant acute side effects. Only mild erythema and transient alopecia were noted over the irradiation fields. At her latest follow-up 18 months after the completion of therapy, no evidence of disease progression has been noted on serial MR scans. Moreover, the patient remains free of any significant late sequelae referable to her treatment.

Our initial clinical experience of ^{68}Ga-DOTATOC-PET–guided target delineation in patients with intracranial meningiomas was published earlier.[4] Twenty-six patients underwent stereotactic CT, MR, and ^{68}Ga-DOTATOC-PET as part of their initial treatment planning. The PTV (PTV$_1$) outlined on CT and contrast MRI was compared with the PTV (PTV$_2$) delineated on PET. The PTV (PTV$_3$) defined with CT, MRI, and PET was actually used for treatment planning. The PTV$_3$ was smaller than PTV$_1$ in nine patients, the same size in seven patients, and

larger in 10 patients. Median PTV$_1$ and PTV$_3$ were 49.6 cc and 57.2 cc, respectively. In all patients, ^{68}Ga-DOTATOC-PET supplied additional information regarding tumor extension. Overall, PTV$_3$ was significantly modified based on Ga-DOTATEC-PET in 19 patients (73%). In one patient, no tumor was identified on CT and MR but was visible on PET.

References

1. Heppeler A, Froidevaux S, Macke HR, et al. Radiometal-labelled macrocyclic chelator-derivatised somatostatin analogue with superb tumour-targeting properties and potential for receptor-mediated internal radiotherapy. *Chem Eur J.* 1999;5(7):1974–1981.
2. Henze M, Schuhmacher J, Hipp P, et al. PET imaging of somatostatin receptors using [68Ga]-DOTA-D Phe^1-Tyr^3-Octreotide (DOTATOC): first results in patients with meningiomas. *J Nucl Med.* 2001;42(7):1053–1056.
3. Hoess A, Debus J, Bendl R, et al. Computerized procedures in 3-dimensional radiotherapy planning. *Radiologe.* 1995;35:583–586.
4. Milker-Zabel S, Zabel-du Bois A, Henze M, et al. Improved target volume definition for fractionated stereotactic radiotherapy in patients with intracranial meningiomas by correlation of CT, MRI and [68Ga]-DOTATOC-PET. *Int J Radiat Oncol Biol Phys.* 2006;65(1):222–227.

MR Spectroscopy-Guided Target Delineation in a Patient with a Recurrent Glioblastoma Multiforme

Case Study

Åse M. Ballangrud, PhD, Stella Lymberis, MD, Kathryn Beal, MD, Philip H. Gutin, MD, Jenghwa Chang, PhD

Patient History

A 30-year-old man presented 6.5 months following surgery and adjuvant chemoradiation for a left parietal glioblastoma multiforme (GBM) with evidence of progressive disease on follow-up imaging studies. On presentation, the patient was without neurologic deficits. His initial treatment consisted of a total radiation dose of 59.4 Gy in 1.8 Gy fractions with concurrent temozolomide chemotherapy.

The patient was enrolled in an institutional review board (IRB)–approved prospective clinical trial combining bevacizumab, a humanized monoclonal antibody to vascular endothelial growth factor, and hypofractionated intensity-modulated stereotactic radiotherapy for patients with recurrent glioma.[1] In this protocol, magnetic resonance (MR) images and magnetic resonance spectroscopy (MRS) images were acquired before and after the first cycle of bevacizumab. Voxels with enhanced metabolite activity were identified on MRS and used to help guide target delineation and treatment planning.

Simulation

The patient was immobilized with a Gill-Thomas-Cosman frame (Integra Radionics, Burlington, MA) in the supine position. Simulation was performed with a PQ-5000 CT-simulator (Philips Medical Systems, Andover, MA). Transaxial 2-mm images were obtained from the top of the head to the base of the skull following contrast administration. The MRS images were acquired on a 1.5-Tesla (T) Excite scanner (GE Healthcare, Waukesha, WI) by using a point-resolve spectroscopy sequence (PRESS) with TE/TR of 144/1000 milliseconds and a voxel size of $10 \text{ mm}^3 \times 10 \text{ mm}^3 \times 10 \text{ mm}^3$. The array of MRS spectra were processed with Functool software (GE Healthcare, Waukesha, WI) and overlaid on the Fluid Attenuated Inversion Recovery (FLAIR) MR images acquired successively with 2-mm spacing and no gap. Both the MR and MRS scans were acquired before the first cycle of bevacizumab and again a few days before the planning CT scan.

Imaging and Target Delineation

The MRS voxels with enhanced metabolic ratio of choline to N-acetylaspartate (Cho/NAA) and choline to creatine (Cho/Cr) were marked by an experienced radiologist on the screen-dumped MRS spectral images. These images were imported into the treatment planning system (BrainLAB, Feldkirchen, Germany) using the method outlined by Chang et al.,[2] and fused to the planning CT. Figure 15b-1A shows an axial slice of the image processed by this coregistration method. Pixels of the FLAIR MR in the MRS box were replaced by voxels of different gray scales representing the Cho-to-Cr ratios (the brighter the image intensity, the higher the Cho-to-Cr ratio). The processed FLAIR was then fused with the T1-weighted MR scans and simulation CT scan using the fusion tools of the treatment planning system.

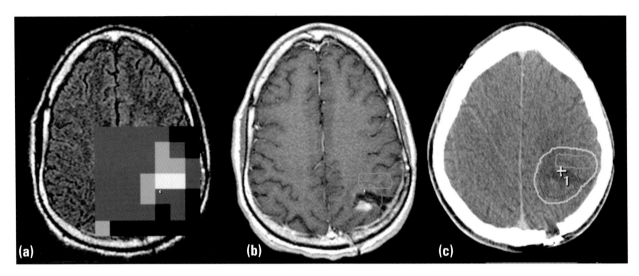

FIGURE 15B-1. Axial images showing **(a)** magnetic resonance spectroscopic (MRS) imaging overlaid on fluid-attenuated inversion recovery image, **(b)** a magnetic resonance (MR) image T1-weighted postcontrast, and **(c)** computed tomography images. The gross tumor volume (pink) and the MRS voxels (green) are shown.

In this patient, the gross tumor volume (GTV) was defined as the contrast-enhancing tumor visualized on the T1-weighted MR acquired both before and after the first cycle of the antibody, and on the planning CT. The clinical target volume (CTV) was defined as the GTV including MR image voxels with elevated metabolite ratios within 1 cm of the GTV. A planning target volume (PTV) was generated by adding a three-dimensional 3-mm margin around the CTV. The GTV, CTV, and PTV were 10.9 cm³, 17.6 cm³, and 58.6 cm³, respectively. Of note, if the MRS voxels had not been included, the PTV would have been 21.4 cm³. A PTV limit of 40 cm³ was set on this IRB protocol because of concerns over possible radiation-induced toxicities. Therefore, the margins used to create the CTV were reduced for this patient, resulting in a final PTV of 33.6 cm³. Figures 15B-1B and 15B-1C illustrate the GTV (pink) and the MRS image voxels (green) with enhanced metabolite ratios, and PTV (orange) on one axial slice of the T1-weighted MR image and the simulation CT scan.

Treatment Planning

The treatment plan consisted of eight non-coplanar intensity-modulated radiation therapy (IMRT) beams delivered using BrainLAB m3 dynamic 3-mm micro-multileaf collimator. A total radiation dose of 30 Gy was delivered in five fractions delivered over 2.5 weeks. The treatment plan was generated with the aim to keep cumulative maximum dose from previous and current radiation treatment to less than 60 Gy for brainstem, chiasm, and optic nerves, and to less than 50 Gy for the retina.

Figure 15B-2 shows the dose distribution of the IMRT plan for (A) axial, (B) coronal, and (C) sagittal view. A total dose of 30 Gy was prescribed to the 100% isodose line. The PTV maximum dose, minimum dose, and dose to 95% of the volume was 106%, 99%, and 102%, respectively. Maximum doses to the brainstem from previous and current radiation plans were 59.9 Gy and 0.6 Gy,

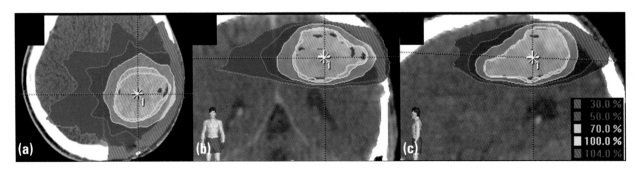

FIGURE 15B-2. Dose distributions from the intensity-modulated radiation therapy plan delivering 30 Gy (=100%) in five fractions are shown on **(a)** axial, **(b)** coronal, and **(c)** sagittal view.

respectively. No dose was delivered to the chiasm or the optic structures in the current treatment plan.

Clinical Outcome

The patient tolerated treatment well without significant acute toxicities. Follow-up MR scans revealed stable disease. He experienced no late toxicities related to his radiation therapy. At approximately 11.5 months post-treatment, the patient developed a local recurrence and underwent re-resection. The pathology was consistent with recurrent GBM.

Our initial experience incorporating MRS imaging into the treatment planning process in a series of 12 recurrent high-grade gliomas was presented earlier.[3] Treatment consisted of intensity-modulated hypofractionated stereotactic radiotherapy combined with bevacizumab chemotherapy. For treatment planning, T1-weighted postcontrast MR and MRS images were acquired before and after the first chemotherapy cycle. Enhancing tumors defined on the second MR or MRS scans were generally smaller than those identified on the pretreatment scans. The MRS scans for seven patients showed voxels with elevated metabolite ratios but not all elevated voxels

were included because of clinical considerations including PTV size, proximity to critical organs, and prior radiation dose. Among these seven cases, the MR- and/or CT-defined CTVs of four patients were increased by 2%, 4%, 15%, and 23% when the MRS imaging voxels were included. The PTV size ranged from 18.6 cc to 57.6 cc, with a median size of 33.2 cc. The PTVs were fully covered by the prescription dose in all but one case because of dose constraints to surrounding critical organs from the prior treatment.

References

1. Gutin PH, Iwamoto FM, Beal K, et al. Safety and efficacy of bevacizumab with hypofractionated stereotactic irradiation for recurrent malignant gliomas. *Int J Radiat Oncol Biol Phys.* 2009;75:156–163.
2. Chang J, Thakur S, Perera G, et al. Image-fusion of MR spectroscopic images for treatment planning of gliomas. *Med Phys.* 2006;33:32–40.
3. Ballangrud AM, Lymberis S, Thakur SB, et al. Feasibility of incorporating magnetic resonance spectroscopy imaging (MRSI) in radiotherapy treatment planning of recurrent gliomas [abstract]. *Int J Radiat Oncol Biol Phys.* 2007;69:S67.

Functional MR-Guided Target Delineation in a Patient with a Cerebral AVM Undergoing SRS

Case Study

Joseph Stancanello, PhD, Carlo Cavedon, PhD,
Federico Colombo, MD, Paolo Francescon, PhD,
Leopoldo Casentini, MD, Francesco Causin, MD

Patient History

A 46-year-old woman presented with a sudden-onset partial seizure involving her right arm and leg, followed by a short episode of loss of consciousness, right hemiparesis, and language impairment. Emergent cerebral computed tomography (CT) revealed an abnormal vascular structure in the left parietal area, with no evidence of acute intracranial hemorrhage or ischemia. After administration of an intravenous steroid and a benzodiazepine, her neurological examination rapidly returned to normal. The patient was subsequently maintained on antiepileptic medication.

Neuroradiological work up included cerebral magnetic resonance (MR) imaging with contrast enhancement that confirmed the presence of a medium-sized cerebral arteriovenous malformation (AVM) with an enlarged draining vein in the left Rolando–parietal area. Digital subtraction angiography (DSA) revealed an arteriolar nidus fed by an enlarged and tortuous Rolando–parietal ascending branch of the middle cerebral artery. The draining vein was directed to the superior sagittal sinus and was markedly enlarged with a pseudoaneurysm at its departure from the nidus (Figure 15C-1). Blood flow velocity through the arteriovenous shunt was increased. A functional MR (fMR) scan was performed and demonstrated that the nidus was in close proximity to the corti-

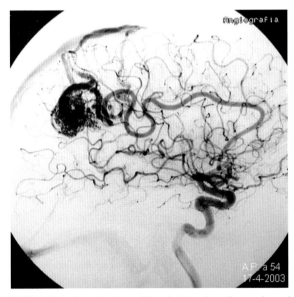

FIGURE 15C-1. Lateral view of the digital subtraction angiography used to identify the arteriovenous malformation.

cal areas involved in contralateral limb motor and sensory function, as well as to language areas.

The patient's case was discussed in our multidisciplinary neuroradiological and neurosurgical conference and, taking into account the absence of prior intracranial hemorrhages, the consensus recommendation was for stereotactic radiosurgery (SRS). We elected to incorporate fMR into the SRS treatment planning process.

Simulation

After fabrication of an immobilization mold to be used during treatment, the patient was imaged on a Somatom Plus 4 CT scanner (Siemens AG, Erlangen, Germany) in the Neuroradiology Department. Radio-opaque contrast was injected to enhance the visualization of the AVM nidus. Axially oriented, 2-mm-thick slices were obtained from the base to the top of the skull. This volume was used for treatment planning and for the generation of digitally reconstructed radiographs used during treatment delivery.

Imaging and Target Delineation

In addition to the planning CT and three-dimensional (3D) rotational angiography (3DRA) for AVM nidus delineation, a T2-weighted MR (T2-MR) scan was acquired for better morphological identification of the patient anatomy and 60 Echo Planar Images (EPI-MRs) were used for the identification of functional organs at risk (fOARs); the EPI-MRs were acquired with and without appropriate stimuli. Because of the peripheral location of the AVM, no critical structures were selected for treatment planning apart from the functional areas identified by fMR. On the basis of the AVM location (left hemisphere), we decided to perform blood oxygen level–dependent analyses of the following tasks: motor function of the right hand and right thumb, language-related areas using a category generation task (CGT), letter generation, and simple question. After the acquisition, the statistical parametric mapping (SPM99) software package (Wellcome Department of Cognitive Neurology, London) was used to perform both image processing and statistical analysis on the raw data.[1] The P value and the minimum number of voxels (n) representing an activation cluster for the motor task were equal to 0.05 (Bonferroni-corrected analysis for false positives) and 20, respectively; for language and understanding related tasks, parameters of P = .001 (uncorrected) and n = 100 were satisfactory for the estimation of activation areas. Different P values were chosen because language tasks tend to produce diffuse activation that would give no activated area with the same parameters as motor tasks.

Treatment Planning

All of the volumes were rigidly registered to the planning CT[2] and imported into the CyberKnife treatment planning system (Accuray, Sunnyvale, CA). Nonrigid registration, though optionally available, was not performed

because of the limited amount of image distortion in the EPI images. However, normalization to the brain atlas usually included in the analysis procedure was not used in this case to avoid the introduction of additional distortion.[2] Spatial registration of the EPI images to the planning CT was achieved through registration to the T2-MR images. Using this collection of data sets, the AVM nidus was delineated on the 3DRA and the fOAR on the functional maps superimposed to the T2 volume. These structures were then superimposed onto the planning CT as a starting point for the optimization process.

The fOARs were used to impose dose constraints similarly to what is done for morphologically delineated OARs. The dose constraints for fOARs closer to the AVM nidus were assigned a higher priority in the optimization process. Dose constraints were set to ensure adequate coverage of the target while maximally sparing the adjacent fOARs.

CyberKnife is capable of pseudo-isocentric or free conformal geometry. A conformal approach was selected in this case. A dose of 19.5 Gy was prescribed to the 75% isodose level in a single fraction (26 Gy maximum dose). The target percentage coverage after the treatment plan optimization was 95%; the conformity and the homogeneity indexes were 1.21 and 1.33, respectively.

To assess the benefit of incorporating fMR imaging into the treatment planning process in this patient, a simulation was performed comparing dose–volume histograms (DVHs) with and without dose constraints within the fMR-identified areas (Figure 15C-2). The maximum dose within the closest functional area (motor - right hand) was 5.4 Gy in the optimized case and 12.8 Gy without dose constraints, which corresponds to a 58% reduction. Figure 15C-3 illustrates a DVH generated with and without dose constraints in adjacent functional areas. The target DVH was practically unaffected, yet the motor area of the right hand was significantly spared. The volume of the motor area exceeding 15% of the maximum dose was reduced from 32% to 0.3% of the activation volume as determined by the functional analysis.

Clinical Outcome

The patient was treated on a CyberKnife with image guidance throughout treatment delivery. She tolerated treatment extremely well and at discharge from our hospital she did not require any medication, except for her prophylactic antiseizure medication. The postradiosurgical period was completely uneventful and the patient immediately returned to work as a director of her own small company. She has not developed any new seizures. She has undergone biannual contrast-enhanced MR scans following treatment that have demonstrated progressive regression of the abnormal vascular components of the

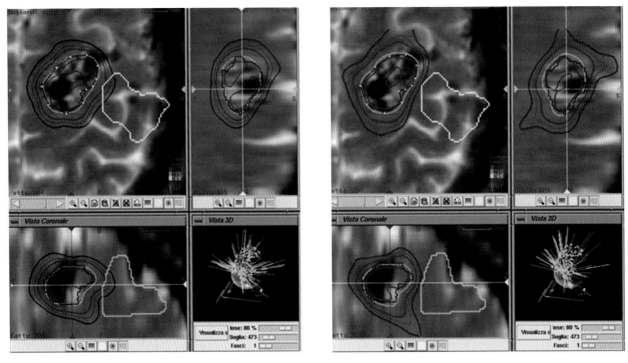

FIGURE 15C-2. Comparison between dose distributions obtained with (right) and without (left) sparing of the motor area of the right hand (yellow-green line) defined by functional magnetic resonance imaging during the optimization process.

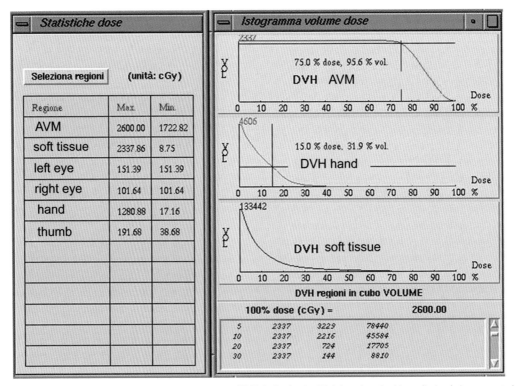

FIGURE 15C-3. Comparison between dose–volume histograms (DVHs) obtained with (above) and without (below) dose constraints assigned to adjacent functional regions. The DVH of the target arteriovenous malformation is practically unaffected, yet the motor area of the right hand is significantly spared by including it into the optimization process.

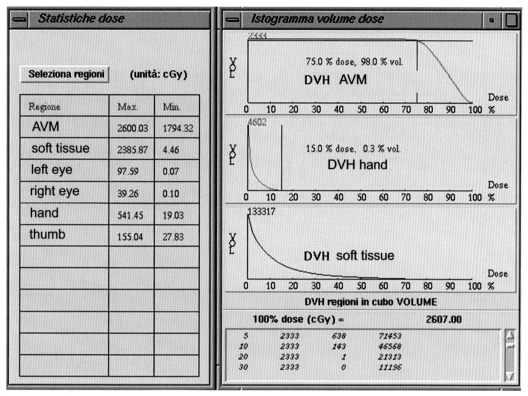

FIGURE 15C-3. (Continued)

AVM. At 24 months, a contrast-enhanced MR scan with angiography has revealed complete obliteration of the AVM nidus. Obliteration confirmation by DSA has been planned for the near future.

Our initial clinical experience integrating fMR into the SRS treatment planning process for cerebral AVM patients was published earlier.[2] Five patients scheduled to undergo SRS were scanned prior to treatment with CT, 3DRA, T2-MR, and fMR imaging. Tasks were chosen based on lesion location by considering those areas that could be potentially near treatment targets. Functional data were superimposed on 3DRA and CT used for treatment planning. Treatment plans studied with and without considering fOARs were significantly different, particularly in terms of the maximum dose and DVHs. Consideration of the fOARs allowed quality indices of treatment plans to remain almost constant or to improve in four of the five cases studied.

References

1. Friston KJ, Ashburner J, Poline JB, et al. Spatial registration and normalization of images. *Hum Brain Mapp.* 1995;2:165–189.
2. Stancanello J, Cavedon C, Francescon P, et al. BOLD fMRI integration into radiosurgery treatment planning of cerebral vascular malformations. *Med Phys.* 2007;34:1176–1184.

Image-Guided SRS in a Patient with Trigeminal Neuralgia Using the CyberKnife System

Case Study

Alan T. Villavicencio, MD, Lee McNeely, MD

Patient History

A 60-year-old man presented with severe, lancinating right V2 trigeminal neuralgia pain that was gradually increasing in frequency and intensity over the past several years. The pain was coming in paroxysms or "clusters" with repeated episodes of a very intense and essentially debilitating pain, triggered by an intraoral stimulation, such as chewing, cutaneous stimulation with cold wind, or touching over the lateral side of the nose or malar region. He rated his pain at 5 to 6 on a 10-point visual analog scale and was taking high doses of gabapentin (4800 mg/daily) and carbamazepine (600 mg/daily), which tremendously interfered with his daily activities as he was severely fatigued.

Clinical and neurological examinations were normal, with light touch sensation preserved in all three trigeminus branches bilaterally. Magnetic resonance (MR) imaging of the brain showed no vascular loops or other local lesions in association with the right-sided trigeminal root entry zone.

In the past, the patient had undergone two radiofrequency neurolysis procedures with some improvement that only lasted 4 and 2 months each time, respectively. Our recommendation was for image-guided stereotactic radiosurgery using the CyberKnife system (Accuray Inc, Sunnyvale, CA).

Simulation

A week before the treatment, the patient underwent computed tomography (CT) simulation on a LightSpeed scanner (GE Healthcare, Waukesha, WI) after fabrication of a customized thermoplastic immobilization mask of the head. A contrast cisternography for precise visualization of the trigeminal nerve within the prepontine cistern was also performed and fused to the CT.

Treatment Planning

The trigeminal nerve was indentified on the CyberKnife planning workstation and a segment of the nerve was marked as the clinical target volume (CTV). A radiosurgery treatment plan was generated consisting of 123 beams collimated to 5 mm prescribing 60 Gy marginal dose (D$_{max}$, 70 Gy) to a 6-mm section of the nerve sparing 2 mm at the dorsal root entry zone and not extending into the gasserian ganglion within the Meckel's cave (Figure 15D-1). The treatment plan was generated through nonisocentric geometry using the 650 node set especially designed for trigeminal neuralgia cases. In the treatment planning process an artificial dose tuning structure was generated to additionally protect the brain stem.

Treatment Delivery

On the day of treatment, the patient was placed in the treatment position and his head was immobilized within his customized thermoplastic mask. Patient setup and target tracking were accomplished by comparing digitally reconstructed radiographs created from the planning CT data set with standard orthogonal cranial x-rays taken after every five beams throughout the treatment. Small patient movements were detected and new target coordinates sent to the robotic arm to adjust the aiming of the linear accelerator. These offsets were reduced to less than 1 mm in the treatment space and less than 1° of rotation

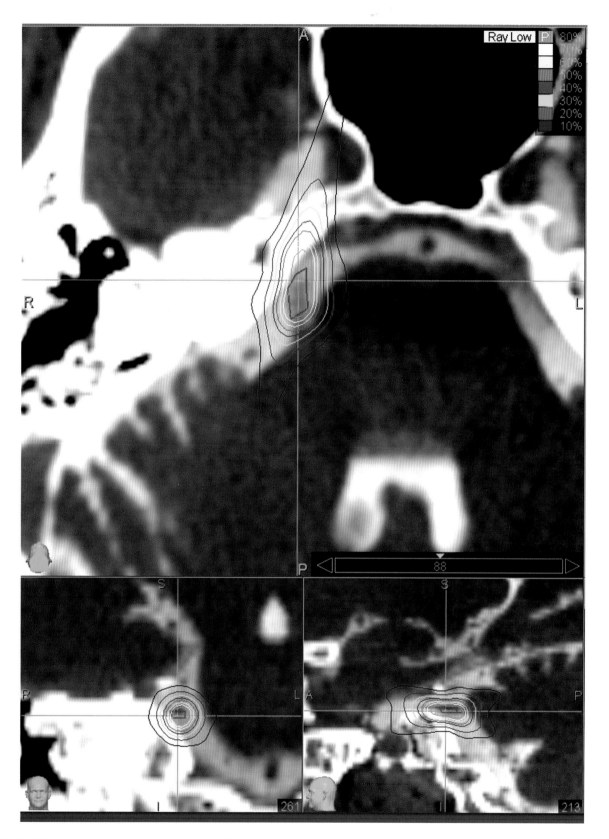

FIGURE 15D-1. Treatment plan: axial (top), coronal (left), and sagittal (right) views. A red line demonstrates the nerve segment contoured as target volume with a short segment near the root entry zone excluded from the target volume. Surrounding isodose lines represent 10% (dark-blue outermost line), 30% (light-blue line), 50% (magenta line), and 80% (orange line at the nerve margin) of the maximum nerve dose of 100%.

before initiation of treatment. The entire treatment took approximately 60 minutes.

Clinical Outcome

The patient tolerated the treatment well and had a substantial improvement of his pain within a few days. He noted minimal lancinating pain, substantial improvement in triggering factors, and no facial numbness at his 3-week follow-up. His pain relief was rated as moderate – 2 on the Boulder-Stanford pain relief scale (> 50% pain relief, and < 90% reduction in use of pain medications).[1] Medications were tapered to 600 mg/daily of gabapentin for the first 6 months after the treatment.

At the most recent follow-up (3 years and 8 months) pain relief was rated as excellent –1 (> 90% pain relief, completely off pain medications); however, the patient developed some mild, nonbothersome facial numbness.

Our preliminary multicenter experience treating trigeminal neuralgia with the CyberKnife system was published earlier.[1] Ninety-five patients were treated between May 2002 and October 2005. Sixty-five (67%) noted excellent pain relief, with a median time to pain relief of 14 days (range, 0.3–180 days). Overall, 45 (47%) experienced posttreatment numbness. The overall complication rate was 18%. At a mean follow-up of 2 years, 47 (50%) of patients were noted to have sustained pain relief and no longer required medications. Radiation dose and length of nerve treated were correlated with better pain relief.

Reference

1. Villavicencio AT, Lim M, Burneikiene S, et al. CyberKnife radiosurgery for trigeminal neuralgia treatment: a preliminary multicenter experience. *Neurosurgery.* 2008;62(3):647–655.

PLANAR IMAGE-GUIDED FRAMELESS IMRT IN A PATIENT WITH RECURRENT NASOPHARYNGEAL CARCINOMA ON A NOVALIS LINEAR ACCELERATOR

CASE STUDY

EDWARD MELIAN, MD, ANIL SETHI, PhD

Patient History

A 53-year-old man with a history of nasopharyngeal carcinoma treated with combined modality cisplatin and 5-fluorouracil chemotherapy and definitive external beam radiotherapy (RT) presented 7 years after completing treatment with progressive headaches and diplopia. On physical exam, he was noted to have reduced facial sensation in all divisions of the left 5th cranial nerve and palsy of the left 6th cranial nerve. He had poor but useable vision in the right eye.

Radiographic workup included a magnetic resonance (MR) scan, which demonstrated recurrent disease in left cavernous sinus extending into the inferior temporal lobe (Figure 15E-1). Positron emission tomography (PET) revealed increased metabolic activity in the left cavernous sinus (maximum standardized uptake value [SUV], 6.2) but no evidence of tumor crossing the midline. In addition, there was no evidence of disease in the neck or distant sites. A biopsy was done trans-sphenoidally confirming recurrent nasopharyngeal carcinoma. Computed tomography (CT) scans of the neck and chest showed no evidence of distant disease.

The patient was discussed at our multidisciplinary head and neck tumor conference. On review, the recurrence was noted to be intimately involved with the left

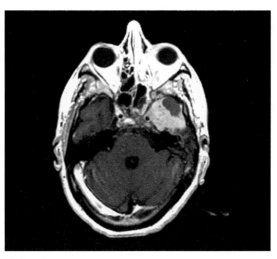

FIGURE 15E-1. Magnetic resonance scan illustrating the recurrent disease in the left cavernous sinus extending into the inferior temporal lobe.

optic nerve. The patient was thus informed that further treatment could put the left optic nerve at risk and may cause left eye blindness, an important concern because of his poor vision on the right. Because further chemotherapy would be palliative at best, he chose to undergo fractionated stereotactic intensity-modulated RT (IMRT). We elected to treat him with daily image guidance on a Novalis linear accelerator (BrainLab AG, Feldkirchen, Germany) using noninvasive frameless radiosurgery.

Simulation

The patient was simulated in the supine position with a fractionated immobilization head frame. First, the patient was fitted with a custom head and neck and shoulder mask. Next, a stereotactic localizer and target positioner box (BrainLAB AG, Feldkirchen, Germany) was placed and a contrast-enhanced CT scan was performed on an AcuSim Big Bore Brilliance 16-slice scanner (Philips Medical Systems, Andover, MA) from the top of the head to the chest. The target positioner box (Figure 15E-2) consists of six embedded localizer rods and serves two purposes. It provides a three-dimensional (3D) patient coordinate system, because the localizer rods appear as an array of index marks on the CT scan that define the exact position of target on every slice. Additionally, the localizer box enables precise patient setup on the treatment table by using infrared (IR) markers and orthogonal kV x-rays.

Treatment Planning

The PET images and thin-sliced (2 mm) MR scans (axial T1, T2, and coronal with contrast) obtained for treatment planning were then fused to the treatment planning CT. The tumor was delineated on each modality and then a composite gross tumor volume (GTV) was created. The GTV was then expanded 3 mm in each direction to create

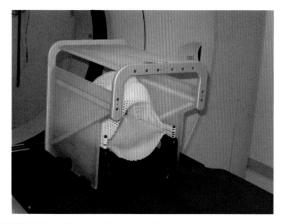

FIGURE 15E-2. Stereotactic head and neck localizer/target positioner box with six embedded rods used for CT scanning.

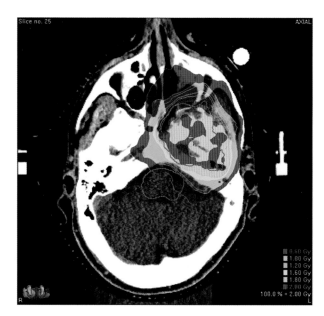

FIGURE 15E-3. Isodose curves superimposed on the planning computed tomography scan on a slice containing the isocenter.

a planning target volume (PTV). The optic chiasm and optic nerves were demarcated as organs at risk (OARs).

A shaped 10-field plan was created to deliver 54 Gy in 30 fractions to the PTV in the BrainScan software (BrainLab AG, Feldkirchen, Germany). Beams were chosen at angles to help avoid the chiasm. The PTV mean dose was 60 Gy with 90% receiving 56 Gy. The GTV received a maximum point dose of 68.4 Gy and a minimum dose of 58 Gy. The optic chiasm maximum dose was 7.2 Gy. The right and left optic nerve maximum doses were 5.4 Gy and 60 Gy, respectively. The PTV coverage at 54 Gy was 100%, and the resulting conformity index was 1.56 (Figure 15E-3).

Treatment Delivery

In the treatment room, the patient was placed in the custom mask and a frameless radiosurgery array (with a unique pattern of six IR markers) was attached (Figure 15E-4a). The IR markers, in conjunction with the IR camera, provide automated patient setup using feedback from the planning system. The Novalis Exactrac system (BrainLAB AG, Feldkirchen, Germany), equipped with a robotic controlled couch with six degrees of freedom (three translation and three rotation) was used for precise patient positioning. Next, a pair of kV x-ray images was acquired and matched (bony-fusion) with digitally reconstructed radiographs generated from the planning system to correct patient positioning and verify alignment with the treatment isocenter (Figure 15E-4b). A variety of tools (manual/auto/region-of-interest fusion, spy-glass, color-blending, etc.) are provided in the software to assess the accuracy of

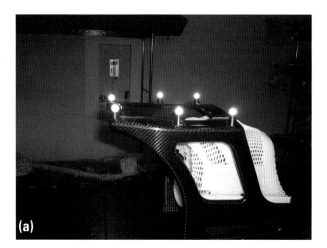

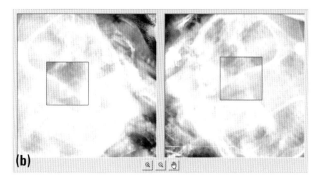

FIGURE 15E-4. Novalis Exactrac work-flow: **(a)** A frameless array with six infrared markers is placed around patient mask to provide initial patient positioning and assist with robotic couch control. **(b)** A pair of orthogonal kV x-rays are taken and fused with digitally reconstructed radiographs to precisely align the target to the isocenter.

fusion. A "snap" x-ray verification option is also available to check patient positioning during treatment.

Clinical Outcome

Overall, the patient tolerated his treatment well and experienced a rewarding decrease in pain by the completion of treatment subsequently no longer requiring pain medication. His diplopia, however, persisted. Initial MR imaging 2 months posttreatment showed a change from a uniform avid tumor enhancement in the left cavernous sinus to a more heterogeneous pattern. The tumor had also markedly retracted medially from the left middle cranial fossa. Follow-up scans over the following year were stable. He subsequently underwent strabismus surgery with resolution of his diplopia.

Two years after completing therapy, however, he represented with worsening headaches and right facial pain. He was found to have right-sided ptosis, a dilated pupil, and palsies of cranial nerves III, IV, and VI. He also had relative deficits in his right cranial nerve V_2 and V_3 distribution. Magnetic resonance imaging demonstrated recurrence in the right cavernous sinus with tumor still controlled on the left side. The patient was generally weak and wheelchair bound. Because of the previous sparing of the chiasm and right optic nerve, it was believed we could treat him again with RT. Because of the severity of symptoms and now poorer performance status, we felt he needed a rapid response to treatment. We recommended a hypofractionated approach (25 Gy in 5 fractions). Care was taken to avoid the previous high-dose region.

Chapter 16

Head and Neck Tumors: Overview

ANDREAS RIMNER, MD, NANCY Y. LEE, MD

Image-guided radiation therapy (IGRT) has experienced an unprecedented surge in use in recent years. This is primarily attributable to the increased availability of fast and high-quality imaging technology as well as the emergence of new and increasingly precise external beam radiation treatment delivery techniques such as intensity-modulated radiation therapy (IMRT). This chapter will focus on the use of image-guided intensity-modulated radiation therapy (IG-IMRT) in the treatment of head and neck cancer, followed by a series of case reports to highlight individual technologies and scenarios. Target delineation, imaging techniques, and dose delivery assurance will be at the center of this discussion.

Head and Neck Cancer Radiotherapy

For locally advanced head and neck cancer, the standard of care is definitive combined chemotherapy and radiation (RT). Acute and long-term toxicity from RT to the head and neck has significantly improved with the development of IMRT. Owing to the increased precision of radiation treatment delivery with IMRT, rates of xerostomia, mucositis, hearing loss, osteoradionecrosis, dysphagia, and feeding tube dependence have decreased as a function of reduced dose to normal tissues, such as the parotid glands, inner ears, mandible, or oral cavity.[1–9]

In addition, the higher conformality of IMRT has the potential of dose escalation by dose painting and delivery of higher doses per fraction to potentially resistant or heavily involved tumor portions, thus increasing the biologically effective dose.[10] Thus, in head and neck cancer, locoregional control of greater than 90% has been achieved with the definitive use of IMRT.[5,7,11,12] Even with concurrent chemotherapy, IMRT has contributed to a change in failure patterns from local failure to predominantly distant failure.[10]

Highly conformal radiation allows for inherent improved dose distribution, decreased dose to normal tissues at risk, and the ability to treat larger volumes of disease without exceeding normal tissue tolerances. However, the risks of being too conformal include geographical misses and, ultimately, locoregional failures. A higher integral dose is a common disadvantage of attempting maximal conformality and may offset the benefits, if modern technology is not prudently adapted and carefully tested.[13] This is especially true in the head and neck region, where target volumes and critical normal structures are extremely closely situated. Smaller treatment volumes and margins pose a greater risk of a "geographic miss" and underdosing leading to marginal recurrences, which makes head and neck cancers particularly challenging targets. Defining the exact tumor location and extent is particularly relevant for this patient population, because locoregional control is critical and most patients have a good chance for cure with local treatment.[14] Similarly important is the accurate delivery of a carefully developed treatment plan. Nowadays, modern imaging technologies including electronic portal imaging devices (EPIDs) and cone-beam computed tomography (CBCT) can be combined with treatment delivery systems in the treatment room for image-guided delivery of RT to increase the level of treatment delivery accuracy.

The complex anatomy of the head and neck requires a high level of anatomical knowledge and a comprehensive understanding of the primary tumor site, patterns of common lymph node involvement, and the inherent biology of the tumor. It is critical to determine the exact extension of the primary tumor by clinical examination and the judicious use of available imaging technologies. A careful clinical examination including flexible endoscopy by the radiation oncologist remains important, as many squamous cell carcinomas of the head and neck have a propensity to spread submucosally or superficially, which may not be fully assessed even with advanced imaging including computed tomography (CT), magnetic resonance (MR) imaging, and positron emission tomography (PET). Especially for early stage disease, it has been shown that no imaging modality is able to accurately depict superficial tumor extension.[15]

Highly focused RT with steep dose gradients near critical structures calls for more accurate patient setup and immobilization, as well as verification of intra- and interfractional patient positioning to avoid missing target structures and to effectively treat the tumor. Optimal immobilization of the patient is therefore paramount to minimize systematic setup errors as well as systematic and random patient motion.[16] In the head and neck region, rigid immobilization with a thermoplastic five-point mask has worked best and has shown the least setup variation.[17] A study from our institution found that the five-point mask was especially accurate in maintaining the head position intrafractionally compared with reproducing the position from one fraction to the next.[18] Whenever the neck is being treated, patients should be positioned in hyperextension to avoid skin folds and minimize the dose to the oral cavity from anteriorly entering beam angles. Random setup uncertainty with this system lies between 3 mm and 7 mm. Motion because of swallowing cannot be eliminated, but likely has only a small influence on the delivered treatment dose, as it is a short-lived process of approximately 1 second corresponding to 0.45% of the total treatment time.[19,20] Swallowing frequency increases with longer treatment time, but was found to decrease the total dose by only 0.5% with the use of conventional opposed lateral fields for larynx cancer.[21]

Imaging can be used for RT guidance during four different stages of the process:

1. Diagnostic imaging of target delineation and planning
2. Simulation imaging
3. Treatment imaging for patient positioning, setup corrections, and treatment verification on the linac
4. Treatment imaging for replanning during RT, when plan adjustments because of changes in the patient's anatomy are needed, also known as adaptive RT.[22]

Image-Guided Target Delineation

The unprecedented precision, control of dose distribution, and conformality available with IMRT mandates high-quality imaging, before treatment and during treatment delivery. In addition, IMRT calls for a higher attention to detail as to selection and delineation of target volumes.[23] Intraobserver, interobserver, and interinstitutional differences in target selection and delineation are likely more significant than the accurate target dose coverage or setup variations and are probably the most important source of uncertainty during RT planning.[24,25] Therefore, close communication between the radiologist and radiation oncologist is essential for accurate assessment of the primary tumor and for identifying nodal regions at high and intermediate risk for metastases. Several imaging technologies

have been explored to aid with the assessment of loco-regional tumor extent for treatment planning purposes, including CT, MR, and PET scanning. All radiological findings in conjunction with clinical observations have to be integrated for treatment planning and target delineation.[11] In postoperative patients, the areas at risk should be discussed with the surgeon to ensure coverage of all areas that appeared suspicious during resection.

As smaller margins are being used because of the ability to more precisely define the patient's position at the time of treatment, it is paramount that the target and avoidance structures are correctly delineated. Weight loss during treatment, rapid decrease in size of the primary tumor, and bulky nodal metastases add to the complexity of treatment. Currently, one determines the gross tumor volume (GTV) based on pretreatment/simulation scans and depends on the quality and reader's interpretation of these images. The GTV is encompassed by a clinical target volume (CTV), which is designed to cover any microscopic extent of disease from the primary tumor or involved lymph node beyond the resolution of imaging and clinical determination, as well as nodal regions at high risk for nodal metastases.[26] A safety margin is added to the CTV to generate the planning target volume (PTV), which should take into account any setup errors and organ motion. The dose is prescribed to the PTV to ensure that the planned prescription dose is actually delivered to the CTV, even in the presence of small geometrical errors.[16] To avoid long-term toxicity, the CTV and PTV may require adjustments in areas of critical normal structures such as the brainstem. The normal tissue constraints used at our institution are listed in Table 16-1. General guidelines for target delineation are described in Table 16-2.

It is beyond the scope of this chapter to describe in detail the target delineation criteria for each subsite of the

TABLE 16–1 General Normal Tissue Guidelines

Normal Tissue Guidelines	Dose Constraints
Spinal cord	$D_{max} \leq 45$ Gy
Brainstem	$D_{max} \leq 50$ Gy (≤ 54 Gy in select cases)
Temporal lobe	$D_{max} \leq 60$ Gy
Optic chiasm	$D_{max} \leq 54$ Gy (≤ 57 Gy in select cases)
Eyes	$D_{max} \leq 45$ Gy
Lens of the eye	$D_{max} \leq 5$ Gy
Inner/middle ear	$D_{max} \leq 50$ Gy
Brachial plexus	$D_{max} \leq 65$ Gy and $D_{05} \leq 60$ Gy
Parotid gland	Mean dose ≤ 26 Gy in at least one gland
Submandibular gland	Mean dose ≤ 39 Gy
Mandible	$D_{max} \leq 70$ Gy
Oral cavity	Mean dose 35 Gy to 40 Gy
Esophagus	Mean dose ≤ 50 Gy
Glottic larynx	Mean dose ≤ 45 Gy

TABLE 16–2 General Target Volume Guidelines

Primary Site	GTV	CTV	PTV
Nasopharynx	Primary tumor + grossly involved lymph nodes	GTV + 5 mm to 10 mm, neck levels IB–V + retropharyngeal lymph nodes	CTV + 5 mm, may be reduced to a minimum of 1 mm near critical structures, e.g., brainstem
Oropharynx	Primary tumor + grossly involved lymph nodes	GTV + 5 mm to 10 mm, neck levels IB–V + retropharyngeal lymph nodes	CTV + 5 mm
Hypopharynx	Primary tumor + grossly involved lymph nodes	GTV + 5 mm to 10 mm, neck levels II–V + retropharyngeal lymph nodes	CTV + 5 mm
Supraglottic and glottic larynx	Primary tumor + grossly involved lymph nodes	GTV + 5 mm to 10 mm, neck levels II–V	CTV + 5 mm
Oral cavity	Primary tumor + grossly involved lymph nodes	GTV + 5 mm to 10 mm, neck levels I–V	CTV + 5 mm
Thyroid	Primary tumor + grossly involved lymph nodes	GTV + 5 mm to 10 mm, neck levels II–VII	CTV + 5 mm
Unknown primary	Mucosal surfaces of the nasopharynx, oropharynx, and hypopharynx + grossly involved lymph nodes	GTV + 5 mm to 10 mm, neck levels II–V + retropharyngeal lymph nodes	CTV + 5 mm, may be reduced to a minimum of 1 mm near critical structures, e.g., brainstem

Notes. CTV = clinical target volume; GTV = gross tumor volume; PTV = planning target volume.

head and neck. We therefore refer the reader to the IMRT literature for more specific instructions on target delineation. At our institution, we define gross tumor and grossly involved lymph nodes as the GTV. The CTV$_1$ consists of the GTV + 5 mm to 10 mm margin. The CTV$_2$ includes subclinical high-risk disease, which typically includes the neck node levels at high risk depending on the site of the primary tumor. The CTV$_3$ may include areas of lesser risk for disease involvement such as the uninvolved contralateral neck.

Errors in target delineation are systematic errors that likely have the most significant effect on outcome, as they equally influence each fraction. The resolution of the imaging modality and partial volume effects between slices have to be considered as additional potential sources for error.[27] Systematic errors are associated with a shift of the delivered dose distribution relative to the PTV, whereas random errors cause blurring of the delivered dose, because their direction varies from one fraction to the other.[16] Random errors, therefore, result in only a small dose decrease at the edge of the tumor.

The optimal number of beams is five to nine beams for most scenarios in head and neck cancer. New delivery systems including tomotherapy and arc therapy are not dependent on specific numbers of beams and beam angles, as they have the potential to deliver radiation from 360°.[28] A typical dose fractionation regimen at our institution consists of 70 Gy to the CTV$_1$ given as 2.12 Gy per fraction, 59.4 Gy to the CTV$_2$ given as 1.8 Gy per fraction, and 54 Gy to the CTV$_3$ given as 1.64 Gy per fraction. For the uninvolved lower neck at low risk for involvement, we commonly match a low anterior neck field at the level of the arytenoid cartilages and deliver 50.4 Gy in 28 fractions.

Computed Tomography

Computed tomography imaging is superior to other modalities in visualizing cortical bony anatomy and detecting calcifications. It has also been found to be a useful tool for identifying necrosis and extranodal extension in lymph node metastases.[29,30] In CT scans of the head and neck region, special attention should be paid to evaluating the invasion or encasement of large vessels and tumor extension to the skull base or prevertebral space, all of which are important criteria for potential surgical ineligibility.[31] Although MR is generally the preferred method for perineural invasion assessment, it is in most cases detectable on modern CT images by loss of the normal fat signal, enlargement of the neuroforamina, or muscle atrophy.[29,32]

Computed tomography is an excellent imaging technology for lymph node staging.[30,33,34] Computed tomography imaging has significantly improved the sensitivity and accuracy of lymph node detection compared with clinical assessment, especially in the clinically N0 setting.[31,35–37] Some areas at risk for nodal spread, such as the retropharyngeal lymph nodes, are not amenable to clinical examination and can only be assessed by imaging.[38] Generally accepted criteria for lymph nodes suspicious for malignancy are listed in Table 16-3.[34,36,37,39] Despite significant efforts to improve the negative predictive value of CT imaging for nodal disease by comparing and combining different imaging modalities, there has not been sufficient evidence to safely exclude clinical or radiographic uninvolved lymph node levels from treatment volumes.[29]

Limitations of CT imaging in the head and neck area include streak artifacts caused by dental implants, which have been found to increase contouring variability,[40] suboptimal detection of small or superficial tumors,

TABLE 16–3 Criteria for Lymph Nodes Suspicious for Malignancy

Nodal size of > 1 cm (> 1.1 cm to 1.5 cm for jugulodigastric lymph nodes)

Clusters of ≥ 3 borderline-sized lymph nodes

Spatial distribution pattern of enlarged lymph nodes

Smaller nodes with spherical rather than ellipsoidal shape

Inhomogeneities, e.g., low central attenuation, suggestive of necrotic centers, contrast enhancement, and demarcation to adjacent normal structures.

and tumors in the oral tongue. In addition, surrounding inflammation or edema can lead to overestimation of the extent of the tumor. Because CT involves the use of ionizing radiation, its use is limited in pregnant women and children. Furthermore, the common use of iodinated contrast agents bears the risk of potential side effects and allergic reactions.[29,41]

Virtual CT simulation with or without intravenous contrast has become established as the single most important and most widely used modality for target delineation, because of its speed, operational efficiency, cost-effectiveness, and the ability to produce thin sections with high resolution.[42] Because helical CT imaging is fast, motion artifacts from swallowing, breathing, tongue motion, or eye movement are limited to a minimum. It is therefore the easiest imaging modality to tolerate with excellent compliance, including imaging of children and patients with dysphagia or respiratory problems.[41] The electron density relative to water as provided by Hounsfield units is the basis for dosimetric calculations and inhomogeneity corrections.[14] No other imaging modality has been able to replace this unique property of CT scanning. Furthermore, CT provides highly accurate geometrical information that is invaluable with highly conformal radiation therapy, particularly in areas of bone, fat, air, and tumor interfaces.[14,43]

Because of significant interobserver variability, efforts have been made to develop standards for the target delineation of the normal, uninvolved head and neck anatomy. Clear definitions for six neck levels and three neck sublevels were initially proposed by the American Head and Neck Society and the Committee for Head and Neck Surgery and Oncology of the American Academy of Otolaryngology – Head and Neck Surgery.[44] These have been continually updated and refined.[45] They were initially translated for the radiation oncology community by the proposal of the so-called Brussels and Rotterdam guidelines.[46,47] Subsequently, consensus guidelines for all major cooperative groups in Europe (DAHANCA, EORTC, GORTEC) and North America (RTOG, NCIC) have been developed and endorsed for delineation of nodal levels in the node-negative, non–surgically violated neck, taking into account the predictable patterns of lymph node drainage and tumor spread in the previously

untreated head and neck region.[23] They are now available on the RTOG Web site (http://www.rtog.org/atlases/hnatlas/main.html).

To date, no such consensus has been developed for the node-positive or postoperative setting. In general, gross lymph nodes and nodes with extracapsular extension are covered with larger CTV contours. The surgical bed should be treated in its entirety. Detailed discussion of neck node level definitions and of which levels need to be covered for each primary subsite is beyond the scope of this chapter. Automated atlas-based delineation to automate the process of target delineation is currently under investigation, but its usefulness in routine practice remains to be proven.[48] In early tests, a small improvement in accuracy and shortened contouring time was noted, but the most significant reason for contour variability remained the interreader variability in interpretation of the images.[27]

Magnetic Resonance Imaging

Magnetic resonance imaging is superior to CT with respect to visualization of soft tissue, as its imaging parameters can be manipulated, so that even soft tissues with similar electron densities can be easily discriminated.[43] It is an excellent tool for determining the extent of disease in the nasopharynx, paranasal sinuses, masticator space, parotid gland, tongue, skull base, retropharyngeal space, and parapharyngeal space.[24,30,43] In addition, MR is able to detect bone marrow involvement,[29] cartilage invasion[49–51] (in particular direct invasion of the thyroid cartilage), and has identified up to 40% more intracranial extension than CT.[52] In nasopharyngeal carcinoma, MR has been found to significantly affect staging in up to 50% of cases compared with CT imaging.[53,54]

Furthermore, MR is superior in detecting perineural invasion (PNI)[55] which represents a complicating factor in the locoregional treatment of head and neck tumors. When extending into the skull base, the tumor is usually considered unresectable. It is associated with increased risk for local recurrence and poor outcome and especially relevant for adenoid-cystic, mucoepidermoid, and nasopharyngeal carcinomas, as well as squamous cell carcinomas of the skin.[29,56–59]

Microscopic metastases and extranodal spread in small lymph nodes remain one of the most challenging scenarios in lymph node staging of the head and neck. King et al. found MR to be equivalent to CT in its sensitivity and specificity for extranodal spread.[60] Extracapsular extension (ECE) or extranodal spread has been found to be an important factor for nodal control, which has significant implications on prognosis and treatment planning.[61] On MR, signs suspicious for ECE include large nodal size, irregular nodal margins on gadolinium-enhanced T1-weighted sequences ("shaggy margins"), and high-intensity signal in the soft tissue around a metastatic node on fat-suppressed T2-weighted sequences ("flare" sign).[62]

Furthermore, MR is a good adjunct method for assessment of invasion of the mandible, especially minimal inner cortex invasion and involvement of the medulla. Computed tomography often fails to detect subtle signs of involvement because of the irregular shape of the inner cortex, dental sockets, dental fillings, or infections.[63–65] One prospective study found MR to have excellent sensitivity and specificity of 93% and 93%, respectively, for mandibular involvement from oral and oropharyngeal squamous cell carcinoma.[63]

Despite much improvement in multiplanar reconstruction of CT images, MR continues to have a particular advantage in determining the craniocaudal tumor extent on true sagittal or coronal slices because of the direct multiplanar image acquisition.[29,30,43] This is especially true for invasion along vertical fascial planes such as the prevertebral, pretracheal, or superficial fascia.[43]

In addition, MR is more useful in patients with tumors that are hypodense on CT, but hyperintense on T1- and intermediate on T2-weighted images such as liposarcomas.[29,65] It may be used as an adjunct or alternative to CT in patients with iodine allergies or with thyroid tumors, where iodinated contrast agents may need to be avoided in order not to interfere with future radio-iodine therapy.

Contraindications for the use of MR include pacemaker or defibrillator implants, claustrophobia, cerebral aneurysm clips, and cochlear implants.[41] Other disadvantages include the costliness of MR scanning[41] and the length of the examination, which can be challenging for head and neck patients with swallowing difficulties, pooling of secretions, and respiratory problems.[67] Because of the length of the examination, MR is prone to motion artifacts. Therefore, its usefulness is limited in restless patients and in the evaluation of moving organs, such as the larynx and hypopharynx.[49]

Many new MR techniques are currently being investigated, including diffusion-weighted imaging, dynamic contrast-enhanced MR, MR spectroscopy (MRS), ultrafast imaging, superparamagnetic iron oxide contrast agents, cine-mode acquisitions, and 3 Tesla (T) scanners. They may allow for even better soft tissue differentiation, account for tumor and/or organ motion, provide clearer distinction between benign and malignant lymph node involvement, and detect mandibular invasion more accurately. They may also facilitate better insight into the biologic state of tumors, including the level of hypoxia, edema, and necrosis, and markers of angiogenesis, such as blood volume, perfusion, microvessel density, and vessel permeability.[43,65,68–74]

Magnetic resonance spectroscopy allows analysis of the tissue composition and metabolic state, which may be used as complementary information to the anatomical detail provided by CT and MR.[75] Also, MRS has the potential to aid with target delineation, as it can reveal tumor areas that may not be contrast-enhancing. It may also have prognostic value and assist in the early recognition of tumor recurrence. It is currently mainly limited by the large voxel size available with a spatial resolution of a maximum of 6 mm to 10 mm.[76] This may continue to improve over the coming years. However, to date, experience with MRS in the head and neck region has been limited, as most MRS studies have looked at brain and prostate cancer.

Mack and colleagues looked at the sensitivity and specificity of ultrasmall superparamagnetic iron oxide particles that are taken up by the reticuloendothelial tissues of normal lymph nodes in the head and neck and found them to be 86% and 100%, respectively. The minimum transverse diameter of the lymph nodes involved ranged from 8 mm to 40 mm.[77]

Magnetic resonance has been used for treatment planning purposes. Initially the attempt was made to superimpose sagittal and coronal planes from MR on radiographs.[78] With CT imaging becoming the standard cross-sectional imaging modality for treatment planning, MR fusion has become more attractive and feasible as an adjunct technique. Magnetic resonance–based GTVs have been found to be smaller, to improve exact tumor extension delineation, and to decrease the interobserver variation in contours compared with GTVs based on CT imaging only, because of fewer artifacts.[52,67] See Chapter 16B for a discussion of the utility of MR-based target delineation in a patient with a nasopharyngeal tumor.

Subsequently, open MR scanners were developed to allow for radiation treatment simulation. Although they initially only used low magnetic fields,[79,80] modern MR simulators now use up to 1.0 T magnetic fields. A prototype of a hybrid 1.5-T MR with an integrated 6-MV linear accelerator for MR-guided IGRT is under construction.[81] However, MR simulators are not widely available at this time.

Because MR does not provide any information about electron density and harbors a potential risk for image distortion, it cannot be directly used for radiation treatment planning and dosimetric calculations.[43] Magnetic resonance image distortions occur because of inhomogeneities in the magnetic field (system-induced) or the patient inside the scanner himself (object-induced). Distortions of up to 10 mm have been reported by most studies, especially significant with increasing distance from the magnetic isocenter in larger fields of view.[82,83] Therefore, MR images have to be evaluated and corrected, if necessary, for any image distortion before treatment planning to avoid systematic errors. Various algorithms and correction methods have been developed to at least partially account for these distortions,[83,84] but there continues to be a lack of optimized software for integration of MR information into treatment planning systems.[82]

Another disadvantage of MR simulators is that digitally reconstructed radiographs (DRRs) cannot be automatically calculated because of the lack of information of bony anatomy; different techniques have been suggested to solve this dilemma, including a contour-based wire frame reconstruction.[85] In contrast to the pelvis or the central nervous system, where most studies have found disagreement of CT- and MR-based dose calculations of 2% or less,[86–88] manual assignment of photon attenuation coefficients for RT planning purposes is neither practicable nor reliable in complex, heterogeneous anatomic areas such as the head and neck. Therefore, image fusion of the MR data set with the planning CT remains the preferred method for MR integration in head and neck treatment planning. Emami and coworkers[53] found that fusion of CT and MR for planning purposes in nasopharyngeal carcinoma revealed that the MR-based target volumes were 74% larger and their shape was more irregular than the targets outlined based on CT alone. Computed tomography and MR appeared to be complementary. Care must be taken to image the patient in the exact treatment position and with the same specifications as for simulation to achieve accurate fusion. The desired sequence, resolution, slice thickness, and region of interest should be predetermined, and the MR obtained close to the time of simulation.[53]

An accurate assessment of the presence or absence of PNI is also critical to tailor therapy accordingly and provide appropriate coverage during target delineation.[89] All involved major cranial nerves need to be traced back to the skull base when one is contouring patients with PNI to avoid locoregional failures that will have very limited salvage options.[57,58] For patients with neck dissection who were found to have ECE, the CTV should be more generous and cover the overlying skin.

Intrinsic susceptibility-weighted, blood oxygenation–level dependent MR for hypoxia imaging has been tested, but was found to not be sufficiently reproducible for RT planning in patients with head and neck cancers.[14]

Positron Emission Tomography

Positron emission tomography scanning depicts metabolically active areas that take up ^{18}F-fluorodeoxyglucose (^{18}F-FDG) and, therefore, allows functional imaging beyond the mere anatomical structure. The detection rate for head and neck primary tumors using PET has been estimated as 88% to 98%.[90–92] Positron emission tomography has an overall higher sensitivity than either CT or MR.[92–94] Also, PET has a higher sensitivity and specificity of up to 96% to 100% for evaluating nodal involvement.[95–98] (Figure 16-1) However, when the sensitivity and specificity of PET in the clinically node-negative neck was compared to the gold standard of a neck dissection, PET

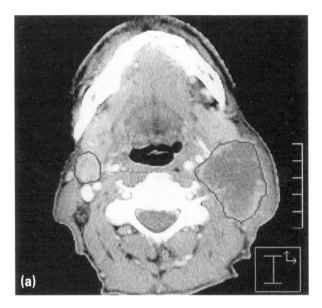

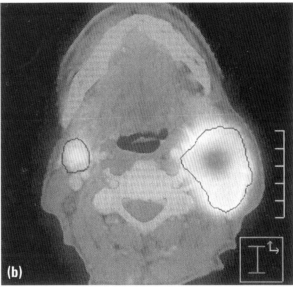

FIGURE 16-1. Example of the use of ^{18}F-fluorodeoxyglucose (^{18}F-FDG) positron emission tomography–computed tomography (PET–CT) for defining the gross tumor volume. **(a)** Axial planning CT scan and **(b)** PET–CT image on the same slice. The blue contours represent the CT-identified lymph nodes. Reproduced with permission from Schwartz et al.[97]

was found to have a high number of false-positive findings and limited sensitivity in detecting micrometastases despite an approximate incidence of 25% to 50% of occult metastases found on pathological specimen.[99,100]

Compared with CT or MR, PET imaging has been found to affect TNM staging in 15% to 36% of patients.[101–105] Whole body PET scanning has the advantage of detecting occult distant metastases that may significantly change the recommended treatment course.[106] It has been found to detect distant metastases or secondary tumors in 24% to 31% of head and neck cancer patients staged with CT or MR leading to a change in management in 15% to 31% of patients.[101,102] It is therefore the staging modality of choice for locally advanced head and neck cancer. It has also been found to be useful in patients with unknown primary tumors in the head and neck region metastatic to the cervical lymph nodes, where PET was able to correctly identify the primary tumor in about 50% (47% to 56%) of cases.[105,107]

Integrated PET–CT, which allows coregistration of anatomic and metabolic information in one session, has been described to have a sensitivity of as high as 98%, a specificity of up to 92%, and an accuracy of up to 96% in patients with head and neck cancer, superior to PET and CT obtained separately.[108,109]

Similar to CT and MR, limitations of PET include poor detection of very small and superficial primary tumors. Evaluation by PET can further be complicated when the tumor is located near tissues with physiologically intense ^{18}F-FDG uptake, including salivary tissues, Waldeyer's ring, muscles, and the larynx, especially when patients speak during the ^{18}F-FDG uptake phase.[14,110] It has also been found to be inferior to MR in the evaluation of parotid neoplasms.[111]

Another drawback of PET imaging is its low spatial resolution of 4 mm to 5 mm, which results in poor anatomic detail. Fortunately, the lack of anatomic detail can be largely overcome by coregistering the PET with a CT. Ciernik and colleagues found PET–CT coregistration to have an accuracy of 2.1 mm or less.[112] In addition, PET imaging involves exposure to radioactive ^{18}F-FDG and possibly iodine, when performed in combination with a CT scan.[1,99]

There is considerable variability in the threshold levels chosen for target delineation in patients with head and neck cancer, and no consensus has been reached so far.[112-114] Several trials have been conducted to investigate the impact of PET–CT versus CT alone for target volume delineation. Eight of nine studies found significant changes with the introduction of PET–CT in the volume of GTV and/or PTV. The results of these studies are summarized in Table 16-4.

Greco and coworkers tested four different methods of GTV delineation based on visual estimation, a 50% maximum standardized uptake value (SUV) threshold, a 2.5 SUV absolute threshold, and an iterative segmentation algorithm that were compared with a reference volume created based on the simulation CT and diagnostic MR data.[114] Visual estimates and tumor volumes were not significantly different from the reference GTV. The 2.5 SUV absolute threshold did not differ from the reference GTVs, but included some 18F-FDG-avidity in normal tissues, such as the laryngeal muscles. The GTVs derived from the 50% maximum SUV threshold technique and iterative segmentation algorithm resulted in significantly smaller target volumes.

Automatic thresholding based on "source-to-background ratios," as it is commonly used in nuclear medicine, has been tested for target delineation.[115,116] This method depends on the size, shape, and contrast of the lesion of interest, and is generally more prone to error in smaller lesions (< 4 mL to 8 mL).[116] Newer gradient-based methods have been developed and have been found to be more accurate, especially in areas with more background noise. In a small series of laryngeal tumors, the gradient-based method estimated the tumor volume more accurately than the "source-to-background ratio" method.[117] These results will have to be validated on a larger scale.

As of now, although highly desirable, no single automated method has emerged as clearly superior to the others. A phase II study to determine the feasibility of PET-based automatic segmentation of the GTV is ongoing.[25] In addition, automated algorithms cannot replace the judicious evaluation of the experienced contouring physician who takes both clinical and radiographic aspects into account for the patient's RT plan.

Gardner and colleagues showed that MR–CT fusion images and combined PET–CT scans, all taken in the treatment position with a thermoplastic mask, allowed for diagnostic image quality and assessment, RT treatment planning and target delineation, and decreased interobserver variability of the parotid gland volumes and GTVs.[118]

The optimal margin width for target delineation based on PET in patients with head and neck cancer remains unclear.[105] Currently, it is common practice to expand the GTV to include all PET-positive disease and to apply standard margins for CTV-to-PTV expansions. Soto and colleagues confirmed that most locoregional failures in a group of 61 patients recurred within the biological target volume defined on a pretherapy PET–CT with all failures occurring within the GTV, indicating that PET–CT provides reliable information for target delineation.[119] In general, this approach includes a larger target volume and may thus be a safer way to avoid marginal failures.[25] To date, the clinical outcome of patients planned on PET–CT scanners in smaller series has been favorable compared with historic controls, although no prospective randomized trials have been published comparing PET–CT based treatments with conventional or CT-based plans.[120] Thus, these results may be subject to many confounders, including improved IMRT techniques, more accurate coverage of regions at risk, and improved systemic therapies. In fact, studies investigating the benefit of IMRT irrespective of the use of PET–CT have shown similar results.[5,11]

Whether ^{18}F-FDG PET has prognostic value remains a subject of great discussion. Whereas some studies have found poorer local control and disease-free survival with higher SUV pretreatment using various cut-offs, others have not been able to identify any predictive value of SUV in the primary tumor or nodal metastases.[6,120-123] A

TABLE 16–4 Head and Neck Cancer: Target Delineation With Positron Emission Tomography–Computed Tomography (PET–CT) Versus CT Alone

Study	Population	N	PET Thresholding Technique	GTV	PTV	Comment/Conclusion
Nishioka et al.[113]	Oropharynx (n = 12) and nasopharynx (n = 9) carcinoma	21	Brain cortex boundary as internal reference	No change in 89% of patients	N/A	PET fusion with MRI–CT: 3 cases of superficial primary tumors not detected by PET; parotid sparing improved in 71% of patients with adjacent PET-negative lymph nodes
Ciernik et al.[112]	Solid tumors (n = 39), including various head and neck primary carcinomas (n = 12)	39	40% of background-subtracted tumor maximum uptake	PET–CT changed GTV ≥ 25% in 6 of 12 patients (50%) (17% ↑GTV; 33% ↓GTV)	20% (± 5%) difference in PTV	Interobserver variability significantly decreased with PET–CT; upstaging with distant metastases in 16% of patients with PET–CT
Wang et al.[191]	Various primary carcinomas of the head and neck	28	SUV > 2.5	CT > PET–CT volumes by 11% to 40% in 9 patients; PET–CT > CT volumes by 14% to 31% in 5 patients	N/A	Staging change in 16 of 28 patients (57%) with PET–CT
Ashamalla et al.[192]	Various primary carcinomas of the head and neck	25	Anatomic biologic halo (thickness 2.02 mm ± 0.21 mm; SUV 2.19 ± 0.28)	PET–CT changed GTV ≥ 25% in 17 of 25 patients (68%)	N/A	Increased concordance (≤ 10% volume discrepancy) and decreased interobserver variability with PET–CT
Newbold et al.[105]	Various primary carcinomas of the head and neck (n = 9 with unknown primary)	18	50% of maximum count density	GTV increased by 74%	PTV increased by 7%.	Upstaging in 8 of 18 patients (44%); identification of primary tumor in 5 of 9 (56%) patients with unknown primary
Guido et al.[193]	Various primary carcinomas of the head and neck	38	50% of tumor maximum	PET–CT < CT volumes in 35 of 38 patients (92%)	PET–CT < CT volumes in 35 of 38 patients (92%), not significant	Staging change in 6 of 38 patients (5 upstaged, 1 downstaged)
Heron et al.[194]	Various primary carcinomas of the head and neck	21	SUV normalized to 18F-FDG liver uptake	PET–CT < CT volumes in all patients for primaries, but not for nodal regions	N/A	3 primary tumors missed on CT, none missed on PET–CT.
El-Bassiouni et al.[195]	Various primary carcinomas of the head and neck	25	Threshold of background-subtracted tumor maximum uptake	PET–CT < CT volumes in 18 of 25 patients (72%); PET–CT > CT volumes in 7 of 25 patients (28%)	Same as GTV	
Scarfone et al.[196]	Various primary carcinomas of the head and neck	6	50% of maximum intensity	PET–CT > CT volumes by 15% (average 3.3 cm³)	N/A	

Notes. CT = computed tomography; 18F-FDG = fluorodeoxyglucose; GTV = gross tumor volume; MRI = magnetic resonance imaging; PET = positron emission tomography; PTV = planning target volume; SUV = standardized uptake value.

phase I study, in which the 18F-FDG-avid tumor volume within the GTV was boosted, found that four out of nine local recurrences were located in the boost volume, which confirms the assumption that these areas represent especially aggressive and resistant tumor subvolumes and the fact that dose escalation to those boost volumes beyond our current abilities is needed. The maximum tolerated dose was not reached and the dose escalation was well-tolerated.[25,119] Boosting such areas, ideally 60% to 80% of the GTV, to 120% to 130% of the prescription dose may theoretically improve the tumor control probability from 50% up to 75% according to a standard linear-quadratic algorithm.[123] Ling et al.[127] referred to this technique as

"dose painting IMRT." Hot spots and dose inhomogeneities within the GTV may in select cases even allow steeper dose gradients toward normal tissue structures, if necessary, to achieve a higher boost dose.[124,125] In the future, "dose painting by numbers," proportional to the intensity of a PET, single photon emission computed tomography (SPECT), or dynamic MR/MRS signal, may become available.[126]

Newer PET developments have focused on the functional abilities of PET and the development of tracers that can demonstrate biological processes within the tumor. This would add valuable information beyond the metabolic activity measured by FDG or the purely anatomical information on CT or MR and could be used for the design of biological target volumes.[126]

Hypoxia is a known poor prognostic factor contributing to radioresistance of a tumor, decreased locoregional control, disease-free survival, and overall survival.[128–130] In one study, pretherapy nodal status and the ratio of mean tumor uptake of ^{18}F-fluoromisonidazole (^{18}F-MISO) over maximum blood signal as an expression of tumor hypoxia were associated with decreased overall survival.[131] Up to 78% of patients with advanced head and neck cancer have been found to have significant hypoxia.[128,131] Causes of hypoxia include tumors outgrowing their blood and oxygen supply, aberrant blood vessel formation as a result of angiogenesis and vasculogenesis, and fluctuation in blood flow because of variation of blood vessel tonus.[10] Hypoxia, in turn, causes cells to be relatively radioresistant, because the lack of oxygen decreases the production of free radicals that mediate radiation-induced DNA damage. Therefore, efforts have been made to specifically target areas of chronic hypoxia with more aggressive treatment, such as dose escalation. In addition, a small, but significant, benefit in locoregional control and survival has been noted with the use of hypoxia cell sensitizers.[132]

Although the gold standard for hypoxia measurements remains P_{O_2} histography with an Eppendorf microelectrode, this method is neither clinically feasible nor practical because of its invasiveness and interobserver variability. Nonetheless, accurate imaging of tumor hypoxia is critical to reliably escalate radiation doses to potentially more resistant subsections of the tumor. Although several markers have been developed to image tumor hypoxia, "there is not, and probably will never be, a single clear 'gold standard' for in vivo hypoxia measurement."[133] Exogenous hypoxia tracers for PET that measure chronic hypoxia include ^{18}F-MISO, Cu(II)-diacetyl-bis-(N4-methylthiosemicarbazone) (Cu-[ATSM]), and ^{18}F-fluoroazomycinarabino-furanoside (^{18}F-FAZA). There have also been attempts to use endogenous markers for biologic hypoxia. These include HIF-1, CA-IX, Glut-1, OPN, and VEGF.[10,134] However, these may be less tumor- and hypoxia-specific than exogenous markers.

^{18}F-MISO is a fluorinated radiotracer commonly used in hypoxia imaging. It was developed from the hypoxic radiosensitizer misonidazole and selectively localizes to areas of hypoxia. Dose escalation to 80 Gy and 84 Gy, respectively, using ^{18}F-MISO- or Cu-(ATSM)–based target delineation has been found to be feasible and achievable using IMRT, meeting all standard normal tissue constraints.[135,136] However, variability of ^{18}F-MISO uptake between the two scans, which were 3 days apart, was considerable, thereby decreasing the reliability of the ^{18}F-MISO signal as a marker for chronic hypoxia.[137] This temporal variability of hypoxia may be the most significant obstacle for hypoxia-targeted radiotherapy, as it raises concerns about the changes in hypoxia that occur

between hypoxia imaging, treatment planning, and treatment initiation. These changes may be attributable to regional subacute blood flow alteration and subsequent redistribution of hypoxia, as well as patient positioning errors. Hypoxia-targeted treatment itself may likely change the intratumoral hypoxia patterns as well and may require multiple rounds of plan adaptation.[138] How to account for treatment-induced changes or other changes in the tumor microenvironment during the treatment course is unclear at this point.

Clear target delineation for tumors with a heterogeneous hypoxic pattern is especially challenging. Busk and colleagues described that hypoxic regions in tumors with patchy hypoxic patterns were overlooked with the use of the hypoxia marker ^{18}F-FAZA because of averaging and thresholding.[138]

Other factors that currently detract from the resolution and reliability of hypoxia imaging by PET include the absence of a specific uptake mechanism for hypoxia tracers, a pathway length of up to greater than 100 μm between the vessels and the target cells, and the slow rate of tracer washout from nonhypoxic tissue areas that is necessary for good contrast development.[138]

^{18}F-FAZA appears to have a better tumor-to-background ratio than ^{18}F-MISO, as it is cleared faster from the blood pool and normal tissues.[128,139] A disadvantage of ^{18}F-MISO PET related to this problem may be the relatively short half-life of ^{18}F of about 110 minutes. Late imaging more than 24 hours postinjection may improve the contrast between hypoxic areas and background signal.[106]

Alternative tracers with longer half lives have been investigated including Cu-(ATSM).[136] Cu-(ATSM) is a copper chelate that is irreversibly reduced in hypoxic tissues and retained, while it is quickly washed out from normoxic tissues. Unfortunately, more recent data from animal models have indicated that Cu-(ATSM) may have too high of an intertumoral variability in uptake to be a routinely used hypoxia tracer.[140] Other markers that have been studied, but are not routinely used yet because of problems with low sensitivity and specificity include radiolabeled amino acids, such as O-(2-^{18}F]fluoroethyl)-L-tyrosine (FET) and ^{18}F]galacto-RGD to measure angiogenesis by $\alpha_v\beta_3$ expression[141]; deoxy-^{18}F-fluorothymidine (FLT), which is taken up by proliferating cells in DNA synthesis[142]; markers of EGFR expression[143]; and 1-^{11}C]-acetate (ACE), which is taken up into the lipid pool in cells with high lipid synthesis rate.[144] In a phase I study, ACE correctly detected metastatic carcinoma in 20 of 21 lymph nodes and resulted in larger tumor volumes than FDG–PET. The ACE-based tumor volumes were 51% larger than FDG-based contours.[144] However, additional work is required to confirm these early results and to establish the role of these new tracers.[106,144] See Chapters 16A, 16C, and 16D for illustrations of PET-based target delineation in patients with head and neck cancers.

Image-Guided Treatment Delivery

Image guided–IMRT involves the acquisition of pretreatment or intratreatment diagnostic quality imaging in the treatment room and comparison of the images with the target delineation in the treatment plan. The perfect image guidance system should provide three-dimensional (3D) soft tissue information, and efficient and rapid image acquisition and comparison, as well as an efficient adaptation and intervention in response to the level of congruence found.[145]

The goal of IG-IMRT is to minimize systematic daily patient setup errors, which is crucial because of the close margins and steep dose gradients associated with IMRT. Absolute certainty about patient positioning is also critical in the setting of re-irradiation near critical structures or hypofractionated treatments to still allow adequate protection of normal tissues. This is particularly relevant in areas of critical organs, such as the brainstem, optic chiasm, or spinal cord. Besides variation in target delineation, systematic daily setup errors may stem from the patient's weight loss, tumor shrinkage, organ motion during treatment, geometric setup errors on the machine table, and equipment tolerances.[27] Previous data suggest that three to five repeat images followed by weekly verification films should be sufficient to minimize systematic setup errors.[146] Random errors should be taken into account by expanding the CTV with sufficient margin to obtain the PTV.[16,145]

Routine use of IG-IMRT for patients on treatment may be used to determine if and when replanning should be performed. This may be especially relevant in patients with bulky disease at presentation, as they may undergo greater changes than smaller tumors while on treatment. Weight loss has been shown to cause an increase in radiation dose to the spinal cord that now can be quantified more specifically because of the ability to image frequently during treatment.[19,147,148]

Imaging at the time of treatment has become increasingly available through the use of planar EPIDs (see Chapter 16E) and built-in kilovoltage (kV) imaging capabilities on linear accelerators. These devices can be used with CBCT.[149] This allows for frequent verification of patient and tumor position between fractions and even during radiation delivery to minimize intrafractional motion.[24]

Planar Imaging

Two-dimensional (2D) imaging is quick and offers close to real-time verification of the target position and its variation. It also allows for on- or off-line correction based on fiducials or surrogates.[150] As such, it has been shown to be useful for evaluating setup errors, verifying margin adequacy, and comparing immobilization devices.[17,150,151]

Initially, planar electronic portal imaging devices (EPIDs) used the megavoltage (MV) treatment beam for portal imaging. Two-dimensional MV imaging usually requires the use of fiducial markers and has been tested in head and neck cancer.[152] However, specifically in the head and neck region, 2D MV imaging with a well-planned correction protocol alone may be sufficient, as bony landmarks can be reliably used for positioning of target and critical structures.[24,153] Therefore, fiducial markers are not routinely used in head and neck cancer. Although isocenter positioning is generally very accurate as shown by daily orthogonal MV portal imaging, there is much greater variability in shoulder position, leading to an underdosing error of less than 95% of the prescribed dose.[154] Although weekly MV portal images for setup verification remain the standard at many institutions, more advanced, easy-to-use on-treatment imaging techniques are rapidly leading to a more frequent use of image guidance on treatment.

Kilovoltage imaging is made possible by attaching a separate imaging unit to the treatment machine. Although it makes for a more expensive machine, the image quality is higher than for MV images. Kilovoltage imaging is especially useful with the use of fiducials or reliable bony anatomy markers.

One study with 14 patients found no significant differences between 2D kV and MV radiographs when applied in a variety of sites. However, for the neck region and particularly the larynx, kV localization was associated with a reduced setup error rate compared with MV images.[155] A study from our institution using an orthogonal onboard kV imaging unit (OBI) for head and neck cancer found that translational setup errors were –0.1 cm ± 0.3 cm in the anterior–posterior, 0.0 cm ± 0.2 cm in the right–left, and –0.2 cm ± 0.3 cm in the superior–inferior directions, with rotational errors less than 3°. Intrafractional errors were small and random.[18] A clear and systematic approach and protocol for portal imaging with clear guidelines for setup error corrections may make it possible to reduce the CTV–PTV margins to 3 mm to 4 mm.[151] At our institution, we routinely use 2D kV imaging for all patients undergoing re-irradiation to the same region.

Volumetric Imaging

Volumetric imaging, though more time-consuming, includes significantly more information on soft tissue structures, target volumes without surrogates, or fiducial markers and can be overlaid with the treatment plan to verify dose distributions. There are various technologies that allow the acquisition of CBCTs. They include MV CTs obtained on the linear accelerator or on integrated MV CT systems, such as tomotherapy units; a separate CT scanner in the treatment room that is aligned with the linear accelerator; a C-arm CT scanner; or an onboard kV CT.[149]

Similar to portal imaging, MV-based CBCT uses the treatment beam for generating a CBCT by performing a full-gantry rotation around the patient. The advantage is that no additional hardware or dedicated machine is required and that the imaging and treatment beam are easily aligned, because the images are generated by the treatment beam.[149] With daily MV CT and automatic deformable registration techniques it has been shown that the volume of the parotid glands decreased by 21% at a rate of 0.7% per day during RT. The parotid glands appeared to lose more volume during the earlier phase of RT and moved 5.3 mm toward the center of the patient overall.[156]

Helical tomotherapy has been explored for similar use with the added advantage of high mechanical stability of the helical scanner and a high accuracy with an error of less than 1 mm or 1°.[157] The MV CT scan can also be coregistered with the planning CT scan for automation of target localization and patient positioning. In addition, CT detectors can measure the delivered dose and reconstruct it using the exit dose, which has the potential to be used for in vivo dosimetry and adaptive planning.[149] The disadvantages of 3D MV imaging are that soft tissue contrast is poor compared with kV imaging; however, high-Z artifacts are usually not as problematic as in kV imaging. Chapter 16F provides an illustration of the use of helical tomotherapy in a patient with advanced tonsillar cancer.

Kilovoltage-based cone-beam imaging and subsequent 3D reconstruction is becoming increasingly common (see Chapter 16G). It provides exquisite soft tissue resolution and excellent bone definition on the treatment machine with an image quality close to diagnostic helical CT.[158] It therefore allows target localization and setup correction based on the actual tumor rather than on surrogate bony landmarks, thus reducing systematic and random errors to a minimum. However, the image quality has not quite reached the quality of dedicated diagnostic scanners because of the fact that onboard kV imaging uses onboard flat-panel detectors that are subject to greater scatter, mechanical instability, and organ motion during imaging.[149] Some systems are attached to the linear accelerator orthogonal to the gantry, which allows for stereoscopic planar imaging when one is combining kV imaging with the onboard unit and MV imaging with the EPID. Others are attached in line with the gantry, which allows imaging in the axis of the treatment beam.

Repeat volumetric imaging and replanning has been shown to be essential in reducing the volume of normal tissue doses in head and neck cancer.[148] Rescanning of patients on days 11, 22, and 33 of their treatment in a CT scanner revealed that rotational and translational variation of the skull, mandible, and cervical spine position is overall small during treatment progression, but with a significant range of random variation of up to 21° or 16 mm, respectively, especially in the positioning of the mandible and lower cervical spine.[158] Barker and coworkers obtained kV CT images on 14 head and neck cancer patients three times per week on an integrated CT–linear accelerator system. The GTV, external contour, and parotid glands significantly changed in their shape and geometry over the course of a definitive external RT treatment. The GTVs decreased asymmetrically by a median of 1.8% per treatment day to a median total relative loss of 69.5% of the initial GTV; this decrease was most significant during the second half of the treatment. A medial shift of the parotid glands by a median of 3.1 mm correlating with patient's weight loss was observed as well.[147]

How frequently imaging for target position verification should be applied is not clear at this point. Although it may appear tempting to verify the target position with every treatment, it may not be necessary or cost-efficient for every standard fractionation treatment regimen.[145] Frequent imaging may also cause the workload of treatment planning staff, physicians, and radiation therapists to grow exponentially and reach a level that is not justifiable for small clinical improvement.[160] Unfortunately, it is challenging to measure the improvement in clinical outcome, as there is likely never going to be a randomized trial comparing IMRT with IG-IMRT. However, one should not forget that perfect geometric positioning of the tumor and the patient are not the only factors in the cure for cancer. Instead, a better understanding of the natural history, biology, and tumor response to treatment are of great importance and will also improve target delineation and planning.

Another concern is the increase in integral dose to the patient from frequent imaging. Several authors found that the patient dose is lower and image quality better with kV imaging compared to MV imaging.[161] Also, kV imaging has been found to provide superior visualization of soft tissue.[145] Even so, the dose from daily kV CBCT can accumulate up to about 300 cGy, delivering 5 cGy to 8 cGy per fraction, over the course of a fractionated treatment.[162] For a 2-Gy-per-fraction prescription of an IMRT plan, Perks and coworkers found up to 1 cGy peripheral dose per scan at 20 cm from the central axis outside the CBCT volume.[163] An attempt to reduce dose from OBI using digital tomosynthesis has been presented by Wu and colleagues. In contrast to CBCT, which uses a full 360° gantry rotation, this technique involves limited gantry rotation angles to create a stack of slices but is comparable to CBCT in the level of positioning variation for head and neck IMRT.[164] Long-term data are needed to measure the impact of this slight increase in low-dose radiation on long-term sequelae and second malignancy rates.[160]

In the future, advanced imaging using MR or PET may allow tracking of biological and physiological characteristics on treatment and dose distributions adjusted in real time.[24] Whether all these advances in on-line imaging with their theoretical advantages will translate into improved clinical outcomes remains to be proven.[145]

Future Directions

Adaptive IGRT

Cone-beam CT not only allows for more accurate daily setup of the patient, but also provides information on soft tissue and tumor size changes during treatment. It thereby facilitates the identification of the time point during treatment at which the change in anatomy is significant enough to warrant replanning.

As mentioned previously, Barker and coworkers found in a pilot study from M.D. Anderson Cancer Center that the GTV, external contour, and parotid glands significantly changed in shape and geometry over the course of a definitive external RT treatment.[147] Hansen and colleagues looked at a series of locally advanced head and neck tumors and found reduced coverage of the target volumes in 92% of patients and a dose reduction of up to 7.4 Gy to the CTV. They also identified an increase in D_{max} to the spinal cord in all patients of up to 15.4 Gy above the prescribed dose and a dose increase to the brainstem in 85% of patients because of tumor shrinkage or weight loss. This was demonstrated on a new hybrid IMRT plan on the basis of a second CT scan during treatment, which was performed based on the clinical judgment of the treating physician[148] (Figure 16-2). Similar increases in dose to the parotid glands and the spinal cord were identified by MV CT on a tomotherapy unit by Han et al.[165] In contrast to these studies, Mechalakos et al. described a case of a recurrent neck mass with an unusually high decrease of 45% tumor volume.[166] Weekly kV CBCTs were obtained and research treatment plans were developed. In the absence of setup errors, the tumor volume shrinkage led to a decrease in dose to the spinal cord because of decreased scatter from the overlying tissue. Dose to the PTV, mandible, and oral cavity slightly increased in this case. The authors concluded that replanning in this case was necessary, not because of dose distribution changes, but only because of setup errors and suboptimal immobilization after the significant tumor response. Such significant changes in the anatomy are commonly seen in head and neck radiation oncology. They raise the question of developing and adjusting an adaptive treatment plan that takes these changes into account.[147]

Treatment planning based on a kV CBCT is readily available with several software packages allowing quick determination of the dose distributions delivered. It is therefore an attractive option for adaptive replanning. Its feasibility has been tested in phantoms and in patients. It

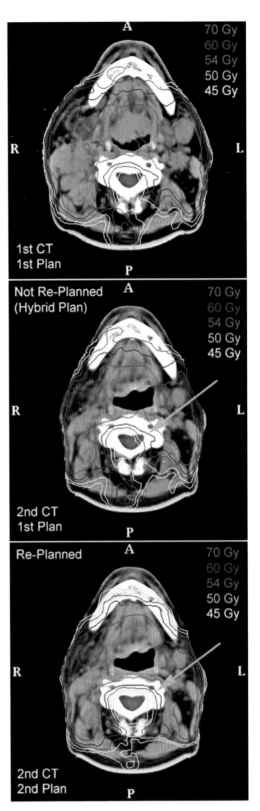

FIGURE 16-2. Illustration of the use of multiple computed tomography (CT) scans during the course of treatment. The upper image shows the planning CT scan with isodose curves overlaid. The middle image was obtained after 22 fractions, and shows the dosimetric effect of patient weight loss. The lower image shows the new dose distribution after replanning. Reproduced with permission from Hansen et al.[147]

was found to carry a dosimetric error of up to 3% in inhomogeneous phantoms with good agreement of isodose distributions and differences of less than 2 mm between CBCT-based plans and diagnostic CT-based plans.[167] Others have also described agreement of CBCT-based dosimetric prediction and conventional CT-based planning within 3%.[168,169] Tanyi and coworkers found the use of volumetric OBI imaging to lead to an increased demand of adaptive replanning of up to 23% of patients on study that were replanned at least once because of changes in tumor size, weight loss, and systematic setup errors. The need for replanning was higher in conventional fractionation regimens than in hypofractionated treatment courses. In more than 91% of repeat plans there was a discrepancy between the new and the original plan of greater than 5% for 10% or more of the target volume and critical normal structures, respectively. The mean dose to the parotid gland was decreased by 23.5% in a case presentation after replanning in week 5.[170] The best timing for planning of an adaptive RT plan is under investigation. A cutoff of greater than 30% decrease in the volume of the GTV has been suggested, but currently no clear guidelines exist.[170]

Intensity deformation algorithms that adjust the designed radiation treatment plan to the anatomic changes during RT near real time may allow us to circumvent the labor intensity of multiple rounds of replanning.[171] Deformable registration of kV- and MV-based CBCTs has been tested.[171,172] It involves several steps including accurate image registration, measures of anatomy changes, deformation of dose accumulation to the time point of image registration, automatic recontouring, or deformation of contours.[172] However, the development of deformable registration methods is much more challenging than comparing dose distributions that assume rigid and homogeneous transformations.[173] Current automatic online adaptive RT methods have limitations when patient position and target shapes change significantly, and more work in this direction is clearly necessary before it can be implemented in routine clinical use.[174] These methods are therefore not yet able to obviate the need for reliable and reproducible immobilization.

It may not be possible to completely eliminate geometrical errors that would allow margins to be reduced to zero. There will remain a certain level of CTV variability as well as errors in the imaging system detection, organ motion between image verification and treatment, and accuracy of the setup corrections.[16] The PTV margins, however, have potential to be further reduced to an absolute minimum (e.g., 3 mm) with the use of daily imaging and subsequent setup correction.[175]

Image-guided RT will not only improve the accuracy of setup and treatment delivery, but will also be a critical part of translating diagnostic functional and molecular imaging into a treatment outcome improvement. Functional imaging has already changed our way of thinking about tumor biology and will continue to affect RT planning and delivery.[126] The integration of imaging molecular and functional changes over time has been termed "theragnostic imaging." It may be used to modulate and adapt radiotherapy to the live processes and changes within a tumor undergoing treatment. Early attempts to image specific pathways, such as hypoxia inducible factor (HIF)-1α transcriptional activity with PET, have been successful in preclinical experiments.[176] Such approaches open the door to unprecedented individualization of tumor treatment based on signal transduction pathways that are activated or inactivated in any given tumor. Epidermal growth factor receptor (EGFR) expression and pathways represent another potential marker for theragnostic imaging in head and neck cancer.

"Dose painting by numbers" with automated dose escalation to areas of unfavorable expression of markers such as hypoxia tracer ^{18}F-MISO as surrogates for more radioresistant tumor subsites has been successfully tested for feasibility, with a potential increase in local tumor control from 55.9% to 70.2%.[177,178] However, further validation of functional imaging targets is needed before these can be routinely used for targeted treatment delivery. Also, the relationship between the signal intensity of a given surrogate marker and the required optimal additional boost dose remains to be investigated. As seen in the area of hypoxia imaging, the temporal stability of the detected signals is crucial. It is unclear at this point how acute changes in hypoxia will affect the overall sensitivity of tumor subsites.[126]

Image-guided RT may allow dose escalation and decreased dose to normal tissue because of even smaller margins as we are able to better define the target location, thus improving the therapeutic ratio. In some sites, including the brain, spine, and lung, single-dose stereotactic body radiation has already shown some early successes. To what degree a hypofractionated approach can also be translated to the head and neck region remains to be seen.[145] Nonetheless, IGRT at the very least provides the treating physician with greater freedom to choose a fractionation regimen that previously may not have been possible because of excessive dose to normal tissues.

Newer technologies for photon delivery such as intensity-modulated arc therapy (IMAT) are currently being implemented. The advantages of delivering the entire treatment in a single 360° gantry rotation in less than 2 minutes possibly include even higher conformality, easier plan optimization because of the absence of beam numbers and angles, and very high efficiency in treatment delivery. Because it can be installed on a regular linear accelerator, it provides very high flexibility in usage of the machine. Quality assurance tests of the RapidArc IMAT system (Varian Medical Systems, Palo Alto, CA) have demonstrated that the dose distribution and delivery is very reliable with good agreement of the dose 1% or less compared with stationary mode or open field, even with modulation of gantry rotation range and speed, dynamic leaf motion, and dose rates.[179] The dose distribution has been found to be comparable or even slightly superior to tomotherapy because of the ability to deliver non-coplanar arcs with IMAT.[28] If used at a resolution of 2.5 mm or less, the dosimetric accuracy of RapidArc plans was found to be acceptable in a series of six oropharynx cases using a Monte Carlo algorithm.[180] The disadvantage of IMAT is that the multileaf collimator (MLC) leaves have to move across the target volume several times during the treatment to achieve complex dose distributions. This may require a total treatment time of greater than 2 minutes to achieve a satisfying quality level of the dose distribution. Bortfeld and Webb have therefore suggested inclusion of the total treatment time as a variable into treatment planning systems for IMAT to strike the right balance between quality and efficiency. Other factors that have to be accounted for in the treatment planning of IMAT are the finite MLC leaf speed and acceleration, the speed and acceleration of the gantry rotation in itself and relative to the MLC motion, and dose rate.[181] The radiation delivery from 360° spreads out low dose levels over large tissue volumes, thus potentially increasing the integrated dose.

Protons carry the promise of being able to treat tumors with high conformality and in very close proximity to critical structures without delivering a significant dose to structures at risk, such as the spinal cord, the optic nerves, the chiasm, or the brain. Mean doses to organs at risk can be decreased by up to 62%.[175,182] Studies comparing photon and proton plans for paranasal sinus tumors and advanced head and neck tumors found that protons were more powerful in preserving normal tissue dose constraints with acceptable target coverage and homogeneity.[183–184] However, long-term data are not available yet. Early results suggest that local control rates are comparable to photon radiation with minimal toxicity.[185,186] Intensity-modulated proton therapy (IMPT) is likely going to be the next step in developing the use of protons even further. Preliminary studies have already shown the advantage of IMPT over photon IMRT in higher conformality, thus sparing normal tissue and improving target coverage while using fewer beams.[187,188] Particle radiation using carbon ions is another field of interest because of its high linear energy transfer. It has been found to provide high local control rates with low toxicities for melanomas and adenoid-cystic carcinomas of the head and neck in a dose escalation study.[189]

Conclusions

The rapid advancements in IGRT in recent years have allowed us to visualize patient anatomy in exquisite and unprecedented detail. The development of IMRT has given us the ability to conform dose with a high level of precision, even too high at times, so that we need to build in "safety margins" for the uncertainties that we were unable to measure. This has changed with the advent of IGRT, which enables us to image the tumor and surrounding tissue in near real-time. With improved understanding of the uncertainties, we will be able to decrease margin widths. In addition, we are likely going to move from targeting purely structural abnormalities of cancer to increasingly targeting pathophysiological processes. Much is to be expected from new tracers for proliferation, angiogenesis, hypoxia, receptor status, gene expression levels, and apoptosis, to name a few.[190] The ever-advancing field of medical physics is already providing us with extraordinary tools of dose delivery and verification. We are likely going to see another revolution with the increasing availability of real-time imaging during treatment, arc therapy, and proton and particle radiation. A better understanding of the underlying biology of head and neck tumors will guide us in the selection of our targets for radiation therapy.

References

1. Ahn PH, Garg MK. Positron emission tomography/computed tomography for target delineation in head and neck cancers. *Sem Nuc Med.* 2008;38:141–148.
2. Eisbruch A, Levendag PC, Feng FY, et al. Can IMRT or brachytherapy reduce dysphagia associated with chemoradiotherapy of head and neck cancer? The Michigan and Rotterdam experiences. *Int J Radiat Oncol Biol Phys.* 2007;69, S40–S42.
3. Eisbruch A, Schwartz M, Rasch C, et al. Dysphagia and aspiration after chemoradiotherapy for head-and-neck cancer: which anatomic structures are affected and can they be spared by IMRT? *Int J Radiat Oncol Biol.* 2004; 60:1425–1439.
4. Lee NY, de Arruda FF, Puri DR, et al. A comparison of intensity-modulated radiation therapy and concomitant boost radiotherapy in the setting of concurrent chemotherapy for locally advanced oropharyngeal carcinoma. *Int J Radiat Oncol Biol Phys.* 2006;66:966–974.
5. Daly ME, Lieskovsky Y, Pawlicki T, et al. Evaluation of patterns of failure and subjective salivary function in patients treated with intensity modulated radiotherapy for head and neck squamous cell carcinoma. *Head Neck.* 2007;29:211–220.
6. Kam MKM, Leung SF, Zee B, et al. Prospective randomized study of intensity-modulated radiotherapy on salivary gland function in early-stage nasopharyngeal carcinoma patients. *J Clin Oncol.* 2007;25:4873–4879.
7. Wolden SL, Chen WC, Pfister DG, et al. Intensity-modulated radiation therapy (IMRT) for nasopharynx cancer: update of the Memorial Sloan-Kettering experience. *Int J Radiat Oncol Biol Phys.* 2006;64:57–62.
8. Gomez DR, Zhung JE, Gomez J, et al. Intensity-modulated radiotherapy in postoperative treatment of oral cavity cancers. *Int J Radiat Oncol Biol Phys.* 2009;73:1096–1103.

9. Ben-David MA, Diamante M, Radawski JD, et al. Lack of osteo-radionecrosis of the mandible after intensity-modulated radiotherapy for head and neck cancer: likely contributions of both dental care and improved dose distributions. *Int J Radiat Oncol Biol Phys.* 2007;68:396–402.

10. Lee NY, Le QT. New developments in radiation therapy for head and neck cancer: intensity-modulated radiation therapy and hypoxia targeting. *Sem Oncol.* 2008; 35:236–250.

11. Lee N, Xia P, Fischbein NJ, et al. Intensity-modulated radiation therapy for head-and-neck cancer: the UCSF experience focusing on target volume delineation. *Int J Radiat Oncol Biol Phys.* 2003;57:49–60.

12. De Arruda FF, Puri DR, Zhung J, et al. Intensity-modulated radiation therapy for the treatment of oropharyngeal carcinoma: The Memorial Sloan-Kettering Cancer Center experience. *Int J Radiat Oncol Biol Phys.* 2006;64:363–373.

13. Bernier J, Bentzen SM. Radiotherapy for head and neck cancer: latest developments and future perspectives. *Curr Opin Oncol.* 2006;18:240–246.

14. Newbold K, Partridge M, Cook G, et al. Advanced imaging applied to radiotherapy planning in head and neck cancer: a clinical review. *Br J Radiol.* 2006;79:554–561.

15. Daisne JF, Duprez T, Weynand B, et al. Tumor volume in pharyngolaryngeal squamous cell carcinoma: comparison at CT, MR imaging, and FDG PET and validation with surgical specimen. *Radiology.* 2004;233:93–100.

16. Van Herk M. Errors and margins in radiotherapy. *Sem Rad Oncol.* 2004;14:52–64.

17. Gilbeau L, Octave-Prignot M, Loncol T, et al. Comparison of setup accuracy of three different thermoplastic masks for the treatment of brain and head and neck tumors. *Radiother Oncol.* 2001;58:155–162.

18. Mechalakos JG, Hunt MA, Lee NY, et al. Using an onboard kilovoltage imager to measure setup deviation in intensity-modulated radiation therapy for head-and-neck patients. *J Appl Clin Med Phys.* 2007;8:2439.

19. Hong TS, Tome WA, Chappell RJ, et al. The impact of daily setup variations on head-and-neck intensity-modulated radiation therapy. *Int J Radiat Oncol Biol Phys.* 2005;61:779–788.

20. Astreinidou E, Bel A, Raaijmakers CPJ, et al. Adequate margins for random setup uncertainties in head-and-neck IMRT. *Int J Radiat Oncol Biol Phys.* 2005;61:938–944.

21. Hamlet S, Ezzell G, Aref A. Larynx motion associated with swallowing during radiation therapy. *Int J Radiat Oncol Biol Phys.* 1994;28:467–470.

22. Kubicek GJ, Machtay M. New advances in high-technology radiotherapy for head and neck cancer. *Hem Onc Clin N Am.* 2008;22:1165–1180.

23. Gregoire V, Levendag P, Ang KK, et al. CT-based delineation of lymph node levels and related CTVs in the node-negative neck: DAHANCA, EORTC, GORTEC, NCIC, RTOG consensus guidelines. *Radiother Oncol.* 2003;69:227–236.

24. Greco C, Ling CC. Broadening the scope of image-guided radiotherapy (IGRT). *Acta Oncol.* 2008;47:1193–1200.

25. Eisbruch A, Gregoire V. Balancing risk and reward in target delineation for highly conformal radiotherapy in head and neck cancer. *Sem Radiat Oncol.* 2009;19:43–52.

26. Eisbruch A, Foote RL, O'Sullivan B, et al. Intensity-modulated radiation therapy for head and neck cancer: emphasis on the selection and delineation of the targets. *Sem Radiat Oncol.* 2002; 12:238–249.

27. Rasch C, Steenbakkers R, Van Herk M. Target definition in prostate, head, and neck. *Sem Radiat Oncol.* 2005;15:136–145.

28. Cao D, Holmes TW, Afghan MKN, et al. Comparison of plan quality provided by intensity-modulated arc therapy and helical tomotherapy. *Int J Radiat Oncol Biol Phys.* 2007;69:240–250.

29. Alberico RA, Husain SHS, Sirotkin I. Imaging in head and neck oncology. *Surg Oncol Clin N Am.* 2004;13:13–35.

30. Yousem DM, Som PM, Hackney DB, et al. Central nodal necrosis and extracapsular neoplastic spread in cervical lymph nodes: MR imaging versus CT. *Radiology.* 1992;182:753–759.

31. Atula TS, Varpula MJ, Kurki TJI, et al. Assessment of cervical lymph node status in head and neck cancer patients: palpation, computed tomography and low field magnetic resonance imaging compared with ultrasound-guided fine-needle aspiration cytology. *Eur J Radiol.* 1997;25:152–161.

32. Curtin HD, Williams R, Johnson J. CT of perineural tumor extension: Pterygopalatine fossa. *Am J Roentgenol.* 1985;144: 163–169.

33. Stevens MH, Harnsberger HR, Mancuso AA. Computed tomography of cervical lymph nodes. Staging and management of head and neck cancer. *Arch Otolaryngol.* 1985;111:735–739.

34. Curtin HD, Ishwaran H, Mancuso AA, et al. Comparison of CT and MR imaging in staging of neck metastases. *Radiology.* 1998;207:123–130.

35. Lenz M, Kersting-Sommerhoff B, Gross M. Diagnosis and treatment of the NO neck in carcinomas of the upper aerodigestive tract: current status of diagnostic procedures. *Eur Arch Otorhinolaryngol.* 1993;250:432–438.

36. Van Den Brekel MWM. Lymph node metastases: CT and MRI. *Eur J Radiol.* 2000;33:230–238.

37. Merritt RM, Williams MF, James TH, et al. Detection of cervical metastasis: a meta-analysis comparing computed tomography with physical examination. *Arch Otolaryngol Head Neck Surg.* 1997;123:149–152.

38. Lell M, Baum U, Greess H, et al. Head and neck tumors: imaging recurrent tumor and post-therapeutic changes with CT and MRI. *Eur J Radiol.* 2000;33:239–247.

39. Gor DM, Langer JE, Loevner LA. Imaging of cervical lymph nodes in head and neck cancer: the basics. *Radiol Clin N Am.* 2006;44:101–110.

40. O'Daniel JC, Rosenthal DI, Garden AS, et al. The effect of dental artifacts, contrast media, and experience on interobserver contouring variations in head and neck anatomy. *Am J Clin Oncol.* 2007;30:191–198.

41. Som PM. The present controversy over the imaging method of choice for evaluating the soft tissues of the neck. *Am J Neuroradiol.* 1997;18:1869–1872.

42. Sherouse GW, Bourland JD, Reynolds K, et al. Virtual simulation in the clinical setting: some practical considerations. *Int J Radiat Oncol Biol Phys.* 1990;19:1059–1065.

43. Khoo VS, Joon DL. New developments in MRI for target volume delineation in radiotherapy. *Br J Radiol.* 2006;79: S2–S15.

44. Robbins KT, Medina JE, Wolfe GT, et al. Standardizing neck dissection terminology. Official report of the Academy's Committee for Head and Neck Surgery and Oncology. *Arch Otolaryngol Head Neck Surg.* 1991;117:601–605.

45. Robbins KT, Shaha AR, Medina JE, et al. Consensus statement on the classification and terminology of neck dissection. *Arch Otolaryngol Head Neck Surg.* 2008;134:536–538.

46. Gregoire V, Coche E, Cosnard G, et al. Selection and delineation of lymph node target volumes in head and neck conformal radiotherapy. Proposal for standardizing terminology and procedure based on the surgical experience. *Radiother Oncol.* 2000;56:135–150.

47. Nowak PJCM, Wijers OB, Lagerwaard FJ, et al. A three-dimensional CT-based target definition for elective irradiation of the neck. *Int J Radiat Oncol Biol Phys.* 1999;45:33–39.

48. Commowick O, Gregoire V, Malandain G. Atlas-based delineation of lymph node levels in head and neck computed tomography images. *Radiother Oncol.* 2008;87:281–289.

49. Rumboldt Z, Gordon L, Bonsall R, et al. Imaging in head and neck cancer. *Curr Treat Options Oncol.* 2006;7:23–34.

50. Becker M, Burkhardt K, Dulguerov P, et al. Imaging of the larynx and hypopharynx. *Eur J Radiol.* 2008;66:460–479.

51. Castelijns JA, Gerritsen GJ, Kaiser MC, et al. Invasion of laryngeal cartilage by cancer: comparison of CT and MR imaging. *Radiology.* 1988;167:199–206.

52. Chung NN, Ting LL, Hsu WC, et al. Impact of magnetic resonance imaging versus CT on nasopharyngeal carcinoma: primary tumor target delineation for radiotherapy. *Head Neck.* 2004;26:241–246.

53. Liao XB, Mao YP, Liu LZ, et al. How does magnetic resonance imaging influence staging according to AJCC staging system for nasopharyngeal carcinoma compared with computed tomography? *Int J Radiat Oncol Biol Phys.* 2008;72:1368–1377.

54. Emami B, Sethi A, Petruzzelli GJ. Influence of MRI on target volume delineation and IMRT planning in nasopharyngeal carcinoma. *Int J Radiat Oncol Biol Phys.* 2003;57:481–488.

55. Nemzek WR, Hecht S, Gandour-Edwards R, et al. Perineural spread of head and neck tumors: how accurate is MR imaging? *Am J Neuroradiol.* 1998;19:701–706.

56. Garden AS, Weber RS, Morrison WH, et al. The influence of positive margins and nerve invasion in adenoid cystic carcinoma of the head and neck treated with surgery and radiation. *Int J Radiat Oncol Biol Phys.* 1995;32:619–626.

57. Mendenhall WM, Amdur RJ, Williams LS, et al. Carcinoma of the skin of the head and neck with perineural invasion. *Head Neck.* 2002;24:78–83.

58. Sham JST, Cheung YK, Choy D, et al. Cranial nerve involvement and base of the skull erosion in nasopharyngeal carcinoma. *Cancer.* 1991;68:422–426.

59. Fagan JJ, Collins B, Barnes L, et al. Perineural invasion in squamous cell carcinoma of the head and neck. *Arch Otolaryngol Head Neck Surg.* 1998;124:637–640.

60. King AD, Tse GMK, Yuen EHY, et al. Comparison of CT and MR imaging for the detection of extranodal neoplastic spread in metastatic neck nodes. *Eur J Radiol.* 2004;52:264–270.

61. Vergeer MR, Doornaert P, RenLeemans C, et al. Control of nodal metastases in squamous cell head and neck cancer treated by radiation therapy or chemoradiation. *Radiother Oncol.* 2006;79:39–44.

62. Kimura Y, Sumi M, Sakihama N, et al. MR imaging criteria for the prediction of extranodal spread of metastatic cancer in the neck. *Am J Neuroradiol.* 2008;29:1355–1359.

63. Bolzoni A, Cappiello J, Piazza C, et al. Diagnostic accuracy of magnetic resonance imaging in the assessment of mandibular involvement in oral-oropharyngeal squamous cell carcinoma: a prospective study. *Arch Otolaryngol Head Neck Surg.* 2004;130:837–843.

64. Shaha AR. Preoperative evaluation of the mandible in patients with carcinoma of the floor of mouth. *Head Neck.* 1991;13:398–402.

65. Van Cann EM, Rijpkema M, Heerschap A, et al. Quantitative dynamic contrast-enhanced MRI for the assessment of mandibular invasion by squamous cell carcinoma. *Oral Oncol.* 2008;44:1147–1154.

66. Patel SC, Silbergleit R, Talati SJ. Sarcomas of the head and neck. *Topics Magn Res Imaging.* 1999;10:362–375.

67. Toonkel LM, Soila K, Gilbert D, et al. MRI assisted treatment planning for radiation therapy of the head and neck. *Magn Reson Imaging.* 1988;6:315–319.

68. Leach MO, Brindle KM, Evelhoch JL, et al. The assessment of antiangiogenic and antivascular therapies in early-stage clinical trials using magnetic resonance imaging: issues and recommendations. *Br J Cancer.* 2005;92:1599–1610.

69. Wang J, Takashima S, Takayama F, et al. Head and neck lesions: characterization with diffusion-weighted echo-planar MR imaging. *Radiology.* 2001;220:621–630.

70. Wycliffe ND, Grover RS, Kim PD, et al. Hypopharyngeal cancer. *Topics Magn Reso Imaging.* 2007;18:243–258.

71. Star-Lack JM, Adalsteinsson E, Adam MF, et al. In vivo 1H MR spectroscopy of human head and neck lymph node metastasis and comparison with oxygen tension measurements. *Am J Neuroradiol.* 2000;21:183–193.

72. Anzai Y, Prince MR. Iron oxide-enhanced MR lymphography: the evaluation of cervical lymph node metastases in head and neck cancer. *J Magn Res Imaging.* 1997;7:75–81.

73. Friedrich KM, Matzek W, Gentzsch S, et al. Diffusion-weighted magnetic resonance imaging of head and neck squamous cell carcinomas. *Eur J Radiol.* 2008;68:493–498.

74. Neeman M, Provenzale JM, Dewhirst MW. Magnetic resonance imaging applications in the evaluation of tumor angiogenesis. *Sem Radiat Oncol.* 2001;11:70–82.

75. Harrison RM. Imaging in radiotherapy treatment planning and delivery. *Br J Radiol.* 2006;79:S1.

76. Payne GS, Leach MO. Applications of magnetic resonance spectroscopy in radiotherapy treatment planning. *Br J Radiol.* 2006;79:S16–S26.

77. Mack MG, Balzer JO, Straub R, et al. Superparamagnetic iron oxide-enhanced MR imaging of head and neck lymph nodes. *Radiology.* 2002;222:239–244.

78. Potter R, Heil B, Schneider L, et al. Sagittal and coronal planes from MRI for treatment planning in tumors of brain, head and neck: MRI assisted simulation. *Radiother Oncol.* 1992;23:127–130.

79. Weber DC, Wang H, Albrecht S, et al. Open low-field magnetic resonance imaging for target definition, dose calculations and

set-up verification during three-dimensional CRT for glioblastoma multiforme. *Clin Oncol.* 2008;20:157–167.

80. Mizowaki T, Nagata Y, Okajima K, et al. Development of an MR simulator: experimental verification of geometric distortion and clinical application. *Radiology.* 1996;199:855–860.

81. Lagendijk JJW, Raaymakers BW, Raaijmakers AJE, et al. MRI/linac integration. *Radiother Oncol.* 2008;86:25–29.

82. Khoo VS, Dearnaley DP, Finnigan DJ, et al. Magnetic resonance imaging (MRI): considerations and applications in radiotherapy treatment planning. *Radiother Oncol.* 1997;42:1–15.

83. Fransson A, Andreo P, Potter R. Aspects of MR image distortions in radiotherapy treatment planning. *Strahlen Onkol.* 2001;177:59–73.

84. Tanner SF, Finnigan DJ, Khoo VS, et al. Radiotherapy planning of the pelvis using distortion corrected MR images: the removal of system distortions. *Phys Med Biol.* 2000;45:2117–2132.

85. Chen L, Nguyen TB, Jones E, et al. Magnetic resonance-based treatment planning for prostate intensity-modulated radiotherapy: creation of digitally reconstructed radiographs. *Int J Radiat Oncol Biol Phys.* 2007;68:903–911.

86. Schad LR, Bluml S, Hawighorst H, et al. Radiosurgical treatment planning of brain metastases based on a fast, three-dimensional MR imaging technique. *Magn Res Imaging.* 1994;12:811–819.

87. Lee YK, Bollet M, Charles-Edwards G, et al. Radiotherapy treatment planning of prostate cancer using magnetic resonance imaging alone. *Radiother Oncol.* 2003;66:203–216.

88. Chen L, Price RA Jr, Wang L, et al. MRI-based treatment planning for radiotherapy: dosimetric verification for prostate IMRT. *Int J Radiat Oncol Biol Phys.* 2004;60:636–647.

89. Lee KJ, Abemayor E, Sayre J, et al. Determination of perineural invasion preoperatively on radiographic images. *Otolaryngol Head Neck Surg.* 2008;139:275–280.

90. Hannah A, Scott AM, Tochon-Danguy H, et al. Evaluation of 18F-Fluorodeoxyglucose positron emission tomography and computed tomography with histopathologic correlation in the initial staging of head and neck cancer. *Ann Surg.* 2002;236:208–217.

91. Paulus P, Sambon A, Vivegnis D, et al. 18FDG-PET for the assessment of primary head and neck tumors: clinical, computed tomography, and histopathological correlation in 38 patients. *Laryngoscope.* 1998;108:1578–1583.

92. Greven KM, Williams DW III, Frederick McGuirt W Sr, et al. Serial positron emission tomography scans following radiation therapy of patients with head and neck cancer. *Head Neck.* 2001;23:942–946.

93. Kutler DI, Wong RJ, Kraus DH. Functional imaging in head and neck cancer. *Curr Oncol Rep.* 2005;7:137–144.

94. Wong WL, Chevretton EB, McGurk M, et al. A prospective study of PET-FDG imaging for the assessment of head and neck squamous cell carcinoma. *Clin Otolaryngol Allied Sci.* 1997;22:209–214.

95. Kau RJ, Alexiou C, Laubenbacher C, et al. Lymph node detection of head and neck squamous cell carcinomas by positron emission tomography with fluorodeoxyglucose F 18 in a routine clinical setting. *Arch Otolaryngol Head Neck Surg.* 1999;125:1322–1328.

96. Adams S, Baum RP, Stuckensen T, et al. Prospective comparison of 18F-FDG PET with conventional imaging modalities (CT, MRI, US) in lymph node staging of head and neck cancer. *Eur J Nucl Med.* 1998;25:1255–1260.

97. Schwartz DL, Ford E, Rajendran J, et al. FDG-PET/CT imaging for preradiotherapy staging of head-and-neck squamous cell carcinoma. *Int J Radiat Oncol Biol Phys.* 2005;61:129–136.

98. Ng SH, Yen TC, Chang JTC, et al. Prospective study of [18F] fluorodeoxyglucose positron emission tomography and computed tomography and magnetic resonance imaging in oral cavity squamous cell carcinoma with palpably negative neck. *J Clin Oncol.* 2006;24:4371–4376.

99. Stoeckli SJ, Steinert H, Pfaltz M, et al. Is there a role for positron emission tomography with 18F-fluorodeoxyglucose in the initial staging of nodal negative oral and oropharyngeal squamous cell carcinoma. *Head Neck.* 2002;24:345–349.

100. Schöder H, Carlson DL, Kraus DH, et al. 18F-FDG PET/CT for detecting nodal metastases in patients with oral cancer staged N0 by clinical examination and CT/MRI. *J Nucl Med.* 2006;47:755–762.

101. Goerres GW, Schmid DT, Grätz KW, et al. Impact of whole body positron emission tomography on initial staging and therapy in patients with squamous cell carcinoma of the oral cavity. *Oral Oncol.* 2003;39:547–551.

102. Ha PK, Hdeib A, Goldenberg D, et al. The role of positron emission tomography and computed tomography fusion in the management of early-stage and advanced-stage primary head and neck squamous cell carcinoma. *Arch Otolaryngol Head Neck Surg.* 2006;132:12–16.

103. Koshy M, Paulino AC, Howell R, et al. F-18 FDG PET-CT fusion in radiotherapy treatment planning for head and neck cancer. *Head Neck.* 2005;27:494–502.

104. Veit-Haibach P, Luczak C, Wanke I, et al. TNM staging with FDG-PET/CT in patients with primary head and neck cancer. *Eur J Nucl Med Mol Imaging.* 2007;34:1953–1962.

105. Newbold KL, Partridge M, Cook G, et al. Evaluation of the role of 18FDG-PET/CT in radiotherapy target definition in patients with head and neck cancer. *Acta Oncol.* 2008;47:1229–1236.

106. Garcia C, Flamen P. Role of positron emission tomography in the management of head and neck cancer in the molecular therapy era. *Curr Opin Oncol.* 2008;20:275–279.

107. Aassar OS, Fischbein NJ, Caputo GR, et al. Metastatic head and neck cancer: role and usefulness of FDG PET in locating occult primary tumors. *Radiology.* 1999;210:177–181.

108. Branstetter BF IV, Blodgett TM, Zimmer LA, et al. Head and neck malignancy: is PET/CT more accurate than PET or CT alone? *Radiology.* 2005;235:580–586.

109. Schöder H, Yeung HWD, Gonen M, et al. Head and neck cancer: clinical usefulness and accuracy of PET/CT image fusion. *Radiology.* 2004;231:65–72.

110. Greven KM. Positron-emission tomography for head and neck cancer. *Sem Radiat Oncol.* 2004;14:121–129.

111. McGuirt WF, Keyes JW Jr, Greven KM, et al. Preoperative identification of benign versus malignant parotid masses: a comparative study including positron emission tomography. *Laryngoscope.* 1995;105:579–584.

112. Ciernik IF, Dizendorf E, Baumert BG, et al. Radiation treatment planning with an integrated positron emission and computer tomography (PET/CT): a feasibility study. *Int J Radiat Oncol Biol Phys.* 2003;57:853–863.

113. Nishioka T, Shiga T, Shirato H, et al. Image fusion between 18FDG-PET and MRI/CT for radiotherapy planning of oropharyngeal and nasopharyngeal carcinomas. *Int J Radiat Oncol Biol Phys.* 2002;53:1051–1057.

114. Greco C, Nehmeh SA, Schoder H, et al. Evaluation of different methods of 18F-FDG-PET target volume delineation in the radiotherapy of head and neck cancer. *Am J Clin Oncol.* 2008;31:439–445.

115. Daisne JF, Sibomana M, Bol A, et al. Tri-dimensional automatic segmentation of PET volumes based on measured source-to-background ratios: influence of reconstruction algorithms. *Radiother Oncol.* 2003;69:247–250.

116. Jarritt PH, Carson KJ, Hounsell AR, et al. The role of PET/CT scanning in radiotherapy planning. *Br J Radiol.* 2006;79:S27–S35.

117. Geets X, Lee JA, Bol A, et al. A gradient-based method for segmenting FDG-PET images: methodology and validation. *Eur J Nucl Med Mol Imaging.* 2007;34:1427–1438.

118. Gardner M, Halimi P, Valinta D, et al. Use of single MRI and 18F-FDG PET-CT scans in both diagnosis and radiotherapy treatment planning in patients with head and neck cancer: advantage on target volume and critical organ delineation. *Head Neck.* 2009;31:461–467.

119. Soto DE, Kessler ML, Piert M, et al. Correlation between pretreatment FDG-PET biological target volume and anatomical location of failure after radiation therapy for head and neck cancers. *Radiother Oncol.* 2008;89:13–18.

120. Vernon MR, Maheshwari M, Schultz CJ, et al. Clinical outcomes of patients receiving integrated PET/CT-guided radiotherapy for head and neck carcinoma. *Int J Radiat Oncol Biol Phys.* 2008;70:678–684.

121. Brun E, Kjellén E, Tennvall J, et al. FDG PET studies during treatment: prediction of therapy outcome in head and neck squamous cell carcinoma. *Head Neck.* 2002;24:127–135.

122. Allal AS, Dulguerov P, Allaoua M, et al. Standardized uptake value of 2-[18F] gluoro-2-deoxy-D-glucose in predicting outcome in head and neck carcinomas treated by radiotherapy with or without chemotherapy. *J Clin Oncol.* 2002;20:1398–1404.

123. Schwartz DL, Rajendran J, Yueh B, et al. FDG-PET prediction of head and neck squamous cell cancer outcomes. *Arch Otolaryngol Head Neck Surg.* 2004;130:1361–1367.

124. Tome WA, Fowler JF. Selective boosting of tumor subvolumes. *Int J Radiat Oncol Biol Phys.* 2000;48:593–599.

125. Vineberg KA, Eisbruch A, Coselmon MM, et al. Is uniform target dose possible in IMRT plans in the head and neck? *Int J Radiat Oncol Biol Phys.* 2002;52:1159–1172.

126. Bentzen SM. Theragnostic imaging for radiation oncology: dose-painting by numbers. *Lancet Oncol.* 2005;6:112–117.

127. Ling CC, Humm J, Larson S, et al. Towards multidimensional radiotherapy (MD-CRT): biological imaging and biological conformality. *Int J Radiat Oncol Biol Phys.* 2000;47:551–560.

128. Rischin D, Fisher R, Peters L, et al. Hypoxia in head and neck cancer: studies with hypoxic positron emission tomography imaging and hypoxic cytotoxins. *Int J Radiat Oncol Biol Phys.* 2007;69:S61–S63.

129. Brizel DM, Sibley GS, Prosnitz LR, et al. Tumor hypoxia adversely affects the prognosis of carcinoma of the head and neck. *Int J Radiat Oncol Biol Phys.* 1997;38:285–289.

130. Brizel DM, Dodge RK, Clough RW, et al. Oxygenation of head and neck cancer: changes during radiotherapy and impact on treatment outcome. *Radiother Oncol.* 1999;53:113–117.

131. Rajendran JG, Schwartz DL, O'Sullivan J, et al. Tumor hypoxia imaging with [F-18] fluoromisonidazole positron emission tomography in head and neck cancer. *Clin Cancer Res.* 2006;12:5435–5441.

132. Overgaard J, Horsman MR. Modification of hypoxia-induced radioresistance in tumors by the use of oxygen and sensitizers. *Sem Radiat Oncol.* 1996;6:10–21.

133. Arbeit JM, Brown JM, Chao KSC, et al. Hypoxia: importance in tumor biology, noninvasive measurement by imaging, and value of its measurement in the management of cancer therapy. *Int J Radiat Oncol Biol Phys.* 2006;66:699–757.

134. Giaccia A, Siim BG, Johnson RS. HIF-1 as a target for drug development. *Nat Reviews Drug Disc.* 2003;2:803–811.

135. Lee NY, Mechalakos JG, Nehmeh S, et al. Fluorine-18-labeled fluoromisonidazole positron emission and computed tomography-guided intensity-modulated radiotherapy for head and neck cancer: a feasibility study. *Int J Radiat Oncol Biol Phys.* 2008;70:2–13.

136. Chao KSC, Bosch WR, Mutic S, et al. A novel approach to overcome hypoxic tumor resistance: Cu-ATSM-guided intensity-modulated radiation therapy. *Int J Radiat Oncol Biol Phys.* 2001;49:1171–1182.

137. Nehmeh SA, Lee NY, Schroder H, et al. Reproducibility of intratumor distribution of 18F-Fluoromisonidazole in head and neck cancer. *Int J Radiat Oncol Biol Phys.* 2008;70:235–242.

138. Busk M, Horsman MR, Overgaard J. Resolution in PET hypoxia imaging: voxel size matters. *Acta Oncol.* 2008;47:1201–1210.

139. Piert M, Machulla HJ, Picchio M, et al. Hypoxia-specific tumor imaging with 18F-fluoroazomycin arabinoside. *J Nucl Med.* 2005;46:106–113.

140. Yuan H, Schroeder T, Bowsher JE, et al. Intertumoral differences in hypoxia selectivity of the PET imaging agent 64Cu(II)-diacetyl-bis(N4-methylthiosemicarbazone). *J Nucl Med.* 2006;47:989–998.

141. Beer AJ, Haubner R, Sarbia M, et al. Positron emission tomography using [18F]Galacto-RGD identifies the level of integrin alpha(v)beta3 expression in man. *Clin Cancer Res.* 2006;12:3942–3949.

142. Salskov A, Tammisetti VS, Grierson J, et al. FLT: measuring tumor cell proliferation in vivo with positron emission tomography and 3'-Deoxy-3'-[18F]Fluorothymidine. *Sem Nucl Med.* 2007;37:429–439.

143. Pal A, Glekas A, Doubrovin M, et al. Molecular imaging of EGFR kinase activity in tumors with 124 I-labeled small molecular tracer and positron emission tomography. *Mol Imaging Biol.* 2006;8:262–277.

144. Sun A, Soٰrensen J, Karlsson M, et al. 1-[11C]-acetate PET imaging in head and neck cancer—a comparison with 18F-FDG-PET: implications for staging and radiotherapy planning. *Eur J Nucl Med Mol Imaging.* 2007;34:651–657.

145. Ling CC, Yorke E, Fuks Z. From IMRT to IGRT: frontierland or neverland? *Radiother Oncol.* 2006;78:119–122.

146. Bortfeld T, van Herk M, Jiang SB. When should systematic patient positioning errors in radiotherapy be corrected? *Phys Med Biol.* 2002;47:N297–N302.

147. Barker JL Jr, Garden AS, Ang KK, et al. Quantification of volumetric and geometric changes occurring during fractionated radiotherapy for head-and-neck cancer using an integrated CT/linear accelerator system. *Int J Radiat Oncol Biol Phys.* 2004;59:960–970.

148. Hansen EK, Bucci MK, Quivey JM, et al. Repeat CT imaging and replanning during the course of IMRT for head-and-neck cancer. *Int J Radiat Oncol Biol Phys.* 2006;64:355–362.

149. Verellen D, De Ridder M, Tournel K, et al. An overview of volumetric imaging technologies and their quality assurance for IGRT. *Acta Oncol.* 2008;47:1271–1278.

150. Prisciandaro JI, Frechette CM, Herman MG, et al. A methodology to determine margins by EPID measurements of patient setup variation and motion as applied to immobilization devices. *Med Phys.* 2004;31:2978–2988.

151. Van Lin ENJT, Van Der Vight L, Huizenga H, et al. Set-up improvement in head and neck radiotherapy using a 3D off-line EPID-based correction protocol and a customised head and neck support. *Radiother Oncol.* 2003;68:137–148.

152. Van Asselen B, Dehnad H, Raaijmakers CPJ, et al. Implanted gold markers for position verification during irradiation of head-and-neck cancers: a feasibility study. *Int J Radiat Oncol Biol Phys.* 2004;59:1011–1017.

153. Herman MG. Clinical use of electronic portal imaging. *Semin Radiat Oncol.* 2005;15:157–167.

154. Court LE, Wolfsberger L, Allen AM, et al. Clinical experience of the importance of daily portal imaging for head and neck IMRT treatments. *J Appl Clin Med Phys.* 2008;9:26–33.

155. Pisani L, Lockman D, Jaffray D, et al. Setup error in radiotherapy: on-line correction using electronic kilovoltage and megavoltage radiographs. *Int J Radiat Oncol Biol Phys.* 2000;47:825–839.

156. Lee C, Langen KM, Lu W, et al. Evaluation of geometric changes of parotid glands during head and neck cancer radiotherapy using daily MVCT and automatic deformable registration. *Radiother Oncol.* 2008;89:81–88.

157. Mackie TR, Kapatoes J, Ruchala K, et al. Image guidance for precise conformal radiotherapy. *Int J Radiat Oncol Biol Phys.* 2003;56:89–105.

158. Létourneau D, Wong JW, Oldham M, et al. Cone-beam-CT guided radiation therapy: technical implementation. *Radiother Oncol.* 2005;75:279–286.

159. Ahn PH, Ahn AI, Lee CJ, et al. Random positional variation among the skull, mandible, and cervical spine with treatment progression during head-and-neck radiotherapy. *Int J Radiat Oncol Biol Phys.* 2009;73:626–633.

160. Dawson LA, Sharpe MB. Image-guided radiotherapy: rationale, benefits, and limitations. *Lancet Oncol.* 2006;7:848–858.

161. Walter C, Boda-Heggemann J, Wertz H, et al. Phantom and in-vivo measurements of dose exposure by image-guided radiotherapy (IGRT): MV portal images vs. kV portal images vs. cone-beam CT. *Radiother Oncol.* 2007;85:418–423.

162. Ding GX, Coffey CW. Radiation dose from kilovoltage cone beam computed tomography in an image-guided radiotherapy procedure. *Int J Radiat Oncol Biol Phys.* 2009;73:610–617.

163. Perks JR, Lehmann J, Chen AM, et al. Comparison of peripheral dose from image-guided radiation therapy (IGRT) using kV cone beam CT to intensity-modulated radiation therapy (IMRT). *Radiother Oncol.* 2008;89:304–310.

164. Wu QJ, Godfrey DJ, Wang Z, et al. On-board patient positioning for head-and-neck IMRT: comparing digital tomosynthesis to kilovoltage radiography and cone-beam computed tomography. *Int J Radiat Oncol Biol Phys.* 2007;69:598–606.

165. Han C, Chen YJ, Liu A, et al. Actual dose variation of parotid glands and spinal cord for nasopharyngeal cancer patients during radiotherapy. *Int J Radiat Oncol Biol Phys.* 2008;70:1256–1262.

166. Mechalakos J, Lee N, Hunt M, et al. The effect of significant tumor reduction on the dose distribution in intensity-modulated radiation therapy for head and neck cancer: a case study. *Med Dosim.* 2009;34(3):250–255.

167. Yoo S, Yin FF. Dosimetric feasibility of cone-beam CT-based treatment planning compared to CT-based treatment planning. *Int J Radiat Oncol Biol Phys.* 2006;6:1553–1561.

168. Ding GX, Duggan DM, Coffey CW, et al. A study on adaptive IMRT treatment planning using kV cone-beam CT. *Radiother Oncol.* 2007;85:116–125.

169. Yang Y, Schreibmann E, Li T, et al. Evaluation of on-board kV cone beam CT (CBCT)-based dose calculation. *Phys Med Biol.* 2007;52:685–705.

170. Tanyi JA, Fuss MH. Volumetric image-guidance: does routine usage prompt adaptive re-planning? An institutional review. *Acta Oncol.* 2008;47:1444–1453.

171. Mohan R, Zhang X, Wang H, et al. Use of deformed intensity distributions for on-line modification of image-guided IMRT to account for interfractional anatomic changes. *Int J Radiat Oncol Biol Phys.* 2005;61:1258–1266.

172. Lu W, Olivera GH, Chen Q, et al. Deformable registration of the planning image (kVCT) and the daily images (MVCT) for adaptive radiation therapy. *Phys Med Biol.* 2006;51:4357–4374.

173. Ostergaard Noe K, De Senneville BD, Elstrom UV, et al. Acceleration and validation of optical flow based deformable registration for image-guided radiotherapy. *Acta Oncol.* 2008;47:1286–1293.

174. Court LE, Tishler RB, Petit J, et al. Automatic online adaptive radiation therapy techniques for targets with significant shape change: a feasibility study. *Phys Med Biol.* 2006;51:2493–2501.

175. Feng M, Eisbruch A. Future issues in highly conformal radiotherapy for head and neck cancer. *J Clin Oncol.* 2007;25:1009–1013.

176. Serganova I, Doubrovin M, Vider J, et al. Molecular imaging of temporal dynamics and spatial heterogeneity of hypoxia-

inducible factor-1 signal transduction activity in tumors in living mice. *Cancer Res.* 2004;64:6101–6108.

177. Thorwarth D, Eschmann SM, Paulsen F, et al. Hypoxia dose painting by numbers: a planning study. *Int J Radiat Oncol Biol Phys.* 2007;68:291–300.

178. Alber M, Paulsen F, Eschmann SM, et al. On biologically conformal boost dose optimization. *Phys Med Biol.* 2003;48: 763–774.

179. Ling CC, Zhang P, Archambault Y, et al. Commissioning and quality assurance of RapidArc radiotherapy delivery system. *Int J Radiat Oncol Biol Phys.* 2008;72:575–581.

180. Gagne IM, Ansbacher W, Zavgorodni S, et al. A Monte Carlo evaluation of RapidArc dose calculations for oropharynx radiotherapy. *Phys Med Biol.* 2008;53:7167–7185.

181. Bortfeld T, Webb S. Single-Arc IMRT? *Phys Med Biol.* 2009; 54:N2–N9.

182. Mock U, Georg D, Bogner J, et al. Treatment planning comparison of conventional, 3D conformal, and intensity-modulated photon (IMRT) and proton therapy for paranasal sinus carcinoma. *Int J Radiat Oncol Biol Phys.* 2004;58:147–154.

183. Lomax AJ, Goitein M, Adams J. Intensity modulation in radiotherapy: photons versus protons in the paranasal sinus. *Radiother Oncol.* 2003;66:11–18.

184. Cozzi L, Fogliata A, Lomax A, et al. A treatment planning comparison of 3D conformal therapy, intensity modulated photon therapy and proton therapy for treatment of advanced head and neck tumours. *Radiother Oncol.* 2001;61: 287–297.

185. Slater JD, Yonemoto LT, Mantik DW, et al. Proton radiation for treatment of cancer of the oropharynx: early experience at Loma Linda university medical center using a concomitant boost technique. *Int J Radiat Oncol Biol Phys.* 2005;62: 494–500.

186. Chan AW, Liebsch NJ. Proton radiation therapy for head and neck cancer. *J Surg Oncol.* 2008;97:697–700.

187. Steneker M, Lomax A, Schneider U. Intensity modulated photon and proton therapy for the treatment of head and neck tumors. *Radiother Oncol.* 2006;80:263–267.

188. Taheri-Kadkhoda Z, Björk-Eriksson T, Nill S, et al. Intensity-modulated radiotherapy of nasopharyngeal carcinoma: a comparative treatment planning study of photons and protons. *Radiat Oncol.* 2008;3:4.

189. Mizoe JE, Tsujii H, Kamada T, et al. Dose escalation study of carbon ion radiotherapy for locally advanced head-and-neck cancer. *Int J Radiat Oncol Biol Phys.* 2004;60:358–364.

190. Nimmagadda S, Ford EC, Wong JW, et al. Targeted molecular imaging in oncology: focus on radiation therapy. *Semin Radiat Oncol.* 2008;18:136–148.

191. Wang D, Schultz CJ, Jursinic PA, et al. Initial experience of FDG-PET/CT guided IMRT of head-and-neck carcinoma. *Int J Radiat Oncol Biol Phys.* 2006;65:143–151.

192. Ashamalla H, Guirguis A, Bieniek E, et al. The impact of positron emission tomography/computed tomography in edge delineation of gross tumor volume for head and neck cancers. *Int J Radiat Oncol Biol Phys.* 2007;68:388–395.

193. Guido A, Fuccio L, Rombi B, et al. Combined 18F-FDG-PET/CT imaging in radiotherapy target delineation for head-and-neck cancer. *Int J Radiat Oncol Biol Phys.* 2009;73:759–763.

194. Heron DE, Andrade RS, Flickinger J, et al. Hybrid PET-CT simulation for radiation treatment planning in head-and-neck cancers: a brief technical report. *Int J Radiat Oncol Biol Phys.* 2004;60:1419–1424.

195. El-Bassiouni M, Ciernik IF, Davis JB, et al. [18FDG] PET-CT-based intensity-modulated radiotherapy treatment planning of head and neck cancer. *Int J Radiat Oncol Biol Phys.* 2007;69:286–293.

196. Scarfone C, Lavely WC, Cmelak AJ, et al. Prospective feasibility trial of radiotherapy target definition for head and neck cancer using 3-dimensional PET and CT imaging. *J Nucl Med.* 2004;45:543–552.

^{18}F-FDG PET-Guided Target Delineation in a Patient with Hypopharyngeal Carcinoma

Case Study

Indira Madani, MD, PhD, Wilfried De Neve, MD, PhD

Patient History

A 65-year-old man presented with a 2-month history of odynophagia. On physical examination, multiple non-tender right jugulodigastric lymph nodes were noted. Direct laryngoscopy demonstrated a tumor arising in the right pyriform sinus involving the right arytenoid; there was no fixation of the true vocal cords. A computed tomography (CT) scan of the head and neck region revealed a 3.5 cm by 4 cm by 3 cm tumor mass in the right pyriform sinus with involvement of the right arytenoid. Two pathological right level II lymph nodes were noted, the largest measuring 2.5 cm. Biopsy of the primary tumor demonstrated invasive poorly differentiated squamous cell carcinoma. The remainder of the workup revealed no distant metastases.

A selective lymph node dissection on the right side was performed revealing two involved level II nodes, of which one had evidence of extracapsular extension. Pathology was consistent with squamous cell carcinoma. The tumor was thus staged as a T2N2bM0 hypopharyngeal cancer and the patient was enrolled on an in-house phase I clinical trial designed to homogenously escalate dose limited to the 18-fluorodeoxyglucose positron emission tomography (^{18}F-FDG PET)–defined subvolume within the gross tumor volume (GTV). Focal dose escalation was performed as an upfront simultaneously integrated boost (SIB) by using intensity-modulated radiotherapy (IMRT).

Simulation

For planning CT and ^{18}F-FDG PET imaging, the patient was positioned and immobilized with a thermoplastic mask and neck support. All images were acquired in the treatment position. Contrast-enhanced CT scanning of the head and neck region and thorax was performed with 2 mm and 5 mm adjacent slices inside and outside the macroscopic tumor region, respectively. Positron emission tomography imaging was performed within 1 week after the planning CT on a Siemens Exact HR+ camera (CTI, Knoxville, TN) operating in three-dimensional (3D) mode using an axial field of view of 26.675 cm (two bed positions, with 3.9 cm overlap between the two bed positions). The PET images were reconstructed with an ordered subset expectation maximization (OSEM) algorithm after Fourier rebinning.

Imaging and Target Delineation

All targets and organs at risk (OARs) were outlined on each CT image. Two GTVs were outlined for radiotherapy (RT) planning: the anatomical imaging (CT)-based GTV (GTV$_{CT}$) and biological imaging (PET)-based GTV (GTV$_{PET}$) (Figure 16A-1). The PET transmission scans were manually coregistered with planning CT images on our treatment planning system, (Pinnacle version 6.2b, Philips Medical Systems, Andover, MA). The GTV$_{PET}$

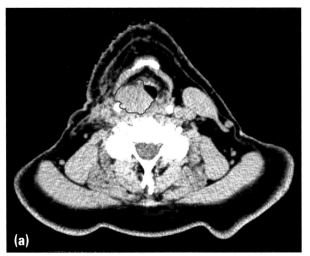

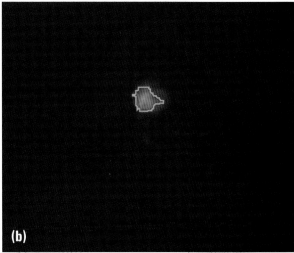

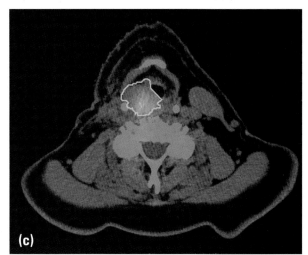

FIGURE 16A-1. Axial computed tomography (CT) **(a)**, 18-fluorodeoxy-glucose positron emission tomography (18F-FDG PET) slices, **(b)** indication of FDG-PET axial slices, and their fusion **(c)** illustrating the target volumes delineation for the presented case: *red*: the CT-based gross tumor volume (GTV$_{CT}$); *green*: the PET-based gross tumor volume (GTV$_{PET}$); *light blue*: the union gross tumor volume (GTV$_{union}$).

resulted from automatic segmentation of the 18F-FDG PET images based on the source-to-background ratio. The union GTV (GTV$_{union}$) encompassed both the GTV$_{CT}$ and the GTV$_{PET}$ (Figure 16A-1). The union clinical target volume (CTV$_{union}$) resulted from 3D expansion of the GTV$_{union}$ by adding a 1.5-cm margin with adjustment to exclude uninvolved bones and air cavities. In delineation of the elective neck CTV, international consensus guidelines were followed (Figure 16A-2).[1] For the CTVs of the elective neck and the CTV$_{union}$, a margin of 3 mm was added to generate the respective planning target volumes (PTVs). The PET-based PTV (PTV$_{PET}$) resulted from expansion of the GTV$_{PET}$ by a 3-mm margin. The volumes of contoured targets were for GTV$_{PET}$ = 6.8 cc; PTV$_{PET}$ = 18.4 cc; GTV$_{union}$ = 17.4 cc; and CTV$_{union}$ = 149.9 cc.

The following structures were outlined as OARs: the spinal cord, brainstem, parotid glands, and mandible. The spinal cord itself and the brainstem were expanded by 5-mm and 3-mm margins, respectively, to obtain the respective planning OAR volumes (PRVs). The following nonanatomical structures were automatically generated

for optimization purposes: PTV$_{whbu}$ and PTV$_{optim}$. Subtraction of a 6-mm-wide build-up region from the PTV resulted in the PTV without build-up (PTV$_{whbu}$). To create the PTV$_{optim}$, a structure used in optimization, the PRV of the spinal cord as well as all PTVs to which a higher dose was prescribed, were subtracted from the PTV$_{whbu}$.

Treatment Planning

The beam configuration used to treat this patient was based on a class solution of six nonopposing coplanar beams with a single isocenter at beam angles 45°, 75°, 165°, 195°, 285°, and 315°. The IMRT treatment plans were optimized by using an in-house developed extension of the GRATIS software package.[2] For every beam, the in-house developed Anatomy Based Segmentation Tool generated initial beam segments based on all PTVs, taking into account the presence of the spinal cord and the distance from the target structures to the skin.[3] Both parotids were not included into the tool as an organ of avoidance. Segment weight and leaf position optimiza-

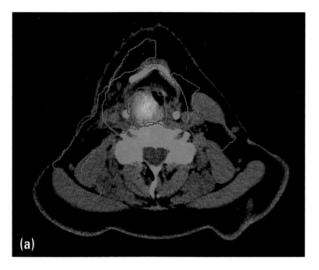

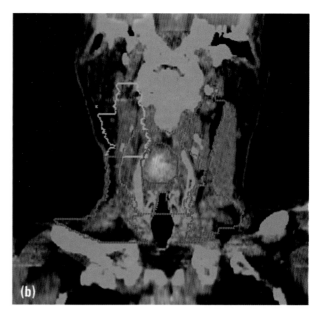

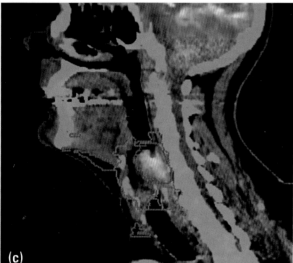

FIGURE 16A-2. Fused axial **(a)**, coronal **(b)**, and sagittal **(c)** 18-fluorodeoxyglucose positron emission tomography (^{18}F-FDG PET) and computed tomography (CT) slices illustrating the target volume delineation for the presented case: *blue*: PET-based planning target volume (PTV$_{PET}$); *pink*: the union clinical target volume (CTV$_{union}$); *orange*: the clinical target volume of resected lymph nodes with extracapsular extension receiving 66 Gy; *purple*: the clinical target volume of the elective neck receiving 56 Gy.

tion was performed with the in-house developed Segment Outline and Weight Adapting Tool. The optimization algorithm involves a biophysical objective function.[4,5] When the treatment plan fulfilled the acceptance criteria, the CRASH (combine, reorder and step and shoot) tool resulted in a prescription file for the linear accelerator.[6]

The IMRT was delivered in two phases. During the first phase the dose was escalated to a focal region defined by ^{18}F-FDG PET within the GTV to 30 Gy in 10 fractions. The second phase consisted of a standard IMRT delivered in 22 fractions of 2.16 Gy. This resulted in a total physical dose of 77.52 Gy delivered in 32 fractions to the ^{18}F-FDG PET–positive subvolume. The prescription featured multiple dose levels delivered simultaneously (Table 16A-1).

TABLE 16A–1 Prescription Dose Levels to the PTVs

	Dose per Fraction, Gy			
	Fractions 1–10	Fractions 11–32	Total Dose, Gy	NID$_{2Gy}$, Gy
PTVPET = focal dose escalation	3.0	2.16	77.5	86.7
PTV69 = macroscopic tumor + enlarged lymph nodes	2.16	2.16	69.1	72.5
PTV66 = resected lymph nodes with capsule rupture	2.06	2.06	65.9	67.2
PTV56 = elective lymph nodes	1.75	1.75	56.0	51.1

Notes. NID$_{2Gy}$ = normalized isoeffective dose, equivalent to the dose delivered in 2.0 Gy fractions based on the linear-quadratic equation, with α/β = 10, β = 0.035, and a potential doubling time of 4 days; PTV = planning target volume; PTV$_{56}$ = PTV receiving 56 Gy; PTV$_{66}$ = PTV receiving 66 Gy; PTV$_{69}$ = PTV receiving 69 Gy; PTV$_{PET}$ = PET-based PTV.

TABLE 16A–2 Dose–Volume Constraints for Organs at Risk and Corresponding PRVs

Organ at Risk	Dose–Volume Constraint
Spinal cord, PRV	$D_{50} < 45$ Gy and $V_{\geq 50} < 5\%$
Brainstem, PRV	$D_{50} < 50$ Gy and $V_{\geq 60} < 5\%$
Parotid gland	$V_{\geq 27} < 50\%$
Mandible	$V_{\geq 70} < 5\%$

Notes. D_{50} = dose level on the DVHs above which is exposed 50% of the contoured volume; PRV = planning risk volume; $V_{\geq 27}$ = relative volume of the parotid receiving at least 27 Gy; $V_{\geq 50}$ = relative volume of the spinal cord receiving at least 50 Gy; $V_{\geq 60}$ = relative volume of the brainstem receiving at least 60 Gy; $V_{\geq 70}$ = relative volume of the mandible receiving at least 70 Gy. Hard dose–volume constraints are in bold.

A median dose of 69 Gy in 32 fractions of 2.16 Gy was prescribed to the PTV encompassing the CTV$_{union}$ further called PTV$_{69}$. The dose levels of 66 Gy and 56 Gy were prescribed respectively to the regions of resected lymph nodes with extracapsular extension and elective lymph nodes. The PTV$_{PET}$ was the target for focal dose escala-tion. The aim was to deliver a dose greater than 65.5 Gy to 95% or more of the volume of PTV$_{69}$ minus PTV$_{PET}$ and to restrict doses exceeding 73.8 Gy to less than 7% of the volume of the PTV$_{69}$ minus PTV$_{PET}$. Proportionally similar dose–volume constraints were applied to other PTVs. Dose inhomogeneity calculated as $(D_2 - D_{98})/D_{50}$ had to be less than 12% in PTV$_{69}$ and PTV$_{PET}$. The total physical dose for PTV$_{PET}$ was 77.52 Gy. D_2, D_{50}, and D_{98} are dose levels on the dose–volume histograms (DVHs) above which lay 2%, 50%, and 98% of the contoured volume, respectively. Dose–volume constraints to OARs are shown in Table 16A-2. Isodose distributions for the whole treatment are shown in Figure 16A-3. The DVHs for the first and second phases of IMRT as well as for the whole treatment are presented in Figure 16A-4.

Treatment Delivery

Intensity-modulated RT treatment was delivered via a step-and-shoot technique with 6-MV photons on a Sli 18 linear accelerator (Elekta AB, Stockholm, Sweden). To

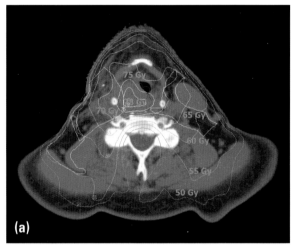
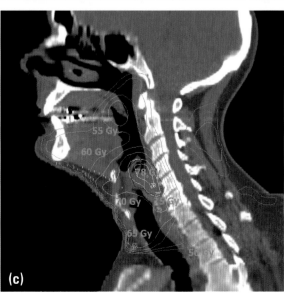
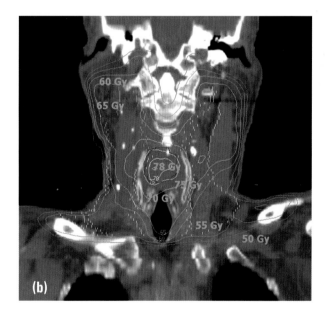

FIGURE 16A-3. Isodose distributions summed for the whole treatment for the presented case in the axial (a), coronal (b), and sagittal (c) planes. A total median dose of 77.5 Gy is prescribed to the positron emission tomography (PET)-based planning target volume (PTV$_{PET}$): *blue*: PTV$_{PET}$; *red*: the planning target volume receiving 69 Gy (PTV$_{69}$); *green*: the planning target volume of resected lymph nodes with extracapsular extension receiving 66 Gy (PTV$_{66}$); *yellow*: the planning target volume of the elective neck receiving 56 Gy (PTV$_{56}$).

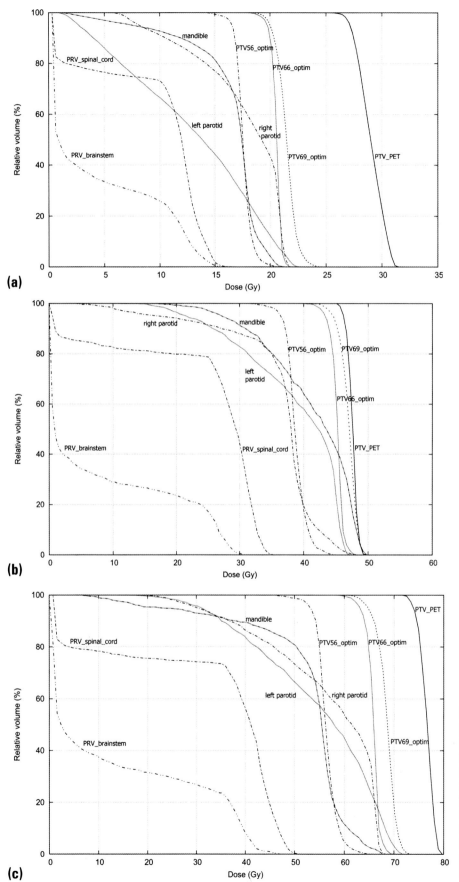

FIGURE 16A-4. Dose–volume histograms for the target volumes and organs at risk for the presented case: **(a)** the first phase of intensity-modulated radiation therapy (IMRT); **(b)** the second phase of IMRT; **(c)** the sum of the two phases of IMRT. A median dose of 30 Gy is prescribed to the positron emission tomography (PET)-based planning target volume (PTV$_{PET}$) in the first phase of IMRT. A total median dose of 77.5 Gy is prescribed to the PTV$_{PET}$.

reduce the systematic errors, electronic portal images were acquired during the first 4 days of treatment. The average setup error was corrected and weekly electronic portal imaging was performed.

Clinical Outcome

Treatment was completed without interruption in 45 days. During week 5, the patient developed grade 3 dysphagia and mucositis requiring percutaneous gastrostomy (PEG) tube placement. A complete response was observed on physical examination and CT 3 months after the completion of treatment. The patient remained free of disease at his latest follow-up (36 months posttreatment). His complaints were limited to grade 2 xerostomia (partial but persistent dryness of the mouth) and grade 2 skin fibrosis. The PEG tube was removed at 6 months follow-up.

Our initial clinical experience with PET-guided, focal dose escalation using a SIB IMRT technique was presented earlier.[7] This phase I trial included two planned dose levels: 25 Gy (level I) and 30 Gy (level II) delivered in 10 fractions. Forty-one patients were enrolled, with 23 in dose level I and 18 at dose level II; 39 patients completed the planned therapy. Two cases of dose-limiting toxicity occurred in level I (grade 4 dermatitis and grade 4 dysphagia). One treatment-related death in level II halted the study. Completed responses were observed in 18 (86%) and 13 (81%) of dose level I and II patients, respectively. At a median follow-up of 14 months, the 1-year actuarial local control rates in level I and II

patients were 85% and 87%, respectively. Corresponding 1-year overall survivals were 82% and 54%. In four of nine patients, the site of relapse was in the boosted PET-delineated volume.

References

1. Grégoire V, Coche E, Cosnard G, et al. Selection and delineation of lymph node target volumes in head and neck conformal radiotherapy. Proposal for standardizing terminology and procedure based on the surgical experience. *Radiother Oncol.* 2000;56:135–150.
2. Sherouse GW, Thorn J, Novins K, et al. A portable 3D radiotherapy design system. *Med Phys.* 1989;16:466.
3. De Gersem W, Claus F, De Wagter C, et al. An anatomy-based beam segmentation tool for intensity-modulated radiation therapy and its application to head-and-neck cancer. *Int J Radiat Oncol Biol Phys.* 2001;51:849–859.
4. De Gersem W, Claus F, De Wagter C, et al. Leaf position optimization for step-and-shoot IMRT. *Int J Radiat Oncol Biol Phys.* 2001;51:1371–1388.
5. De Neve W, De Gersem W, De Meerleer G, et al. In response to Drs. Vaarkamp and Krasin. *Int J Radiat Oncol Biol Phys.* 2001;49:1519–1520.
6. De Neve W, De Gersem W, Derycke S, et al. Clinical delivery of intensity modulated conformal radiotherapy for relapsed or second-primary head and neck cancer using a multileaf collimator with dynamic control. *Radiother Oncol.* 1999;50:301–314.
7. Madani I, Duthoy W, Derie C, et al. Positron emission tomography-guided, focal-dose escalation using intensity-modulated radiotherapy for head and neck cancer. *Int J Radiat Oncol Biol Phys.* 2007;68:126–135.

MR-Guided Target Delineation in a Patient with Nasopharyngeal Carcinoma

Case Study

Chien-Yu Lin, MD, Joseph Tung-Chieh Chang, MD, PhD

Patient History

A 48-year-old man presented with progressive right-sided tinnitus and hearing impairment for 1 year. More recently, he developed headaches especially at night. No diplopia, facial numbness, or other systemic symptoms were noted. Fiberoptic nasopharyngoscopy revealed a bulky mass in the right-side nasopharynx crossing midline and extending to the right choana. No palpable cervical lymph nodes were noted on physical examination. Biopsy of the nasopharyngeal mass and the right nasal cavity revealed keratinizing squamous cell carcinoma.

A magnetic resonance (MR) scan of the head and neck and an ^{18}F-fluorodeoxyglucose (^{18}F-FDG) positron emission tomography (^{18}F-FDG PET)–computed tomography (CT) scan were performed for staging purposes. Magnetic resonance revealed a bulky nasopharyngeal mass crossing the midline with involvement of adjacent structures on the right side including the parapharyngeal space, nasal cavity, oropharynx, carotid sheath, petrous apex, and clivus bone. Perineural spread along the maxillary nerve via the foramen ovale into right cavernous sinus were also noted (Figure 16B-1). Neck status, according to our scoring system (Table 16B-1), were right retropharyngeal (RP) 4+, left RP 3+, and bilateral level II nodes 2+. ^{18}F-FDG PET–CT revealed increased metabolic activity in the nasopharynx (maximum standardized uptake value [SUV], 6.5, 4+) and in the right RP (max SUV 5.82, 4+) (Figure 16B-2). No distant metastasis was seen.

The inconsistency of left retropharyngeal lymph nodes between MR imaging and ^{18}F-FDG PET–CT was

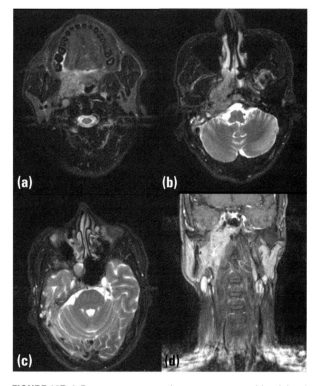

FIGURE 16B-1. Pretreatment magnetic resonance scan with axial and coronal views. (a) Right nasopharyngeal tumor extending inferiorly to right oropharynx with bilateral retropharyngeal lymph node involvement. (b) Tumor extending to right nasal cavity, right parapharyngeal space, right carotid sheath, right petrous apex, and right clivus. (c) Right petrous apex and right cavernous sinus involvement and (d) tumor with perineural spread along maxillary nerve via the foramen ovale into right cavernous sinus.

TABLE 16B–1 Scoring System of Image Findings Based on Our Multidisciplinary Nasopharyngeal Carcinoma Consensus

Scoring	Definition
0+	No evidence of visible lesions
1+	Benign lesions
2+	Probably benign lesions
3+	Probably malignant lesions
4+	Malignant lesions

considered a positive finding because of the limitation of 18F-FDG PET–CT for detecting small-size lymph nodes (left retropharyngeal lymph nodes diameter 7.35 mm). No tissue proof was performed routinely in this area because significant morbidity limited the procedure in clinical practice. Final clinical staging was T4N2M0 by 2002 American Joint Committee on Cancer staging system.

The patient's case was discussed in our multidisciplinary nasopharyngeal carcinoma conference and the consensus recommendation was for concomitant cisplatin chemotherapy and intensity-modulated radiation therapy (IMRT). We elected to use MR imaging to guide target delineation in this patient.

Simulation

The patient was simulated on our departmental GE HISPEED LX/I CT-simulator (GE Healthcare, Waukesha, WI) in the supine position. A customized thermoplastic mask was used to immobilize the patient's neck in hyperextension. The immobilization device was indexed to the CT couch top (extension with carbon fiber frame), which mimics the couch on the treatment unit. Midline marks were drawn on the patient according to the laser during CT-simulation from the cast extending downward to patient's upper trunk to avoid the angulations between the neck and trunk. Transaxial 3.75-mm images were obtained from frontal sinus to the mediastinum.

Imaging and Target Delineation

Targets were defined according to the MR and 18F-FDG PET–CT findings. The gross tumor volumes (GTVs) consisted of the primary tumor and involved RP lymph nodes bilaterally. The clinical target volume (CTV₁) in the initial large field included the nasopharynx, oropharynx, the base of skull with cranial nerve bearing areas, and bilateral whole neck lymphatics with at least 1 cm distance surrounding the GTV (Figure 16B-3). The targets for

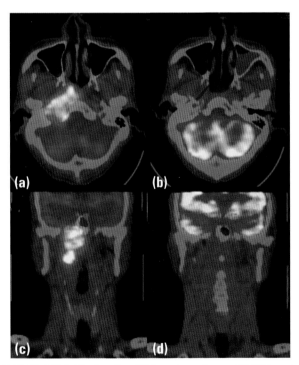

FIGURE 16B-2. The baseline 18F-fluorodeoxyglucose (18F-FDG)–positron emission tomography (PET)–computed tomography (CT) showed increased metabolic lesions at right nasopharynx (a: axial, c: coronal). Three months after chemoradiotherapy, 18F-FDG–PET–CT showed complete remission of primary tumor (b: axial, d: coronal).

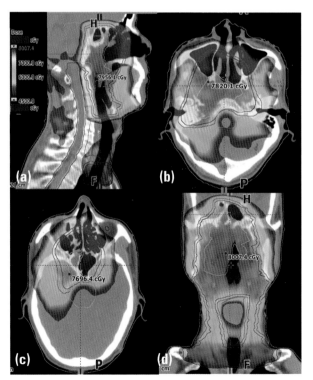

FIGURE 16B-3. Tumor targeting and isodose coverage in the composite plan of the three successive cone-down fields. The target delineation is shown in the initial large field: the gross tumor volume is shown in light blue, the blue line is the clinical target volume, and the red line is the planning target volume (a: sagittal, b-c: axial, d: coronal).

bilateral neck lymphatics were separated below the level of hyoid bone to spare the larynx. A CTV_2 was defined and included GTV, and next echelon lymphatic drainage (bilateral level II). The CTV_3 was generated by placing a 0.5-cm margin around the GTV. Finally, a 3-mm three-dimensional (3D) margin was applied to the three CTVs to generate the planning target volumes (PTVs). Organs at risk (OARs) were also drawn for sparing, including the brainstem, spinal cord, bilateral eyes, and bilateral optic nerves and chiasm.

Although the MR was not fused, it still provided valuable information for target delineation. Magnetic resonance has higher resolution for soft tissue density, so we could define the gross tumor extension more precisely, such as retropharyngeal lymph node metastasis, bone marrow replacement, perineural spreading, muscle swelling or invasion by tumor, paranasal sinusitis, or tumor invasion. Additionally, coronal and sagittal MR views are very useful for target delineation in three dimensions, especially for tracking the route of perineural spreading.

Treatment Planning

Intensity-modulated RT planning was performed with the Eclipse (Varian Medical Systems, Palo Alto, CA) treatment planning software. Plan optimization was performed by Helios IMRT inverse treatment planning system. A total dose of 50 Gy in 25 fractions was prescribed to the PTV_1, 60 Gy in 30 fractions to the PTV_2, and 76 Gy in 38 fractions to the PTV_3, using successive cone-down fields. The dose prescription for treatment planning—maximum brain stem dose less than 85% and maximum spinal cord dose less than 70% of the prescription—was achieved. The GTV was required to receive a minimum of 100% of prescription dosage; minimum dose of 95% for the CTVs and 90% for the PTVs, respectively, were required. The maximum dose was limited to less than 110% of the prescription dose. A composite dose distribution of all three plans is shown in Figure 16B-3. The maximum dose constraints (< 0.1 cc volume) of each OAR were: brain stem 60 Gy, spinal cord 50 Gy, right eye 50 Gy, left eye 40 Gy, right optic nerve 70 Gy, left optic nerve 60 Gy, and chiasm 60 Gy.

Clinical Outcome

Overall, the patient tolerated combined treatment well and did not require any unplanned treatment breaks. Acute grade 2 mucositis and dermatitis, as well as grade 3 pharyngitis occurred. Significant tumor regression was noted on nasopharyngoscopy after 28 Gy, and his headaches were improved after 36 Gy. At the end of treatment, a residual prominence was noted in his right nasopharynx. Complete remission of the primary tumor was

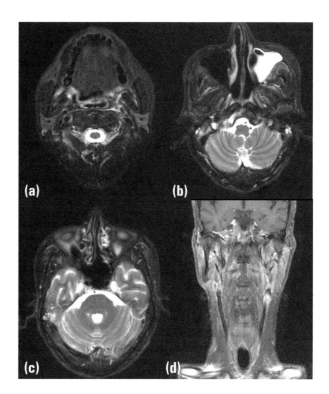

FIGURE 16B-4. Follow-up magnetic resonance scan 1 year after therapy. **(a)** Complete remission of the primary tumor and bilateral involved retropharyngeal lymph nodes. **(b)** Residual density at right clivus bone with strong enhancement in T2-weighted level, favoring inflammation process. Left maxillary sinusitis and bilateral mastoiditis are also noted. **(c)** Complete remission of right cavernous sinus lesion. **(d)** Complete remission of right perineural tumor spread.

suggested with a residual skull base density (score 2+) seen on his first MR, but subsequent imaging revealed further improvement of prior skull base lesions (Figure 16B-4). Scanning with ^{18}F-FDG PET–CT at 3 months posttreatment revealed a complete remission (Figure 16B-2). At his most recent follow-up 13 months posttreatment, he remained without evidence of disease recurrence. No significant late complications have developed, except mild (grade I) xerostomia.

We reported the utility of MR guidance in the staging and planning of nasopharyngeal carcinoma patients undergoing RT earlier.[1] In that study, we focused on 330 patients presenting with cranial nerve palsies treated at our institution between 1979 and 2000. Imaging methods varied over that period, and included conventional tomography in 47 patients, CT in 195, and MR in 88. Upper cranial nerve (II–VI) palsy was noted in 268 patients, lower cranial nerve (IX–XII) palsy in 13, and both in 49. The median dose was 70.2 Gy (range, 63 Gy to 77.5 Gy). A brachytherapy boost was delivered in 156 patients and 139 patients received cisplatin-based chemotherapy.

Five-year actuarial overall and disease-free survival rates for the entire group were 34.4% and 37.8%, respectively. The 5-year disease-free survival of patients staged and planned with conventional tomography, CT, and MR were 21.9%, 36.7%, and 46.9%, respectively ($P = .016$). The difference between CT and MR was also statistically significant ($P = 0.015$). Patients undergoing MR had a significantly better tumor control rate than those undergoing CT or conventional tomography, with a 15% to 30% improvement in local tumor control and survival.

Reference

1. Chang JT, Lin CY, Chen TM, et al. Nasopharyngeal carcinoma with cranial nerve palsy: the importance of MRI for radiotherapy. *Int J Radiat Oncol Biol Phys.* 2005;63:1354–1360.

^{18}F-Fluoromisonidazole PET–Guided Target Delineation in a Patient with Base of Tongue Carcinoma

Case Study

Andreas Rimner, MD, Nancy Y. Lee, MD

Patient History

A 66-year-old man presented with a painless, left-sided neck mass, which had developed over 1.5 months and did not respond to a course of antibiotics. He denied any dysphagia, odynophagia, trismus, otalgia, or decreased range of motion of the neck. On physical examination, a fixed, matted, nontender, left level 2 mass measuring 7 cm and an area of induration in the left base of tongue were noted. On flexible endoscopic examination, the oropharynx appeared normal without any visible tumor. The base of tongue, vallecula, and epiglottis were free of any visible lesions.

Radiographic workup included a magnetic resonance (MR) scan, which confirmed a suspicious, bulky left-sided level 2–3 cervical mass, measuring 3.0 cm by 4.0 cm. A slightly infiltrative minimally exophytic mass was noted arising along the left base of tongue. An ^{18}F-fluorodeoxyglucose positron emission tomography (^{18}F-FDG PET) scan revealed abnormal uptake in the base of tongue extending to the left glosso-tonsillar sulcus and the left tonsillar pillar (standard uptake value [SUV], 7.8). The cervical mass revealed ^{18}F-FDG uptake as well (SUV, 10.6). Direct laryngoscopy and needle biopsy of the base of tongue were positive for poorly differentiated squamous cell carcinoma. The final tumor was thus T1N3M0.

The patient was presented at our multidisciplinary head and neck conference and the consensus recommen-

dation was for concomitant chemoradiation. Because of preexisting moderate to severe hearing loss, concurrent chemotherapy with carboplatin and 5-fluorouracil (5-FU) was recommended. As part of an in-house research study, the patient underwent an ^{18}F-fluoromisonidazole (^{18}F-FMISO) PET–CT scan in addition to our standard workup to identify areas of hypoxia. We present here the potential benefit of incorporating the ^{18}F-FMISO results into the treatment planning of this patient, allowing the potential for dose escalation to hypoxic tumor subregions.

Simulation

The patient was simulated in the supine position and immobilized with an individualized head, neck, and shoulder Aquaplast mask (Orfit Industries, Wijnegem, Belgium). A computed tomography (CT) scan with a 3-mm slice thickness using intravenous contrast was acquired from the top of the skull to midthigh on a Philips AcQSim CT scanner (Philips Medical Systems, Andover, MA). An isocenter was selected, and permanent skin marks were placed. The patient subsequently underwent an ^{18}F-FDG PET–CT scan on the same day as the CT simulation. He was scanned 45 minutes after injection with 15 mCi of ^{18}F-FDG on a GE Discovery LS PET/CT scanner (GE Healthcare, Waukesha, WI) using the same immobilization device and treatment position. Fiducial markers were placed on the immobilization mask to ensure accurate image coregistration.

One day after the CT simulation and the ¹⁸F-FDG PET–CT scan, an additional PET–CT scan using ¹⁸F-FMISO as a tracer for hypoxia was performed on the GE Discovery LS PET–CT scanner. The PET–CT images were acquired approximately 2 hours after intravenous injection of approximately 10 mCi of ¹⁸F-FMISO.

Imaging and Target Delineation

The gross tumor volume (GTV) was delineated on the planning ¹⁸F-FDG PET–CT scan, taking into consideration the clinical examination, as well as the diagnostic MR and PET scan findings (Figure 16C-1a). Note, the ¹⁸F-FMISO images were not used for clinical treatment planning purposes. The GTV contours were then copied to the CT portion of the ¹⁸F-FMISO scan and aligned using the fiducial markers. The CT images of the ¹⁸F-FDG scan were manually aligned with the CT images of the ¹⁸F-FMISO scan and the GTVs were subsequently contoured (Figure 16C-1b and -1c). These were rigidly coregistered using the mutual information registration technique. The hypoxic subvolume was defined as:

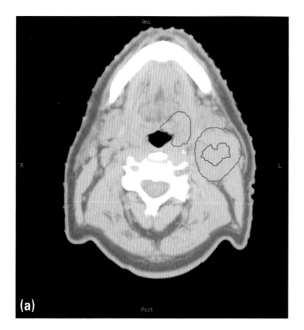

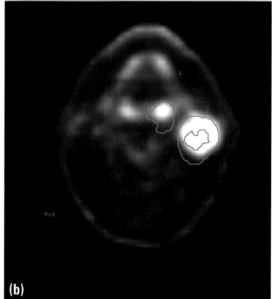

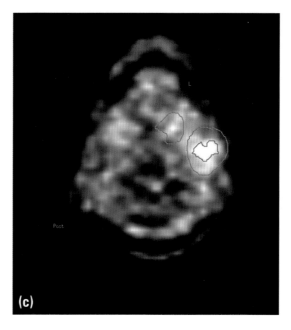

FIGURE 16C-1. (a) Axial planning computed tomography (CT) slice with contours of the gross tumor volumes (GTVs) and hypoxic-GTV (GTV$_h$). **(b)** Axial ¹⁸F-fluorodeoxyglucose positron emission tomography (¹⁸F-FDG PET) slice with contours of the GTVs and GTV$_h$. **(c)** Axial ¹⁸F-fluoromisonidazole (¹⁸F-FMISO) PET slice with contours of the GTVs and GTV$_h$.

$$GTV_h = \frac{^{18}F\text{-}MISO\_GTV_{T:B\geq1.3}}{^{18}FDG\_GTV} \quad (1)$$

using a tumor-to-blood ratio of 1.3 or greater, as per previously published thresholds for tumor hypoxia.[1,2] All target volumes were then transferred and aligned with the treatment planning CT scan.

The clinical target volumes (CTVs) were defined as high-risk and low-risk CTV, based on the risk of microscopic tumor involvement. A 5-mm margin was applied to all CTVs creating corresponding planning target volumes (PTVs), including PTV_{GTV}, $PTV_{high\text{-}risk\ CTV}$, and $PTV_{low\text{-}risk\ CTV}$. The margin was reduced to 3 mm in areas of nearby critical normal structures.

Treatment Planning

An intensity-modulated radiation therapy (IMRT) plan was calculated with a prescribed total dose of 70 Gy to the PTV_{GTV}, 59.4 Gy to the $PTV_{high\text{-}risk\ CTV}$, and 54 Gy to the $PTV_{low\text{-}risk\ CTV}$ (Figures 16C-2a and -3a). A matched, low anterior neck field was treated to a total dose of 50.4 Gy.

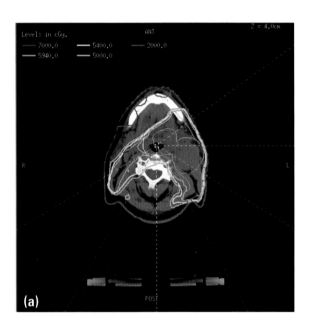
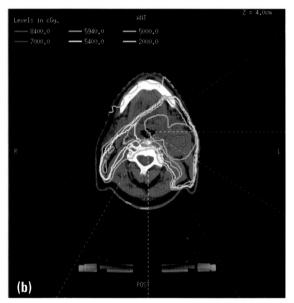
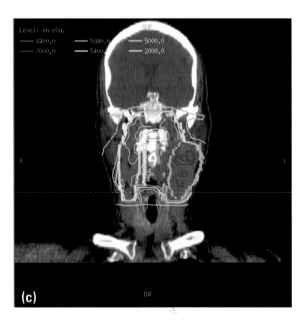

FIGURE 16C-2. (a) Axial computed tomography (CT) slice showing the beam angles of the clinical intensity-modulated radiation therapy (IMRT) plan. **(b)** Axial CT slice showing the beam angles of the hypoxia-guided IMRT plan. **(c)** Coronal slice of hypoxia-guided IMRT plan.

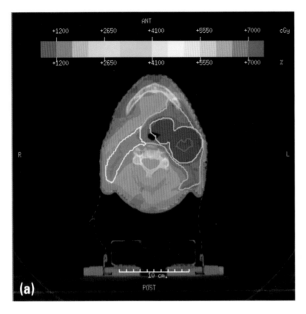 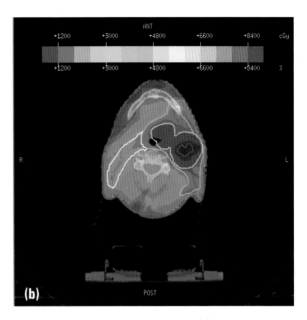

FIGURE 16C-3. (a) Axial color-wash of the intensity-modulated radiation therapy (IMRT) plan used to treat this patient. **(b)** Axial color-wash of hypoxia-guided IMRT plan.

Using the same beam angles as in the previous IMRT plan, a hypoxia dose-painting plan was developed with 20% dose escalation (84 Gy) to the hypoxic subsites of the tumor (GTV$_h$) (Figures 16C-2b, -2c, and -3b). The following avoidance structures were delineated: spinal cord, brainstem, parotid glands, cochleae, oral cavity, mandible, and brachial plexus. The same normal tissue constraints that we routinely use for cancers of the head and neck were applied to both plans (Table 16C-1). All standard tissue constraints were met with the dose-escalated as well as the standard clinical IMRT plan. The patient was treated with 33 daily fractions according to the standard clinical IMRT plan and three cycles of concurrent carboplatin and 5-FU.

TABLE 16C–1 Normal Tissue Constraints

Organ at Risk	Dose Constraint
Cochleae	$D_{max} \leq 50$ Gy
Submandibular glands	$D_{mean} \leq 39$ Gy
Parotid glands	$D_{mean} \leq 26$ Gy
Oral cavity	D_{mean} 30 Gy to 35 Gy
Larynx	Avoid hot spots
Esophagus	Avoid hot spots
Brainstem	$D_{max} \leq 50$ Gy to 54 Gy
Spinal cord	$D_{max} \leq 45$ Gy
Brachial plexus	$D_{max} \leq 65$ Gy; $D_{05} \leq 60$ Gy

Clinical Outcome

The patient tolerated the radiation treatment very well. At the end of treatment, he developed grade 1 dermatitis, grade 1 mucositis, and grade 1 dysphagia. Follow-up CT, PET, and MR scans have shown no evidence of residual or recurrent malignancy. The patient subsequently developed complete obstruction of his cervical esophagus requiring two dilations with one perforation. He remains without evidence of disease 3 years after completion of his therapy.

Our ¹⁸F-FMISO PET–CT planning study in 10 head and neck cancer patients was recently published.[3] In each patient, planning CT, ¹⁸F-FDG PET–CT, and ¹⁸F-FMISO PET–CT scans were obtained and coregistered. Regions of elevated ¹⁸F-FMISO uptake within the ¹⁸F-FDG PET–CT–defined GTV (the GTV$_h$) were targeted for an IMRT boost. In all 10 patients, treatment plans could be generated delivering 84 Gy to the GTV$_h$ and 70 Gy to the GTV without exceeding normal tissue tolerances. In two patients, further dose escalation of 105 Gy to the GTV$_h$ was attempted and found to be possible without exceeding normal tissue tolerances in one patient. This planning study shows that dose escalation to 84 Gy in hypoxic tumor regions is feasible and can be achieved with the same normal tissue constraints. Further studies will have to be conducted to test whether this treatment can be accurately and safely delivered to patients.

References

1. Rajendran JG, Schwartz DL, O'Sullivan J, et al. Tumor hypoxia imaging with [F-18] fluoromisonidazole positron emission tomography in head and neck cancer. *Clin Cancer Res.* 2006;12:5435–5441.
2. Rasey JS, Koh WJ, Evans ML, et al. Quantifying regional hypoxia in human tumors with positron emission tomography of [18F]fluoromisonidazole: a pretherapy study of 37 patients. *Int J Radiat Oncol Biol Phys.* 1996;36:417–428.
3. Lee NY, Mechalakos JG, Nehmeh S, et al. Fluorine-19-labeled fluoromisonidazole positron emission and computed tomography-guided intensity-modulated radiotherapy for head and neck cancer: a feasibility study. *Int J Radiat Oncol Biol Phys.* 2008;70:2–13.

^{18}F-FDG PET–Guided Target Delineation in a Patient with Recurrent Nasopharyngeal Carcinoma

Case Study

Xiao-Kang Zheng, MD, Long-Hua Chen, MD

Patient History

A 46-year-old man with a history of a T3N1M0 nasopharyngeal carcinoma treated with definitive radiation therapy (RT) presented with a 1-month history of headache and spitting bloodstained nasal mucus. Nasopharyngoscopy revealed a tumor on the left lateral wall of the nasopharynx. Biopsy revealed a poorly differentiated squamous cell carcinoma, identical to the histology of the tumor diagnosed 2 years before.

On physical examination, no enlarged neck lymph nodes were noted. Radiographic workup included a chest x-ray, which revealed normal heart and lungs. No bone metastases were noted on single-photon emission computed tomography (SPECT). A liver ultrasound was negative for metastases. The complete blood cell count and biochemical parameters were within normal limits. The final diagnosis was locally recurrent nasopharyngeal carcinoma.

The patient's case was discussed in our department and the consensus recommendation was for definitive re-irradiation combined with concurrent weekly cisplatin chemotherapy. We elected to use ^{18}F-fluorodeoxyglucose positron emission tomography (^{18}F-FDG PET) to help guide target delineation in this patient.

Simulation

The patient was brought to our departmental PET–CT scanner (CT: Light Speed Plus; PET: Advance Nxi, GE Medical System, Milwaukee, WI) and placed in the supine position with customized thermal plastic immobilization. The PET–CT scan was performed from the patient's vertex to his liver. The imaging and data acquisition were performed on an integrated Discovery LS PET–CT system (GE Medical System, Milwaukee, WI).

Imaging and Target Delineation

The PET and CT data sets were then converted to DICOM format and transferred to our CORVUS (version 6.3) treatment planning system (Nomos, Pittsburgh, PA). The PET and CT images were then fused by using the system's automated algorithm.

The complementary features of both PET and CT were used to define the gross tumor volume (GTV). A visual interpretation of the PET images was used to determine the nature of the lesion, and the CT images were used to determine the anatomic boundaries. A focus on PET was considered positive if the activity was significantly greater than the expected background and could not be explained by normal structure or inflammation, according to all information available.

At the vague boundary of the lesion on CT, the GTV was delineated using a qualitative visual assessment of the PET images that was applied with rigorous thresholding to normal tissue.[1] First, the ^{18}FDG PET scans were normalized using the liver as the reference tissue. With this normalization, the liver tissue generally has the greatest uptake of ^{18}F-FDG, except for the brain and a part of the heart. The liver was set in the middle of the 256-level in a linear gray scale. Then, the liver was set at the interface between blue and green in a rainbow color scale for the fused PET–CT images. Thus, the relative intensity of the tumor at the head and neck could be reproducibly compared with the liver activity and appreciated between studies. The GTV boundaries were drawn at the junction between yellow and orange on the rainbow scale. The radiation oncologist then used hard copy PET–CT images to delineate the GTV on the RT planning system. This method of defining the PET–CT–based GTV was previously reported by others[2,3] and is considered to be more accurate and reproducible than the semiquantitative method such as the use of the standardized uptake value (SUV) scales or ^{18}F-FDG intensity levels. We found this method to be better than that we had used previously, in which the 50% ^{18}F-FDG intensity level relative to the tumor maximum was used to delineate the borders of the GTV based on PET–CT.[4] The potential problems of the different methods for the delineation of GTV based on PET–CT have been highlighted by Nestle et al.[5]

In this patient, the CT images revealed thickening at left lateral nasopharyngeal wall with tumor extension to anterior parapharyngeal space, infratemporal fossa, pterygoprocess zone, pterygopalatine fossa, and clivus. However, the boundary of GTV on CT images was vague in some slices (Figure 16D-1), and geographic miss of the

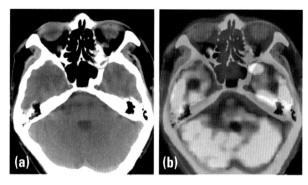

FIGURE 16D-2. Geographic miss of the gross tumor without positron emission tomography (PET) guidance. (a) Gross tumor volume (GTV) delineated on the basis of computed tomography (CT) alone. (b) GTV delineated on the basis of PET–CT.

gross tumor might have taken place without PET guidance (Figure 16D-2). The PET information, in this case, influenced the GTV delineation significantly. The clinical target volume (CTV) was created by expanding the GTV by 6 mm. The estimated position uncertainty was approximately 3 mm.

Treatment Planning

Intensity-modulated RT planning was performed using CORVUS. A dose of 68 Gy in 34 fractions was prescribed to the GTV delineated on the basis of PET–CT, and 63 Gy to the CTV. A satisfactory dosimetric result was achieved (Figure 16D-3). As demonstrated in Figure 16D-3, the isodoses are highly conformal to the PET–CT–guided GTV, with significant dose sparing of the surrounding normal tissues.

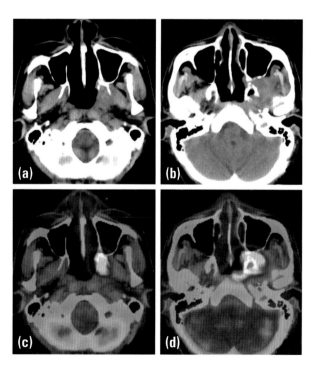

FIGURE 16D-1. Axial computed tomography (CT) slice through the nasopharynx. (a, b) The tumor on left lateral wall of nasopharynx and pterygoprocess zone is evident. The posterior and left side boundary of the tumor are vague. (c, d) Fused positron emission tomography–CT images of the corresponding slices, demonstrating the tumor with clear boundary.

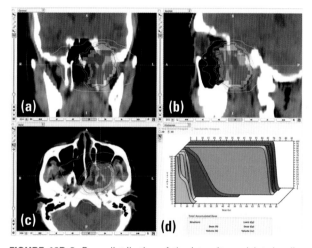

FIGURE 16D-3. Dose distribution of the intensity-modulated radiation therapy plan. (a) Axial, (b) sagittal, and (c) coronal view of dose distribution. (d) Dose–volume histogram of the gross tumor volume (GTV) based on computed tomography alone (purple), GTV that might be missed without the guide of positron emission tomography (red), and the clinical target volume (orange).

Clinical Outcome

The patient tolerated the treatment well and did not require any unplanned treatment breaks. At 18 months posttreatment, no evidence of local-regional or distant disease was found on either imaging or clinical examination. The patient has developed late toxicities including grade 2 xerostomia, grade 3 ipsilateral hearing loss, grade 2 ipsilateral temporal lobe necrosis, and grade 2 trismus.

We recently published our clinical experience using ¹⁸F-FDG PET–guided target delineation in 43 patients with locally recurrent nasopharyngeal carcinoma.[1] All patients underwent ¹⁸F-FDG PET–CT simulation. For each, the GTV was separately contoured with (GTV_{PET-CT}) and without (GTV_{CT}) the addition of PET information. Corresponding PTVs were also generated (PTV_{PET-CT} and PTV_{CT}). Disease metastases were found in four patients following PET–CT imaging. Of the 39 without distant metastases, inadequate coverage of the GTV_{PET-CT} and the PTV_{PET-CT} by the PTV_{CT} occurred in 7 (18%) and 20 (51%) of patients, respectively. This resulted in less than 95% of the GTV_{PET-CT} and the PTV_{PET-CT} receiving 95% or more of the prescribed dose in four (10%) and 13 (33%) of patients, respectively. These results strongly supported the value of ¹⁸F-FDG PET–guided target delineation in these patients.

References

1. Zheng XK, Chen LH, Wang QS, et al. Influence of FDG-PET on computed tomography-based radiotherapy planning for locally recurrent nasopharyngeal carcinoma. *Int J Radiat Oncol Biol Phys.* 2007;69:1381–1388.

2. MacManus M, Hicks R, Bayne M, et al. In regard to Paulino and Johnstone: Use of PET and CT imaging data in radiation therapy planning [*Int J Radiat Oncol Biol Phys.* 2004;59:4–5; letter]. *Int J Radiat Oncol Biol Phys.* 2004;60:1005–1006.

3. Leong T, Everitt C, Yuen K, et al. A prospective study to evaluate the impact of FDG PET on CT based radiotherapy treatment planning for oesophageal cancer. *Radiother Oncol.* 2006;78:254–261.

4. Zheng X-K, Chen L-H, Wang Q-S, Wu H-B. Influence of [18] fluorodeoxyglucose positron emission tomography on salvage treatment decision making for locally persistent nasopharyngeal carcinoma. *Int J Radiat Oncol Biol Phys.* 2006;65:1020–1025.

5. Nestle U, Kremp S, Schaefer-Schuler A, et al. Comparison of different methods for delineation of 18F-FDG PET-positive tissue for target volume definition in radiotherapy of patients with non-small cell lung cancer. *J Nucl Med.* 2005;46:1342–1348.

Electronic Portal Image-Guided Setup in a Patient with Head and Neck Cancer on a Varian Linear Accelerator

Case Study

Felix Y. Feng, MD, Scott Hadley, PhD, Avraham Eisbruch, MD

Patient History

A 68-year-old man with a history of tobacco use presented with sensitivity and discomfort along his right upper jaw. Biopsy of a 2.5-cm indurated lesion along the right maxillary alveolus revealed poorly differentiated squamous cell carcinoma. Additional examination with a flexible laryngoscope was unremarkable. A computed tomography (CT) scan of the neck revealed an expansile soft tissue mass at the level of the right maxillary sinus extending posteriorly into the right maxillary ridge with numerous enlarged right-sided level I and II lymph nodes. Positron emission tomography (PET)–CT showed an fluorodeoxyglucose (^{18}F-FDG)-avid mass along the right maxillary alveolus extending into the right maxillary sinus, the hard and soft palate, across midline, and invading into bone with some suggestion of pterygoid plate invasion. There were ^{18}F-FDG-avid bilateral level I lymph nodes, but no evidence of distant metastatic disease.

The patient underwent right hemimaxillectomy with resection of the pterygoid plate with mid-mandibulotomy, right coronoidectomy, partial excision of the right masseter, right modified radical neck dissection, and a left modified radical neck dissection. He had reconstruction with a right pectoralis major flap. Pathology revealed an invasive poorly differentiated squamous cell carcinoma invading the maxillary bone and maxillary sinus, and overlying the gingival–alveolar ridge. Final margins were free of neoplasm. Examination of the lymph nodes revealed three of 73 lymph nodes positive on the right, in levels I–III, with extracapsular extension at levels I and II, and 0 of 41 lymph nodes involved on the left side. Final staging was pT4N2bM0, stage IVA, squamous cell carcinoma of the maxillary sinus, involving also the alveolar ridge.

The patient was discussed at our multidisciplinary head and neck cancer conference and the consensus opinion was for adjuvant radiation therapy (RT). We elected to treat him with daily electronic portal image guidance to ensure optimal patient setup.

Simulation

Prior to simulation, a customized obturator was fabricated by the dentistry service and left in during the simulation. The patient was positioned with his head in a neutral position, on a head and neck board with head rest. His mouth was open and tongue forward, and a bite block was fashioned out of thermoplastic material and left in place. A five-point thermoplastic mask (Figure 16E-1) was fabricated with a cutout to accept the bite block. Arm pulls were used to bring his shoulders down while the mask was made but were not necessary for treatment.

A contrast-enhanced planning CT was obtained from the vertex through the T6–T7 interspace using our departmental Brilliance Big Bore CT simulator (Philips Medical Systems, Andover, MA; Figure 16E-2), with a

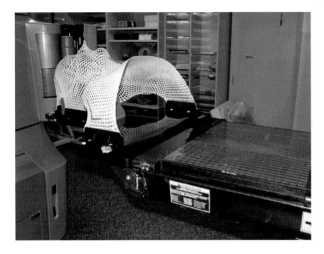

FIGURE 16E-1. Head and neck indexed immobilization board with thermoplastic mask attached. The mask attaches at five points to ensure a good fit and reproducible setup.

slice thickness of 3 mm. To increase in-plane resolution, a smaller field of view was used over the head and neck region and then increased at the shoulders. The mask was marked to facilitate patient setup on the first day of treatment.

Treatment Planning

The planning CT was transferred to our in-house treatment planning system, UMPLAN. The target volumes (CTVs) were contoured, including the tumor bed, levels I–V in the ipsilateral neck, and levels I–IV in the contralateral neck. In the ipsilateral neck, level II was included to the base of skull, whereas in the contralateral neck, level II was only included to the bottom of the transverse process of C1. A 3-mm planning target volume (PTV) margin was added to the targets to account for setup variation with daily image guidance (prior to our routine use of daily image guidance, a 5-mm margin was used). Organs at risk (OARs) were also contoured, including the spinal

cord, parotid glands, noninvolved oral cavity, larynx, pharyngeal constrictors, esophagus, and mandible. Because targets were defined to the base of skull ipsilaterally, the ear and temporal lobe were also delineated as OARs on that side.

An intensity-modulated RT (IMRT) plan was generated. Nine equally-spaced coplanar beams were set, starting with the gantry at 0°. The tumor bed and ipsilateral neck were prescribed 60 Gy and the contralateral neck 54 Gy, all in 30 fractions. The cost function was aimed at attaining a dose homogeneity of 99% to 107% in the targets. The OARs were incorporated into the cost function with the stipulation that, except for the spinal cord, target coverage had priority over OAR sparing. The plan was to clinically define an electron boost to ipsilateral levels I–II (sites of extracapsular lymph nodal metastasis) using 9 MeV electrons prescribed to d_{max} after completion of the IMRT plan.

Once the plan was approved, the fields were sequenced by using a step-and-shoot technique for delivery, and downloaded to the treatment delivery database. An additional quality assurance (QA) plan was derived from the patient plan and downloaded for the requisite IMRT QA. Digitally reconstructed radiographs (DRRs) were generated for patient setup, and match anatomy templates added. Bony anatomy was used as a surrogate for positioning the target and OARs. Because the high-dose targets were closest to the superior portion of the neck, this region, around C2, was preferentially matched to the DRR on a daily basis. For the lateral DRR, the anterior aspect of the spinal canal was defined, along with a straight line from the base of skull to the hard palate. The straight line was used to qualitatively assess the tilt of the head and quantitatively measure the cranial–caudal positioning of the patient. The anterior image used a single line along the spinous processes to verify the lateral position, and individual spinous processes to verify cranial–caudal position (Figure 16E-3).

Treatment Delivery

Treatment was delivered via a Varian 2100 EX linear accelerator fitted with a 120-leaf Millennium multileaf collimator (MLC) and an aS500 amorphous silicon megavoltage (MV) detector (Varian Medical Systems, Palo Alto, CA). The immobilization device used for the head and neck was attached to the end of the treatment couch, allowing the area to be treated to be suspended over the isocenter. The patient was positioned on the treatment table and the mask was carefully fitted to attempt to reproduce the head tilt position. The reference marks placed during CT simulation were placed on the linac isocenter. The patient was translated from the CT reference position to the isocenter location as determined from the isocenter placement in the treatment plan.

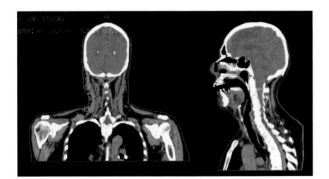

FIGURE 16E-2. Coronal and sagittal computed tomography image of the patient in treatment position. Arm pulls move the shoulders down to allow lateral beams access to the neck. The head is neutral to slightly tilted back to move the jaw out of the path of anterior beams.

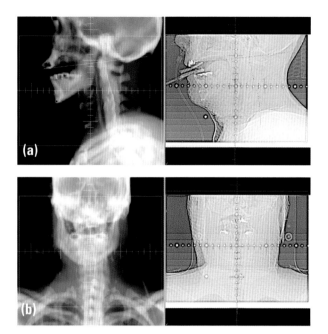

FIGURE 16E-3. Lateral (a) and anterior (b) digitally reconstructed radiographs and megavoltage (MV) portal images used for daily alignment. Match anatomy templates are displayed and aligned to bony anatomy on the MV image to calculate the necessary couch shift to correct positioning errors.

Setup imaging started with the lateral MV image to assess the tilt of the head by using the match anatomy from the anterior aspect of the vertebral bodies, along with a straight line from the base of skull to the hard palate. The lateral image was used to set position in the anterior–posterior direction and the cranial–caudal direction. The anterior image was used to set the lateral and cranial–caudal positioning of the patient and verify the cranial–caudal positioning (Figure 16E-3). Even with excellent immobilization, a daily imaging protocol with a 3-mm threshold for adjustment is needed to support our facility's standard 3-mm PTV margin. A shift in any direction less than or equal to the threshold is not applied for that day's treatment to avoid the situation where an attempt to correct a small error actually introduces a larger one (Figure 16E-4). The on-line matching software calculates the necessary couch movements that are then applied before treatment starts. If any shift is larger than 1 cm, a new set of films is acquired to verify the new position.

Clinical Outcome

During treatment, the patient developed mild mucositis and skin erythema, which both resolved within 3 weeks of treatment. He also developed odynophagia which resolved within 3 weeks of treatment. He additionally developed moderate xerostoma, but this has continued to improve during follow-up. Follow-up PET–CT scans performed 3 months after completion of RT revealed no evidence of disease. He continues to do well.

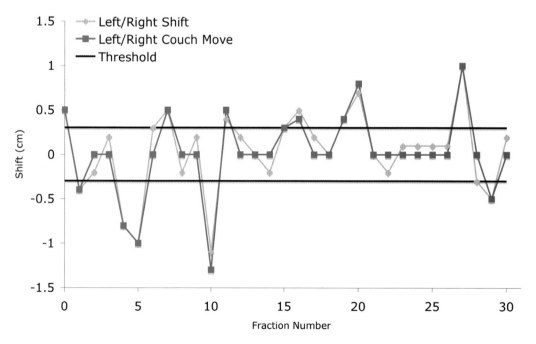

FIGURE 16E-4. Daily positioning errors for the 30 fraction treatment shown in blue and applied couch shift shown in red. Positioning errors less than or equal to the 3-mm threshold were not applied.

MVCT-Guided IMRT Using the Helical Tomotherapy System in a Patient with Tonsillar Carcinoma

Case Study

Ke Sheng, PhD, Paul W. Read, MD, PhD

Patient History

A 75-year-old woman presented with a 3 cm by 3 cm left jugulodigastric mass without an obvious primary mucosal lesion on physical examination. Computed tomography (CT) of the neck revealed two pathologic level II lymph nodes. A fine needle aspirate of these nodes demonstrated squamous cell carcinoma.

The patient subsequently underwent examination under anesthesia with direct laryngoscopy, rigid esophagoscopy, and directed biopsies of the left tonsil, right and left base of tongue, and nasopharynx. Pathology was consistent with a less than 2-cm squamous cell carcinoma in the left tonsillectomy specimen. All other biopsies were normal. Immunohistochemistry (IHC) of the tumor revealed it to be p16 positive, indicative of a human papilloma virus (HPV)-associated tumor; epidermal growth factor receptor was not overexpressed. Metastatic workup, including a chest x-ray and liver function tests, was negative. Her tumor was thus staged as T1N2bM0, stage IVA.

Given her advanced age, low volume of disease burden, and favorable IHC profile, our recommendation was for definitive radiation therapy (RT) alone without chemotherapy or surgery. We elected to treat her with daily image guidance using helical tomotherapy (TomoTherapy Inc, Madison, WI).

Simulation

The patient was simulated in the supine position on a single-slice PQ1000 CT scanner (Picker, Cleveland, OH) with a slice thickness of 3 mm and a pixel size of 0.94 mm. A customized head and neck aquaplast mask and head rest were fabricated for immobilization and attached to the S-plate, which secured to the tabletop (CIVCO, Kalona, IA). Fiducial markers on the bilateral angle of the mandible and the chin were placed on the aquaplast mask with laser guidance for isocenter management. The patient was simulated with fluoride trays in place to absorb low energy electron scatter from her dental fillings during treatment.

Treatment Planning

Target volumes and normal structures were contoured on an AcQSIM workstation (Picker, Cleveland, OH) by a head and neck cancer radiation oncologist. The gross tumor volume (GTV) included the left tonsillar fossa and the two pathologic left level II lymph nodes. Two clinical target volumes (CTVs) were delineated: CTV_1 included the GTV with a 1 cm to 1.5 cm expansion to cover potential microscopic spread and CTV_2 consisted of the bilateral uninvolved cervical and retropharyngeal lymphatics. Both CTV_1 and CTV_2 were enlarged by 3 mm symmetrically to create two planning target volumes (PTVs), namely PTV_1 and PTV_2, respectively.

The CT images and target volumes were exported to the tomotherapy planning station (TomoTherapy, Madison, WI) using the DICOM protocol. The pixel size resolution was increased to 1.88 mm so the dose calculation could be handled by the memory of the cluster, which was 32 GB in a total of 16 nodes. A 2.5-cm jaw size was selected and the pitch was 0.25 (i.e., it would take four revolutions of the gantry to cover 2.5 cm in the superior-inferior direction).

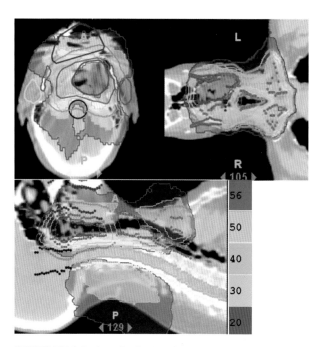

FIGURE 16F-1. Isodose distribution of the TomoTherapy plan overlaid on axial, coronal, and sagittal computed tomography slices. Color bars show corresponding isodose levels.

A dose of 56 Gy in 2 Gy per fraction was prescribed to 95% of the PTV$_1$ and 50.4 Gy in 1.8 Gy per fraction was prescribed to the PTV$_2$. The isodose lines of the approved treatment plan are shown in Figure 16F-1. The dose–volume histogram (DVH) is shown in Figure 16F-2. Patient-specific quality assurance was performed on a phantom to verify the multileaf collimator motion and its synchronization to the gantry rotation. The measured and calculated dose agreed within 3% in the homogeneous region and the isodoses agreed to within 3 mm in distance.

Final boost fields were computed with three-dimensional (3D) conformal techniques on the DAC Pinnacle treatment planning workstation (Philips Medical Systems, Andover, MA). A dose of 12 Gy in 2 Gy per fraction was used to boost the GTV with a 3-mm margin

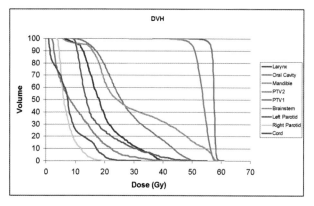

FIGURE 16F-2. Dose–volume histogram of the TomoTherapy plan.

using a left anterior and left posterior wedge pair. Six-MV photons were used for both fields. The GTV thus received a total dose of 68 Gy. The mean doses in the composite plan were 11.23 Gy and 26.69 Gy for right and left parotid glands, respectively.

Treatment Delivery

Initial patient setup in the treatment room was performed by using the mobile lasers with the shifts specified at treatment planning and fiducial markers placed at the time of simulation. Megavoltage CT (MVCT) was performed to image 12 cm (6 cm superior and inferior of the isocenter) with a slice thickness of 4 mm and in-slice resolution of 0.78 mm. The MVCT images were registered to the planning kVCT to determine the positioning error. The registration shown in Figure 16F-3 was initially done by automatic bony anatomy matching and then manually adjusted by an oncologist. A new set of fiducial markers was placed after the first day of MVCT registration to guide the following treatments. Daily MVCT was performed on the patients for all 28 fractions. The result of image registration and the corresponding shift is demonstrated in Figure 16F-3. Except for the first fraction of treatment, all daily shifts were less than 5 mm in any given direction. The treatment time (beam-on time) was 544 seconds.

Patient interfractional response was also monitored by daily MVCT. A significant reduction in the local tissue volume started to appear 2 weeks after the first fraction of radiation and continued to progress though the end of the treatment. Figure 16F-4 shows the "local weight" of the patient defined as the volume within 5 cm superior–inferior of the isocenter as measured from the MVCT. The nearly linear loss of "local weight" may contribute

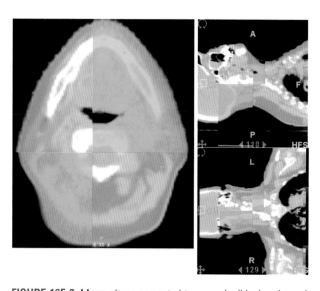

FIGURE 16F-3. Megavoltage computed tomography (blue) registered to the planning kilovoltage computed tomography (gray) to correct daily positioning error.

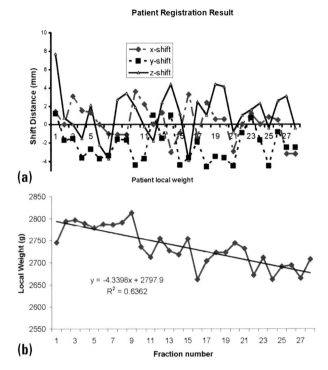

(a)

(b)

FIGURE 16F-4. (a) Daily patient shifts in three Cartesian coordinates based on megavoltage computed tomography (MVCT) and kilovoltage computed tomography (kVCT) coregistration. (b) Change of "local weight" measured by the volume of the MVCT 5 cm superior and inferior to the isocenter.

to a higher parotid dose than the treatment plan as they became closer to the target.

Clinical Outcome

The patient tolerated treatment well; however, she developed the following acute toxicities: grade 3 mucositis limited to the left oropharynx, grade 2 dermatitis, grade 2 nausea, loss of taste, and a 14-pound weight loss representing 7% of her initial body weight. She was able to tolerate a soft diet with liquid nutritional supplementation and she did not require a feeding tube. At the completion of therapy she had no visible or palpable disease and was classified as having a complete clinical response. Four weeks after completion of therapy she underwent a neck CT scan, which revealed no evidence of the primary tumor and resolution of her pathologic nodal disease

and she was classified as having a complete radiographic response.

The patient returned for routine scheduled follow-up appointments over the next 3 years and has remained free of local-regional and distant disease recurrence. Apart from mild late xerostomia (grade 1) and altered taste, she denies any otalgia, dysphagia, odynophagia, cough, shortness of breath, or hoarseness. Of note, she enjoys an excellent quality of life.

Our analysis of daily MVCT guidance in patients with head and neck cancer was recently published.[1] We analyzed the magnitude of setup errors corrected with helical tomotherapy MVCT on a daily or weekly basis and their impact on the delivered dose to the tumor and organs at risk were evaluated in six patients with cancer of the nasal cavity and four patients with nasopharyngeal cancer treated with 25 to 33 fractions. Each patient had MVCT-guided repositioning for all treatment fractions. Dose–volume histograms and equivalent uniform dose (EUD) for the PTV and normal tissues were calculated for hypothetical situations where no image guidance or once-weekly image guidance was performed.

The mean total setup error without image guidance was 3.6 mm ± 1.0 mm, which was reduced to 1.7 mm ± 0.6 mm if weekly image guidance was performed. Geometric uncertainties from the absence of image guidance resulted in a reduction of the mean PTV EUD dose by 2.1% ± 1%, which could be reduced to 1.4% ± 1% with weekly image guidance. The EUD of the normal tissues increased 1.8 Gy ± 2 Gy and 0.8 Gy ±1.3 Gy without or with weekly image guidance. Without daily image guidance, the mean patient position uncertainty has relatively small impacts on the mean PTV and normal tissue dosimetry, which can be further reduced approximately by half using weekly image guidance. On the other hand, because of a large variance, with low probability, substantial deviation from the original planned dosimetry may occur without image guidance, supporting the use of daily MVCT in these patients.

Reference

1. Sheng K, Chow MC, Hunter G, et al. Is daily CT image guidance necessary for nasal cavity and nasopharyngeal radiotherapy: an investigation based on helical tomotherapy. *J Appl Clin Med Phys.* 2008;9:2686.

KV CBCT-Guided IMRT Using the Elekta Synergy System in a Patient with Tonsillar Carcinoma

Case Study

Vivek K. Mehta, MD, Tony P. Wong, PhD

Patient History

A 60-year-old man presented with a 3-month history of a slowly enlarging mass in his anterior right neck. A fine needle aspiration biopsy was attempted, but was nondiagnostic. A computed tomography (CT) scan of the neck revealed a right anterior neck lymph node measuring 4 cm by 3 cm by 2 cm, and no other abnormalities. Excisional biopsy of the lymph node was performed and pathology demonstrated a 5.2 cm by 3.2 cm lymph node that was completely replaced with squamous cell carcinoma, without evidence of extracapsular extension. A CT scan of the chest revealed no abnormalities.

The patient underwent a panendoscopy. Blind biopsies of the base of tongue, nasopharynx bilaterally, left tonsil, and bilateral turbinates were all negative. Although the right tonsil appeared normal grossly, a tonsillectomy was performed. Pathology demonstrated that the tonsil was nearly completely replaced with a 2.8-cm poorly differentiated squamous cell carcinoma. The tumor invaded the underlying skeletal muscle, and was present at the deep and peripheral margins. The tumor was staged as T2N2aM0 (stage IVA).

Our consensus recommendation was for adjuvant chemoradiotherapy. We elected to treat the patient with kilovoltage (kV) volumetric image-guided intensity-modulated radiotherapy (IMRT) by using an Elekta Synergy linear accelerator (Elekta AB, Stockholm, Sweden).

Simulation

The Type-S Overlay Board; Type-S head, neck, and shoulder thermoplastic immobilization mask; and the Silverman head and neck supports (CIVCO, Kalona, IA) were used for patient positioning and immobilization. The patient was first aligned on the couch by using the tracking lasers in the CT room, with the tragal notch as a reference anatomical landmark. With a straight patient alignment in the superior–inferior direction, the patient's shoulders were then pulled down with straps before the mask was made. The CT scan origin and setup alignment reference points were marked on the mask. The CT image was acquired with a slice thickness of 3 mm by using a HiSpeed CT scanner (GE Healthcare, Waukesha, WI).

Treatment Planning

Treatment planning was performed with the XiO Treatment Planning System, version 4.4 (Elekta-CMS, Maryland Heights, MO). The clinical target volumes (CTVs) and organs at risk (OARs) were contoured on individual CT slices. The CTV_1 was the volume of positive margin after the resection. The CTV_2 was the reminder of the faucial arch and the ipsilateral neck. The CTV_3 was the contralateral neck and CTV_4 was the bilateral lower neck and supraclavicular region. The OARs consisted of the parotids, oral cavity, spinal cord, and brainstem. A uniform margin of 5 mm was added to the CTV and each OAR generating the planning target volume (PTV) and planning OAR volume (PRV), respectively.

The planning target volumes in the right tonsil and bilateral upper neck region had prescription doses of 66 Gy, 60 Gy, and 54 Gy over 30 fractions and the bilateral lower neck had a prescription dose of 50.4 Gy over 28 fractions. The planning target volumes were named

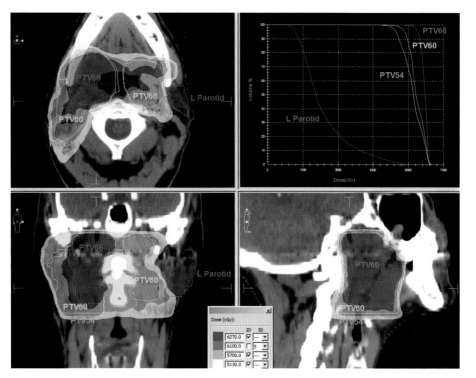

FIGURE 16G-1. The dose distribution highlighting 95% of the prescription doses to planning target volume— 66 Gy (PTV$_{66}$), PTV$_{60}$, and PTV$_{54}$ in the right tonsil and bilateral upper neck region from the seven-field intensity-modulated radiotherapy plan are shown in the transverse plan (upper left), coronal plan (lower left), and the sagittal plan (lower right), along with the dose-volume histogram for the PTV and left parotid (upper right).

PTV$_{66}$ for CTV$_1$, PTV$_{60}$ for CTV$_2$, PTV$_{54}$ for CTV$_3$, and PTV$_{50}$ for CTV$_4$. A treatment plan was generated with a seven-field IMRT to treat the right tonsil and bilateral upper neck region matching with an anterior–posterior (AP) field to treat the lower neck. All the PTVs received at least 95% of the prescription doses to a minimum of 97% their volumes. The maximum doses to the PRV for the spinal cord and brainstem were 45 Gy and 50 Gy, respectively. The mean dose to the left parotid was limited to 24 Gy. Figure 16G-1 shows the dose distribution of 95% of the prescription doses to the PTV$_{66}$, PTV$_{60}$, and PTV$_{54}$ in the right tonsil and bilateral upper neck region from the seven-field IMRT beams and the dose volume histogram for the PTV and left parotid.

After plan approval, the planning CT image data set, structure contours, and treatment isocenter were then exported to the X-ray Volumetric Imaging (XVI) system of the Synergy linear accelerator for cone-beam CT (CBCT)-based image-guided treatment.

Treatment Delivery

The patient was positioned on the treatment couch with the Type-S head extension attached on the superior end of the couch. He was immobilized with the same head rest and thermoplastic head, neck, and shoulder mask that were fabricated during simulation. For the first four treatment days, on-line correction for setup error was performed. After the patient setup using lasers and markers on the mask, a CBCT scan was performed to verify setup accuracy. Setup errors were then calculated based on anatomical structures with image registration between the planning CT and CBCT as shown in Figure 16G-2. Translational setup errors were corrected by shifting the couch in the AP, lateral–medial (ML), and superior–inferior (SI) directions using the auto couch shift feature of the linac. Setup errors for the first four fractions were recorded after each treatment delivery.

The systematic and random errors were calculated to determine if a correction of systematic error should be made. A treatment isocenter shift is made on the fifth fraction to correct for the systematic error if the random error is less than the action level of 3 mm. Table 16G-1 shows the systematic and random errors based on the first four treatments for this patient. After the systematic error was corrected on the fifth fraction, a CBCT scan was obtained prior to treatment to ensure that setup accuracy in all directions was within the 3-mm action level. With the new treatment isocenter, the patient's setup was then verified weekly with CBCT to ensure the setup accuracy and to access any anatomical changes because of tumor response to radiation or weight loss. The systematic and random errors in the AP, ML, and SI direction of the subsequent treatments (after the systematic error was corrected) were 1 mm, 0 mm, and 1 mm; and 0.3 mm, 0.8 mm, and 0.9 mm, respectively. Should the systematic and random errors exceed 3 mm in any direction for the subsequent treatment after the treatment isocenter shift, the daily on-line strategy may be used instead.

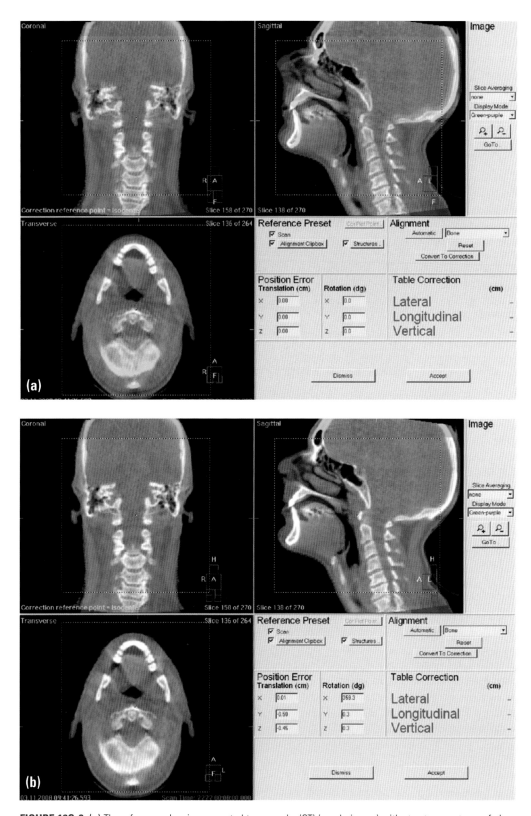

FIGURE 16G-2. (a) The reference planning computed tomography (CT) (purple image) with structure contours of planning target volume—66 Gy (PTV$_{66}$; shown in red), PTV$_{60}$ (green), and PTV$_{54}$ (brown) and the cone beam CT (CBCT) scan (green image) for the first fraction before three-dimensional (3D) image registration. (b) The translation errors of 1 mm, 5 mm, and 4.5 mm in the medial–lateral, superior–inferior, and anterior–posterior directions after 3D image registration based on bony anatomical structures. Rotation errors were well within 1°.

TABLE 16G–1 Systematic and Random Errors Based on the Patient Setup for the First Four Fractions

Direction	Systematic Error, mm	Random Error, mm
Medial–lateral	0	0.5
Superior–inferior	−5	0.8
Anterior–posterior	−5	0.7

Clinical Outcome

The patient tolerated treatment well. The patient experienced the usual side effects of skin reaction and mucosal reaction in the oropharynx. All of these effects were moderate. There were no unplanned treatment interruptions in his course of radiation treatment. The patient also received all of his concurrent chemotherapy without dose reductions or delays. The patient was seen 9 months after completion of therapy. He does not complain of xerostomia and he reports improvement in his taste and swallowing function. He has not experienced any late toxicity to date and remains clinically without evidence of disease.

We recently reviewed our initial clinical experience using kV CBCT imaging to verify setup in patients with a variety of malignancies.[1] In this study, we specifically addressed the utility of a second (post-shift) CBCT. A total of 2651 CBCT scans were acquired in 122 patients. Overall, 11 patients had head and neck or brain tumors. In this group, 115 initial CBCT scans were performed and six post-shift CBCT scans were obtained. All six post-shift CBCT scans revealed residual errors of 2 mm or less. Similar findings were seen in patients with thoracic, abdominal, and pelvic tumors. We concluded that a post-shift CBCT was not needed for the majority of our patients using our current patient immobilization techniques.

Reference

1. Ye J, Wong T, Cao D, Afghan M, Shepard D, Mehta V. Is it necessary to acquire post shift verification cone beam CT? *Int J Radiat Oncol Biol Phys.* 2008:72(1):S648–S649.

Real-Time Reverse Subtraction Video-Guided Setup and Intrafraction Monitoring in a Patient with Head and Neck Cancer

Case Study

Joseph K. Salama, MD, Karl Farrey, MS

Patient History

A 60-year-old man presented with 1 month of right-sided sinus headaches. After a course of antibiotics did not relieve his symptoms, he subsequently developed diplopia and pain behind his right eye. Head and neck magnetic resonance (MR) imaging and computed tomography (CT) scans revealed a 3.5-cm mass replacing the clivus, destroying the anterior and posterior cortex and invading into the cavernous sinuses encasing the carotid arteries bilaterally. Extension into the nasopharynx was also visualized with tumor abutting the right posterior choanae. A positron emission tomography (PET) scan demonstrated increased metabolic activity only within the clival soft tissue mass. A biopsy was performed and was consistent with poorly differentiated carcinoma, and distinctly not sinonasal undifferentiated carcinoma or nasopharyngeal carcinoma.

The patient was evaluated by a head and neck surgeon and was not deemed to be technically resectable with a good functional outcome. After discussion in our multidisciplinary head and neck oncology conference, our consensus recommendation was for neoadjuvant chemotherapy followed by concurrent chemotherapy and radiotherapy (RT), delivered on an alternate-week schedule.[1] We elected to treat the patient by using real-time reverse subtraction video to optimize patient setup and monitor intrafraction motion.

Simulation

A CT simulation was performed before induction chemotherapy to define the patient's disease burden in the treatment position. He was placed supine on the simulator couch. A head rest was used and 50 cc alpha cradle (Smithers Medical Products Inc, North Canton, OH) was used to customize his head position. A lite cast was fashioned about the patient's head to ensure reproducible setup and proper immobilization. Shoulder pulls were used to provide traction on the patient's arms and adequately expose the neck for treatment. Thin (3-mm) CT slices were obtained from above the calvarium to the carina with our Brilliance Big Bore scanner (Philips Medical Systems, Andover, MA). Following neoadjuvant chemotherapy, the procedure was repeated.

Treatment Planning

The preinduction, postinduction planning CTs and the diagnostic MR were transferred to Pinnacle (Koninklijke Philips Electronics NV, Amsterdam, Netherlands) and fused. Per the International Commission on Radiation Units and Measurements (ICRU) Task Group 50 recommendations, the gross tumor volume (GTV) and the organs at risk (OARs) were contoured. The GTV was expanded 7 mm posteriorly and 1.5 cm in all other directions creating planning target volume 1 (PTV_1).

Additionally, as the primary tumor invaded the nasopharynx increasing the risk for microscopic cervical nodal involvement, levels II, III, IV, and V were included bilaterally along with the PTV_1 creating the PTV_2. The OARs including both eyes, optic nerves, the optic chiasm, brain, brainstem, spinal cord, both parotids, and larynx were also contoured.

The planning software placed the isocenter in the geometric center of PTV_1. Two separate plans were calculated, the first to irradiate PTV_2 to 50.4 Gy followed by a boost to PTV_1 with a dose of 21.6 Gy. These volumes were to be treated sequentially. Nine coplanar gantry angles ($200°$, $240°$, $280°$, $320°$, $0°$, $40°$, $80°$, $120°$, and $160°$) were selected. Using a direct machine parameter optimization algorithm, an optimal solution was calculated. A plan with acceptable target coverage and normal tissue constraints was created and approved.

Following plan approval, dose verification with Mapcheck (Sun Nuclear Corporation, Melbourne, FL) was performed. Overall, 99.2% of the points were in agreement with the initial plan and 98.5% with the boost plan based on a 3% per 3 mm distance-to-agreement criterion. Digital reconstructed radiographs (DRRs) were created for both megavoltage (MV) and kilovoltage (kV) treatment setup. Specific anatomic regions (orbits, C1, C2, mandible, sphenoid, and sella) were outlined to aid in quick analysis of the kV images.

Treatment Delivery

Because of the close and immediate proximity of the PTV to the brain stem, daily kilovoltage (kV) imaging was performed. Prior to the first fraction, with the patient in the treatment position, kV imaging was performed in the anterior–posterior (AP) and lateral positions using the On Board Imaging (OBI) system (Varian Medical Systems, Palo Alto, CA). Once appropriate shifts were made by the attending physician, and the patient's setup was judged acceptable, reference video images were captured from the anterior, right, and left directions. These images were obtained by using video cameras permanently mounted in the treatment room next to the left and right lateral lasers and on the ceiling directly above the foot of the patient support apparatus (Figure 16H-1).[2] Subsequently, treatment was delivered. For each subsequent treatment, the patient's initial positioning was directed with a real-time reverse subtraction video positioning system.

Reference video images were first captured following physician approval of pretreatment radiographic imaging. Custom software was used to acquire and archive these video images. Real-time subtraction images were then obtained by subtracting the patient images in the correct position from the live video. A computer and monitor within the treatment room allowed the thera-

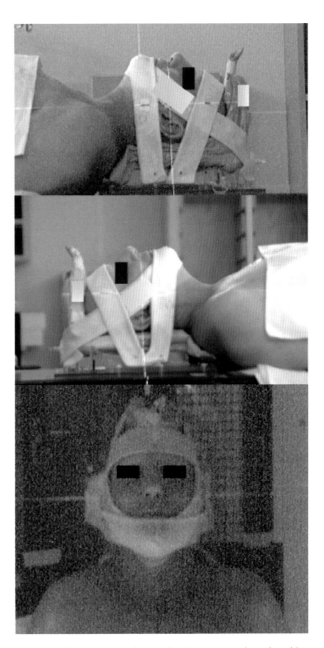

FIGURE 16H-1. Reference images for the reverse subtraction video imaging system. Note that three reference images (right lateral, left lateral, and anterior–posterior) are taken.

pists to view these images, updated at a rate of 15 frames per second, revealing patient misalignment in multiple views, and interactively return the patient to the reference (correct treatment) position. Therapists were trained to try to match areas of anatomy not readily deformed with the custom immobilization as well as having high pixel counts, notably the nose, chin, and ear. Areas not in alignment were highlighted with contrast-rich features of white and gray shades. As the position became more exact, the outlines became thinner, and, finally, as each pixel registered with the reference image, became a featureless gray image. The utility of this system relies on

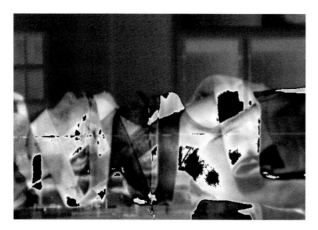

FIGURE 16H-2. Reverse subtraction video image showing a large misalignment of the patient. The reference image in white guides the therapists toward proper alignment.

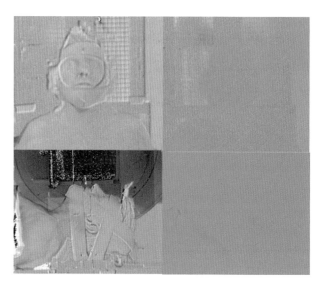

FIGURE 16H-3. Reverse subtraction video images. In the left column, the patient is in close but not perfect alignment in both the anterior and lateral views. This is demonstrated by the white shadows on the right side of the patient's mask and the dark shadows on the left side of the mask. On the right side, the patient alignment is correct, with the reference image completely subtracting out the real-time image leaving only faint shades of gray.

the fact that small positioning errors (0.5 mm and 0.5°) are easily detected by eye. The imaging system has been shown to be sensitive to changes in position of approximately 0.1 mm.[2]

Our video system has many advantages over conventional x-ray imaging. First, daily accurate patient positioning is achieved without the use of ionizing radiation. Second, the system is quick, requiring approximately 1 minute, which is shorter than the time needed for many other image-guided devices. Furthermore, it is intuitive and allows rapid identification of setup errors, and ease of use. As shown in Figures 16H-2 and 16H-3, the reference image can be used to guide and fine-tune a patient's initial setup.

An additional benefit for this system is the ability for it to be used not only for daily patient positioning, but also to analyze patient motion during each fraction. During the patient's treatment course, he was constantly observed by the treating therapists. When alignment deviated from the optimal, corrective instructions were communicated to the patient as shown in Figure 16H-4.

Clinical Outcome

The patient tolerated his treatment well. His cranial nerve deficits and intractable headaches resolved 2 weeks into therapy. He continues on treatment currently and will be monitored closely following completion of his therapy for treatment response and potential late toxicities.

Our initial clinical experience using video-based image-guided setup and intrafraction monitoring in patients with head and neck cancer was published earlier.[3] In a prospective study on patients with head and neck cancer, use of this video imaging system was found to reduce

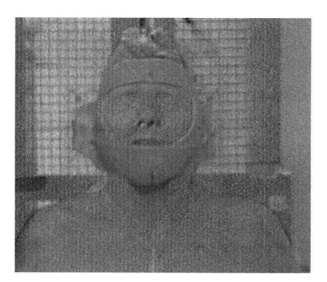

FIGURE 16H-4. During treatment the reverse subtraction video imaging is used to monitor intrafraction motion. In this image, the patient's head is turned slightly to the right, as illustrated by the white shadows appearing on the left side of the patient's mask. Corrective instructions are communicated during treatment to the patient to correct these issues as treatment continues.

the standard deviation of setup error from 3.5 mm using conventional radiographic imaging to 1.2 mm. The extra time required to use the system was found to be approximately 1 minute.

References

1. Salama JK, Stenson KM, Kistner EO, et al. Induction chemo-therapy and concurrent chemoradiotherapy for locoregionally advanced head and neck cancer: a multi-institutional phase II trial investigating three radiotherapy dose levels. *Ann Oncol.* 2008;19:1787–1794.

2. Milliken BD, Rubin SJ, Hamilton RJ, et al. Performance of a video-image-subtraction-based patient positioning system. *Int J Radiat Oncol Biol Phys.* 1997;38:855–866.

3. Johnson LS, Milliken BD, Hadley SW, et al. Initial clinical experience with a video-based patient positioning system. *Int J Radiat Oncol Biol Phys.* 1999;45:205–213.

Chapter 17

Lung Cancer: Overview

Elizabeth Kidd, MD, Daniel Low, PhD, Jeffrey Bradley, MD

Image-guided radiation therapy (IGRT) represents a new era of radiation oncology, using advanced imaging techniques to better aid in target definition and treatment planning, and onboard imaging to localize and position the patient's tumor at the planned location. Such technologies provide the potential for more conformal dose distributions and improved patient outcomes.

For patients with lung cancer, IGRT offers particular advantages. Historically, lung cancer has been associated with poor rates of local control following radiation therapy (RT). Some of the main reasons for this relate to (1) geographic miss because of the inability to detect all areas of disease for staging and subsequent RT treatment planning, (2) geographic miss because of respiratory motion, relating both to adequately defining the full extent of disease for treatment planning and developing a treatment plan that accounts for the motion so the full course of radiation is appropriately delivered to the tumor, and (3) inadequate radiation dose prescription because of the potential toxicity to surrounding normal tissues. All three of these issues are directly and indirectly aided by the use of IGRT in patients with non–small cell lung cancer (NSCLC).

Image-guided RT offers significant potential for improving lung cancer RT. Image-guided RT aids in more accurate target delineation, in particular with ^{18}F-fluorodeoxyglucose positron emission tomography (^{18}F-FDG PET). Four-dimensional (4D) CT simulation helps define the extent of lung tumor movement caused by respiration, facilitating more accurate treatment planning. Onboard imaging systems including real-time kilovoltage fluoroscopy, cone-beam computed tomography (CT), and megavoltage CT, help ensure the tumor is accurately aligned with the treatment plan. Additionally, performing a cone-beam CT (CBCT) scan before each individual treatment decreases positional uncertainty and may allow for tighter margins. With smaller target volumes, less normal tissues are at risk, allowing for the possibility of dose escalation. Other imaging modalities, such as single positron emission computed tomography (SPECT), can also aid the process of sparing more normal lung tissues. Furthermore, stereotactic body RT (SBRT) for lung cancer, delivering highly conformal high doses of radiation in a limited number of fractions with image guidance before each treatment, demonstrates the advantages and applications of IGRT in patients with NSCLC (Table 17-1). The multiple uses of imaging to guide RT represent a major breakthrough in lung cancer treatment.

Image-Guided Target Delineation
Positron Emission Tomography

In the era of intensity-modulated RT (IMRT) and more conformal targeting, accurately defining areas of disease becomes critically important, as tissues outside the target volume will not receive therapeutic radiation doses. ^{18}F-FDG PET represents an essential tool for lung cancer RT planning, by aiding in accurately defining all areas of disease. Variability in tumor contouring among radiation oncologists is known to be a factor that may adversely affect treatment planning and delivery.[1] A significant decrease in inter- and intraobserver variation in tumor contouring, in particular for lung cancer, has been shown by incorporating functional imaging, such as ^{18}F-FDG PET fusion.[2–4] It has been estimated that approximately 60% of lung cancer patients undergoing imaging with ^{18}F-FDG PET have potential changes in target volume and/or dose distribution parameters.[5]

^{18}F-FDG PET greatly aids in staging lung cancer patients. Pieterman and colleagues reported that ^{18}F-FDG PET has better sensitivity and specificity than CT for detecting involved mediastinal lymph nodes and changed the stage in more than half the patients evaluated, decreasing it in one third and increasing the stage in the other two thirds.[6] The superior specificity and sensitivity of ^{18}F-FDG PET has been further confirmed in a metaanalysis involving 39 studies, which found that ^{18}F-FDG PET was significantly more accurate than CT in identifying lymph node

TABLE 17–1 Lung Stereotactic Body Radiation Therapy Local Control Rates

Study	Years of Study	Disease Type	Number of Patients	Dose/ Fractionation	Median Follow-Up	Local Control
Baumann et al.[64]	1996–2003	Stage I NSCLC	138	30 Gy to 48 Gy, 2 to 4 fractions	33 months	88%
McGarry et al.[65]	1/2000–1/2003	Stage I NSCLC	47	24 Gy to 72 Gy, 8 Gy to 24 Gy/fraction	~24 months	79%
Onishi et al.[66]	4/1995–2/2003	Stage I NSCLC	245	18 Gy to 75 Gy, 1 to 22 fractions	24 months	91.9%
Timmerman et al.[67]	2/2000–6/2002	Stage I NSCLC	37	24 Gy to 60 Gy, 8 to 20 Gy/fraction	15.2 months	84%
Uematsu et al.[69]	10/1994–6/1999	Stage I NSCLC	50	50 Gy to 60 Gy, 5 to 10 fractions	36 months	94%
Zimmermann et al.[68]	12/2000–10/2003	Stage I NSCLC	30	24 Gy to 37.5 Gy, 3 to 5 fractions	18 months	93%

Note. NSCLC – non–small cell lung cancer.

involvement ($P < .001$), and from all the studies ^{18}F-FDG PET had a median sensitivity of 85% and a median specificity of 90%.[7] Besides aiding in identifying involved lymph nodes and areas of tumor, ^{18}F-FDG PET is also useful for distinguishing atelectasis from tumor. Other studies have suggested that integrated ^{18}F-FDG PET–CT is more accurate for tumor and lymph node staging in NSCLC than CT alone or ^{18}F-FDG PET alone.[8] ^{18}F-FDG PET has also been shown to have superior reliability, compared with CT, for distinguishing benign versus malignant solitary pulmonary nodules.[9] The additional information about the extent of tumor and nodal involvement provided by ^{18}F-FDG PET and ^{18}F-FDG PET–CT greatly improves RT treatment planning for lung cancer. Moreover, some studies have shown that more than 50% of lung cancer treatment plans are modified by a coregistered ^{18}F-FDG PET imaging study, compared with the use of CT-based treatment planning alone.[10] Figure 17-1 shows some example images of where ^{18}F-FDG PET revealed new areas of disease. The use of ^{18}F-FDG PET to guide target delineation in a patient with lung cancer is discussed in Chapter 17A.

Besides providing useful anatomic information, the functional aspects of ^{18}F-FDG PET also provide significant prognostic information for lung cancer, which can also aid RT planning. Maximal lung tumor standardized uptake value (SUV) has been shown to be correlated with radiation treatment response.[11] Additionally, a meta-analysis involving 13 studies found that the SUV of the primary lung tumor has prognostic value with a higher value correlating with an increased risk of recurrence.[12] The prognostic value of high ^{18}F-FDG uptake within the primary NSCLC tumor suggests the possible utility of dose-painting or boosting particular subvolumes of the lung tumor with higher doses of radiation.

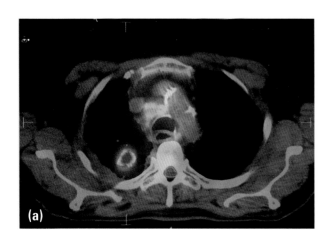 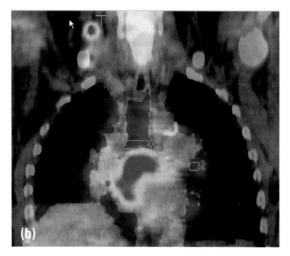

FIGURE 17-1. Examples of ^{18}F-fluorodeoxyglucose positron emission tomography (^{18}F-FDG PET) demonstrating previously undetected areas of disease that caused the radiation treatment plan to be changed. **(a)** A patient with a presumed stage I (T1N0M0) non–small cell lung cancer before an ^{18}F-FDG PET that revealed a paratracheal lymph node and T1N2M0 disease. **(b)** An example of where an ^{18}F-FDG PET scan revealed supraclavicular lymph node involvement.

Single Photon Emission Computed Tomography

Another imaging modality that has value for NSCLC is SPECT. Rather than highlighting areas of cancer that should be targeted with radiation, SPECT can help identify the most functional areas of lung tissue so they can be avoided. SPECT lung imaging relies on injected radiolabeled microspheres becoming trapped in lung capillaries. The microsphere concentration is related to regional pulmonary blood flow.[13] SPECT lung perfusion has been shown to correlate with lung function.[14] Two different groups have shown that SPECT-guided IMRT can effectively reduce the radiation dose delivered to the highly functional lung regions.[15] Figure 17-2 illustrates an IMRT treatment plan comparison with and without SPECT-based planning. This novel use of SPECT to guide NSCLC radiation treatment planning could potentially reduce treatment-related toxicity, such as radiation pneumonitis, and may allow for further dose escalation.

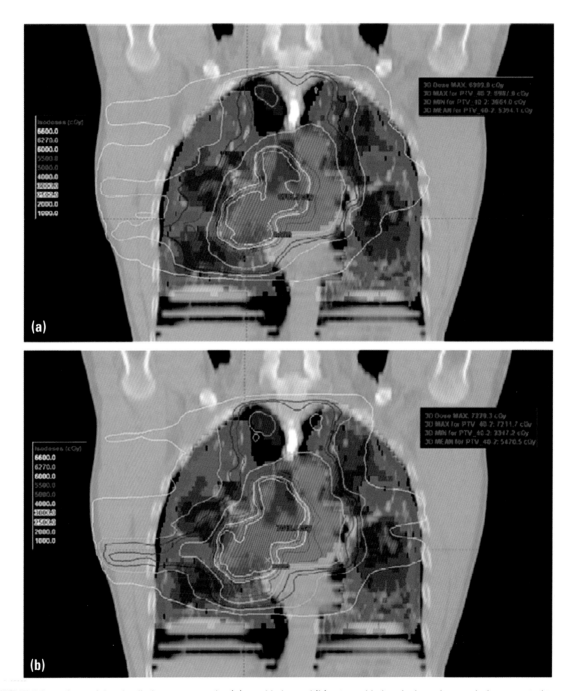

FIGURE 17-2. Intensity-modulated radiation treatment plan (a) considering and (b) not considering single positron emission computed tomography (SPECT) image-based lung perfusion. SPECT shows the most to least functional lung regions as red, orange, yellow, and green. (From Mcguire SM et al. *Int J Radiat Oncol Biol Phys.* 2006;66(5):1543–1552. Permission granted from Elsevier.)

Four-Dimensional Computed Tomography

Tumor motion is another obstacle to treating patients with NSCLC that is aided by advances in imaging. Numerous studies have reported that lung tumors can substantially vary in position during quiet breathing, thereby causing issues for treatment delivery and loss of tumor coverage.[16–20] Four-dimensional (4D) CT simulation provides a means to measure lung tumor motion and thereby improve target coverage. A 4D CT scan is similar to a traditional 3D scan, except the patient support table moves at a much slower speed during which each region of tissue is repeatedly and rapidly imaged during the breathing cycle. The resultant images are then sorted to user-specified breathing phases. This imaging is typically conducted with multislice CT scanners (i.e., 16- or 64-slice scanners). Additionally, a breathing cycle measurement system (e.g., spirometry or a bellows mechanism) is attached to the patient to provide respiratory phase information. During the acquisition of images, each slice is tagged with respiratory phase information. Following completion of the 4D scan, all slices of the same respiratory phase are binned together, and a composite CT is created for each phase. The images can be replayed as a movie, giving the impression of tumor and organ motion. Internal motion is not actually followed in real-time by 4D CT, but instead it creates an approximate model.[21] Four-dimensional CT provides an estimation of how much a particular lung tumor moves to determine what type of target volume modification is necessary to account for that motion.

Four-dimensional CT simulation creates a large scan data set. To reduce the amount of image data that the treatment planner needs to review, the maximum intensity projection (MIP) technique was introduced as a simple means of extracting the motion information.[22] To create an MIP, each voxel in the complete 4D CT data collection is set to the highest density it had during the entire respiratory cycle. The MIP thus creates a representation of the entire volume through which the lung tumor transversed during the respiratory cycle. The International Commission on Radiation Units and Measurements (ICRU) Report 62 introduced the concept of internal target volume (ITV), which can be used to account for tumor motion, such as observed with a MIP.

The increased use of 4D CT has expanded our understanding of lung tumor motion. In a recent 4D CT study, Liu and colleagues found that more than 50% of tumors moved more than 5 mm during treatment and 10.8% moved more than 1 cm, whereas some tumors (particularly lesions close to the diaphragm) move as much as 3 cm to 4 cm.[23] Other groups have found a statistically significant difference in the amount of movement between lower and upper lobe tumors, with lower lobe tumors displaying more movement.[24] Seppenwoolde and coworkers also reported that the amplitude of tumor movement was greatest in the cranio–caudal direction for tumors situated in the lower lobes and not attached to rigid structures, such as the chest wall and vertebrae.[25] With 4D CT helping to show the extent of lung tumor motion, the applications of this technique for guiding lung radiation became more extensive.

Despite the advantages of 4D CT, there are also some limitations. For example, 4D CT does not take into account movements not associated with breathing, such as cardiac motion.[21] Additionally, 4D CT represents a sampling of the tumor motion and does not actually track the tumor in real time. If the patient has an irregular breathing pattern, the 4D CT may have artifacts and may not be representative of the patient's breathing and tumor location at the time of treatment. One group found that lung tumor volume decreased by 20% to 71% over the 7 weeks of radiation, leading to significantly increased tumor mobility, particularly in the superior–inferior and anterior–posterior directions, which may suggest the initial ITV is not appropriate for the full course of treatment.[26]

Radiation treatment planning and delivery can be performed using a few methods including ITV, breath-hold, linear accelerator gating, or tumor tracking. Ideally, the selected method is individualized to the patient's tumor motion magnitude and the regularity of their breathing pattern. The ITV method is the most straightforward method to use and works well for tumors that move 5 mm or less. For tumors that move more than 5 mm, one could choose to deliver RT while a patient holds his or her breath, if the patient is able to hold their breath for approximately 15 seconds. Alternatively, linear accelerator beam gating may be used to turn the radiation beam "off" and "on" during treatment when the tumor is outside or inside a selected gating window, respectively. Commercially available breath-hold and gating technology includes Active Breathing Control (ABC; Elekta AB, Stockholm, Sweden) and Real-time Position Management (RPM; Varian Medical Systems Inc, Palo Alto, CA). An example case of a patient treated with the Varian RPM system is presented in Chapter 17E.

Tumor tracking, a more advanced form of 4D treatment, follows the tumor at all times and allows for irradiation of the tumor in motion. At this time, the Accuray CyberKnife (Accuray Inc, Sunnyvale, CA) and Novalis BrainLAB (BrainLAB, Feldkirchen, Germany) are the only commercially available technologies that employ tumor tracking. Image-guided RT, regardless of which of these respiratory motion management methods is employed, is used to verify that the tumor position at the time of treatment corresponds to the planning images. The use of metallic fiducial markers is helpful, particularly when gating or tracking, to verify that the tumor position is within the planned location both before and during beam delivery. Metallic fiducial markers are visible on both kV x-ray and CT and should ideally be placed within or adjacent to the tumor target. See Chapter 11 for further discussion of the technologies and research focused on motion management in patients with lung cancer undergoing RT.

Image-Guided Treatment Delivery

The sharp dose fall-offs that surround target volumes when using highly conformal RT necessitates accurate target delineation during treatment planning and accurate target alignment during treatment. In-room imaging allows for verification of tumor alignment to the planned treatment position, just before treatment. Historically, imaging has consisted of weekly port films, but with the use of more conformal treatment plans and the additional challenge of tumor motion, many clinical situations require more accurate and more frequent imaging.

Kilovoltage Onboard Imaging Systems

Kilovoltage onboard imaging (OBI) systems rotate with the gantry, allowing kV images to be taken from any gantry angle around the patient. Onboard imaging allows the user to conduct a match of the two-dimensional kV image and a two-dimensional projection through the CT simulation data set, termed a digitally reconstructed radiograph (DRR). Many commercial RT treatment units can now provide 3D soft tissue imaging immediately before, during, or after radiation delivery, thereby improving the localization of the target. In particular, some systems allow for a kV CBCT to be taken, permitting a comparison of the 3D CBCT data set with the 3D CT simulation data set. The 3D volumetric imaging and alignment reduces interfraction geometric uncertainties and thereby allows for reduction in the planning target volume (PTV) margin. The Varian Trilogy (Varian Medical Systems, Palo Alto, CA) and Elekta Synergy (Elekta AB, Stockholm, Sweden) are two examples of treatment machines with integrated kV imaging systems capable of producing CBCT images.

Image-guided information can be applied in different ways. Image registration is an important tool for the measurement of tumor positioning errors. Registration can be applied to fiducial markers, bony landmarks, tumors, or other visual cues. Mageras and Mechalakos compared residual errors from registration methods, showing the advantages of CBCT over weekly or daily radiographs and how much smaller residual errors were when alignment was conducted using the tumor rather than bony anatomy.[27] Whether the image-guided corrections are applied immediately or before a later fraction are decisions that are made by the treating physician and/or institution. On-line corrections use images that are evaluated before each treatment and adjustments occur just before the delivery of each fraction. This on-line correction allows for the possibility of reducing both systematic and random uncertainties, but can be time consuming. Having automated control of the treatment couch facili-

tates incorporating this procedure into clinical routine. With off-line corrections, images are collected during the course of radiation therapy but no immediate change is applied. After a small number of fractions, the systematic positioning error is calculated and a correction is applied for future fractions.

Cone-beam CT can be useful in different treatment situations. In one study comparing CBCT and electronic portal imaging device (EPID) images for patients with lung cancer, CBCT showed significantly larger setup errors and, if CBCT had not been used, more than 50% of patients would have had a setup error larger than 5 mm.[28] Bissonnette and colleagues evaluated the geometric accuracy of lung cancer treatments using daily CBCT and on-line couch adjustments.[29] They evaluated three different situations: (1) early stage NSCLC treated with SBRT, (2) locally advanced NSCLC with manual couch adjustment, and (3) locally advanced NSCLC with remote controlled couch adjustment. Imaging revealed that 3D positioning errors greater than 5 mm occurred in 54.5% of all fractions. Cone-beam CT reduced these systematic and random positional errors to less than 2 mm for the SBRT patients. For the locally advanced patients, significant postcorrection improvements were seen with the remote-controlled couch, in comparison with the manual couch. Improving random and systematic positional errors with daily CBCT could potentially allow for margin reductions and dose escalation.

Purdie and associates evaluated the accuracy of localization with CBCT for T1–T2 NSCLC patients to be treated with SBRT.[30] With this study, they found that pretreatment CBCT reduced the average residual positioning error to less than 2 mm. Additionally, they noted an average difference of 6.8 mm between the target and bony anatomy, suggesting that bony anatomy is not a good surrogate of the target for localization. Other studies have also compared the accuracy of bony anatomy versus target volume registration for hypofractionated lung cancer treatments, and also found that isocenter positions can differ by more than 5 mm, suggesting that target-based registration is more appropriate than bony-anatomy–based registration.[31]

At the Siteman Cancer Center, all lung SBRT patients are treated with a protocol using CBCT and fluoroscopy. The fluoroscopy image is superimposed onto a projection of the tumor boundary (including a margin for motion, if appropriate). When the patient has been correctly positioned, the fluoroscopic tumor shadow should project within the tumor boundary. Figure 17-3 shows a CBCT and fluoroscopic images from a lung SBRT treatment.

Image-guided RT using CBCT is fairly straightforward to introduce into the clinical setting. Because the goal of CBCT imaging is to localize the tumor or markers, and not to diagnose or detect new tumors, the imaging dose can be substantially lower than a diagnostic CT. Fox and

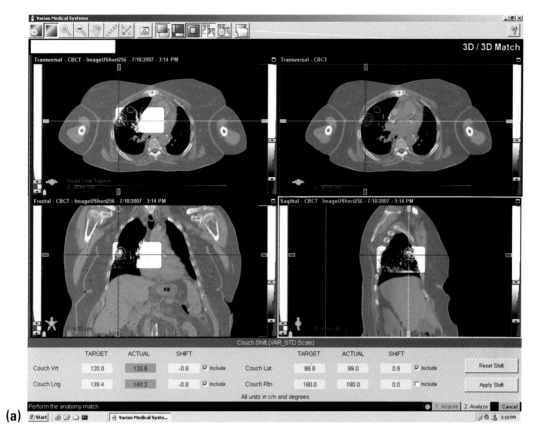

(a)

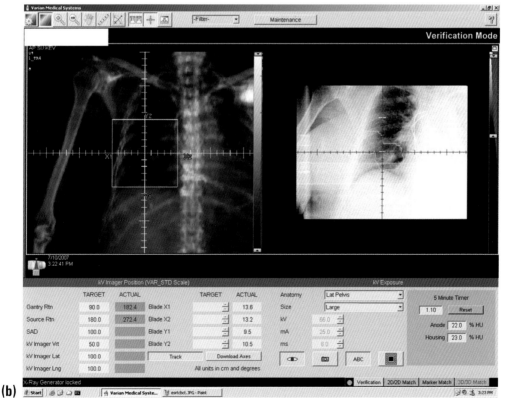

(b)

FIGURE 17-3. Image-guided lung stereotactic body radiation therapy, **(a)** Treatment planning computed tomography (CT) and superimposed cone-beam CT (smaller box) registration for the three-dimensional (3D) to 3D match. **(b)** Fluoroscopy-based verification that the lung tumor lies within the planning target volume.

coworkers noted that the average IGRT procedure time significantly decreased over the first year in use and each therapist showed improvement in reducing IGRT procedure time.[32] With routine use, IGRT may be performed within 3 to 4 minutes with minimal disruption to the clinical treatment process. Example cases of patients with lung cancer treated with daily CBCT for tumor localization are presented in Chapters 17D and 17E.

Tomotherapy

Tomotherapy (TomoTherapy Inc, Madison, WI) involves an integrated technology combining a helical megavoltage (MV) CT with a linear accelerator specifically designed for delivering IMRT using a slit geometry. There have been some small feasibility studies showing how helical tomotherapy can be used for lung SBRT with the pretreatment MVCT providing good target visualization.[33-35] A phase I dose escalation study involving patients with stage I–IV NSCLC demonstrated lower than expected rates of pneumonitis and esophagitis when they were treated with hypofractionated, image-guided tomotherapy.[36]

It has been suggested that helical tomotherapy with MVCT image guidance can be easily integrated into routine clinical practice. One of the larger tomotherapy studies, involving 37 thoracic tumors along with 113 other types of tumors, found that the average time on the tomotherapy treatment table was 24.8 minutes with an average of 10.7 minutes being devoted to treatment, and the average correction vector after MV-CT registration was 6.9 mm.[37] Additionally, the average radiation dose from the tomotherapy MVCT is about 1.5 cGy per image, and the dose is greatest when the anatomic thickness is the smallest and the CT pitch is set to the lowest value.[38] An example case of a patient with lung cancer treated with helical tomotherapy is presented in Chapter 17C.

Other research involving lung cancer and tomotherapy relate to dealing with tumor motion and adaptive planning. For example, slow MVCT may be a reasonable substitute for determining an ITV for nongated moving lung tumors.[39] Ramsey and coworkers suggested that the gross tumor volume (GTV) could be reduced by 60% to 80%

during the course of lung cancer tomotherapy treatment, with the greatest benefit being for tumors larger than 25 cm³, and that this would decrease the volume of ipsilateral lung receiving 20 Gy by an average of 21%.[40] Additional research is still needed on the applicability of these techniques.

CyberKnife

The CyberKnife system (Accuray Inc, Sunnyvale, CA) has a compact 6-MV linear accelerator mounted on a robotic arm with six degrees of freedom that can be programmed to deliver radiation to a tumor from multiple angles. Additionally, the treatment room contains two orthogonal kV x-ray imaging systems. CyberKnife requires fiducial markers that are placed in or close to the tumor. The kV imaging system takes repeated orthogonal images of the implanted fiducial markers to verify tumor position and alignment for treatment. If the images indicate displacement of the fiducial markers, the robotic arms of the linear accelerator will adjust to track tumor motion. The CyberKnife robotic arm can move at a speed of several centimeters per second, and Cyberknife was the first clinical RT system to use real-time motion compensation.[41]

Several small studies have shown that CyberKnife is tolerable and feasible for treating stage I NSCLC or lung metastasis with hypofractionated image-guided radiation.[42-44] Le and coworkers conducted a single fraction dose escalation study for T1–T2 NSCLC or solitary lung metastasis and found that doses greater than 20 Gy were associated with higher local control, but patients who have received prior thoracic radiotherapy have increased risk of toxicity for doses greater than 25 Gy.[45] Table 17-2 summarizes the results of the CyberKnife studies involving lung cancer. This system can be used to effectively treat early stage NSCLC or lung metastasis, but the optimal dosing and fractionation are still in the early phases of investigation. An example of a patient with lung cancer treated with the CyberKnife system is presented in Chapter 17B.

Another area of CyberKnife research is the use of different types of fiducial markers. Depending on the location of the tumor, the requirement that the markers be

TABLE 17–2 Data From CyberKnife Lung Cancer Studies

Study	Disease Type	Number of Patients	Dose/ Fractionation	Median Follow-Up	Local Control
Brown et al.[42]	Stage I NSCLC	59	15 Gy to 67.5 Gy, 1 to 5 fractions	Longest follow-up = 36 months	90%
Collins et al.[43]	Stage I NSCLC	20	42 Gy to 60 Gy, 3 fractions	25 months	100%
Coon et al.[44]	Stage I and recurrent NSCLC, metastasis	51	60 Gy, 3 fractions	12 months recurrent 62%	85% stage I 92% metastasis
Le et al.[45]	Stage I NSCLC, metastasis	32	15 Gy to 30 Gy, 1 fraction	18 months	91% > 20 Gy 54% < 20 Gy

Note. NSCLC – non–small cell lung cancer.

placed in or near the tumor can create a challenge for placing a marker while not causing a pneumothorax, especially because many patients with thoracic tumors might already have compromised lung function. One group examined three different methods of marker placement: (1) intravascular coil placement, (2) percutaneous intrathoracic, and (3) percutaneous extrathoracic placement, and all were found to be safe and efficacious.[46] The use of endovascular coils placed in the subsegmental pulmonary artery branches in close proximity to the tumor is another technique that has been investigated, which may be particularly useful for patients who cannot tolerate standard transthoracic percutaneous marker placement.[47] Anantham and colleagues have also shown the feasibility of electromagnetic navigation bronchoscopy-guided fiducial placement for peripheral lung tumors.[48] The expansion of methods for placing fiducial markers has expanded the clinical scenarios where CyberKnife can be used.

CyberKnife relies on fiducial markers for image guidance of the radiation treatment, but respiratory and tumor motion represent a separate issue. Synchrony, the optic motion tracking system of CyberKnife, uses a complex system of cameras, motion-tracking software, fiberoptic sensing technology, infrared emitters, and a special tight-fitting elastic patient vest. While a patient is under treatment with CyberKnife, the Synchrony system continually identifies patient breathing movement in conjunction with the internally placed fiducial markers. This information is then used to update the treatment delivery. Synchrony has also been shown to be useful in the treatment of early stage NSCLC or lung metastasis.[49,50] Initially, the tumor tracking method was not used routinely in clinical practice because of heavy computing requirements and hardware limitations, but this has improved with the latest software and equipment updates.

Novalis BrainLAB

Novalis BrainLAB (BrainLAB, Feldkirchen, Germany) is an integrated IGRT system for target localization, setup correction, and delivery of high-precision stereotactic radiosurgery. The system requires implanted fiducials and infrared-reflecting markers placed on the patient's skin. The skin markers are visible by two infrared (IR) cameras and one video camera mounted on the ceiling of the treatment room. A kV imaging system images the implanted fiducial markers and is fully integrated with the IR tracking system. The isocenter is determined by the special relationship between the kV system and the IR tracking system. This system allows patient and treatment couch movement to be controlled by real-time tracking of the IR markers. The kV system always requires a surrogate to identify the target, either bony structures or radio-opaque implanted markers. As the kV system operates independently of the treatment machine, image acquisition can be performed during treatment, allowing real-time assessment of target motion to cope with intrafractional organ motion.[51]

Compared with the other IGRT technologies, there is a more limited number of studies of the Novalis BrainLAB system and lung cancer. Some preliminary studies have shown that image-guided hypofractionated treatment of early stage primary NSCLC or lung metastasis can be safely and effectively carried out with the BrainLAB system.[52-56] Table 17-3 summarizes Novalis BrainLAB studies involving lung cancer. The Novalis IGRT system can be used for lung SBRT, but additional research is still needed on its full application.

Future Directions

Growing evidence supports the feasibility of and potential benefit to dose escalation in patients with NSCLC.[57-63] Increasing interest is also focused on the expanded role of SBRT in lung cancer.[64-69] Stereotactic body RT has outcomes that appear similar to surgery, with local control rates greater than 85%.[66,70] Image-guided RT is critical to ensure optimal target coverage and sparing of surrounding normal tissues in patients with lung cancer who are treated with escalated doses using conventionally

TABLE 17-3 Data From Novalis BrainLAB Studies Involving NSCLC

Study	Disease Type	Number of Patients	Dose/ Fractionation	Median Follow-Up	Local Control
Chen et al.[52]	NSCLC stage I–IV, metastasis	85	50 Gy to 52 Gy, 4 Gy to 5 Gy/ fraction	18.5 months	72% newly diagnosed 57% recurrent
Ernst-Stecken et al.[53]	Stage I NSCLC, metastasis	21 patients 39 tumors	35 Gy to 40 Gy, 7 Gy to 8 Gy/ fraction	6.3 months	87%
McCammon et al.[54]	Primary, recurrent, metastatic lung and liver	165 lung 81 liver (65 primary or recurrent; 181 metastatic)	15 Gy to 60 Gy, 3 fractions	8.2 months	89.3% > 54 Gy 59% 36 Gy to 53.9 Gy 8.1% < 36 Gy

Note. NSCLC – non–small cell lung cancer.

fractionated and hypofractionated regimens. Consequently, the role of IGRT, for image-guided target and normal tissue delineation as well as image-guided treatment delivery, is expected to grow significantly in the coming years.

Imaging a lung tumor before each treatment with IGRT leads to the possibility of modifying treatment plans during the course of radiation, or adaptive radiation therapy (ART). Harsolia and colleagues evaluated different lung tumor treatment plans, including 3D conformal, 4D-union (similar to an ITV plan), 4D-offline adaptive with single correction, and 4D-online adaptive with daily correction.[71] They found the ART techniques provided better PTV coverage than the other techniques. Additionally, the 4D plans decreased the amount of irradiated normal tissue, compared with the 3D-conformal plan, and thereby resulted in a lower mean lung dose and V_{20}, with both 4D adaptive plans showing the greatest decreases. Implementing ART raises many other issues, such as after what dose is it appropriate to modify treatment margins, what are the thresholds for knowing when adaptive treatment should be applied, and how can adaptive replanning be efficiently integrated into the clinical setting. Although IGRT creates the possibility of further reducing tumor margins as treatment progresses, ART planning using IGRT data is topic that needs further research.

References

1.. Weiss E, Hess CF. The impact of gross tumor volume (GTV) and clinical target volume (CTV) definition on the total accuracy in radiotherapy theoretical aspects and practical experiences. *Strahlenther Onkol.* 2003;179:21–30.

2. Caldwell CB, Mah K, Ung YC, et al. Observer variation in contouring gross tumor volume in patients with poorly defined non-small-cell lung tumors on CT: the impact of 18FDG-hybrid PET fusion. *Int J Radiat Oncol Biol Phys.* 2001;51:923–931.

3. Fox JL, Rengan R, O'Meara W, et al. Does registration of PET and planning CT images decrease interobserver and intraobserver variation in delineating tumor volumes for non-small-cell lung cancer? *Int J Radiat Oncol Biol Phys.* 2005;62:70–75.

4. Steenbakkers RJ, Duppen JC, Fitton I, et al. Reduction of observer variation using matched CT-PET for lung cancer delineation: a three-dimensional analysis. *Int J Radiat Oncol Biol Phys.* 2006;64:435–448.

5. Guha C, Alfieri A, Blaufox MD, et al. Tumor biology-guided radiotherapy treatment planning: gross tumor volume versus functional tumor volume. *Semin Nucl Med.* 2008;38:105–113.

6. Pieterman RM, van Putten JW, Meuzelaar JJ, et al. Preoperative staging of non-small-cell lung cancer with positron-emission tomography. *N Engl J Med.* 2000;343:254–261.

7. Gould MK, Kuschner WG, Rydzak CE, et al. Test performance of positron emission tomography and computed tomography for mediastinal staging in patients with non-small-cell lung cancer: a meta-analysis. *Ann Intern Med.* 2003;139:879–892.

8. Lardinois D, Weder W, Hany TF, et al. Staging of non-small-cell lung cancer with integrated positron-emission tomography and computed tomography. *N Engl J Med.* 2003;348:2500–2507.

9. Fletcher JW, Kymes SM, Gould M, et al. A comparison of the diagnostic accuracy of 18F-FDG PET and CT in the characterization of solitary pulmonary nodules. *J Nucl Med.* 2008;49:179–185.

10. Bradley J, Thorstad WL, Mutic S, et al. Impact of FDG-PET on radiation therapy volume delineation in non-small-cell lung cancer. *Int J Radiat Oncol Biol Phys.* 2004;59:78–86.

11. Borst GR, Belderbos JS, Boellaard R, et al. Standardised FDG uptake: a prognostic factor for inoperable non-small cell lung cancer. *Eur J Cancer.* 2005;41:1533–1541.

12. Berghmans T, Dusart M, Paesmans M, et al. Primary tumor standardized uptake value (SUVmax) measured on fluorodeoxyglucose positron emission tomography (FDG-PET) is of prognostic value for survival in non-small cell lung cancer (NSCLC): a systematic review and meta-analysis (MA) by the European Lung Cancer Working Party for the IASLC Lung Cancer Staging Project. *J Thorac Oncol.* 2008;3:6–12.

13. Klumper A, Zwijnenburg A. Dual isotope (81Krm and 99Tcm) SPECT in lung function diagnosis. *Phys Med Biol.* 1986;31:751–761.

14. Osborne D, Jaszczak RJ, Greer K, et al. SPECT quantification of technetium-99m microspheres within the canine lung. *J Comput Assist Tomogr.* 1985;9:73–77.

15. McGuire SM, Zhou S, Marks LB, et al. A methodology for using SPECT to reduce intensity-modulated radiation therapy (IMRT) dose to functioning lung. *Int J Radiat Oncol Biol Phys.* 2006;66:1543–1552.

16. Ekberg L, Holmberg O, Wittgren L, et al. What margins should be added to the clinical target volume in radiotherapy treatment planning for lung cancer? *Radiother Oncol.* 1998;48:71–77.

17. Guerrero T, Zhang G, Segars W, et al. Elastic image mapping for 4-D dose estimation in thoracic radiotherapy. *Radiat Prot Dosimetry.* 2005;115:497–502.

18. Ross CS, Hussey DH, Pennington EC, et al. Analysis of movement of intrathoracic neoplasms using ultrafast computerized tomography. *Int J Radiat Oncol Biol Phys.* 1990;18:671–677.

19. Stevens CW, Munden RF, Forster KM, et al. Respiratory-driven lung tumor motion is independent of tumor size, tumor location, and pulmonary function. *Int J Radiat Oncol Biol Phys.* 2001;51:62–68.

20. Yu CX, Jaffray DA, Wong JW. The effects of intra-fraction organ motion on the delivery of dynamic intensity modulation. *Phys Med Biol.* 1998;43:91–104.

21. Park C, Zhang G, Choy H. 4-Dimensional conformal radiation therapy: image-guided radiation therapy and its application in lung cancer treatment. *Clin Lung Cancer.* 2006;8:187–194.

22. Napel S, Rubin GD, Jeffrey RB Jr. STS-MIP: a new reconstruction technique for CT of the chest. *J Comput Assist Tomogr.* 1993;17:832–838.

23. Liu HH, Balter P, Tutt T, et al. Assessing respiration-induced tumor motion and internal target volume using four-dimensional computed tomography for radiotherapy of lung cancer. *Int J Radiat Oncol Biol Phys.* 2007;68:531–540.

24. Shimizu S, Shirato H, Kagei K, et al. Impact of respiratory movement on the computed tomographic images of small lung tumors in three-dimensional (3D) radiotherapy. *Int J Radiat Oncol Biol Phys.* 2000;46:1127–1133.

25. Seppenwoolde Y, Shirato H, Kitamura K, et al. Precise and real-time measurement of 3D tumor motion in lung due to breathing and heartbeat, measured during radiotherapy. *Int J Radiat Oncol Biol Phys.* 2002;53:822–834.

26. Britton KR, Starkschall G, Tucker SL, et al. Assessment of gross tumor volume regression and motion changes during radiotherapy for non-small-cell lung cancer as measured by four-dimensional computed tomography. *Int J Radiat Oncol Biol Phys.* 2007;68:1036–1046.

27. Mageras GS, Mechalakos J. Planning in the IGRT context: closing the loop. *Semin Radiat Oncol.* 2007;17:268–277.

28. Borst GR, Sonke JJ, Betgen A, et al. Kilo-voltage cone-beam computed tomography setup measurements for lung cancer patients; first clinical results and comparison with electronic portal-imaging device. *Int J Radiat Oncol Biol Phys.* 2007;68:555–561.

29. Bissonnette J-P, Purdie T, Higgins J, et al. Cone-beam computed tomographic image guidance for lung cancer radiation therapy. *Intl J Radiat Oncol Biol Phys.* 2009;73:927–934.

30. Purdie TG, Bissonnette JP, Franks K, et al. Cone-beam computed tomography for on-line image guidance of lung stereotactic radiotherapy: localization, verification, and intrafraction tumor position. *Int J Radiat Oncol Biol Phys.* 2007;68:243–252.

31. Biancia CD, Guan Y, Yorke E, et al. SU-FF-J-43: Use of kilo-voltage cone beam CT (kV-CBCT) for hypofractionated image-guided radiation therapy (HF-IGRT) of lung tumors. *Med Phys.* 2007;34:2377–2378.

32. Fox TH, Elder ES, Crocker IR, et al. Clinical implementation and efficiency of kilovoltage image-guided radiation therapy. *J Am Coll Radiol.* 2006;3:38–44.

33. Baisden JM, Romney DA, Reish AG, et al. Dose as a function of lung volume and planned treatment volume in helical tomotherapy intensity-modulated radiation therapy-based stereotactic body radiation therapy for small lung tumors. *Int J Radiat Oncol Biol Phys.* 2007;68:1229–1237.

34. Fuss M, Shi C, Papanikolaou N. Tomotherapeutic stereotactic body radiation therapy: techniques and comparison between modalities. *Acta Oncol.* 2006;45:953–960.

35. Hodge W, Tome WA, Jaradat HA, et al. Feasibility report of image guided stereotactic body radiotherapy (IG-SBRT) with tomotherapy for early stage medically inoperable lung cancer using extreme hypofractionation. *Acta Oncol.* 2006;45:890–896.

36. Adkison JB, Khuntia D, Bentzen SM, et al. Dose escalated, hypofractionated radiotherapy using helical tomotherapy for inoperable non-small cell lung cancer: preliminary results of a risk-stratified phase I dose escalation study. *Technol Cancer Res Treat.* 2008;7:441–448.

37. Sterzing F, Schubert K, Sroka-Perez G, et al. Helical tomotherapy. Experiences of the first 150 patients in Heidelberg. *Strahlenther Onkol.* 2008;184:8–14.

38. Shah AP, Langen KM, Ruchala KJ, et al. Patient dose from megavoltage computed tomography imaging. *Int J Radiat Oncol Biol Phys.* 2008;70:1579–1587.

39. Smeenk C, Gaede S, Battista JJ. Delineation of moving targets with slow MVCT scans: implications for adaptive non-gated lung tomotherapy. *Phys Med Biol.* 2007;52:1119–1134.

40. Ramsey CR, Langen KM, Kupelian PA, et al. A technique for adaptive image-guided helical tomotherapy for lung cancer. *Int J Radiat Oncol Biol Phys.* 2006;64:1237–1244.

41. Chang JY, Dong L, Liu H, et al. Image-guided radiation therapy for non-small cell lung cancer. *J Thorac Oncol.* 2008;3:177–186.

42. Brown WT, Wu X, Wen BC, et al. Early results of CyberKnife image-guided robotic stereotactic radiosurgery for treatment of lung tumors. *Comput Aided Surg.* 2007;12:253–261.

43. Collins B, Vahdat S, Erickson K, et al. Radical cyberknife radiosurgery with tumor tracking: an effective treatment for inoperable small peripheral stage I non-small cell lung cancer. *J Hematol Oncol.* 2009;2:1.

44. Coon D, Gokhale AS, Burton SA, et al. Fractionated stereotactic body radiation therapy in the treatment of primary, recurrent, and metastatic lung tumors: the role of positron emission tomography/computed tomography-based treatment planning. *Clin Lung Cancer.* 2008;9:217–221.

45. Le QT, Loo BW, Ho A, et al. Results of a phase I dose-escalation study using single-fraction stereotactic radiotherapy for lung tumors. *J Thorac Oncol.* 2006;1:802–809.

46. Nuyttens JJ, Prevost JB, Praag J, et al. Lung tumor tracking during stereotactic radiotherapy treatment with the CyberKnife: marker placement and early results. *Acta Oncol.* 2006;45:961–965.

47. Prevost JB, Nuyttens JJ, Hoogeman MS, et al. Endovascular coils as lung tumour markers in real-time tumour tracking stereotactic radiotherapy: preliminary results. *Eur Radiol.* 2008;18:1569–1576.

48. Anantham D, Feller-Kopman D, Shanmugham LN, et al. Electromagnetic navigation bronchoscopy-guided fiducial placement for robotic stereotactic radiosurgery of lung tumors: a feasibility study. *Chest.* 2007;132:930–935.

49. Brown WT, Wu X, Fayad F, et al. CyberKnife radiosurgery for stage I lung cancer: results at 36 months. *Clin Lung Cancer.* 2007;8:488–492.

50. Castelli J, Thariat J, Benezery K, et al. Feasibility and efficacy of cyberknife radiotherapy for lung cancer: Early results. *Cancer Radiother.* 2008;12:793–799.

51. Verellen D, Soete G, Linthout N, et al. Optimal control of set-up margins and internal margins for intra- and extracranial radiotherapy using stereoscopic kilovoltage imaging. *Cancer Radiother.* 2006;10:235–244.

52. Chen Y, Milano M, Roloff G, et al. Novalis stereotactic body radiotherapy for recurrent and newly diagnosed poor risk non-small cell lung cancer (NSCLC). *Int J Radiat Oncol Biol Phys.* 2008;72:S466–S467.

53. Ernst-Stecken A, Lambrecht U, Mueller R, et al. Hypofractionated stereotactic radiotherapy for primary and secondary intrapulmonary tumors: first results of a phase I/II study. *Strahlenther Onkol.* 2006;182:696–702.

54. McCammon R, Schefter TE, Gaspar LE, et al. Observation of a dose-control relationship for lung and liver tumors after stereotactic body radiation therapy. *Int J Radiat Oncol Biol Phys.* 2009;73:112–118.

55. Teh BS, Paulino AC, Lu HH, et al. Versatility of the Novalis system to deliver image-guided stereotactic body radiation therapy (SBRT) for various anatomical sites. *Technol Cancer Res Treat.* 2007;6:347–354.

56. Wurm RE, Gum F, Erbel S, et al. Image guided respiratory gated hypofractionated stereotactic body radiation therapy (H-SBRT) for liver and lung tumors: initial experience. *Acta Oncol.* 2006;45:881–889.

57. Bradley JD, Ieumwananonthachai N, Purdy JA, et al. Gross tumor volume, critical prognostic factor in patients treated with three-dimensional conformal radiation therapy for non-small-cell lung carcinoma. *Int J Radiat Oncol Biol Phys.* 2002;52:49–57.

58. Kong FM, Ten Haken RK, Schipper MJ, et al. High-dose radiation improved local tumor control and overall survival in patients with inoperable/unresectable non-small-cell lung cancer: long-term results of a radiation dose escalation study. *Int J Radiat Oncol Biol Phys.* 2005;63:324–333.

59. Rengan R, Rosenzweig KE, Venkatraman E, et al. Improved local control with higher doses of radiation in large-volume stage III non-small-cell lung cancer. *Int J Radiat Oncol Biol Phys.* 2004;60:741–747.

60. Bradley J, Graham MV, Winter K, et al. Toxicity and outcome results of RTOG 9311: a phase I-II dose-escalation study using three-dimensional conformal radiotherapy in patients with inoperable non-small-cell lung carcinoma. *Int J Radiat Oncol Biol Phys.* 2005;61:318–328.

61. Blackstock A, Socinski M, Bogart J, et al. Induction (Ind) plus concurrent (Con) chemotherapy with high-dose (74 Gy) 3-dimensional (3-D) thoracic radiotherapy (TRT) in stage III non-small cell lung cancer (NSCLC); preliminary report of Cancer and Leukemia Group B (CALGB) 30105. Part I. *Proc Amer Soc Clin Oncol.* 2006;24:18S.

62. Bradley J, Graham M, Suzanne S, et al. Phase I results of RTOG 0117; a phase I/II dose intensification study using 3DCRT and concurrent chemotherapy for patients with inoperable NSCLC. Part I of II. *Proc Amer Soc Clin Oncol.* 2005;23:16S.

63. Lee C, Socinski M, Lin L, et al. High-dose 3D chemoradiotherapy trials in stage III non-small cell lung cancer (NSCLC) at the University of North Carolina: long-term follow up and late complications. Part I. *Proc Amer Soc Clin Oncol.* 2006;24:18S.

64. Baumann P, Nyman J, Lax I, et al. Factors important for efficacy of stereotactic body radiotherapy of medically inoperable stage I lung cancer. A retrospective analysis of patients treated in the Nordic countries. *Acta Oncol.* 2006;45:787–795.

65. McGarry RC, Papiez L, Williams M, et al. Stereotactic body radiation therapy of early-stage non-small-cell lung carcinoma: phase I study. *Int J Radiat Oncol Biol Phys.* 2005;63:1010–1015.

66. Onishi H, Araki T, Shirato H, et al. Stereotactic hypofractionated high-dose irradiation for stage I nonsmall cell lung carcinoma: clinical outcomes in 245 subjects in a Japanese multiinstitutional study. *Cancer.* 2004;101:1623–1631.

67. Timmerman R, Papiez L, McGarry R, et al. Extracranial stereotactic radioablation: results of a phase I study in medically inoperable stage I non-small cell lung cancer. *Chest.* 2003;124:1946–1955.

68. Zimmermann FB, Geinitz H, Schill S, et al. Stereotactic hypofractionated radiation therapy for stage I non-small cell lung cancer. *Lung Cancer.* 2005;48:107–114.

69. Uematsu M, Shioda A, Suda A, et al. Computed tomography-guided frameless stereotactic radiotherapy for stage I non-small cell lung cancer: a five-year experience. *Int J Radiat Oncol Biol Phys.* 2001;51:666–670.

70. Timmerman RD, Park C, Kavanagh BD. The North American experience with stereotactic body radiation therapy in non-small cell lung cancer. *J Thorac Oncol.* 2007;2:S101–S112.

71. Harsolia A, Hugo GD, Kestin LL, et al. Dosimetric advantages of four-dimensional adaptive image-guided radiotherapy for lung tumors using online cone-beam computed tomography. *Int J Radiat Oncol Biol Phys.* 2008;70:582–589.

^{18}F-FDG PET-Guided Target Delineation in a Patient with Lung Cancer

Case Study

Maria Picchio, MD, Mariangela Caimi, MD, Claudio Landoni, MD, Cinzia Crivellaro, MD, Filippo Alongi, MD, Nadia Di Muzio, MD, Cristina Messa, MD

Patient History

A 67-year-old man with a long history of chronic obstructive pulmonary disease presented with worsening cough and exertional dyspnea. Chest x-ray revealed consolidation in the right hilar region. A contrast-enhanced computed tomography (CT) of the chest demonstrated a 3-cm right peri-hilar lesion with enlarged ipsilateral hilar and mediastinal adenopathy. Fiberoptic bronchoscopy confirmed the presence of a lesion completely occluding the posterior segmental bronchus of the right upper lobe. Endobronchial biopsy and bronchial washings were consistent with squamous cell carcinoma. Bone scan and CT scans of the abdomen, pelvis, and brain were negative for metastases. The tumor was staged as clinical stage T1N2M0 (IIIA).

The patient's case was discussed in our multidisciplinary oncology conference and the consensus recommendation was for neoadjuvant vinorelbine followed by a reevaluation. After six cycles of chemotherapy, a repeat whole-body CT revealed stable disease. The patient was then referred for definitive radiotherapy (RT). We elected to use ^{18}F-fluorodeoxyglucose positron emission tomography (^{18}F-FDG PET) to restage the patient and to guide target delineation.

Simulation

The ^{18}F-FDG PET–CT study was performed on a Discovery STE scanner (GE Healthcare, Waukesha, WI) 1 hour after the injection of 370 MBq of the PET tracer. The patient was immobilized in the supine position on the PET–CT couch using a foam cradle extending from the shoulders to the pelvis. ^{18}F-FDG PET–CT revealed a focal and pathological uptake corresponding to the tumor mass and another area of increased ^{18}F-FDG uptake in the ipsilateral hilum. Unlike the prior chest CT, which noted enlarged mediastinal lymphadenopathy (maximum diameter, 1.4 cm), no increased metabolic activity was identified in the mediastinum (Figures 17A-1 and 17A-2).

Imaging and Target Delineation

Positron emission tomography and CT images were subsequently used to delineate the target volumes. The PET images were used to define a biological target volume (BTV). The BTV was contoured by an expert nuclear medicine physician and consisted of the metabolically active tumor mass including the primary tumor and the ipsilateral hilar lymph nodes (Figures 17A-3 and 17A-4). The CT images and the BTV contours were then transferred via the network to the planning computer to define the remaining target volumes and the organs at risk (OARs).

The gross tumor volume (GTV) was then defined by using the BTV. The GTV included the primary tumor as well as the right hilar lymph nodal lesions characterized by increased ^{18}F-FDG uptake. A clinical target volume (CTV) was created with an isotropic expansion of 0.5 cm around the GTV. Then, an isotropic margin of 1.5 cm was applied to the CTV to generate the planning target volume

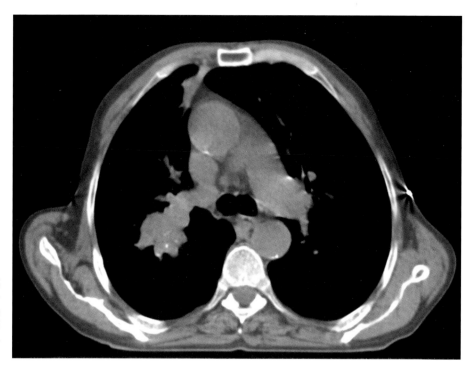

FIGURE 17A-1. Pretreatment chest computed tomography (CT) demonstrating a pulmonary lesion in the right posterior para-hilar region and ipsilateral mediastinal lymphadenopathy.

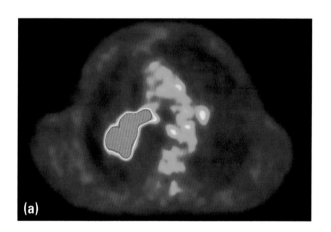 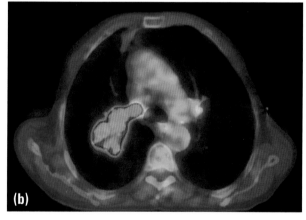

(a)   (b)

FIGURE 17A-2. Axial positron emission tomography (PET) **(a)** and PET–computed tomography (PET–CT) **(b)** slices after the completion of neoadjuvant chemotherapy demonstrating uptake in the right lung and ipsilateral hilum. No uptake is noted in the mediastinum.

(PTV). We elected not to include the mediastinum in the target volume, because of the well-described high negative predictive value of ^{18}F-PET–CT in lymph nodal staging.

Treatment Planning

Helical tomotherapy planning was performed with the Hi-Art software (TomoTherapy Inc, Madison, WI). The dose constraints for each OAR surrounding the PTV were previously determined based on normal tissue complication probability (NTCP) analysis. A dose of 70.2 Gy in 39 daily fractions (five fractions/week) was prescribed to the PTV. Optimization of tomotherapy treatments is

different from that of "conventional" IMRT inverse planning. The inverse planning system seeks the best solution by changing the shape and the weight of a large number of segments (typically thousands). In tomotherapy, three main parameters can be set by the operator: field width, pitch, and modulation factor. Briefly, field width is the fixed field dimension in the cranial–caudal direction (to be chosen among 1 cm, 2.5 cm, and 5 cm); pitch is the ratio between the couch translation during one gantry rotation and the field width; the modulation factor is the ratio between maximum and average beam intensity. The goal was to deliver more than 98% of the prescribed dose to more than 95% of the PTV while maintaining the highest

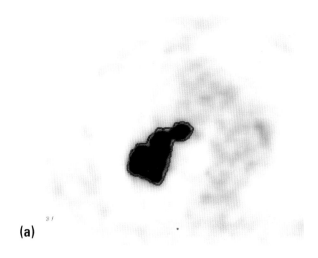
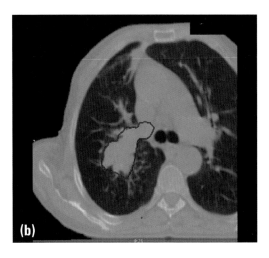

FIGURE 17A-3. (a) Positron emission tomography transaxial image with delineation of the biological target volume (BTV), used for treatment planning. **(b)** Corresponding computed tomography image with superimposed BTV.

FIGURE 17A-4. Axial computed tomography (CT) slice **(a)** showing final volumes used for treatment planning. The gross tumor volume (GTV), clinical target volume (CTV), and planning target volume (PTV) are shown in orange, light blue, and red, respectively. **(b)** Anterior and **(c)** lateral digitally reconstructed radiographs with the PTV superimposed.

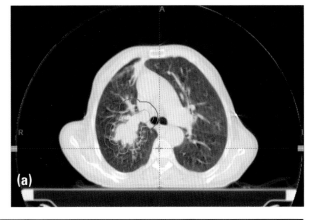
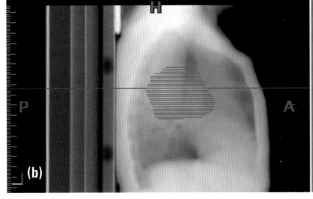
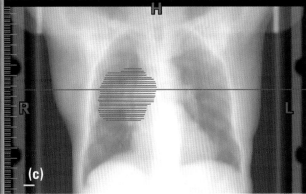

possible dose homogeneity as well as to maintain dose to OARs lower than the dose constraints.

Treatment Delivery

Setup was assessed before each fraction by means of megavoltage (MV) CT image guidance of the tomotherapy unit (TomoTherapy Inc, Madison, WI). After patient positioning and MVCT acquisition these images were matched with the planning kilovoltage (kV) CT through automatic bone matching. This fusion was followed by physician adjustments to optimize the image alignment based on fixed organs close to the PTV, such as vertebral body or large vessels in the mediastinum.

A significant and progressive reduction of the primary tumor compared with the previously defined GTV was

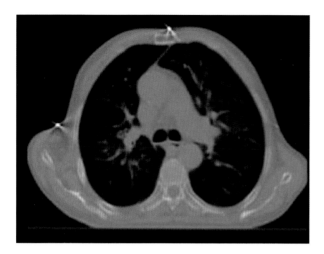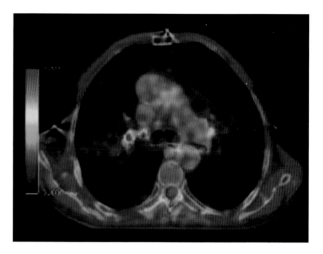

FIGURE 17A-5. A positron emission tomography–computed tomography (PET-CT) study obtained during treatment illustrating a marked reduction of the tumor mass and metabolic activity. The treatment could be "adapted" based on the new metabolically active tumor.

observed with daily MVCT during the first 28 fractions. A new ^{18}F-FDG PET–CT study was performed during treatment, to evaluate the evolution of the disease. The F-FDG PET–CT acquisition protocol and image analysis followed the same criteria used for the pretreatment F-FDG PET–CT study. Based on the metabolic and morphologic tumor response, we decided to modify the plan during the radiation course, adapting the remaining dose to the reduced dimension of the lesion on MVCT images obtained at 50.4 Gy. New CTV and PTV contours were defined based on a second BTV identified from the second ^{18}F-FDG PET–CT scan. A significant reduction of ^{18}F-FDG uptake was detected at right-lung hilum (Figure 17A-5) and the mediastinal lymph nodes were still metabolically normal. The remaining 11 fractions were delivered to a smaller PTV, potentially reducing further effects on healthy tissues. Furthermore, F-FDG PET–CT showed a disease progression in a lung nodule, located posterolaterally to the primary right lung lesion.

Clinical Outcome

The patient tolerated treatment well and did not require any unplanned treatment breaks. A followup PET–CT study performed 1 month after the end of treatment confirmed a good local response and the progression of metastatic disease in the right lung, previously described. The patient remained free of local disease recurrence but died 7 months later because of progressive brain metastases.

Our initial experience using ^{18}F-FDG PET–CT-guided target delineation in 21 advanced non–small cell lung cancer patients was published earlier.[1] The CTV contoured based on CT alone (CTV_{CT}) and on the coregistered F-FDG PET–CT (CTV_{PET-CT}) were compared in each patient, with a differences of greater than 25% considered clinically significant. Of 18 evaluable patients, a CTV change, after inclusion of the F-FDG PET–CT data, was observed in 10 patients (55%): larger in seven (range, 33% to 279%) and smaller in three (range, 26% to 34%), mainly because of the inclusion or exclusion of lymph nodal disease and better definition of tumor extent. In the remaining eight patients, CTV changes less than 25% were noted.

Reference

1. Messa C, Ceresoli GL, Rizzo G, et al. Feasibility of ^{18}FDG-PET and co-registered CT on clinical target volume definition of advanced non-small cell lung cancer. *Q J Nucl Med Mol Imaging.* 2005;49:259–266.

Four-Dimensional SBRT Using the CyberKnife Synchrony System in a Patient with Early Stage Lung Cancer

Case Study

Joost Jan Nuyttens, MD, PhD, Noelle van der Voort van Zyp, MD, Mischa Hoogeman, PhD

Patient History

A 78-year-old man presented with increasing shortness of breath and a 3-cm mass noted on a chest x-ray. A computed tomography (CT) scan of the chest demonstrated a 3.7-cm left middle lobe mass. As the diagnosis could not be confirmed by bronchoscopy, a positron emission tomography (PET)–CT scan was obtained. A solitary hotspot was observed in the left middle lobe corresponding to the location of the tumor on the CT scan. Pathology was obtained by transthoracic biopsy and revealed an adenocarcinoma.

The patient had a history of two anteroseptal myocardial infarctions and a ventricular ejection fraction of 40%. His forced expiratory volume in one second (FEV_1) was 75% of the predicted value and his diffusion capacity was 74%. A ventilation/perfusion scan was performed and revealed that the right lung contributed 60% of his ventilation/perfusion capacity and the left lung contributed 40%. Because of his poor cardiac function and mediocre lung function, he was considered to be medically inoperable. He was subsequently referred to our hospital for curative intent stereotactic body radiotherapy (SBRT). We elected to treat him with four-dimensional (4D) tumor-tracking using the CyberKnife Synchrony (Accuray Inc, Sunnyvale, CA).

Simulation

Before simulation, the patient was referred to an interventional radiologist for the placement of fiducial markers, which are required to track the tumor with the 4D tumor-tracking capabilities of the Cyber-Knife. Recently, new software has become commercially available that allows direct soft tissue tracking of tumors visible on orthogonal chest x-rays. In this patient, fiducials were placed using the intravascular coil method,[1,2] which involves placement of five vascular embolization coils (Tornado 4/3, Cook, Bloomington, IN) into small subsegmental pulmonary endbranches within or adjacent to the tumor. The pulmonary artery catheter was inserted via the femoral vein in the groin under local anesthesia with electrocardiogram monitoring. After coil insertion, the patient was observed for a few hours to detect any postprocedural bleeding. No complications occurred during or after the procedure in this patient.

One week later, the patient underwent CT simulation. He was placed in the prone position on a vacuum mattress. Intravenous contrast was injected during exhalation and the scan was obtained on our departmental wide-bore multislice CT simulator (Sensation Open, Siemens AG, Erlangen, Germany). The patient was scanned from his teeth to the middle of his abdomen. The transaxial imaging had a slice thickness of 1.5 mm.

Treatment Planning

The planning CT data set was transferred to the On-Target Treatment Planning System (Accuray, Sunnyvale, CA). The tumor and organs at risk (OARs) were then contoured. The gross tumor volume (GTV) was contoured using the lung window and consisted of the visualized tumor. The planning target volume (PTV) was derived by adding a 5-mm margin to the GTV in three dimensions. In this patient, the OARs consisted of both lungs, the heart, and the spinal cord.

Inverse treatment planning was performed with a 30-mm cone and the final plan consisted of 102 noncoplanar beams. The PTV (outer line) was treated with a dose of 60 Gy in three fractions and the dose was prescribed to the 80% isodose line (Figure 17B-1). Doses to normal tissues (lungs, heart, spinal cord, etc.) were deemed to be acceptable. Two opposite orthogonal (45°) digitally reconstructed radiographs (DRRs) were generated for the 4D tumor tracking.

Treatment Delivery

The CyberKnife is a frameless image-guided radiotherapy (RT) system involving a compact 6-MV linear accelerator mounted on a robotic arm, which possesses six degrees of freedom.[3,4] The imaging system consists of two diagnostic x-ray sources mounted to the ceiling paired with amorphous silicon detectors that are used to acquire live digital radiographic images of the tumor, patient, or fiducial markers. The Synchrony subsystem enables 4D real-time tracking of tumors that move with respiration. Briefly, Synchrony combines noncontinuous x-ray imaging of internal fiducial markers, with a continuously updated external breathing signal. A correlation model that relates the external breathing signal with the motion of the internal fiducial markers provides a real-time update of the beam position.[5-7]

In the treatment room, the patient was placed in the prone position on the couch in the vacuum mattress. Three light-emitting diodes (LEDs) were placed on the patient's back to provide the external breathing signal. The motion of these LEDs caused by respiration was registered by a camera array (Figure 17B-2). The patient alignment was conducted by the image-guidance

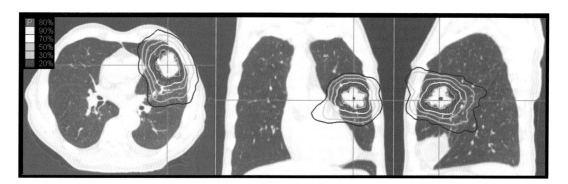

FIGURE 17B-1. The dose distribution in the three planes. The planning target volume is shown in red. The dose is prescribed to the 80% isodose line (pink).

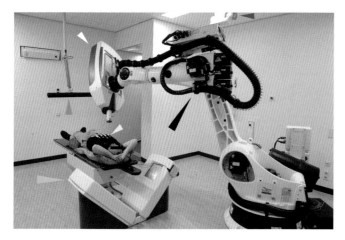

FIGURE 17B-2. Patient positioned on the CyberKnife unit. White arrow: linear accelerator; black arrow: robot; red arrow: one of the two x-ray tubes; green arrow: two flat panels; blue arrow: Synchrony camera; yellow arrow: three light-emitting diodes.

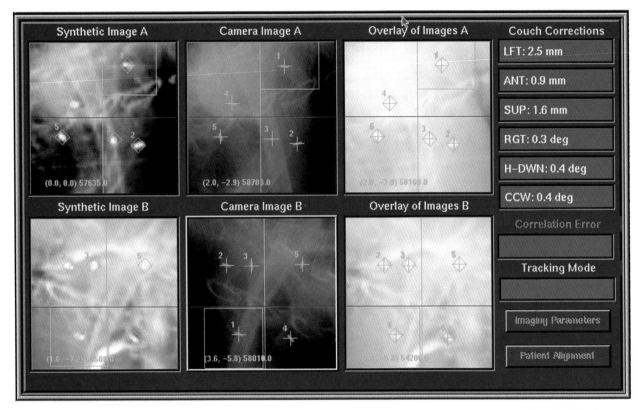

FIGURE 17B-3. A screen capture demonstrating the alignment of the tumor with the use of the markers. The first column shows the digitally reconstructed radiographs (DRRs). The markers on the DRRs are highlighted in the green cubes. In the second column, the two orthogonal images of the patient are displayed. The green crosses are placed by the therapist on the markers, and, as a result, the required couch corrections and shifts in all directions are shown in the fourth column. An overlay of the DRR and the camera image is presented in the third column.

system and the remotely controlled treatment couch, such that the extent of the respiratory motion was within the translational limits of the robot. The tumor was localized by reconstructing the 3D position of the fiducial markers, which are automatically segmented in the x-ray images. The reconstructed position was compared with the position in the planning CT scan (Figure 17B-3). Just before the start of the irradiation, the correlation model was built by acquiring approximately eight x-ray image pairs at different phases of the breathing cycle (Figure 17B-4). The Synchrony system made a correlation model that relates the movement of the fiducial markers and the LEDs. Nonlinear models were used to account for hysteresis in the tumor trajectory. By the model, the linear accelerator could continuously track the motion of the tumor via the motion of the LEDs. The correlation model was validated and updated throughout the treatment by acquiring x-ray image pairs every 1 to 6 minutes.

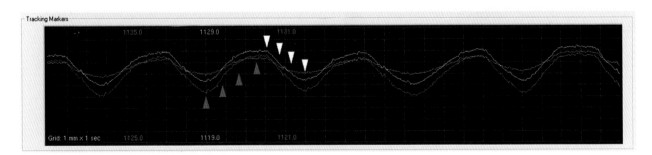

FIGURE 17B-4. The breathing cycle of the patient as shown on the treatment console and the timing of imaging to enable four-dimensional real-time tumor tracking. The green, red, and blue lines show the motion of the light-emitting diodes (LED) lights, captured by the Synchrony camera and represent together the breathing cycle of the patient; the red and white arrows show the moment at which the imaging should be taken during inhalation and expiration to enable four-dimensional real-time tumor tracking.

After each image pair acquisition, the correlation model error was displayed on the system console. If the correlation model error was larger than 5 mm a system interruption was generated and the operator had to build a new model. At our clinic, a new model was built when the correlation model error exceeded 3 mm twice in a row. This ensures accurate real-time tumor tracking, for which the 3D correlation model error was on average 1.2 mm. The patient was asked to breathe freely for the whole procedure.

Clinical Outcome

The patient tolerated treatment very well. Three weeks after treatment, his weight increased by 3 kilograms. Clinical examination and CT scans of the chest at 2, 6, 12, 18, 24, 30, and 36 months posttreatment showed an excellent response and local control of the tumor. The patient had no respiratory or other chest complaints but needed a pacemaker at 18 months after treatment. Figure 17B-5 shows the tumor before the treatment and the clinical result after 1, 2, and 3 years, respectively. There is no evidence of tumor progression locally or distally at the most recent date of follow-up.

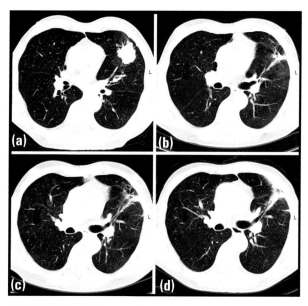

FIGURE 17B-5. Axial computed tomography images of the tumor before treatment (**a**) and the clinical result after (**b**) 1 year, (**c**) 2 years, and (**d**) 3 years.

Our initial clinical experience using 4D tumor-tracking in 70 medically inoperable early stage lung cancer patients was recently published.[8] Thirty-nine patients had T1 tumors; 31 had T2 tumors. Patients received either 45 Gy or 60 Gy delivered in three fractions. Markers were placed in all patients. At a median follow-up of 15 months, the 2-year actuarial local control was 96% in the patients receiving 60 Gy and 78% in those treated with 45 Gy. All four local recurrences occurred in patients with T2 tumors. Overall and cause-specific actuarial survival rates were 62% and 85%, respectively. Grade 3 toxicity was noted in two patients after marker placement and in seven patients after treatment.

References

1. Nuyttens JJ, Prevost JB, Praag J, et al. Lung tumor tracking during stereotactic radiotherapy treatment with the Cyber-Knife: marker placement and early results. *Acta Oncol.* 2006;45: 961–965.
2. Prevost JB, Nuyttens JJ, Hoogeman MS, et al. Endovascular coils as lung tumour markers in real-time tumour tracking stereotactic radiotherapy: preliminary results. *Eur Radiol.* 2008;18:1569–1576.
3. Adler JR Jr, Murphy MJ, Chang SD, et al. Image-guided robotic radiosurgery. *Neurosurgery.* 1999;44:1299–1306.
4. Chang SD, Adler JR. Robotics and radiosurgery—the cyberknife. *Stereotact Funct Neurosurg.* 2001;76:204–208.
5. Murphy MJ. Tracking moving organs in real time. *Semin Radiat Oncol.* 2004;14:91–100.
6. Hara W, Soltys SG, Gibbs IC. CyberKnife robotic radiosurgery system for tumor treatment. *Expert Rev Anticancer Ther.* 2007;7:1507–1515.
7. Seppenwoolde Y, Berbeco RI, Nishioka S, et al. Accuracy of tumor motion compensation algorithm from a robotic respiratory tracking system: a simulation study. *Med Phys.* 2007;34:2774–2784.
8. van der Voort van Zyp NC, Prevost JB, Hoogeman MS, et al. Stereotactic radiotherapy with real-time tumor tracking for non-small cell lung cancer: clinical outcome. *Radiother Oncol.* 2009;91:296–300.

Hypofractionated IGRT Using the Helical Tomotherapy System in a Patient with Inoperable Lung Cancer

Case Study

Jarrod B. Adkison, MD, Ranjini Tolakanahalli, PhD, Deepak Khuntia, MD

Patient History

A 63-year-old woman presented to the emergency room with a suspected chronic obstructive pulmonary disease (COPD) exacerbation and possible pulmonary embolus. Workup included computed tomography (CT) angiography of the chest, which revealed a spiculated 2.6-cm left upper lobe mass, a 2.3-cm necrotic aorto-pulmonary window lymph node, and a 2-cm left hilar lymph node. Transbronchial biopsy of the hilar node was consistent with squamous cell carcinoma. Complete staging included magnetic resonance (MR) imaging of the brain and positron emission tomography (PET). These scans confirmed only the disease noted on chest CT; no sites of metastatic disease were noted. Pulmonary function testing demonstrated a FEV_1 of 1.24 L (59% predicted), FVC of 2.09 L (72% predicted), and DLCO at 67% predicted. Her tumor was thus staged as T1N2M0 (stage IIIA).

The patient was evaluated in our multidisciplinary lung cancer clinic. She was not deemed to be a good surgical candidate because of her underlying poor pulmonary function and locally advanced disease. She elected to enroll on our phase I dose-escalated hypofractionated image-guided radiotherapy (IGRT) using helical tomotherapy protocol for patients with inoperable lung cancer.

Simulation

The patient was placed in a custom-made double-vacuum BodyFIX system (Medical Intelligence, Munich, Germany) to ensure accurate patient positioning and to mini-mize patient motion during treatment. Vacuum suction was applied to adhere the cover sheet tightly to the patient restricting tumor motion caused by respiration. Her arms were placed above her head using a wing-board. Intravenous contrast was delivered during the planning CT scan to allow visualization of the vasculature. A free-breathing planning CT of the chest was performed with a slice thickness of 2.5 mm using helical CT. A thoracic four-dimensional CT (4D CT) scan was then obtained on our departmental GE Lightspeed CT scanner (GE Healthcare, Waukesha, WI) coupled with the Varian Real Position Management (RPM) Gating system (Varian Medical Systems, Palo Alto, CA). Maximum intensity projection (MIP) images were generated from the 4D CT data set using GE Advantage 4D CT software (GE Healthcare, Waukesha, WI).

Treatment Planning

The planning CT and the MIP images were transferred to the Pinnacle treatment planning system (Philips Medical Systems, Andover, MA). Automatic and subsequent manual registration techniques ensured proper fusion of the MIP and planning CT.

The primary left upper lobe tumor and involved regional adenopathy were contoured as the gross tumor volume (GTV). The organs at risk (OARs) contoured included the heart, esophagus, spinal cord, and uninvolved lung. An internal target volume (ITV) was delineated on the MIP images generated from the 4D CT[1] and expanded by 6 mm to form the clinical target volume (CTV), based on prior histopathological studies in squamous cell carcinoma.[2] A 2-mm expansion was then added to the CTV to generate the planning target volume (PTV), as prior phantom studies evaluating automatic registration of megavoltage (MV) to kilovoltage (kV) CT images in helical tomotherapy have demonstrated total uncertainty within approximately 1 mm.[3]

The dose per fraction specified by the protocol is based on the relative normalized tissue mean dose ($RNTD_{mean}$), which is the ratio of the mean normalized tissue dose (assuming conventional 2-Gy fractions) of lung to the normalized prescription PTV dose. Higher volume of normal lung irradiated and higher dose per fraction result in higher $RNTD_{mean}$, allowing stratification of patients into bins based on pneumonitis risk. In each dose bin, the starting dose was determined by the $RNTD_{mean}$ predictive of less than 20% grade 2 pneumonitis based on previously reported multiinstitutional data incorporated into a normal tissue complication probability model.[4] The patient's total prescribed dose was determined to be 63.25 Gy with dose per fraction equal to 2.53 Gy, because her $RNTD_{mean}$ was in the range of 0.18 to 0.239.

A highly conformal treatment plan was generated using the Hi-Art treatment planning system (Tomo-Therapy Inc, Madison, WI; Figure 17C-1). Ninety-eight percent of the PTV received the prescription dose determined by bin assignment. A field width of 2.5 cm and a

modulation factor of 3.1 were used. A pitch of 0.215 was used to avoid thread artifacts.[5] The maximum normalized tissue dose (NTD) to esophagus and spinal cord were 58.7 Gy_3 and 27.4 Gy_3, respectively, assuming an α–β ratio of 3 and conventional 2 Gy fractionation. The NTD mean dose to the residual lungs was 10.71 Gy_3.

Treatment Delivery

The patient was placed in the custom-made BodyFIX immobilization device (Medical Intelligence, Schwab-munchen, Germany; Figure 17C-2). A MVCT was obtained after the patient was lined up to the starting coordinates marked at the time of simulation. Automatic registration (bone plus soft tissue technique) of MVCT to planning kV CT images preceded manual registration by the physician before treatment. This process took approximately 5 minutes. The appropriate shifts were made to achieve the localization determined by the registration (Figure 17C-3). Typical shifts ranged from 8 mm to 10 mm superior–inferior and 3 mm to 4 mm in the left–right and anterior–posterior directions.

Treatment was delivered using the Hi-Art tomotherapy system, which delivers coplanar intensity-modulated radiation therapy using the simultaneous movement of the couch and the gantry. The binary multileaf collimator allowed for the modulation of the fanbeam. The beam-

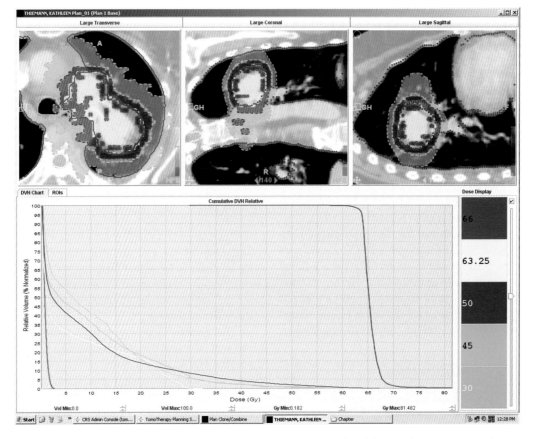

FIGURE 17C-1. Dose distribution and dose–volume histograms of the target and organs at risk of the tomotherapy treatment plan.

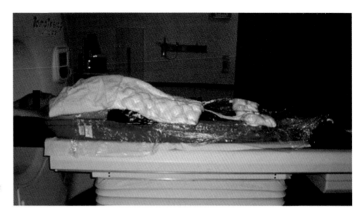

FIGURE 17C-2. BodyFIX immobilization device used to reduce setup uncertainty and target motion during treatment.

on time was 274.7 seconds with an actual time of about 6 minutes.

Clinical Outcome

The patient tolerated treatment well with no acute pulmonary or esophageal toxicity. She subsequently received three cycles of carboplatin and paclitaxel chemotherapy completed 4 months after RT. On follow-up scans, her tumor demonstrated progressive regression such that by 9 months, she achieved a complete response. Apart from only mild radiographic evidence of posttreatment changes consistent with grade 1 pneumonitis, she has not developed any chronic toxicity. She remains free of disease recurrence 2.5 years following treatment.

Our initial clinical experience using hypofractionated image-guided RT in non-small cell lung cancer patients was recently published.[6] Forty-six patients judged not to be surgical candidates with stage I–IV disease were included. The RT was delivered via helical tomotherapy and was limited to the primary site and clinically proven or suspicious lymph nodal regions without elective nodal irradiation. Patients were placed in one of five dose "bins," all treated with 25 fractions, with dose per fraction ranging from 2.28 Gy to 3.22 Gy. In each bin, the starting dose was determined by the relative normalized tissue mean dose modeled to result in less than 20% grade 2 pneumonitis.

Overall, treatment was well tolerated, with no grade 3 acute pneumonitis or esophageal toxicities observed. Pneumonitis rates were 70% grade 1 and 13% grade 2. Multivariate analysis identified mean lung NTD and adjuvant chemotherapy following RT to be independent risk factors for grade 2 pneumonitis. Only 7 patients (15%) required narcotic analgesics for esophagitis. Overall, 17% of patients had an in-field complete response, 43% a partial response, 26% stable disease, and 6.5% in-field progression. At a median follow-up of 8.1 months, median survival was 18 months, with a 2-year overall survival of 46.8%.

References

1. Underberg RW, Lagerwaard FJ, Slotman BJ, et al. Use of maximum intensity projections (MIP) for target volume generation in 4DCT scans for lung cancer. *Int J Radiat Oncol Biol Phys.* 2005;63:253–260.

2. Giraud P, Antoine M, Larrouy A, et al. Evaluation of microscopic tumor extension in non-small-cell lung cancer for three-dimensional conformal radiotherapy planning. *Int J Radiat Oncol Biol Phys.* 2000;48:1015–1024.

3. Boswell S, Tome W, Jeraj R, et al. Automatic registration of megavoltage to kilovoltage CT images in helical tomotherapy: an evaluation of the setup verification process for the special case of a rigid head phantom. *Med Phys.* 2006;33:4395–4404.

4. Kwa SL, Lebesque JV, Theuws JC, et al. Radiation pneumonitis as a function of mean lung dose: an analysis of pooled data of 540 patients. *Int J Radiat Oncol Biol Phys.* 1998;42:1–9.

5. Kissick MW, Fenwick J, James JA, et al. The helical tomotherapy thread effect. *Med Phys.* 2005;32:1414–1423.

6. Adkison JB, Khuntia D, Bentzen SM, et al. Dose escalated hypofractionated radiotherapy using helical tomotherapy for inoperable non-small cell lung cancer: preliminary results of a risk-stratified phase I dose escalation study. *Technol Cancer Rest Treat.* 2008;7:441–447.

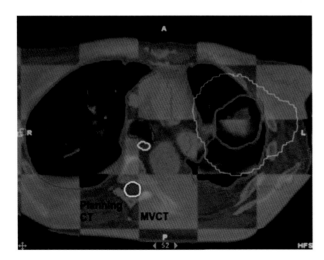

FIGURE 17C-3. Daily megavoltage computed tomography (CT) images acquired before each treatment fraction were used to line up to the target precisely relative to the original planning kilovoltage CT.

Chapter 17D

Deep Inspiration Breath-Hold kV CBCT-Guided SBRT Using the Varian Trilogy System in a Patient with Stage I Lung Cancer

Case Study

Ildiko Csiki, MD, PhD, Misun Hwang, BS, Wyndee Kirby, MS, Jostin B. Crass, MS, George X. Ding, PhD, Charles Coffey, PhD, Bo Lu, MD, PhD

Patient History

A 70-year-old man with a 90 pack-year smoking history and prior asbestos exposure presented with a right lung lesion, incidentally noted on a magnetic resonance (MR) scan performed during a workup for an abdominal aneurysm. A subsequent chest computed tomography (CT) scan revealed a 2.1 cm by 1.7 cm spiculated mass in the right lower lobe (RLL). A positron emission tomography (PET) scan was performed and demonstrated intense uptake in the RLL nodule highly suggestive of malignancy without evidence of metastasis. Bronchoscopic biopsy was nondiagnostic; however, a CT-guided fine-needle aspiration demonstrated squamous cell carcinoma.

The patient was initially evaluated for surgical resection but, because of his extensive cardiac history and poor pulmonary function, he was felt to be medically inoperable and, therefore, stereotactic body radiation therapy (SBRT) was proposed. We elected to treat him with deep inspiration breath-hold (DIBH) kilovoltage (kV) cone beam CT (CBCT) guidance on a Varian Trilogy linear accelerator (Varian Medical Systems, Palo Alto, CA).

Simulation

Before simulation, we confirmed that that patient was a good candidate for our DIBH technique by ensuring that

he was able to hold his breath for at least 35 seconds. On the day of the simulation, the patient was immobilized using a custom mold (vacuum lock) to ensure reproducibility of each treatment. He was then instructed to perform a DIBH. The steps included: (1) taking a deep breath, (2) exhaling, and (3) taking another deep breath and holding it. We have found from previous procedures that tumors generally move no more than 3 mm in the superior–inferior and lateral–medial direction with this technique. A DIBH planning CT was then obtained in the treatment position on our departmental Large Bore CT simulator (Philips Medical Systems, Andover, MA) and the patient was marked. The DIBH CT volume was such that the potential number of combinations of treatment and gantry angles for treatment planning was maximized while holding the scan time to less than 35 seconds. The CT scan extent consisted of the entire thoracic cavity with an additional 5 cm for treatment planning purposes, for a total scan length of 30 cm. Intravenous contrast was also used during the CT scan.

Treatment Planning

The planning DIBH CT data set was then transferred to the Eclipse planning system (Varian Medical Systems, Palo Alto, CA). Images were reviewed in the axial, coronal, and sagittal planes. Contouring and planning were then performed on the DIBH CT in accordance with the Japanese Clinical Oncology Group protocol 0403. Four fractions of 12 Gy for a total of 48 Gy were prescribed.

The gross tumor volume (GTV) consisted of all visualized tumor on the DIBH CT scan. The clinical tumor volume (CTV) consisted of GTV contoured on lung window. The planning target volume (PTV) consisted of 0.5-cm margin added to the CTV along the anterior–posterior and medial–lateral axis and 1 cm added along the superior–inferior axis. Thus, the margin around the GTV was a combination of internal and setup margin. The organs at risk (OARs) consisted of left and right lung, spinal cord, esophagus, and large airways.

A single isocenter was placed in the center of the PTV. Ten fields (four non-coplanar and six coplanar) were selec0ted to deliver an optimized treatment plan with a prescribed PTV dose of 12 Gy to the 67% isodose line to maintain dose homogeneity within the target (Figure 17D-1). The doses to normal tissues were reviewed and found acceptable. The lung volume receiving 20 Gy (V_{20}) was 4.7% and the right lung V_{20} was 11.7% (Figure 17D-2). To ensure that the patient would never need to hold his breath more than 35 seconds, a dose rate of 600 monitor units (MU) per minute was used and several beams (two non-coplanar and two coplanar) were split as needed to reduce the MU setting to 350 or less. Additionally, digitally reconstructed radiographs (DRRs) were produced from the DIBH CT scan to aid in patient positioning and alignment.

Treatment Delivery

Quality assurance checks were performed by the physics groups to ensure accurate dose delivery. Additionally, before the first treatment the patient was positioned on the

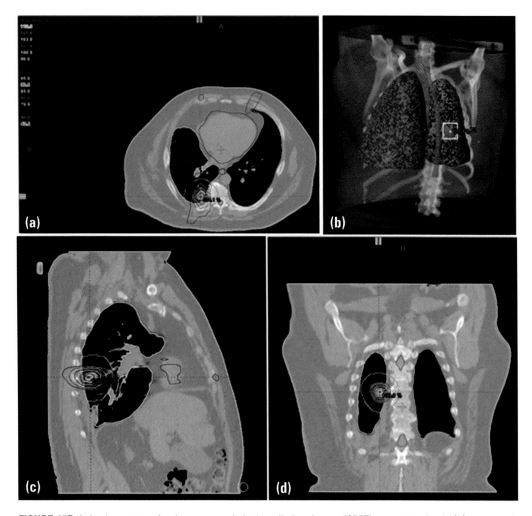

FIGURE 17D-1. Isodose curves for the stereotactic body radiation therapy (SBRT) treatment plan in (a) transversal, (c) sagittal, and (d) coronal views on breath-hold planning CT showing contours for spinal cord, esophagus, trachea, right and left lungs (organs at risk [OARs]), and gross tumor volume (GTV). This slice contains the isocenter. Panel (b) represents a three-dimensional bone digitally reconstructed radiograph with OARs and GTV shown.

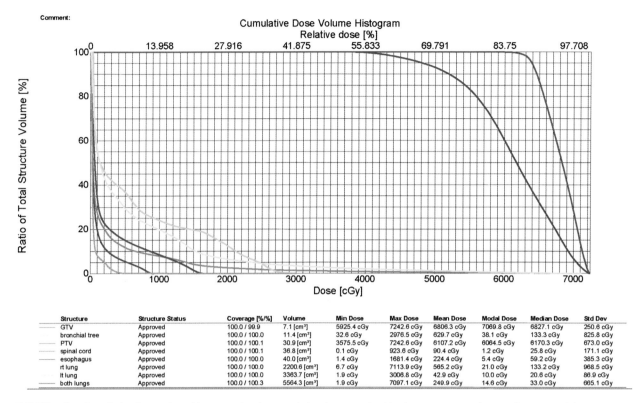

FIGURE 17D-2. Cumulative dose–volume histogram showing cumulative doses received by the gross tumor volume and organs at risk.

Structure	Structure Status	Coverage [%/%]	Volume	Min Dose	Max Dose	Mean Dose	Modal Dose	Median Dose	Std Dev
GTV	Approved	100.0 / 99.9	7.1 [cm³]	5925.4 cGy	7242.6 cGy	6806.3 cGy	7069.8 cGy	6827.1 cGy	250.6 cGy
bronchial tree	Approved	100.0 / 100.0	11.4 [cm³]	32.6 cGy	2976.5 cGy	629.7 cGy	38.1 cGy	133.3 cGy	825.8 cGy
PTV	Approved	100.0 / 100.1	30.9 [cm³]	3575.5 cGy	7242.6 cGy	6107.2 cGy	6064.5 cGy	6170.3 cGy	673.0 cGy
spinal cord	Approved	100.0 / 100.1	36.8 [cm³]	0.1 cGy	923.6 cGy	90.4 cGy	1.2 cGy	25.8 cGy	171.1 cGy
esophagus	Approved	100.0 / 100.0	40.0 [cm³]	1.4 cGy	1681.4 cGy	224.4 cGy	5.4 cGy	59.2 cGy	385.3 cGy
rt lung	Approved	100.0 / 100.0	2200.6 [cm³]	6.7 cGy	7113.9 cGy	565.2 cGy	21.0 cGy	133.2 cGy	968.5 cGy
lt lung	Approved	100.0 / 100.0	3363.7 [cm³]	1.9 cGy	3006.8 cGy	42.9 cGy	10.0 cGy	20.6 cGy	86.9 cGy
both lungs	Approved	100.0 / 100.3	5564.3 [cm³]	1.9 cGy	7097.1 cGy	249.9 cGy	14.6 cGy	33.0 cGy	665.1 cGy

linac couch using his skin marks and all table and gantry angles were checked for collisions.

On the first day of treatment and every day thereafter, the patient was coached to perform a DIBH. Subsequently, a CBCT acquisition was obtained in three breath-hold segments. Each breath-hold lasted approximately 30 seconds, thus interrupting the acquisition twice. Once the CBCT acquisition was complete, the images were used to align the patient. Using the On-Board Imaging (OBI) software (version 1.3, Varian Medical Systems, Palo Alto, CA), the contoured target (GTV) from the planning CT was mapped onto the CBCT. The CBCT image was manually adjusted to align the tumor with the GTV contour from the planning CT (Figure 17D-3). Patient alignment was accomplished by shifting the treatment couch in the lateral, vertical, and longitudinal directions, based on calculated shifts from the OBI software.

Confirmation of CBCT-based shifts was performed by acquiring anterior and lateral breath-hold projection radiographs. Additionally, portal images were obtained for each beam. To ensure that the patient would not have to remain for very long times in the treatment position, megavoltage portal images were obtained for only half of the beams during the first treatment. The remainder of the megavoltage portal images was obtained during the second treatment. The total treatment time ranged between 45 minutes and 90 minutes.

Clinical Outcome

Treatment was well tolerated without any significant acute toxicity. Before treatment, the patient was experiencing activity-limiting shortness of breath while walking around the house. Afterward, he reported that his functional status was limited primarily by preexisting back and hip pain. However, he was feeling well overall and after a cardiology follow-up visit he planned to begin to walk on the treadmill.

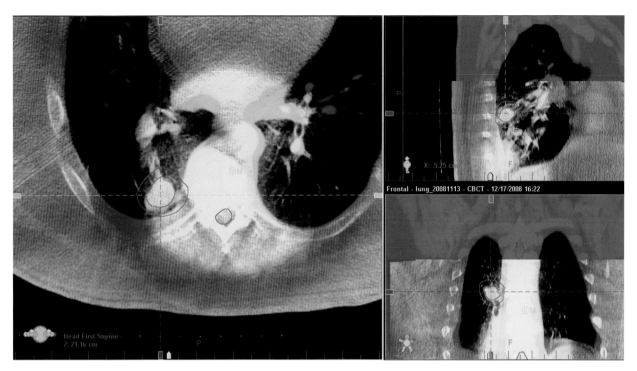

FIGURE 17D-3. Deep-inspiration breath-hold cone-beam CT (CBCT) superimposed on a reference CT used for planning. The tumor can be seen on three reconstructed planes from a CBCT acquisition. The tumor position (not bony anatomy) was used for patient positioning before each treatment. Red: CBCT; blue: planning CT. Left: CBCT axial slice through isocenter. Upper right: sagittal reconstruction from CBCT through isocenter. Lower right: coronal reconstruction from CBCT through isocenter. CBCT reconstructed images as seen on the four-dimensional treatment console screen, with tumor position. The planning CT is turned off, while the tumor contour is visible.

Respiratory Gated kV CBCT-Guided SBRT Using the Varian Trilogy System in a Patient with Stage I Lung Cancer

Case Study

Ajay Sandhu, MD, Steve B. Jiang, PhD

Patient History

A 70-year-old woman with a history of prior lung cancer was noted to have a new lung nodule on follow-up imaging. Her oncologic history dates back 4 years when she was diagnosed with a stage IIIA (T1N2M0) adenocarcinoma of the left lung. She was treated with a left upper lobectomy and mediastinal lymph node dissection followed by adjuvant radiation therapy (RT) to a total dose of 52 Gy.

She was closely followed and had no evidence of disease recurrence until a follow-up CT scan demonstrated a 5-mm nodule in her right lower lobe. This was closely monitored. A positron emission tomography (PET) scan obtained at the same time was negative.

A repeat CT scan 3 months later revealed that the nodule had increased in size to 8 mm. Serial CT scans showed this nodule to further increase in size to 1.17 cm (Figure 17E-1). A repeat PET scan performed at that time was positive in her right lower lobe with a standardized uptake value (SUV) of 3.2. There was no evidence of enlarged hilar or mediastinal adenopathy. Biopsy of this lesion was consistent with squamous cell carcinoma, suggesting that this lesion represented a new primary lesion and not a recurrence of her prior lung cancer.

The patient was presented at our multidisciplinary lung cancer tumor board and, because of her significant comorbidities, including poor pulmonary function and cardiac disease, she was felt to be medically inoperable. The consensus recommendation was for stereotactic body radiotherapy (SBRT). We elected to treat her with daily kilovoltage (kV) cone beam CT (CBCT) guidance using a Trilogy linear accelerator (Varian Medical Systems, Palo Alto, CA).

Simulation

On the day of simulation, the patient was carefully positioned in the exact geometric alignment that would be used for the actual delivery of treatment. She was placed on a chest board with her arms overhead. A Vac Lok (CIVCO Medical Solutions, Kalona, IA) and index bar were used to ensure the highest possible accuracy in day-to-day positioning. A respiratory gated plan and treatment delivery was deemed appropriate, because of the desire to spare as much lung volume as possible and to more accurately define and treat the target volume. A four-dimensional (4D) CT scan was acquired from the supraclavicular to below the diaphragm following a free-breathing CT scan. Breathing signals used to sort 4D CT images were generated using the Real-time Position Management (RPM) System (Varian Medical Systems Inc, Palo Alto, CA), by monitoring the patient's abdominal surface motion in the anterior–posterior direction.

An interval of the breathing cycle (30% to 70% breathing phases) was defined as gating window for planning the gated treatment, based on remaining target motion in the gating window. To obtain a regular and reproducible breathing pattern, which is required to ensure the quality of 4D CT images as well as the gated treatment, a pair of video goggles was used to coach the patient's breathing. Through the video goggles, the patient could see her own breathing waveform produced by the RPM system.

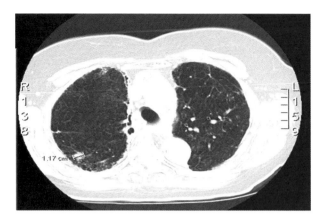

FIGURE 17E-1. Diagnostic computed tomography scan illustrating new right lower lobe lesion.

This approach forms a closed feedback loop, allowing the patient to control her breathing following certain instructions. Near the bottom of the breathing waveform where the end-of-exhale phase is, two horizontal lines formed the gating window. The patient was instructed to place the breathing curve in between two lines when she breathed out. This way, a constant end-of-exhale tumor position, where the gating window is, could be maintained.

Treatment Planning

The planning 4D CT data set was transferred to the Eclipse treatment planning system (Varian Medical Systems, Palo Alto, CA). The gross tumor volume (GTV) and clinical target volume (CTV) were contoured after the planning CT slices and diagnostic images were reviewed. The GTV consisted of all visualized tumor on the planning and diagnostic scans. The 4D CT scans obtained at the time of simulation were used to delineate an internal target volume (ITV), by combining GTVs from all breathing phases in the gating window via a technique called maximum intensity projection (MIP). The ITV was expanded by 5 mm to 7 mm, generating a planning target volume (PTV), accounting for the setup uncertainties. Normal tissues including the lungs and spinal cord were contoured on individual CT slices. The planning goals including dose specifications and normal tissue dose constraints were approved for producing the optimal treatment plan. Isodose lines and dose–volume histograms (DVHs) were reviewed and approved. The final prescription was 48 Gy delivered over four fractions (12 Gy/fraction) biweekly. The treatment plan used in this patient is shown in Figure 17E-2.

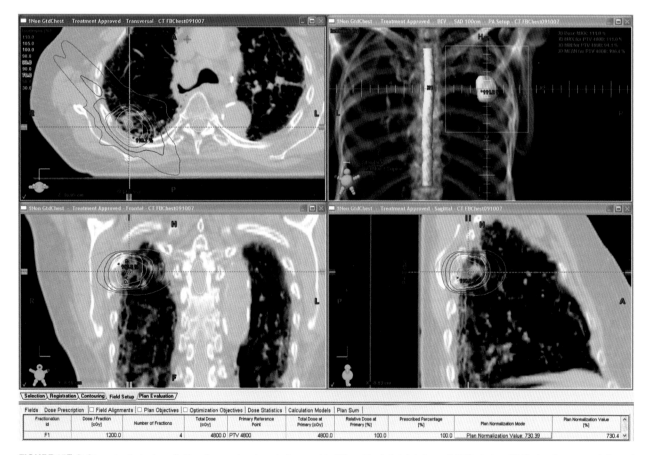

FIGURE 17E-2. Stereotactic body radiation therapy treatment plan used in this patient. A total dose of 48 Gy in four 12-Gy fractions was delivered twice weekly.

Treatment Delivery

The same breath-coaching technique used at simulation was also used during treatment to ensure a constant end-of-exhale tumor position when the beam was turned on. For patient setup, a CBCT scan using the On-Board Imager (OBI; Varian Medical Systems, Palo Alto, CA) was acquired under coached free breathing. The CBCT image generated a smeared GTV, which can be used to approximate the ITV. This approximate ITV was matched to the gated ITV (combined GTVs in the gating window) by aligning the upper edges (where end-of-exhale tumor position was). Corresponding patient shifts were applied. Fluoroscopy was used to verify the proper setup and operation of the gating system before treatment. If everything was correct, the gated treatment was then delivered using RPM. In this patient, gating added approximately 10 minutes on top of the normal treatment delivery time.

Clinical Outcome

The patient tolerated her treatment well without significant acute sequelae. She remains free of tumor recurrence

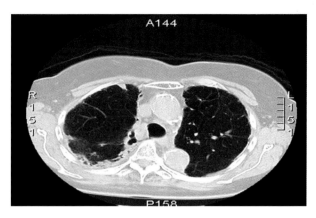

FIGURE 17E-3. Follow-up computed tomography scan illustrating radiographic changes corresponding to the high-dose-treated region but no evidence of disease recurrence.

at 1 year posttreatment with no acute or late toxicity. She is able to perform normal activities with no compromise on her lung functions from her pretreatment baseline. A recent follow-up scan showed subclinical radiographic changes corresponding to high-dose-treated zone but no evidence of disease recurrence (Figure 17E-3).

Chapter 18

Breast Cancer: Overview

J. Keith DeWyngaert, PhD, Gabor Jozsef, PhD, Stella Lymberis, MD, Stewart Becker, PhD, Silvia C. Formenti, MD

Tangent-directed fields, with or without intensity-modulated radiation therapy (IMRT), remain the standard treatment technique for whole breast radiotherapy (RT). As such, planar x-rays may provide adequate and sufficient information for evaluating the integrity of the patient setup. The dose distribution has been shown to be relatively insensitive to changes of 3° to 4° in the gantry angle or collimator angles for both three-dimensional (3D) and IMRT planning.[1–3] However, for courses of therapy directed at a circumscribed target within the breast, such as in partial breast irradiation (PBI) using simultaneous integrated boost (SIB) or concomitant boost techniques, additional anatomical information is desirable. In these settings image-guided radiation therapy (IGRT) provides information on the extent of margins to expand the target in creating a clinical target volume (CTV) and a planning target volume (PTV).[4–16]

Two main challenges hamper the progress in partial breast and tumor bed boost irradiation: (1) the accurate definition of the target, and (2) the accurate, reproducible delivery of the dose. Each will be discussed in the sections that follow.

Target Definition

The definition of CTV to encompass the postsurgical site and the tumor bed, in breast-conserving radiation therapy is derived from imaging information obtained by multiple sources, including mammography, ultrasound, computed tomography (CT), magnetic resonance (MR) imaging, and radiography of surgical clips positioned around the cavity. It is not unusual for combinations of these methods to be used to try to better define the target and follow any changes in volume through the course of therapy. Although the CTV is assumed to remain constant throughout treatment, it is well-known that the shape and volume of the tumor bed, and by extension of the CTV, are time-dependent, varying with time postsurgery. The ramifications of this remains to be understood

with regard to the optimal timing for acquiring a planning image set or adjustments made during the course of therapy.[17]

Planar x-rays have long been the standard for monitoring patient positioning with respect to the treatment fields for breast RT. Portal images have been utilized to examine both intrafraction and interfraction motion.[18] The addition of metallic clips inserted into the tumor bed site may also improve the accuracy of the process of evaluation and correction of the patient's position.

Cone beam CT (CBCT) is a method of generating images for CT reconstruction using rotational large field cone beams instead of slit beams as in conventional CT imaging. These images may be generated using either kilovoltage (kV) or megavoltage (MV) x-rays and both are used in clinical practice. The advantage of this technology is in the high definition of anatomic and geometric imaging information brought to evaluate both the patient's position on the treatment couch and the target of the treatment. It must be realized that an exact match between the planned image set and the newly acquired CBCT image set is impossible because the imaged tissue is not a rigid structure and soft tissue can deform with positioning or rotation. However, it may be possible that subtle changes in anatomic relationships of the soft tissues in the field of CBCT can be dismissed for small targets or targets without proximal critical structures. Finally, CBCT has advanced from full rotational imaging to partial rotation acquisition. Although in either case there may be clearance concerns for C-arm linacs, our group has demonstrated full rotational imaging capability for patients lying in the prone position.[19]

Image-Guided Target and Tissue Delineation

Two-Dimensional Ultrasound

Ultrasound provides real-time guidance for breast biopsy or needle localization procedures and is widely used in breast diagnostic procedures. Breast ultrasound is highly specific in differentiating solid from fluid-filled structures. In the diagnostic setting, two-dimensional (2D) conventional ultrasound remains the standard approach despite its lacking the spatial orientation information of three dimensions.[20]

There have been several reports regarding the use of 2D ultrasound for the localization of the postsurgical cavity both for improved targeting during interstitial brachytherapy of the breast[21] and for the accurate delivery of electron boost treatment.[22,23] In addition, 2D ultrasound has also been used with fused CT images for interstitial breast brachytherapy. A computer-generated image of an implant template was applied virtually to serial CT scans of a patient's breast. Intraoperative ultrasound was used to check the real-time position of the after-loading needles in reference to the chest wall and posterior border of the target volume. No adjustments of needles were required in any of the 11 patients. There was excellent agreement of the target volume coverage between the virtual implant and the actual CT image of the implant.[24]

Information obtained from 2D ultrasound has been compared with that from surgical clips in the estimation of the postsurgical cavity in two studies, both of which reported that 2D ultrasound resulted in inferior volumes compared with that originated from surgical clips. In both series, clips volumes were estimated by using orthogonal radiographs. Rabinovitch and colleagues compared 2D images to the clips methods in defining the lumpectomy cavity for breast boost treatment planning in 29 women and found that 2D ultrasound significantly underestimated the volume of the cavity compared with clips.[25] Ringash et al. also compared 2D ultrasound to clips for tumor bed localization. The results in 52 women demonstrated that ultrasound mean tumor bed volumes were 24 cc, compared with 38 cc when derived from surgical clips. In addition, they defined as "marginal" a plan that included the clips within a less than 1-cm margin and as "inadequate" a plan with any clip outside the field. In their experience the former occurred in 28% of patients and the latter in 7%.[26] See Chapter 18A for a case study illustrating the use of ultrasound for target delineation in a patient with early stage breast cancer.

One disadvantage of 2D ultrasound is that the volume is estimated from the maximum of each of the three dimensions, an expansion unlikely to represent the actual complex and irregular shapes of the postoperative cavity. Techniques that provide 3D visualization such as 3D ultrasound or CT more accurately describe irregular 3D shapes. Another confounder is the fact that the obtained image is affected by the angle at which the probe is held.

In summary, although 2D ultrasound is better than clinical localization of the target for direct electron boost fields, the problems with conformity to the target and spatial accuracy make this technique inadequate when more complex 3D conformal photon planning techniques are used.

Three-Dimensional Ultrasound

High-resolution 3D ultrasound, has been more widely used clinically in recent years.[27,28] Because of the real-time image and volume reconstruction capacity it is commonly used in diagnostic radiology procedures including breast biopsies and ultrasound-guided lumpectomies.[29-31] In addition, there has been interest to apply 3D ultrasound in the radiation therapy treatment planning for breast cancer treatment. However, because the breast tissue can change shape during sonographic imaging with pressure of the probe, accurate registration of images between ultrasound and CT has been difficult.

Nevertheless, 3D ultrasound localization of the tumor bed appears superior to 2D ultrasound and, if coregistered with a planning CT, it provides additional information on the size and location of the tumor bed to be integrated into complex RT planning.

A study by Coles et al.[32] first evaluated the accuracy of a 3D ultrasound compared with CT for measuring volume and spatial location using a breast phantom. Coregistration was performed by using a 3D tracked pointer with a series of infrared-emitting diodes enabling the position of point locations to be recorded. After analysis with the phantom, a clinical trial was conducted using 3D ultrasound examinations in 40 patients undergoing breast RT. Based on the availability of the imaging information, the localization of the tumor bed from these scans was compared with 2D ultrasound and CT, surgical clips and CT, and CT alone in 32 of 40, 14 of 40 and five of 40 patients, respectively. The mean surgery-to-imaging interval was 44 days (range, 23–86 days). A CT–ultrasound registration was achieved in all cases. The postoperative cavity was visualized in all cases with 3D ultrasound, and was graded as highly visible in 53%, visible in 30%, and subtle in 17% of the cases. Three-dimensional ultrasound better localized the tumor bed compared with 2D ultrasound. Although the study had overall small numbers, the data suggest that 2D and 3D ultrasound result in smaller tumor bed volume estimation than volume estimation via clips.[32]

Researchers at the Vancouver Island Health Authority developed a 3D ultrasound imaging system that references to room coordinates and to the CT isocenter. They evaluated coregistration of 3D ultrasound to planning CT images in the treatment planning of partial breast RT, specifically comparing seroma contouring consistency among three radiation oncologists. Three-dimensional ultrasound and CT coregistration was accurate within 2 mm or less in 19 of 20 (95%) breast cancer patients studied. Seroma clarity scores for CT and 3D ultrasound were equivalent in only 25% of cases. The CT seroma clarity was reduced with dense breast parenchyma ($P = .035$), small seroma volume ($P < .001$), and small volume of excised breast tissue (P = .01) whereas ultrasound seroma clarity was not affected by these factors. Ultrasound was associated with improved interobserver consistency compared with CT in eight of 20 (40%) cases. Of these eight cases, seven had low CT seroma clarity scores and four had heterogeneously to extremely dense breast parenchyma. In conclusion, in cases of poor CT seroma clarity and dense breast tissue, 3D ultrasound images enhanced contouring of the breast seroma target, with improved interobserver consistency.[33]

Computed Tomography

The advent of IMRT and image-guided therapy planning has forced the adoption of CT planning for most anatomic sites, including breast. The need for accurate geometric as well as density information warrants CT imaging as the foundation for planning. This data may be augmented by MR or ultrasound, which are often outside the radiation oncology department, wheraes CT simulators are readily available in most departments. For breast conservation RT, CT provides the general landscape of chest anatomy,

including important information about the residual seroma associated with the postsurgical cavity. Postoperative architectural distortion may not be clearly circumscribed and can lead to operator-based variations in tumor bed delineation, particularly in women with high breast densities.[34,35] Petersen et al. evaluated in 30 patients the pattern of tumor bed contouring amongst three radiation oncologists[34]. The concordance among the group demonstrated a conformity index of 0.61. Agreement was dependent upon the clarity of the seroma as well as location, density of the breast parenchyma, and presence of reference calcifications within the breast. It has been proposed that a standard set of guidelines could improve consistency among observers. An example of CT images of a patient positioned in both the prone and supine positions is presented in Figure 18-1.

Surgical Clips

Implanted markers have been used extensively in the prostate as fiducial markers. This approach has also been tested in the breast, to help identify the postsurgical

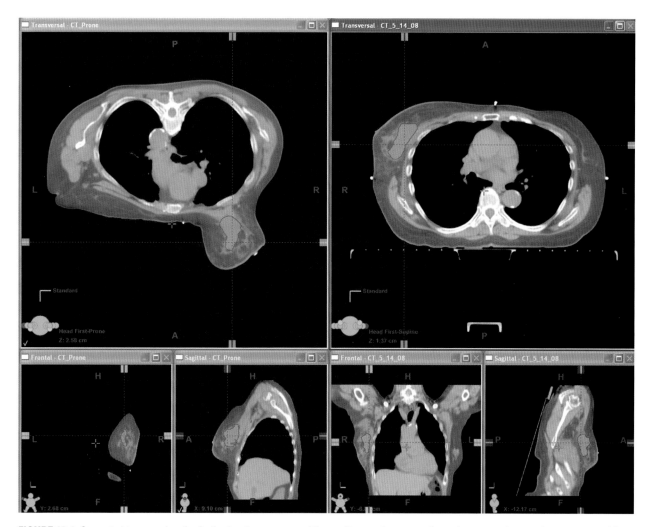

FIGURE 18-1. Computed tomography slice indicating the seroma position and breast changes as the patient moves from supine to prone position.

tumor bed, generally in conjunction with CT imaging.[36-44] The expectation is that these markers represent the boundaries of the surgical site and will be visible on film or electronic planar imaging as an aid to patient positioning. With the introduction of kV imaging, the clips may be more easily visualized and combined with automatic matching protocols to determine patient offsets. In addition, clips placed in tissue surrounding the cavity may prove a more reliable surrogate for the treatment site as the seroma volume changes during treatment.

Buehler et al. studied the ability to image the surgical clips considering different imaging angles and different clip sizes.[37] Generally they reported that the different clips were difficult to recognize, particularly the smaller ones. The interference between clips and density and anatomy of the breast makes it difficult to image each clip individually. Thomas et al. explored which combination of clip sizes, materials, and imaging technique best suited tumor bed localization.[43] Comparing kV or MV planar imaging versus CBCT, they did not find a single candidate that provided adequate visibility for planar imaging with minimal CT artifact. They concluded that a small tantalum clip worked well for floor-mounted x-rays as well as isocentric kV and MV imaging; however, a medium titanium clip would be acceptable for kV imaging but not for MV imaging. The advantage of tantalum clips for MV imaging has been originally recognized by others.[45]

Another study found that kV imaging of clips had a residual error of only 2.4 mm compared with room lasers or the chest wall references for landmarks, which produced errors of 7.1 mm and 5.4 mm, respectively.[38] The residual clip error of 2.4 mm is approaching the limits of the system considering that couch rotations were not included and that the breast tissue may exhibit interfraction variability in shape and form.

A concern regarding the dependence on clips for target localization over a course of therapy is that of marker migration or tissue deformation owing to changes in the postsurgical cavity.[32,46] To eliminate migration as a variable, Harris et al.[47] sutured markers into the wall of the excision cavity. It should be noted that with this approach the gross tumor volume (GTV), determined only by the markers, was a factor of 10 smaller than that of similar studies that used a combination of markers and seroma to define the target volume.[44] Single marker movements up to 7 mm were observed over the course of treatment. These are believed to result from anatomic changes during the resolution of the surgical cavity. Many studies have documented the change with time in the volume of the seroma formed after surgical excision.[17,42,44,48-51] Kim et al. reviewed several series reporting these changes and questioned whether the changes in seroma volume reflect a change in the tissue around the surgical site or rather the organized hematoma/seroma when the cavity fills with new solid tissue as the fluid component resolves.[17]

The work by Harris and colleagues have suggested that the tissue surrounding the tumor bed is moving.[47]

Magnetic Resonance Imaging

The role for MR in planning breast radiation treatment remains undefined. However, for partial breast treatment or for concomitant or integrated boost treatment MR imaging may provide additional information to help define the tumor bed.[52-54]

Ahn et al. used a dedicated coil, developed to fit around the breast with the patient lying in the prone position.[52] They showed that high-quality images could be obtained with a dedicated coil without respiratory artifact with the patient in the prone position. In another study the patient was positioned supine and the postsurgical site was classified based on the proximity of the cavity to the chest wall. They reported that 53% of the postsurgical cavities were in contact with the chest wall, suggesting that perhaps in these cases part of the chest needs to be included in the PTV.

Studies comparing the postsurgical sites defined by CT and MR have indicated that the MR-defined postsurgical site tends to be significantly larger than the CT-defined site.[55,56] Figure 18-2 is an example of CT and MR images for a patient scanned in the prone position for both sets of data. Owing to the different positioning tables and patient arm positions, the breast hangs quite differently between the two imaging studies. Kirby et al. used clips inserted at the time of surgery to guide the fusion of the MR and CT images of 30 patients imaged in the prone position and found a median conformity index (overlap of the CT and MR volumes to the combined total CT+MR volume) of 53%.[55] The median increase in volume of the tumor bed from CT to MR was 44.8%. However, once the CTV was defined as tumor bed + 1.5 cm 3D expansion, and was limited by 5 mm from the skin surface and posteriorly by the chest wall, the percentage increase dropped to 10.3%. Applying boundaries that restrict the expansion of the tumor bed resulted in a closer match between the CTV defined by CT versus that defined by MR. Partial breast RT to a CT-defined PTV in the prone position using minitangents covered the CTV with the 95% isodose surface in 26 of 30 cases. This may support the use of minitangents to achieve a more conformal non-coplanar field arrangement.

Image-Guided Treatment Delivery

Planar Imaging

For years, planar MV images have been the standard for evaluating the integrity of the patient setup. In breast RT, these consist of portal images, although they could also be orthogonal beams for the purpose of evaluating the treatment isocenter.[57] The era of electronic portal imaging devices (EPIDs) has streamlined the process, expediting

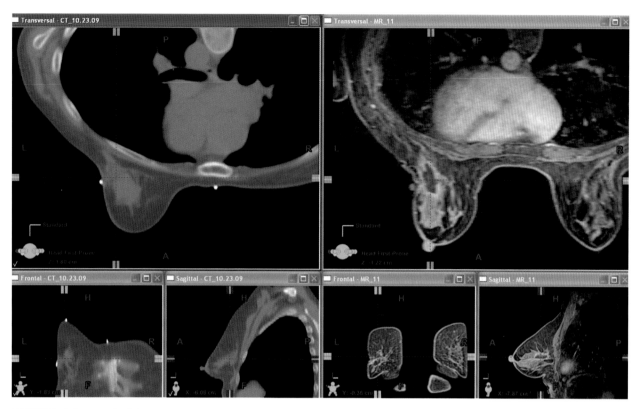

FIGURE 18-2. Images of left breast showing the postsurgical edema on computed tomography (CT) image (left panel) and T1-magnetic resonance (MR) image (right panel). The MR series was acquired with the standard breast MR patient table whereas the CT image reflects the setup and table support used for prone breast radiation therapy.

image acquisition, evaluation, and eventual introduction of adjustments of the patient position. Planar images enable the user to correct for patient positioning with three to six degrees of freedom. This range depends on software and table properties. Standard patient treatment tables allow up to four degrees of freedom (x, y, z, and yaw or couch rotation), whereas some commercially available systems are able to correct for pitch and roll. Several studies have shown that these small rotations in gantry or collimator angle generally have an insignificant effect upon the dose distribution.[1–3]

Electronic portal imaging has been utilized to evaluate intrafraction respiratory motion as well as interfraction and systematic setup variances.[18,58–62] The ability to take snapshot images in rapid succession distinguishes electronic portal imaging from CBCT. These studies have demonstrated that respiratory motion of the breast tissue is negligible when the patient is positioned prone. This has been further confirmed through CT and MR studies.[52,59] The respiratory motion of breast tissue when prone is comparable to that measured supine (in the 2 mm to 3 mm range). However, George et al.[63] considered the effect of respiratory motion upon IMRT dose distributions and found that the PTV coverage becomes degraded as a consequence of heavy breathing, a problem that was not encountered for prone positioning. Interfraction variability is of greater concern than intrafraction variations.

An advantage of kV imaging to assist in isocenter verification is the reduced patient exposure compared with that of MV portal images (typically 1 to 3 monitor units). Either standard tangent angles may be used to compare the isocenter location against the chest wall and breast tissue or a pair of orthogonal beams may be imaged for localization. Orthogonal (anterior–posterior [AP] and lateral) images inherently use the same coordinate system as the treatment table making it simpler to correct for errors in patient positioning compared with using oblique opposed images. When a nontangent beam arrangement is used for treatment, such as in supine partial breast[64] or SIB treatments with multiple fields[7,9–12,41] a pair of orthogonal images is the appropriate tool for monitoring patient setup. However, AP and lateral MV images could represent considerable additional dose over the course of the treatment to the lung and heart that can be reduced through the use of kV imaging.[57] A limitation of kV images is the lack of information about the entire treated field and the surrounding breast tissue, hampering judgments on daily variations in position.

Cone-Beam Computed Tomography

The advantage of CBCT in RT is that a scan can be obtained right before the treatment with the patient in the treatment position, through an x-ray source and detector array attached to the treatment machine. Despite the fact that image quality is inferior to that of the past generation diagnostic CT, bony structures, cavities, and structures with distinct density differences from their environments are clearly visible. The quality of CBCT is about equivalent to that of the 1980s CT scanners—perfectly adequate to align the planning CT images with those obtained at CBCT scans. The process generates the information to perform a set of treatment couch shifts and rotations, by which the patient, or rather the table, moves in 3D to match the originally planned position (Figure 18-3). The use of CBCT imaging in patients undergoing breast irradiation is illustrated in Chapter 18C.

The alignment, however, is not just based on matching to rigid reference structures. Small differences can occur by slight differences in the geometry of deformable body structures, or by functional changes such as breathing. Furthermore, the exact definition of the soft tissue structures is sometimes difficult because of the different imaging techniques.

Intrafraction movement—primarily breathing—is not analyzed clinically as yet with CBCT because of the time constraints associated with obtaining the images. However, phantom measurements have been performed by registering a four-dimensional (4D) or gated and an ungated CBCT to overcome image degradation by breathing and reconstructing breathing phases.[65,66] As already mentioned, several studies have used portal imaging techniques for intrafraction movement evaluation during irradiation of the breast.[18,58–60,67–69]

For whole breast irradiation, the standard technique is the "tangent field technique": a set of parallel oblique beams, whose posterior field edge is tangent to the chest wall. Planar x-ray images from the "beams-eye-view" suffice most of the time to align the patient correctly. In treatment techniques irradiating only a target in the breast—partial breast, SIB, tumor bed boosts—CBCT provides additional anatomical information for achieving accurate setup, and has been a valuable evaluation tool of the accuracy as well as a method for following anatomical changes during the course of RT.

For whole breast and nodal treatment in the supine position, the patient is usually lying on an elevated angled board, with her arms reproducibly immobilized by holding onto pegs positioned above the head. This board is not used for whole breast or partial breast prone treatment. In the prone position, the patient lies on a special board with an opening that allows the treated breast to hang freely[12]

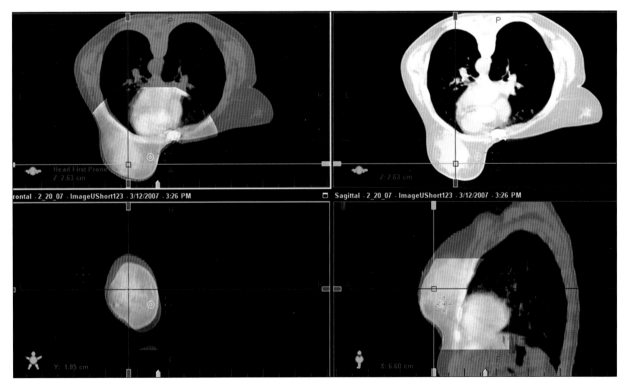

FIGURE 18-3. Cone-beam computed tomography CBCT (blue) acquired prior to treatment is shown overlaid on computed tomography (CT) images (orange) during a course of partial breast radiation therapy. The images were taken using a Varian 21EX unit (Varian Oncology Systems, Palo Alto, CA) equipped with onboard imaging.

and the arms are again positioned above the head. The elevated position of the patient and the elbows protruding out of treatment couch could limit the rotation of the x-ray source attached to the gantry. Fortunately, a full rotation is generally possible. Nevertheless, Buehler et al. showed that an 80° rotation can suffice if clips are used in the target for delineation and localization.[37]

The use of clips implanted in the surgical bed during surgery is somewhat controversial. Although it increases visibility on planar x-rays, it also leads to artifacts in both the planning CT and the CBCT. The artifact can be decreased by: (a) choosing clips with more radiotransparent material such as the medium or small tantalum clips as Thomas et al.[43] recommended for CBCT and (b) by using artifact-suppressing reconstruction algorithms or clip recognition software, such as the one reported by Kim et al.[39] The possible migration of the clips can also be of concern, as the surgical cavity changes its size with time.

In the presence of clip(s), alignment can be performed based on their location(s). For example, results of setup accuracies with clip alignment and CBCT in PBI demonstrated a positional error of the clip of about 7 mm (the method of the initial setup is not specified), which can be reduced to less than 2 mm.[39] If clips are not used, alignment of the planning and CBCT can be based on anatomical structures such as the ribs or lungs, or by using as a reference the external surface or the seroma (tumor bed). Although the seroma size may change over time, the delivery of PBI over the brief period interval of a week has persuaded our group at the New York University to perform the alignment based on the seroma boundaries.

Several studies involving alignment without using clips have been published. Jain et al., Fatunase et al., and White et al. reported results along the three principal directions in the supine position.[69–71] Fatunase et al. used bony anatomy, whereas White et al. used ipsilateral lung and external contours for alignment. All three methods demonstrated smaller than 7-mm changes, measured as the 3D distance of the shifts.

Fewer CBCT studies on the prone position have been reported. Our group showed the feasibility of CBCT in the prone position[19] and reported very similar shifts as Fatunase et al.'s supine study,[72] suggesting that setup errors are comparable in the two positions.

Target Delineating and Dosimetric Consequences

The role of the expansion of the CTV to generate the PTV is to create a margin of volume that accounts for setup uncertainties. Because IGRT provides a quantitative measure of these uncertainties (shifts), one can calculate the extent of the necessary margins. However, the terminology for reporting and analyzing the shifts is not yet standardized. Some authors denote the total shift (root of the square sum of the shifts in three orthogonal directions) as the vector sum. Frequently, the root mean

squares (RMS) of the shifts in each direction are calculated instead of the average, as the averages are (and should be) close to zero. In addition, the terms systematic and random errors are used according to the definition of van Herk.[73] The population systematic error (Σ) is defined as the standard deviation of the average shifts calculated for each individual patient. Population random errors are the average of the standard deviations of the shifts for every patient.

Several formulas for margin calculation are listed in the work by van Herk.[73] Among them the most frequently used (and the most conservative) formula is: $2.5^{*}\Sigma + 0.7^{*}\sigma$, where Σ and σ are the systematic and random errors, respectively. Using CBCT data, the resulting margins by Fatunase et al.[70] in supine and Jozsef et al.[72] in prone position were found to be comparable: 1.2 cm in the AP direction. The originally empirically designed margin around the outlined tumor bed was 1.5 cm to 2 cm for prone PBI, which appears to be sufficient to account for setup errors. However, because the calculated margins in these studies are different in the three principal directions a possibility for applying nonuniform margins should be investigated.

Another issue concerns the size and shape evolution of the seroma over time. Instead of CBCTs, the studies of these changes are performed by using diagnostic CTs before, during, and after the treatment, an adequate approach for accelerated PBI delivered over a week period. However, when the information for a boost is applied over a period of several weeks of whole breast irradiation, significant changes in volume may occur. Sharma et al.[51] found a seroma volume change in the range of 40% and Tersteeg et al.[42] reported even larger decreases (62%) of the seroma volume after an average 37 days of treatment.

Cone-beam CT information to determine the daily setup error permits us to estimate the consequent dosimetric errors.[69,74] A simple approach we tested[74] applied the shifts from CBCT to reposition the isocenter on the planning CT for prone PBI. The PTV (tumor bed expanded by 1.5-cm margin) coverage decreased by an average of 4.8%, while the tumor bed retained full coverage and the lung and heart dose remained low. A similar approach was adopted by Jain et al. for supine treatments, who registered the CBCT image to the planning CT in their treatment planning program.[69] These investigators also observed loss of the PTV coverage, and warned about possible loss of the tumor coverage if the tumor is adjacent to the chest wall.

Cone-beam CT images can also be exported to the planning software, and treatment plans can be evaluated using those images. However, in this case, different conversion tables between CBCT Hounsfield units (HU) to electron density have to be established for each applied technique and region,[75] although Yang et al.[76] and Yoo et al.[77] judged that the existing difference may be acceptable. As of now, we are not aware of reports on dosimetric error modeling programs for breast irradiation.[69]

Importantly, CBCT itself, however, delivers some dose to the patients. Monte-Carlo calculations predicted 2 cGy to 2.5 cGy for a pelvis or lung CBCT procedure, and 5 cGy or more in head and neck cases.[78] Other studies emphasized the fact that the dose to the bones can be approximately three times higher because of the increased role of photoelectric effect for the kV energies used in CBCT.[79] The exact nature of this dose deposition is technique dependent and is worthy of further investigation.

MVCT: Tomotherapy

Tomotherapy units include MVCT capabilities with the same rotating linac used for treatment. Therefore, it is natural to obtain an MVCT before fractions for accurate alignment. The alignment accuracy for partial breast treatments in the supine position was reported by Langen et al.[80] to be about 2 mm, averaged over 50 MVCTs. Dosimetric consequences of uncorrected setup errors were calculated by Goddu et al.[81] with a conclusion that about a 14% dose difference can occur in the superficial region, but at depth of greater than 5 mm the error is less than 3%. Their treatment planning methodology seemed to be insensitive to setup errors up to about 7 mm. The dose from the MVCT has been reported as approximately 2 cGy per fraction.[82] See Chapter 18B for a case study illustrating the use of MVCT imaging in a patient with breast cancer.

Video-Based Surface Mapping

Video surface imaging is a system in which the surface of the breast is imaged and used to align the patient for daily setup. Each treatment day, the patient's breast is imaged in the treatment position. The imaged surface is then compared with a reference surface obtained by digital reconstruction of the images from CT simulation. The comparison generates an alignment shift for the therapist to perform. The process of imaging the surface of the breast falls under two categories: (a) discrete marker tracking and (b) whole surface shape matching.

Discrete marker-based tracking uses five to 10 markers, placed directly on the breast surface. These markers are then tracked using infrared cameras. This technique captures the entire surface shape. Marker matching has the advantage of enabling the user to directly compare daily scans to the reference image. The difference between the markers from scan to scan is rapidly computed to produce a rigid-body shift. This technique, however, does not have the ability to capture shape changes in the whole breast or changes attributable to the effect of breathing. Conversely, whole breast surface mapping can track changes in the contour of the breast and breathing motion. Although this provides a detailed view of the breast, it can

generate conflicting information as far as shifts are concerned. Changes in contours do not always correspond well to rigid shifts especially when the entire breast is imaged. Generally this problem may be addressed by focusing only on the region of the breast closest to the seroma.

In contrast to the additional dose contributed to the breast and other parts of the body[83,84] from daily CBCT and kV imaging, video-based techniques do not use ionizing radiation. Therefore, they can be used repeatedly without additional dose to the patient. As of yet, the correspondence between the movement of the seroma and the surface of the breast has not been well characterized. Preliminary data suggest that surface mapping can be accurate to 3 mm[38,85,86] (see Chapter 18D).

Future Directions

Adaptive IGRT

Breast tissue is inherently deformable and as such localization and positioning of patients typically focuses on one or a few anatomical elements such as chest wall, skin surface, seroma, or clips. Adaptive IGRT therapy in this context has been limited to the ability to accumulate the dose to structures and then adapt subsequent treatments by introducing appropriate PTV expansion margins. For postsurgical tumor bed targeting, such as concomitant, SIB, or partial breast radiation therapy, CBCT may offer the ability to visualize and directly target using both seroma and chest wall as references for registration. Several investigators have considered the effects of these daily positioning adjustments on dose by applying the 3D offsets determined from CBCT or MVCT imaging to the original treatment plan and simulating the effect of this movement by summing the dose.[70,74,81] Goddu et al. ascertained setup errors using video surface mapping, determined frequency distributions, and applied these weighted offsets to whole breast treatment with helical tomotherapy.[81] When the patient was offset relative to the isocenter in a posterior–medial direction, the breast PTV coverage was compromised, owing to the sharp drop off of dose at the chest wall. For accelerated PBI, both Fatunase et al. (supine positioning) and DeWyngaert et al.[70,74] (prone positioning) showed some compromise for the PTV volume but concluded that the target volume coverage did not degrade. Fatunase and coworkers limited the value of CBCT in supine positioned patients to women with large breasts and to specific anatomic situations requiring tight margins.

Finally, if the seroma represents an accurate marker or target surrogate for accelerated PBI, concomitant boost, or SIB treatment, then modifications should be made to the plan in accordance with changes to the seroma.[17] Issues about whether the surrounding tissue at risk (CTV) is shrinking or is the seroma being replaced with new tissue remain unsolved. Moreover, results from Harris et al. demonstrate that the changes in volume and shape of the excision wall are not uniform for each patient. They have defined indices to use to help determine when changes occur, directed toward the use of adaptive radiation therapy.[47]

Feature Analysis

It may be possible to make predictions regarding the appropriateness of IGRT-based treatments by analyzing individual patient features. For example, it may be possible to quickly determine if a patient is a suitable candidate for accelerated PBI at the time of simulation without creating a plan, by determining if the dose constraints can be met. Kron et al. have modeled this approach through a volume comparison of the seroma to the breast volume using a few measurements taken from the CT images.[87] Our group has applied a process of feature analysis in evaluating preferences for patient positioning (prone vs supine)[88,89] for both whole breast and IGRT-based treatments.

References

1. Yang J, Ma C, Wang L, et al. Effect of collimator and couch angle change on breast IMRT dose distributions. *J Appl Clin Med Phys.* 2009;10:3058.
2. Das IJ, Cheng CW, Fosmire H, et al. Tolerances in setup and dosimetric errors in the radiation treatment of breast cancer. *Int J Radiat Oncol Biol Phys.* 1993;26:883–890.
3. Harron EC, McCallum HM, Lambert EL, et al. Dosimetric effects of setup uncertainties on breast treatment delivery. *Med Dosim.* 2008;33:293–298.
4. McCormick B. Partial-breast radiation for early staged breast cancers: hypothesis, existing data, and a planned phase III trial. *J Natl Compr Canc Netw.* 2005;3:301–307.
5. Oliver M, Chen J, Wong E, et al. A treatment planning study comparing whole breast radiation therapy against conformal, IMRT and tomotherapy for accelerated partial breast irradiation. *Radiother Oncol.* 2007;82:317–323.
6. Vicini F, Winter K, Wong J, et al. Initial efficacy results of RTOG 0319: three-dimensional conformal radiation therapy (3D-CRT) confined to the region of the lumpectomy cavity for stage I/ II breast carcinoma. *Int J Radiat Oncol Biol Phys.* 2009; Nov 10 [Epub ahead of print].
7. Guerrero M, Li XA, Earl MA, et al. Simultaneous integrated boost for breast cancer using IMRT: a radiobiological and treatment planning study. *Int J Radiat Oncol Biol Phys.* 2004;59:1513–1522.
8. Hurkmans CW, Meijer GJ, van Vliet-Vroegindeweij C, et al. High-dose simultaneously integrated breast boost using intensity-modulated radiotherapy and inverse optimization. *Int J Radiat Oncol Biol Phys.* 2006;66:923–930.
9. McDonald MW, Godette KD, Whitaker DJ, et al. Three-year outcomes of breast intensity-modulated radiation therapy with simultaneous integrated boost. *Int J Radiat Oncol Biol Phys.* 2009; Sep 21 [Epub ahead of print].
10. Singla R, King S, Albuquerque K, et al. Simultaneous-integrated boost intensity-modulated radiation therapy (SIB-IMRT) in the treatment of early-stage left-sided breast carcinoma. *Med Dosim.* 2006;31:190–196.
11. van der Laan HP, Dolsma WV, Maduro JH, et al. Three-dimensional conformal simultaneously integrated boost technique for breast-conserving radiotherapy. *Int J Radiat Oncol Biol Phys.* 2007;68:1018–1023.
12. DeWyngaert JK, Jozsef G, Mitchell J, et al. Accelerated intensity-modulated radiotherapy to breast in prone position: dosimetric results. *Int J Radiat Oncol Biol Phys.* 2007;68:1251–1259.
13. Formenti SC. External-beam partial-breast irradiation. *Semin Radiat Oncol.* 2005;15:92–99.
14. Formenti SC. External-beam-based partial breast irradiation. *Nat Clin Pract Oncol.* 2007;4:326–327.
15. Formenti SC, Gidea-Addeo D, Goldberg JD, et al. Phase I-II trial of prone accelerated intensity modulated radiation therapy to the breast to optimally spare normal tissue. *J Clin Oncol.* 2007;25:2236–2242.
16. Formenti SC, Rosenstein B, Skinner KA, Jozsef G. T1 stage breast cancer: adjuvant hypofractionated conformal radiation therapy to tumor bed in selected postmenopausal breast cancer patients—pilot feasibility study. *Radiology.* 2002;222:171–178.
17. Kim LH, Vicini F, Yan D. What do recent studies on lumpectomy cavity volume change imply for breast clinical target volumes? *Int J Radiat Oncol Biol Phys.* 2008;72:1–3.
18. Mitchell J, Formenti SC, DeWyngaert JK. Interfraction and intrafraction setup variability for prone breast radiation therapy. *Int J Radiat Oncol Biol Phys.* 2009; Nov 10 [Epub ahead of print].
19. Becker SJ, Jozsef G, DeWyngaert JK, Formenti S. Cone-beam CTs of the prone breast. *Int J Radiat Oncol Biol Phys.* 2007;69:S721.
20. Yang W, Dempsey PJ. Diagnostic breast ultrasound: current status and future directions. *Radiol Clin North Am.* 2007;45:845–861, vii.
21. DeBiose DA, Horwitz EM, Martinez AA, et al. The use of ultrasonography in the localization of the lumpectomy cavity for interstitial brachytherapy of the breast. *Int J Radiat Oncol Biol Phys.* 1997;38:755–759.
22. Leonard C, Harlow CL, Coffin C, et al. Use of ultrasound to guide radiation boost planning following lumpectomy for carcinoma of the breast. *Int J Radiat Oncol Biol Phys.* 1993;27:1193–1197.
23. Haba Y, Britton P, Sinnatamby R, et al. Can ultrasound improve the accuracy of delivery of electron boost treatment following breast conserving surgery? *Eur J Cancer.* 2001;37:38.
24. Vicini FA, Jaffray DA, Horwitz EM, et al. Implementation of 3D-virtual brachytherapy in the management of breast cancer: a description of a new method of interstitial brachytherapy. *Int J Radiat Oncol Biol Phys.* 1998;40:629 635.
25. Rabinovitch R, Finlayson C, Pan Z, et al. Radiographic evaluation of surgical clips is better than ultrasound for defining the lumpectomy cavity in breast boost treatment planning: a prospective clinical study. *Int J Radiat Oncol Biol Phys.* 2000;47:313–317.

26. Ringash J, Whelan T, Elliott E, et al. Accuracy of ultrasound in localization of breast boost field. *Radiother Oncol.* 2004;72:61–66.

27. Downey DB, Fenster A, Williams JC. Clinical utility of three-dimensional US. *Radiographics.* 2000;20:559–571.

28. Sahiner B, Chan HP, Roubidoux MA, et al. Malignant and benign breast masses on 3D US volumetric images: effect of computer-aided diagnosis on radiologist accuracy. *Radiology.* 2007;242:716–724.

29. Kuban DA, Dong L, Cheung R, et al. Ultrasound-based localization. *Semin Radiat Oncol.* 2005;15:180–191.

30. Cannon JW, Stoll JA, Salgo IS, et al. Real-time three-dimensional ultrasound for guiding surgical tasks. *Comput Aided Surg.* 2003;8:82–90.

31. Cash CJ, Coles CE, Treece GM, et al. Breast cancers: noninvasive method of preoperative localization with three-dimensional US and surface contour mapping. *Radiology.* 2007;245:556–566.

32. Coles CE, Cash CJ, Treece GM, et al. High definition three-dimensional ultrasound to localise the tumour bed: a breast radiotherapy planning study. *Radiother Oncol.* 2007;84:233–241.

33. Berrang TS, Truong PT, Popescu C, et al. 3D ultrasound can contribute to planning CT to define the target for partial breast radiotherapy. *Int J Radiat Oncol Biol Phys.* 2009;73:375–383.

34. Petersen RP, Truong PT, Kader HA, et al. Target volume delineation for partial breast radiotherapy planning: clinical characteristics associated with low interobserver concordance. *Int J Radiat Oncol Biol Phys.* 2007;69:41–48.

35. Wong EK, Truong PT, Kader HA, et al. Consistency in seroma contouring for partial breast radiotherapy: impact of guidelines. *Int J Radiat Oncol Biol Phys.* 2006;66:372–376.

36. Benda RK, Yasuda G, Sethi A, et al. Breast boost: are we missing the target? *Cancer.* 2003;97:905–909.

37. Buehler A, Ng SK, Lyatskaya Y, et al. Evaluation of clip localization for different kilovoltage imaging modalities as applied to partial breast irradiation setup. *Med Phys.* 2009;36:821–834.

38. Gierga DP, Riboldi M, Turcotte JC, et al. Comparison of target registration errors for multiple image-guided techniques in accelerated partial breast irradiation. *Int J Radiat Oncol Biol Phys.* 2008;70:1239–1246.

39. Kim LH, Wong J, Yan D. On-line localization of the lumpectomy cavity using surgical clips. *Int J Radiat Oncol Biol Phys.* 2007;69:1305–1309.

40. Leonard CE, Tallhamer M, Johnson T, et al. Clinical experience with image-guided radiotherapy in an accelerated partial breast intensity-modulated radiotherapy protocol. *Int J Radiat Oncol Biol Phys.* 2009; May 19 [Epub ahead of print].

41. Penninkhof J, Quint S, Boer H, et al. Surgical clips for position verification and correction of non-rigid breast tissue in simultaneously integrated boost (SIB) treatments. *Radiother Oncol.* 2009;90:110–115.

42. Tersteeg RJ, Roesink JM, Albregts M, et al. Changes in excision cavity volume: prediction of the reduction in absolute volume during breast irradiation. *Int J Radiat Oncol Biol Phys.* 2009;74:1181–1185.

43. Thomas CW, Nichol AM, Park JE, et al. An anthropomorphic phantom study of visualisation of surgical clips for partial

breast irradiation (PBI) setup verification. *Radiother Oncol.* 2009;90:56–59.

44. Oh KS, Kong FM, Griffith KA, et al. Planning the breast tumor bed boost: changes in the excision cavity volume and surgical scar location after breast-conserving surgery and whole-breast irradiation. *Int J Radiat Oncol Biol Phys.* 2006;66:680–686.

45. Jozsef G, Luxton G, Formenti SC. Application of radiosurgery principles to a target in the breast: a dosimetric study. *Med Phys.* 2000;27:1005–1010.

46. Kass R, Kumar G, Klimberg VS, et al. Clip migration in stereotactic biopsy. *Am J Surg.* 2002;184:325–331.

47. Harris EJ, Donovan EM, Yarnold JR, et al. Characterization of target volume changes during breast radiotherapy using implanted fiducial markers and portal imaging. *Int J Radiat Oncol Biol Phys.* 2009;73:958–966.

48. Kader HA, Truong PT, Pai R, et al. When is CT-based postoperative seroma most useful to plan partial breast radiotherapy? Evaluation of clinical factors affecting seroma volume and clarity. *Int J Radiat Oncol Biol Phys.* 2008;72:1064–1069.

49. Prendergast B, Indelicato DJ, Grobmyer SR, et al. The dynamic tumor bed: volumetric changes in the lumpectomy cavity during breast-conserving therapy. *Int J Radiat Oncol Biol Phys.* 2009;74:695–701.

50. Weed DW, Yan D, Martinez AA, et al. The validity of surgical clips as a radiographic surrogate for the lumpectomy cavity in image-guided accelerated partial breast irradiation. *Int J Radiat Oncol Biol Phys.* 2004;60:484–492.

51. Sharma R, Spierer M, Mutyala S, et al. Change in seroma volume during whole-breast radiation therapy. *Int J Radiat Oncol Biol Phys.* 2009;75:89–93.

52. Ahn KH, Hargreaves BA, Alley MT, et al. MRI guidance for accelerated partial breast irradiation in prone position: imaging protocol design and evaluation. *Int J Radiat Oncol Biol Phys.* 2009;75:285–293.

53. Tendulkar RD, Chellman-Jeffers M, Rybicki LA, et al. Preoperative breast magnetic resonance imaging in early breast cancer: implications for partial breast irradiation. *Cancer.* 2009;115:1621–1630.

54. Whipp EC, Halliwell M. Magnetic resonance imaging appearances in the postoperative breast: the clinical target volume-tumor and its relationship to the chest wall. *Int J Radiat Oncol Biol Phys.* 2008;72:49–57.

55. Kirby AM, Yarnold JR, Evans PM, et al. Tumor bed delineation for partial breast and breast boost radiotherapy planned in the prone position: what does MRI add to x-ray CT localization of titanium clips placed in the excision cavity wall? *Int J Radiat Oncol Biol Phys.* 2009;74:1276–1282.

56. Sabine B, Giovanna D, Peter P, et al. Open low-field magnetic resonance (MR) versus CT scanner (CT) imaging in breast radiotherapy treatment planning:. *Int J Radiat Oncol Biol Phys* 2005;63:S232–S233.

57. Wang X, Du W, Smith SA, et al. The radiation exposure from portal images during the course of breast radiotherapy. *Am J Clin Oncol.* 2008;31:345–351.

58. Smith RP, Bloch P, Harris EE, et al. Analysis of interfraction and intrafraction variation during tangential breast irradiation

with an electronic portal imaging device. *Int J Radiat Oncol Biol Phys.* 2005;62:373–378.

59. Morrow NV, Stepaniak C, White J, et al. Intra- and interfractional variations for prone breast irradiation: an indication for image-guided radiotherapy. *Int J Radiat Oncol Biol Phys.* 2007;69:910–917.

60. Mitchell JD, DeWyngaert JK, Formenti SC. Interfraction setup variability for prone breast radiotherapy. *Int J Radiat Oncol Biol Phys.* 2007;69:S710–S711.

61. Truong PT, Berthelet E, Patenaude V, et al. Short communication: setup variations in locoregional radiotherapy for breast cancer: an electronic portal imaging study. *Br J Radiol.* 2005;78:742–745.

62. Kinoshita R, Shimizu S, Taguchi H, et al. Three-dimensional intrafractional motion of breast during tangential breast irradiation monitored with high-sampling frequency using a real-time tumor-tracking radiotherapy system. *Int J Radiat Oncol Biol Phys.* 2008;70:931–934.

63. George R, Keall PJ, Kini VR, et al. Quantifying the effect of intrafraction motion during breast IMRT planning and dose delivery. *Med Phys.* 2003;30:552–562.

64. Baglan KL, Sharpe MB, Jaffray D, et al. Accelerated partial breast irradiation using 3D conformal radiation therapy (3D-CRT). *Int J Radiat Oncol Biol Phys.* 2003;55:302–311.

65. Leng S, Zambelli J, Tolakanahalli R, et al. Streaking artifacts reduction in four-dimensional cone-beam computed tomography. *Med Phys.* 2008;35:4649–4659.

66. Sonke JJ, Zijp L, Remeijer P, van Herk M. Respiratory correlated cone beam CT. *Med Phys.* 2005;32:1176–1186.

67. Lawson JD, Fox T, Elder E, et al. Early clinical experience with kilovoltage image-guided radiation therapy for interfraction motion management. *Med Dosim.* 2008;33:268–274.

68. Huh SJ, Han Y, Park W, Yang JH. Interfractional dose variation due to seromas in radiotherapy of breast cancer. *Med Dosim.* 2005;30:8–11.

69. Jain P, Marchant T, Green M, et al. Inter-fraction motion and dosimetric consequences during breast intensity-modulated radiotherapy (IMRT). *Radiother Oncol.* 2009;90:93–98.

70. Fatunase T, Wang Z, Yoo S, et al. Assessment of the residual error in soft tissue setup in patients undergoing partial breast irradiation: results of a prospective study using cone-beam computed tomography. *Int J Radiat Oncol Biol Phys.* 2008;70:1025–1034.

71. White EA, Cho J, Vallis KA, et al. Cone beam computed tomography guidance for setup of patients receiving accelerated partial breast irradiation. *Int J Radiat Oncol Biol Phys.* 2007;68:547–554.

72. Jozsef G, Lymberis SC, DeWyngaert KJ, Formenti SC. Prospective study of cone-beam CT (CBCT) guidance for prone accelerated partial breast irradiation (APBI). *Int J Radiat Oncol Biol Phys.* 2009;75:S571–S572.

73. van Herk M. Errors and margins in radiotherapy. *Semin Radiat Oncol.* 2004;14:52–64.

74. DeWyngaert J, Lymberis S, Addeo D, et al. CBCT enabled reconstruction of inter-fraction variation of dose distribution for partial breast irradiation. *Int J Radiat Oncol Biol Phys.* 2008;72:S514.

75. Richter A, Hu Q, Steglich D, et al. Investigation of the usability of cone-beam CT data sets for dose calculation. *Radiat Oncol.* 2008;3:42.

76. Yang Y, Schreibmann E, Li T, et al. Evaluation of on-board kV cone beam CT (CBCT)-based dose calculation. *Phys Med Biol.* 2007;52:685–705.

77. Yoo S, Yin FF. Dosimetric feasibility of cone-beam CT-based treatment planning compared to CT-based treatment planning. *Int J Radiat Oncol Biol Phys.* 2006;66:1553–1561.

78. Downes P, Jarvis R, Radu E, et al. Monte Carlo simulation and patient dosimetry for a kilovoltage cone-beam CT unit. *Med Phys.* 2009;36:4156–4167.

79. Ding GX, Duggan DM, Coffey CW. Accurate patient dosimetry of kilovoltage cone-beam CT in radiation therapy. *Med Phys.* 2008;35:1135–1144.

80. Langen KM, Buchholz DJ, Burch DR, et al. Investigation of accelerated partial breast patient alignment and treatment with helical tomotherapy unit. *Int J Radiat Oncol Biol Phys.* 2008;70:1272–1280.

81. Goddu SM, Yaddanapudi S, Pechenaya OL, et al. Dosimetric consequences of uncorrected setup errors in helical tomotherapy treatments of breast-cancer patients. *Radiother Oncol.* 2009;93:64–70.

82. Shah AP, Langen KM, Ruchala K, et al. Patient-specific dose from megavoltage CT imaging with a helical tomotherapy unit. *Int J Radiat Oncol Biol Phys.* 2007;69:S193–S194.

83. Peng LC, Yang CC, Sim S, et al. Dose comparison of megavoltage cone-beam and orthogonal-pair portal images. *J Appl Clin Med Phys.* 2007;8:10–20.

84. Chow JC. Cone-beam CT dosimetry for the positional variation in isocenter: a Monte Carlo study. *Med Phys.* 2009;36:3512–3520.

85. Baroni G, Ferrigno G, Orecchia R, Pedotti A. Real-time optoelectronic verification of patient position in breast cancer radiotherapy. *Comput Aided Surg.* 2000;5:296–306.

86. Riboldi M, Gierga DP, Chen GT, Baroni G. Accuracy in breast shape alignment with 3D surface fitting algorithms. *Med Phys.* 2009;36:1193–1198.

87. Kron T, Willis D, Miller J, et al. A spreadsheet to determine the volume ratio for target and breast in partial breast irradiation. *Australas Phys Eng Sci Med.* 2009;32:98–104.

88. Chang J, Zhao X, Wong E, et al. A support vector machine (SVM) classifier enables prediction of optimal setup, prone versus supine, in left breast cancer patients. *Int J Radiat Oncol Biol Phys.* 2009;75:S218–S219.

89. Lymberis SC, Parhar P, Yee D, et al. Results of prospective trial to determine optimal patient positioning prone vs. supine for whole breast radiation. *Int J Radiat Oncol Biol Phys.* 2008;72:S509.

Three-Dimensional Ultrasound-Guided Target Delineation and Treatment Delivery Using the Clarity Ultrasound System in a Patient with Breast Cancer

Case Study

Ruth Heimann, MD, PhD, Daphne Hard, RT(R)(T), CMD, BS

Patient History

A 72-year-old woman presented with an abnormal left breast screening mammogram. Stereotactic core biopsy demonstrated an invasive ductal carcinoma that was moderately differentiated, estrogen receptor (ER)–positive, progesterone receptor (PR)–positive, and HER2/neu–negative. Following consultation in our Breast Multidisciplinary Clinic, the patient opted for breast conservation and underwent a local excision and sentinel lymph node biopsy. Pathology revealed a T1 moderately differentiated invasive ductal carcinoma. All margins of excision and two sentinel lymph nodes were negative. Metastatic workup consisted of chest x-ray and a complete metabolic panel, both of which were negative.

The patient was offered the option of accelerated partial breast radiation therapy (RT) on a clinical trial, or whole breast RT followed by an electron boost. She opted for the standard whole breast RT, delivered using an intensity-modulated RT approach. We elected to use the Clarity three-dimensional (3D) ultrasound (US) System (Resonant Medical, Montreal, Canada; Figure 18A-1) to assist both target delineation and treatment delivery during the electron boost phase of her treatment.

Simulation

A few days before start of the electron boost treatments, the patient was simulated for the boost using a dedicated computed tomography (CT) simulator (AcQsim, Philips Medical Systems, Andover, MA). It is important to initiate the treatment planning close in time to the actual start of the boost treatments because significant changes may occur over time in the geometry of the lumpectomy cavity.[1–3]

The patient was placed in the supine position with her arms above the head using a carbon fiber breast board (CIVCO Medical Solutions, Kalona, IA). A custom Vac-Lok (CIVCO Medical Solutions) was used for patient comfort and reproducibility. The Vac-Lok was indexed to the breast board, which was subsequently indexed to the CT couch top. The patient was set up to the simulation isocenter used for the whole breast treatment. The simulation isocenter is the basis for defining the image coordinates within the Clarity system. The radiation oncologist next outlined the estimated boost volume based on clinical palpation, scar location, and prior imaging. The clinically estimated field was traced with radio-opaque wires. Radio-opaque markers were also placed on the surgical

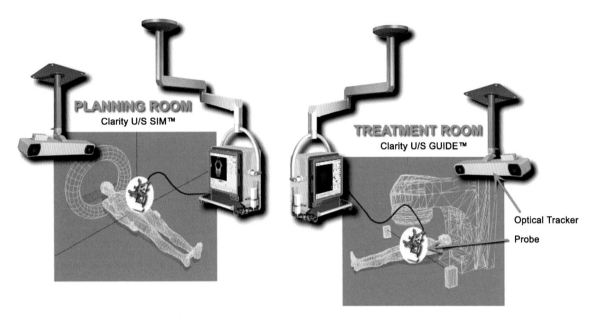

FIGURE 18A-1. The components of the three-dimensional Clarity ultrasound (US) system: planning—Clarity US Sim includes the linear probe tracked by the optical tracker registered to the simulation images acquired with the computed tomography scanner in the simulator; treatment—US Guide includes the linear probe, the optical tracker, and the workstation for the daily setup verification in the treatment room. (Courtesy of Resonant Medical Systems.)

incision and in close proximity to the nipple. Transaxial 3-mm images were obtained from the sternal notch to below the diaphragm. The cavity visibility and depth were determined from the CT scan.

Immediately following the CT simulation, the patient alignment with the lasers was again confirmed and 3D US images were acquired. A linear breast probe and high viscosity gel to assure minimal probe pressure were used. The Clarity US Sim system was designed such that the probe is being tracked with an optical tracker overhanging from the ceiling as seen in Figure 18A-1 and registers the US images to the isocenter and the CT scan. The patient was scanned throughout the entire surgical cavity and special attention was given to include the chest wall. The inclusion of the chest wall and skin were used to verify and optimize the quality of the US–CT fusion.

Imaging and Target Delineation

The Simulation CT and US Sim images were transferred to the Clarity and the treatment planning workstations (Pinnacle, Philips Medical Systems, Andover, MA). The US and CT data sets were automatically registered. Both the CT and US images were used for target delineation. The US Sim complements the CT, allows improved contouring, or delineation, and enhances the radiation oncologist's ability to define the target volumes.

In the Clarity system, the US cavity was defined as a reference positioning volume (RPV). This RPV is the image-guided radiotherapy (IGRT) reference volume and

is used during treatment to localize and find the displacement of the cavity from the planning simulation to the treatment times and to guide the therapists in repositioning the patient for treatment. The cavity clinical target volume (CTV) was defined by the radiation oncologist and it included the cavity defined on CT based on tissue density, clips, and the RPV defined on US. The CT, US, and fused US–CT images are shown in Figure 18A-2.

Treatment Planning

The electron boost planning target volume (PTV) was created by expanding the CTV by 8 mm, and was verified to include the surgical incision. A 3D treatment plan was designed consisting of an *enface* 9-MeV electron beam prescribed to the 90% isodose. The plan, structures, isocenter, beams, and block geometry were transferred to the Clarity workstation. The relationship between the block and the US volume (RPV) were again verified as well as prescription depths coverage of the entire volume in 3D as seen in Figure 18A-3. The RPV and cut out were approved and automatically sent to the US Guide workstation in the treatment room to be used for daily image-guided position verification.

Treatment Delivery

The patient was treated daily to the boost PTV volume. The US Guide system was used to verify the accurate targeting of the lumpectomy cavity from a real time beam's

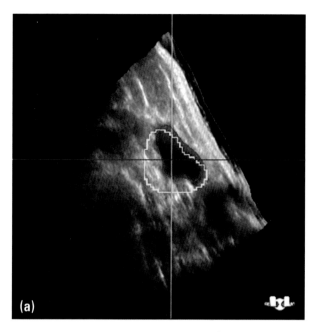

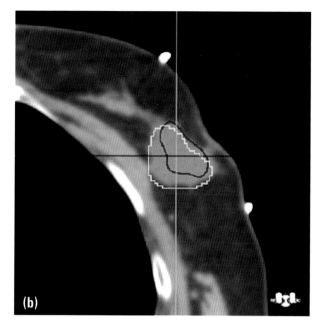

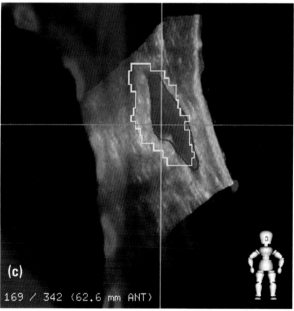

FIGURE 18A-2. The lumpectomy cavity outlined on **(a)** the three-dimensional (3D) ultrasound (US) images (red), **(b)** the treatment planning computed tomography (CT) scan (yellow), and **(c)** the fused 3D US–CT images. Note the good alignment of the chest wall in the fused image.

eye view, as well as depth (Figure 18A-3B and -3C). A daily 3D US was performed in the treatment room using an identical probe that was used at simulation, which was being tracked by the ceiling optical tracker in the treatment room (Figure 18A-1). The daily US images were compared with the reference US scan (RPV) done at simulation that was registered to the simulation CT. The position of the cavity was compared with the RPV and adjustments were made in the patient position to reproduce the simulated position and plan. Figure 18A-3B shows an example of a daily US with adequate match to the RPV, minimal displacement, adequate distance to block, and good coverage at depths over the entire volume, not needing any position adjustment. Figure 18A-3C shows a more substantial

displacement bringing the cavity too close to the block edge, therefore compromising the dosimetric coverage.

Clinical Outcome

The patient tolerated treatments well and completed them without interruptions and with minimal skin toxicity. She was without evidence of disease and had excellent cosmesis at 9 months of follow-up.

Our initial clinical experience using the Clarity 3D US system for optimizing tumor bed localization and treatment delivery was recently presented.[3] Thirty-seven patients with breast cancer underwent a set of two CT scans, one at simulation and one before their electron

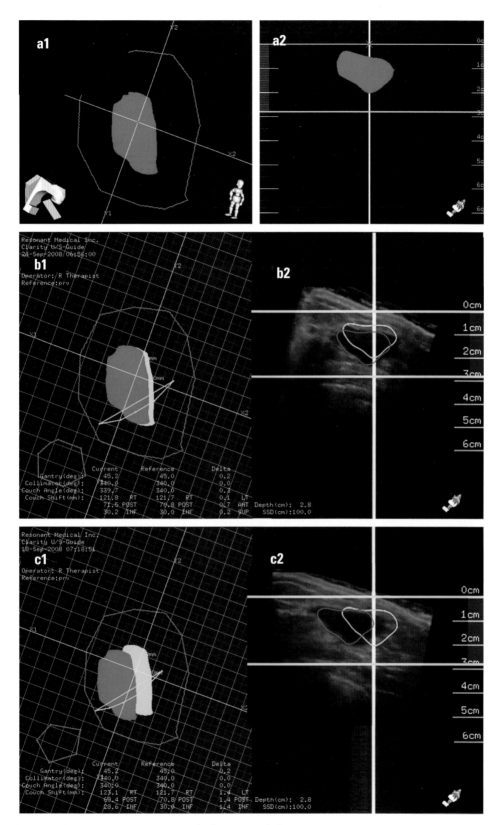

FIGURE 18A-3. Treatment planning and three-dimensional (3D) ultrasound (US)-guided treatment delivery of the electron boost treatments: **(a1)** reference position volume (RPV; red) in beam's eye view within block geometry (blue); **(a2)** RPV viewed in relation to prescription depth; **(b)** a daily 3D US (green) with minimum displacement compared with the RPV (red) not necessitating patient position adjustment (**b1** = beam's eye view; **b2** = depth verification); **(c)** a daily image showing a displacement compared with the RPV needing patient position adjustment (**c1** = beam's eye view; **c2** = depth verification). Nipple (purple) and lumpectomy scar (light blue) were also digitized.

boost. Each CT was immediately followed by a coregistered 3D US. The tumor bed was contoured independently on the CT and US, and compared to evaluate spatial and temporal differences. The patients were divided into two groups based on whether they received RT alone (Group A; n = 22 patents) or chemotherapy before RT (Group B; n = 15 patients).

The tumor bed was visible on either US or CT in 95% of Group A and 80% of Group B patients. Overall, US-defined tumor bed volumes were smaller than CT-defined volumes by an average of 30%. Group B tumor bed volumes were an average of 69% smaller than those in Group A. The difference in tumor bed volume displacements as detected by paired CT versus paired US for Group A were 0.7 mm, 1.0 mm, and 0.0 mm in the anterior–posterior (AP), left–right (LR), and superior–inferior (SI) directions, respectively, and 0.3 mm, 0.6 mm, and 1.2 mm for Group B. The displacements predicted by the two modalities were not significantly different within either Group A or Group B. We thus concluded that tumor bed volumes were well visualized throughout treatment for the major-

ity of patients, with or without chemotherapy. Moreover, clinically insignificant differences in the displacements calculated by paired CT versus paired US demonstrates the feasibility of using 3D US for day-to-day positioning in these patients.

References

1. Jacobson G, Betts V, Smith B. Change in volume of lumpectomy cavity during external-beam irradiation of the intact breast. *Int J Radiat Oncol Biol Phys.* 2006;65:1161–1164.
2. Oh KS, Kong FM, Griffith KA, et al. Planning the breast tumor bed boost: changes in the excision cavity volume and surgical scar location after breast-conserving surgery and whole-breast irradiation. *Int J Radiat Oncol Biol Phys.* 2006;66:680–686.
3. Wong P, Heimann R, Hard D, et al. A multi-institutional comparison study evaluating the use of 3D-ultrasound for defining the breast tumor bed for IGRT in chemotherapy versus non-chemotherapy patients. *Int J Radiat Oncol Biol Phys.* 2008;72:S179–S180.

MVCT-Guided Patient Setup Using the Helical Tomotherapy System in a Patient with Early Stage Breast Cancer

Case Study

Yi Rong, PhD, James S. Welsh, MS, MD

Patient History

A 65-year-old woman presented with a suspicious left breast nodule on a routine screening mammogram. An ultrasound-guided needle biopsy was performed, revealing sclerosing adenosis with extensive stromal sclerosis but further evaluation was recommended because of a moderate degree of suspicion for associated malignancy. A subsequent biopsy revealed low-grade adenosquamous carcinoma. The tumor size was 1 cm and surgical margins were negative but focally close. Because of the confirmation of malignancy and the close margins, a re-excision was performed along with sentinel lymph node biopsy. The re-excision revealed no residual carcinoma and, thus, the final pathological diagnosis was a stage T1BN0 adenosquamous carcinoma of the left breast.

Although systemic therapy was not thought warranted because adenosquamous carcinomas can behave locally aggressively, adjuvant whole breast radiotherapy (RT) was recommended. We elected to treat her with daily image-guided intensity-modulated RT with a simultaneous integrated boost using the Helical Tomotherapy system (Tomotherapy Inc, Madison, WI).

Simulation

The patient was immobilized in the supine position using VacLok immobilization devices (CIVCO, Kalona, IA) and simulated using a Philips Brilliance CT (Philips Medical Systems, Andover, MA). Transaxial imaging with a slice thickness of 3 mm was performed from a few slices above patient's clavicles to a few slices below her diaphragm (to include the level markers that were placed inferior to the diaphragm to avoid respiratory motion).

Treatment Planning

Two target volumes were contoured in this patient: a gross tumor volume (GTV) consisting of the lumpectomy cavity and the anatomical breast tissue as the clinical target volume (CTV). The GTV was expanded by 1 cm to yield a lumpectomy planning target volume (PTV). Organs at risk (OARs) in this patient included the contralateral breast, heart, lung(s), and spinal cord. The delineations of all structures are shown in Figure 18B-1.

To avoid overdosing OARs, such as lungs, heart, contralateral breast, and spinal cord, we formerly created a large dosimetric block covering the entire body except the involved breast and set it as a "directional" block in the "Sensitive Structure Constraints" module. However, this method not only adds extra work for the dosimetrist but also raises questions about how to properly design this block. If the block is drawn too close to the chest wall, dose coverage will be degraded for the involved breast, whereas if the block is too tight in the axillary and infra-axillary region, unwanted dose can be dumped into the ipsilateral lung, mediastinum, and heart.

We now set all the contoured OARs as directional blocks rather than attempting to create a large, ill-defined

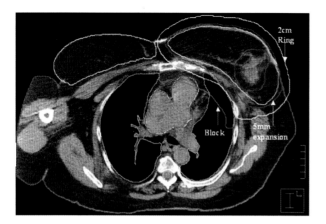

FIGURE 18B-1. Delineations of all structures including organs at risk (such as lumpectomy planning target volume (red), left breast (light orange), right breast (green), heart (pink), lungs (orange), and spinal cord (cyan) and three structures that were used to help with planning block (light blue), 5-mm expansion on the left breast (dark blue), and 2-cm ring (yellow).

dosimetric block. The dose distribution of the newer method appears to be at least equivalent to that of our prior approach, if not better. Additionally, we also draw a banana-shaped block along the interior aspect of the chest wall, as shown in Figure 18B-1, to further push the dose away from the lung and heart. Finally, we created a 2-cm ring around the 5-mm expansion of the intact breast to help confine the dose.

In this patient, a dose of 59.92 Gy was prescribed to the lumpectomy PTV and 50.4 Gy to the left breast in 28 fractions. The planning objectives included limiting the hot spot in the lumpectomy to be less than 105% for 95% PTV coverage, the 5% volume of the ipsilateral lung to no more than 30 Gy, and the maximum dose to the heart less than 25 Gy, even for this left-sided case. The pitch value was set to be 0.287 to minimize the thread artifact. A modulation factor of 2 and a field width of 2.5 cm were used to minimize the treatment delivery time while maintaining a highly conformal dose distribution.

The TomoTherapy planning system uses an adaptive convolution/superposition method and IMRT technique with 6-MV photon beams for every patient. It allows users to set one "hard constraint" in the "prescription" module for optimization and we normally set this to be the prescription dose given to 95% of a chosen PTV volume. In the presented example, the lumpectomy PTV was set to be the hard constraint (the one that is given the highest weight during optimization) instead of the whole breast PTV. Figures 18B-2 and 18B-3 show the dose–volume histogram (DVH) and isodose map from the final treatment plan. A uniform dose coverage for both the left breast and lumpectomy PTV was achieved as seen in the figures, with an acceptably low dose to the heart and lungs. The lumpectomy PTV received an average dose of 60.93 Gy with a minimum of 59.26 Gy and a maximum of 62.69 Gy (thus meeting the less-than-105% hotspot objective), while the left breast PTV received an average

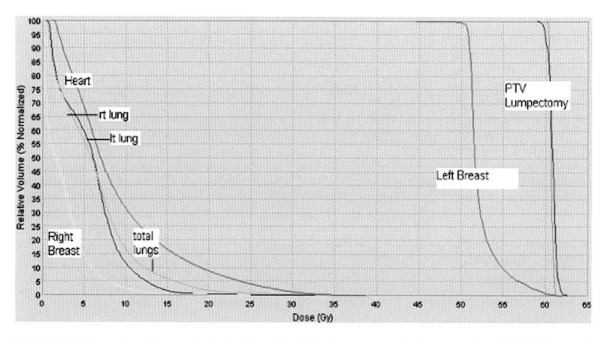

FIGURE 18B-2. Dose–volume histograms for treatment targets including the lumpectomy planning target volume (PTV), left breast, and avoided organs, such as heart, right breast, and lungs in a typical breast helical tomotherapy plan with hard constraint set at 95% volume of the lumpectomy PTV.

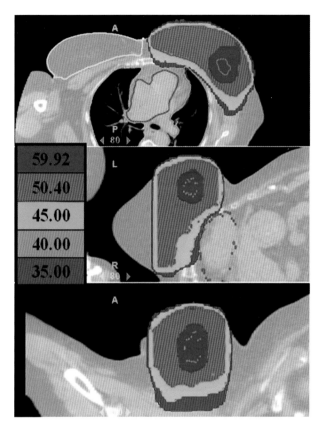

FIGURE 18B-3. Five isodose levels of 59.92 Gy (lumpectomy planning target volume [PTV] prescription), 50.4 Gy (left breast prescription), 45Gy, 40Gy, and 35Gy for a left breast tomotherapy plan with the hard constraint set to the lumpectomy PTV.

of 52.46 Gy with a $V_{110\%}$ = 8% (because the lumpectomy is directly enclosed within the breast) and a minimum of 44.79 Gy. In this plan, 5% of ipsilateral lung received 12.6 Gy and 5% of heart volume received 23.5 Gy. The maximum dose to the heart was 38 Gy, and only 5% of the contralateral breast received a maximum of 7.6 Gy. Detailed information of dose distribution is shown in Table 18B-1.

TABLE 18B–1 Plan Quality for a Left-Sided Whole Breast Irradiation with a Simultaneous In-Field Boost

Index	Dose
Lumpectomy PTV volume receiving 105% of PD	0%
Lumpectomy PTV volume receiving 95% of PD	100%
% Dose received by 95% of lumpectomy PTV	59.98 Gy
Index breast volume receiving 110% of PD	8%
Index breast volume receiving 95% of PD	99.9%
Dose received by 95% of index breast	50.8 Gy
Dose received by 5% of ipsilateral lung	12.6 Gy
Dose received by 5% of heart	23.5 Gy
Max dose to heart	38 Gy
Dose received by 5% of contralateral breast	7.6 Gy

Notes. PD = prescription dose (PD = 59.92 Gy for lumpectomy PTV and PD = 50.4 Gy for the index breast); PTV = planning target volume.

Treatment Delivery

Quality assurance (QA) was performed by a physicist before bringing the patient into the vault for treatment to ensure that the actual treatment would be within +3% of what was planned. On the day of treatment, the patient was positioned on the treatment couch in her customized immobilization device. A megavoltage computed tomography (MVCT) image was then obtained with a 4-MV fan beam rather than the 6-MV beam used for treatment. This process takes approximately 90 to 120 seconds. The MVCT images were then superimposed onto the simulation kilovoltage CT (kVCT) images with the corresponding contours. The lumpectomy cavity, from both image sets, was used to guide patient positioning. Limited field of view imaging can reduce MVCT time and is routinely employed in patients for whom the setup is not especially challenging (which represent the vast majority). However, in this patient, a full view scan was utilized.

Initially we had concerns about respiratory motion but early in our experience we realized that the MVCT is spread out over several breaths, thereby providing a "smeared-out" image representing a free-breathing CT, an observation similar to what has been described for lung tomotherapy. Because we have observed that these MVCT images match up very well with the kVCT simulation images and contours (as shown in Figure 18B-4), we are now more confident that respiratory motion is not as problematic as we initially feared.

The time for an individual treatment fraction duration was 372.6 seconds. The overall treatment time including setup, MVCT, readjustment, and treatment was typically less than 20 minutes.

Clinical Outcome

This presented patient, as with the majority of patients treated in this fashion, had relatively mild skin reactions. In our experience with approximately 200 breast cancer patients, we have observed that this skin reaction is generally less intense than what was previously seen with tangent fields, perhaps because of the improved dose homogeneity. There is especially less moist desquamation in the inframammary fold and axilla. To date, with a median follow-up of about 2 years and some patients out over 3 years, no patients have had any late sequelae or unusual cosmetic effects. Cosmesis is generally excellent but of course depends most on the quality of the surgical intervention. None of the patients have recurred locally in this brief interval. Subjectively, the reduction in course length by about a week seems to benefit the patients in terms of fatigue.

We have presented our initial observations with hypofractionated breast and chest wall irradiation using simultaneous in-field boost intensity-modulated RT delivered

kVCT	MVCT	Fusion

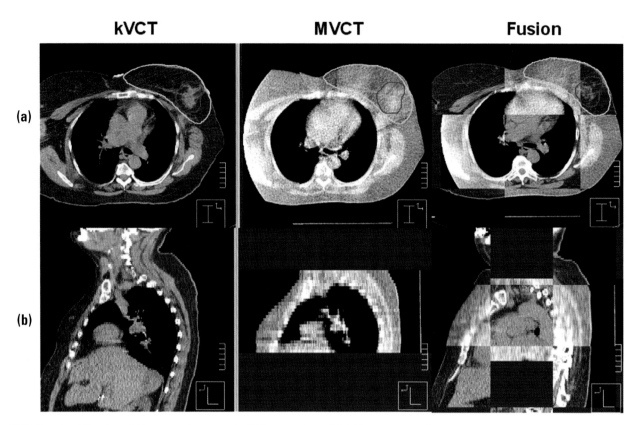

FIGURE 18B-4. Kilovoltage (kV) computed tomography (CT), megavoltage (MV) CT, and kV–MV CT fusion images for left breast and lungs in (a) transverse and (b) sagittal views.

with the Tomotherapy system.[1] We have found that excellent dose distributions can be achieved with this approach through a careful selection of treatment planning parameters. Dose homogeneity to the whole breast and simultaneously targeted lumpectomy region appears superior to conventional "tangents" with minimal hot or cold spots. Dose–volume histogram analysis reveals effective reduction of high dose to surrounding OARs, although a greater volume of these nontarget organs receive low dose compared with what is typical with tangent beams. Pretreatment MVCT imaging has proven invaluable in aiding setup and engenders greater confidence that the planned IMRT dose distributions are truly being delivered.

In some situations, MVCT can provide visual feedback when a seroma or overall breast volume has changed since simulation, thereby identifying cases where replanning might be indicated. Treatment is brief, typically requiring 6 to 9 minutes. Further refinements of this technique and formal prospective clinical evaluation are underway.

Reference

1. Rong Y, Fahner T, Welsh JS. Hypofractionated breast and chest wall irradiation using simultaneous in-field boost IMRT delivered via helical tomotherapy. *Technol Cancer Res Treat.* 2008;7:433–439.

KV CBCT-Guided Treatment Delivery Using the Elekta Synergy System in a Patient with Breast Cancer

Case Study

Leonard Kim, MS, A. Mus. D, Yasmin Hasan, MD

Patient History

A 76-year-old woman underwent routine screening mammography, which demonstrated an irregular, spiculated mass with associated heterogeneous calcifications at the four o'clock position in the anterior right breast. Needle-localized, excisional biopsy was performed revealing grade 2 invasive ductal carcinoma with associated high-grade ductal carcinoma in situ. The cancer measured 0.9 cm, and margins were positive. No angiolymphatic invasion was noted. The tumor was estrogen receptor– and progesterone receptor–positive. Staging radiographic studies included a chest x-ray and a bone scan, which were both negative for metastatic disease.

The patient then underwent right partial mastectomy and sentinel lymph node biopsy. No residual carcinoma was noted in the partial mastectomy specimen, and the sentinel lymph node evaluation revealed no regional disease. The patient's breast cancer was thus Stage I (T1bN0M0) and, as she elected to pursue breast-conserving therapy, adjuvant irradiation to the breast was recommended to reduce the risk of recurrence.

During her radiation oncology consultation, adjuvant radiation therapy (RT) options were thoroughly discussed including standard whole breast irradiation for approximately 6 and a half weeks, hypofractionated regimens of approximately 3 weeks, and accelerated partial breast irradiation (APBI) including the NSABP B-39 trial for which she would have been eligible. The patient declined the NSABP study and, because of logistical constraints, she was offered APBI off-protocol. The patient was informed that technical and anatomical parameters evaluated with computed tomography (CT) simulation would determine her candidacy for APBI and which type of APBI would be most suitable (intracavitary brachytherapy, interstitial brachytherapy, or external beam).

An initial planning CT was acquired 29 days after surgery, at which time an alpha cradle (Smithers Medical Products, North Canton, OH) was fabricated for immobilization. On the basis of this CT, the patient was determined to be eligible for external beam APBI. We elected to treat her with kilovoltage (kV) cone beam CT (CBCT) image guidance using the Synergy (Elekta, Stockholm, Sweden).

Simulation

Five days before treatment, a Brilliance Big Bore CT simulator (Philips Medical Systems, Andover, MA) was used to guide placement of a midline setup point and determine the lateral shift from this point to the treatment isocenter. Three days before treatment, the patient underwent a portal imaging and CBCT session on the treatment machine. Because of the size of the patient and lateral target position, it was impossible to acquire a CBCT of the patient in treatment position while also allowing the couch rotations called for by the treatment plan. To acquire the CBCT without collision, the couch would have to have been approximately centered in the lateral dimension, whereas to deliver treatment without collision, the couch needed to be positioned laterally. It was therefore decided that localization CBCT scans would not be acquired in the treatment position. It was found that CBCTs could be consistently acquired when the couch was 10 cm medial of its final treatment position, so that position was established for image acquisition.

An additional CT was acquired on the first day of treatment, 54 days after surgery and 25 days after the initial planning CT. The latter CT showed the seroma volume had shrunk from 81 cc in the initial CT to 28 cc. There was also a volume reduction of the whole breast of approximately 4% between the two CTs. Because of the observed change in seroma volume, it was decided that automatic, gray-scale–based registration of the seroma was inappropriate for image guidance. Also, because the seroma in the latter CT was difficult to visualize in places (Figure 18C-1) and had changed asymmetrically relative to the clinical target volume (CTV) and surrounding anatomy (Figure 18C-2), manual localization of the seroma was similarly rejected. The whole breast, including the chest wall and skin surface, was thus chosen as the reference structure for localization. It should be noted that posttreatment analysis showed our fears to be overstated and that manual registration of the seroma would have in fact produced excellent CTV localization.

Treatment Planning

The physician's contour of the seroma was expanded by 15 mm and then trimmed 5 mm away from the skin surface to generate the CTV. The CTV was expanded in three dimensions (3D) by 10 mm to generate the planning target volume (PTV). A 3D conformal treatment plan using four non-coplanar, 6-MV beams with couch rotations of

up to 30° was generated. A total dose of 3850 cGy in 10 twice-daily fractions (385 cGy/fraction) was prescribed to the PTV.

Treatment Delivery

Imaging, reconstruction, and registration were performed by using an Elekta Synergy with the XVI software. The patient was laser-localized to the setup point, and the couch was moved laterally to a position 10-cm medial of the presumed isocenter. In this position, a CBCT was acquired using a 200° arc, which is sufficient for image reconstruction of a small field-of-view scan. Because the seroma was not being directly localized, but rather larger structures such the breast surface and chest wall, a comparatively low-dose technique was used: 120 kV, 40 mA, 10 milliseconds per frame. The bowtie filter was not used, and images were reconstructed at medium resolution.

Because of the 10-cm gap between them, the planning and CBCT images were first approximately registered manually. Automatic gray-scale–based registration of the whole breast then followed. This registration was checked, particularly at the skin surface, which had appeared stable relative to the CTV in CT images (Figures 18C-1 and 18C-2), and was adjusted as needed. The resulting couch move, comprising the remaining 10-cm lateral shift as well as actual setup error correction, was applied. The couch was rotated, and the treatment was delivered.

Posttreatment analysis of the CBCT images showed a systematic setup error of nearly 2 cm posteriorly before correction. Without online image guidance, the percentage of CTV receiving 90% of the prescription dose would have been 8% less than planned.

After the patient had completed treatment, in-house, gray-scale–based, deformable registration software was

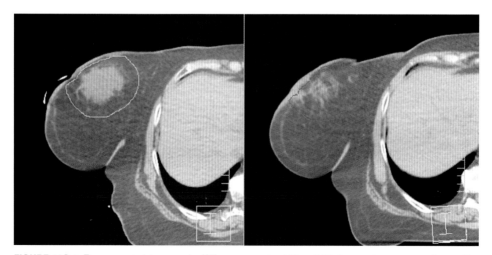

FIGURE 18C-1. Two computed tomography (CT) scans acquired 29 and 54 days postsurgery are shown. The earlier CT was used for planning, and the latter CT was acquired on the first day of treatment. The near-disappearance of the seroma in the later CT renders it difficult for use in image guidance.

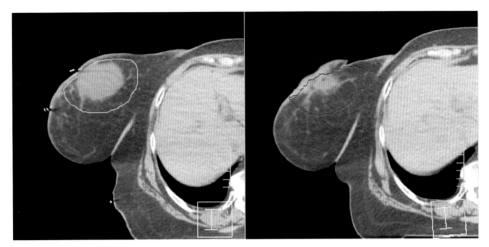

FIGURE 18C-2. A different slice of the same computed tomography (CT) scan. Here the seroma is visible in the latter CT, but its asymmetric shrinkage should be taken into account during image guidance. In addition, deformable registration shows that, despite the dramatic change in the seroma, the CTV remains comparatively stable.

used to assess whether the seroma shrinkage observed in the latter CT would have significantly affected the original, planned CTV. Despite the change in the seroma, the extent of the CTV was seen to be relatively unaffected (Figures 18C-1 and 18C-2). It would thus have been inappropriate to modify the treatment plan to irradiate a smaller volume on the basis of the observed seroma shrinkage.[1,2]

Clinical Outcome

Treatment was well-tolerated, and the patient experienced only minimal tenderness and edema in the lower–inner aspect of the right breast toward the end of the 5-day treatment course as was expected. She reported no fatigue, symptoms of infection, or other acute toxicity. The patient was seen most recently in follow-up 15 months posttreatment and had no clinical or mammographic evidence of disease recurrence. She did have some mild hyperpigmentation in the treated region of the right breast but no pain, edema, necrosis, induration, symptomatic seroma, volume reduction, or telangiectasia. Her cosmetic outcome was rated as good. The patient continues to receive antiestrogen therapy under the care of her medical oncologist.

References

1. Kim L, Vicini F, Yan D. What do recent studies on lumpectomy cavity volume change imply for breast clinical target volumes? [editorial]. *Int J Radiat Oncol Biol Phys.* 2008;72:1–3.
2. Kim L, DeCesare S, Vicini F, Yan D. Effect of lumpectomy cavity volume change on the clinical target volume for accelerated partial breast irradiation: a deformable registration study. *Int J Radiat Oncol Biol Phys.* 2010;78:1121–1126.

Video-Guided Patient Positioning and Localization Using the AlignRT System in a Patient with Breast Cancer

Case Study

Douglas A. Miller, MD, Eric E. Klein, PhD

Patient History

A 35-year-old G_1P_1 premenopausal woman presented with a nonpalpable 12-mm spiculated mass with adjacent microcalcifications in the lower outer quadrant of her left breast on a routine screening mammogram. Needle core biopsy was positive for malignancy. The patient subsequently underwent a lumpectomy and sentinel node biopsy. Pathology revealed a 9-mm infiltrating ductal carcinoma, histological grade 2, estrogen- and progesterone-receptor–positive. Surgical margins were all negative. Two sentinel lymph nodes were also negative for malignancy. Preoperative computed tomography (CT) scans of the chest, abdomen, and pelvis, along with a bone scan, were negative for metastatic disease. The pathologic stage for this patient's breast cancer was thus T1bN0M0, stage I.

Postoperatively, the patient received four cycles of adjuvant docetaxel and cyclophosphamide, to be followed by 5 years of tamoxifen. Whole breast irradiation, along with a boost to the lumpectomy cavity, was recommended following her chemotherapy to decrease her risk of local recurrence. We elected to use the AlignRT system (VisionRT, London, UK) to aid in both patient setup and breast localization during her treatment.

Simulation

The patient underwent a multislice computed tomography (CT) simulation using the Big-Bore (85-cm) scanner (Philips Medical Systems, Andover, MA). Before scanning, a custom solid foam immobilization form (alpha cradle; Smithers Medical Products, North Canton, OH)

was created with the patient in the treatment position. The cradle contains a strategic elevation (built within) to level the sternum parallel to the table. The patient was positioned supine, with both arms elevated above the head and neck slightly extended. At our center, wooden hand-grips are incorporated into the cradle for position reproducibility, unless patient discomfort limits comfortable arm extension. In this case, a left hand grip was not used (Figure 18D-1A). The clinically defined breast volume, including superior, medial, lateral, and inferior port edges were defined by the physician, including identification of the lumpectomy incision. A 3-cm radial margin was marked around the lumpectomy incision to serve as the initial reference for the lumpectomy cavity boost volume (Figure 18D-1B, -1C) Transaxial imaging with a slice thickness of 3 mm was performed from the base of skull to 4 cm below the inferior port edge. No intravenous or oral contrast was used. Of note, the AlignRT system is not installed in the CT simulator room. The nominal images for daily localization are extracted from the CT-acquired external contours, as detailed in the following sections.

Treatment Planning

The planning CT images were transferred to our Pinnacle workstation (Philips Medical Systems, Andover, MA) for contouring. Normal structures, including the external skin surface, left and right lungs, heart, and spinal cord, were contoured by dosimetry staff for calculation of dose–volume histogram (DVH) statistics. The external contour is specifically used for daily localization with

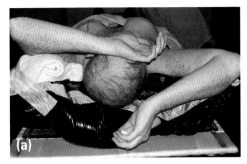 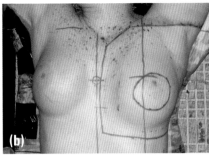 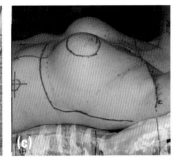

FIGURE 18D-1. (a) Cranial–caudal view of patient arm positioning. Hand grips are used for reproducibility according to patient comfort. (b) Anterior view of patient setup for whole breast radiation therapy. Please note medial, superior, and inferior port borders. The boost volume is delineated on the left breast by the innermost contour. (c) Lateral view of patient setup for whole breast radiation therapy. The lateral port edge typically follows the mid- or posterior axillary line to cover the lateral breast and axillary tail.

AlignRT. The lumpectomy cavity, including any internal surgical clips, was contoured by the treating physician to determine the most appropriate *en face* electron energy and prescription depth-dose for the boost treatment.

Medial and lateral tangential fields were designed according to target volumes determined at the time of simulation. For this patient, the medial and lateral tangential fields used 9° table rotations and 5° collimator rotations to achieve a nondivergent superior field border. The field dimensions were 14.5 cm by 24.5 cm and 14.2 cm by 23.5 cm for the medial and lateral tangents, respectively, and nearly "beam-split" along the chest wall. Each tangential beam used an optimized field-in-field technique with five control points to compensate for breast tissue density and reduce the breast apex hot spot. The prescription for the tangential fields was 46 Gy in 2-Gy fractions, using equally weighted 6-MV photons with no bolus. The dose was prescribed to a specified weight point anterior to the central axis at middepth. The boost field was designed to cover the cavity volume. The boost prescription was 14 Gy in 2-Gy fractions using a single *en face* 9-MeV electron beam, prescribed to the 90% depth dose (2.1 cm).

The completed plan, after physician review and approval, was exported to our record and verify system for delivery on an Precise linear accelerator (Elekta AB, Stockholm, Sweden; Figure 18D-2). Before treatment

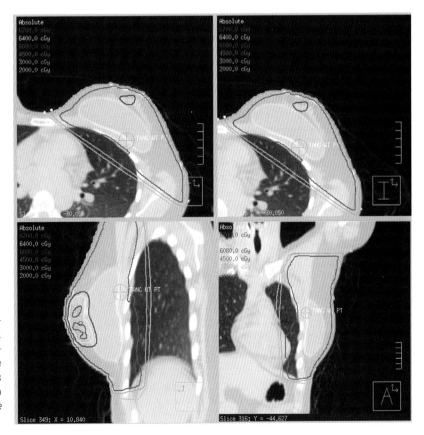

FIGURE 18D-2. Treatment plan with isodose levels in the axial (top panels), coronal (bottom left), and sagittal planes (bottom right). The prescription was 46 Gy delivered in 2-Gy fractions to the entire breast using medial and lateral tangents followed by a 16 Gy boost in 2-Gy fractions to the lumpectomy cavity delivered with *en face* electrons.

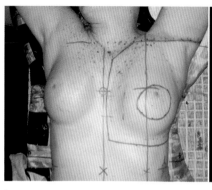 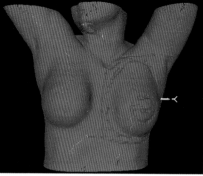 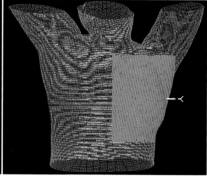

FIGURE 18D-3. Region of interest defined on AlignRT. The clinician-defined whole breast volume (left panel) is transferred from the treatment planning system as an external surface contour to the AlignRT system via the Digital Imaging and Communications in Medicine (DICOM) protocol (center panel), where the target region of interest is defined using AlignRT for patient positioning (right panel).

delivery, megavoltage portal images were taken using the treatment field parameters and compared with the treatment planning generated digital reconstructed radiographs for accuracy. The electron boost was verified directly using a light field for accuracy and compared with the treatment planning generated digital composite radiograph.

In preparation for use of the AlignRT system (version 4.0.268), the external body surface contour was exported by the treatment planning software via the Digital Imaging and Communications in Medicine (DICOM) protocol to the AlignRT software to generate a reference surface topogram. The clinician-defined region of interest, the entire breast volume with an appropriate margin (Figure 18D-3), was recorded to serve as the reference structure for alignment and assessment of daily patient positioning.

Treatment Delivery

Patient positioning was verified using several techniques. Daily patient setup, performed using laser-guided superficial skin fiducials and the AlignRT system, was supplemented by weekly portal imaging. Once the patient was placed in the alpha cradle according to simulation specifications, the isocenter was verified using anterior–posterior (AP) and lateral skin fiducials, and the source-to-skin distance was affirmed. The patient was then ready for positioning with the AlignRT system.

AlignRT is a stereoscopic system that acquires video images to capture the dynamic surfaces of the subject's skin and reconstruct the surface using proprietary software. The system uses two ceiling-mounted pods, each pod with two 3D cameras, to reconstruct a surface image acquired from the projection of 10,000 to 20,000 3D points spanning a volume of 650 mm (across couch) by 1000 mm (along couch) by 350 mm (vertically). The cameras can take single-frame images or perform con-

tinuous data acquisition (7.5 frames/sec) for monitoring. The three-dimensional matching software aligns a daily image with the reference and calculates the couch shifts to correct the patient's position. The patient's reference topogram is recalled using the AlignRT software, and a new treatment topogram is captured using the 3D cameras, which project a bright speckle pattern across the patient for several seconds. The acquired topogram is generated and compared with the reference topogram using the system's software to produce three planar translations required for precise reproduction of the patient's expected position (Figure 18D-4). We chose not to include table angulation in this process. All orthogonal shifts (in millimeters) were applied to this patient, and a second image acquisition and analysis using AlignRT was performed for verification. The entire process took less than 3 minutes, and was repeated if necessary until the suggested shifts were less than 5 mm in any one plane. As an added benefit, the AlignRT software was used to calculate the volume of tissue within a specified distance from the reference topogram and to localize regions of the breast that deviate beyond this threshold (Figure 18D-5).

With the patient's position verified using daily external surface fiducials and AlignRT (in addition to weekly portal imaging), treatment specific couch rotations to the treatment isocenter were applied according to the treatment plan specification for each field.

Clinical Outcome

The patient tolerated her treatment without any significant acute toxicity. She developed confluent erythema of the breast which was managed with topical emollients and quickly resolved following therapy. No supplemental pain medication was required. The patient is scheduled to return to our clinic in 6 weeks for a posttreatment evaluation. She will soon start tamoxifen and undergo her first posttreatment bilateral mammogram.

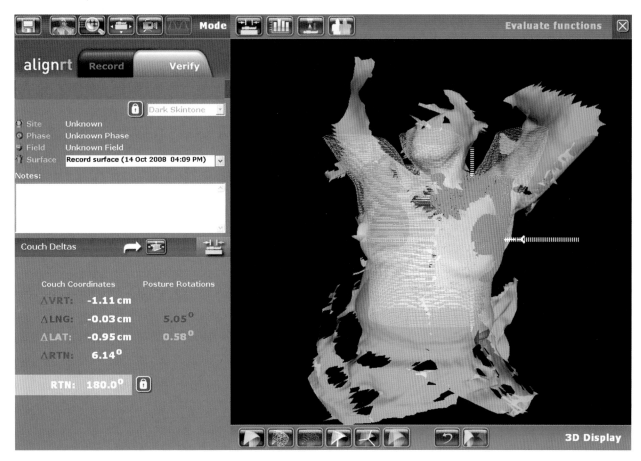

FIGURE 18D-4. The reference topogram (pink) with clinician-defined region of interest is compared with the acquired treatment topogram (green). The data sets are analyzed using the AlignRT software to calculate couch shifts required to reproduce expected patient position.

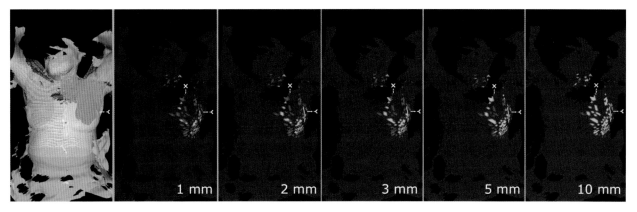

FIGURE 18D-5. Breast position varies between treatments. AlignRT localizes regions of the breast that deviate beyond a user-defined threshold compared with the initial reference topogram. From left to right, the location of breast position above (red), below (blue), and within (green) a specified threshold for variation between topograms of 1 mm, 2 mm, 3 mm, 5 mm, and 10 mm. For this treatment, the majority of breast tissue fell within 10 mm from the initial reference, with the greatest breast position deviation localized to the upper-inner quadrant.

KV CT-Guided Radiotherapy Using the Siemens CT-on-Rails System in a Patient with Early Stage Breast Cancer

Case Study

Natalya V. Morrow, PhD, Julia White, MD, X. Allen Li, PhD

Patient History

A 57-year-old woman presented with an abnormal finding in the right breast on a routine screening mammogram. Ultrasound (US)-guided core biopsy was performed and confirmed the presence of estrogen receptor–positive, progesterone receptor–negative, human epidermal growth factor 2–negative invasive tubular carcinoma. The patient underwent breast conservation surgery with an excision of an approximately 1-cm mass with a negative margin. Additionally, the sentinel axillary lymph nodes were negative.

The patient was discussed at our multidisciplinary breast oncology conference and the recommendation was for four cycles of adriamycin and cyclophosphamide followed by radiotherapy (RT). We elected to treat her with image-guided whole breast RT using the Siemens computed tomography (CT)-on-Rails System (CTVision, Siemens AG, Erlangen, Germany).

Simulation

On the day of simulation, the patient was placed on an in-house–designed prone breast board with the arms stabilized in an alpha cradle (Smithers Medical Products, North Canton, OH; Figure 18E-1). She was positioned prone with the contralateral breast situated away from the possible treatment angles to limit the exposure. The ipsilateral breast was allowed to hang away from the body through an opening in the Plexiglas support. A helical scan in the treatment position from T1 to L4 was obtained by using a large-bore LightSpeed CT scanner (GE Healthcare, Waukesha, WI).

Treatment Planning

The planning CT data set was transferred to the XiO treatment planning system (Elekta-CMS, Maryland Heights, MO). Contours of the breast, lumpectomy, and lung were delineated on individual CT slices. The whole right breast was planned with three-dimensional conformal RT using medial and lateral tangent fields at gantry angles of 70° and 257°, respectively. Appropriate multileaf collimator shaping was used to achieve dose homogeneity and normal tissue sparing. The dose to the isocenter was 50 Gy delivered over 25 fractions in 2-Gy fractions, providing a dose of 47.5 Gy to 95% of the targeted breast volume. The whole breast treatment was then followed by a boost to the planning target volume (PTV; i.e., the lumpectomy cavity plus 1.5-cm margin for microscopic diseases and an additional 1.0 cm margin for setup uncertainty) for a total dose to the isocenter of 62 Gy. The approved plan was transferred to the Lantis record-and-verify software (Siemens AG, Erlangen, Germany) and treatment console. The CT images and isocenter location information were exported to a software package for the registration with daily treatment CT (Adaptive Targeting, Siemens AG, Erlangen, Germany). Anterior–posterior (AP) and right lateral digitally reconstructed radiographs (DRRs) were generated for patient setup verification.

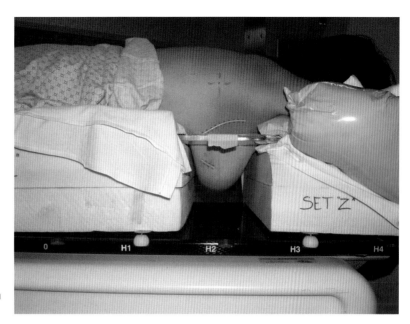

FIGURE 18E-1. Patient setup in prone position with the ipsilateral breast hanging away from the body.

Treatment Delivery

In the treatment room, the patient was placed in the prone position based on the setup points from simulation. During the boost stage, CT-based image guidance was performed for five consecutive fractions as part of an in-house study that enrolls patients with prone breast irradiation to be treated on a linac (Primus, Siemens AG, Erlangen, Germany) and CT-on-Rails combination. While on the linac couch, three BBs were placed to identify the

isocenter on the CT scan. The treatment table was then rotated 180° and the patient was scanned by the fan-beam kilovoltage (kV) CT. The daily CT was first automatically registered based on bony anatomy with the treatment planning CT. Then the registration was adjusted manually to achieve alignment of the surgical cavity (or at least three surgical clips) with the planning CT and inclusion of all clips in the boost PTV (Figure 18E-2). The table was returned to the treatment position, and the patient

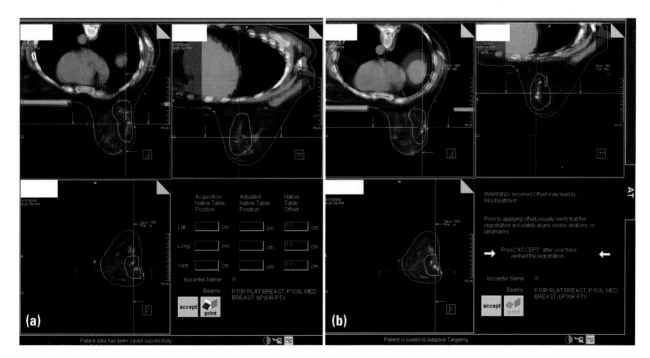

FIGURE 18E-2. The registration reflecting original setup to the BBs (a) and the final manual registration to optimize target volume coverage (b). Treatment computed tomography (CT): gray-scale layer; planning CT: orange layer and the contours.

setup to the original isocenter. The patient was then repositioned based on the shifts determined from the registration of the treatment and planning CTs using the Adaptive Targeting software package prior to the delivery of the planned treatment.

To verify the CT-based repositioning and to compare with the conventional setup method based on two-dimensional (2D) images, orthogonal portal images were taken before and after the CT-based repositioning. The treatment isocenter was delineated on the 2D images by the tungsten rod tray inserted during imaging. The 2D images were subsequently aligned with DRRs based on the chest wall and the breast external contour (Figure 18E-3). The difference between the planning isocenter (from DRRs) and the treatment isocenter (from the portal images) were noted in vertical and longitudinal directions. The shifts determined from the 2D portal images were strongly correlated to the respective shifts determined from the daily CT registration (correlation coefficient of 0.8 and 1.0 for vertical and longitudinal directions, respectively; see Figure 18E-4).

The CT showed that the soft breast tissue can be easily distorted and this distortion can affect the position of clips and the lumpectomy cavity. It is necessary to perform a manual registration based on soft tissue agreement to achieve good coverage and the alignment based solely on the positions of clips may not be adequate. Reflecting the difficult nature in the breast treatment setup,

rotation of the torso as well as rotation and distortion of the soft breast tissue can be easily seen in the daily CT images and can be corrected if necessary (Figures 18E-2 and 18E-3a) by repositioning or replanning the patient. The CT provides a distinct advantage over the 2D portal images in visualizing these rotations and distortions. In addition, the diagnostic image quality of the fan beam CT allowed us to clearly visualize the seroma and clips that are usually not visible with the 2D images.

Clinical Outcome

The patient tolerated treatment well without significant acute sequelae. She was most recently seen approximately 11 months posttreatment and at that time remained without evidence of recurrence or significant late sequelae.

Preliminary results of our in-house study (described in the "Treatment Delivery" section and which included this patient) were recently presented.[1] To date, four patients undergoing prone breast irradiation have been enrolled. Computed tomography imaging was acquired for five consecutive fractions. As noted previously, rotation of the torso as well as rotation and distortion of the soft breast tissue were easily seen in the CT images. The magnitude of shifts determined based on CT registration varied between patients, with the smallest average shift of 0 mm ± 3 mm and the largest of -18 mm ± 3 mm. The shifts determined from CT registration and from portal images

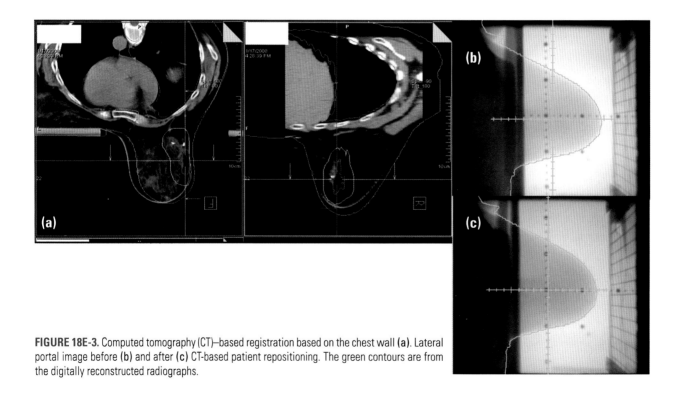

FIGURE 18E-3. Computed tomography (CT)–based registration based on the chest wall (a). Lateral portal image before (b) and after (c) CT-based patient repositioning. The green contours are from the digitally reconstructed radiographs.

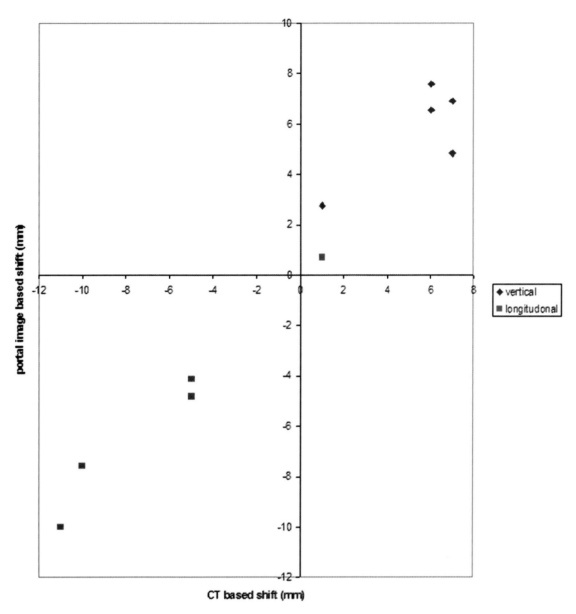

FIGURE 18E-4. Comparison between shifts obtained from registration of two-dimensional portal images with digitally reconstructed radiographs and daily three-dimensional computed tomography (CT) with planning CT. Correlation coefficients of 0.8 and 1.0 were obtained for the vertical and longitudinal directions, respectively.

were strongly correlated. The clips within the lumpectomy site were not identifiable on portal imaging and could not serve as surrogates for cavity identification. The large patient variability and the interfractional variability support the use of 3D image guidance for accurate and reproducible treatment delivery in prone breast treatment.

Reference

1. Morrow NV, White J, Rownd JJ, et al. IGRT with CT-on-Rails for prone breast irradiation. *Int J Radiat Oncol Biol Phys.* 2008; 72:S522.

Chapter 19

GASTROINTESTINAL TUMORS: OVERVIEW

MARY FENG, MD, ALBERT C. KOONG, MD, PhD, EDGAR BEN-JOSEF, MD

Image-guided radiation therapy (IGRT) has an important and growing role in the planning and treatment of gastrointestinal (GI) tumors. Advanced imaging techniques, including positron emission tomography (PET) and magnetic resonance (MR) imaging, have been increasingly applied to radiation therapy (RT) planning in a variety of GI tumors, including esophageal,[1,2] rectal,[3] and anal[4,5] carcinomas. Moreover, multiple in-room IGRT technologies have been explored in the treatment of these tumors.[6,7]

In this chapter, IGRT approaches for optimizing both target delineation and treatment delivery are highlighted in two important GI tumor sites, namely the pancreas and liver. Image-guided RT applications in other tumor sites are illustrated in the accompanying case studies.

Image-Guided Target Delineation

Accurate definition of the gross tumor volume (GTV) for pancreatic and liver tumors is essential for optimal RT planning. Accurate measurement of tumor volume is also essential in assessing response to treatment. The various imaging modalities used are reviewed in this chapter, including computed tomography (CT), MR, and PET, as well as the appropriate margins needed to encompass surrounding microscopic disease.

Pancreas Tumors: Defining the GTV

A dual-phase thin-section helical CT scan performed after administration of intravenous and oral contrast is the optimal technique used for detecting and staging pancreatic cancer. Following intravenous contrast administration, scans are obtained in the pancreatic phase and portal venous phase. The pancreatic parenchymal phase is ideal for detection of pancreatic cancer because of its superior tumor-to-parenchymal contrast difference and is also essential for evaluation of adjacent arterial involvement to determine resectability.[8] The portal venous phase is essential to evaluate the liver for metastases, which would be most evident on this phase, and also to assess for adjacent venous encasement, occlusion, or thrombosis.[9] Multiplanar and three-dimensional (3D) reconstructed images are useful in determining the extent of pancreatic cancer, vascular encasement, and ductal obstruction.

Pancreatic cancer is most commonly seen as a hypoattenuating mass in the pancreas showing less enhancement than the normal adjacent pancreatic parenchyma. In approximately 10% of cases, pancreatic cancer is isoattenuating on CT scan and detection of tumor in these cases is based on indirect signs such as bile duct or pancreatic duct obstruction or deformity of pancreatic contour.[10] The sensitivity of multidetector CT in the detection of pancreatic cancer varies from 76% to 92%, with lesser sensitivities reported for tumors 2 cm or smaller and with older-generation scanners.[11–13]

Accurate measurement of tumor size on CT is difficult mainly because of the infiltrative growth pattern of pancreatic cancer, raising the possibility that the measured hypodense tumor seen on CT could underestimate the true tumor size. On the other hand, tumor size could also be overestimated on CT because of inclusion of the adjacent desmoplastic reaction induced by the tumor and any resulting inflammation around the tumor secondary to pancreatitis induced by ductal obstruction.[14,15] With these limitations, it is surprising to note the relatively good correlation reported between tumor size on pathological examination and on CT.[14–16] Ballard et al. compared CT tumor size with measurements on pathological specimens in 29 patients.[16] In this study from 1995, only a minority received intravenous contrast, and sections were obtained at (relatively large) 5-mm to 10-mm intervals. In tumors 2 cm to 5 cm in size, 86% of the radiographic estimates were within 1 cm of the correct size and the correlation factor was $R^2 = 0.87$. Computed tomography overestimated all smaller tumors by at least 1.5 cm to 2 cm, and underestimated the larger ones by 2.5 cm. Underestimation occurred in two diffuse mucinous tumors that involved the entire length of the pancreas. Furukawa et al.[14] found good correlation ($R^2 = 0.65$) between tumor size on dynamic CT and histopathological examination. However, a greater discrepancy in measurement was noted in larger tumors (> 4 cm). The pancreatic parenchymal phase should be used for delineation of gross tumor volume (GTV) as the correlation of image size with resected specimens size is highest in this phase compared with the precontrast or portal venous phase.[15] If there are any changes of pancreatitis associated with pancreatic cancer because of ductal obstruction, a follow-up CT scan after resolution of inflammatory changes, if the clinical situation permits such delay, can help better delineate the GTV.

Multiphase contrast-enhanced MR has been reported to be at least equivalent or even superior to dual-phase helical CT for detection of pancreatic cancer.[13,17] The sequences that are most helpful are the T1-weighted fat-suppressed, and gadolinium-enhanced postcontrast T1 gradient echo (GRE) sequences, with the tumor being seen as hypointense to adjacent pancreatic parenchyma on the precontrast and in the arterial and venous phase following intravenous contrast administration. Magnetic resonance cholangiopancreatography (MRCP) sequences in coronal and oblique projections are essential to evaluate for pancreatic ductal obstruction.

Published comparisons of MR and CT with histopathology are scarce. Ichikawa and coworkers reported that the frequency of agreement between tumor size measurement on imaging and tumor size on pathology was superior with dynamic MR (76%) compared with helical CT (57%).[12] Tumor size was underestimated by helical CT in eight patients and by dynamic MR in four patients and tumor size was overestimated by both helical CT and dynamic MR in one patient. In all seven patients with tumor-associated pancreatitis, the contrast between tumor and tumor-associated pancreatitis was better on dynamic MR than dynamic CT. MR appeared to be superior to CT in correctly identifying retroperitoneal extension and portal venous involvement. However, none of these differences reached statistical significance. Others have also not been able to demonstrate superiority of MR over CT in establishing vascular involvement.[13,18]

It is not clear how modern day MR and CT scans compare in defining the size and shape of pancreatic tumors. Both technologies have evolved significantly in recent years. In 1999, Sheridan and colleagues studied 33 consecutive surgical candidates.[19] Magnetic resonance imaging included fast spin-echo (TR/TE 4000/91), fat-suppressed T1-weighted spin-echo (500/15), and T1-weighted breath-hold GRE fast low-angle shot (100/4; flip angle, 80°) images before and after the administration of gadopentetate dimeglumine. Helical CT used 5-mm collimation with a pitch of 1:1.5–1.7; images were obtained 20 seconds and 65 to 70 seconds after injection of 150 mL of contrast material. Results were correlated with surgery in 25 patients. Although MR and helical CT performed equally well in lesion detection, MR was significantly better in the assessment of resectability.

More recently, Mehmet Erturk et al. compared dynamic contrast-enhanced multirow detector CT (MDCT) with and without multiplanar reformatted images (MPR) and MR for the detection and assessment of locoregional extension of pancreatic adenocarcinoma.[20] Twenty-four patients with and 21 without pancreatic adenocarcinoma were studied and scan results were compared with surgical findings. Multirow detector CT with MPR imaging was superior to MDCT without MPR imaging and to comprehensive MR employing 2D sequences and MRCP for both the detection and assessment of locoregional extension of pancreatic adenocarcinomas.

In unresectable cases of pancreatic cancer, it is unlikely that MR provides additional benefit compared with CT in delineating the GTV. Although MR has superior tissue contrast resolution, it also has similar limitation as CT scan in estimating tumor size, with MR also not being able to definitively differentiate pancreatic tumor from adjacent fibrosis and inflammatory changes. Currently, contrast-enhanced MR has a role as a problem-solving tool in pancreatic cancer imaging for detection of small tumors when helical CT scan reveals equivocal results or in patients when CT is contraindicated.[21]

The role of fusion PET–CT imaging in the evaluation of patients with pancreatic cancer has been recently reported in the literature. Farma and coworkers reported that PET–CT has increased sensitivity in detection of metastasis compared with PET alone or CT alone (87%, 61%, and 57%, respectively).[22] Moreover, PET–CT changed management in 11% of patients with the detection of two occult liver lesions, two peritoneal implants, two supraclavicular lymph nodes, and one peri-esophageal lymph node not seen on CT. However, there have been no reports correlating tumor size measurements on PET with those on CT or pathological assessment to evaluate whether PET provides any additional benefit in GTV delineation.

Pancreas Tumors: Defining the CTV

Traditionally, the clinical target volume (CTV) for pancreatic cancer has included the regional lymphatics. Recently, some groups have begun omitting regional lymphatics for the sake of increasing tolerability and the intensity of chemotherapy. Investigators at the University of Michigan became interested in combining full-dose gemcitabine with radiation to simultaneously maximize both systemic and radiosensitizing effects. To reduce toxicity, the fields were designed to encompass the primary tumor only, without prophylactic lymph node irradiation. It was thought that the majority of the benefit from RT would come from controlling the primary tumor, and that the combined effects of gemcitabine and incidental irradiation would eradicate clinically occult disease in regional nodes.

We have recently examined our experience to determine if these assumptions were correct. Between 1999 and 2005, 77 patients with unresectable nonmetastatic pancreas cancer were treated with full-dose gemcitabine and RT. The planning target volume (PTV) was limited to the GTV plus 1 cm. The total dose ranged from 24 Gy to 42 Gy. Pretreatment, treatment-planning, and follow-up CT scans were reviewed systematically. In-field failure was defined as disease progression within the 80% isodose volume. Although the local progression rate was high (34% at 1 year), the vast majority occurred within the GTV. Of the 15 patients who first progressed locally, 12 progressed within the GTV, two progressed within the GTV and in-field lymph node metastases, and only one patient experienced a marginal peripancreatic lymph node failure. Thus, it appears that when RT is combined with a potent radiosensitizer such as gemcitabine, the regional lymphatics may be safely excluded without excess marginal failures. The potential advantage of the resultant smaller PTV is better integration with more intensive systemic therapy and/or a more intensive radiation dose schedule.

Liver Tumors: Defining the GTV

Computed tomography and MR are the dominant imaging modalities used for characterization and evaluation of liver tumors. The advent of MDCT has improved hepatic imaging considerably by enabling scans to be acquired during a single breath hold, with thinner slices, enabling multiplanar reformatting. Computed tomography evaluation of the liver is based on two basic parameters: attenuation differences and differential enhancement. Because soft tissues have similar attenuation coefficients, the soft-tissue contrast of CT is inherently limited. Dynamic contrast-enhanced CT takes advantage of the differential enhancement of liver lesions and the surrounding hepatic parenchyma, thus providing valuable diagnostic information.

State-of-the-art CT scanning of the liver involves acquisition of three contrast phases: arterial hepatic, portal venous, and delayed equilibrium. As most hepatocellular carcinomas (HCCs) are hypervascular, they typically display intense heterogeneous enhancement during the arterial phase. During the portal venous phase, these tumors are typically hypodense compared with the liver parenchyma, because of rapid "washout" of contrast.[23,24] Intrahepatic cholangiocarcinoma (IHC), on the other hand, typically shows delayed and prolonged enhancement. The most common pattern of enhancement of IHC is rimlike peripheral enhancement in both arterial and portal venous phases with retention of contrast material during late equilibrium phase.[25,26]

Liver metastases are typically hypodense compared with the surrounding liver parenchyma on unenhanced CT, but may occasionally be isodense.[27] The enhancement patterns of liver metastases on dynamic contrast-enhanced CT depend on their vascularity. Hypervascular liver metastases that derive their blood supply from the hepatic arteries often show ring enhancement during the arterial phase.[28,29] Most liver metastases, however, are best depicted on portal venous phase images as hypodense areas compared with the enhancing surrounding liver parenchyma.[30,31]

Magnetic resonance has inherent excellent soft-tissue contrast that can be further improved by nonspecific and liver-specific contrast agents.[32] Hepatobiliary MR uses a combination of different MR pulse sequences, each of which produces images that provide unique information about the liver and the biliary tree. Recent advances in technology, such as larger gradients, improved surface coils, and parallel imaging techniques, have substantially improved image quality and the speed of image acquisition.[33] Combination of the information from both unenhanced and dynamic contrast-enhanced MR improves detection and characterization of liver lesions. Chapter 19B illustrates the use of MR guidance for target delineation in a patient with hepatocellular carcinoma.

On unenhanced T1-weighted MR, HCC can have a variable appearance. On T2-weighted images HCCs typically show increased signal. The enhancement pattern of HCC on dynamic gadolinium-enhanced MR follows that of triphasic CT, with pronounced heterogeneous enhancement on the arterial phase and delayed washout.[33–35]

Biliary cancers are well depicted on combined MR and MRCP. With the intrinsic high signal from bile, MRCP produces high-quality images of both the intrahepatic and extrahepatic bile ducts. New high-resolution MRCP that acquires very thin sections through the biliary tree can localize the tumor by showing a focal biliary stricture and the associated biliary obstruction. The MR images demonstrate the tumor itself, the extent of liver invasion, and the presence of lymphatic or peritoneal metastases. Typically, biliary tumors show increased enhancement on delayed gadolinium-enhanced images.[28,33,36,37]

Liver metastases are typically hypointense on T1-weighted images and hyperintense on T2-weighted images of unenhanced MR. Hypervascular metastases, such as those arising from melanoma, renal cell carcinoma, neuroendocrine tumors, and thyroid cancer, typically show peripheral ring enhancement on the arterial-phase images. A pattern of peripheral or heterogeneous washout on delayed equilibrium phase is specific for liver metastases and is common in hypervascular metastases.[28,33,38] Hypovascular metastases, such as metastases of colon, lung, and bladder cancers, are best depicted during the portal venous phase. Transient perilesional enhancement may be observed in hypovascular metastases during the arterial phase and may correspond to areas of desmoplastic reaction, peritumoral inflammation, and vascular proliferation.[39,40]

The use of liver-specific contrast agents, such as superparamagnetic iron oxide (SPIO), may further improve the depiction and characterization of hepatic lesions.[41,42] Future directions may include the addition of diffusion-weighted imaging to the routine MR. Diffusion-weighted imaging uses pulse sequences and techniques that are sensitive to microscopic random movement of molecules in response to thermal energy. The healthy liver parenchyma is dark on diffusion-weighted imaging, whereas liver tumors are depicted as high-signal-intensity masses because of their restricted diffusion of water.[33] Diffusion-weighted imaging may increase the detection rate of liver tumors, but its role in the evaluation of the extent of disease has yet to be studied.[43]

FDG-PET has been proved to be highly sensitive in detecting hepatic metastases from various primary sites,[44,45] and is also quite sensitive in detecting IHC,[46] but has low sensitivity for HCC.[47,48] Other PET tracers, such as ^{11}C-acetate, may improve the detection of primary liver lesions, but their clinical role is still limited.[49]

Magnetic resonance has been shown in multiple studies to be superior to CT in the detection and char-

acterization of different liver lesions.[28,50–52] It is not clear, however, how these two modalities compare with each other regarding the extent of disease and definition of tumor borders, which are essential for RT treatment planning. A study comparing GTV contours on triphasic CT with those delineated on MR imaging in 26 patients with hepatic malignancies found concordance of only 73% between the CT- and MR-defined GTVs (Figure 19-1).[53] Concordance was better for liver metastases (81%) and worst for cholangiocarcinoma (64%). The MR volumes for the dominant tumor mass were at least 20% greater than the CT volumes in three tumors, whereas CT volumes were at least 20% greater than the MR in nine tumors. In five of the 10 patients with HCC, there was discrepancy in the number of satellite lesions between the two modalities. No such discrepancy was found in patients with metastases or cholangiocarcinoma. In the absence of pathological correlates, which modality and sequences best represent the GTV remains unknown.

Detailed correlation studies between imaging and pathology in patients with liver tumors are scarce. Kelsey and colleagues found good correlation ($R^2 = 0.8$)

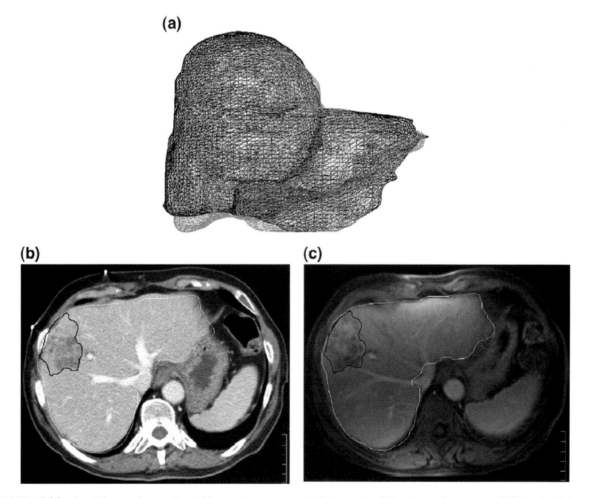

FIGURE 19-1. (a) Overlay of liver meshes constructed from contours on computed tomography (CT) and magnetic resonance (MR) imaging data sets (light gray, CT; black, MR). **(b)** Axial CT slice and **(c)** axial MR slice for a patient with hepatocellular carcinoma, with MR liver contour shown in light gray and MR-determined gross tumor volume shown in dark gray. Reproduced with permission from Voroney JP et al.[53]

between the radiographic and pathological size of 27 resected HCCs smaller than 5 cm. The measurement was performed on the CT series or MR sequences that best depicted tumor margins. The authors calculated that a 0.5-cm or 1.0-cm margin around the radiographic tumor would have encompassed the gross pathologic tumor in 93% and 100% of cases, respectively.[54] On the other hand, another retrospective study of 212 HCC patients found poor correlation between tumor size on preoperative imaging and the pathological tumor size. Tumor size was underestimated by CT in 30% of cases, and overestimated in 40%.[55]

Detailed studies comparing radiographic findings with pathological results are needed to define which imaging modality and phase best correlate with the GTV and extent of microscopic disease. Until such information is available, no solid recommendation can be made as to which modality and sequence to use for GTV delineation and how to delineate it. Currently, several different strategies have been described in the literature. In a French phase II trial of 3D-conformal RT for HCC, the GTV was defined as the contrast-enhancing mass on arterial phase images.[56] In a study of liver stereotactic body RT (SBRT) for primary and metastatic liver lesions, Mendez Romero and coworkers used contrast-enhanced CT with arterial and venous phases for treatment planning.[57] The rim of contrast enhancement was delineated on the images of both phases and summed to construct the CTV. In another study of SBRT for metastatic lesions only, Hoyer et al. used contrast-enhanced CT for target delineation.[58] The visible hypodense tumor volume and the surrounding hypervascular rim were defined as the CTV. Wulf and coworkers used triphasic CT for liver SBRT treatment planning.[59] The CTV was defined as the contrast-enhancing zone plus a 3-mm margin and was delineated on the contrast phase with the largest tumor diameter. Other studies do not provide their definition of GTV, but do mention registration of MR and PET images to the treatment planning CT.[7,60,61]

Liver Tumors: Defining the CTV

The margin needed for microscopic disease extension in patients with liver tumors can be deduced from pathological studies as well as from detailed pattern of failure studies. Shi and colleagues retrospectively examined unfixed resection specimens of 109 patients with solitary HCC who had no evidence of macroscopic metastases or vascular invasion.[62] Micrometastases, defined as tumor nodules smaller than 2 mm, were found in 57 patients. The majority of the micrometastases were intravascular and only a few were satellite micronodules. Intravascular metastases were found as far as 6.10 cm from the main tumor (range, 0.05 cm to 6.10 cm) and the distance of tumor satellite nodules from the primary tumor was 0.10 cm to 0.80 cm. Of note, tumor size predicted for the

presence of micrometastases. Also, there was significantly more spread of the disease along the direction of portal venous flow. For HCC tumors less than or equal to 3 cm, a 1-cm margin would be adequate for 92% of patients for a distal margin and for 100% of patients for a proximal margin. For tumors larger than 3 cm, a margin of 1 cm would be adequate for 91% of patients for a proximal margin, but only for 63% of patients for a distal margin. Therefore, a distal margin of 2 cm seemed to be more appropriate for tumors larger than 3 cm, as this would cover 89% of micrometastases.

In a Japanese retrospective study of 116 patients who underwent hepatic resections for HCCs smaller than 3 cm with three or fewer nodules, 24% were found to have micrometastases. The maximum distance of the micrometastases from the main tumor was 9.5 mm ± 6.2 mm for tumors of the "nonboundary type" (single nodule with extranodular growth, confluent multinodular lesion, or invasive lesion) whereas in the "boundary-type" lesions this distance was 3.1 mm ± 1.4 mm.[63] In another pathological series, the maximum distance of micrometastases from the main tumor was 6 mm for primary tumors that had no macroscopic tumor thrombi or satellites, whereas it was 19 mm for cases with macroscopic vascular involvement or macrometastases.[64] Another report describes micrometastases at a distance of up to 96.9 mm from the dominant nodule.[65]

The optimal resection margin for HCC was studied retrospectively in multiple surgical series, with conflicting results.[63,66–70] Shi and colleagues conducted a prospective study in which 169 patients with single-nodule HCC were randomized to undergo partial hepatectomy aiming grossly at either a narrow (1-cm) or wide (2-cm) resection margin. All 13 recurrences at the liver resection margin occurred in the narrow-margin group.[71]

The best guidance for the optimal GTV-to-CTV margin would be provided by detailed analysis of failure patterns following 3D conformal RT. Most of the recurrences of primary liver malignancies are within the liver,[7,72] but data on the spatial distribution of these recurrences relative to the dose distribution map are, unfortunately, not available. Atrophy of the irradiated area within the liver and compensatory regeneration of other regions may cause liver volume changes as well as significant deformation.[73] As a result, registration of pre- and posttreatment imaging and exact spatial localization of tumor recurrences may be challenging. In the absence of pattern of failure data, a 1 cm to 2 cm margin is most commonly used.

Motion Considerations

Pancreas

Pancreatic motion remains poorly understood, with a handful of studies based on fluoroscopy and two using MR. Murphy and colleagues at Stanford University reported the results of one patient who had three 2-mm gold fiducials sutured into the tumor at the time of exploratory laparotomy as part of an aborted Whipple procedure.[74] This patient was imaged fluoroscopically for 1 minute each in the anterior–posterior (AP) and lateral directions to assess tumor motion during respiration. The maximal cranial–caudal (CC) movement was found to be 6 mm with breathing, and the lateral deviation 1 mm with aortic pulsation. Gierga and coworkers at the Massachusetts General Hospital (MGH) reported a study of six patients with pancreatic cancer who also underwent invasive marker placement and were observed fluoroscopically for 30 seconds each in the AP and lateral dimensions.[75] The range of CC maximum motion was 6.5 mm to 18 mm, with an average of 4.4 mm to 12 mm. Movement in the AP dimension was much smaller, with a range of maximum values of 6.0 mm to 8.7 mm and a range of average values of 2.5 mm to 6.9 mm. Though simple, these small series provided important initial data regarding pancreatic movement.

In a more advanced study, investigators in Leuven, Belgium, reported their data using dynamic MR to quantify pancreatic motion.[76] No fiducials were placed. Instead, they acquired one image every second for 1 minute in the axial and coronal planes. One reader contoured the pancreatic volume on each image, and the center of gravity on each frame was calculated. The movement over time of this center of gravity was analyzed in 12 patients. A larger degree of movement was found in the CC direction than reported by both the Stanford and MGH groups, at 24 mm ± 16 mm. A few limitations of this study include the use of the center of gravity as a convenient, but not very clinically relevant, focus of analysis, and the lack of information regarding organ deformation. Indeed, it is the motion of tumor borders, rather than a single or a few points in space, such as fiducials or a center of mass, that are most important when one is designing PTV margins. It is inadequacy of coverage of these borders that could potentially lead to marginal misses in the era of highly conformal RT.

The University of Michigan group recently presented the results of a 17-patient study in which they used cine-MR to capture three images per second in sagittal and coronal planes through pancreatic tumors.[77] Similar to the Belgian MR study, tumor range of motion was found to be a mean of 20 mm in the CC direction, and 6 mm to 8 mm in the AP direction. Movement in the lateral direction was negligible. Additionally, tumors did not move *en bloc*. Instead, motion of the tumor borders was not correlated, suggesting deformation. Loo and colleagues at Stanford University also have reported evidence for pancreatic tumor motion and deformation in an analysis of implanted fiducial position from 4D planning CT scans.[78] Thus, if one plans to track tumors, one must account for more than a single point at a time. Instead, several fiducials or the actual tumor borders should be accounted for. The Michigan study also addressed the reproducibility of motion for patients and found high variability in breathing patterns between imaging sessions in addition to the irregularity in breathing patterns during each session. This underscores the importance of continuous imaging during treatment as well as methods to increase reproducibility, such as coaching.

Liver

Liver motion can be quite significant. Initial studies using nuclear imaging of technetium (Tc)-99 compounds found motion in the 11 mm to 14 mm range under normal free breathing.[79,80] A CT-based study found a mean liver movement of 17 mm.[81] In a later study of fluoroscopically monitored intratumoral coil position, 4.9 mm to 30.4 mm of movement was noted in the eight patients studied.[82] Kitamura and colleagues described the motion of gold fiducials implanted near liver tumors and found 9 mm ± 5 mm of motion in the CC direction, with a range of 2 mm to 19 mm.[83]

Image-Guided Treatment Delivery

The major toxicities associated with RT for pancreatic cancer relate to the volume of normal tissue irradiated. One strategy for reducing normal tissue toxicity is to reduce treatment margins around the tumor. However, accurate targeting is essential to ensure that the primary tumor receives the planned radiation dose.

Planning and Daily Setup

A solution to account for respiratory-associated pancreatic tumor motion is to implant fiducial seeds into the pancreatic mass. Typically, these are made of 100% gold and three to five seeds are implanted into the tumor or surrounding adjacent tissues. Various methods of implantation can be used including CT guidance or endoscopic ultrasound guidance. Typically, a patient will present with a newly diagnosed pancreatic mass that needs a biopsy confirmation of cancer. If a biopsy is indicated, the fiducial seeds can be implanted at the same time, immediately after pathologic confirmation of the cancer.

Following fiducial seed implantation, minor shifts in seed position can occur within the first 5 days. For this reason, it is generally recommended to wait at least 5 days before bringing the patient back for treatment planning. This gives the seeds time to settle down into a stable position, ensuring reproducibility of the setup position.

For the treatment planning scan, four-dimensional (4D) CT scans should be utilized whenever possible. A review of the tumor position throughout the respiratory cycle is essential for optimal treatment planning. From these scans, an assessment of the extent of tumor motion is possible. Minn and coworkers reported in an analysis of 20 consecutive RT treatment planning scans for patients with locally advanced pancreatic cancer, the mean extent of motion was greatest in the superior–inferior (SI) direction.[84] Mean pancreatic tumor motions in all directions were as follows: SI 9.2 (range, 0.9–28.8 mm), left–right 3.2 (range, 0.1–13.7 mm), and AP 3.8 (range, 0.2–7.6 mm). In addition, a poor correlation between tumor positions as predicted by the 4D planning CT and actual tumor positions measured during treatment was found. These discrepancies (likely attributable to setup error, drift, etc.) suggest that an additional correction is necessary to account for tumor location during the actual treatment. Real-time or near-real-time imaging of the fiducials is required throughout treatment to make this final correction and to ensure the accuracy of the intended treatment.

Following treatment planning, daily kilovoltage (kV) imaging is useful to assess the position of implanted fiducials relative to the adjacent bony anatomy. Although these landmarks are aligned for some of the fractions, an additional shift is usually required to move the seeds into the correct position. In a preliminary analysis of patients treated in this manner, after alignment to bony anatomy, a secondary shift was required 80% of the time to align the fiducial seeds properly. The magnitude of this secondary shift was greatest in the SI direction with a mean of 4.1 mm (range, 0–19 mm).[85]

Free Breathing

In a cine-MR study performed at the University of Michigan, it was found that if planned from the end-exhale position, margins of 20 mm, 10 mm, 7 mm, and 4 mm must be added in the inferior, anterior, superior, and posterior directions, respectively, to achieve 99% temporal coverage of pancreatic tumors.[77] Estimating and accounting for the magnitude of motion for individual patients is recommended, with the understanding that this can vary between imaging and treatment sessions.

Active Breathing Control

One method used to manage ventilatory motion is to minimize it using breath-hold techniques. Active breathing control (ABC) suspends breathing in a specific point in the respiratory cycle, during which RT can be delivered with very tight PTV margins accounting only for setup variability, because organ motion is essentially eliminated.[86] In liver cancer, ABC has been shown to be feasible and to facilitate dose escalation and normal tissue sparing, with an average decrease in normal tissue complication probability of 4.5% and an average 6-Gy to 8-Gy dose escalation (Figure 19-2).[87-90] Active breathing control is

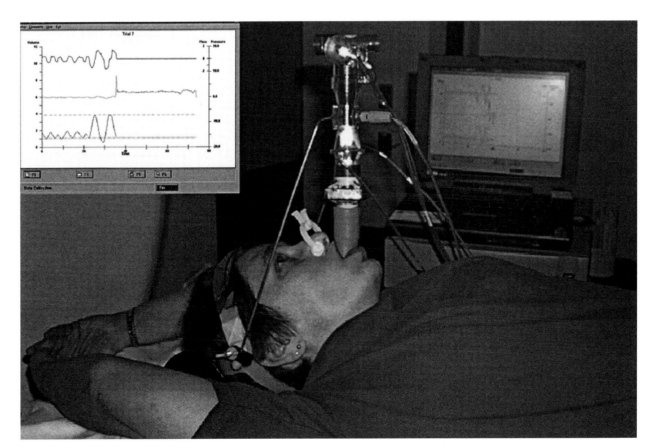

FIGURE 19-2. Active breathing control device (Vmax22LV by Sensormedics, Yorba Linda, CA) with insert of computer screen in top left corner. Reproduced with permission from Dawson LA et al.[87]

standard practice for all patients with liver and pancreatic cancer treated with RT at the University of Michigan who can tolerate the required breath holds.

Respiratory Gating

If respiratory gating is used, fluoroscopic imaging may be used to confirm that the radiation beam is turned on only when the fiducials are in the correct location. The extent of respiratory-associated fiducial seed movement can be recorded and compared with the predicted motion based upon the planning 4D CT scan. In the planning phase, each seed should be contoured with a uniform margin expansion. These structures can be exported and superimposed onto the digitally reconstructed radiographs and are visible on standard portal imaging. In addition, these contours can be superimposed onto fluoroscopic images, which may be taken each day before treatment and the required shifts should be made as appropriate. Typically, these daily images are taken during a breath hold at end-inspiration. Fiducials can also be imaged dynamically during treatment to confirm that the beam is turned on only when the fiducials are in the correct location. This type of dynamic verification of tumor position allows clinicians to be confident in treating pancreatic tumors with minimal margins. Minimizing margin expansions is a major factor in reducing the volume irradiated, which, in turn, reduces both acute and late normal tissue complications. Chapter 19C demonstrates the use of planar imaging and respiratory gating in a patient with pancreatic cancer.

Future Directions

Electromagnetic Transponders

Targeting of tumors can also be accomplished without traditional imaging methods. Calypso Medical Beacon Transponders (Calypso Medical Technologies, Seattle, WA) are a relatively new way to obtain real-time information on tumor location during treatment. It has been used mostly for prostate cancer,[91–99] but several groups are now investigating the use for other types of cancers including pancreas, lung, and breast. These transponders are 1.85 mm by 8.5 mm and are composed of a passive inner electronic circuit and encapsulation material. This inner circuit makes the transponder appear opaque when viewed with standard imaging techniques such as ultrasound, CT, or planar x-ray. The electronic circuit of the transponder is secured within a biocompatible glass vial with adhesive. The glass vial housing is then hermetically sealed to form a cylinder with rounded ends.

The transponders are externally stimulated using an electromagnetic source, and the resulting resonant signals are detected and localized by receiver coils. Each transponder responds at a different frequency, so multiple transponders can be tracked simultaneously. The source and receiver coils are housed in an array that has

been engineered to stay in place during RT delivery with minimal impact on the treatment beam (~3% attenuation, ~2 mm buildup, no electromagnetic interference). The array can be positioned in a region above the patient, near isocenter, with its location tracked continuously via an infrared tracking system with submillimeter precision. The combination of array position in the treatment room and transponder position relative to the array yields the actual position of the transponders in the room relative to their intended position. The accuracy of Beacon tracking has been established to be within 0.1 mm. With real-time knowledge of tumor position, gating and tracking could be feasible, and could allow for radiation dose escalation without increasing normal tissue toxicity.

Multiple Instance Geometry Approximation

Currently, when treating patients with RT, physicians define a target and then add a safety margin around this to ensure adequate coverage with radiation in the face of organ motion and setup variation. This entire region, the PTV, is treated to the same dose as the actual clinical target. Nearby organs at risk receive unnecessary radiation, and this is likely responsible for a significant portion of RT-induced morbidity. A more appropriate PTV would take not only the range of target positions into consideration, but also the proportion of time spent in each position. At the University of Michigan, multiple instance geometry approximation (MIGA) incorporates the weighted distribution of target position into inverse planning optimization and dose calculation.[100] This method has been previously tested in breast and head and neck cancers.[101,102] Recently, MIGA was compared with treatment using ABC, and there was no difference in the ability to spare normal tissue or to escalate target dose.[103]

Conclusions

Image-guided RT represents a significant technological advance to minimize treatment-related toxicities and may allow for radiation dose escalation. Proper use of radiographic studies to define the GTV and CTV in pancreatic and liver tumors is crucial to construct the smallest possible targets yet avoid marginal recurrences. Understanding and accounting for tumor motion in treatment planning and delivery are also important. Several motion management strategies are available. The choice of system requires a joint decision among all members of the team, including physicians, physicists, therapists, and dosimetrists.

References

1. Zhong X, Yu J, Zhang B, et al. Using 18F-fluorodeoxyglucose positron emission tomography to estimate the length of gross tumor in patients with squamous cell carcinoma of the esophagus. *Int J Radiat Oncol Biol Phys.* 2009;73:136–141.

2. Leong T, Everitt C, Yuen K, et al. A prospective study to evaluate the impact of FDG-PET on CT-based radiotherapy treatment planning for oesophageal cancer. *Radiother Oncol.* 2006;78: 254–261.

3. O'Neill BD, Salerno G, Thomas K, et al. MR vs CT imaging: low rectal cancer tumor delineation for three-dimensional conformal radiotherapy. *Br J Radiol.* 2009;82:509–513.

4. Nguyen BT, Joon DL, Khoo V, et al. Assessing the impact of FDG-PET in the management of anal cancer. *Radiother Oncol.* 2008;87:376–382.

5. Grigsby PW. FDG-PET/CT: new horizons in anal cancer. *Gastroenterol Clin Biol.* 2009;33:456–458

6. Fuss M, Salter BJ, Cavanaugh SX, et al. Daily ultrasound-based image-guided targeting for radiotherapy of upper abdominal malignancies. *Int J Radiat Oncol Biol Phys.* 2004;59:1245–1256.

7. De Ridder M, Tournel K, Van Nieuwenhove Y, et al. Phase II study of preoperative helical tomotherapy for rectal cancer. *Int J Radiat Oncol Biol Phys.* 2008;70:728–734.

8. Lu DS, Vedantham S, Krasny RM, et al. Two-phase helical CT for pancreatic tumors: pancreatic versus hepatic phase enhancement of tumor, pancreas, and vascular structures. *Radiology.* 1996;199:697–701.

9. Fletcher JG, Wiersema MJ, Farrell MA, et al. Pancreatic malignancy: value of arterial, pancreatic, and hepatic phase imaging with multi-detector row CT. *Radiology.* 2003;229:81–90.

10. Prokesch RW, Chow LC, Beaulieu CF, et al. Isoattenuating pancreatic adenocarcinoma at multi-detector row CT: secondary signs. *Radiology.* 2002;224:764–768.

11. Bluemke DA, Cameron JL, Hruban RH, et al. Potentially resectable pancreatic adenocarcinoma: spiral CT assessment with surgical and pathologic correlation. *Radiology.* 1995;197:381–385.

12. Ichikawa T, Haradome H, Hachiya J, et al. Pancreatic ductal adenocarcinoma: preoperative assessment with helical CT versus dynamic MR imaging. *Radiology.* 1997;202:655–662.

13. Schima W, Fugger R, Schober E, et al. Diagnosis and staging of pancreatic cancer: comparison of mangafodipir trisodium-enhanced MR imaging and contrast-enhanced helical hydro-CT. *AJR Am J Roentgenol.* 2002;179:717–724.

14. Furukawa H, Takayasu K, Mukai K, et al. Computed tomography of pancreatic adenocarcinoma: comparison of tumor size measured by dynamic computed tomography and histopathologic examination. *Pancreas.* 1996;13:231–235.

15. Aoki K, Okada S, Moriyama N, et al. Accuracy of computed tomography in determining pancreatic cancer tumor size. *Jpn J Clin Oncol.* 1994;24:85–87.

16. Ballard RB, Hoffman JP, Guttman MC, et al. How accurate is size measurement of pancreas cancer masses by computed axial tomography (CT) scanning? *Am Surg.* 1995;61:686–691.

17. Irie H, Honda H, Kaneko K, et al. Comparison of helical CT and MR imaging in detecting and staging small pancreatic adenocarcinoma. *Abdom Imaging.* 1997;22:429–433.

18. Romijn MG, Stoker J, van Eijck CH, et al. MRI with mangafodipir trisodium in the detection and staging of pancreatic cancer. *J Magn Reson Imaging.* 2000;12:261–268.

19. Sheridan MB, Ward J, Guthrie JA, et al. Dynamic contrast-enhanced MR imaging and dual-phase helical CT in the preoperative assessment of suspected pancreatic cancer: a comparative study with receiver operating characteristic analysis. *AJR Am J Roentgenol.* 1999;173:583–590.

20. Mehmet Erturk S, Ichikawa T, Sou H, et al. Pancreatic adenocarcinoma: MDCT versus MRI in the detection and assessment of locoregional extension. *J Comput Assist Tomogr.* 2006; 30:583–590.

21. Schima W, Ba-Ssalamah A, Kolblinger C, et al. Pancreatic adenocarcinoma. *Eur Radiol.* 2007;17:638–649.

22. Farma JM, Santillan AA, Melis M, et al. PET/CT fusion scan enhances CT staging in patients with pancreatic neoplasms. *Ann Surg Oncol.* 2008;15:2465–2471.

23. Monzawa S, Ichikawa T, Nakajima H, et al. Dynamic CT for detecting small hepatocellular carcinoma: usefulness of delayed phase imaging. *AJR Am J Roentgenol.* 2007;188:147–153.

24. Saar B, Kellner-Weldon F. Radiological diagnosis of hepatocellular carcinoma. *Liver Int.* 2008;28:189–199.

25. Valls C, Guma A, Puig I, et al. Intrahepatic peripheral cholangiocarcinoma: CT evaluation. *Abdom Imaging.* 2000;25:490–496.

26. Kim NR, Lee JM, Kim SH, et al. Enhancement characteristics of cholangiocarcinomas on multiphasic helical CT: emphasis on morphologic subtypes. *Clin Imaging.* 2008;32:114–120.

27. Kanematsu M, Kondo H, Goshima S, et al. Imaging liver metastases: review and update. *Eur J Radiol.* 2006;58:217–228.

28. Larson RE, Semelka RC, Bagley AS, et al. Hypervascular malignant liver lesions: comparison of various MR imaging pulse sequences and dynamic CT. *Radiology.* 1994;192:393–399.

29. Oliver JH III, Baron RL, Federle MP, et al. Hypervascular liver metastases: do unenhanced and hepatic arterial phase CT images affect tumor detection? *Radiology.* 1997;205:709–715.

30. Soyer P, Poccard M, Boudiaf M, et al. Detection of hypovascular hepatic metastases at triple-phase helical CT: sensitivity of phases and comparison with surgical and histopathologic findings. *Radiology.* 2004;231:413–420.

31. Sheafor DH, Frederick MG, Paulson EK, et al. Comparison of unenhanced, hepatic arterial-dominant, and portal venous-dominant phase helical CT for the detection of liver metastases in women with breast carcinoma. *AJR Am J Roentgenol.* 1999;172:961–968.

32. Hussain SM, Semelka RC. Hepatic imaging: comparison of modalities. *Radiol Clin North Am.* 2005;43:929–947

33. Low RN. Abdominal MRI advances in the detection of liver tumours and characterisation. *Lancet Oncol.* 2007;8:525–535.

34. Kelekis NL, Semelka RC, Worawattanakul S, et al. Hepatocellular carcinoma in North America: a multiinstitutional study of appearance on T1-weighted, T2-weighted, and serial gadolinium-enhanced gradient-echo images. *AJR Am J Roentgenol.* 1998;170:1005–1013.

35. van den Bos IC, Hussain SM, Dwarkasing RS, et al. MR imaging of hepatocellular carcinoma: relationship between lesion size and imaging findings, including signal intensity and dynamic enhancement patterns. *J Magn Reson Imaging.* 2007;26:1548–1555.

36. Vogl TJ, Schwarz WO, Heller M, et al. Staging of Klatskin tumours (hilar cholangiocarcinomas): comparison of MR cholangiography, MR imaging, and endoscopic retrograde cholangiography. *Eur Radiol.* 2006;16:2317–2325.

37. Manfredi R, Barbaro B, Masselli G, et al. Magnetic resonance imaging of cholangiocarcinoma. *Semin Liver Dis.* 2004;24:155–164.

38. Semelka RC, Helmberger TK. Contrast agents for MR imaging of the liver. *Radiology.* 2001;218:27–38.

39. Danet IM, Semelka RC, Leonardou P, et al. Spectrum of MRI appearances of untreated metastases of the liver. *AJR Am J Roentgenol.* 2003;181:809–817.

40. Semelka RC, Hussain SM, Marcos HB, et al. Perilesional enhancement of hepatic metastases: correlation between MR imaging and histopathologic findings-initial observations. *Radiology.* 2000;215:89–94.

41. Reimer P, Jahnke N, Fiebich M, et al. Hepatic lesion detection and characterization: value of nonenhanced MR imaging, superparamagnetic iron oxide-enhanced MR imaging, and spiral CT-ROC analysis. *Radiology.* 2000;217:152–158.

42. Kim MJ, Kim JH, Chung JJ, et al. Focal hepatic lesions: detection and characterization with combination gadolinium- and superparamagnetic iron oxide-enhanced MR imaging. *Radiology.* 2003;228:719–726.

43. Low RN, Gurney J. Diffusion-weighted MRI (DWI) in the oncology patient: value of breathhold DWI compared to unenhanced and gadolinium-enhanced MRI. *J Magn Reson Imaging.* 2007;25:848–858.

44. Kinkel K, Lu Y, Both M, et al. Detection of hepatic metastases from cancers of the gastrointestinal tract by using noninvasive imaging methods (US, CT, MR imaging, PET): a meta-analysis. *Radiology.* 2002;224:748–756.

45. Bipat S, van Leeuwen MS, Comans EF, et al. Colorectal liver metastases: CT, MR imaging, and PET for diagnosis—meta-analysis. *Radiology.* 2005;237:123–131.

46. Breitenstein S, Apestegui C, Clavien PA. Positron emission tomography (PET) for cholangiocarcinoma. *HPB (Oxford).* 2008;10:120–121.

47. Khan MA, Combs CS, Brunt EM, et al. Positron emission tomography scanning in the evaluation of hepatocellular carcinoma. *J Hepatol.* 2000;32:792–797.

48. Trojan J, Schroeder O, Raedle J, et al. Fluorine-18 FDG positron emission tomography for imaging of hepatocellular carcinoma. *Am J Gastroenterol.* 1999;94:3314–3319.

49. Ho CL, Chen S, Yeung DW, et al. Dual-tracer PET/CT imaging in evaluation of metastatic hepatocellular carcinoma. *J Nucl Med.* 2007;48:902–909.

50. Semelka RC, Martin DR, Balci C, et al. Focal liver lesions: comparison of dual-phase CT and multisequence multiplanar MR imaging including dynamic gadolinium enhancement. *J Magn Reson Imaging.* 2001;13:397–401.

51. Yamashita Y, Mitsuzaki K, Yi T, et al. Small hepatocellular carcinoma in patients with chronic liver damage: prospective comparison of detection with dynamic MR imaging and helical CT of the whole liver. *Radiology.* 1996;200:79–84.

52. Semelka RC, Shoenut JP, Ascher SM, et al. Solitary hepatic metastasis: comparison of dynamic contrast-enhanced CT and MR imaging with fat-suppressed T2-weighted, breath-hold T1-weighted FLASH, and dynamic gadolinium-enhanced FLASH sequences. *J Magn Reson Imaging.* 1994;4:319–323.

53. Voroney JP, Brock KK, Eccles C, et al. Prospective comparison of computed tomography and magnetic resonance imaging for liver cancer delineation using deformable image registration. *Int J Radiat Oncol Biol Phys.* 2006;66:780–791.

54. Kelsey CR, Schefter T, Nash SR, et al. Retrospective clinicopathologic correlation of gross tumor size of hepatocellular carcinoma: implications for stereotactic body radiotherapy. *Am J Clin Oncol.* 2005;28:576–580.

55. Huo TI, Wu JC, Lui WY, et al. Reliability of contemporary radiology to measure tumour size of hepatocellular carcinoma in patients undergoing resection: limitations and clinical implications. *Scand J Gastroenterol.* 2004;39:46–52.

56. Mornex F, Girard N, Beziat C, et al. Feasibility and efficacy of high-dose three-dimensional-conformal radiotherapy in cirrhotic patients with small-size hepatocellular carcinoma non-eligible for curative therapies—mature results of the French Phase II RTF-1 trial. *Int J Radiat Oncol Biol Phys.* 2006;66:1152–1158.

57. Mendez Romero A, Wunderink W, Hussain SM, et al. Stereotactic body radiation therapy for primary and metastatic liver tumors: a single institution phase I-II study. *Acta Oncol.* 2006;45:831–837.

58. Hoyer M, Roed H, Traberg Hansen A, et al. Phase II study on stereotactic body radiotherapy of colorectal metastases. *Acta Oncol.* 2006;45:823–830.

59. Wulf J, Guckenberger M, Haedinger U, et al. Stereotactic radiotherapy of primary liver cancer and hepatic metastases. *Acta Oncol.* 2006;45:838–847.

60. Dawson LA, Eccles C, Craig T. Individualized image guided iso-NTCP based liver cancer SBRT. *Acta Oncol.* 2006;45:856–864.

61. Kavanagh BD, Schefter TE, Cardenes HR, et al. Interim analysis of a prospective phase I/II trial of SBRT for liver metastases. *Acta Oncol.* 2006;45:848–855.

62. Shi M, Zhang CQ, Zhang YQ, et al. Micrometastases of solitary hepatocellular carcinoma and appropriate resection margin. *World J Surg.* 2004;28:376–381.

63. Ueno S, Kubo F, Sakoda M, et al. Efficacy of anatomic resection vs nonanatomic resection for small nodular hepatocellular carcinoma based on gross classification. *J Hepatobiliary Pancreat Surg.* 2008;15:493–500.

64. Zhou XP, Quan ZW, Cong WM, et al. Micrometastasis in surrounding liver and the minimal length of resection margin of primary liver cancer. *World J Gastroenterol.* 2007;13:4498–4503.

65. Lai EC, You KT, Ng IO, et al. The pathological basis of resection margin for hepatocellular carcinoma. *World J Surg.* 1993;17:786–790.

66. Shimada K, Sakamoto Y, Esaki M, et al. Role of the width of the surgical margin in a hepatectomy for small hepatocellular carcinomas eligible for percutaneous local ablative therapy. *Am J Surg.* 2008;195:775–781.

67. Lise M, Bacchetti S, Da Pian P, et al. Prognostic factors affecting long term outcome after liver resection for hepatocellular carcinoma: results in a series of 100 Italian patients. *Cancer.* 1998;82:1028–1036.

68. Poon RT, Fan ST, Ng IO, et al. Significance of resection margin in hepatectomy for hepatocellular carcinoma: a critical reappraisal. *Ann Surg.* 2000;231:544–551.

69. Yamanaka N, Okamoto E, Toyosaka A, et al. Prognostic factors after hepatectomy for hepatocellular carcinomas. A univariate and multivariate analysis. *Cancer.* 1990;65:1104–1110.

70. Ng IO, Lai EC, Fan ST, et al. Prognostic significance of pathologic features of hepatocellular carcinoma. A multivariate analysis of 278 patients. *Cancer.* 1995;76:2443–2448.

71. Shi M, Guo RP, Lin XJ, et al. Partial hepatectomy with wide versus narrow resection margin for solitary hepatocellular carcinoma: a prospective randomized trial. *Ann Surg.* 2007;245: 36–43.

72. Tse RV, Hawkins M, Lockwood G, et al. Phase I study of individualized stereotactic body radiotherapy for hepatocellular carcinoma and intrahepatic cholangiocarcinoma. *J Clin Oncol.* 2008;26:657–664.

73. Ahmadi T, Itai Y, Onaya H, et al. CT evaluation of hepatic injury following proton beam irradiation: appearance, enhancement, and 3D size reduction pattern. *J Comput Assist Tomogr.* 1999;23:655–663.

74. Murphy MJ, Martin D, Whyte R, et al. The effectiveness of breath-holding to stabilize lung and pancreas tumors during radiosurgery. *Int J Radiat Oncol Biol Phys.* 2002;53:475–482.

75. Gierga DP, Chen GT, Kung JH, et al. Quantification of respiration-induced abdominal tumor motion and its impact on IMRT dose distributions. *Int J Radiat Oncol Biol Phys.* 2004;58:1584–1595.

76. Bussels B, Goethals L, Feron M, et al. Respiration-induced movement of the upper abdominal organs: a pitfall for the three-dimensional conformal radiation treatment of pancreatic cancer. *Radiother Oncol.* 2003;68:69–74.

77. Feng M, Balter JM, Normolle DP, et al. Characterization of pancreatic tumor motion using cine MRI: surrogates for tumor position should be used with caution. *Int J Radiat Oncol Biol Phys.* 2009 Jul 1;74(3):884–891.

78. Loo BW, Thorndyke BR, Maxim PG, et al. Determining margin for target deformation and rotation in respiratory motion-tracked stereotactic radiosurgery of pancreatic cancer. *Int J Radiat Oncol Biol Phys.* 2005;63:S31–S31.

79. Harauz G, Bronskill MJ. Comparison of the liver's respiratory motion in the supine and upright positions: concise communication. *J Nucl Med.* 1979;20:733–735.

80. Weiss PH, Baker JM, Potchen EJ. Assessment of hepatic respiratory excursion. *J Nucl Med.* 1972;13:758–759.

81. Balter JM, Ten Haken RK, Lawrence TS, et al. Uncertainties in CT-based radiation therapy treatment planning associated with patient breathing. *Int J Radiat Oncol Biol Phys.* 1996;36:167–174.

82. Balter JM, Dawson LA, Kazanjian S, et al. Determination of ventilatory liver movement via radiographic evaluation of diaphragm position. *Int J Radiat Oncol Biol Phys.* 2001;51: 267–270.

83. Kitamura K, Shirato H, Seppenwoolde Y, et al. Tumor location, cirrhosis, and surgical history contribute to tumor movement in the liver, as measured during stereotactic irradiation using a real-time tumor-tracking radiotherapy system. *Int J Radiat Oncol Biol Phys.* 2003;56:221–228.

84. Minn Y, Schellenberg D, Maxin P, et al. Pancreatic tumor motion on a single planning 4D-CT does not correlate with intrafraction tumor motion during treatment. *Am J Clin Oncol.* 2009;32(4):364–368.

85. Chang DT; personal communication; July 1, 2009.

86. Wong JW, Sharpe MB, Jaffray DA, et al. The use of active breathing control (ABC) to reduce margin for breathing motion. *Int J Radiat Oncol Biol Phys.* 1999;44:911–919.

87. Dawson LA, Brock KK, Kazanjian S, et al. The reproducibility of organ position using active breathing control (ABC) during liver radiotherapy. *Int J Radiat Oncol Biol Phys.* 2001;51:1410–1421.

88. Ten Haken RK, Balter JM, Marsh LH, et al. Potential benefits of eliminating planning target volume expansions for patient breathing in the treatment of liver tumors. *Int J Radiat Oncol Biol Phys.* 1997;38:613–617.

89. Balter JM, Brock KK, Litzenberg DW, et al. Daily targeting of intrahepatic tumors for radiotherapy. *Int J Radiat Oncol Biol Phys.* 2002;52:266–271.

90. Balter JM, Brock KK, Lam KL, et al. Evaluating the influence of setup uncertainties on treatment planning for focal liver tumors. *Int J Radiat Oncol Biol Phys.* 2005;63:610–614.

91. Kitamura K, Shirato H, Seppenwoolde Y, et al. Three-dimensional intrafractional movement of prostate measured during real-time tumor-tracking radiotherapy in supine and prone treatment positions. *Int J Radiat Oncol Biol Phys.* 2002;53: 1117–1123.

92. Litzenberg DW, Willoughby TR, Balter JM, et al. Positional stability of electromagnetic transponders used for prostate localization and continuous, real-time tracking. *Int J Radiat Oncol Biol Phys.* 2007;68:1199–1206.

93. Shirato H, Shimizu S, Kitamura K, et al. Four-dimensional treatment planning and fluoroscopic real-time tumor tracking radiotherapy for moving tumor. *Int J Radiat Oncol Biol Phys.* 2000;48:435–442.

94. Willoughby TR, Kupelian PA, Pouliot J, et al. Target localization and real-time tracking using the Calypso 4D localization system in patients with localized prostate cancer. *Int J Radiat Oncol Biol Phys.* 2006;65:528–534.

95. Quigley MM, Mate TP, Sylvester JE. Prostate tumor alignment and continuous, real-time adaptive radiation therapy using electromagnetic fiducials: clinical and cost-utility analyses. *Urol Oncol.* 2009;27(5):473–482.

96. Kupelian P, Willoughby T, Mahadevan A, et al. Multi-institutional clinical experience with the Calypso System in localization and continuous, real-time monitoring of the prostate gland during external radiotherapy. *Int J Radiat Oncol Biol Phys.* 2007;67:1088–1098.

97. Kupelian PA, Willoughby TR, Reddy CA, et al. Impact of image guidance on outcomes after external beam radiotherapy for localized prostate cancer. *Int J Radiat Oncol Biol Phys.* 2008; 70:1146–1150.

98. Kupelian PA, Willoughby TR, Reddy CA, et al. Hypofractionated intensity-modulated radiotherapy (70 Gy at 2.5 Gy per fraction) for localized prostate cancer: Cleveland Clinic experience. *Int J Radiat Oncol Biol Phys.* 2007;68:1424–1430.

99. Langen KM, Willoughby TR, Meeks SL, et al. Observations on real-time prostate gland motion using electromagnetic tracking. *Int J Radiat Oncol Biol Phys.* 2008;71:1084–1090.

100. McShan DL, Kessler ML, Vineberg K, et al. Inverse plan optimization accounting for random geometric uncertainties with a multiple instance geometry approximation (MIGA). *Med Phys.* 2006;33:1510–1521.

101. Lin A, Moran JM, Marsh RB, et al. Evaluation of multiple breathing states using a multiple instance geometry approximation (MIGA) in inverse-planned optimization for locoregional breast treatment. *Int J Radiat Oncol Biol Phys.* 2008 Oct 1;72(2):610–616.

102. Feng M, Vineberg KA, Lam KL, et al. Can we replace PTV expansions with a model of set-up uncertainty in IMRT for head and neck cancer? *Int J Radiat Oncol Biol Phys.* 2006;66: S102.

103. Feng M, Oh KS, Vineberg KA, et al. Multiple instance geometry approximation (MIGA) using individualized tumor motion data is equivalent to best breath hold method in IMRT for unresectable pancreatic cancer. *Int J Radiat Oncol Biol Phys.* 2008;72:S255.

^{18}F-FDG PET–Guided Target Delineation in a Patient with Esophageal Cancer

Case Study

Suneel N. Nagda, MD, John C. Roeske, PhD

Patient History

A 67-year-old man presented with a 3-month history of increasing odynophagia and substernal chest pain exacerbated by meals. Esophagogastroduodenoscopy (EGD) was performed and revealed an esophageal mass extending from 30 cm to 40 cm from the incisors. Two separate biopsies, taken at 33 cm and 35 cm, both revealed poorly differentiated, infiltrating adenocarcinoma.

Computed tomography (CT) of the chest and abdomen, ^{18}F-fluorodeoxyglucose positron emission tomography (^{18}F-FDG PET), and endoscopic ultrasound (EUS) were performed for staging purposes. Computed tomography revealed distal esophageal thickening without mediastinal adenopathy (Figure 19A-1). ^{18}F-FDG PET revealed increased metabolic activity in the distal esophagus (maximum standardized uptake value [SUV] 5.0) and in the right superior mediastinum (SUV 4.5; Figure 19A-2). No distant activity was seen. Software fusion of the ^{18}F-FDG PET and CT images demonstrated that the mediastinal activity corresponded with a small (9 mm short axis) right paratracheal/paraesophageal lymph node on CT (Figure 19A-3). This lymph node did not meet size criteria for enlarged mediastinal

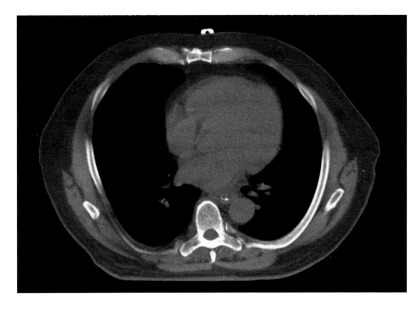

FIGURE 19A-1. Axial computed tomography slice through the thoracic esophagus. Esophageal thickening representing the tumor is evident.

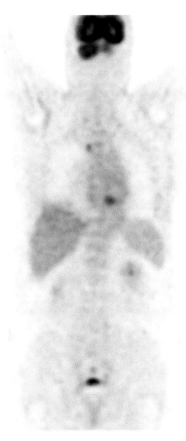

FIGURE 19A-2. Coronal positron emission tomography slice demonstrating uptake in the lower esophagus, as well as the right superior mediastinum corresponding to the malignant paratracheal lymph node.

A 14-mm malignant-appearing node was seen in the paratracheal area at approximately 23 cm from the incisors. A fine-needle aspiration of the lymph node was performed and pathology was consistent with a poorly differentiated adenocarcinoma. Final clinical staging was T2N1M0.

The patient's case was discussed in our multidisciplinary gastrointestinal (GI) oncology conference and the consensus recommendation was for neoadjuvant chemoradiotherapy followed by restaging and evaluation for transthoracic esophagectomy. The operating surgeon stated that the involved right paratracheal lymph node would not be removed at the time of surgery. We elected to use the ¹⁸F-FDG PET scan to help guide target delineation in this patient.

Simulation

The patient was brought to the department's AcQSim CT simulator (Philips Medical Systems, Andover, MA) and placed in the supine position with his arms above his head. He was immobilized by using a foam cradle extending from shoulders to pelvis. The immobilization device was indexed to the CT couch top, which mimics the couch on the treatment unit. Immediately before the scan, a teaspoon of radio-opaque paste was administered orally. Transaxial 5-mm images were obtained from base of skull to the top of pelvis.

Imaging and Target Delineation

The simulation CT and ¹⁸F-FDG PET were imported into the Focal (version 4.34) workstation (Elekta-CMS, Maryland Heights, MO). ¹⁸F-FDG PET images were registered to the planning CT data set using the system's automated algorithm (Figure 19A-4). Manual adjustments were made to fine-tune the registration. The ¹⁸F-FDG

adenopathy and was not identified on the initial read of the CT.

The EUS revealed that the primary tumor penetrated into the muscularis propria layer of the esophageal wall without penetration through the wall. Two 4-mm lymph nodes were seen within 5 mm of the tumor.

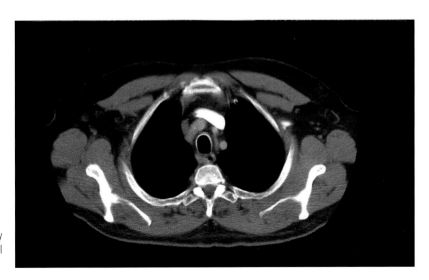

FIGURE 19A-3. Axial computed tomography slice highlighting the small right paratracheal lymph node.

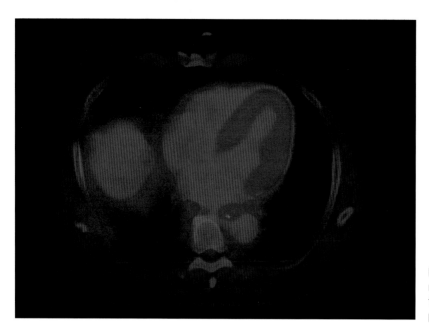

FIGURE 19A-4. Fused positron emission tomography–computed tomography images obtained from the Focal workstation at the level of the primary tumor.

PET window level settings were then adjusted to display a SUV threshold of 2.5 or greater. With the EGD, EUS, and ^{18}F-FDG PET findings, the primary esophageal tumor as well as malignant paratracheal were contoured as the gross tumor volume (GTV). The clinical target volume (CTV) was created by expanding the primary tumor GTV by 0.7 cm radially and 4 cm longitudinally (Figure 19A-5). The normal esophagus around the paratracheal lymph node was also included because of presumed mucosal and submucosal lymphatic drainage from the primary. Finally, a 0.8-cm three-dimensional margin was applied to the CTV to generate the planning target volume (PTV$_1$; Figure 19A-6) Boost volumes around the gross tumor in the esophagus (PTV$_2$) and the paratracheal lymph node (PTV$_3$) were also generated. The final target volumes were highly influenced by the ^{18}F-FDG PET detection of the malignant paratracheal lymph node and certainly would have been smaller without PET imaging.

Treatment Planning

Three-dimensional conformal RT (3DCRT) planning was performed. A dose of 45 Gy in 25 fractions was prescribed to the PTV$_1$, 50.4 Gy in 28 fractions to the PTV$_2$, and 64.8 Gy in 36 fractions to the PTV$_3$ using successive cone-down fields. The PTV$_3$ boost dose was higher than traditional dosing as the lymph node was not going to be removed during surgery. The PTV$_1$ was treated with anterior–posterior (AP–PA) and opposed oblique (right posterior oblique [RPO], and left posterior oblique [LPO]) fields with the oblique fields weighted lightly to minimize the dose delivered to normal lung parenchyma as patient was to have future surgery. The percentage volume of normal bilateral lung receiving 20 Gy or greater (V$_{20}$) was 27%. The boost volumes (PTV$_2$ and PTV$_3$) were treated with oblique fields to ensure that the maximum cumulative spinal cord dose remained below 45 Gy.

Clinical Outcome

The patient tolerated neoadjuvant therapy extremely well and did not require any unplanned treatment breaks. He underwent a restaging ^{18}F-FDG PET and CT scan 4 weeks posttherapy, which demonstrated that the previous activity seen in the mediastinum and distal esophagus was no longer present. Additionally, by CT, the involved paratracheal lymph nodes appeared smaller. The patient subsequently underwent a transthoracic esophagectomy and final pathology revealed residual adenocarcinoma of the gastro–esophageal junction. Ten lymph nodes removed were negative for metastatic disease. Final pathologic staging was pT2N0. At 46 months following therapy, the patient remains without disease recurrence on imaging and by clinical examination. No significant late significant sequelae have developed.

Our initial experience evaluating ^{18}F-FDG PET–guided target delineation in 22 patients with esophageal cancer was recently reported.[1] For purposes of this study, the tumor epicenter was determined to be the axial slice containing the greatest tumor burden based on CT, endoscopy, and ultrasound. The GTV epicenter was derived from the original GTV by reducing it superiorly and inferiorly, but not radially, to yield a 1-cm-long subsection of the tumor at the epicenter. The PET scans were then coregistered to the simulation CT scan. The PET volumes were delineated at various threshold levels

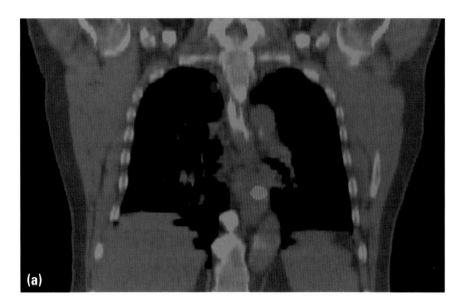

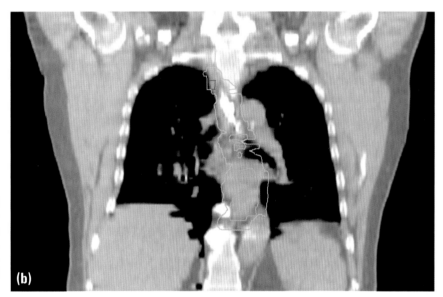

FIGURE 19A-5. (a) Coronal view of the fused positron emission tomography–computed tomography (CT) images with a threshold standardized uptake value of 2.5. **(b)** Coronal view of the planning CT illustrating the gross tumor volume and clinical target volume.

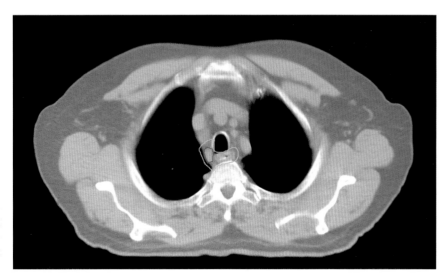

FIGURE 19A-6. Axial computed tomography slice showing the clinical target volume with inclusion of the right paratracheal lymph node and normal adjacent esophagus.

(SUV ≥ 2, ≥ 2.5, ≥ 3, ≥ 3.5; $\geq 40\%$, $\geq 45\%$, and $\geq 50\%$ of the maximum SUV) at the level of the GTV epicenter, according to previously published methods.[2] The ratio of the PET to GTV-epicenter volumes were then determined.

Of the 21 patients studied, the average maximum SUV was 10.6 (range, 4.1–25.4) and the mean GTV epicenter was 26 cc (range, 5 cc – 60 cc). Mean conformality indices were different and greatest for SUV ≥ 2.5. The mean PET-to-GTV epicenter volume ratios ranged from 0.39 to 2.82 across all thresholds, being closest to 1 at the SUV ≥ 2.5 level. These results suggest that a PET SUV threshold of approximately 2.5 yields the highest conformality index and best approximates the CT volume at the tumor epicenter.

Reference

1. Vali F, Nagda S, Hall W, et al. Comparison of standardized uptake value-based positron emission tomography and computed tomography target volumes in esophageal cancer patients undergoing radiotherapy. *Int J Radiat Oncol Biol Phys.* 2010 Nov 15; 78(4):1057–1063.

2. Hong R, Halama J, Bova D, et al. Correlation of PET standard uptake value and CT window-level thresholds for target delineation in CT-based radiation treatment planning. *Int J Radiat Oncol Biol Phys.* 2007 Mar 1;67(3):720–726.

MR-Guided Target Delineation in a Patient with Hepatocellular Carcinoma

Case Study

Charles Cho, MD, Mark Lee, MD, Laura Dawson, MD

Patient History

A 42-year-old man with a history of cirrhosis secondary to hepatitis B and human immunodeficiency virus (HIV) infection presented with an abnormal liver lesion on annual surveillance ultrasound along with an elevated alpha-fetoprotein (AFP) of 300 µg/L. Clinically, he had a Child-Pugh score of A5 and was asymptomatic at the time of presentation.

Additional radiographic studies included a triphasic computed tomography (CT) scan of the abdomen and pelvis, which revealed a cirrhotic liver with coarse hepatic attenuation and a nodular contour. An ill-defined hypoattenuated mass was noted in the right lobe of the liver spanning segments 6 and 7, measuring 2.8 cm by 2.2 cm by 3.0 cm. There was no obvious visible arterial enhancement or arterial venous shunting with washout, making it difficult to determine the tumor boundaries. The hepatic veins were patent without evidence of thrombus and no significant lymphadenopathy was identified.

As the CT did not clearly demonstrate the tumor, a magnetic resonance (MR) scan of the liver was obtained, which demonstrated an infiltrative mass with low T1 signal and high T2 signal within the posterior right hepatic lobe, measuring 5.8 cm by 6.5 cm. The mass demonstrated early arterial enhancement with washout on the portal venous phase.

Although no biopsy was performed, a clinical diagnosis of hepatocellular carcinoma (HCC) was made based on the patient's elevated AFP, known cirrhosis, and arterial enhancement on imaging, characteristic for HCC.

The patient was initially referred for transarterial chemoembolization, but was felt not to be a candidate because of his chronic neutropenia. Similarly, he was not a candidate for radiofrequency ablation because of the large size of the lesion. The patient was thus referred for treatment with conformal hypofractionated radiotherapy (RT) on an in-house phase II study. We elected to use MR imaging to help guide target delineation in this patient.

Simulation

Diaphragmatic motion under conditions of free breathing, abdominal compression, and active breathing control (ABC) to immobilize the liver in end-exhalation was assessed, by using kilovoltage (kV) fluoroscopy. ABC liver immobilization was chosen in this patient, as it reduced cranio–caudal liver motion from 26 mm seen with free breathing to less than 2 mm with repeat breath holds. The liver motion was 8 mm with abdominal compression. For patients treated with either free breathing or abdominal compression, cine MR is also useful in assessing the motion of the liver tumor in three planes (cranio–caudal, left–right, anterior–posterior), over longer time periods (several minutes), without any radiation exposure to the patient.

With the patient in a Vac-Lok (Bionix, Toledo, OH) body mold for immobilization, a computed tomography (CT) simulation was performed on a Discovery Hybrid PET–CT (GE Healthcare, Waukesha, WI). This scan was obtained in exhale ABC breath hold, with the patient in the supine position and both arms placed overhead. Trans-axial 3-mm CT images were obtained from the level of the carina to the femoral heads. Intravenous contrast at a rate of 5 cc per second was administered and the images were obtained at 25 seconds for the arterial images and at 60 seconds for the venous images.

Imaging and Target Delineation

Following conventional CT simulation, MR simulation was performed on a 1.5-Tesla Sigma Twin Speed scanner (GE Healthcare, Waukesha, WI). The patient was immobilized in the treatment position and repeat-exhale breath holds were used for liver immobilization. Intravenous contrast was administered and the images obtained at 15 seconds (arterial phase) and approximately 4 minutes (delayed venous phase). Extensive tumor thrombus extending to the right atrium was seen, consistent with rapid disease progression. Clinically, the patient was noted to have developed bilateral leg edema and fatigue. His AFP had also rapidly risen to 1490 µg/L.

The CT and MR simulation images were imported into the Pinnacle (Philips Medical Systems, Andover, MA) treatment planning software. The MR images were registered to the planning CT data set using mutual infor-

mation and manual adjustments to ensure the best rigid registration of the livers, with a priority in optimally registering the portion of the liver that contained the tumor (Figure 19B-1). The arterial contrast-enhancing HCC was contoured as the gross tumor volume (GTV; from the arterial contrast CT and MR) whereas the portal vein thrombus (GTV_PVT) was contoured separately from the venous contrast MR image. Fusion of the multiphase CT and MR images allowed better delineation of the primary tumor and thrombosis, as perfusion defects could be distinguished from tumor with MR, and the venous phases of imaging could be used for delineation of the tumor thrombus and arterial phase imaging was used for the primary tumor delineation.

A clinical target volume (CTV) was then created by expanding the GTV by 5 mm in all directions, within the liver contour. No CTV was created for the GTV_PVT as there is likely no microscopic extension of disease beyond the vessel wall. A planning target volume (PTV) was generated by adding a margin of 5 mm to the GTV creating a GTVPTV. A 5-mm PTV margin was also added to the

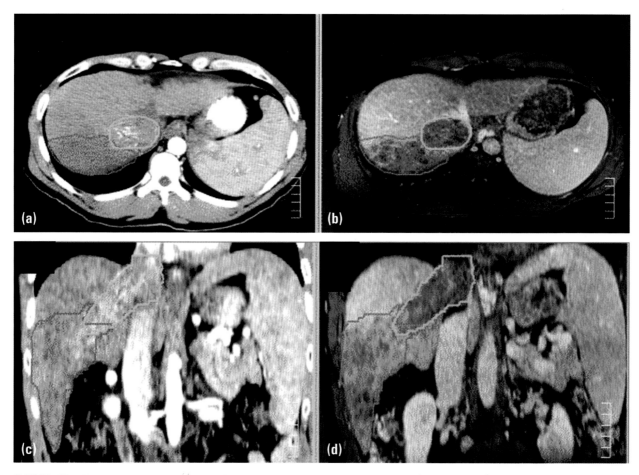

FIGURE 19B-1. Fusion of the magnetic resonance (MR) imaging of the liver with the primary computed tomography (CT) data set: arterially enhancing images obtained with active breathing control in end exhalation in axial (a) and coronal (c) planes, and venous phase MR images in axial (b) and coronal (d) planes that delineate the primary tumor and the tumor thrombus. The gross tumor volume is outlined in red with tumor thrombus outlined in green.

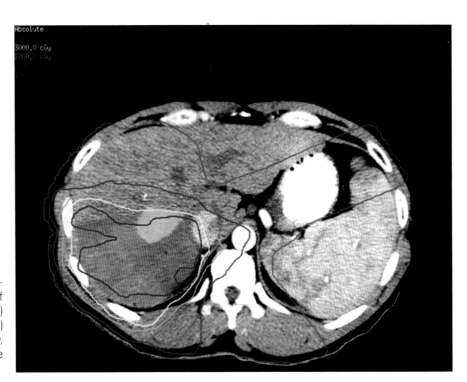

FIGURE 19B-2. Axial planning computed tomography slice with contours of the gross tumor volume (red colorwash) and tumor thrombus (green colorwash) and various isodose lines (blue 33 Gy, yellow 30 Gy, orange 27 Gy, purple 20 Gy, brown 10 Gy, in six fractions).

CTV and GTV_PVT. The PTV was used to account for residual geometric uncertainty in tumor position in this patient whose liver was immobilized using ABC breath hold and in whom daily image guidance using kV fluoroscopy and cone-beam CT (CBCT) was used during treatment delivery.

Treatment Planning

Intensity-modulated radiation therapy (IMRT) was used for treatment planning (Figure 19B-2). A dose of 30 Gy in six fractions was delivered to the PTV surrounding the GTV (GTVPTV) and the PTV surrounding the GTV_PVT. A dose of 27 Gy in six fractions was delivered to the PTV surrounding the CTV. A nonopposed five-field beam arrangement was used to minimize dose to the uninvolved normal liver. The dose constraints used for treatment planning included the spinal cord planning organ at risk volume (PRV) less than 27 Gy, duodenum less than 33 Gy maximum dose to 0.5 cc, stomach less than 32 Gy maximum dose to 0.5 cc, small bowel less than 34 Gy maximum dose to 0.5 cc, and large bowel less than 36 Gy maximum dose to 0.5 cc, in six fractions.

Clinical Outcome

Overall, the patient tolerated treatment very well. Symptomatically, he experienced mild nausea that required the use of prochlorperazine on an as-needed basis temporarily. His treatment was interrupted for a period of 1 week after completing four (20 Gy) of a planned six (30 Gy) fractions because of an elevation in liver enzymes that was attributed to the rapid progression of his hepatocellular carcinoma. After 1 week, the liver indices had improved significantly, which was attributed to a treatment effect, and he went on to receive the last two fractions of radiotherapy and complete his treatment as prescribed.

Initial follow-up imaging with a CT of the abdomen and pelvis 1 month posttreatment revealed stability of the thrombus and the primary tumor compared with the baseline diagnostic CT. A subsequent CT image 3 months following treatment revealed that the treated HCC had decreased in size and the right hepatic venous and inferior venous thrombi had decreased in caliber. There was a corresponding reduction in serum AFP level from 1499 μg/L to 146 μg/L. Clinically, the patient had complete resolution of his leg edema and renormalization of his elevated liver enzymes (to < 2X ULN). The patient was started on sorafenib 8 months following therapy because of development of thoracic metastases. At the time of most recent follow-up, 12 months following radiation therapy, there was no evidence of progression of HCC in the liver and liver function remained stable.

We have recently published several comprehensive reviews regarding the role of RT in patients with HCC tumors.[1-3] Moreover, our initial clinical experience using hypofractionated RT in HCC patients on an in-house dose escalation trial was recently presented.[4] In that study, 31 patients unsuitable for standard therapies were treated with hypofractionated regimens. Doses from 24 Gy to 54 Gy in six fractions were delivered to patients with both large and small HCC and Child-Pugh liver function class A. Most patients (53%) had portal vein thrombus. Overall, treatment was well tolerated with no dose-limiting toxicity seen following treatment, although five patients had a decline in their liver function at 3 months. However, these patients had large tumors, and three experienced rapid tumor progression most likely contributing to the decline in liver function. The median survival of the entire group was 11.7 months, higher than expected with similar untreated historical controls.

References

1. Dawson LA. The evolving role of radiation therapy in hepatocellular carcinoma. *Cancer Radiother.* 2008;12:96–101.
2. Krishnan S, Dawson LA, Seong J, et al. Radiotherapy for hepatocellular carcinoma: an overview. *Ann Surg Oncol.* 2008;15:1015–1024.
3. Tse RV, Guha C, Dawson LA. Conformal radiotherapy for hepatocellular carcinoma. *Crit Rev Oncol Hematol.* 2008;67:113–123.
4. Tse RV, Kim JJ, Hawkins M, et al. Phase I study of individualized stereotactic body radiotherapy for hepatocellular carcinoma and intrahepatic cholangenic sarcoma. *J Clin Oncol.* 2008;26(4):657–664.

KV Planar Image-Guided Tumor Localization in a Pancreatic Cancer Patient Treated with Respiratory-Gating Using the Varian Trilogy System

Case Study

Daniel T. Chang, MD, Albert C. Koong, MD, PhD

Patient History

A 63-year-old woman presented to the local emergency room with a 1-week history of nausea, gray-colored stool, dark urine, and painless jaundice. She also noticed a 15-pound weight loss over the preceeding 3 weeks. An abdominal computed tomography (CT) scan revealed a hypodense mass in the head of the pancreas with pancreatic and common bile duct dilation.

Further radiographic workup included a pancreatic protocol CT scan, which revealed a 4 cm by 3.5 cm mass in the head of the pancreas, with complete encasement of the superior mesenteric artery (Figure 19C-1). An endoscopic retrograde cholangiopancreatography (ERCP) was performed, and a biliary stent was placed into the common bile duct, which relieved the jaundice. An endoscopic ultrasound revealed a hypoechoic lesion in the head of the pancreas, measuring 3.8 cm by 4.4 cm. Fine needle aspiration biopsies revealed malignant cells consistent with adenocarcinoma. During this procedure, in anticipation of radiotherapy (RT), four gold fiducial markers were implanted into and around the tumor.

The patient's case was discussed at a multidisciplinary gastrointestinal oncology conference and the consensus recommendation was for initial treatment with gemcitabine-based chemotherapy followed by chemoradiotherapy using concurrent capecitabine and intensity-modulated RT (IMRT). We elected to treat her with respiratory gating using daily image guidance.

Simulation

The patient was immobilized in an alpha cradle in the supine position. A high-resolution biphasic (arterial and venous phase) CT scan was performed with images acquired at end expiration. In addition to intravenous contrast, oral contrast was administered. Transaxial 1.25-mm images were obtained from the mid-sternum to the pubis. The patient also underwent a four-dimensional (4D) CT scan to capture organ motion throughout the respiratory cycle. Positron emission tomography (PET) images were obtained 90 minutes following ^{18}F-fluorodeoxyglucose (^{18}F-FDG) injection.

Treatment Planning

^{18}F-FDG PET–CT images were registered to the arterial CT data set using the automated DICOM coordinate matching algorithm. The ^{18}F-FDG PET window level settings were then adjusted to display a standardized uptake value (SUV) threshold of 2.5 or greater. In addition, the CT image sets from the phases of the 4D CT at each end

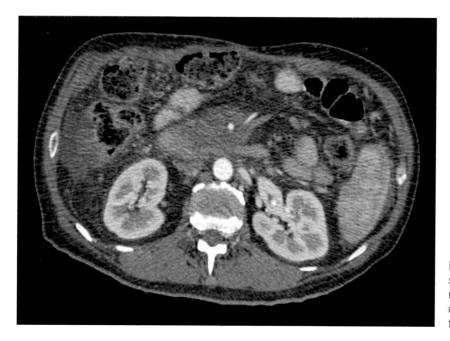

FIGURE 19C-1. Axial computed tomography slice through the upper abdomen showing a mass in the pancreatic head. The mass encases the superior mesenteric artery, and is therefore unresectable.

of the gating window, centered around end-expiration, were registered to the arterial phase CT scan to account for tumor motion. The gating window was custom-defined for this patient after manual inspection of the tumor motion throughout the breathing cycle and defining the phases during which the tumor appeared to be the most immobile. The gross tumor volume (GTV) was defined as the visible gross primary tumor seen on the arterial phase CT and ^{18}F-FDG PET scan (Figure 19C-2).

The clinical target volume-1 (CTV$_1$) was defined as the GTV and the regional lymph nodes (peripancreatic, celiac, superior mesenteric, porta hepatic, retroperitoneal). The internal target volume-1 (ITV$_1$) was created by adjusting the CTV$_1$ to encompass the tumor and nodal regions on the respiratory phases corresponding to both ends of the gating window. The ITV$_1$ was expanded an additional 5 mm for setup uncertainty to generate a planning target volume-1 (PTV$_1$). The ITV$_2$ was defined as the GTV only as seen on the arterial phase CT and the gating window 4D CT phases. A similar 5-mm expansion was added for the PTV$_2$ (Figure 19C-3). The normal surrounding structures, including duodenum, stomach, kidneys, liver, and spinal cord, were also contoured. In addition, the fiducial seeds were contoured, and a 5-mm expansion was added.

A treatment plan was created using Eclipse (Varian Medical Systems, Palo Alto, CA) to deliver 45 Gy to PTV$_1$ (1.8 Gy/fraction) and an additional 9 Gy to PTV$_2$ (1.8 Gy/fraction). The total dose prescribed to PTV$_2$ was thus 54 Gy. The plans were optimized so that 95% of the PTV received the prescription dose (Figure 19C-4). The dose constraints to the normal structures were as follows: maximum dose to the duodenum less than 55 Gy, volume receiving 50 Gy or above (V$_{50}$) of the duodenum less than 10%, V$_{45}$ of the stomach less than 15%, V$_{20}$ of each kidney less than 50%, V$_{30}$ of the liver less than 40%, and the maximum dose of the spinal cord less than 45 Gy.

Treatment Delivery

The patient was treated on a Varian Trilogy linear accelerator equipped with kilovoltage (kV) On-Board Imaging (OBI; Varian Medical Systems, Palo Alto, CA). Before each fraction, orthogonal kV images were obtained during end-expiration. Isocenter shifts were made to align the bony anatomy with the digitally reconstructed radiograph (DRR). Typically, on this static image, the position of the implanted fiducials are also visualized and confirmed to be in the correct position based on the projection of the fiducial contours onto the DRR by making additional isocenter shifts for the seeds to be centered within the projected fiducial contours. Fluoroscopy was then used to verify this seed positioning. The expanded fiducial contours were projected onto the fluoroscopic images to note the correct position. Final shifts are applied under fluoroscopic imaging to confirm that the respiratory-associated motion of the fiducials occurs in concert with the gated radiation treatment such that the beam is "on" when the seeds migrate into the projected fiducial contours with expiration and the beam is "off" when the seeds migrate outside the projected contours with inspiration (Figure 19C-5). After this final verification step was performed for both orthogonal isocenter angles, the radiation treatment was given, and this process was repeated at the beginning of each daily treatment.

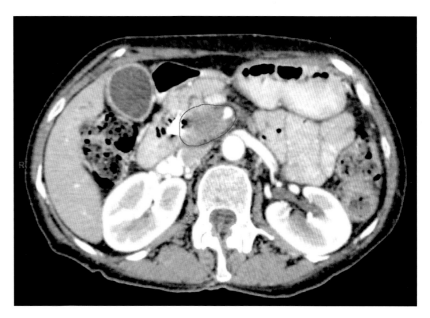

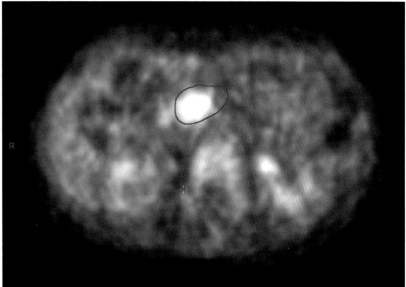

FIGURE 19C-2. Coregistered ¹⁸F-fluorode-oxyglucose positron emission tomography and computed tomography image showing the hypermetabolic region corresponding to the pancreatic mass. The gross tumor volume is contoured in brown.

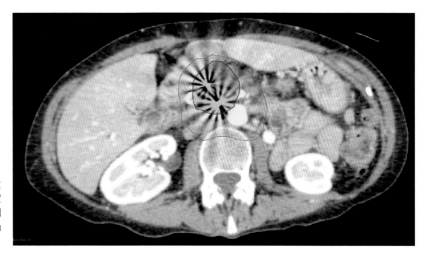

FIGURE 19C-3. Planning target volume-1 (PTV$_1$; green colorwash) and planning target volume-2 (PTV$_2$; red colorwash) on the planning computed tomography scan. Two fiducial markers are seen within the PTV$_2$.

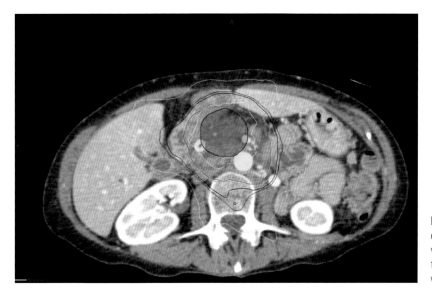

FIGURE 19C-4. Composite isodose plan generated to deliver 45 Gy to the planning target volume-1 (PTV$_1$; green colorwash) and 54 Gy to the planning target volume-2 (PTV$_2$; red colorwash) sequentially.

Clinical Outcome

The patient tolerated the treatment well with grade 2 diarrhea, nausea, and grade 1 vomiting, all of which were well-controlled with standard antidiarrheal and antinausea medication. At 3 months post-RT, an ^{18}F-FDG PET scan revealed a significant decrease in metabolic activity of the primary tumor with no evidence of metastases. A follow-up pancreatic protocol CT scan showed no significant change in the tumor. Further follow-up imaging scans showed continued stability of the tumor, and at 9 months following therapy, the patient remains without progressive disease clinically or radiographically. No significant late toxicities have developed.

We recently analyzed interfractional uncertainty comparing pancreatic tumor position using bony anatomy and implanted fiducial markers in five pancreatic adenocarcinoma patients undergoing IMRT with respiratory gating.[1] Daily kV orthogonal images were obtained to verify patient positioning, and isocenter shifts were made initially to match bony anatomy. A final shift to the fiducial seeds was made under fluoroscopic guidance to confirm location of the pancreatic tumor during the respiratory-gated phase. In a total of 140 fractions analyzed, the mean absolute shift to the fiducial markers after aligning the bony anatomy was 1.6 mm (range, 0–9 mm), 1.8 mm (range, 0–13 mm) and 4.1 mm (range, 0–19 mm) in the anterior–posterior, left–right, and superior–inferior directions, respectively. The mean interfractional vector shift distance was 5.5 mm (range, 0–19.3 mm). In 28 of 140 fractions (20%), no fiducial shift was required after alignment to bony anatomy.

Reference

1. Jayachandran P, Minn AY, Van Dam J, et al. Interfractional uncertainty in the treatment of pancreatic cancer with radiation. *Int J Radiat Oncol Biol Phys.* 2010; 76(2):603–607.

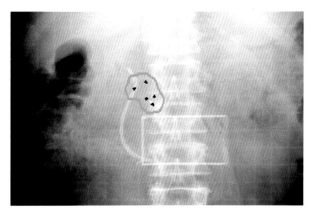
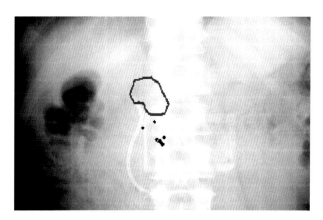

FIGURE 19C-5. Amplitude gating using fluoroscopy: The gating window is based on the seed position. In the right image, during inspiration, the seeds migrate outside the projected fiducial contour, which turns red to indicate beam "off." In the left image, during expiration, the seeds migrate into the projected fiducial contour, which turns green to indicate beam "on."

Image-Guided Hypofractionated Radiotherapy Using the RTRT System in a Patient with Hepatocellular Carcinoma

Case Study

Hiroshi Taguchi, MD, Masayori Ishikawa, PhD, Hiroki Shirato, MD

Patient History

A 64-year-old man with a history of hepatitis C viral infection and multiple other comorbidities presented with a 6.5-cm liver mass consistent with a primary hepatocellular carcinoma on routine follow-up abdominal computed tomography (CT) imaging.

In light of his multiple significant comorbidites (ischemic heart disease and diabetes-induced renal failure), surgical resection and liver transplantation were not considered. Transarterial chemoembolization using iodized oil was performed twice over a 3-month period but did not effectively eradicate the tumor. The residual tumor was too large for radiofrequency ablation or percutaneous ethanol injection. At that time, the PIVKA-II (protein-induced by vitamin K absence or antagonist II) level was 85 mAU/mL. His alpha-fetoprotein level was not elevated.

We thus elected to treat the patient with image-guided hypofractionated radiotherapy (RT) using the Real-Time Tumor Tracking (RTRT) system (Mitsubishi Co Ltd, Tokyo, Japan).

Simulation

Before simulation, a gold fiducial marker was inserted transcutaneously by an interventional radiologist under ultrasound guidance. An effort was made to place the gold marker within 3 cm of the tumor. The tip of the needle was verified not to be in any of the vessels or the bile tract by applying negative pressure. Under fluoroscopic guidance using a guide-wire, the introducer of the gold marker was inserted. After the guide-wire was removed, a 2.0-mm gold marker was inserted from the end of the introducer. To absorb blood resulting from bleeding induced by the procedure, gelatin sponges were also inserted.

After confirmation of reproducibility of the marker position the patient was taken to our multislice CT simulator (Aquilion, Toshiba Corporation, Tokyo, Japan) and placed in the supine position without any molds or shells. Transaxial imaging at end expiration with a slice thickness of 1 mm was performed to include the entire liver. Intravenous contrast was used to aid in visualization of the tumor.

Treatment Planning

Planning CT images were transferred to our departmental treatment planning system XiO (Elekta-CMS, Maryland Heights, MO) and the tumor and organs at risk (OARs) were contoured. The gross tumor volume (GTV) consisted of all visualized tumor on the planning CT scan. The GTV was 161 cc. A 5-mm expansion was used to create the clinical target volume (CTV). The planning target volume (PTV) was generated by adding 5 mm in all directions around the CTV. The OARs consisted of the liver, stomach, duodenum, colon, lung, and spinal cord.

A single isocenter was placed manually ensuring that the implanted fiducial marker would be in the visible area (i.e., within 50 mm from the isocenter) of the RTRT system. Six non-coplanar static beams (table angles: 0°, 90°) were used for treatment planning and the prescribed total dose was 40 Gy in eight fractions.

Gantry angles were 15° and 330° at the table angle 90°, 283°, 165°, 205°, and 245°, respectively (Figure 19D-1).

Maximum, minimum, and mean dose to GTV was 42 Gy, 32 Gy, and 40 Gy, respectively. Doses to OARs were reviewed and judged to be acceptable, with the mean liver dose of 13 Gy. After plan approval, the CT image data set, isocenter location, and couch information of each beam were exported to the computer of the RTRT system. Anterior–posterior (AP) and right lateral digitally reconstructed radiographs (DRRs) were generated for patient setup.

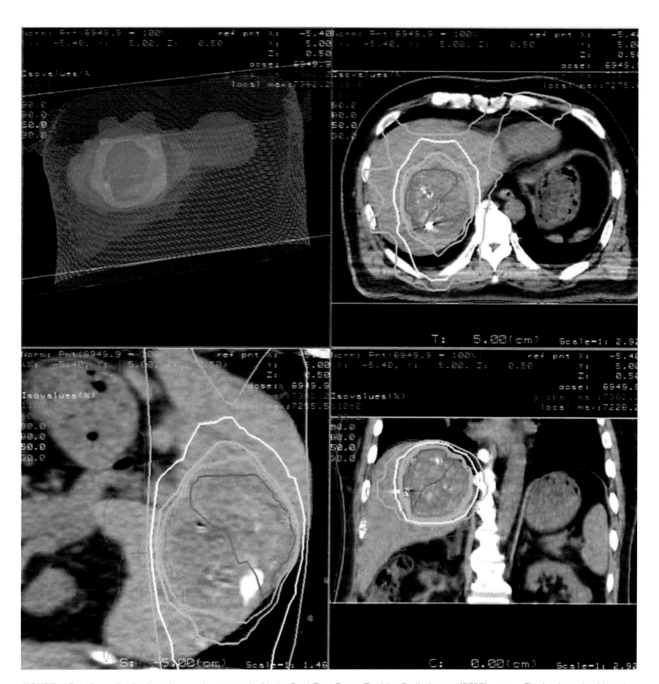

FIGURE 19D-1. Dose distribution of the patient treated with the Real-Time Tumor-Tracking Radiotherapy (RTRT) system. The implanted gold marker is visible on the transaxial and coronal reconstructed images. Blue, green, light blue, white, and orange lines represent 100%, 90%, 80%, 50%, and 30% of the prescribed dose of 40 Gy in eight fractions.

Treatment Delivery

Before bringing the patient into the vault for treatment, additional quality assurance (QA) was performed by the physics staff. A matrix method was used to calibrate the coordinates of the RTRT system relative to the linear accelerator (MHCL-15, Mitsubishi Electronics, Tokyo, Japan).

The patient was then positioned using optical guidance on the treatment couch. As additional QA for patient setup, a pair of orthogonal kilovoltage images was obtained. These images were compared with the DRRs to confirm correct patient positioning grossly. By briefly switching on the x-ray sources, the operator confirmed that (1) the implanted marker was visible using the two selected fluoroscopic cameras, (2) the reference markers coincided with their planned coordinates, and (3) the moving tumor marker passed through its planned position. If necessary, the patient couch was adjusted by remote control from outside the treatment room.

Treatment was delivered on a linear accelerator using 6-MV photons. During treatment, the fluoroscopic camera was used to provide real-time (intrafraction) monitoring of the gold marker. The RTRT system was switched on and started to search automatically for the marker in the x-ray images. Once the computer recognized the tumor marker, a black square was centered on the marker. This square followed the movement of the marker in real time. The image recognition system automatically interlocks the linac when the quality of the match is poor. The three-dimensional (3D) coordinates of the tumor marker were then calculated from the pair of images 30 times a second. The linac was enabled during the period that the detected location of the tumor marker was within the accepted volume as defined by the "allowed displacement" values (Figure 19D-2). For this patient, if an internal displacement of greater than 2.0 mm were to occur, treatment would be stopped and the patient repositioned. Treatment was completed within a 1-hour time slot. The trajectory of the marker position was stored in the computer.

Clinical Outcome

Overall, treatment was well tolerated, without any significant acute toxicities. At 3 months posttreatment, the tumor diameter was reduced in size. The PIVKA-II level decreased to 22 mAU/mL at 6 months and was less than 10 mAU/mL 9 months posttreatment. At that time, a follow-up magnetic resonance (MR) image of the liver revealed a near complete response.

No elevation in liver function tests was noted during or following treatment. A transient, small gastric

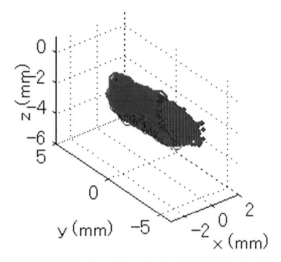

FIGURE 19D-2. The three-dimensional path of the implanted gold marker near the tumor during treatment. The red dots represent the irradiated tumor position, the blue dots represent the not-irradiated tumor position. Some overlap is caused by filtering in this analysis.

ulcer was noted 21 months following therapy. Of note, the total dose to the gastric wall in this region was estimated to be less than 8 Gy to 12 Gy. From the transient clinical course and its shape, it was felt not to be related to the treatment (Figure 19D-3). A CT scan performed 3 years posttreatment demonstrated no evidence of disease recurrence. [Dr. Roeske: No Figure 4 was provided. 2 views of Figure 3 show before and after. Should ref. to Fig. 4 be eliminated?] No new liver tumors have been detected in subsequent follow-up ultrasound, CT, or MR examinations. The patient was seen most recently approximately 7 years after RTRT treatment, at which time he remained without any complaints referable to the liver and had no liver dysfunction.

Our clinical experience using the RTRT system in patients with hepatocellular carcinoma was published earlier.[1] From 2001 to 2004, 18 lesions (mean diameter, 36 mm) in 15 patients were treated. All tumors were treated with a hypofractionated schedule with tight margins for setup and organ motion using a 2-mm fiducial marker implanted in the liver. The most commonly used dose was 48 Gy in eight fractions. With a mean follow-up period of 20 months (range, 3–57 months), the 2-year overall survival rate was 39%. Two-year local control rates were 83% for initial RTRT but was 92% after allowance for re-irradiation using RTRT. Significant sequelae were uncommon, with only one patient developing a transient grade 3 gastric ulcer and two patients with transient grade 3 increases in liver function tests.

344 / Image-Guided Radiation Therapy: A Clinical Perspective

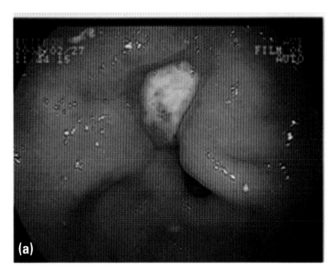 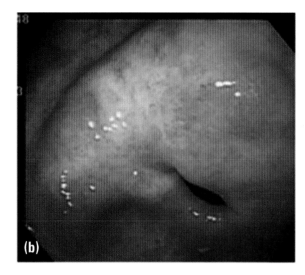

FIGURE 19D-3. (a) A gastric ulcer developed on the stomach wall at 21 months after the treatment (left side). It was felt not to be consistent with a radiation-induced ulcer; no inflammatory change around the ulcer was seen. (b) One year later, the ulcer was no longer present.

Reference

1. Taguchi H, Sakuhara Y, Hige S, et al. Intercepting radiotherapy using a real-time tumor-tracking radiotherapy system for highly selected patients with hepatocellular carcinoma unresectable with other modalities. *Int J Radiat Oncol Biol Phys.* 2007;69: 376–380.

KV Planar Image-Guided SBRT Using the CyberKnife System in a Patient with Recurrent Pancreatic Cancer

Case Study

Chris Lominska, MD, Frank Xia, PhD, Nadim Nasr, MD, Gregory Gagnon, MD

Patient History

A 69-year-old woman presented with vague abdominal complaints. Abdominal computed tomography (CT) revealed a 7-cm multiloculated cyst in the tail of the pancreas. Endoscopic ultrasound-guided fine-needle aspiration was performed revealing an elevated carcinoembryonic antigen level, consistent with a mucinous cystic neoplasm.

The patient subsequently underwent a distal pancreatectomy with splenectomy. The pathology was consistent with invasive ductal pancreatic adenocarcinoma, with associated intraductal papillary mucinous neoplasm and a positive pancreatic margin. Lymph node evaluation was negative. A completion pancreatectomy was performed with no evidence of residual malignancy.

She then underwent adjuvant radiotherapy (RT) to the pancreatic bed and regional nodes using a three-field (anterior–posterior [AP] and right and left lateral) technique. Treatment was performed with concurrent capecitabine. The patient declined further treatment after 4140 cGy secondary to significant gastrointestinal toxicity.

The patient did well until 1 year following her diagnosis when she developed a 2-cm recurrent mass involving the superior mesenteric artery (SMA) on a surveillance abdominal CT scan. No other sites of disease involvement were detected. The recurrent lesion was not amenable to surgery secondary to SMA involvement. Salvage gemcitabine was offered; however, she declined further chemotherapy. Given her localized disease recurrence, we elected to treat the patient with image-guided stereotactic body RT (SBRT) using the CyberKnife (Accuray Inc, Sunnyvale, CA).

Simulation

The patient was simulated in the supine position with arms at her sides, a pillow under her head and angled sponge under her knees. A treatment planning 1.25-mm fine-cut positron emission tomography (PET)–CT scan was performed (Figure 19E-1) using a Biograph 6 (Siemens AG, Erlangen, Germany) with 14.9 mCi of ^{18}F-fluorodeoxyglucose (^{18}F-FDG). Because the target volume was not felt to exhibit significant motion with respiration because of its location and vessel involvement, fiducial placement and respiratory tracking were not performed in this case.

Treatment Planning

The PET and CT images were fused and the PET-positive gross tumor volume (GTV) was contoured, as well as a high-risk adjacent prevertebral lymph node region clinical target volume (CTV). Organs at risk (OARs) were contoured including the spinal cord, kidneys, small bowel, and stomach. No expansion was applied to create the planning target volume (PTV).

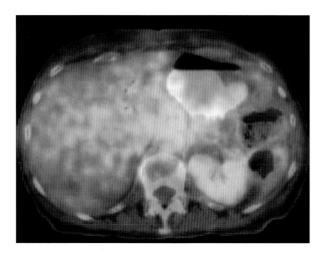

FIGURE 19E-1. Treatment planning positron emission tomography–computed tomography scan, demonstrating tumor recurrence in the region of the superior mesenteric artery with a maximum standardized uptake value of 6.5.

The images with contoured targets and OARs were transferred to the CyRIS MultiPlan treatment planning system (Accuray Inc, Sunnyvale, CA). A nonisocentric treatment technique was selected, using a 20-mm collimator for treatment. Inverse planning was performed for a prescription dose of 2500 cGy in five fractions to the prevertebral high-risk area and 3000 cGy in five fractions to the PET-positive GTV (Figure 19E-2). Treatment was prescribed to the 62.5% isodose line for the prevertebral high-risk area and to the 75% isodose line for the GTV. The prescribed isodose lines encompassed 99.8% and 99.6% of the high-risk CTV and the PET-positive GTV, respectively. A total of 226 beams were employed, with total treatment monitor units equaling 49,986. Doses to the OARs were reviewed and deemed to be within an

acceptable range. Specifically, the maximum point dose to the bowel was less than 3000 cGy, and maximum point dose to the spinal cord was 1310 cGy.

Treatment Delivery

After being placed on the treatment couch in the supine position, the patient was aligned with reference to the CT planning scan using the Xsight spine tracking system (Accuray Inc, Sunnyvale, CA). This system obtains orthogonal images taken from portals mounted on the treatment machine and compares them to digitally reconstructed radiographs (DRRs) from the planning CT scan. During treatment, the Xsight imaging system provided real-time, orthogonal x-ray images of the patient to verify treatment. Computers provided tracking of reference spinal points along the x-, y-, and z-axes and rotations about each axis. For setup purposes, the overlaid images were required to be within 1 mm on the x-, y-, and z-axes and 1° of rotation (Figure 19E-3). Dynamic tracking data were then automatically transmitted for positioning and pointing of the compact 6-megavoltage (MV) linear accelerator mounted on the robotic arm capable of delivering multiple, nonisocentric, non-coplanar radiation beams. Imaging occurred every minute and the robot corrected the position of the x-ray source for intrafraction positional variation.

Treatment was delivered over 5 consecutive days. Treatment delivery was divided into three paths through which the robot moved, each made up of discrete stopping points or nodes. Each node is a potential platform for dose delivery, with actual doses ranging from 0 cGy to 67 cGy per node. Path one consisted of 106 nodes (10 of which were null nodes not delivering any dose) that delivered 257 cGy with an output of 4953 monitor units (MU). Path two consisted of 86 nodes (five null nodes)

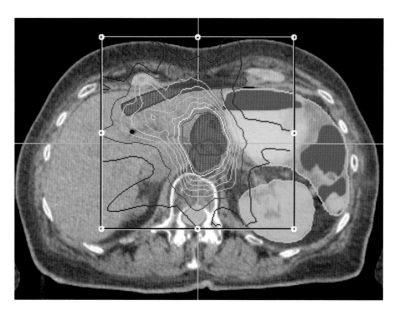

FIGURE 19E-2. Inverse treatment plan with isodose lines and contoured target volumes and organs at risk. The overlapping target volumes consist of the gross tumor volume (GTV; highly positron emission tomography–avid primary site), with the prevertebral clinical target volume (CTV; which separated from the GTV inferiorly) felt to represent a high-risk nodal area. The prescription was 500 cGy to the CTV and 600 cGy to the GTV for five fractions to a total dose of 25 Gy and 30 Gy, respectively. Treatment was prescribed to the 75% (orange) isodose line.

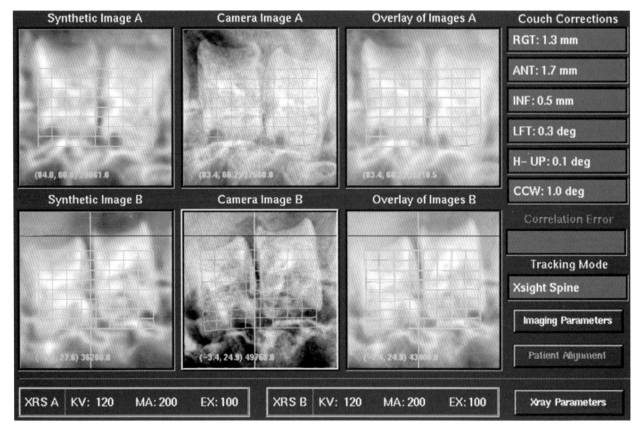

FIGURE 19E-3. Paired synthetic images along with the setup images and overlay grid. The associated couch corrections are shown in the x,y,z coordinates, as well as the rotational corrections for roll, pitch, and yaw, respectively.

delivering 271 cGy with an output of 3940 MU. The final path consisted of 34 nodes (five null nodes) delivering 72 cGy with an output of 1104 MU.

The mean patient setup time was 20 minutes, with a mean treatment time of 54 minutes, resulting in an average total time of 74 minutes. Approximately 45 paired orthogonal images were taken during each treatment. A total of 253 paired orthogonal images were taken during the delivery of the five treatment fractions for an estimated additional dose of 25.3 cGy.

Treatment was delivered with concurrent capecitabine. Because of her history of poor tolerance of abdominal radiotherapy, she was treated with daily prophylactic oral ondansetron.

Clinical Outcome

Overall, treatment was well tolerated without any significant acute side effects. At 6 months posttreatment, a PET–CT scan demonstrated a good but partial metabolic response to therapy (Figure 19E-4). Eight months after treatment the patient developed fatigue and shortness of breath. A CT scan of the abdomen was performed showing no evidence of recurrent tumor; however, ascites and pleural effusions were detected. The cytology was strongly suggestive of recurrent malignancy. The patient underwent a course of palliative chemotherapy. She died of her disease shortly thereafter.

Our initial experience with image-guided SBRT in locally recurrent previously irradiated pancreatic cancer

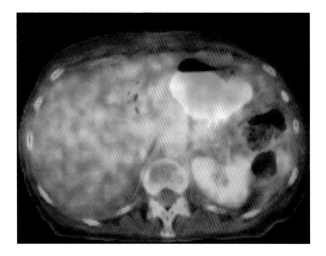

FIGURE 19E-4. Six-month follow-up positron emission tomography scan. Both the area and the maximum standardized uptake value (now 5) of the lesion have decreased.

patients was recently presented.[1] Between June 2002 and July 2007, 28 patients were treated after failing definitive chemoradiation (20 patients) or surgery followed by adjuvant chemoradiation (eight patients). Prior radiation consisted of a median dose of 50.4 Gy. Stereotactic body RT was performed using the CyberKnife system with a median dose of 22.5 Gy (range, 20 Gy to 30 Gy) prescribed to the 75% isodose line in three to five fractions. Of 24 evaluable patients, the median survival was 5.3 months (range, 1–27 months). Seven patients (25%) lived more than 8 months posttreatment. Treatment was well tolerated with only two patients experiencing serious gastrointestinal toxicity (one peripancreatic abscess,

one bowel obstruction). Both patients were treated with three fractions. Local control was achieved in six patients, local control with distant progression in six patients, and local and distant progression in two patients. The two surviving patients remained locally controlled at 3 and 8 months.

Reference

1. Lominska CE, Nasr NM, Silver NL, Gagnon GJ. Salvage stereotactic radiosurgery for locally recurrent previously irradiated pancreatic cancer [abstract]. *Int J Radiat Oncol Biol Phys.* 2008;72(Suppl 1):S276–S277.

Chapter 20

Genitourinary Tumors: Overview

Arthur J. Iglesias, MD, Dayssy A. Diaz, MD,
Radka Stoyanova, PhD, Alan Pollack, MD, PhD

The imaging tools available for target delineation and, hence, image guidance, have evolved substantially over the past 10 years. In particular, the development of intensity-modulated radiation therapy (IMRT) and the ability to control dose deposition has forced us to be ever more aware of how dose is distributed between the target(s) and normal tissues. This has fueled a revolution in image-guided radiotherapy (IGRT), in terms of both treatment planning and delivery. Prostate cancer is a model for the early adoption of image-guided methods.

From the application of computed tomography (CT)-based planning to conformal radiotherapy (RT) emerged the recognition that delivering higher RT doses to the prostate afforded a greater chance of remaining disease-free.

Multiple retrospective and the notable phase II dose escalation trial from Memorial Sloan-Kettering Cancer Center set the stage for a series of phase III trials demonstrating substantial gains in freedom from biochemical failure (FFBF) going from 70 Gy to nearly 80 Gy (Table 20-1).

A meta-analysis found a significant FFBF benefit for dose escalation when all of the trials ($P < .0001$) were considered.[1] This benefit was significant for National Comprehensive Cancer Network low- ($P = .007$), intermediate- ($P < .0001$), and high- ($P < .0001$) risk groups, although no difference was found for overall survival ($P = .69$) or disease-specific survival ($P = .41$). All of the trials had less than 10 years of follow-up, which is probably not sufficient for survival endpoints.

TABLE 20–1 Freedom from Biochemical Failure (FFBF) and Toxicity of Dose Escalation Randomized Trials[1]

		M.D. Anderson		MRC RT01		Dutch Trial		Zietmann	
		LD Arm	HD Arm	LD Arm	HD Arm	LD Arm	HD Arm	LDArm	HD Arm
	Follow-up, years	10		5		7		5	
	Definition FFBF	Phoenix		Nadir +2 (modified)		Phoenix		ASTRO	
	EBRT dose (Gy)	70	78	64	74	68	78	70.2	79.2
	Patients no.	150	151	410	401	301	333	197	195
	FFBF, %	50	73	60	71	45	56	61.4	80.4
Late GU toxicity	Grade 2 or greater, %	8	13	8	11	41	40	18	20
Late GU toxicity	Grade 3 or greater, %	5	4	2	4	12	13	2	1
Late GI toxicity	Grade 2 or greater, %	13	26	24	33	25	35	8	17
Late GI toxicity	Grade 3 or greater (%)	1	7	6	10	6	4	1	1

Notes. EBRT = external beam radiotherapy; GI = gastrointestinal; GU = genitourinary; HD = high dose; LD = low dose.

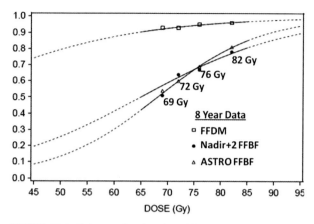

FIGURE 20-1. Eight-year freedom from failure rates using fitted logistic regression. Data are adjusted for pretreatment initial prostate-specific antigen, Gleason score, and T-stage.

Eade et al. described the dose response for more than 1500 men treated with three-dimensional (3D)-conformal RT or IMRT at Fox Chase Cancer Center from 1998 to 2002, demonstrating that there are continued gains of approximately 2.2% FFBF for every 1-Gy increase, even beyond 80 Gy, using either the Nadir+2 or the American Society for Radiation Oncology (ASTRO) definitions of biochemical failure (Figure 20-1).[2] These data, combined with biopsy data, indicate that lower RT doses do not completely eradicate disease—cells are left beyond that may take years to proliferate such that biochemical failure is identified.[3,4] The need for RT doses in the 80-Gy and higher range in 1.8-Gy to 2.0-Gy fraction equivalents is clear from multiple pieces of evidence. Image guidance affords an opportunity to address this problem head-on and improve patient outcome without increasing toxicity.

Associated toxicity is the main concern when dose escalation is used. Results from randomized trials have not shown any significant difference in late genitourinary (GU) toxicity[5-7]; however, the results are conflicting regarding associated gastrointestinal (GI) toxicity. Whereas the M.D. Anderson trial[6] and MRC RT01[5] showed a significantly increased incidence of grade 2 and higher GI toxicity, the Dutch trial[7] did not. The trend of higher GI reactions with dose escalation was reflected in the meta-analysis by Viani et al.[1]

At the root of enhancing the capability to maximize RT dose to the target structures and minimize toxicity to the organs at risk in patients with prostate cancer is image guidance in the planning and radiation delivery processes. These approaches are outlined here with an emphasis on magnetic resonance (MR) imaging for the planning phase and fiducial markers in the delivery phase.

The focus of this chapter is on patients with prostate cancer treated with definitive or postoperative RT. The potential utility of IGRT in patients with bladder cancer is illustrated in Chapter 20J.

Image-Guided Target Delineation and Planning

Magnetic Resonance and Computed Tomography Anatomy

The prostate is an exocrine gland that surrounds the prostatic urethra. The normal adult gland measures approximately 4 cm by 3 cm by 3 cm, and weighs 15 to 20 grams.[8] The size of the prostate generally increases with age and, according to Zackrisson et al.,[9] up to 85% of healthy men aged older than 40 years have prostate volumes higher than 20 cc. Five anatomical prostatic zones are recognized: (1) anterior fibromuscular stroma, (2) periurethral glandular tissue, (3) transition zone, (4) central zone, and (5) peripheral zone.[8]

Inconsistencies in CT contouring are the result of poor definition of the prostate relative to adjacent structures and wide variation in anatomic position relative to the pelvic bones.[10] The prostate tends to blend in with muscle, making it unclear where the prostate borders are relative to the levator ani muscle, the rectum (particularly inferiorly near the prostatic apex), and the bladder wall superiorly. Magnetic resonance imaging considerably resolves these boundaries and makes accurate contouring of the prostate more consistent[11,12] (see Chapter 20A). In addition, MR is less sensitive to imaging artifacts (Figure 20-2A) and allows better delineation of treatment volumes. Magnetic resonance–based prostate volumes are more aligned with ultrasound volumes[13]; CT prostate volumes are about 30% to 40% larger than MR volumes.[14,15] However, current planning algorithms are based on CT, making CT–MR fusion the best approach to define the prostate, seminal vesicles, and pelvic lymph node regions.

Fusion of CT and MR is fraught with potential problems that could lead to significant errors if not performed appropriately. The CT should be used primarily and the MR only used as a reference because of the inherent problems with the accuracy of the fusion. The position of the prostate on MR may be substantially different from that on the CT because of bladder and rectal filling. Such differences are influenced by the MR being performed at a different time (not in sequence with the CT) and in many cases on a concave tabletop (instead of a flat table on the CT simulator). If possible, the conditions should be replicated on the MR as much as possible. Patients should be given strict instructions on diet to minimize gas and should perform an enema before going for both the MR and CT. It would be best if a radiation simulation therapist were present at the MR and the MR equipped with lasers, ensuring that patient position and bowel and bladder filling are similar. In many instances this will not be possible and the fusion will be complicated as a result.

Fusion of MR and CT is based on soft tissue and not the bones. If there are considerable differences in bladder and rectal filling, the fusion will be inaccurate.

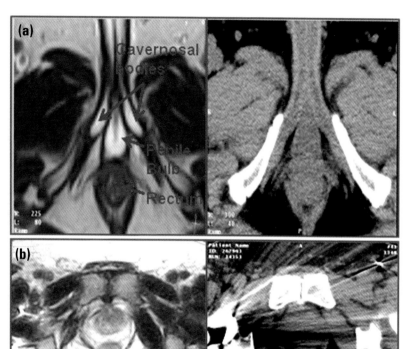

FIGURE 20-2. Magnetic resonance (MR)–computed tomography (CT) fusion for treatment planning. (a) Magnetic resonance and CT of a patient with right hip replacement. Magnetic resonance is less sensitive to the imaging artifact caused by the artificial hip and allows for better delineation of treatment volumes. (b) The penile bulb, cavernosal bodies, and rectum (marked with arrows) are clearly delineated on the MR.

The random error for CT–MR registration along the three spatial directions is estimated to be on the order of 0.5 mm and around 0.4° in rotation (standard deviation) for each axis.[16] One way to minimize fusion error is to place fiducials in the prostate before the MR, obtain T2* MR sequences and then fuse on the fiducial markers.[17]

Because MR is better than CT in determining extracapsular extension and seminal vesicle involvement, the clinical target volume (CTV) may be modified more accurately by using MR to include additional margin for subclinical spread in these areas.

The seminal vesicles (SV) are paired organs located in the connective tissue lodged between the urinary bladder and the rectum lateral to the ampulla of the vas deferens. Seminal vesicles can vary in size and differences in dimension between the right and left SV have been reported.[18,19] According to surgical specimen reports, the length is about 31 mm ± 10.3 mm,[18] which is concordant with reported results on ultrasound.[9]

The angle between the seminal vesicles and the horizontal plane (normally 50° to 60°) changes with bladder and rectal filling.[20] Seminal vessel contouring, similar to that of prostate contouring, is better delineated on MR because of enhanced anatomic detail.[21]

The bulb of the penis is formed by the elongation of the corpus spongiosum after the separation of the corpora cavernosa to form the crura of the penis. The bulb of the penis is attached superiorly to the inferior surface of the urogenital diaphragm.[22] It is best visualized on

T2-weighted (T2w) MR images as an oval-shaped, hyperintense midline structure (Figure 20-2B).[22,23] Although the penile bulb can also be identified on CT imaging and transverse transrectal ultrasound, MR is best for the superior and inferior aspects. Contouring should stop inferiorly when the bulb loses the lateral bulging aspects of the corpus spongiosum.

As summarized by Van der Wielen et al.,[24] the sparing of the penile bulb, corporal bodies, and neurovascular structures has sometimes been associated with increased preservation of erectile function, but results have been mixed.[23,25] Intensity-modulated RT reduces the dose received by the penile bulb, as shown by some authors.[26,27] Regarding the relationship between the penile bulb dose and the development of erectile dysfunction, some studies have not shown any significant association between the dose received and the development of erectile dysfunction,[28] whereas Merrick et al. found a significant relationship between the doses received by the proximal penis and the incidence of erectile dysfunction[29] and Roach et al. advocates keeping the penile bulb dose to less than 52.5 Gy.[30]

The prostatic apex is not recognizable on CT. The rectum blends into the apex posteriorly and urogenital diaphragm inferiorly. These structures are clearly visualized on T2w MR.[31] If one uses CT alone, the apex location may be estimated to be about 1.0 cm to 1.5 cm superior to the bulb of the penis. It is best to overestimate the inferior location of the apex in the absence of MR.

The use of adjuvant and salvage RT for selected prostatectomy patients has increased. The prostate bed borders are more clearly seen on MR, but CT provides a reasonable estimation. As mentioned previously, there are problems with MR–CT fusion and the MR should only be used as a guide. If clips are present in the bed, these may be helpful. The prostate bed CTV consensus guidelines have been described by Michalski et al.[32]

Prostate Imaging for Identification of Tumor Location by Biopsy

Presently, the clinically acceptable method for the diagnosis of prostate cancer is transrectal ultrasound (TRUS)–guided biopsy. However, TRUS cannot reliably visualize cancer foci, with up to 40% of tumors being isoechoic.[33] Because TRUS-guidance does not reliably direct the biopsy needle to the tumor location, a gridlike systematic biopsy of the gland is routinely performed in addition to biopsy of suspicious hypoechoic areas. Even with these additional samples, this technique misses up to 23% of cancers at the time of first biopsy.[34] If imaging could localize prostate tumors more accurately, then the biopsy needle would be directed more specifically to the site of dominant tumor lesions, which would be useful in confirming tumor location for RT planning.

Functional MR to Localize Dominant Tumor Locations

Several alternatives of gray-scale ultrasound for visualization of prostate cancer have been considered. The principal modalities competing with MR have been contrast-enhanced ultrasound (CEUS), and positron emission tomography (PET) performed with ^{18}F-fluorocholine and ^{11}C-choline.[35,36] Three-dimensional (3D) CEUS studies with whole-mount pathology correlation are lacking; thus, the ability of CEUS to localize cancer in 3D remains uncertain. The reported ^{18}F-fluorocholine and ^{11}C-choline PET studies have shown an inferior sensitivity to MR.

Magnetic resonance is the most promising noninvasive technique for utilization in the clinic for detecting prostate cancer. Accuracy of cancer detection with MR varies according to the use of either whole-mount prostate histology or TRUS biopsies as a reference standard. Differences in the methodology are also a source of variability. At present, whole-mount prostate histology is regarded as a gold standard and is the focus of the summary below.

Multiparameter MR, including T2w, T1 noncontrast, T1 dynamic contrast-enhanced MR (DCE-MR), MR proton spectroscopy (MRS), and diffusion-weighted MR (DWI) sequences have been shown to improve the sensitivity and specificity of tumor localization (Figure 20-3).

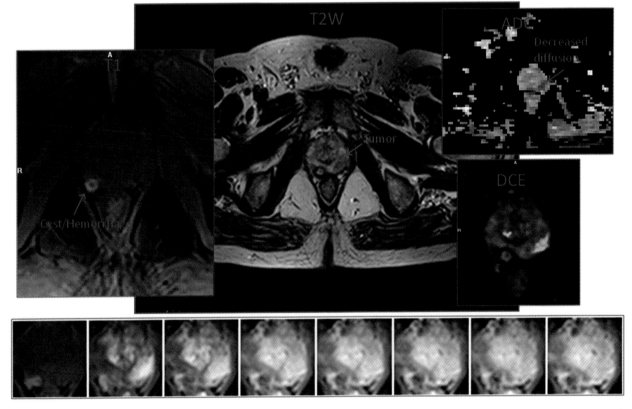

FIGURE 20-3. Multiparametric magnetic resonance (MR) imaging of the prostate. Center: T2-weighted MR. From top (counterclockwise): T1 image noncontrast; T1-dynamic contrast-enhanced (DCE) series (pre- and postcontrast); DCE area overlaid on the T2w MR; apparent diffusion coefficient map.

Magnetic resonance T2w provides an excellent depiction of the prostatic anatomy with regions of healthy peripheral zone prostate tissue demonstrating higher signal intensity than prostate cancer. The observed reduction in MR image signal intensity is attributed to a loss of the normal glandular (ductal) morphology in regions of prostate cancer. However, other benign pathologies such as inflammation, benign prostatic hyperplasia (BPH), blood, and prior irradiation also cause a loss of ductal morphology and low signal intensity on T2w MR. Additionally, infiltrating prostate cancer does not always cause a reduction in normal glandular morphology and, therefore, will not be hypointense on T2w MR. Because of these confounding factors, T2w MR alone can localize cancer larger than 0.5 cc in volume with only 65% to 74% sensitivity and low specificity.[37] Other studies also report quite variable sensitivity (50% to 83%) and specificity (21% to 88%). Utilizing an endorectal coil improves MR's sensitivity to 78%, but the specificity still remains poor (55%).

Magnetic resonance proton spectroscopy, DWI, and DCE-MR have been used to image the prostate to determine tumor location and extent. Localization accuracies of greater than 80% may be achieved by combining these methods.[38] Each has shown promise when combined with T2w MR. The technique that has consistently showed high sensitivity and specificity and has the greatest potential in our opinion for broader clinical application is DCE-MR.

Magnetic resonance proton spectroscopy imaging provides metabolic information specific to the prostate through detection of the cellular metabolites citrate, creatine, and choline.[39] The sensitivity and specificity of MRS alone and combined with T2w MR are 68% and 85% and 82% (59%–94%) and 88% (80%–95%), respectively. However, the technique is tricky and artifacts are common.

Diffusion-weighted MR is an imaging technique that is sensitive to random thermal movement of water molecules and provides a determination of stiffness. Diffusion-weighted MR measures apparent diffusion coefficient (ADC) values, which are significantly lower in tumor than in normal prostate because of the restriction of water displacement. Respective ADC cutoff values of 0.0014 mm^2/sec and 0.0016 mm^2/sec yield sensitivities of 82% and 95% and specificities of 85% and 65% for localizing tumor.[40] There have been gains in DWI, indicating that it may have a more general role in localizing tumor volumes that dictate outcome.

Dynamic contrast-enhanced MR imaging of patients with prostate cancer has also demonstrated potential for discriminating between normal and cancerous tissues.[41,42] Greater and earlier enhancement is seen in tumor tissue versus normal tissue (Figure 20-4). Dynamic contrast-enhanced MR is a measure of tissue vascularity and angiogenesis. There are varying sensitivity and specificity assessments of DCE-MR, depending upon what is used as the "gold standard"—biopsy or prostatectomy samples—and

how many partitions (bilateral, quadrants, sextants, etc.) of the prostate are correlated. Specificity has been notably high at close to or greater than 90% in a number of studies,[43,44] and sensitivity has been 65% to greater than 80%. A high sensitivity may not be desired because we are not interested in identifying all tumors, just those that have a high probability of requiring escalated RT doses to eradicate. In summary, DCE-MR, in our opinion, has the greatest likelihood of being broadly adapted in RT treatment planning to facilitate higher RT doses to subvolumes in the prostate.[45]

At the University of Miami, all patients who are a candidate for MR with contrast undergo diagnostic and simulation 3.0T MR of the prostate and pelvis using a body coil. Currently the sequences include T2w, T1 noncontrast, T1 DCE-MR, and DWI. The acquisition details are: resolution 0.7 mm^3 by 0.7 mm^3 by 2.5 mm^3; rectangular field of view: 360 mm by 264 mm; slice thickness: 2.5 mm; 72 slices.

Functional MR in the Postprostatectomy "Salvage" Setting

Magnetic resonance performed for a rising prostate-specific antigen (PSA) postprostatectomy identifies residual disease in the prostate bed (Figures 20-5 and 20-6) in the majority of cases when scrutinized by radiologists who are experts in the field.[46] The use of DCE-MR compliments T2w MR and the localization of residual disease is simplified. Recurrences present as lobulated masses with intermediate signal intensity on T2w images, slightly higher than that of muscle or fibrosis and they enhance early after intravenous injection of contrast medium.[47] Two recent studies on 51 and 72 patients, with a mean PSA level of 1.9 ng/mL (range, 0.1–6 ng/mL) and 1.23 ng/mL (range, 0.2–8.8 ng/mL), respectively, found sensitivities and specificities of 48% to 61.4% and 52% to 82.1% for T2 imaging alone. In the same patients, DCE imaging either alone or in combination with T2 imaging significantly improved sensitivity and specificity to 84.1% to 88% and 89.3% to 100%, respectively.[48,49] There is emerging evidence for a dose response in patients treated with salvage RT[50,51] and the MR data suggest that there may be bulkier tumor in the prostate bed than previously suspected.

ProstaScint Imaging

ProstaScint (Eusa Pharma [USA] Inc, Langhorne, PA) uses a radiolabeled monoclonal antibody (^{111}In capromab pendetide) that targets an epitope of the prostate-specific membrane antigen.[52] This imaging modality has been most often used for newly diagnosed patients at high risk for lymph node involvement and for patients with increasing PSA. A multicenter study reported by Hinkle et al. examined 51 patients at high risk for lymph node involvement.[53] When the results were compared with the

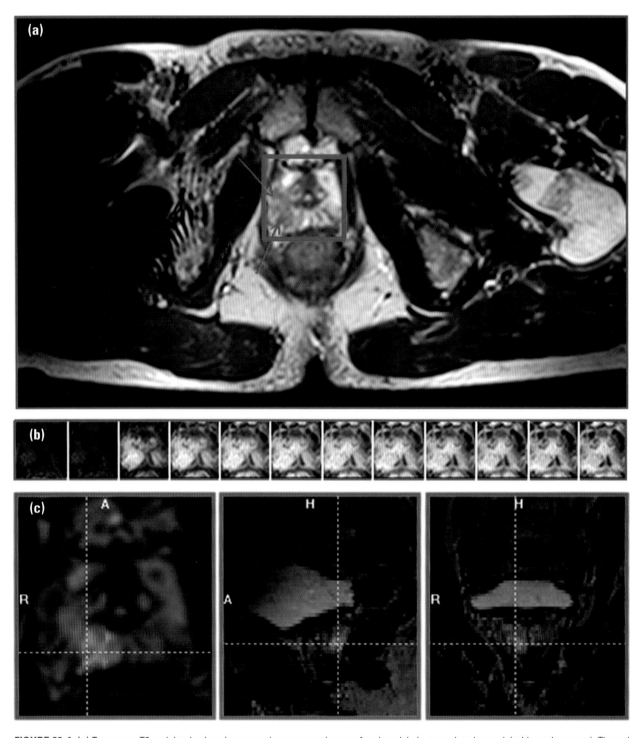

FIGURE 20-4. (a) Transverse T2-weighted spin-echo magnetic resonance image of male pelvis (note patient has a right hip replacement). The red box surrounds the prostate. The arrows indicate a hypointense area in the right peripheral zone suspicious for tumor. **(b)** Prostate area in the series of T1-weighted gradient echo sequence images, following contrast administration. **(c)** Axial, coronal, and sagittal T2w views of the prostate overlaid with a color three-dimensional dynamic contrast-enhanced (DCE) map depicting the area of the tumor.

pathological findings, high specificity, sensitivity, accuracy, and positive predictive value were found (86%, 75%, 81%, and 79%, respectively) compared with a combined accuracy of CT and MR of only 48%.

Ultrasound and single-photon emission CT (SPECT)–CT fused images were used for treatment planning in a study performed by Ellis et al.[54]; the patients received seed implant dose escalation to intraprostatic and periprostatic

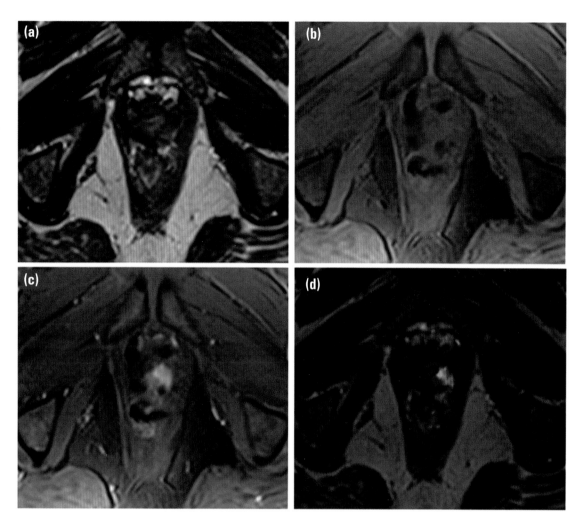

FIGURE 20-5. Transverse magnetic resonance (MR) images in a 56-year-old man 4 years after radical prostatectomy. Prostate-specific antigen level prior to salvage radiotherapy was 6.8 ng/mL. **(a)** T2-weighted (6000/112) fast spin-echo; **(b)** T1-weighted (5.08/2.3) gradient echo images precontrast. Note the artifacts created by surgical clips, which are only visible on the dynamic study because gradient-echo images are more sensitive to susceptibility artifacts. **(c)** Postcontrast dynamic MR images show early enhancement suggesting recurrent cancer in the left midgland. **(d)** Color dynamic contrast-enhanced map depicting the area of the tumor, overlaid with the T2-weighted MR. The recurrent cancer was not clearly seen on the T2-weighted images.

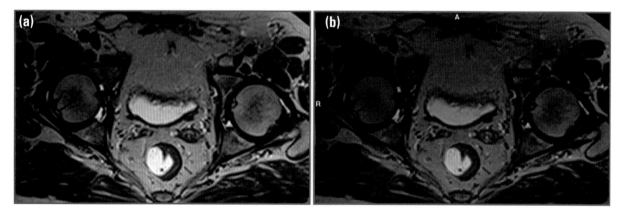

FIGURE 20-6. Transverse magnetic resonance (MR) images in a 71-year-old man 4 years after radical prostatectomy. Prostate-specific antigen level prior to salvage radiotherapy (RT) was 0.3 ng/mL. **(a)** T2-weighted MR with abnormal low intensity in the left seminal vesicle. **(b)** Color dynamic contrast enhanced map depicting the area of the left seminal vesicle, overlaid with the T2-weighted MR.

biological target volumes identified by SPECT–CT uptake (Chapter 20B). This group found a significant relationship between the SPECT–CT findings of ^{11}C-methionine (MET) and the FFBF, which suggests that SPECT–CT might be used as tool for prognosis of high-risk patients. However, further randomized studies are required to establish a benefit from the use of this immunoscintography tool.

Prostascint imaging has also been tested in the postsurgical setting; however, multiple studies have not established the test to be a predictor of clinical outcome.[55–58]

Volume and Field Delineation

In primary RT, the standard definition of gross tumor volume (GTV) is the entire prostate gland. This is actually incorrect, because the prostate gland is used as a means for estimating the CTV, not the GTV. In our practice, the GTV is defined on functional MR as being the areas of distinct tumor involvement. The CTV, therefore, is the prostate ± SV volume plus consideration of additional margin in areas where the GTV is perceived to contribute to a risk of extension beyond the gland. The CTV_1 for low- and intermediate-risk (T1–T2) patients includes the prostate ± proximal SV ($\leq$ 10 mm). In high-risk patients, the CTV_1 includes at least 50% of the SV, in addition to the prostate and any extraprostatic extension. In the high-risk patients, the CTV_2 is comprised of the distal portions of the SVs and the CTV_3 is comprised of the periprostatic

tissue, periseminal vesicle, external iliac, obturator, and internal iliac lymph nodes.[59] The planning target volume (PTV) is defined as the CTV with a margin to account for physical uncertainties including setup reproducibility and inter- and intrafraction organ motion.[60]

For postprostatectomy patients, CTV guidelines have been suggested by both the EORTC[61] and RTOG[32] (Figure 20-7). Table 20-2 shows a comparison of both guidelines comparing anatomical boundaries.

University of Miami Simulation Technique and Sequence

1. Magnetic resonance (3 Tesla/body coil) of the prostate and pelvis with T2, T1 plain, and T1 with DCE and DWI sequences in 2.5-mm slices throughout the pelvis. This is a diagnostic as well as a simulation scan, which should be obtained at 2.5-mm cuts.
2. Placement of fiducial markers (tracking beacons or gold seed fiducials).
3. Wait a minimum of 7 days for fiducial marker position to stabilize.
4. A limited 2.5-mm slice thickness MR-simulation is encouraged at this point to facilitate MR–CT fusion using T2* and T2w sequences.
5. Computed tomography simulation at 2.5-mm slices throughout the pelvis in supine position with legs in an immobilization device.
6. Computed tomography–MR fusion based on soft tissue and fiducials if step 4 is performed.

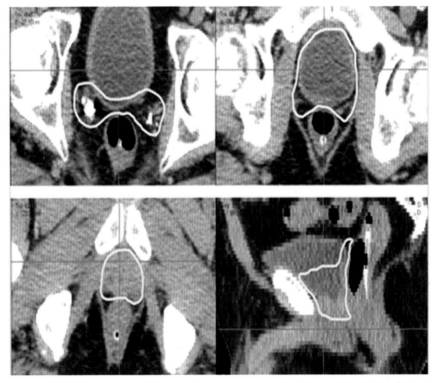

FIGURE 20-7. Axial and sagittal computed tomography views with consensus contours for patients with apical positive margins and biochemical recurrence. Reproduced with permission from Michalski et al.[32]

TABLE 20–2 Comparison of EORTC Guidelines and RTOG Guidelines

Limits	RTOG (2009)	EORTC (2007)
Caudal	8 mm to 12 mm below vesicourethral anastomosis	Including the apex (15 mm from the penile bulb)
Cranial	Level of cut end of vas deferens or 3 cm to 4 cm above top of symphysis	Bladder neck
Anterior	Caudal: posterior edge of pubic bone	
Cranial: posterior 1 cm to 2 cm of bladder wall		Including the anastomosis and the urethral axis
Posterior	Caudal: anterior rectal wall	Up to, but not including, the outer rectal wall
Laterally	Caudal: levator ani muscles, obturator internus	
	Cranial: sacrorectogenitopubic fascia	Up to the neurovascular bundles
Additional margins		CTV will include 5-mm margin in all directions; supplementary 5 mm in the posterior and lateral directions in the presence of incompletely resected ECE; supplementary 5 mm in the direction of microscopically involved tumor margins

Notes. CTV = clinical target volume; ECE = extracapsular extension.

Image-Guided Treatment Delivery

Adjusting for Prostate Interfractional Motion

Interfractional motion occurs during the daily setup of patients and can result in decreased dose to the PTV and increased dose to normal tissues. This is related to both setup error and prostate motion. Uncertainties may be systematic or random. Systematic errors do not change, they are reproducible, and they always occur in the same direction and magnitude. Random errors vary daily and they are not reproducible.[62]

The prostate is not a fixed organ and can change location from day to day.[63–66] The amount of prostate motion also varies from patient to patient and ranges in extent and is on average about 5 mm. Motion in the anterior–posterior dimension is usually greatest and in the lateral dimensions usually lowest. Correcting for interfractional motion is essential.

The impact of rectal distension on treatment dose and patient outcomes has been well-studied. A study by de Crevoisier et al.[67] in 2005 analyzed the effect of an increased rectal cross-sectional area on biochemical control rates and 2-year prostate biopsy results. In half of patients with a median increased rectal cross-sectional area (CSA) greater than 11.2 cm^2, there was a 25% reduction in freedom from failure rates 6 years after RT. On biopsy 2 years after RT, there was a statistically significant increased risk of positive cores on logistic analysis, correlating with decreased local control. Similar results were found by Heemsbergen et al.[68] in patients with an increased risk of geographical miss (anorectal volume > 90 mm^3 and > 25% of on treatment time diarrhea) and increased risk of SV involvement of greater than 25%. However, the effects of rectal distension can be mitigated by the use of daily image guidance.[69]

Ultrasound

Ultrasound has been used for to adjust for interfractional motion of the prostate for IMRT since the late 1990s[70] (Chapter 20C). Because it is inexpensive and widely available, ultrasound is a desirable technique for confirmation of daily positioning of patients receiving IMRT. In the early invocation of the technology, the therapists performing the alignments had to make judgments that contributed to variability that has been demonstrated in several reports to be greater than that seen with fiducial marker alignments.[71–74] Ultrasound has been shown to have greater systematic and random variation in daily setup and increased interuser (radiation therapist) variability compared with other methods.[71,72,75,76] However, if done under the strictest conditions, ultrasound is highly correlated with CT.[77]

Poor ultrasound image quality can be caused by increased distance from the probe to the isocenter, lack of bladder filling, increased tissue thickness anterior to the bladder, and bowel gas.[75] The pressure of the ultrasound itself has been reported to change prostate position by up to 5 mm.[75,78] Newer 3D ultrasound technology and methods of application are anticipated to reinvigorate the role of ultrasound in prostate alignments for RT.

Gold Seed Fiducials

Gold seed fiducials are currently the most commonly employed method to correct for interfractional motion employed. Although patients do require an extra outpatient procedure, they tolerate the insertion well.[79] The most common reported side effects are hematuria (15%) and rectal bleeding (4%). Patients report that their pain is less than that of diagnostic biopsy, even without local anesthesia. Fiducial marker alignment daily before each treatment has been shown to reduce variability and, consequently, may be used to reduce margins and increase dose.[80]

Three or four 2.0-mm gold seeds are implanted into the prostate with the location of placement essential; seeds need to be placed to represent the relevant anatomy, especially near the prostate–rectal interface. Although there is a concern over migration of gold seeds, this has not played out in multiple studies.[81,82] At the Princess Margaret Hospital, there was no significant migration of gold seeds in 6 years.[83] When markers do migrate, they move systematically and uniformly as a group, rarely more than 1 mm.[84] The use of androgen deprivation may cause uneven shrinkage of the prostate and change interseed distances. Gold seed fiducials can then be imaged daily via portal imaging, cone-beam CT (CBCT), or in-room CT scans.

The prostate moves independently relative to the bones. Using implanted fiducial marker margins of 5 mm to 7 mm, to less than 3 mm, have been advocated[84]; compared with the 7 mm to 11 mm margins advocated with the use of daily electronic portal imaging.[85] Similar results have been seen in multiple studies, although with various recommended PTV margins.[80,86–88]

Gold seed fiducial placement is an accurate and relatively inexpensive method of correcting for daily prostate and possibly even prostate bed motion.[89] At the University of Miami, we use a PTV expansion of 5 mm everywhere, except posteriorly where the margin is 4 mm. These margins are reasonable, particularly with the use of volumetric modulated arc therapy treatments of less than 3 minutes. Langen et al.[90] have shown that the chance for prostate displacement increases over time.

Cone-Beam Computed Tomography

Cone-beam CT is the reconstruction of 3D volumes from a series of two-dimensional (2D) projection images, performed on the patient on the treatment table. Cone-beam CT imaging of the prostate is mainly used for correction of interfractional motion. Megavoltage (MV) CBCT uses conventional radiation equipment allowing a common isocenter between imaging and treatment. The measures obtained by the use of CBCT are highly accurate, with the greatest displacement usually observable in the anterior–posterior (AP) axis.[65,91]

As reported by Morin et al.,[92] CBCT on the average delivers 0.6 cGy to 1.2 cGy per MV CBCT monitor unit (MU); MV CBCT and MV helical CT doses are slightly higher than for kilovoltage (kV) CBCT.[92] The MV CBCT dose is 5 cGy to 15 cGy[93] and 1.5 cGy to 12 cGy with the use of helical MV CBCT.[94]

Cone-beam CT appears to be associated with less variability than ultrasound.[95] However, therapists must still make subjective decisions[96] and it is likely that alignment to points using fiducial markers has less variability over-

all. The two techniques may be combined to assess bladder and rectal filling. A broad comparison of MV CBCT with other imaging modalities was done by Bylund et al.,[65] who compared the results obtained by their study with published studies using electromagnetic transponders,[97] ultrasound,[72] seed implants,[72] and CT-on-rails as imaging guidance methods; finding a close measurement to the reported with CT-on-rails, which, as it is known, provides the best definition for image guidance.

In postprostatectomy patients, ultrasound localization should be avoided.[98] Using in-room CT or CBCT, surgical clips (when present) may be used similarly to intraprostatic fiducial markers to confirm the localization of the prostatic bed. There is no proven advantage to using clips or fiducial markers in the postprostatectomy setting; CBCT provides excellent images of the bed and is probably adequate.[99]

Adjusting for Intrafractional Motion

Patients and targets may exhibit a relatively slow drift in the posterior and inferior directions that does not correct over time. These shifts have been correlated with pelvic muscle relaxation,[90] moving rectal content,[100] or bladder filling (most often when the patient is prone). On the other hand, transient target motion is sudden, often in the anterior and superior directions, tends to resolve on its own, and may be caused by peristalsis or gas.

There are many methods to ascertain the position of the prostate during radiation treatment. Previous studies have used fluoroscopy,[63,101–103] MR,[104–106] ultrasound,[107] and electromagnetic tracking.[90] Padhani et al. imaged the prostate using cine MR in 55 patients.[104] In 7 minutes of acquisition by imaging every 10 seconds, they observed movement in 29% of patients, with 16% having movements that were greater than 5 mm. Throughout most of the series, the maximal tumor motion occurred in the anterior direction.[101,104,107–110] Respiratory motion has also been analyzed in prostate RT and has been shown to be more pronounced in the prone position[111] and when patients are immobilized in thermoplastic shells.[112] Electromagnetic transponder tracking has allowed for the observation of real-time intrafraction motion during RT with very high accuracy.

The clinical effect of intrafraction motion is beginning to be elucidated; however, there are no consensus data. Li et al.[113] looked at the dosimetric effect of intrafraction motion by using electromagnetic transponder tracking devices (Calypso; Calypso Medical Technologies Inc, Seattle, WA) and found that 2 mm are sufficient when one is aligning the patient with electromagnetic transponders pretreatment.

Electromagnetic Tracking Transponders

Electromagnetic tracking transponders or beacons (Calypso) allow real-time tracking of the prostate during RT (see Chapters 20H and 20K). Transponders measuring 8 mm by 1.85 mm are transrectally or transperineally implanted into the prostate under ultrasound guidance. There are two placed at the base and two at the left apex. The beacons contain an array of alternating-current magnetic coils that emit a resonant signal detected by receiver coils on a moveable four- dimensional electromagnetic array or plate. A magnetic field of current is created between the array and transponder whereby a signal is detected, allowing for real-time tracking of prostatic motion. The transponders signal their position relative to that obtained on the planning CT at 10 Hz.[114] Patients are set up based on skin marks, then the couch is adjusted based on beacon readings until the patient is aligned to 0.0 mm ± 0.5 mm. The system continuously monitors the current beacon-projected isocenter compared with the intended isocenter. This information is used to stop the treatment if a predetermined threshold is exceeded. For example, a threshold of 5 mm or greater in the superior–inferior–lateral axis or changes of 4 mm or more in the anterior–posterior axis warranted treatment interruption and repositioning of the patient as adopted in the data reported by Bittner et al.[115] The threshold used in our institution is 3 mm. A temporary change noted in transponder that is less than 1 second requires no correction as normal anatomical function changes may account for these and are known to self-correct.

The beacons cause a significant artifact on MR. If the beacons are being used, an MR before placement is important. One should take note that if MR is used in follow-up, the beacons will interfere substantially with such assessments.

Image-Guided Stereotactic Body Radiation Therapy

Studies have theorized that the α–β ratio for prostate cancer may be as low as 1.5 Gy and, therefore, therapeutic ratio would be significantly improved with hypofractionation.[116] Preliminary results using SBRT with conventional linear accelerators or CyberKnife (Accuray Inc, Sunnyvale, CA) have been favorable[117–120] (see Chapter 20F). Target tracking with gold seeds is commonly used with CyberKnife being the most robust system for intrafractional tracking of the target and adjusting the radiation beams in near real-time. If the system detects a significant variation in the position of the intraprostatic markers, a pause in treatment occurs and the treatment couch is repositioned. The system compares the intrafraction images to the DRRs that were created at the time of treatment planning. A retrospective review of 21 patients performed by Xie et al.[121] looked at intrafraction prostate motion using stereoscopic imaging by confirming fiducial marker position during treatment. Variation obtained from imaging in a period of successive couch movements

represents a data set. A 2-mm variation was noted in 5% of the data sets within 30 seconds of treatment; the percentage increases with progression of time. The group found that an approximate tracking range of 40 seconds between imaging was sufficient to confirm intraprostatic treatment motion.

Future Directions

Image-guided RT has provided tools for the accurate delineation and targeting of prostate cancer. However, advances in technology are occurring at a rapid pace. The incorporation of functional imaging into treatment planning and delivery promises to further improve patient outcomes. directions to address on the IGRT field. One very promising area is in the imaging of hypoxia. Hypoxic areas are known to be highly radioresistant; therefore, pinpointing the location of these areas could lead to targeted boosts to overcome radioresistance. Blood oxygenated level–dependent MR (BOLD-MR) is a new tool that proposes to locate these hypoxic areas through the identification of paramagnetic deoxyhemoglobin, which allows the detection of pO2 within, and in tissues adjacent to, perfused vessels[122,123].

Hoskin et al.[124] compared the results obtained with pimonidazole staining of pathology specimens of 24 prostate cancer patients versus BOLD-MR findings in the same patients. The results showed sensitivity as high as 95% when there was a high percentage of tumor per grid; however, the specificity was low (36%). Moreover, the BOLD imaging reflects primarily acute hypoxia in contrast to chronic hypoxia attributable to the distance from the red blood cells from the chronic hypoxic areas. However, studies have shown a good approximation of BOLD-MR imaging with global hypoxic areas.[125] Therefore, BOLD-MR is an imaging method with high sensitivity that would allow the easy identification of hypoxic areas; however, further work is still required to have more accurate results.

Another very promising area that is on the verge of being applied on a broad clinical level is the use of lymphotropic superparamagnetic particles to detect lymph node involvement in the pelvis. Lymphotropic nanoparticle MR is a new imaging method that allows the identification of lymph node metastases. These particles are injected into the patient with posterior absorption by the macrophages in the lymph nodes, producing a hypointense signal in the normal nodes because of accumulation of the metabolite. In contrast, metastatic lymph nodes express a hyperintense signal,[123] highlighting the metastatic nodes. This imaging modality has the potential to identify micrometastases as small as 2 mm,[126] providing valuable information for treatment planning and selection of candidate patients for salvage therapy.[127]

References

1. Viani GA, Stefano EJ, Afonso SL. Higher-than-conventional radiation doses in localized prostate cancer treatment: a meta-analysis of randomized, controlled trials. *Int J Radiat Oncol Biol Phys.* 2009;74:1405–1418.

2. Eade TN, Hanlon AL, Horwitz EM, et al. What dose of external-beam radiation is high enough for prostate cancer? *Int J Radiat Oncol Biol Phys.* 2007;68:682–689.

3. Vance W, Tucker SL, de Crevoisier R, et al. The predictive value of 2-year posttreatment biopsy after prostate cancer radiotherapy for eventual biochemical outcome. *Int J Radiat Oncol Biol Phys.* 2007;67:828–833.

4. Zelefsky MJ, Yamada Y, Fuks Z, et al. Long-term results of conformal radiotherapy for prostate cancer: impact of dose escalation on biochemical tumor control and distant metastases-free survival outcomes. *Int J Radiat Oncol Biol Phys.* 2008;71:1028–1033.

5. Dearnaley DP, Sydes MR, Graham JD, et al. Escalated-dose versus standard-dose conformal radiotherapy in prostate cancer: first results from the MRC RT01 randomised controlled trial. *Lancet Oncol.* 2007;8:475–487.

6. Kuban DA, Tucker SL, Dong L, et al. Long-term results of the M. D. Anderson randomized dose-escalation trial for prostate cancer. *Int J Radiat Oncol Biol Phys.* 2008;70:67–74.

7. Peeters ST, Heemsbergen WD, Koper PC, et al. Dose-response in radiotherapy for localized prostate cancer: results of the Dutch multicenter randomized phase III trial comparing 68 Gy of radiotherapy with 78 Gy. *J Clin Oncol.* 2006;24:1990–1996.

8. Coakley FV, Hricak H. Radiologic anatomy of the prostate gland: a clinical approach. *Radiol Clin North Am.* 2000;38: 15–30.

9. Zackrisson B, Hugosson J, Aus G. Transrectal ultrasound anatomy of the prostate and seminal vesicles in healthy men. *Scand J Urol Nephrol.* 2000;34:175–180.

10. McLaughlin PW, Evans C, Feng M, et al. Radiographic and anatomic basis for prostate contouring errors and methods to improve prostate contouring accuracy. *Int J Radiat Oncol Biol Phys.* 2010;76(2):369–378.

11. Debois M, Oyen R, Maes F, et al. The contribution of magnetic resonance imaging to the three-dimensional treatment planning of localized prostate cancer. *Int J Radiat Oncol Biol Phys.* 1999;45:857–865.

12. Milosevic M, Voruganti S, Blend R, et al. Magnetic resonance imaging (MRI) for localization of the prostatic apex: comparison to computed tomography (CT) and urethrography. *Radiother Oncol.* 1998;47:277–284.

13. Smith WL, Lewis C, Bauman G, et al. Prostate volume contouring: a 3D analysis of segmentation using 3DTRUS, CT, and MR. *Int J Radiat Oncol Biol Phys.* 2007;67:1238–1247.

14. Roach M III, Faillace-Akazawa P, Malfatti C, et al. Prostate volumes defined by magnetic resonance imaging and computerized tomographic scans for three-dimensional conformal radiotherapy. *Int J Radiat Oncol Biol Phys.* 1996;35:1011–1018.

15. Rasch C, Barillot I, Remeijer P, et al. Definition of the prostate in CT and MRI: a multi-observer study. *Int J Radiat Oncol Biol Phys.* 1999;43:57–66.

16. van Herk M, de Munck JC, Lebesque JV, et al. Automatic registration of pelvic computed tomography data and magnetic resonance scans including a full circle method for quantitative accuracy evaluation. *Med Phys.* 1998;25:2054–2067.

17. van Lin EN, Futterer JJ, Heijmink SW, et al. IMRT boost dose planning on dominant intraprostatic lesions: gold marker-based three-dimensional fusion of CT with dynamic contrast-enhanced and 1H-spectroscopic MRI. *Int J Radiat Oncol Biol Phys.* 2006;65:291–303.

18. Gofrit ON, Zorn KC, Taxy JB, et al. The dimensions and symmetry of the seminal vesicles. *J Robotic Surg.* 2009;3:29–33.

19. Banner MP, Hassler R. The normal seminal vesiculogram. *Radiology.* 1978;128:339–344.

20. Secaf E, Nuruddin RN, Hricak H, et al. MR imaging of the seminal vesicles. *AJR Am J Roentgenol.* 1991;156:989–994.

21. Villeirs GM, Van Vaerenbergh K, Vakaet L, et al. Interobserver delineation variation using CT versus combined CT + MRI in intensity-modulated radiotherapy for prostate cancer. *Strahlenther Onkol.* 2005;181:424–430.

22. Wallner KE, Merrick GS, Benson ML, et al. Penile bulb imaging. *Int J Radiat Oncol Biol Phys.* 2002;53:928–933.

23. Perna L, Fiorino C, Cozzarini C, et al. Sparing the penile bulb in the radical irradiation of clinically localised prostate carcinoma: a comparison between MRI and CT prostatic apex definition in 3DCRT, Linac-IMRT and Helical Tomotherapy. *Radiother Oncol.* 2009;93:57–63.

24. van der Wielen GJ, Mulhall JP, Incrocci L. Erectile dysfunction after radiotherapy for prostate cancer and radiation dose to the penile structures: a critical review. *Radiother Oncol.* 2007;84:107–113.

25. Buyyounouski MK, Horwitz EM, Uzzo RG, et al. The radiation doses to erectile tissues defined with magnetic resonance imaging after intensity-modulated radiation therapy or iodine-125 brachytherapy. *Int J Radiat Oncol Biol Phys.* 2004;59:1383–1391.

26. Kao J, Turian J, Meyers A, et al. Sparing of the penile bulb and proximal penile structures with intensity-modulated radiation therapy for prostate cancer. *Br J Radiol.* 2004;77:129–136.

27. Brown MW, Brooks JP, Albert PS, et al. An analysis of erectile function after intensity modulated radiation therapy for localized prostate carcinoma. *Prostate Cancer Prostatic Dis.* 2007;10:189–193.

28. Macdonald AG, Keyes M, Kruk A, et al. Predictive factors for erectile dysfunction in men with prostate cancer after brachytherapy: is dose to the penile bulb important? *Int J Radiat Oncol Biol Phys.* 2005;63:155–163.

29. Merrick GS, Butler WM, Wallner KE, et al. Erectile function after prostate brachytherapy. *Int J Radiat Oncol Biol Phys.* 2005;62:437–447.

30. Roach M, Winter K, Michalski JM, et al. Penile bulb dose and impotence after three-dimensional conformal radiotherapy for prostate cancer on RTOG 9406: findings from a prospective, multi-institutional, phase I/II dose-escalation study. *Int J Radiat Oncol Biol Phys.* 2004;60:1351–1356.

31. Villeirs GM, De Meerleer GO. Magnetic resonance imaging (MRI) anatomy of the prostate and application of MRI in radiotherapy planning. *Eur J Radiol.* 2007;63:361–368.

32. Michalski JM, Lawton C, El Naqa I, et al. Development of RTOG consensus guidelines for the definition of the clinical target volume for postoperative conformal radiation therapy for prostate cancer. *Int J Radiat Oncol Biol Phys.* 2010;76:361–368.

33. Shinohara K, Wheeler TM, Scardino PT. The appearance of prostate cancer on transrectal ultrasonography: correlation of imaging and pathological examinations. *J Urol.* 1989;142:76–82.

34. Roehl KA, Antenor JA, Catalona WJ. Serial biopsy results in prostate cancer screening study. *J Urol.* 2002;167:2435–2439.

35. Testa C, Schiavina R, Lodi R, et al. Prostate cancer: sextant localization with MR imaging, MR spectroscopy, and 11C-choline PET/CT. *Radiology.* 2007;244:797–806.

36. Pallwein L, Mitterberger M, Pelzer A, et al. Ultrasound of prostate cancer: recent advances. *Eur Radiol.* 2008;18:707–715.

37. Coakley FV, Kurhanewicz J, Lu Y, et al. Prostate cancer tumor volume: measurement with endorectal MR and MR spectroscopic imaging. *Radiology.* 2002;223:91–97.

38. Mazaheri Y, Shukla-Dave A, Hricak H, et al. Prostate cancer: identification with combined diffusion-weighted MR imaging and 3D 1H MR spectroscopic imaging—correlation with pathologic findings. *Radiology.* 2008;246:480–488.

39. Heerschap A, Jager GJ, van der Graaf M, et al. Proton MR spectroscopy of the normal human prostate with an endorectal coil and a double spin-echo pulse sequence. *Magn Reson Med.* 1997;37:204–213.

40. Mazaheri Y, Hricak H, Fine SW, et al. Prostate tumor volume measurement with combined T2-weighted imaging and diffusion-weighted MR: correlation with pathologic tumor volume. *Radiology.* 2009;252:449–457.

41. Padhani AR, Gapinski CJ, Macvicar DA, et al. Dynamic contrast enhanced MRI of prostate cancer: correlation with morphology and tumour stage, histological grade and PSA. *Clin Radiol.* 2000;55:99–109.

42. Turnbull LW, Buckley DL, Turnbull LS, et al. Differentiation of prostatic carcinoma and benign prostatic hyperplasia: correlation between dynamic Gd-DTPA-enhanced MR imaging and histopathology. *J Magn Reson Imaging.* 1999;9:311–316.

43. Girouin N, Mege-Lechevallier F, Tonina Senes A, et al. Prostate dynamic contrast-enhanced MRI with simple visual diagnostic criteria: is it reasonable? *Eur Radiol.* 2007;17:1498–1509.

44. Schmuecking M, Boltze C, Geyer H, et al. Dynamic MRI and CAD vs. choline MRS: where is the detection level for a lesion characterisation in prostate cancer? *Int J Radiat Biol.* 2009;85:814–824.

45. Futterer JJ, Heijmink SW, Scheenen TW, et al. Prostate cancer localization with dynamic contrast-enhanced MR imaging and proton MR spectroscopic imaging. *Radiology.* 2006;241:449–458.

46. Sella T, Schwartz LH, Swindle PW, et al. Suspected local recurrence after radical prostatectomy: endorectal coil MR imaging. *Radiology.* 2004;231:379–385.

47. Pucar D, Hricak H, Shukla-Dave A, et al. Clinically significant prostate cancer local recurrence after radiation therapy occurs at the site of primary tumor: magnetic resonance imaging and step-section pathology evidence. *Int J Radiat Oncol Biol Phys.* 2007;69:62–69.

48. Casciani E, Polettini E, Carmenini E, et al. Endorectal and dynamic contrast-enhanced MRI for detection of local recurrence after radical prostatectomy. *AJR Am J Roentgenol.* 2008;190:1187–1192.

49. Cirillo S, Petracchini M, Scotti L, et al. Endorectal magnetic resonance imaging at 1.5 Tesla to assess local recurrence following radical prostatectomy using T2-weighted and contrast-enhanced imaging. *Eur Radiol.* 2009;19:761–769.

50. King CR, Kapp DS. Radiotherapy after prostatectomy: is the evidence for dose escalation out there? *Int J Radiat Oncol Biol Phys.* 2008;71:346–350.

51. Bernard JR Jr, Buskirk SJ, Heckman MG, et al. Salvage radiotherapy for rising prostate-specific antigen levels after radical prostatectomy for prostate cancer: dose-response analysis. *Int J Radiat Oncol Biol Phys.* 2010;76:735–740.

52. Brassell SA, Rosner IL, McLeod DG. Update on magnetic resonance imaging, ProstaScint, and novel imaging in prostate cancer. *Curr Opin Urol.* 2005;15:163–166.

53. Hinkle GH, Burgers JK, Neal CE, et al. Multicenter radioimmunoscintigraphic evaluation of patients with prostate carcinoma using indium-111 capromab pendetide. *Cancer.* 1998;83:739–747.

54. Ellis RJ, Zhou EH, Fu P, et al. Single photon emission computerized tomography with capromab pendetide plus computerized tomography image set co-registration independently predicts biochemical failure. *J Urol.* 2008;179:1768–1773; discussion 1773–1774.

55. Koontz BF, Mouraviev V, Johnson JL, et al. Use of local (111) in-capromab pendetide scan results to predict outcome after salvage radiotherapy for prostate cancer. *Int J Radiat Oncol Biol Phys.* 2008;71:358–361.

56. Nagda SN, Mohideen N, Lo SS, et al. Long-term follow-up of 111In-capromab pendetide (ProstaScint) scan as pretreatment assessment in patients who undergo salvage radiotherapy for rising prostate-specific antigen after radical prostatectomy for prostate cancer. *Int J Radiat Oncol Biol Phys.* 2007;67:834–840.

57. Proano JM, Sodee DB, Resnick MI, et al. The impact of a negative (111)indium-capromab pendetide scan before salvage radiotherapy. *J Urol.* 2006;175:1668–1672.

58. Liauw SL, Weichselbaum RR, Zagaja GP, et al. Salvage radiotherapy after postprostatectomy biochemical failure: does pretreatment radioimmunoscintigraphy help select patients with locally confined disease? *Int J Radiat Oncol Biol Phys.* 2008;71:1316–1321.

59. Pollack A, Hanlon AL, Horwitz EM, et al. Dosimetry and preliminary acute toxicity in the first 100 men treated for prostate cancer on a randomized hypofractionation dose escalation trial. *Int J Radiat Oncol Biol Phys.* 2006;64:518–526.

60. Halperin EC, Perez CA, Brady LW. *Perez and Brady's Principles and Practice of Radiation Oncology.* Philadelphia PA: Lippincott, Williams & Wilkins; 2007.

61. Poortmans P, Bossi A, Vandeputte K, et al. Guidelines for target volume definition in post-operative radiotherapy for prostate cancer, on behalf of the EORTC Radiation Oncology Group. *Radiother Oncol.* 2007;84:121–127.

62. Korreman S, Rasch C, McNair H, et al. The European Society of Therapeutic Radiology and Oncology-European Institute of

Radiotherapy (ESTRO-EIR) report on 3D CT-based in-room image guidance systems: a practical and technical review and guide. *Radiother Oncol.* 2010.

63. Vigneault E, Pouliot J, Laverdiere J, et al. Electronic portal imaging device detection of radioopaque markers for the evaluation of prostate position during megavoltage irradiation: a clinical study. *Int J Radiat Oncol Biol Phys.* 1997;37:205–212.

64. Chandra A, Dong L, Huang E, et al. Experience of ultrasound-based daily prostate localization. *Int J Radiat Oncol Biol Phys.* 2003;56:436–447.

65. Bylund KC, Bayouth JE, Smith MC, et al. Analysis of interfraction prostate motion using megavoltage cone beam computed tomography. *Int J Radiat Oncol Biol Phys.* 2008;72:949–956.

66. Rosewall T, Chung P, Bayley A, et al. A randomized comparison of interfraction and intrafraction prostate motion with and without abdominal compression. *Radiother Oncol.* 2008;88:88–94.

67. de Crevoisier R, Tucker SL, Dong L, et al. Increased risk of biochemical and local failure in patients with distended rectum on the planning CT for prostate cancer radiotherapy. *Int J Radiat Oncol Biol Phys.* 2005;62:965–973.

68. Heemsbergen WD, Hoogeman MS, Witte MG, et al. Increased risk of biochemical and clinical failure for prostate patients with a large rectum at radiotherapy planning: results from the Dutch trial of 68 Gy versus 78 Gy. *Int J Radiat Oncol Biol Phys.* 2007;67:1418–1424.

69. Kupelian PA, Willoughby TR, Reddy CA, et al. Impact of image guidance on outcomes after external beam radiotherapy for localized prostate cancer. *Int J Radiat Oncol Biol Phys.* 2008;70:1146–1150.

70. Lattanzi J, McNeeley S, Pinover W, et al. A comparison of daily CT localization to a daily ultrasound-based system in prostate cancer. *Int J Radiat Oncol Biol Phys.* 1999;43:719–725.

71. Langen KM, Pouliot J, Anezinos C, et al. Evaluation of ultrasound-based prostate localization for image-guided radiotherapy. *Int J Radiat Oncol Biol Phys.* 2003;57:635–644.

72. Scarbrough TJ, Golden NM, Ting JY, et al. Comparison of ultrasound and implanted seed marker prostate localization methods: implications for image-guided radiotherapy. *Int J Radiat Oncol Biol Phys.* 2006;65:378–387.

73. Trichter F, Ennis RD. Prostate localization using transabdominal ultrasound imaging. *Int J Radiat Oncol Biol Phys.* 2003;56:1225–1233.

74. Artignan X, Smitsmans MH, Lebesque JV, et al. Online ultrasound image guidance for radiotherapy of prostate cancer: impact of image acquisition on prostate displacement. *Int J Radiat Oncol Biol Phys.* 2004;59:595–601.

75. Serago CF, Chungbin SJ, Buskirk SJ, et al. Initial experience with ultrasound localization for positioning prostate cancer patients for external beam radiotherapy. *Int J Radiat Oncol Biol Phys.* 2002;53:1130–1138.

76. Fuss M, Salter BJ, Cavanaugh SX, et al. Daily ultrasound-based image-guided targeting for radiotherapy of upper abdominal malignancies. *Int J Radiat Oncol Biol Phys.* 2004;59:1245–1256.

77. Feigenberg SJ, Paskalev K, McNeeley S, et al. Comparing computed tomography localization with daily ultrasound during image-guided radiation therapy for the treatment of prostate cancer: a prospective evaluation. *J Appl Clin Med Phys.* 2007;8:2268.

78. Pinkawa M, Pursch-Lee M, Asadpour B, et al. Image-guided radiotherapy for prostate cancer. Implementation of ultrasound-based prostate localization for the analysis of inter- and intrafraction organ motion. *Strahlenther Onkol.* 2008;184:679–685.

79. Igdem S, Akpinar H, Alco G, et al. Implantation of fiducial markers for image guidance in prostate radiotherapy: patient-reported toxicity. *Br J Radiol.* 2009;82:941–945.

80. Gauthier I, Carrier JF, Beliveau-Nadeau D, et al. Dosimetric impact and theoretical clinical benefits of fiducial markers for dose escalated prostate cancer radiation treatment. *Int J Radiat Oncol Biol Phys.* 2009;74:1128–1133.

81. Kupelian PA, Willoughby TR, Meeks SL, et al. Intraprostatic fiducials for localization of the prostate gland: monitoring intermarker distances during radiation therapy to test for marker stability. *Int J Radiat Oncol Biol Phys.* 2005;62:1291–1296.

82. Poggi MM, Gant DA, Sewchand W, et al. Marker seed migration in prostate localization. *Int J Radiat Oncol Biol Phys.* 2003;56:1248–1251.

83. Chung PW, Haycocks T, Brown T, et al. On-line aSi portal imaging of implanted fiducial markers for the reduction of interfraction error during conformal radiotherapy of prostate carcinoma. *Int J Radiat Oncol Biol Phys.* 2004;60:329–334.

84. Schallenkamp JM, Herman MG, Kruse JJ, et al. Prostate position relative to pelvic bony anatomy based on intraprostatic gold markers and electronic portal imaging. *Int J Radiat Oncol Biol Phys.* 2005;63:800–811.

85. Tinger A, Michalski JM, Cheng A, et al. A critical evaluation of the planning target volume for 3-D conformal radiotherapy of prostate cancer. *Int J Radiat Oncol Biol Phys.* 1998;42:213–221.

86. Beltran C, Herman MG, Davis BJ. Planning target margin calculations for prostate radiotherapy based on intrafraction and interfraction motion using four localization methods. *Int J Radiat Oncol Biol Phys.* 2008;70:289–295.

87. Alonso-Arrizabalaga S, Brualla Gonzalez L, Rosello Ferrando JV, et al. Prostate planning treatment volume margin calculation based on the ExacTrac X-Ray 6D image-guided system: margins for various clinical implementations. *Int J Radiat Oncol Biol Phys.* 2007;69:936–943.

88. Nederveen AJ, Dehnad H, van der Heide UA, et al. Comparison of megavoltage position verification for prostate irradiation based on bony anatomy and implanted fiducials. *Radiother Oncol.* 2003;68:81–88.

89. Schiffner DC, Gottschalk AR, Lometti M, et al. Daily electronic portal imaging of implanted gold seed fiducials in patients undergoing radiotherapy after radical prostatectomy. *Int J Radiat Oncol Biol Phys.* 2007;67:610–619.

90. Langen KM, Willoughby TR, Meeks SL, et al. Observations on real-time prostate gland motion using electromagnetic tracking. *Int J Radiat Oncol Biol Phys.* 2008;71:1084–1090.

91. Ryan D, Rivest C, Riauka TA, et al. Prostate positioning errors associated with two automatic registration based image guidance strategies. *J Appl Clin Med Phys.* 2009;10:3071.

92. Morin O, Gillis A, Descovich M, et al. Patient dose considerations for routine megavoltage cone-beam CT imaging. *Med Phys.* 2007;34:1819–1827.

93. Pouliot J, Bani-Hashemi A, Chen J, et al. Low-dose megavoltage cone-beam CT for radiation therapy. *Int J Radiat Oncol Biol Phys.* 2005;61:552–560.

94. Meeks SL, Harmon JF Jr, Langen KM, et al. Performance characterization of megavoltage computed tomography imaging on a helical tomotherapy unit. *Med Phys.* 2005;32:2673–2681.

95. Gayou O, Miften M. Comparison of mega-voltage cone-beam computed tomography prostate localization with online ultrasound and fiducial markers methods. *Med Phys.* 2008;35:531–538.

96. Moseley DJ, White EA, Wiltshire KL, et al. Comparison of localization performance with implanted fiducial markers and cone-beam computed tomography for on-line image-guided radiotherapy of the prostate. *Int J Radiat Oncol Biol Phys.* 2007;67:942–953.

97. Kupelian P, Willoughby T, Mahadevan A, et al. Multi-institutional clinical experience with the Calypso System in localization and continuous, real-time monitoring of the prostate gland during external radiotherapy. *Int J Radiat Oncol Biol Phys.* 2007;67:1088–1098.

98. Paskalev K, Feigenberg S, Jacob R, et al. Target localization for post-prostatectomy patients using CT and ultrasound image guidance. *J Appl Clin Med Phys.* 2005;6:40–49.

99. Tran PK, Haworth A, Foroudi F, et al. Prospective development of an individualised predictive model for treatment coverage using offline cone beam computed tomography surrogate measures in post-prostatectomy radiotherapy. *J Med Imaging Radiat Oncol.* 2009;53:574–580.

100. van Herk M, Remeijer P, Rasch C, et al. The probability of correct target dosage: dose-population histograms for deriving treatment margins in radiotherapy. *Int J Radiat Oncol Biol Phys.* 2000;47:1121–1135.

101. Shimizu S, Shirato H, Kitamura K, et al. Use of an implanted marker and real-time tracking of the marker for the positioning of prostate and bladder cancers. *Int J Radiat Oncol Biol Phys.* 2000;48:1591–1597.

102. Nederveen AJ, van der Heide UA, Dehnad H, et al. Measurements and clinical consequences of prostate motion during a radiotherapy fraction. *Int J Radiat Oncol Biol Phys.* 2002;53:206–214.

103. Kitamura K, Shirato H, Shimizu S, et al. Registration accuracy and possible migration of internal fiducial gold marker implanted in prostate and liver treated with real-time tumor-tracking radiation therapy (RTRT). *Radiother Oncol.* 2002;62:275–281.

104. Padhani AR, Khoo VS, Suckling J, et al. Evaluating the effect of rectal distension and rectal movement on prostate gland position using cine MRI. *Int J Radiat Oncol Biol Phys.* 1999;44:525–533.

105. Mah D, Freedman G, Milestone B, et al. Measurement of intra-fractional prostate motion using magnetic resonance imaging. *Int J Radiat Oncol Biol Phys.* 2002;54:568–575.

106. Ghilezan MJ, Jaffray DA, Siewerdsen JH, et al. Prostate gland motion assessed with cine-magnetic resonance imaging (cine-MRI). *Int J Radiat Oncol Biol Phys.* 2005;62:406–417.

107. Huang E, Dong L, Chandra A, et al. Intrafraction prostate motion during IMRT for prostate cancer. *Int J Radiat Oncol Biol Phys.* 2002;53:261–268.

108. Antolak JA, Rosen II, Childress CH, et al. Prostate target volume variations during a course of radiotherapy. *Int J Radiat Oncol Biol Phys.* 1998;42:661–672.

109. Melian E, Mageras GS, Fuks Z, et al. Variation in prostate position quantitation and implications for three-dimensional conformal treatment planning. *Int J Radiat Oncol Biol Phys.* 1997;38:73–81.

110. Stroom JC, Kroonwijk M, Pasma KL, et al. Detection of internal organ movement in prostate cancer patients using portal images. *Med Phys.* 2000;27:452–461.

111. Dawson LA, Litzenberg DW, Brock KK, et al. A comparison of ventilatory prostate movement in four treatment positions. *Int J Radiat Oncol Biol Phys.* 2000;48:319–323.

112. Malone S, Crook JM, Kendal WS, et al. Respiratory-induced prostate motion: quantification and characterization. *Int J Radiat Oncol Biol Phys.* 2000;48:105–109.

113. Li HS, Chetty IJ, Enke CA, et al. Dosimetric consequences of intrafraction prostate motion. *Int J Radiat Oncol Biol Phys.* 2008;71:801–812.

114. Noel C, Parikh PJ, Roy M, et al. Prediction of intrafraction prostate motion: accuracy of pre- and post-treatment imaging and intermittent imaging. *Int J Radiat Oncol Biol Phys.* 2009;73:692–698.

115. Bittner N, Butler WM, Reed JL, et al. Electromagnetic tracking of intrafraction prostate displacement in patients externally immobilized in the prone position. *Int J Radiat Oncol Biol Phys.* 2010;77(2):490–495.

116. Brenner DJ, Martinez AA, Edmundson GK, et al. Direct evidence that prostate tumors show high sensitivity to fractionation (low alpha/beta ratio), similar to late-responding normal tissue. *Int J Radiat Oncol Biol Phys.* 2002;52:6–13.

117. Abdel-Wahab M, Pollack A. Radiotherapy: encouraging early data for SBRT in prostate cancer. *Nat Rev Urol.* 2009;6:478–479.

118. Friedland JL, Freeman DE, Masterson-McGary ME, et al. Stereotactic body radiotherapy: an emerging treatment approach for localized prostate cancer. *Technol Cancer Res Treat.* 2009;8:387–392.

119. King CR, Brooks JD, Gill H, et al. Stereotactic body radiotherapy for localized prostate cancer: interim results of a prospective phase II clinical trial. *Int J Radiat Oncol Biol Phys.* 2009;73:1043–1048.

120. Tang CI, Loblaw DA, Cheung P, et al. Phase I/II study of a five-fraction hypofractionated accelerated radiotherapy treatment for low-risk localised prostate cancer: early results of pHART3. *Clin Oncol (R Coll Radiol).* 2008;20:729–737.

121. Xie Y, Djajaputra D, King CR, et al. Intrafractional motion of the prostate during hypofractionated radiotherapy. *Int J Radiat Oncol Biol Phys.* 2008;72:236–246.

122. Howe FA, Robinson SP, McIntyre DJ, et al. Issues in flow and oxygenation dependent contrast (FLOOD) imaging of tumours. *NMR Biomed.* 2001;14:497–506.

123. John SS, Zietman AL, Shipley WU, et al. Newer imaging modalities to assist with target localization in the radiation

treatment of prostate cancer and possible lymph node metastases. *Int J Radiat Oncol Biol Phys.* 2008;71:S43–S47.

124. Hoskin PJ, Carnell DM, Taylor NJ, et al. Hypoxia in prostate cancer: correlation of BOLD-MRI with pimonidazole immunohistochemistry-initial observations. *Int J Radiat Oncol Biol Phys.* 2007;68:1065–1071.

125. Padhani AR, Krohn KA, Lewis JS, et al. Imaging oxygenation of human tumours. *Eur Radiol.* 2007;17:861–872.

126. Harisinghani MG, Barentsz J, Hahn PF, et al. Noninvasive detection of clinically occult lymph-node metastases in prostate cancer. *N Engl J Med.* 2003;348: 2491–2489.

127. Ross RW, Zietman AL, Xie W, et al. Lymphotropic nanoparticle-enhanced magnetic resonance imaging (LNMRI) identifies occult lymph node metastases in prostate cancer patients prior to salvage radiation therapy. *Clin Imaging.* 2009;33:301–305.

MR-Guided Target Delineation in a Patient with Prostate Cancer

Case Study

Mark K. Buyyounouski, MD, MS, Eric M. Horwitz, MD

Patient History

A 74-year-old man presented with an elevated and rising prostate-specific antigen (PSA). His PSA rose to a level of 11.4 ng/mL from 6 ng/mL 1 year before and 4 ng/mL 2 years before. A repeat PSA was 13 ng/mL. On digital rectal examination (DRE), firm nodularity was noted on the right side of the prostate with a flattened right lateral sulci suggesting extracapsular extension at the level of the apex and midgland. The median raphe was intact and the seminal vesicles were nonpalpable.

He was recommended to undergo a transrectal ultrasound-guided prostate biopsy that demonstrated a 39-cc prostate but was otherwise unremarkable. Surgical pathology revealed prostatic adenocarcinoma, Gleason score 4 + 4 = 8 involving 80% of tissue from the right base lateral, 95% of tissue from the right apex lateral, 70% of tissue from the right base medial, 80% of tissue from the left base lateral, and 60% of tissue from the left base medial. There was also Gleason 4 + 3 = 7 adenocarcinoma involving 30% of tissue from the right apex medial, 60% of tissue from the right mid-medial, and 30% of tissue from the right mid-lateral. Specimens from the left apex lateral, left apex medial, left mid-lateral, and left mid-medial were benign. Computed tomography (CT) scans of the abdomen and pelvis demonstrated no suspicious adenopathy and a bone scan was negative for osseous metastases. The patient was staged as clinical stage III (T3AN0M0) adenocarcinoma of the prostate.

Our consensus recommendation was for external beam radiotherapy (RT) with intensity-modulated RT (IMRT) and daily image-guided prostate localization. Because of the high-risk nature of his disease, he was also recommended to receive long-term adjuvant androgen-deprivation therapy. We elected to use magnetic resonance (MR) imaging to guide target delineation.

Simulation

The patient underwent CT simulation using our department's Light Speed scanner (GE Healthcare, Waukesha, WI). Before scanning, the patient was placed in the supine position, immobilized in a cast, with a comfortable full bladder and empty rectum. Immediately after the CT, the patient was taken to the MR suite where a second scan was performed using a 1.5 Tesla (T) Signa EXCITE scanner (GE Healthcare, Waukesha, WI). The patient was placed in the same position as before, and the same immobilization device was used. Contrast was not used for either scanning modality.

Imaging and Target Delineation

Though not evident on physical exam or CT, there was clear involvement of the seminal vesicles on the T2-weighted MR scan. The seminal vesicles normally appear with heterogeneous high-signal intensity on T2-weighted MR (Figure 20A-1, lower panels, dashed arrow). In this patient, the bilateral seminal vesicle appears dark, which is characteristic of involvement with prostate cancer (Figure 20A-1, upper panels, solid arrow). This finding has important implications for treatment planning.

The structures outlined for treatment planning included the prostate, seminal vesicles, rectum (entire contents) from the ischial tuberosities to the sigmoid flexure, bladder (entire contents), femurs down to the

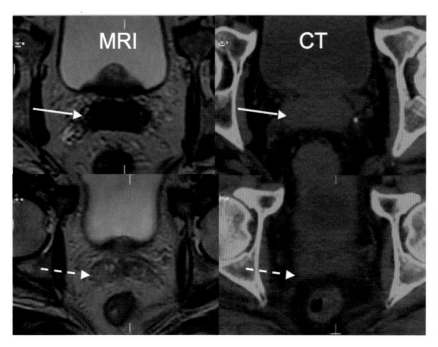

FIGURE 20A-1. Magnetic resonance (MR) image and computed tomography images on axial slices through the seminal vesicles. The seminal vesicles normally have a high-intensity, heterogeneous signal on T2-weighted MR as shown in the lower panel. However, in this patient, the seminal vesicles appear dark (upper panel) indicating prostate cancer involvement.

superior aspect of the lesser trochanter, and the external contour. The penile bulb and corporal bodies were outlined for reference; no dose constraints were placed on these structures. The CT images were used to outline the external contour and femoral heads. All other contours, including the bladder, rectum, prostate, seminal vesicles, and lymph nodes were outlined by using the MR images.

Treatment Planning

The maxim of RT is to deliver dose to the tumor. Generally, for most prostate cancers that are clinically localized, this means ensuring the clinical target volume (CTV) consists of the prostate and proximal portions of the seminal vesicles (which can have microscopic involvement up to a few millimeters). High-risk patients, such as the one described here, should also receive treatment to the distal seminal vesicles and regional lymph nodes, delivered in sequential or concurrent technique. At Fox Chase Cancer Center, high-risk patients are prescribed 80 Gy in 40 fractions to the prostate and proximal seminal vesicles and 56 Gy to the distal seminal vesicles and regional lymph nodes at 1.4 Gy per fraction concurrent with treatment to the prostate. The proximal seminal vesicles are defined as the proximal 1 cm and the distal seminal vesicles as the remainder.

On the basis of the MR findings during simulation showing involvement of the bilateral seminal vesicles,

the IMRT dose prescription was modified to ensure the entire seminal vesicles received the full prescription dose (80 Gy in 40 fractions). Thus, the CTV included the prostate and entire seminal vesicles. The planning target volume (PTV) consisted of the CTV plus an 8-mm margin, except posteriorly where the margin was 3 mm to 5 mm as measured on a slice-by-slice basis.

The prostate and seminal vesicle planning criteria were that 95% of the PTV received 100% of the prescription dose, and that the minimum distance from the posterior edge of the prostate to the prescription isodose was 4 mm to 8 mm on all CT slices. Care was also taken to limit the volume of bladder and rectum irradiated. For the rectum, the dose was limited such that the volume receiving 65 Gy (V_{65}) was less than 17%, and the V_{40} was less than 35%. Additionally, the 50% isodose line was contained within the posterior edge of the rectum on all slices. Similarly, the bladder constraints were V_{65} less than 25%, and V_{40} less than 50%.

Clinical Outcome

The patient tolerated treatment well experiencing the usual side effect of increased number of bowel movements and mild urinary frequency that responded well to Flomax. He is still receiving long-term androgen-deprivation therapy and has an undetectable PSA. His acute side effects resolved after 3 months.

ProstaScint-Guided Target Delineation in a Patient with Prostate Cancer Undergoing Interstitial Brachytherapy

Case Study

Rodney J. Ellis, MD, Deborah A. Kaminsky, DPh

Patient History

A 62-year-old man presented with a prostate-specific antigen (PSA) level of 29.69 ng/mL on a routine screening evaluation. Digital rectal exam (DRE) was unremarkable. Ultrasound-guided transrectal prostate biopsy was performed and identified a Gleason 3 + 3 adenocarcinoma in the left lateral mid-gland, involving 5% of a single positive sextant biopsy core. His presenting baseline American Urology Association (AUA) prostate symptom score was 12 and his Sexual Health Inventory Score for Men (SHIM) returned at 13, consistent with moderate baseline erectile difficulty. Radiographic workup, including a bone scan as well as pelvic and prostate magnetic resonance (MR) imaging, was negative for metastatic disease. The tumor was thus staged as T1cNxM0, stage II, and classified as intermediate risk.[1]

Because of the patient's marked PSA elevation, an ^{111}In-labeled capromab pendetide (ProstaScint, EUSA Pharma, Oxford, United Kingdom) scan was obtained, along with a computed tomography (CT) scan of the pelvis for single photon emission CT (SPECT)–CT fusion. The SPECT and CT data sets were manually aligned, utilizing bone marrow activity, vascular uptake, and bony anatomy using MIM image fusion software (MIM Vista, Cleveland, OH). ProstaScint imaging demonstrated no evidence of metastatic disease. However, bilateral intraprostatic monoclonal antibody (MoAB) uptake was noted. A focal area of concentration was present in the left mid-gland, extending from the anterior to posterior portion of the prostate. A separate, less focally active lesion was also present in the right posterior prostatic apex, as shown in Figure 20B-1.

With confirmation of the localized disease status, and moderate- to low-grade Gleason score, definitive radiotherapy (RT) was recommended, consisting of a combination of three-dimensional external beam RT (EBRT; total dose, 45 Gy) followed by interstitial brachytherapy. Pelvic lymph nodes were excluded from the EBRT volume because of the ProstaScint results (negative for nodal involvement) and the moderate to low tumor grade (Gleason 3 + 3) on diagnostic biopsy. We elected to use ProstaScint imaging to help guide target delineation during the brachytherapy phase of his treatment. .

Imaging and Target Delineation

Before the initiation of EBRT, the patient presented to the radiation oncology brachytherapy suite for a transrectal ultrasound (TRUS) volume study. With the patient in a dorsal lithotomy position, with slight hyperflexion of the hips using operating room stirrups, a Foley catheter was placed into the bladder to enable urethra localization. The TRUS probe was positioned, utilizing a B-K 7.5 MHz transducer and ultrasound (US) unit (B-K Medical, Herlev, Denmark). Ultrasound images were obtained in 0.5-cm increments from the base to apex of the prostate using the attached Surepoint stabilizer/stepping unit (C.R. Bard, Murray Hill, NJ), and captured in the Rosses (Rosses Medical Systems, Columbia, MD) brachytherapy treatment planning system.

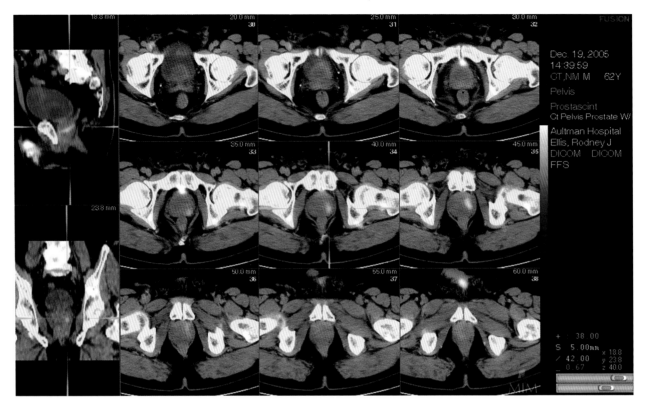

FIGURE 20B-1. Indium-111 capromab pendetide single photon emission computed tomography (SPECT)–CT image fusion. Left upper and lower panels show sagittal and coronal pelvic planes, followed by a series of transverse axial cuts at 5-mm increments from the prostate base to the apex. The green crosshairs in the center image identify the isocenter of the fusion images placed within the dominant biological target volume (BTV-1) in the left mid-gland. A second lesion (BTV-2) is also present in the right prostatic apex, most notably in the last panel.

The size and shape of the rectum, urethra, and prostate were localized, showing a 66.9-cc prostate volume. Axial images were generated encompassing the prostate and periprostatic tissue, extending from 5 mm above to 5 mm below the prostate volume. By matching similar slices from base to apex between the fused SPECT–CT image set and the US volume study, two biological target volumes (BTV) were manually transferred to the corresponding US images within the treatment planning system, defining a dominant left mid-gland BTV (BTV-1) and a right apex (BTV-2) dose escalation target.

Treatment Planning

An interstitial brachytherapy boost was prescribed to be delivered 4-weeks after completion of EBRT. The pretreatment planning dose–volume histogram (DVH) is shown in Figure 20B-2 and axial treatment planning images are shown in Figure 20B-3. The pretreatment plan prescribed a total activity of 31.62 mCi (0.31 mCi/iodine-125 seed). An iodine-125 brachytherapy dose of 110 Gy was prescribed to the periphery of the prostate gland, using a modified peripheral loading technique with 5-mm margins. Peripheral loading modification was utilized to provide dose escalation (165 Gy) to intraprostatic BTV-1 and BTV-2.

Brachytherapy Procedure

Validation of SPECT–CT uptake was performed by transperineal biopsy directed to each BTV immediately before the brachytherapy implant procedure, using the clinician's correlated histopathology and marker placement protocol.[2] Utilizing a general anesthetic in the brachytherapy suite, the patient was prepped and draped for implant in the usual sterile fashion. The B-K 7.5 maximal MHz US transducer probe was positioned and attached to the stabilizing device. As in simulation, a Foley catheter was placed into the bladder with dilute Hypaque in the Foley bulb. The patient was positioned under fluoroscopy for further visualization of the operative field.

After localization of the prostate volume within the treatment planning template, and utilizing the TRUS needle guide, an 18-gauge C.R. Bard gun and needle system was directed transperineally to the region of interest defined as BTV-1 within the left side of the prostate gland. A biopsy tissue sample measuring 18 mm was withdrawn, processed and sent to pathology. The biopsy needle was withdrawn, and a preloaded needle containing a gold fiducial marker, measuring 2 cm in length by 0.33 mm, was similarly guided through the biopsy needle track, with placement of the marker into the biopsy tissue void,

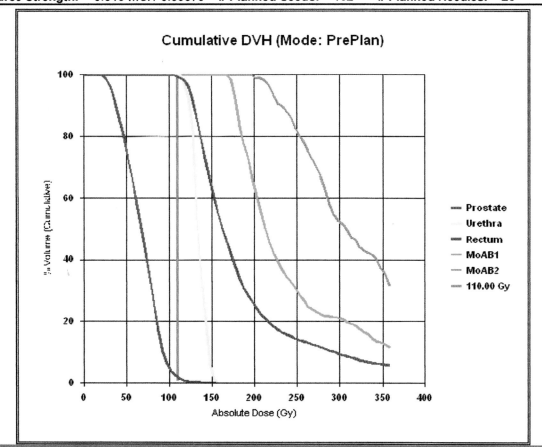

VolumePlan	Dose Volume Histogram (Pre Volume)			Rosses Medical Systems, Inc.

Patient ID: Print Date: 11:43 AM- Thu, March 09, 2006
Name: Physician: - Implant Date: 1/10/2006
Age (years): - Stage: - PSA (ng/ml): - Gleason: - Hormones: - TURP: -
Implant Type: Boost Prescribed Dose (Gy): 110 Seed Type: Thera_Beb_I125S06
Source Strength: 0.310 mCi / 0.39370 # Planned Seeds: 102 # Planned Needles: 26

Value	Prostate	Urethra	Rectum	MoAB1	MoAB2
Volume	66.98 cc	0.43 cc	9.32 cc	5.99 cc	0.85 cc
D90	127.50 Gy	122.50 Gy	37.50 Gy	177.50 Gy	232.50 Gy
D100	92.50 Gy	112.50 Gy	17.50 Gy	167.50 Gy	197.50 Gy
V90	99.99%	100.00%	6.32%	100.00%	100.00%
V100	99.31%	100.00%	1.40%	100.00%	100.00%
V150	45.83%	0.00%	0.00%	100.00%	100.00%
V200	18.44%	0.00%	0.00%	41.97%	93.17%
D80	137.567				

FIGURE 20B-2. Dose–volume histograms from the pretreatment plan show a prostate V100 of 99.31%, prostate V150 of 45.3%, and prostate V200 of 18.4%. The urethral V100 is 100% (constraints include no portion of the urethra to receive either 150% or 200% of prescribed dose). The rectal V100 is 1.4%. Both biological target volumes, labeled MoAB-1 (BTV-1) and MoAB-2 (BTV-2) V100 and V150 are planned to receive 100% of the prescribed dose.

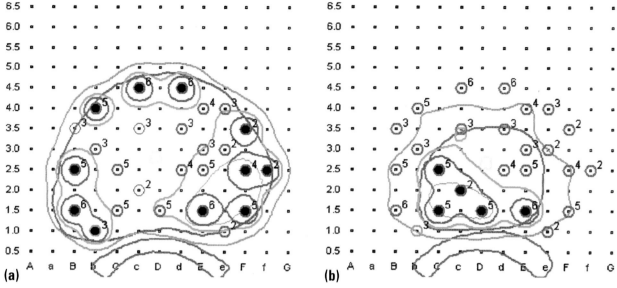

FIGURE 20B-3. Mid- and apical axial treatment plan images of the prostate. (a) Mid-gland axial image from the preplan ultrasound volume study with the prostate in red, urethra in yellow, and rectum in brown. The biological target volume (BTV-1) located in the left mid-gland is outlined in green, showing additional seeds (in black) placed to escalate dose to 150% of prescription dose. The prescribed dose (100%) to the entire prostate is outlined in dark blue, 150% in green, and 200% in brown. (b) Apical gland axial image from the preplan ultrasound volume study showing the prostate outlined in red, urethra in yellow, and rectum in brown. The biological target volume (BTV-2) located in the right lower apex of the gland is outlined in light blue, showing additional seeds (in black) placed to escalate dose to 150% of the prescription dose. The prescribed dose (100%) to the entire prostate is outlined in dark blue, 150% in green, and 200% in brown.

establishing in vivo marking of BTV-1. A biopsy was then directed to BTV-2 and a second gold fiducial marker was placed, as before.

An intraoperative volume study was then completed. The SPECT–CT–identified BTV regions were manually transferred to the intraoperative US images within the brachytherapy planning system. Intraoperative structural volumes are shown in Table 20B-1. The final intraoperative treatment planning prescription dose resulted in a 26 needle implant of 94 seeds, for a total activity of 28.9 mCi. A dose–volume histogram was generated, in addition to a 3D isodose distribution. Intraoperative BTV biopsy, treatment planning, and seed implant were completed in approximately 45 minutes.

TABLE 20B–1 Interstitial Brachytherapy Dose Quality Indicators: Iodine-125 Brachytherapy Dosimetric Parameters, Structure Volumes, and Percent Dose Estimates as Determined by Intraoperative Ultrasound Treatment Planning and Postoperative Computed Tomography (CT)–Based Dosimetry Analysis Dose–Volume Histogram

Dosimetric Parameter	Intraoperative Volume, cc	Intraoperative Treatment Plan	Postoperative Volume, cc	Postoperative Dosimetry
Prostate V100	58.6	98.7%	51.1	91.3%
Prostate V150	58.6	43.6%	51.1	55.8%
Prostate V200	58.6	16.7%	51.1	24.0%
BTV-1 V100	5.8	100.0%	6.2	100.0%
BTV-1 V150	5.8	92.9%	6.2	92.7%
BTV-2 V100	0.5	100.0%	0.6	100.0%
BTV-2 V150	0.5	100.0%	0.6	99.7%
Rectum V100	9.1	1.4%	29.0	7.2%
Urethra V100	0.4	100.0%	0.3	91.7%
Prostate D90	58.6	127.5%	51.1	102.5%

Notes. V100, V150, and V200 dosimetric parameters are expressed as a percentage of prescription dose (100%, 150%, and 200%, respectively) by structure volume. The intraoperative treatment plan is expressed as a total percentage of the prescription dose during intraoperative modeling by structure volume; postoperative dosimetry is reported by CT dosimetric evaluation at 1-month posttreatment. D90 values are expressed as a percentage of the prescription dose (110 Gy) to the prostate. BTV = biologic target volume.

Before the patient's 1-month return for postoperative CT dosimetry, both intraoperative SPECT–CT–directed BTV biopsies were reported positive for adenocarcinoma. Interestingly, the dominant left prostatic lesion identified by SPECT–CT (BTV-1) demonstrated Gleason score of 7 (3 + 4) involving 25% of the core; in contrast to the Gleason score of 6 (3 + 3) involving 5% found in the diagnostic biopsy. In this manner, the SPECT–CT–guided transperineal biopsy results established an upgrading of the patient's risk status to high-risk, based on the standard Sloan-Kettering classification schema.[1] Had these data been available at the time of initial consultation, we would have considered expanding the EBRT field to include pelvic lymph nodes and/or perhaps adding neoadjuvant hormone therapy. The patient's intraoperative and postoperative dosimetric values are shown in Table 20B-1.

Clinical Outcome

The patient tolerated RT without significant acute sequelae. Follow-up included DRE and PSA tests at 3-month intervals. At 3 months following RT, his PSA value was 7.32 ng/mL. His DRE remained unremarkable; other than for a reduced prostate volume, which remained enlarged (+1) and rubbery, but free of palpable nodularity. At that time, the patient reported slight transient increases (+11) in his AUA score (23, without use of an alpha blocker) while his SHIM score remained stable (14). He was provided samples of sildenafil citrate to treat his preexisting symptom of moderate erectile dysfunction.

At his most recent follow-up, 2-years posttreatment, his PSA nadir was 1.9 ng/mL. Although he remains clinically free of disease by the Phoenix criteria, he remains at high risk for failure and requires close surveillance.[3]

Our clinical experience using ProstaScint-guided target delineation in prostate cancer patients undergoing interstitial brachytherapy was recently published.[4] A total of 239 stage T1C–T3BNxM0 prostate cancer patients underwent pretreatment ProstaScint imaging. Intraprostatic BTVs based on the SPECT–CT imaging were targeted to receive a 150% dose escalation during interstitial brachytherapy. Overall, 150 patients underwent brachytherapy alone and 89 received EBRT plus brachytherapy. Neoadjuvant hormonal therapy was administered to 50 patients. At a median follow-up of 47.2 months (range, 24.8–96.1 months), the 7-year actuarial biochemical disease-free survival (bDFS) based on the American Society for Therapeutic Radiology and Oncology (ASTRO) Consensus definition was 88.0%. The ASTRO-defined bDFS rates for low-, intermediate-, and high-risk patients were 96.0%, 87.0%, and 72.5%, respectively.

References

1. Potters L, Cha C, Oshinsky G, et al. Risk profiles to predict PSA relapse-free survival for patients undergoing permanent prostate brachytherapy. *Cancer J Sci Am.* 1999;5:301–305.
2. Ellis RJ, Kaminsky DA, Zhou H, et al. Molecular image validation utilizing the correlation of histopathology and marker placement system (CHAMPS) protocol. *Int J Radiat Oncol Biol Phys.* 2006;66:S360.
3. Roach M III, Hanks G, Thames H Jr, et al. Defining biochemical failure following radiotherapy with or without hormonal therapy in men with clinically localized prostate cancer: recommendations of the RTOG-ASTRO Phoenix Consensus Conference. *Int J Radiat Oncol Biol Phys.* 2006;65:965–974.
4. Ellis RJ, Zhou H, Kim EY, et al. Biochemical disease-free survival rates following definitive low-dose-rate prostate brachytherapy with dose escalation to biologic target volumes identified with SPECT/CT capromab pendetide. *J Brachytherapy.* 2007;6:16–25.

Ultrasound-Guided Target Localization Using the Clarity System in a Patient with Prostate Cancer

Case Study

Fabio Cury, MD, William Parker, MSc, Nicholas Rene, MD

Patient History

A 75-year-old man underwent a routine prostate-specific antigen (PSA) test, yielding a level of 6.97 ng/mL prompting a transrectal biopsy. Digital rectal examination revealed a normal prostate. The pathology report demonstrated a prostatic adenocarcinoma, Gleason score 7 (3 + 4) in one out of 16 biopsy cores. A repeat PSA was was 9.03 ng/mL. The patient was classified as having an intermediate-risk prostate cancer, according to the Genito-Urinary Radiation Oncologists of Canada (GUROC) consensus.

The patient was offered radical prostatectomy and radiation therapy (RT) as possible curative treatment options. He elected to undergo RT and agreed to enroll in the Radiation Therapy Oncology Group (RTOG) 0126 phase III trial, randomizing patients between 70.2 Gy in 39 fractions and 79.2 Gy in 44 fractions. He was randomized to the experimental arm (79.2 Gy) and treatment was delivered according to our standard practice, using three-dimensional (3D) conformal RT with daily ultrasound (US)-based image guidance.

Simulation

On the day of simulation, the patient was asked to present with an empty rectum and a comfortably full bladder. He was placed in the supine treatment position and a styrofoam block was placed between both ankles and aligned with the frontal room laser, maintaining a con-stant separation between both legs. An urethrogram was performed to assist in defining the prostatic apex during treatment planning. Computed tomography (CT) scan images were obtained on our department Brilliance Big Bore CT (Philips Medical Systems, Cleveland, OH) with 3-mm slice thickness; skin tattoos were used to mark the simulation isocenter.

Immediately after the simulation images were obtained, a transabdominal US scan was performed with the patient in the treatment position and a 3D-US image was acquired with the Clarity System (Resonant Medical, Montreal, Canada). This system consists of two 3D-US units: one in the CT-planning room and one in the treatment room. Both units have ceiling-mounted tracking cameras and US probes with infrared sensors. The probe is tracked in real time during image acquisition by the cameras generating a reconstructed 3D image, which is spatially oriented to the same coordinate system as the CT scan images, and used as a reference for daily correction of organ motion during external beam irradiation.

Treatment Planning

The CT scan images were transferred to the Eclipse treatment planning system (Varian Medical Systems, Palo Alto, CA) and the contouring of target volumes and organs at risk (OARs) was performed by the treating physician according to the RTOG protocol guidelines. Clinical target volume-1 (CTV_1) was defined as the prostate gland and the seminal vesicles, and CTV_2 was the prostate

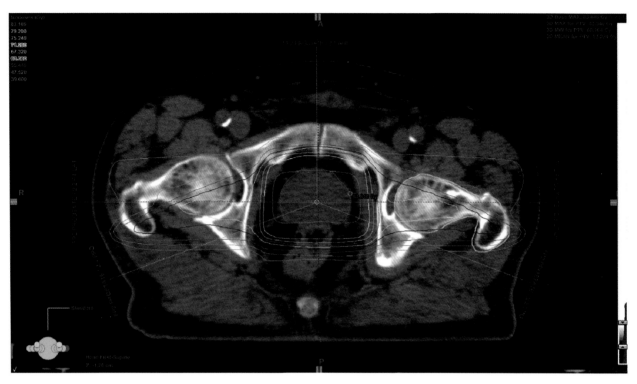

FIGURE 20C-1. Three-dimensional conformal radiation therapy planning for prostate cancer using five-field technique and 18-MV photons. The total dose prescribed was 79.2 Gy in 1.8-Gy fractions.

gland alone. Planning target volumes-1 and -2 (PTV$_1$ and PTV$_2$) were defined as a 7-mm margin around CTV$_1$ and CTV$_2$, respectively, in all directions. The outlined OARs included the rectum, bladder, femoral heads, and penile bulb. A five-field technique planning with gantry at angles 250°, 270°, 0°, 90°, and 110° using 18-MV photons was generated (Figure 20C-1). The doses prescribed to PTV$_1$ and PTV$_2$ were 55.8 Gy and 23.4 Gy, respectively, for a total dose of 79.2 Gy delivered in 1.8-Gy fractions. The planning was found to be satisfactory, meeting the RTOG dose specifications and constraints.

After approval by the treating physician, the plan with the CT images and the reference 3D-US image were sent to the Clarity workstation and coregistered. The Clarity system allows viewing both 3D-US and CT scans coregistered on the same window, with the possibility of switching from one modality to another and comparing for adequate organ positioning (Figure 20C-2). The prostate as seen on the US was contoured, and consistency between both imaging modalities verified. Because in some patients the whole prostate gland cannot be seen on the transabdominal US, mainly because of pubic bone interference, the term "positioning reference volume" (PRV) is used instead of "prostate" to refer to the visible part of the prostate. The treating physician revised the US contours and approved the PRV to be used as the reference for daily correction of organ motion in the treatment room.

Treatment Delivery

For daily treatment, the patient was once again asked to present with an empty rectum and a comfortably full bladder, with no active procedures performed to achieve this status. On the first day of treatment, he was positioned on the linear accelerator treatment couch in the same position as in the simulator. Positioning was then performed with laser guidance. The patient was set up with the isocenter lined up to the skin marks, and the couch was shifted as per the treatment plan such that the center of the PTV was positioned at the isocenter.

Portal images of the five fields were taken in the treatment room to verify field shaping. Immediately afterward, a US scan was performed using the same technique as at simulation by the treating technologist. The image-guidance system displays the acquired scan and the initial US scan (simulation) side-by-side on the same screen (Figure 20C-3A). The technologist positions the PRV contour over the prostate gland visualized in the 3D-US image, and the software automatically displays the distance the couch should be shifted to reposition the prostate to the "ideal" treatment isocenter (Figure 20C-3B), defined from the simulation day isocenter. The couch movements are registered in the system, the patient receives new skin marks at the location of the lasers, and the daily treatment is delivered. The US and repositioning procedure takes approximately 5 minutes in total by trained technologists. As an internal policy, if a

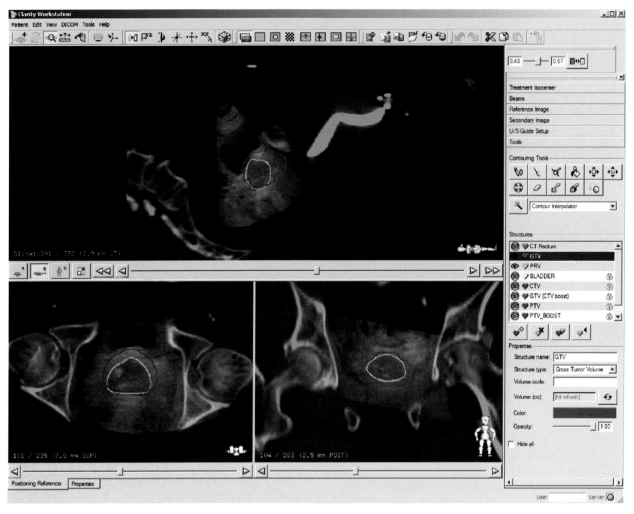

FIGURE 20C-2. Clarity workstation showing computed tomography simulation and transabdominal ultrasound images coregistered during definition of reference volume before treatment delivery.

displacement larger than 2 cm is observed, a radiation oncologist is called to review the procedure. For each one of the 44 treatment days, the patient was positioned at the new skin marks with the lasers, and the US procedure performed afterwards. Couch corrections were performed if differences larger than 0.7 mm were observed.

The daily shifts observed in this patient are displayed in Table 20C-1. The largest corrections were 8.7 mm (lateral), 13.6 mm (anterior–posterior), and 9.1 mm (cranio-caudal). No systematic errors were observed.

Clinical Outcome

The patient tolerated the treatment well without significant acute gastrointestinal or genitourinary toxicity, maintaining his normal lifestyle. He was last seen in follow-up 6 months after the end of his treatment. The worst toxicity observed was grade 1 urinary frequency. His PSA level at that time was 1.80 ng/mL. Rectal examination revealed no evidence of disease.

Our experience using two different US-based verification systems for prostate alignment during external beam RT was published earlier.[1] Comparison was made between a system based on cross-modality verification method (CMVM; BAT, North American Scientific, Chatsworth, CA), which uses two different imaging modalities to assess organ position, and a system based on the intramodality verification method (IMVM; RESTITU, Resonant Medical, Montreal, Canada). A total of 217 CMVM and 217 IMVM displacements were collected within 1 minute of each other in 40 patients with prostate cancer. In 10 patients, IMVM displacements were also compared with those measured with sequential CT scans.

Analysis in the paired CMVM and IMVM displacements demonstrated a significant mean difference of 0.9 mm +/- 3.3 mm in the lateral and 6.0 mm +/- 5.1 mm in the superior–inferior directions ($P < .0001$), whereas no significant difference was seen in the anterior–posterior direction. In contrast, comparison of the CT scan and

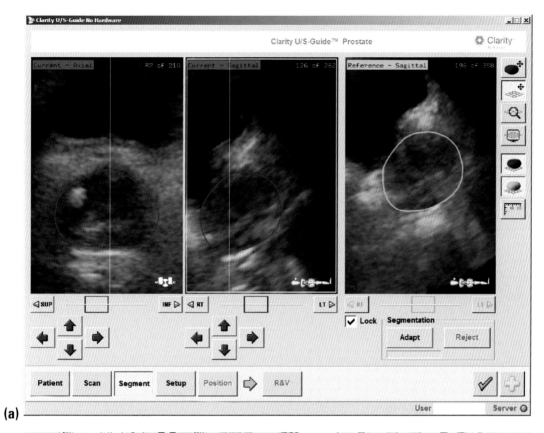

(a)

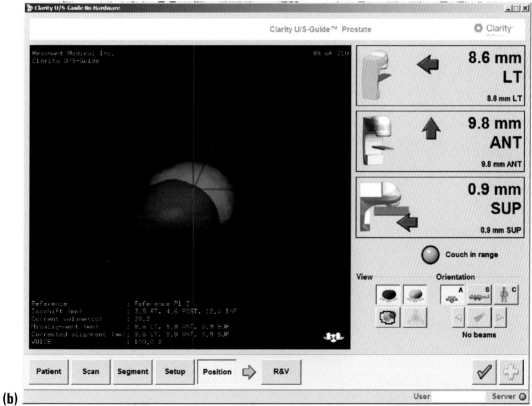

(b)

FIGURE 20C-3. The image-guided radiation therapy system displays the daily (red) and the reference (green) ultrasound scans side-by-side on the same screen (a). After positioning the "positioning reference volume" contour over the prostate gland visualized in the daily image, the software reveals the distance the couch should be shifted to reposition the prostate to the treatment isocenter defined from the simulation day (b).

TABLE 20C–1 Daily Shifts

Session	Misalignment, mm			Session	(cont.)		
	LAT	AP-PA	Sup-Inf		LAT	AP-PA	Sup-Inf
1	0.2	11	−0.4	24	−8.7	9.8	0.9
2	1.5	0.2	−1.3	25	2.8	−0.8	1.5
3	−4.1	2.3	−1.3	26	1.8	−0.7	1.9
4	1.7	−0.3	−2.8	27	−1.3	−13.6	−1.8
5	0.3	−4.6	0.2	28	1.8	2.5	0.3
6	−1.8	−2.5	1.7	29	−1.5	−1.1	3.1
7	5.0	3.0	0.4	30	3.2	3.5	1.7
8	−3.9	0.2	0.4	31	3.2	8.4	−2.2
9	−1.1	−0.6	−1.0	32	1.3	−3.4	9.1
10	−2.2	−2.0	1.7	33	−3.4	−9.3	0.0
11	1.3	−0.6	2.3	34	6.9	1.3	−0.4
12	−2.7	−1.0	1.4	35	4.6	−1.6	5.1
13	−0.2	−0.8	2.2	36	1.2	−0.4	0.2
14	0.6	1.3	−1.6	37	1.5	1.0	6.6
15	−2.5	−6.4	−1.0	38	1.5	−1.1	2.1
16	2.0	−1.9	−0.5	39	−2.7	2.6	0.3
17	0.9	−0.8	1.0	40	1.8	5.7	0.1
18	0.4	−1.9	2.5	41	−0.8	2.0	1.5
19	1.7	3.4	5.4	42	5.1	4.0	−1.0
20	0.3	−4.8	3.5	43	3.7	4.8	3.4
21	−0.1	−1.6	0.7				
22	0.1	−4.1	1.3	Average	0.41	−0.04	1.13
23	−1.7	−2.7	1.4	Median	0.6	−0.6	0.9

Anterior, superior and right shifts are positive.

LAT = lateral; AP = anterior-posterior; Sup-Inf = Superior-Inferior; Rt = right; Ant = anterior; Sup = superior; Lt = left; Post = posterior; Inf = inferior

IMVM-measured displacements revealed no significant differences. Our results suggested that a significant systematic difference exists between the CMVM and IMVM. Because displacements assessed by IMVM are consistent with those assessed by CT, we feel that the IMVM results in a more accurate prostate alignment.

Reference

1. Cury FL, Shenouda G, Souhami L, et al. Ultrasound-based image-guided radiotherapy for prostate cancer: comparison of cross-modality and intra-modality methods for daily localization during external beam radiotherapy. *Int J Radiat Oncol Biol Phys.* 2006;66:1562–1567.

Electronic Portal Image-Guided Setup in a Prostate Cancer Patient with Implanted Fiducial Markers

Case Study

Irene M. Lips, MD, Uulke A. van der Heide, PhD, Marco van Vulpen, MD, PhD

Patient History

A 62-year-old man presented with an elevated prostate-specific antigen (PSA) level (9.2 ng/mL) on routine screening. Digital rectal examination revealed a right-sided palpable nodule with possible extracapsular extension. Ultrasound-guided transrectal biopsies of the prostate were performed. The histopathology was consistent with a Gleason 4 + 4 adenocarcinoma. Metastatic workup, including a bone scan, was negative. No enlarged lymph nodes were noted on contrast-enhanced pelvic computed tomography (CT). A staging pelvic lymphadenectomy was not performed. The tumor was thus staged as T3NxM0.

Based on the European Association of Urology guidelines,[1] the patient was classified as high-risk and our consensus treatment recommendation was for both external beam radiotherapy (RT), to establish local tumor control, and hormonal therapy (before, during, and after RT), to reduce the risk of distant metastases. We elected to treat the patient with image-guided intensity-modulated RT (IMRT) performed by using electronic portal imaging and implanted fiducial markers to ensure optimal prostate localization before each fraction.

Simulation

One week before simulation, three gold fiducial markers (Heraeus GmbH, Hanau, Germany) were implanted in the patient's prostate gland. The three cylindrical markers, with a diameter of 1 mm and a length of 5 mm (Figure 20D-1), were introduced transperineally with two 18-gauge needles placed through a template in a procedure similar to ^{125}I-seed implantation (Figure 20D-2). Through each needle, one or two markers were inserted, at a distance of approximately 2 cm from each other.

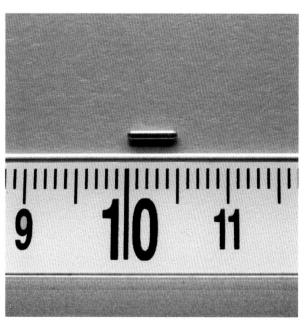

FIGURE 20D-1. Example of a gold fiducial marker used for prostate localization.

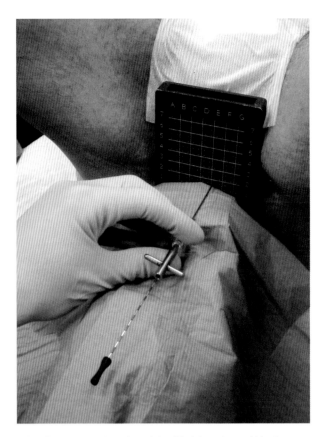

FIGURE 20D-2. Implantation of the fiducial markers within the prostate. Two needles are placed transperineally through a template in a procedure similar to I[125]-seed implantation.

On the day of the procedure, the patient received prophylactic antibiotics (ciproflaxicin 500 mg × 2).

At simulation, the patient was positioned in the supine position with a knee cushion for alignment of his legs. A computed tomography (CT) scan was performed from the fourth lumbar vertebra to the perineum on an Aura CT scanner (Philips Medical Systems, Andover, MA) using 3-mm slices. Magnetic resonance (MR) imaging was also performed on the same day using a 3-Tesla Gyroscan NT Intera (Philips Medical Systems, Andover, MA). Axial T1-weighted and T2-weighted images with 25 slices of 4 mm were obtained using spin echo sequence. Three-dimensional (3D) balanced steady-state free precession images were particularly useful for delineation of the prostate gland. Furthermore, dynamic contrast-enhanced and diffusion-weighted MR imaging was performed to characterize the dominant tumor lesion within the prostate. The patient was instructed to drink 500 cc fluid before imaging.

Treatment Planning

The prostate, dominant lesion, seminal vesicles, and the organs at risk (OARs) were delineated by a physician on the MR images. The clinical target volume (CTV) consisted of the entire prostate and the seminal vesicles.

The structures contoured on the MR images were transferred to the CT by using the transformation and image fusion functionality available in our in-house developed software package, VolumeTool.[2] The images were fused by using automatic rigid registration and a visual verification of registration was done with a linked cursor. The CTV was subsequently expanded by 8 mm to create the planning target volume (PTV). The OARs consisted of the rectum, contoured from the anus up to the recto-sigmoid flexure, and the bladder, which was completely outlined from the bladder neck up to the dome (Figure 20D-3).

The CT data set of the patient was then transferred to the PLATO treatment planning system (Nucletron BV, Veendendaal, Netherlands) and a step-and-shoot five-field IMRT plan was generated, using the following beam angles: 40°, 100°, 180°, 260°, and 320° using 10-MV photons. The prescription dose was to deliver 76 Gy in 35 fractions to the whole PTV, excluding bladder and rectum. Furthermore, at least 99% of the PTV received a dose of 70 Gy. The dominant lesion was enclosed with the 76-Gy isodose. The dose to the rectum was limited ensuring that less than 5% of the rectal volume would receive greater than 72 Gy and less than 50% would receive greater than 50 Gy. For the bladder, the constraint used was that less than 10% would receive greater than 72 Gy (Figure 20D-4). After plan approval, the plan was transferred to the linear accelerator.

Treatment Delivery

Treatment was delivered on an SL-15 linear accelerator (Elekta AB, Stockholm, Sweden) using 10-MV photons.

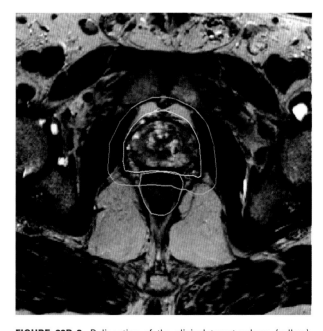

FIGURE 20D-3. Delineation of the clinical target volume (yellow), planning target volume (green), and the rectum (blue) on a transversal T2-weighted magnetic resonance (MR) image.

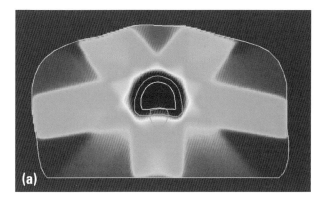

(a)

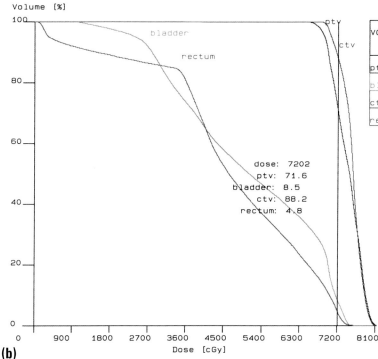

VOI	Vol.	Area		Dose (cGy)	
	(cc)	(%)	Max	Min	Avg.
ptv	252.6	91	8128	6255	7443
bladder	111.2	62	7594	969	5064
ctv	97.6	92	8116	6795	7546
rectum	72.7	56	7570	60	4630

dose: 7202
ptv: 71.6
bladder: 8.5
ctv: 88.2
rectum: 4.8

(b)

FIGURE 20D-4. Transverse image of the dose distribution (a) and dose–volume histograms for the target and the organs at risk (b). The mean dose to the planning target volume was 74 Gy. The percentages of the bladder and rectum volumes receiving greater than 72 Gy were 8.5% and 4.8%, respectively.

Before each fraction, the patient was instructed to drink 500 cc to ensure a full bladder during treatment. For each beam direction, the first segment was used to make a portal image using an iView-GT amorphous silicon flat-panel detector (Elekta AB, Stockholm, Sweden). The fiducial markers were automatically detected on these images with in-house–developed software (Figure 20D-5). Each daily registration was visually inspected by two radiation therapists and manually adjusted as required. The results of this registration were fed into an offline adapted shrinking action level protocol.[3] The translation action level is set to $\alpha / \sqrt{N}$ with α = 6 mm in each direction, N = the number of fractions considered. The maximum number of fractions over which the position deviation is averaged is four. During treatment, one correction in each direction was made. The systematic displacement (± standard deviation) for this patient was 0.3 mm (1.7 mm) in lateral, 0.6 mm (2.1 mm) in cranial–caudal, and 0.04 mm (2.4 mm)

in dorso–ventral directions. No rotational corrections were performed. The IMRT plan required a delivery time of approximately 6 minutes. The total treatment time per fraction, including patient setup and clearing the room after treatment, was approximately 10 minutes.

Clinical Outcome

Overall, the patient tolerated treatment well. He noted no significant genitourinary (GU) or gastrointestinal (GI) side effects during treatment, apart from a mild increase in urinary frequency not requiring medications. At his 3-month follow-up, the patient reported no GU or GI sequelae and has continued with his normal daily activities. At that time, his PSA level was less than 0.1 ng/mL. He was most recently seen in follow-up 15 months posttreatment at which time he remained without any significant late toxicity; his PSA was once again less than 0.1 ng/mL.

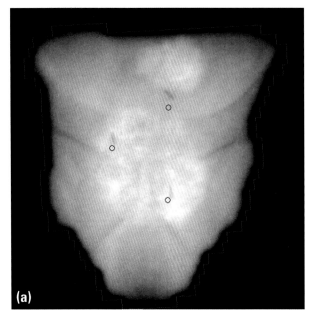
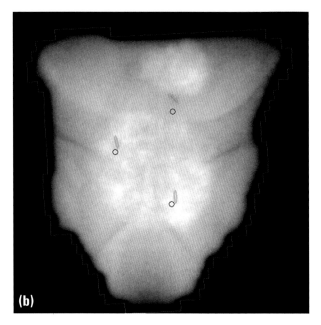

FIGURE 20D-5. Electronic portal images taken from the first segment of the irradiation beam. The actual location of the three fiducial markers can be seen as three dark spots (a) and the location of the three markers based on the planning CT-scan are projected by blue circles. The green ellipses (b) indicate the automatically detected location of the fiducial markers. The position of these green ellipses is visually inspected by two radiographers and manually adjusted as required.

His hormonal treatment is planned for a total of 3 years following IMRT.

Our clinical experience using daily fiducial marker–based prostate position verification in 331 patients with prostate cancer treated with high-dose IMRT (76 Gy in 35 fractions) was recently reported.[4] Acute grade 2 GU and GI toxicities occurred in 47% and 30% of patients, respectively. Only 3% developed acute grade 3 GU toxicity and no acute grade 3 GI toxicity was noted. With a mean follow-up of 47 months, the incidence of grade 2 late GU and GI sequelae was 21% and 9 %, respectively. Grade 3 or higher GU and GI sequelae were noted in 4% and 1% of patients, respectively, with one developing a rectal fistula and a second with severe hemorrhagic cystitis (both grade 4). In a separate analysis of 95 locally advanced prostate cancer patients treated with this approach and a minimum of 3 years of followup,[5] no clinically relevant deterioration in long-term quality of life was noted, except for a persistent decrease in sexual activity.

References

1. Heidenreich A, Aus G, Bolla M, et al. EAU guidelines on prostate cancer. *Eur Urol.* 2008;53:68–80.
2. Bol GH, Kotte ANTJ, van der Heide UA, et al. Simultaneous multi-modality ROI delineation in clinical practice. *Comput Methods Programs Biomed.* 2009;96:133–140.
3. Van der Heide UA, Kotte AN, Dehnad H, et al. Analysis of fiducial marker-based position verification in the external beam radiotherapy of patients with prostate cancer. *Radiother Oncol.* 2007;82:38–45.
4. Lips IM, Dehnad H, van Gils CH, et al. High-dose intensity-modulated radiotherapy for prostate cancer using daily fiducial marker-based position verification: acute and late toxicity in 331 patients. *Radiat Oncol.* 2008;3:15–19.
5. Lips IM, van Gils CH, van der Heide UA, et al. Health-related quality of life 3 years after high-dose intensity-modulated radiotherapy with gold fiducial marker-based position verification. *BJU Int.* 2009;103(6):762–767.

KV Planar Imaging-Guided IMRT Using the Novalis Shaped-Beam System in a Patient with Intermediate Risk Prostate Cancer

Case Study

Richard Garza, MD, Anil Sethi, PhD

Patient History

A 74-year-old man was found to have an abnormal digital rectal examination on routine annual examination. His physician palpated a less-than 1-cm nodule in the left prostatic apex with a corresponding prostate-specific antigen (PSA) level of 4.6 ng/mL. A transrectal ultrasound-guided biopsy of the prostate was performed and pathological review revealed adenocarcinoma Gleason score 4 + 3 and 3 + 4 involving all 12 sampled cores. The percentage of core involvement ranged from 11% to 46%. Metastatic staging workup included a contrast-enhanced computed tomography (CT) scan of the abdomen and pelvis as well as a whole body bone scan. No radiographic evidence of pathologic lymphadenopathy or skeletal metastasis was noted on these examinations.

His initial urologist recommended a radical retropubic prostatectomy with lymphadenectomy or alternatively a combination of external-beam radiation therapy (RT) with a brachytherapy boost. After consultation with his cardiologist because of his history of a viral cardiomyopathy and an ejection fraction of 20%, he chose to avoid any surgical process involving general anesthesia or androgen-deprivation therapy. He subsequently presented to our department for consultation, at which time we offered him noninvasive treatment options. He ultimately chose external-beam intensity-modulated RT (IMRT) without androgen-deprivation therapy. We elected to treat him

with daily image guidance using the Novalis Shaped-Beam System (BrainLab AG, Feldkirchen, Germany).

Simulation

One week before simulation, the patient underwent ultrasound-guided transrectal placement of two 0.75-mm thin and 2-cm long Visicoil fiducial markers (IBA Dosimetry America, Bartlett, TN)—one into each lobe of the prostate. Careful attention was given to place the fiducials along the length of the prostate approximately 0.5 cm from the prostate base.

On the day of simulation, the patient was placed in the supine position in our dedicated wide-bore multislice CT simulator (Philips Medical Systems, Andover, MA) (Figure 20E-1). A stock triangular sponge was positioned under his knees to stabilize the pelvis and legs. A set of six infrared (IR) markers was placed on his abdomen in a V-shaped pattern. Attention was paid to ensuring that all markers would be visible to an IR camera mounted in the treatment room. A urethrogram was performed with 50 cc of iodine contrast to identify the urethral apex and a large red rubber nelation-style catheter was used to evacuate excess air from the rectum. No intravenous or oral contrast was used. After confirmation of an undistended rectum on the CT scout images, transaxial slices were acquired with a slice thickness of 0.5 cm through the pelvis and 0.3 cm at the level of the prostate.

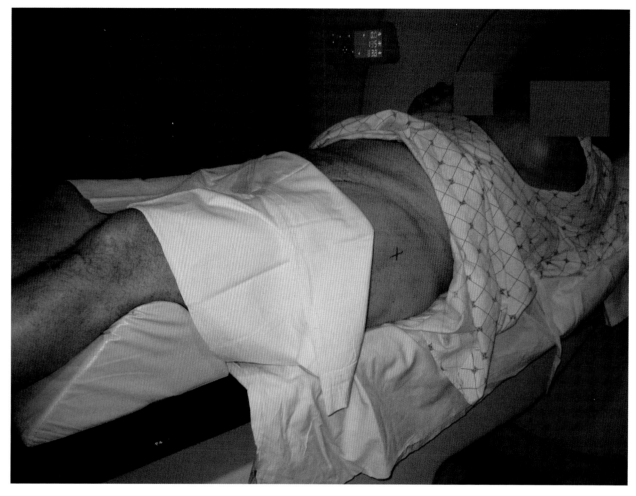

FIGURE 20E-1. Patient immobilized with sponge foam under the knees.

Treatment Planning

The planning CT image set was transferred to the Brain-lAB treatment planning system (BrainScan 5.31, Brainlab AG, Feldkirchen, Germany). The CT image data set was first localized by identifying each of the six IR markers placed on patient's abdomen during simulation. The two implanted fiducial markers were next identified on the image data. (Figure 20E-2). Organs at risk (OARs), namely, the bladder, rectum, and the bilateral femora, were then contoured. The clinical tumor volume (CTV) consisted solely of the prostate. A 0.75-cm three-dimensional (3D) expansion (in all directions except 0.5 cm posteriorly) was used to generate the planning target volume (PTV). Seven coplanar beams with an isocenter at the center of the CTV and gantry angles of 210°, 260°, 310°, 0°, 50°, 100°, and 150° were selected to deliver an optimized IMRT treatment plan. A PTV dose of 78 Gy in 2-Gy daily fractions was prescribed to the isodose line covering 98% of the PTV (Figure 20E-3). Dose–volume histograms (DVHs) were reviewed and doses to PTV and OARs were judged to be acceptable. After plan approval,

the treatment parameters were exported to the Multi-Access (Elekta-IMPAC, Sunnyvale, CA) record and verify system.

Treatment Delivery

At the treatment unit, several quality assurance (QA) steps were performed before treatment delivery. As part of Novalis morning warm-up, the room lasers were checked for coincidence with the linac isocenter. An isocenter pointer containing an embedded 5-mm tungsten ball was attached to the end of the table. The pointer rod was moved to the 3D point in space where all lasers intersected. A therapist then performed the Winston-Lutz test to determine the linac isocentricity with respect to the gantry, collimator, and couch rotations. A 10-mm cone was used to irradiate a piece of XV film placed 10 cm below the tungsten ball. The procedure was repeated for nine gantry and table angle combinations and the film was developed and scanned. The RIT (Radiological Imaging Technology, Colorado Springs, CO) film analysis software was used (stereotactic cone alignment) to analyze

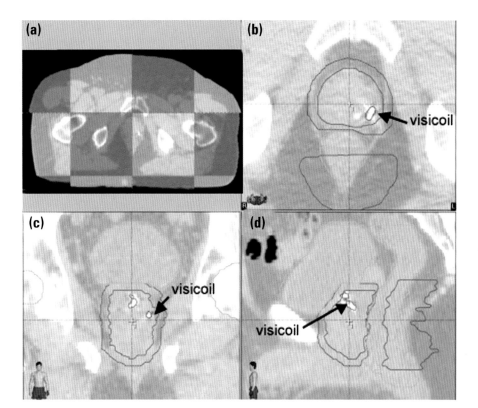

FIGURE 20E-2. Results of mutual information–based image fusion in BrainScan 5.1 **(a)**. Implanted fiducials identified in the three orthogonal image sets **(b, c, d)**.

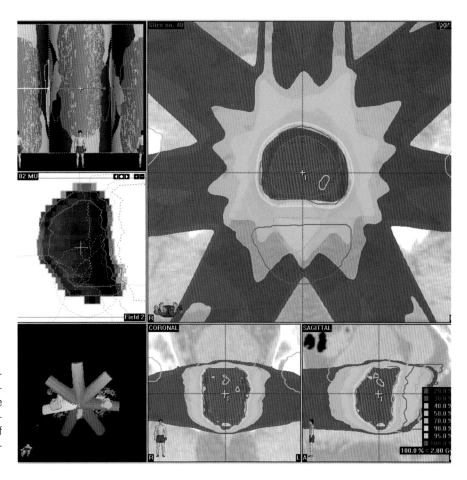

FIGURE 20E-3. Axial, sagittal, and coronal image planes through the planning target volume (PTV) showing dose conformity of a seven-field intensity-modulated radiotherapy plan. A dose of 78 Gy was prescribed to the 98% isodose line covering the PTV.

the film. The distance between the centroids of the tungsten ball and radiation field provided a measure of machine isocentricity (typically less than 0.5 mm average). Next, the Exactrac IR (Brainlab AG, Feldkirchen, Germany) system was calibrated with the isocenter calibration phantom tool, ensuring that the 3D coordinates for the machine isocenter had been accurately defined in the Novalis Exactrac coordinate system.

For treatment, the patient was brought into the linac room and positioned supine on the table with appropriate immobilization devices. Infrared markers were placed on his abdomen at preset locations and used to guide the Exactrac IR camera in positioning the patient to the desired isocenter. Orthogonal x-ray images were then taken with the patient in treatment position and fused with digitally reconstructed radiographs (DRRs) generated by the treatment planning system. The implanted fiducial markers were next identified on the x-ray images and used to fuse them with the DRRs. This fusion provided the necessary shifts to align the patient to the isocenter. As illustrated in Figure 20E-4 and Table 20E-1, there was a total of six shifts generated by the Exactrac software: three translations (x, y, z) and three rotations (around the major axis). After these correction shifts, a second set of verification x-ray images were taken and fused to DRRs to verify that the shifts had been carried out correctly. As an additional QA step, a set of orthogonal AP and lateral setup x-rays (portal images) were taken in this position and compared with DRRs to verify patient setup. These two independent QA steps ensure that the patient is in the correct position before turning on the radiation beam.

Treatment was delivered on a Brainlab Novalis linear accelerator using 6-MV photons at a dose rate of 400 monitor units per minute. During treatment, the optical camera was used to provide real-time (intrafraction) setup monitoring. If a displacement of greater than 0.5 mm were to occur, treatment would be stopped and the patient repositioned. Treatment was completed within a 1-hour time slot.

Clinical Outcome

Overall, treatment was well-tolerated. The patient reported only minor (grade 1) acute genitourinary symptoms starting during week 4 and persisting at the same level until 2 weeks posttreatment. He was seen in follow-up 3 months posttreatment and was noted to have a PSA one half of his pretreatment PSA and reported no bowel or bladder toxicities. His most recent PSA was less than 1 ng/mL. Clinically, he remained sexually potent and continued with his same baseline mild nocturia.

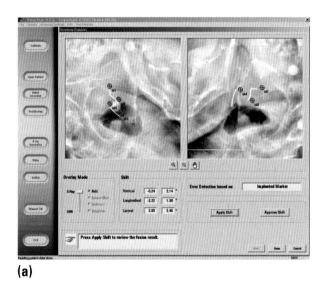
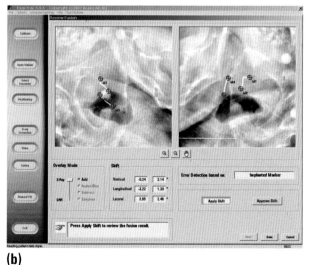

(a) **(b)**

FIGURE 20E-4. Illustration of using the Brainlab ExacTrac robotic table positioning system. (a) Stereoscopic images identifying the fiducial markers in the treatment position within treatment parameters. No shifts are necessary. (b) Stereoscopic images targeting the fiducial markers with residual shifts indicating excellent alignment.

TABLE 20E–1 Daily Shifts and Rotations as Produced by the Exactrac System

Date	Shift [mm]			Angle [°]		
	Lat.	Long.	Vert.	Lat.	Long.	Vert.
Nov 7, 2008	11.38	0.60	−12.19	0.2	4.0	0.4
Nov 10, 2008	11.79	3.58	−16.56	−2.6	3.4	0.3
Nov 11, 2008	14.16	3.42	−19.95	−2.1	4.9	2.1
Nov 12, 2008	12.15	−0.83	−5.82	2.6	3.4	2.0
Nov 13, 2008	14.06	1.88	−6.29	0.6	4.2	1.1
Nov 14, 2008	17.36	−1.60	−1.50	1.7	5.2	0.9
Nov 14, 2008	23.24	−5.68	2.67	−0.5	0.3	0.1
Nov 17, 2008	10.03	−1.20	−1.77	1.6	3.1	0.8
Nov 18, 2008	9.50	−1.84	−9.28	−0.1	3.3	0.5
Nov 19, 2008	12.19	0.07	−5.35	2.2	4.3	1.6
Nov 20, 2008	14.68	−0.34	−8.97	1.6	3.8	1.1
Nov 21, 2008	12.87	−1.04	−9.22	0.8	2.9	0.2
Average	13.50	1.85	8.36	1.3	3.4	0.8
Standard Deviation	4.44	1.73	4.45	0.8	1.2	0.5

KV Planar Imaging-Guided SBRT Using the CyberKnife System in a Patient with Localized Prostate Cancer

Case Study

Christopher R. King, MD, PhD

Patient History

A 68-year-old man presented with an elevated prostate-specific antigen (PSA) level of 4.9 ng/mL (with a 20% free fraction), increased from 3.9 ng/mL 2 years earlier. Digital rectal examination was negative. Transrectal ultrasonography (TRUS) revealed a 56-cc prostate and no hypoechoic lesions. A 10-core biopsy showed 2 foci of adenocarcinoma on the right (both Gleason score 3 + 3), each less than 1 mm, and some atypia on the left.

Because of previous abdominal surgery for diverticulitis, he was not considered a good surgical candidate. The patient had wanted permanent brachytherapy but a planning TRUS in the dorsal lithotomy position revealed significant pubic arch interference. He opted to participate in our image-guided stereotactic body radiotherapy (SBRT) trial using the CyberKnife system (Accuray Inc, Sunnyvale, CA).

Simulation

Before simulation, three gold fiducial markers were placed within the prostate with TRUS image guidance. A noncontrast treatment planning CT scan was obtained within 2 hours following marker placement. Before the planning scan, the patient was asked to void his bladder, but no particular instructions were given regarding his bowels. He was immobilized in the supine position with the aid of a customized alpha cradle mold. The planning CT scan was obtained at 1.25 mm indexing from roughly 15 cm above the iliac crest to 15 cm below the ischium.

Treatment Planning

The prostate and seminal vesicles as well as the following organs at risk (OARs) were contoured: the penile bulb, rectum, bladder, femoral head/neck, and testes. The prostate volume was 62 cc based on the planning CT. The planning target volume (PTV) in this patient was obtained by a 5-mm three-dimensional (3D) expansion of the prostate, with a 3-mm expansion posteriorly. Given his low-risk features, the seminal vesicles were not included. Treatment planning was performed using MultiPlan system (Accuray Inc, Sunnyvale, CA).

A unique aspect of our CyberKnife SBRT prostate approach is the inclusion of the testes as OARs in the treatment planning process.[1] Often ignored in prostate radiotherapy is the incidental dose to the testes. Doses as low as 3 Gy to 4 Gy can result in iatrogenic hypogonadism in older men with all of its associated morbidities, as well as confound PSA-based outcomes. The CyberKnife is able to use many noncoplanar treatment beams to achieve excellent dose conformality, including some beams aimed directly through the testes. By contouring the testes and identifying them as an avoidance structure, one will significantly reduce the dose to the testes to that from internal scatter only.

We illustrate this issue with a patient whose treatment plan was generated first without avoidance of beams incident (or exiting) through the testes and then after turning those beams off (Figure 20F-1). Without this testes constraint, the mean dose to the testes is 6.6 Gy (range, 1.2 Gy to 14.1 Gy). For comparison, the mean dose to the testes

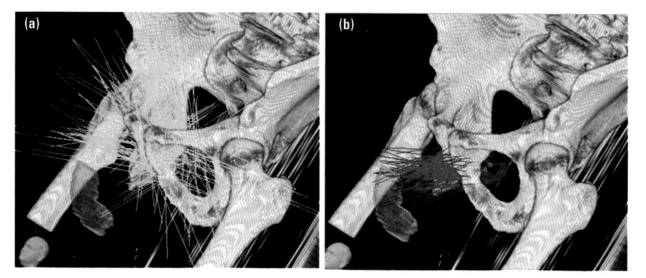

FIGURE 20F-1. Image captured from the CyberKnife treatment planning software for a patient with localized prostate cancer who received stereotactic body radiation therapy. Panel (a) illustrates the beams actually used to treat this patient. Panel (b) illustrates those beams with a direct path through the testes (contoured in translucent green) that needed to be turned off before the final plan optimization.

from internal scatter with a course of 3D conformal external beam radiotherapy to the prostate is about 3% (or 2.4 Gy from a course of 78 Gy with 18-MV photons). Further reductions could be achieved with the use of a testicular shield. After exclusion of beams passing through the testes, the internal scatter dose is reduced to only 1.3 Gy (Figure 20F-2). It is important to note that exclusion of beams passing through the testes does not degrade the

quality of the optimized dosimetry. An illustration of comparative plans through the midaxial plane is shown in Figure 20F-2.

The treatment plan was optimized using a single fixed collimator of 40 mm and achieved our dose–volume goals as illustrated in Figure 20F-3. The plan was normalized to the 87% isodose line covering 95% of the PTV. The prescribed dose was 36.25 Gy in five fractions of 7.25 Gy.

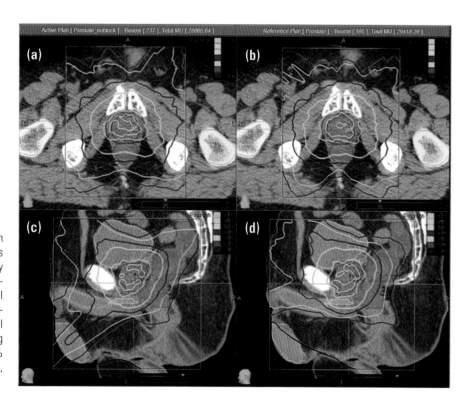

FIGURE 20F-2. Comparison between optimized plans with all available beams and after excluding beams that directly irradiated the testes. Panel (a): midprostate axial, and panel (c): midsagittal planes with all beam. Panel (b): midprostate axial, and panel (d): midsagittal planes after excluding beams passing through the testes. Shown are the 87% (plan normalization) and the 90%, 50%, 30%, 15%, 10%, and 3% isodose lines.

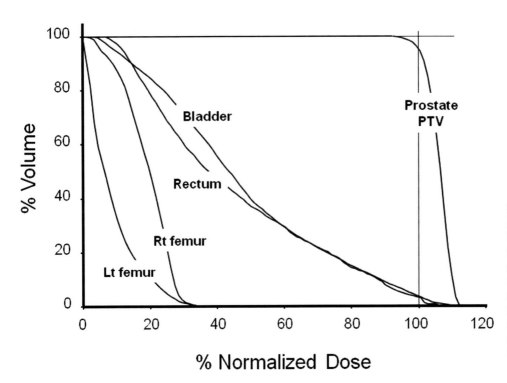

FIGURE 20F-3. Dose–volume histogram achieved with the CyberKnife for a typical patient with prostate cancer on our stereotactic body radiation therapy trial. This plan achieved our goals in terms of planning target volume (PTV) coverage as well as sparing of the rectum, bladder, and femoral head/neck.

Treatment Delivery

Before treatment, the patient was asked to void his bladder primarily for comfort as the duration of treatment is approximately 1 hour. No particular instructions were given regarding his bowels. At initial setup and during treatment, an orthogonal pair of digital kilovoltage (kV) x-ray images was acquired varying intervals ranging roughly from 20 to 60 seconds and alignment of the fiducials with the planning CT scan was made. The isocenter of the beam was adjusted with the robotic arm in 6-D to account for any displacement of the target during treatment delivery. We currently deliver hypofractionated prostate SBRT every other day. Our findings suggest less rectal toxicity using this approach compared with daily treatment.[2]

The total number of paired kV images was approximately 200 for the entire course, and, therefore, the cumulative dose delivered to the entire aperture field from this was estimated to be 50 cGy, bringing the total mean testicular dose (including internal scatter) to about 2 Gy. The contribution to testicular dose from the image-guided system could be reduced or eliminated with smaller aperture fields.

Clinical Outcome

The patient tolerated his treatment well without significant acute toxicity. He has seen a fall in his PSA to 0.66 ng/mL at 6 months after treatment, 0.29 at 1 year, 0.17 at 2 years, 0.1 at 3 years, 0.2 at 4 years, and 0.1 at 4.5 years. His testosterone level at 4.5 years was 527 ng/mL. He has reported being well-satisfied with his urinary and bowel symptoms at last follow-up. He has, however, suffered from erectile dysfunction and is no longer able to have adequate erections for intercourse despite the use of medications.

Our initial clinical experience using CyberKnife-based SBRT in 41 low-risk prostate cancer patients was recently published.[2] All patients received 36.25 Gy in five 7.25 Gy fractions. No patient developed grade 4 acute or late rectal or urinary toxicity (Table 20F-1). Two developed late grade 3 urinary toxicity; none developed late rectal toxicity. Patients treated with an every-other-day schedule

TABLE 20F–1 Late Urinary and Rectal Toxicity on the Radiation Therapy Oncology Group (RTOG) Grade Scale After Prostate CyberKnife Stereotactic Body Radiation Therapy

Late Toxicity	RTOG Grade				
	0	I	II	III	IV
Urinary, % (no. patients)	30% (11)	41% (15)	24% (9)	5% (2)	-
Rectal, % (no. patients)	51% (20)	33% (13)	15% (6)	-	-

Note. Adapted from King CR et al.[2]

experienced less severe late rectal toxicity (0% vs 38%; P = .0035) than those treated on five consecutive days. Of 32 patients with a minimum of 12 months follow-up, 25 (78%) had a PSA nadir of 0.4 ng/mL or less. Patients will be followed continually to assess long-term biochemical control and toxicity.

References

1. King CR, Lo A, Kapp DS. Testicular dose from prostate Cyberknife: a cautionary note [letter]. *Int J Radiat Oncol Bio Phys.* 2009;73:636–637.
2. King CR, Brooks JD, Gill H, et al. Stereotactic body radiotherapy for localized prostate cancer: interim results of a prospective phase II clinical trial. *Int J Radiat Oncol Biol Phys.* 2009;73:1043–1048.

MV CBCT-Guided IMRT on a Siemens Oncor Linear Accelerator in a Patient with Prostate Cancer

Case Study

John E. Bayouth, PhD, Ryan T. Flynn, PhD, Mark C. Smith, MD

Patient History

A 74-year-old man presented with mild urinary obstructive symptoms and a prostate-specific antigen (PSA) level of 4.2 ng/mL. On digital rectal examination, a palpable nodule was appreciated on the right side of the prostate gland. Ultrasound-guided biopsies were obtained and pathology revealed Gleason grade 7 (3 + 4) adenocarcinoma, involving 40% of the tissue examined from the right side of the gland. Biopsies from the left were negative. Bone scan and computed tomography (CT) scans of the abdomen and pelvis were negative for metastases.

Treatment options were discussed with the patient, and he elected to receive a short course (8 months) of androgen-deprivation therapy and external beam radiation therapy (RT). We chose to treat him using magnetic resonance (MR) guidance for target delineation and daily megavoltage (MV) cone-beam CT (CBCT) for target localization on a Siemens Oncor (Siemens AG, Erlangen, Germany) linear accelerator.

Simulation

The patient was simulated using CT and MR imaging modalities, with both devices housed in our department directly across the hall from one another. The planning CT scan was acquired on a Biograph 40 positron emission tomography (PET)–CT simulator (Siemens AG, Erlangen, Germany) with the patient supine, with his pelvis immobilized using a Vac-Lok (CIVCO Medical Solutions, Kalona, IA) device, and aligned on the CT couch with external lasers coincident with external markers. A spiral CT scan without contrast was obtained from the superior edge of L5 to the midfemurs and reconstructed with 2-mm slice thickness. Because the diameter of the reconstructed field of view of the CT scan varies while one is using using 512-by-512 pixels, the resulting size of each voxel within the simulation CT was approximately 1 mm by 1 mm by 2 mm.

Immediately following the CT scan, the patient was transferred across the hall to the MR scanner. Once again, he was aligned using external marks with the same immobilization system as the planning CT scan. Magnetic resonance image acquisition of prostate cancer patients with RT immobilization systems is feasible on a 3-Tesla (3T) scanner without the use of an endorectal coil using the combination of spine matrix and flexible matrix coils (Trio TIM system, Siemens AG, Erlangen, Germany). Magnetic resonance images were acquired with a T2 sequence without contrast, using TR/TE = 2000/122 ms; 1 mm by 1 mm by 2 mm resolution in parallel imaging mode with an acceleration factor of 2 providing a coverage of ~34 cm in 6:44 minutes.

Acquired images were corrected for image distortion by using the vendor-supplied three-dimensional (3D) distortion correction algorithm. Imaging techniques and repositioning of the patient introduced registration errors within the uncertainty inherent in the imaging voxel size and provided superior contrast for prostate delineation, as shown in Figure 20G-1. Note the increased clarity by which the base and apex of the prostate can be defined using the MR data set. Computed tomography and MR

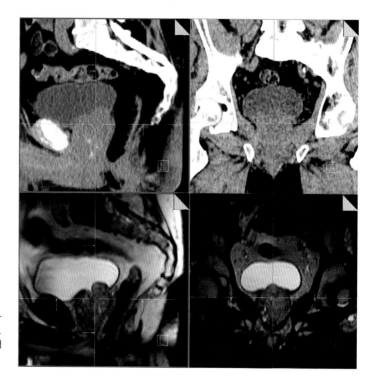

FIGURE 20G-1. Simulation images of prostate. Top row: Computed tomography scan through sagittal and coronal view. Bottom row: Magnetic resonance scan through sagittal and coronal view.

images were registered via rigid-body registration determined by mutual information and fused with the treatment planning system.

Treatment Planning

The patient's prostate, seminal vesicles, and planning target volumes (PTVs) were contoured by the physician using the CT and MR data sets. There were two PTVs: PTV_{54} and PTV_{74}. The PTV_{54} included the prostate and seminal vesicles, plus a 4-mm posterior margin, and a 6-mm margin in all other directions for microscopic tumor extension, patient motion, and setup uncertainty. The PTV_{74} included the prostate only, plus a similar margin as for the PTV_{54}. The prescribed dose to PTV_{54} was set such that the dose received by 97% of the PTV or higher (D_{97}) was 54 Gy, to be delivered in 27 fractions of 2 Gy each. The prescribed dose to PTV_{74} was set such that D_{97} was 74 Gy, to be delivered in a 10-fraction boost with 2 Gy delivered per fraction.

The organs at risk (OARs) were contoured by the dosimetrist and consisted of the bladder, rectum, symphysis pubis, and femoral heads. These organs were segmented for two purposes: (1) for setting dose goals and limits in the treatment planning process, and (2) as structures to visualize during the patient target localization process during treatment delivery. The rectum and bladder dose requirements were: 50% of the volume receives less than 50 Gy, 30% of the volume receives less than 60 Gy, and 15% of the volume receives less than 70 Gy. The maximum femoral head dose was required to be less than 50 Gy. The

treatment plan was generated with the Pinnacle[3] linear accelerator treatment planning system (Philips Medical Systems, Andover, MA) using the direct machine parameter optimization (DMPO) algorithm. A total of seven therapeutic (nonimaging) beams were used for delivery, with gantry angles of 240°, 280°, 320°, 0°, 40°, 80°, and 120°.

Because daily MV CBCT imaging was planned and an additional dose (~10 cGy/CBCT scan) would thus be received by both the target and OARs, this added dose was considered in the treatment planning process using the imaging dose incorporation (IDI) method.[1-4] With the IDI method, the imaging dose that is expected to be delivered throughout a patient's treatment course is calculated and considered an unchangeable base dose. This is computed by adding to the treatment plan a 200° arc beam with the 13 cm by 27.4 cm field size and 15 MU. Once this dose is computed, the inverse planning process is then performed such that the prescription goals and dose limits to critical structures are satisfied, with the *a priori* knowledge of the dose delivered by the imaging arc beam.

The resulting dose distribution is shown in Figure 20G-2, where the impact of the imaging dose is obscured by the much larger doses delivered by the treatment beams when IDI is utilized. Figure 20G-3 shows dose–volume histograms (DVHs) both with (solid lines) and without the use of IDI. The DVHs demonstrate that the imaging dose is substantial and delivers unwanted doses if delivered to the patient but not included in the treatment plan (dashed lines).

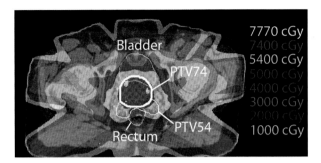

FIGURE 20G-2. Axial dose distribution with planning target volumes, rectum, and bladder.

Treatment Delivery

The patient was treated on a Siemens Oncorlinear accelerator. Clinically, the initial patient alignment was performed using a five-point setup by visually placing skin-mark tattoos with a laser alignment system pointing to the isocenter of the linear accelerator. The daily MV CBCT imaging protocol was selected before the treatment planning process to be a 15 monitor unit (MU) acquisition. The longitudinal field size of the imaging beam was selected to be 13 cm to enclose the entire PTV, and the maximum lateral field size of 27.4 cm was used. The 200° acquisition arc was set to the default of default of 270° to 110°. Because the gantry rotation speed was restricted to one revolution per minute, the image acquisition took approximately 40 seconds. At each integer gantry angle the MV CBCT system acquired a planar image, resulting in a raw projection data set of 200 discrete images. The choices of the MV CBCT protocol and the field size parameters are based on the clinical preference of the physician. At our institution,

5-, 10-, and 15-MU imaging protocols are typically used for head and neck, thoracic, and pelvic cases, respectively.

Image acquisition is integrated with reconstruction and review of the MV CBCT images within the Adaptive Targeting (AT) application. The image reconstruction process began within seconds of the beginning of image acquisition, so that the reconstructed image appeared within 5 seconds of the completion of image acquisition or 45 seconds total when reconstructing a 256 by 256 pixel image with 3-mm slice thickness. Alternatively, images can be reconstructed at different resolutions (128 × 128 pixel to 512 × 512 pixel), slice thickness (1 mm to 10 mm), or with an array of reconstruction kernels. The reconstruction kernels are optimized for Gaussian smoothing or edge enhancement for a range of anatomical sizes. A cupping artifact correction is applied to the images which is optimized for head and neck or pelvic cases. Finally, the user can specify the field length to be imaged (which can be asymmetric) as well as the desired number of monitor units, consistent with that used during the treatment planning process. Because we are able to incorporate the imaging dose into the treatment plan, using IDI as described above, we use as many as 15 MU to better visualize soft tissue. Although this feature is not utilized in our practice, the system will reconstruct reasonable images with as few as 3 MU if one only intends to align to the bony anatomy.

The CBCT images acquired in our patient are shown in the AT application Figure 20G-4. The AT application registers the simulation CT image (above) with the MV CBCT image (below) using a rigid body mutual information algorithm. An image fusion slider allows the user to blend the two image sets, while visualizing the contours drawn on the simulation CT on either image set.

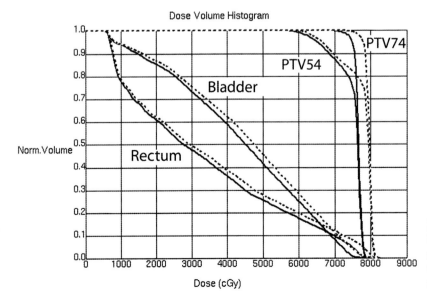

FIGURE 20G-3. Dose–volume histograms (DVH) for the planning target volumes (PTVs), bladder, and rectum. The solid and dotted lines are DVHs with and without the use of image dose incorporation in the treatment planning process.

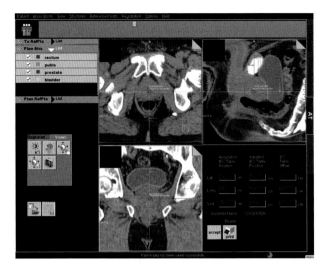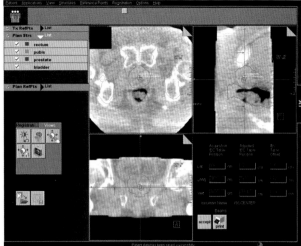

FIGURE 20G-4. Adaptive Targeting application for megavoltage cone-beam computed tomography images.

The user may also adjust the registration manually, seeing the contours and images move in real time. The manual adjustment may be necessary if the patient is experiencing significant nonrigid body deformation, which results from significant changes to bladder or rectal content. Typically the prostate–rectal interface and prostate–bladder interface are used to determine anterior–posterior and superior–inferior displacements, respectively. The prostate gland is used to determine the left–right displacement.

Figure 20G-4 shows a subtle change in rectal content, which results in prostate alignment being slightly different from alignment with the pelvic bones, as seen by the position of the contours around the symphysis pubis. On this treatment day, the patient position correction required a shift of 3 mm to the right, 2 mm superior, and 4 mm anterior with respect to the patient. The AT application indicated this in both absolute and relative table positions, and allowed us to make this shift from the treatment console without re-entering the treatment vault. Once the shift is reviewed by the physician and performed by the technologists, the daily treatment fraction is delivered.

This patient was a participant in an institutional review board–approved study involving improved MV CBCT technology. His CBCT was obtained with an imaging beam line (IBL), which has no flattening filter and generates a beam with a carbon, rather than tungsten, target. This results in a greater fluence of kV-range x-rays than the standard 6-MV treatment beam line (TBL).[5] Image quality is improved when the IBL is used because the flat panel detector response is more optimal for kV than for MV range x-rays.[6,7] The patient was also imaged with the combination of the IBL and an improved flat panel detector system using a sintered pixelated array (SPA) scintillator. This system has increased x-ray detection efficiency relative to the conventional system, and the epoxy separating the scintillator pixels forces visible light to stay inside the SPA pixel it is created in rather than scattering to a neighbor pixel, which reduces blurring and enhances image quality.

Megavoltage CBCT images of the patient with each of these imaging approaches are shown in Figure 20G-5, with Figure 20G-5a showing the simulation CT for comparison. In all cases except the simulation CT patient received a nearly equivalent imaging dose (~10 cGy at isocenter) with the imaging dose incorporated into the treatment plan. These images show an evolution of image quality from the conventional MV CBCT using the TBL (b), the impact of higher abundance of lower energy photons created by the IBL (c), and the contrast improvement

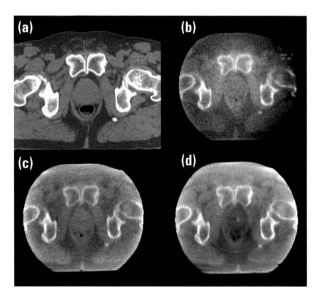

FIGURE 20G-5. Kilovoltage computed tomography, treatment beam line, imaging beam line (IBL), and IBL plus sintered pixelated array images.

with a more efficient SPA detector (d). This patient was imaged for several days with the TBL and for the remaining treatment fractions with the IBL. Because the IBL can also be modeled with Pinnacle,[3] the imaging dose attributable to both TBL and IBL was included in the treatment planning process through IDI.[3]

Clinical Outcome

Clinically, the patient tolerated treatment well. He reported increased urinary frequency and decreased force of stream resulting in an increase in his Flomax dose to 0.8 mg daily. He also reported hot flashes secondary to hormone therapy. However, there were no unexpected side effects during treatment. One month after completing RT, the patient reported feeling well. He was able to decrease his Flomax dose to 0.4 mg daily. He reported no significant bowel or skin issues. His PSA was undetectable.

Megavoltage CBCT has been used extensively at our institution for daily image guidance, with more than 25,000 treatment fractions imaged. We investigated the dosimetric impact of correcting or ignoring mean shifts and extreme shifts for a population of prostate cancer patients using MV CBCT.[8] After an extreme shift was made, mean prostate D_{95} increased from 87.7% to 99.1% of planned dose, while significant differences were not observed after a mean shift but rectal V_{50} and V_{70} improved significantly. We also found clinically significant dosimetric changes in prostate dose, caused by

interfraction motion, are created on various days, but can be corrected with couch translation.

References

1. Morin O, Gillis A, Descovich M, et al. Patient dose considerations for routine megavoltage cone-beam CT imaging. *Med Phys.* 2007;34:1819–1827.
2. Gayou O, Parda DS, Johnson M, et al. Patient dose and image quality from mega-voltage cone beam computed tomography imaging. *Med Phys.* 2007;34:499–506.
3. Flynn RT, Hartmann J, Bani-Hashemi A, et al. Dosimetric characterization and application of an imaging beam line with a carbon electron target for megavoltage cone beam computed tomography. *Med Phys.* 2009;36:2181–2192.
4. Miften M, Gayou O, Reitz B, et al. IMRT planning and delivery incorporating daily dose from mega-voltage cone-beam computed tomography imaging. *Med Phys.* 2007;34:3760–3767.
5. Pouliot J, Bani-Hashemi A, Chen J, et al. Low-dose megavoltage cone-beam CT for radiation therapy. *Int J Radiat Oncol Biol Phys* 2005;61:552–560.
6. Faddegon BA, Wu V, Pouliot J, et al. Low dose megavoltage cone beam computer tomography with an unflattened 4 MV beam from a carbon target. *Med Phys.* 2008;35:5777–5786.
7. Beltran C, Lukose R, Gangadharan B, et al. Image quality and dosimetric property of an investigational imaging beam line MV-CBCT. *J Appl Clin Med Phys* 2009;10:37–48.
8. Bylund KC, Bayouth JE, Smith MC, et al. Analysis of interfraction prostate motion using megavoltage cone beam CT. *Int J Radiat Oncol Biol Phys.* 2009;73:1284–1285.

Image-Guided SBRT Using the Varian Trilogy and Calypso 4D-Localization System in a Patient with Early Stage Prostate Cancer

Case Study

Constantine A. Mantz, MD, Eduardo Fernandez, MD, PhD

Patient History

A 72-year-old man presented with an elevated prostate-specific antigen (PSA) level of 5.1 ng/mL on a routine annual physical exam. A PSA obtained 1 year before was 3.9 ng/mL. Digital rectal examination (DRE) revealed a smooth prostate without a discrete nodule or induration. Transrectal ultrasound demonstrated no hypoechoic lesions. A total of 12 biopsies were obtained, and Gleason score 3 + 3 adenocarcinoma was identified in the right apex and left midgland. The percentage volume involvement of both positive cores was 10%. Radiographic staging studies included computed tomography (CT) scans of the abdomen and pelvis as well as a bone scan; all were negative for metastatic disease. The tumor was therefore staged as T1cN0M0 and classified as low-risk because no high-risk clinical or pathologic features were present.

After consideration of his various treatment options, the patient elected to enroll in our institution's phase II study of image-guided hypofractionated stereotactic body radiation therapy (SBRT) for low-risk, localized prostate cancer using the Trilogy (Varian Medical Systems, Palo Alto, CA) and the Calypso four-dimensional (4D) localization system (Calypso Medical Technologies Inc, Seattle, WA).

Simulation

Before planning imaging, the patient underwent transrectal placement of three Calypso beacon transponders under ultrasound guidance by the urologist. The transponders were implanted within the peripheral zone of the prostate and distributed such that one transponder each was placed at the right base, left base, and apex with at least 1.5 cm spacing between them.

On postimplant day 5, CT and magnetic resonance (MR) imaging were performed. Patient preparation consisted of over-the-counter laxatives the evening before and nothing by mouth after midnight. On the morning of simulation, the patient underwent an enema approximately 2 hours before imaging, a regimen repeated before each treatment fraction. Supine immobilization was achieved through use of a customized Vac-Lok device (CIVCO Solutions, Kalona, IA) placed under his lower torso, pelvis, and thighs. A stereotactic body frame was not used. The CT data set of the pelvis was acquired with 1.25-mm slice thickness without contrast. Subsequently, a T2-weighted pelvic MR was performed using an abdominal phased array coil with 2.0-mm slice thickness.

Treatment Planning

The CT and MR image sets were coregistered for target and organ-at-risk (OAR) volume delineations. The clinical target volume (CTV) consisted of the prostate only. A planning target volume (PTV) was created by a uniform expansion of the CTV by 3 mm in all dimensions, but was truncated at the outer aspect of the anterior rectal wall in cases where the PTV overlapped the rectal volume. The rectum was contoured as a solid structure, including all intraluminal contents from the sigmoid flexure to the ischial tuberosities. The bladder was also outlined as a solid structure inclusive of all contents from the dome to the bladder neck. The urethra, as visualized on MR, was contoured from the bladder neck to the prostatic apex. The femoral heads were delineated from the level of the acetabula to just inferior to the greater trochanters. The penile bulb was outlined from its origin inferior to the urogenital diaphragm and then anteriorly for 2 cm toward the corpora cavernosa.

A total dose of 36.25 Gy in five fractions was prescribed to the PTV. The OAR dose–volume constraints for SBRT on this protocol were appropriated from our institution's conventional fractionation limits and converted for hypofractionated therapy using biological effective dose formalisms. Intensity-modulated treatment planning was performed using the XiO planning system (Computerized Medical Systems, Inc, St Louis, MO). The treatment plan consisted of eight intensity-modulated fields arranged isocentrically in a nonopposing, coplanar orientation. Each field consisted of 10 intensity levels. The isodoses of this plan overlaid on the CT scan are shown in Figure 20H-1.

Treatment Delivery

Treatment was delivered according to an every-other-day schedule over 10 calendar days. Total setup and treatment time was roughly 30 minutes per fraction. Setup procedures consisted of initial target localization using the Calypso system followed by verification and assessment using kilovoltage cone-beam CT (CBCT) imaging on the On-Board Imager (Varian Medical Systems, Palo Alto, CA; Figure 20H-2). The CBCT images were compared to the planning CT images to assess (1) transponder displacement, (2) excessive filling of the bladder and rectum, and (3) target deformation. The first problem has not been encountered. The second and third problems are managed by having the patient void and repeating the setup. Following this assessment, the Calypso system was then re-engaged, and treatment was started. During Calypso real-time tracking, an excursion threshold of 3 mm in all dimensions (lateral, anterior–posterior and superior–inferior) was assigned. If the system detected any target movement beyond this limit, the treatment beam was immediately stopped and then resumed once the target was detected within the assigned threshold. If the target did not return with the assigned threshold by 3 minutes, then the treatment couch was remotely adjusted so that the target's position was zeroed again, and treatment was resumed.

For this patient, treatment was interrupted because of target drift beyond the prescribed threshold during the second, fourth, and fifth fractions. Interruptions were observed at 3 and 16 minutes during the second fraction, at 5 minutes during the fourth fraction, and at 18 and 22 minutes during the fifth fraction. In all instances, the target returned spontaneously within the prescribed

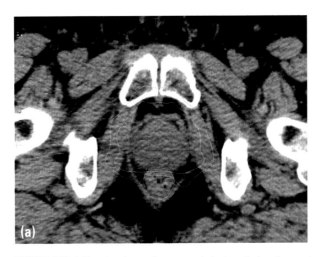
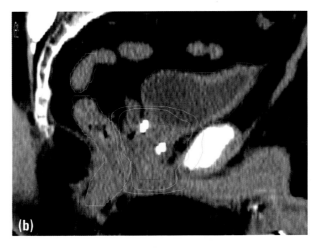

FIGURE 20H-1. Hypofractionated stereotactic body radiation therapy treatment plan for low-risk prostate cancer. Isodose lines: 100% (red), 75% (yellow), and 50% (green). Planning target volume (red), rectum (aqua), and bladder (magenta) are also demonstrated **(a)**. Note two of three implanted Calypso beacons are visible in the sagittal image **(b)**.

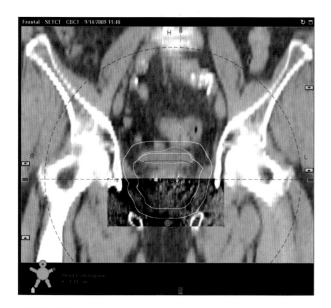

FIGURE 20H-2. Verification of daily setup using cone beam computed tomography (CBCT). A coronal slice through the CBCT scan is shown. Highlighted in the central region is the overlay of the planning CT scan. Alignment of the transponders between the two scans shows good agreement.

threshold within 3 minutes, and no table corrections were necessary. No significant target drifts were noted during the first and third fractions.

Clinical Outcome

Overall, the SBRT treatment was well tolerated, without any significant acute side effects. Urinary symptoms were first observed after the third fraction and consisted of grade 2 frequency and urgency as well as grade 2 dysuria, requiring medication for symptomatic control. These side effects began to resolve within 2 weeks of the completion of treatment. The patient never reported hematuria, incontinence, or significant obstructive symptoms. Acute gastrointestinal toxicity was limited to slight discomfort with bowel movements not requiring medication for relief, which resolved within 4 weeks of completing treatment.

At 18 months posttreatment, no chronic urinary or rectal toxicities have been observed. The patient has had an excellent biochemical response to treatment. Serum PSA levels declined to 1.6 ng/mL at 3 months, 0.4 ng/mL at 6 months, 0.3 ng/mL at 12 months, and 0.2 ng/mL at 18 months. At his most recent follow-up, the patient was experiencing no late urinary or gastrointestinal sequelae.

Our initial clinical experience with image-guided hypofractionated SBRT in 58 patients with prostate cancer (clinical stage T1C-2A; PSA ≤ 10 ng/mL; Gleason score ≤ 6; prostate volume < 60 cc; and an International Prostate Symptom Score < 18) performed on a Varian Trilogy with daily CBCT image guidance and Calypso 4D intra-fraction monitoring was recently presented.[1] The SBRT PTV was generated by a 3-mm uniform expansion of the prostate volume. A total dose of 36.25 Gy was prescribed in five 7.25-Gy fractions, delivered on an every-other-day schedule.

At 1 month posttreatment, grade 1–2 urinary frequency, dysuria, and retention were reported by 43.1%, 15.5%, and 18.9% of patients, respectively. At 6 months, grade 1 urinary frequency, dysuria, and retention rates were 16.7%, 0%, and 6.7%, respectively. No patient reported grade 3 or higher urinary toxicity at any time. Rectal toxicity was uncommon: at 6 months, three patients reported grade 1 proctitis and one patient noted grade 1 rectal bleeding, which resolved without intervention. Mean PSA measurement for the entire cohort demonstrated a rapid decline over the first 6 months from a pretreatment mean value of 7.6 ng/mL (range, 3–10 ng/mL) to a 6-month posttreatment mean value of 1.0 ng/mL (range, 0–3.5 ng/mL). No biochemical failures were noted. Patients are continuing to be followed for biochemical outcome and toxicities.

Reference

1. Mantz C, Fernandez E, Zucker I, et al. A phase II trial of Trilogy-based prostate SBRT: report of favorable toxicity and early biochemical outcomes [abstract]. *Int J Radiat Oncol Biol Phys.* 2008;72:S311.

MVCT-Guided Hypofractionated IMRT Using Helical Tomotherapy in a Patient with Prostate Cancer Following Prostatectomy

Case Study

Cesare Cozzarini, MD, Claudio Fiorino, PhD,
Sara Broggi, PhD, Nadia Di Muzio, MD

Patient History

A 63-year-old man presented with an elevated prostate-specific antigen (PSA) level of 8.2 ng/mL. Workup revealed a clinical stage T2a, Gleason score 3 + 3 adenocarcinoma. He underwent an extended bilateral pelvic lymphadenectomy and radical retropubic prostatectomy. Pathology demonstrated a Gleason score 3 + 4 adenocarcinoma bilaterally, extracapsular invasion, and a positive left posterior–lateral surgical margin. The seminal vesicles were negative. Eighteen pelvic lymph nodes were removed and none had evidence of metastatic disease. The tumor was thus staged as pT3a R1 N0, C1 according to the American Staging System. His postoperative PSA, measured 6 weeks postsurgery, was 0.01 ng/mL.

Based on the extracapsular extension and involved surgical margin, our consensus recommendation in this patient was for early adjuvant radiotherapy (RT) to the prostatic bed. Neither adjuvant hormonal therapy nor pelvic nodal RT was prescribed. We elected to treat him on an in-house phase I–II study of hypofractionated RT delivered with daily megavoltage computed tomography (MVCT) guidance using the helical TomoTherapy system (TomoTherapy Inc, Madison, WI).

Simulation

The patient was simulated in the supine position. A Combifix positioning device (CIVCO Inc, Kalona, IA) was used to keep his leg position as reproducible as possible, as leg position reproducibility has been found to be very important in minimizing setup errors. The patient was scanned using a GE High Speed NXIi CT scanner (GE Healthcare, Waukesha, WI) from L2 to approximately 5 cm below the anus, with a slice thickness of 4 mm. No intravenous or oral contrast was used. The patient, whose postoperative urinary continence was more than satisfactory, was instructed to empty his rectum and to keep his bladder as full as possible during simulation; the patient was also instructed to reproduce these conditions during treatment.

Treatment Planning

Images were subsequently sent to our Eclipse (version 7.4) treatment planning system (Varian Medical Systems, Palo Alto, CA) for contouring. The clinical target volume (CTV_1) included the prostatic fossa and the lower bladder neck. The seminal vesicle bed was not included. Clinical data, location of surgical clips, bony structures, and the anterior rectal wall were used to guide the contouring of the CTV_1, which extended inferiorly to about 1 cm to 1.5 cm from the caudal limit of the ischiatic tuberosities. A planning target volume (PTV_1) was generated by automatic expansion (cranial–caudal 1 cm; elsewhere 0.8 cm) of CTV_1. Body, rectum, bladder, femoral heads, and femurs were contoured as avoidance structures. The rectum was contoured from the anus to the point where the rectum turns into the sigmoid. Additional "helper" regions were contoured to better guide the inverse optimization; a caudal region was contoured just inferior to the PTV_1, increasing the dose gradient in the cranial–caudal direction, reducing the dose to the penile bulb.

After the contouring was completed, images and contours were sent to the TomoTherapy HiArt planning station, a dedicated treatment planning system based on an inverse planning optimization approach with a convolution–superposition dose calculation algorithm. A field width of 2.5 cm, a pitch of 0.3, and a modulation factor of 2 were used in the plan, as the only user-selectable parameters for dose planning.

The total dose specified on our phase I–II trial was 58 Gy in 20 fractions (2.9 Gy/fraction). The goal of the optimization process was to deliver greater than 95% of the prescribed dose to greater than 95% of the PTV (Figure 20I-1), while keeping dose homogeneity as high as possible. Concerning the rectum and bladder, no attempts were made to reduce the dose in the overlap region between these organs and PTV, whereas the dose was reduced as

much as possible outside the PTV. With respect to rectum sparing, the resulting plans were expected to largely satisfy the dose–volume constraints normally used in 3D conformal RT. Strict constraints were not defined for the bladder, because of the variability of its filling. Femoral heads were set to receive a maximum dose less than 35 Gy, reducing the fraction receiving more than 20 Gy (Figure 20I-1). No hot spots (> 50 Gy) were allowed outside the PTV.

As can be seen from Figures 20I-1 and 20I-2, excellent PTV coverage (V_{95} = 99%) and high homogeneity of dose distribution were achieved (SD = 0.60), No hot spots were noted; indeed, the maximum dose within the PTV was 60.6 Gy. The mean dose to the rectum was 19 Gy with a V_{40} of 13.5%. The mean bladder dose was 25 Gy. This excellent result was in part attributable to the ability of the patient to maintain a "full" bladder (volume 259.87 cc). Femoral heads and femurs were also efficiently spared with a maximum dose of 23 Gy, while keeping the fraction of both receiving greater than 15 Gy below 8% (Figure 20I-1).

Treatment Delivery

Before starting treatment, the patient underwent a dosimetry verification, verifying the accuracy and agreement between calculated and measured dose distribution. The dose distribution was checked in a coronal plane passing through the central irradiated region. Microionization chambers (Exradin A1SL, 0.056 cc, Standard Imaging,

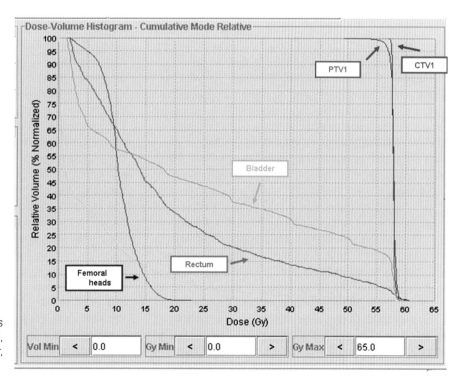

FIGURE 20I-1. Dose–volume histograms (DVH) of the clinical target volume (CTV_1), planning target volume (PTV_1), bladder, rectum, and femoral heads.

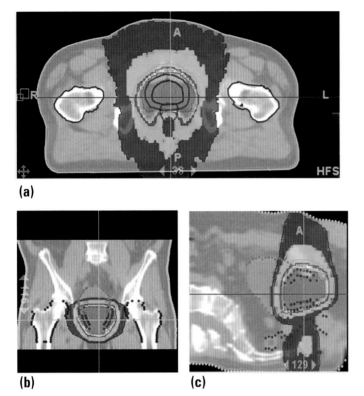

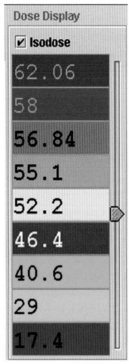

(a)

(b)   (c)

FIGURE 20I-2. Dose distributions in the final treatment plan overlaid on the planning computed tomography scan in (a) axial, (b) coronal, and (c) sagittal views.

Middleton, WI) were positioned in appropriate locations to measure absolute doses in some points in the high-dose homogeneous area included in the chosen coronal plane, and in the area corresponding to the rectum. Properly calibrated EDR2 films (Eastman Kodak, Rochester, NY) were used to measure the dose distribution in the same plane. The measured dose distribution was finally compared with calculated one. Gamma analysis using a 3%/3 mm criteria was applied. Film analysis software implemented in the dedicated TomoTherapy planning station was used for this analysis.

On each treatment day, the patient was placed in the supine position and instructed to keep the rectum and bladder "feeling" as close as possible to the state at planning CT scan (i.e., rectum empty and bladder full). Daily MVCT scans were obtained and registered with planning CT images (Figure 20I-3) and positioning adjustments were assessed to correct daily setup error. Registration was based on a rigid-body approach (three translational and three rotational degrees of freedom). The images were first automatically registered by the radiographer, and then, as necessary, manual adjustments were applied by the physician. Fully automatic registration was carried out by Mutual Information algorithm (MI, also called full-image technique) or a variation of MI called extracted feature fusion, in which the registration parameters are determined by the optimization of a similarity measure that depends only on those voxels in the reconstructed

image with values above a threshold, typical corresponding to bone or bone and tissue.

A daily correction of setup errors without any action level was applied to better investigate setup error fluctuations by monitoring all fractions. The average shifts were: lateral 0.28 mm (SD = 1.99), range: −3.9 mm to + 3.9 mm; longitudinal −4.1 mm (SD = 2.79), range: −6.7 mm to + 4.5 mm; vertical 6.9 mm (SD = 1.92), range: 2.4 mm to 10.7 mm. This approach guaranteed the minimization of the systematic setup error within 3 mm for each direction with the residual systematic error mainly attributable to the intrinsic uncertainty of the fusion as well as any intrafraction patient motion. In Figure 20I-3, a daily MVCT scan is shown with the accepted registration with the corresponding planned CT scans. Fluctuations of rectum or bladder volumes were not taken into account during the image-guide procedure. In other words, no attempt was made to compensate for potential CTV_1 movement caused by variable rectum or bladder filling as it is unclear what is the real impact of bladder and rectum motion on CTV_1 in patients postoperatively irradiated; it is, however, important to underline that, because of the careful instructions given to the patient, the motion of rectum and bladder next to the CTV_1 compared with bony structures was small. Correction of setup error only was considered safer in terms of CTV_1 irradiation, because a reduction of margins was not considered a clinically significant goal for these patients.

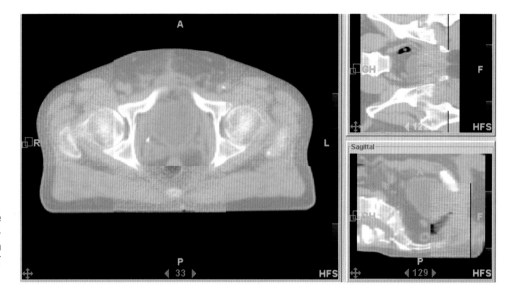

FIGURE 20I-3. An example of a daily megavoltage computed tomography (CT) scan fused with the planning CT scan.

Clinical Outcome

The patient tolerated treatment well, without any significant gastrointestinal (GI) acute sequelae. During treatment, he complained only of mild (grade 1) acute genitourinary (GU) toxicity, mainly urinary urgency and dysuria, both of which resolved within 1 month following the completion of treatment.

At his most recent follow-up (3 years posttreatment), the patient had an undetectable PSA level and no evidence of disease recurrence, on both radiographic and physical examinations. With respect to sexual function, the patient, who noted intermittent nocturnal erections following surgery, reported a partial recovery of erectile function, albeit not firm enough for intercourse.

We recently reported our clinical experience of hypofractionated adjuvant RT delivered using helical tomotherapy with daily MVCT image guidance.[1] Fifty patients were enrolled in our in-house phase I–II trial and received 58 Gy in 20 fractions. Our primary endpoint was to verify a risk of toxicity and biochemical failure not exceeding that observed in 153 of our own patients treated with conventionally fractionated RT. Median patient follow-up was 25 months. Acute grade 2-3 GU and acute grade 2 intestinal toxicities were similar (12% vs 15.6% and 4% vs 7%, respectively), while acute grade 2 proctitis was 0% and 9% in the hypofractionated and convent-ional RT groups. Corresponding late GI toxicities were 0% and 8.5%, respectively. The incidence of late urethral stricture, 8% (hypofractionated) and 9% (conventional), was comparable to that seen in the surgery alone series. Patients are currently being followed to assess biochemical response.

Reference

1. Cozzarini C, Fiorino C, Di Muzio N, et al. Hypofractionated adjuvant radiotherapy with helical tomotherapy after radical prostatectomy: planning data and toxicity results of a phase I-II study. *Radiother Oncol.* 2008;88:26–33.

KV CBCT-Guided IMRT Using a Varian Linear Accelerator in a Patient with Localized Bladder Cancer

Case Study

Ludvig Paul Muren, MSc, PhD, Jimmi Søndergaard, MD,
Anne Vestergaard, MSc, Jørgen Petersen, MSc, Pauliina Wright, MSc,
Ulrik V. Elstrøm, MSc, Cai Grau, MD, PhD, Morten Høyer, MD, PhD

Patient History

A 78-year-old man presented to his general practitioner with new-onset hematuria. After several treatment attempts for urinary infection, diagnostic work-up by an urologist including computed tomography (CT) urography and transurethral resection of the bladder revealed a unifocal, mobile 2.5 cm by 2.5 cm transitional cell muscle-invasive tumor arising on the left bladder wall. Papillomatoid changes were also noted throughout the entire bladder. No enlarged regional lymph nodes were noted on abdominal–pelvic CT. A chest CT was also performed and was negative. The tumor was thus staged as T2N0M0 (stage II).

Although the patient was medically fit, he had earlier undergone surgery for an abdominal aortic aneurysm with complications as well as a left nephrectomy for a renal cell carcinoma. The patient was discussed at our multidisciplinary uro-oncological team conference and our consensus recommendation was for curative radiotherapy (RT).[1,2] We elected to treat the patient with daily kilovoltage (kV) cone-beam CT (CBCT) guidance (Varian Medical Systems, Palo Alto, CA).

Simulation

Before CT simulation, an experienced surgeon performed flexible cystoscopy to localize the bladder tumor. An oil-soluble contrast medium containing iodized ethyl esters of fatty acids of poppy seed oil (Lipiodol-ultra fluid, Laboratoire Guerbet, France) was injected through a contrast injection therapy needle (Interject, Boston Scientific Corporation, Natick, MA) around the tumor into the mucosa.[3] The patient experienced only mild discomfort from the procedure.

One week later, the patient underwent CT simulation using a spiral CT scanner (Siemens Somatom Plus 4, Siemens AG, Erlangen, Germany), acquiring images with 3-mm slice thickness (6 mm/second; Figure 20J-1) from the promontory to 2 cm below the trochanter minor. The scan was performed without contrast as the patient had only one functioning kidney. The images were reconstructed with 512 by 512 pixels and 3-mm interslice distance. During the scanning procedure—as well as during all subsequent treatment sessions—the patient was immobilized in supine position using a heel and knee fixation system. The patient was instructed to empty his bladder immediately before the CT scanning as well as the treatment sessions.[4–8]

Treatment Planning

Organ delineation for treatment planning was performed in collaboration between the treating radiation oncologist and a diagnostic radiologist, using the Eclipse treatment planning system (Varian Medical Systems, Palo

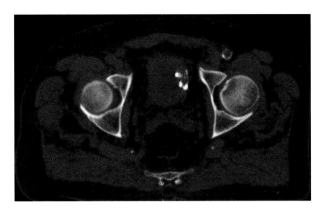

FIGURE 20J-1. An axial slice from the planning computed tomography scan of the patient through the tumor and the Lipiodol volumes.

Alto, CA). Two planning target volumes (PTVs) were contoured: PTV_{60}, which included the bladder with margins, and PTV_{48}, which included both the bladder and relevant lymph nodes with margins. The bladder was outlined as the bladder wall plus the contents of the bladder. The lymph nodes were included from the level of the sacral promontory, with the internal iliacs included to the obturator fossa and the external iliacs to the level of the femoral heads. The pararectal and presacral lymph nodes below the sacroiliac joint were excluded. Isotropic wide bladder-to-PTV margins were used to account for the considerable geometrical uncertainties present in bladder cancer (superior: 25 mm; inferior: 15 mm; lateral: 20 mm; anterior: 25 mm; and posterior: 20 mm). Between the lymph nodes and the PTV_{48}, an isotropic 10-mm margin was used to account for delineation and geometrical uncertainties.[9,10]

The bowel, rectum, and femoral heads were considered organs at risk (OARs) in this patient. For the bowel, we first outlined the bowel volume as all segments of contrast and noncontrast enhanced small intestines and colon as visualized on the planning scan (superior border 12 mm above the PTV_{48}). In addition, we outlined the bowel cavity, i.e., the space where the bowel is free to move. For the rectum, the rectosigmoid flexure was used as the superior–cranial limit and the anal verge as the inferior-caudal limit. Both the bowel and rectum were outlined, including their respective walls and entire contents. The femoral heads were outlined from the most cranial part to the inferior part of minor trochanter on both sides.

Treatment optimization was performed using the Eclipse/ARIA treatment planning system (Varian Medical Systems, Palo Alto, CA). For optimization purposes, we defined four additional volumes: $oPTV_{60}$, $oPTV_{48}$, oBowel, and oRectum. The $oPTV_{60}$ was a copy of the PTV_{60} but modified to be at least 5 mm within the skin surface. Similarly, the $oPTV_{48}$ was a copy of the PTV_{48} modified to be at least 5 mm within the skin surface and also with the $oPTV_{60}$ subtracted so that only one dose level could be

prescribed to the entire volume. The oBowel was defined as the contents of the bowel more than 5 mm from the PTV_{60} and the PTV_{48} in the cranial–caudal extension of the target volumes. The oRectum was the part of the rectum with at distance of more than 8 mm from the PTV_{48}. The PTV constraints were hard whereas the constraints on the rectum and bowel were soft.

A simultaneous integrated boost (SIB) technique was used consisting of a six-field beam arrangement (all 15 MV) with the following gantry angles: 45°, 82°, 168°, 192°, 278°, and 315°. A collimator angle of 5° was used for all beams to reduce the dosimetric impact of the tongue-and-groove effects. Our optimization strategy was to increase the priorities to $oPTV_{60}$ and the $oPTV_{48}$ until at least 99% of the PTV_{60} was covered by 95% of 60 Gy and at least 99% of the PTV_{48} was covered by 95% of 48 Gy while keeping the global maximum less than 107% of 60 Gy. Next, the soft constraints to oBowel and oRectum were adjusted as much as possible—while respecting the target coverage criteria—so that the 50-Gy isodose line did not circumscribe the whole circumference of the rectum on any CT slice level and the V_{35} was less than or close to 20% for the bowel. A smoothing factor of 60 was used for all fields. The resulting plan is shown in Figure 20J-2.

Treatment Delivery

The patient was treated on a Varian Clinac iX equipped with a Millennium MLC-120 multileaf collimator (MLC) and an On-Board Imager kV imaging system (OBI v. 1.4, Varian Medical Systems, Palo Alto, CA). Intensity modulation was performed using the sliding window technique. The SIB IMRT plan was delivered in 30 fractions (2 Gy daily, 5 days a week), to a total dose of 48 Gy to the PTV_{48} and 60 Gy to the PTV_{60}.[9]

During treatment, the patient was scheduled for daily kV CBCT scanning (using the OBI system) before beam delivery (Figure 20J-3). As the patient was part of our recently completed pilot study of Lipiodol-based image-guided RT, the CBCT scans were used for bony anatomy correction only. The variation in the bony anatomy setup corrections throughout the course of treatment is presented in Figure 20J-4, showing that the daily set-up corrections removed a considerable systematic component for this patient. Overall, the average correction was 4 mm, 5 mm, and 10 mm in the lateral, longitudinal, and vertical directions, respectively.

As part of our investigations of the Lipiodol agent, we retrospectively outlined the separate Lipiodol volumes in both the planning CT scan and the CBCT scans, using a fixed Hounsfield units (HU) interval (200 to 2500) for all the CBCT scans. For this patient, the volume was reduced from roughly 4 cm^3 at the beginning of treatment to less than 3 cm^3 at the end of the treatment course ($R^2 = 0.71$ for a linear regression between

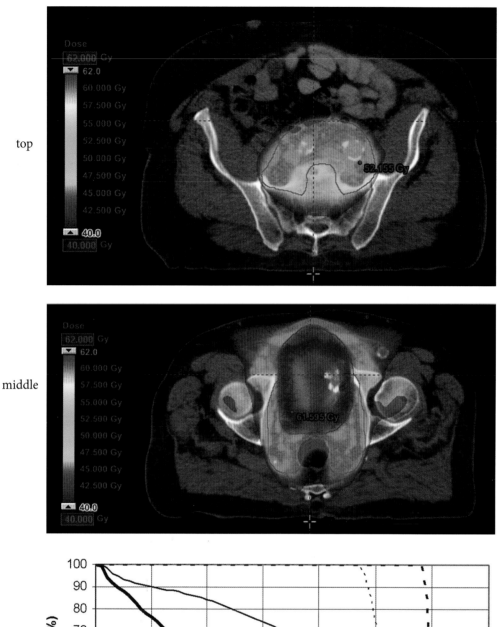

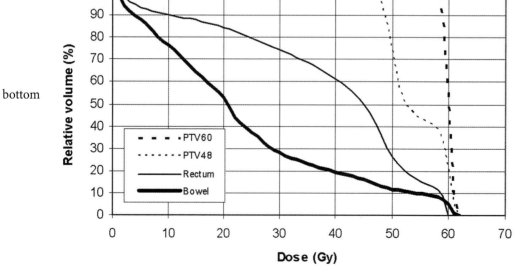

FIGURE 20J-2. The simultaneous integrated boost intensity-modulated radiotherapy treatment plan used in this patient, with the dose distributions on axial slices at the lymph node level (top) and through the center of the bladder (middle) as well as the dose–volume histograms for the targets and organs at risk. The outlined bowel and rectum volumes had absolute volumes of 799 cm³ and 104 cm³, respectively.

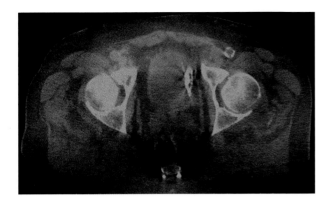

FIGURE 20J-3. The cone-beam computed tomography scan acquired before the first treatment fraction at the level of the Lipiodol.

Lipiodol volume and time). In a subsequent retrospective analysis, the Lipiodol volume in the CBCTs was matched to the Lipiodol volume in the planning scan. The resulting difference in setup correction based on the Lipiodol volumes versus bony anatomy is displayed in Figure 20J-5, illustrating an average difference of 2 mm in the lateral direction and −3 mm in the vertical direction. The difference was within ±5 mm in all three directions in only 11 of the 27 fractions analyzed.

On the five initial treatment days, the patient underwent a second CBCT scan after treatment delivery. These scans were used to estimate the residual or intrafractional movement of the Lipiodol volume (i.e., the tumor), by performing a match against the planning volume of Lipiodol. Intrafractional motion of the Lipiodol motion for this patient was found to be in the range of 5 mm to 10 mm (Figure 20J-6). Although we are currently investigating the precision in the Lipiodol-based match, these

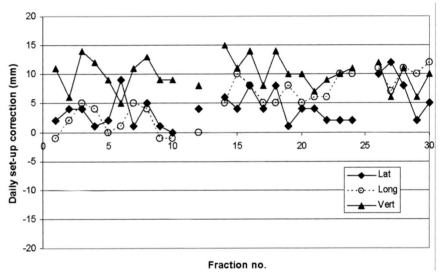

FIGURE 20J-4. The variation in bony anatomy–based daily setup correction during the course of treatment. Three of the cone-beam computed tomography scans were not included in this analysis for technical reasons.

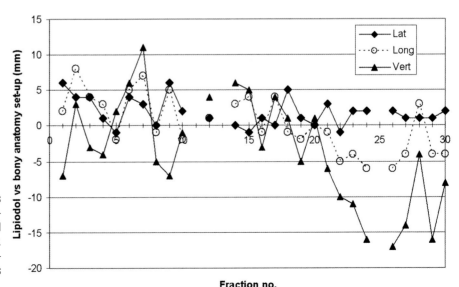

FIGURE 20J-5. Retrospective analysis of the difference in daily setup corrections when based on the Lipiodol contrast volume versus bony anatomy. Three of the cone-beam computed tomography scans were not included in this analysis for technical reasons.

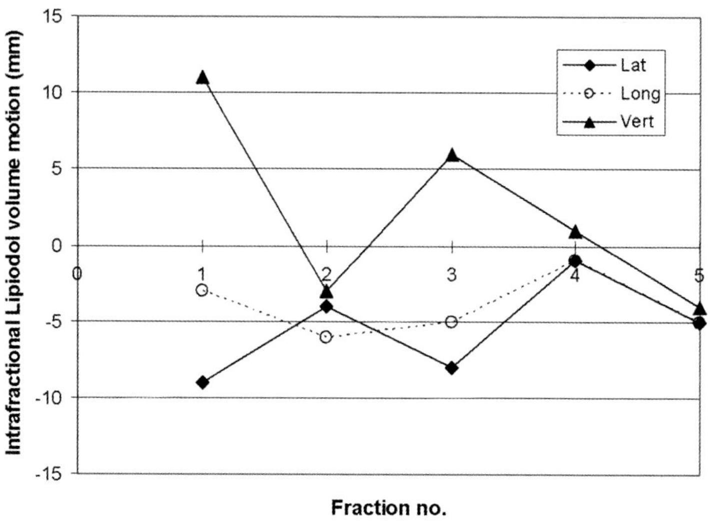

FIGURE 20J-6. Intrafractional motion of the Lipiodol contrast volume observed in the five initial treatment fractions.

findings are calling for increased awareness of bladder filling procedures when one is pursuing bladder IGRT with reduced margins.[7,11–17]

Clinical Outcome

The patient tolerated the treatment well without any significant acute sequelae. No treatment interruptions were required. Compared to baseline measures, the treatment-induced morbidity consisted of a grade 2 diarrhea (halfway during treatment) that was treated with antidiarrheal medications, and a grade 1 flatulence. One year post-RT, the patient is alive and without recurrence having only mild (grade 1) gastrointestinal late effects. The bladder function is unchanged, i.e., the patient has frequency/urgency grade 2 (as before RT) but no bladder incontinence.

Reference

1. Sengelöv L, von der Maase H. Radiotherapy in bladder cancer. *Radiother Oncol.* 1999;52:1–14.
2. Muren LP, Smaaland R, Dahl O. Conformal radiotherapy of urinary bladder cancer. *Radiother Oncol.* 2004;73:387–398.
3. Dudouet P, Portalez D, Lhez J, et al. Trans-rectal ultrasonography (TRUS) with lipiodol injection for localization of the prostatic apex before radiotherapy planning. *Radiother Oncol.* 2001;61:135–141.
4. Muren LP, Smaaland R, Dahl O. Organ motion, set-up variation and treatment margins in radical radiotherapy of urinary bladder cancer. *Radiother Oncol.* 2003;69:291–304.
5. Fokdal L, Honore H, Hoyer M, et al. Impact of changes in bladder and rectal filling volume on organ motion and dose distribution of the bladder in radiotherapy for urinary bladder cancer. *Int J Radiat Oncol Biol Phys.* 2004;59:436–444.
6. Meijer GJ, Rasch C, Remeijer P, et al. 3D analysis of delineation errors, setup errors and organ motion during radiation therapy of bladder cancer. *Int J Radiat Oncol Biol Phys.* 2003;55:1277–1287.
7. Redpath AT, Muren LP. An optimisation algorithm for determination of treatment margins around moving and deformable targets. *Radiother Oncol.* 2005;77:194–201.
8. Muren LP, Redpath AT, Lord H, et al. Image-guided radiotherapy of bladder cancer: bladder volume variation and its relation to margins. *Radiother Oncol.* 2007;84:307–313.
9. Søndergaard J, Høyer M, Petersen JB, et al. The normal tissue sparing obtained with simultaneous treatment of pelvic lymph nodes and bladder using intensity-modulated radiotherapy. *Acta Oncol.* 2009;48:238–244.
10. Muren LP, Redpath AT, McLaren D, et al. A concomitant tumour boost in bladder irradiation: patient suitability and the potential of intensity-modulated radiotherapy. *Radiother Oncol.* 2006;80:98–105.
11. Lotz HT, Pos FJ, Hulshof MC, et al. Tumor motion and deformation during external radiotherapy of bladder cancer. *Int J Radiat Oncol Biol Phys.* 2006;64:1551–1558.
12. Redpath AT, Muren LP. CT-guided intensity-modulated radiotherapy for bladder cancer: isocentre shifts, margins and their impact on target dose. *Radiother Oncol.* 2006;81:276–283.
13. Pos FJ, Hulshof M, Lebesque J, et al. Adaptive radiotherapy for invasive bladder cancer: a feasibility study. *Int J Radiat Oncol Biol Phys.* 2006;64:862–868.
14. Burridge N, Amer A, Marchant T, et al. Online adaptive radiotherapy of the bladder: small bowel irradiated-volume reduction. *Int J Radiat Oncol Biol Phys.* 2006;66:892–897.
15. Wright P, Redpath AT, Høyer M, et al. The normal tissue sparing potential of adaptive strategies in radiotherapy of bladder cancer. *Acta Oncol.* 2008;47:1382–1389.
16. Redpath AT, Wright P, Muren LP. The contribution of on-line correction for rotational organ motion in image-guided radiotherapy of the bladder and prostate. *Acta Oncol.* 2008;47:1367–1372.
17. McBain CA, Green MM, Stratford J, et al. Ultrasound imaging to assess inter- and intra-fraction motion during bladder radiotherapy and its potential as a verification tool. *Clin Oncol (R Coll Radiol).* 2009;21:385–393.

Real-Time Target Localization and Tracking Using the Calypso System in a Patient with Prostate Cancer Undergoing IMRT

Case Study

Jeffrey R. Olsen, MD, Parag J. Parikh, MD

Patient History

A 78-year-old man was noted on annual screening to have an increase in prostate-specific antigen (PSA) from 3 ng/mL to 7.2 ng/mL. Physical examination revealed a diffusely enlarged prostate with no nodules, and a prostate needle biopsy demonstrated adenocarcinoma at the right apex in 1 of 12 cores, with a Gleason grade of 3 + 3 = 6.

After a thorough discussion of active surveillance and definitive treatment options, the patient elected to pursue external beam radiotherapy (RT). We elected to treat with real-time target localization and tracking using the Calypso four-dimensional (4D) localization system (Calypso Medical Technologies, Seattle, WA).

Simulation

The patient's history was reviewed to ensure no implanted medical devices and lack of ferrous internal hardware, as well as minimal abdominal obesity, to allow localization and tracking. A magnetic resonance (MR) scan was obtained of the prostate to aid in target delineation *before* placement of Beacon transponders, to avoid MR artifacts.

The patient was then brought to the operating room for transponder placement while sedated using monitored anesthesia care. He was placed in the dorsal lithotomy position, and three transponders were introduced via a transperineal approach, with rectal ultrasound guidance. With a template placed against the perineum, transponders were inserted into the left base, right base–midgland, and left apex of the prostate. Care was taken to obtain sufficient spacing between transponders, for idealized tracking geometry.

Computed tomography (CT) simulation was scheduled for 1 week after fiducial placement, to allow for resolution of prostate edema, and to avoid transponder migration that might otherwise occur between simulation and treatment. A CT simulation of the pelvis was performed on our Big Bore scanner (Philips Medical Systems, Andover, MA) with the patient supine, with a full bladder, and utilizing a small rectal tube to minimize gas dilation. Alpha Cradle (Smithers Medical Products, Canton, OH) was used for patient immobilization. The three transponders were contoured at the time of simulation, and the isocenter was placed at their center.

Treatment Planning

The planning CT and MR images were imported into the Pinnacle treatment planning software (Philips Medical Systems, Andover, MA), and fused utilizing prostate soft tissue anatomy contoured on both the CT and MR scans, with manual, rigid image registration. Visual verification of images was then performed by the attending physician

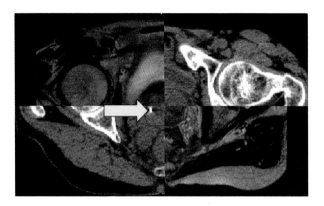

FIGURE 20K-1. Checkerboard axial image of the fused magnetic resonance and computed tomography (CT) scans, to demonstrate adequacy of image registration. The final contoured prostate is shown in red. A Calypso Beacon transponder placed at the right base of the prostate is seen on this CT slice (yellow arrow).

in the axial, coronal, and sagittal planes (Figure 20K-1). The clinical target volume (CTV) was generated by contouring the prostate on the CT and MR fused images. Organs at risk (OARs) were also contoured, including the bladder, rectum, and penile bulb. A uniform 5-mm expansion was used surrounding the CTV, creating a planning target volume (PTV).

A five-field segmental multileaf collimator (SMLC)–based intensity-modulated RT (IMRT) plan was generated with a planning goal of 97.5% PTV coverage by the prescription dose. The prescribed dose was 77.4 Gy in 43 daily fractions using 18-MV photons on a Varian 2100EX linear accelerator (Varian Medical Systems, Palo Alto, CA). The positions of the three transponders and their relationship to the isocenter were entered into the Calypso 4D Localization System located at the treatment linac.

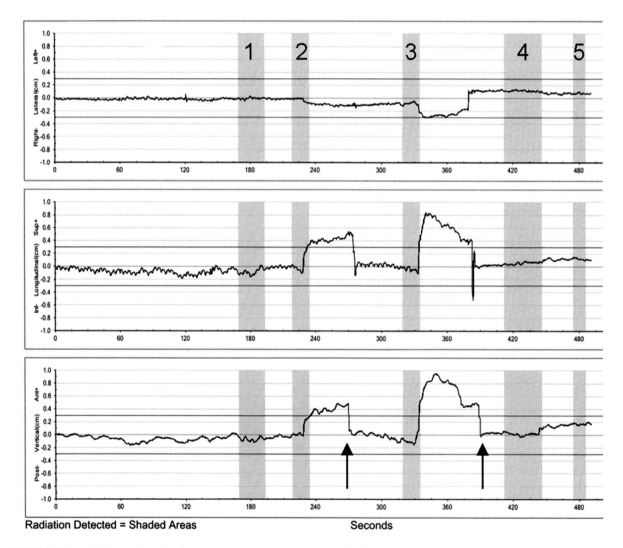

FIGURE 20K-2. Real-time tracking data for one treatment, including right–left (top), superior–inferior (middle), and anterior–posterior (bottom) tracking data. The tracking limits were set at ±0.3 cm for each axis, and are displayed as solid horizontal lines. The shaded regions illustrate the time when the treatment beam was turned on for each of the five planned fields (numbered on top graph). Therapists held delivery and then repositioned the patient (solid arrows) after the second and third beams because of intrafraction prostate motion.

Treatment Delivery

Before each treatment, the patient was placed in the supine position within his Alpha Cradle mold and shifts were made to align his skin marks with the room lasers. The Calypso System 4D Electromagnetic Array was placed above the patient's pelvis for detection of the transponder positions. Optical targets in the top of the array are monitored by the Calypso optical subsystem (three infrared cameras mounted to the ceiling of the RT suite) and used to determine the position of the array relative to the linear accelerator isocenter. Before each treatment, the patient was shifted in "localize" mode, so that the location of the centroid of the three beacons was within 3 mm of the planned position in each of the x, y, and z dimensions. The initial rotation and the geometric residual (measure of changes of the intertransponder distances) were checked before each treatment, and not allowed to vary more than 10° and 0.2 cm, respectively. If the intertransponder distances had changed, then the patient would undergo repeat CT simulation. If the geometric residual had exceeded 10°, then the patient would be repositioned in the alpha cradle.

The system was then placed in "tracking" mode and the therapists began treatment. Radiation delivery during each treatment session was manually paused for at least 15 seconds if the patient's prostate position was noted to deviate more than 3 mm in any direction during treatment. If the deviation persisted beyond 15 seconds, the patient was repositioned. The system provides real-time graphs of the prostate position, translation limits, and radiation beam-on information. An example of a treatment delivery pause, followed by couch repositioning is shown in Figure 20K-2. A summary report of the prostate position in this patient during beam-on time, as well as during the whole treatment fraction, was exported to the record-and-verify system (Mosaiq 1.6, IMPAC Medical Systems, Sunnyvale, CA) for daily review and approval by the attending physician (Figure 20K-3). Therapy was paused during 10 of 43 fractions (23%). The prostate was out of the 3-mm thresholds for 0% to 21% of any given fraction, but only 0% to 3% of the beam-on time.

Clinical Outcome

Treatment was well tolerated, with the patient experiencing only mildly increased urinary frequency, which did not require any medications for management. He has recently completed therapy and is scheduled for his first posttreatment follow-up in the near future.

We recently published an analysis of the accuracy of pre- and posttreatment imaging and intermittent imaging as predictors of prostate motion during the course of RT in 35 patients (1157 fractions) undergoing continuous tracking using the Calypso system.[1] Predictions of prostate motion away from the isocenter were modeled for a pre- and posttreatment imaging schedule and for multiple intermittent intrafraction imaging schedules and compared with actual continuous tracking data. The endpoint was drift of the prostate beyond a certain radial

Intertransponder Distances	Planned	Measured
Apex to Left Base (cm):	2.58	2.53
Right Base to Left Base (cm):	3.05	3.07
Apex to Right Base (cm):	2.28	2.08

	Limit	Measured
Geometric Residual (cm):	0.20	0.09
Rotation about Lateral Axis (deg):	10.0	−5.5
Rotation about Longitudinal Axis (deg):	10.0	−3.7
Rotation about Vertical Axis (deg):	10.0	2.8

Summary of Target Excursions Outside of Tracking Limits

Direction	Tracking Limit	Total Tracking Time			Tracking while Radiation Detected		
		Time	Percent	Max Excur	Time	Percent	Max Excur
Left	0.30 cm	0 sec	0%	0.14 cm	0 sec	0%	0.14 cm
Right	0.30 cm	4 sec	1%	0.31 cm	0 sec	0%	0.22 cm
Superior	0.30 cm	90 sec	18%	0.83 cm	2 sec	2%	0.41 cm
Inferior	0.30 cm	1 sec	0%	0.53 cm	0 sec	0%	0.16 cm
Anterior	0.30 cm	90 sec	18%	0.95 cm	1 sec	1%	0.51 cm
Posterior	0.30 cm	0 sec	0%	0.17 cm	0 sec	0%	0.15 cm
Total		97 sec	20%		3 sec	3%	

FIGURE 20K-3. A report is generated after each fraction, illustrating the planned and measured intertransponder distances, as well as the setup rotations about the lateral, longitudinal, and vertical axes, with rotational tolerance limits of 10°. The report includes a summary of intrafraction motion, illustrating that the total time the prostate was out of tracking limits was 20% of the total fraction (bottom left). Because of intrafraction repositioning, target motion that exceeded the tracking limit was minimized to 3% while the radiation beam was on (bottom right).

displacement for a duration of more than 30 seconds, 1 minute, and 2 minutes. The sensitivity of pre- and post-treatment imaging in determining 30 seconds of intra-fraction prostate motion greater than 3 mm, 5 mm, or 7 mm for all fractions was low, with values of 53%, 49%, and 39%, respectively. The sensitivity of intermittent imaging improved with increasing sampling rate. Our results suggest that pre- and posttreatment imaging is not a sensitive method of assessing intrafraction prostate motion, and that intermittent imaging is sufficiently sensitive only at a high sampling rate. These findings support the value of continuous, real-time tracking in these patients.

Reference

1. Noel C, Parikh PJ, Roy M, et al. Prediction of intra-fraction prostate motion: accuracy of pre- and post-treatment imaging and intermittent imaging. *Int J Radiat Oncol Biol Phys.* 2009;73: 692–698.

Chapter 21

Gynecologic Tumors: Overview

Loren K. Mell, MD, John C. Roeske, PhD, Arno J. Mundt, MD

Radiation toxicity remains one of the most significant barriers to effective treatment of gynecologic cancers. Compared with modern techniques, conventional approaches are known to result in both insufficient target coverage and excessive normal tissue irradiation,[1–5] compromising the therapeutic benefit of radiotherapy (RT). Precision RT techniques, such as intensity-modulated RT (IMRT), have been studied intensively in patients with gynecologic patients over the past decade to confront this problem.[6–14] The development of IMRT and other novel approaches, however, has been beset by inaccuracies in target delineation[15–20] and patient setup,[21,22] and uncertainties in target position because of tumor regression, inter- and intrafraction motion, and normal tissue changes.[23–29] Uncertainties in target location in gynecologic cancers have generally necessitated wide three-dimensional (3D) planning margins to ensure adequate target coverage, counteracting the gains achieved by highly conformal techniques.

Image-guided RT (IGRT) technologies are increasingly providing opportunities for improved target definition and daily localization, enabling greater sophistication in RT delivery for gynecologic cancers. Ideally, the combination of IGRT and conformal RT will allow improved treatment accuracy, limiting toxicity and improving outcomes for women with gynecologic cancer.

Image-Guided Target Delineation

External Beam Radiotherapy

Historically, external beam RT (EBRT) for gynecologic cancer predominantly used planar x-ray technology and skeletal landmarks to design beam portals. This approach, however, has been shown to result in inadequate target coverage and excess normal tissue irradiation compared with 3D planning.[1,2] Computed tomography (CT) provides more accurate and customized target delineation and, because of its wide availability, has become the standard imaging technique for modern RT simulation and planning. However, more sophisticated imaging technologies such as magnetic resonance (MR) imaging and positron emission tomography (PET) are increasingly being used to augment target delineation, via fusion with the simulation CT. For example, in a recent survey of radiation oncologists, 19% and 36% were using MR and PET, respectively, for gynecologic cancer treatment planning (Figure 21-1).[30] These technologies permit greater soft tissue contrast and convey important metabolic or functional information about the tumor and normal tissues.

Although MR is not routinely incorporated into EBRT planning for gynecologic cancer,[30] many studies have found MR imaging to be useful in guiding target delineation[16,18,19,31–33] (Chapter 21A). Many experts now recommend the routine use of MR to guide EBRT planning for intact cervical cancer.[20] Compared with CT, MR provides superior soft tissue definition, permitting better delineation of pelvic tumors.[16,31] Magnetic resonance is also superior to physical examination for assessing uterine involvement and tumor response, as well as better predicts local control and disease-free survival.[32,34,35] For assessing nodal metastasis, routine MR and CT have similar accuracy.[36]

Studies of ultrasmall particles of iron oxide (USPIO) to improve nodal assessment with MR have found that USPIO-enhanced MR increased the sensitivity of MR imaging, without loss of specificity, in endometrial and cervical cancers.[37,38] A meta-analysis demonstrated that MR enhanced with superparamagnetic iron-oxide nanoparticles has a sensitivity of 88% and specificity of 96%, compared with 63% and 93% for unenhanced MR.[39] Taylor et al. used USPIO-enhanced MR imaging to guide nodal delineation and found that a 7-mm margin with slight modifications was sufficient to encompass 99% of pelvic nodes (Figure 21-2).[17]

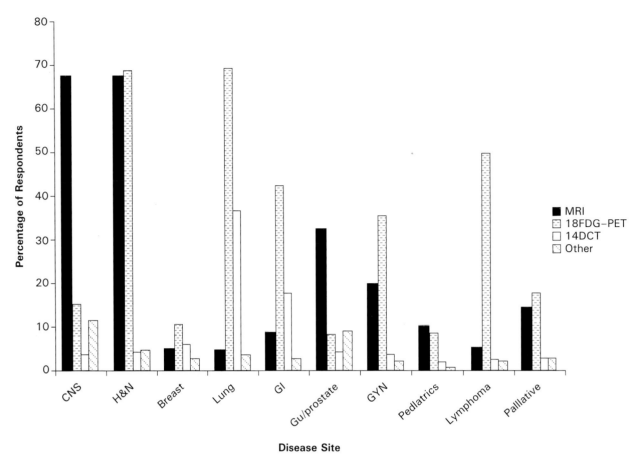

FIGURE 21-1. Prevalence of advanced imaging utilization for radiation therapy target delineation, by disease site, from a 2009 survey of radiation oncologists in the United States. CNS = central nervous system; 4DCT = four-dimensional computed tomography; [18]FDG, 2 = ^{18}F-fluoro-2-deoxyglucose; GI = gastrointestinal; GU = genitourinary; H&N = head and neck; MRI = magnetic resonance imaging; Other = functional MRI, MR spectroscopy, single-photon emission CT, and/or non-FDG PET; PET = positron emission tomography. Reproduced with permission from Simpson et al.[30]

Numerous studies in cervical cancer have demonstrated that ^{18}F-fluorodeoxyglucose (^{18}F-FDG) PET (or PET–CT) detects cervical abnormalities and occult nodal disease with higher sensitivity than MR or CT alone.[40–42] Moreover, several reports have also shown that ^{18}F-FDG PET abnormalities are correlated with poorer outcomes.[40,43,44] Others have found ^{18}F-FDG PET improves diagnosis and staging of endometrial[45] and vaginal cancer.[46] However, although ^{18}F-FDG PET may be a useful tool to guide nodal clinical target volume (CTV) delineation for RT planning purposes, it may not have sufficient negative predictive value to obviate lymph node sampling or lymphadenectomy for patients with preoperative imaging negative for nodal metastasis.[47,18]F-FDG-PET can be used to measure tumor volume and even monitor response during treatment of cervical cancer.[48,49] For patients with para-aortic lymph node metastases, ^{18}F-FDG PET may be useful to delineate the gross disease, which can be safely boosted to 59.4 Gy using IMRT (Figure 21-3)[50–51] (see Chapter 21B).

Several studies have investigated applications of advanced imaging technologies. Dynamic contrast-enhanced

(DCE) MR can identify regions of tumor hypoxia[52] and [1]H-magnetic resonance spectroscopy (MRS) can be useful to differentiate tumor from normal tissue.[53] Studies have also investigated PET with alternative tracers, such as ^{11}C-choline, ^{11}C-methionine, and [60]Cu diacetyl-bis(N4-methylthiosemicarbazone) ([60]Cu-ATSM), to identify metabolic abnormalities or hypoxia.[54–57] Roeske et al. found that single-photon emission CT (SPECT) could be a useful adjunct for IMRT planning by imaging active bone marrow, which could be selectively avoided.[58] Mell et al. have combined ^{18}F-FDG PET with quantitative MR fat fraction maps to image structural and functional properties of bone marrow to design bone marrow–sparing IMRT plans.[59] To date, limited data exist to support the routine use of these sophisticated imaging approaches for RT planning in patients with gynecologic cancer and further study is required to define their role (see Chapter 21D).

Image-Guided Brachytherapy

The current standard for intracavitary brachytherapy in cervical cancer is to prescribe dose to a single point, designated as Point A by the International Commission on

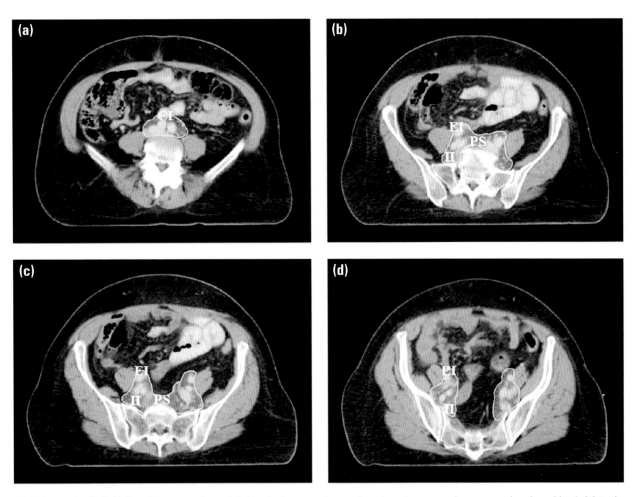

FIGURE 21-2. (a-d). Guidelines for target volume definition in the gynecology patients based on magnetic resonance imaging with administration of iron oxide particles. CI = common iliacs; EI = external iliacs; II = internal iliacs; PS = presacrals. Reproduced with permission from Taylor et al.[17]

Radiation Units and Measurements (ICRU) and defined using two-dimensional (2D) imaging.[60] Doses to organs at risk (OARs) are also traditionally represented by a single point, despite evidence that these points neither represent the maximum dose nor correlate with acute or long-term toxicity.[61,62] Many investigators have reported advantages of 3D imaging and volumetric dosimetry over conventional imaging modalities and standard

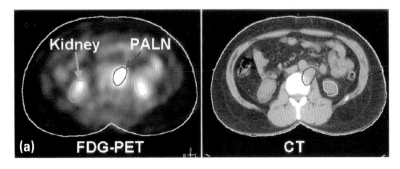

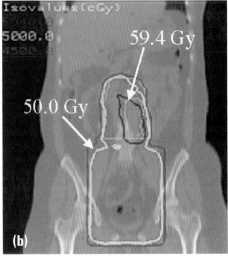

FIGURE 21-3. Positron emission tomography (PET)-guided extended field intensity-modulated radiation therapy (IMRT) planning in a patient with cervical cancer. **(a)** Axial PET and computed tomography images showing a positive para-aortic lymph node. **(b)** Composite IMRT plan showing dose distribution for para-aortic region and whole pelvis. Reproduced with permission from Mutic et al.[50]

point-dose dosimetry for gynecologic brachytherapy[4,5,63] (see Chapter 21B). Both CT and ultrasound are useful and relatively inexpensive imaging techniques that can guide and improve brachytherapy.[5,64–67] More recently, however, MR and PET have received attention as a means of augmenting brachytherapy planning.

T2-weighted contrast-enhanced MR using a pelvic coil provides excellent soft tissue resolution and differentiation between tumor and normal tissues. Tumor shows increased signal intensity on T2-weighted images, allowing better differentiation from normal tissues and more accurate assessment of parametrial and uterine extension.[18,33] Despite the advantages of MR-based planning, a 2007 survey found that the majority of radiation oncologists still use CT or planar imaging for brachytherapy planning.[68] Underutilization of MR may be attributable in part to the lack of availability of MR-compatible applicators and on-site MR units.

Comparisons of CT versus MR have found that CT overestimates tumor width, leading to distortion of the high-risk CTV (HR-CTV) and discrepancies in the volume treated to the prescription dose.[19] In addition,

MR-guided brachytherapy planning can improve dose delivery to the bladder and rectal walls compared with conventional techniques.[61] Fusing the CT and MR at the initial brachytherapy planning session allows for superior target delineation. If MR with each implant insertion is infeasible, CT may be used during subsequent implants for OAR definition, relying on the initial MR for GTV and HR-CTV delineation.[69] High rates of local control and low toxicity have been reported using MR-guided approaches in patients with cervical cancer.[70–73] Although the majority of research in MR-guided brachytherapy has focused on cervical cancer, promising results have also been reported in recurrent endometrial[74] and inoperable uterine[75] cancers.

Investigators at Washington University have conducted several studies on PET-guided intracavitary brachytherapy for cervical cancer, demonstrating the feasibility and dosimetric advantages of this approach over conventional techniques (Figure 21-4).[76,77] The procedure involves scanning patients after both intravenous delivery of ^{18}F-FDG and insertion of tubes containing ^{18}F-FDG into the tandem and colpostats. The PET image is then transferred to the 3D

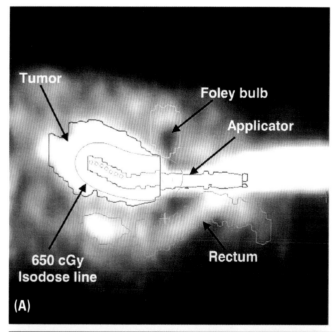

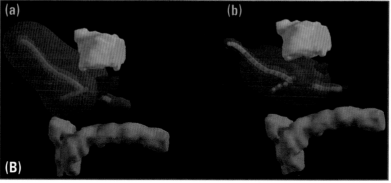

FIGURE 21-4. (A) Positron emission tomography (PET)-assisted brachytherapy planning in a patient with cervical cancer. Reproduced from Malyapa et al.[77] with permission. **(B)** Final implant without **(a)** and with **(b)** optimization to the PET-defined tumor volume in a patient with locally advanced cervical cancer. Bladder, yellow; PET tumor volume, red; rectum, brown. Target isodose surface (6.5 Gy) is in purple. Reproduced with permission from Lin et al.[78]

planning system where volumes are delineated. Lin et al. evaluated the utility of serial PET scans in 11 cervical cancer patients undergoing high-dose-rate (HDR) brachytherapy.[78] A standard brachytherapy plan designed to deliver 6.5 Gy to Point A was compared with plans designed to conform the 6.5 Gy isodose surface to the PET-defined volume. Although no difference in target coverage was observed between the optimized and nonoptimized plans at the initial insertion, target coverage was significantly improved during later insertions using PET-based adaptive plans. No differences were observed in normal tissue sparing using the adapted plans. Outcome data are awaited to assess the potential benefits of PET-guided brachytherapy.

To standardize and evaluate image-based dosimetry for cervical cancer brachytherapy, both the Group Européen de Curiethérapie–European Society for Therapeutic Radiology and Oncology (GEC-ESTRO) and North American IGBT Working Group have published recommendations for MR-guided brachytherapy in cervical cancer.[64,72,73] The nomenclature that has been adopted worldwide for image-guided brachytherapy (IGBT) is based on work primarily performed by GEC-ESTRO (Figure 21-5).[79,80]

Current recommendations for IGBT are to contour gross tumor volume (GTV), HR-CTV, intermediate-risk CTV (IR-CTV), and OARs including bladder, rectum, sigmoid colon, and small bowel. The HR-CTV should include the entire cervix as well as any macroscopic disease that persists in the parametria, uterus, rectum, bladder, or vagina (but not to cross these anatomic boundaries without clear rationale). The prescription goal is 80 Gy to 95 Gy to the HR-CTV. The IR-CTV should include tumor extension at diagnosis or a 1-cm extension around the HR-CTV, with the intent to deliver 60 Gy to this volume.

Recommendations for reporting and quality assurance (QA) include calculation and reporting of the minimum dose to 90% and 100% of the contoured target volume (D_{90}, D_{100}). In addition, for evaluation within a single treatment scheme, the volume encompassed by the 100% isodose line (V_{100}) should also be calculated. The V_{150} and V_{200} should be calculated to determine volumes of tissue exceeding the prescription dose. For OARs, reporting of the ICRU reference points to bladder and rectum should continue for comparison with the dose–volume

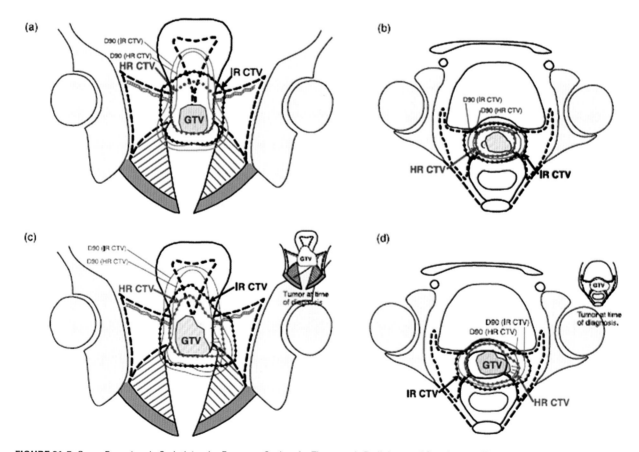

FIGURE 21-5. Group Européen de Curiethérapie–European Society for Therapeutic Radiology and Oncology working group concepts and terms used for image-guided brachytherapy. Schematic diagram with coronal (**a,c**) and transverse (**b,d**) sections of an optimized treatment plan for limited (**a,b**) and advanced (**c,d**) disease with partial remission after external irradiation. GTV = gross tumor volume; HR CTV = high-risk clinical target volume; IR CTV = intermediate-risk clinical target volume. Reproduced with permission from Haie-Meder et al.[72]

histogram (DVH) data. The minimum dose received by the maximally irradiated contiguous 0.1 cm³, 1 cm³, and 2 cm³ of the bladder, rectum, sigmoid, and small bowel, respectively, should also be calculated and reported. Dose should be expressed as bioequivalent doses given at 2 Gy per fraction, using the linear quadratic radiobiologic model (EQD_2), to standardize for different dose rates (e.g., low-dose rate [LDR], HDR, and pulse-dose rate [PDR]).[81] Total doses should be expressed including the dose from external beam radiation. Provisional dose–volume constraints for OARs (converted to EQD_2) are to maintain the bladder below 85 Gy to 90 Gy and the rectum and sigmoid below 75 Gy. There has been validation for the recommendations for rectum, but there is a weaker basis for recommendations for bladder, sigmoid, and vagina.[82–85]

Application of IGBT with dose adaptation and escalation has been reported, demonstrating an increase in local control by 20% and a 7% decrease in grades 3 and 4 morbidity demonstrating that these techniques hold promise for increased local control and survival.[71] Despite these promising results, IGBT awaits more general adoption, reproducibility, systematic utilization, and reporting to replace the current ICRU standard.

Image-Guided Treatment Delivery

A strong rationale exists to use in-room IGRT technologies to guide the delivery of RT in gynecologic cancer. It is widely known that accurate positioning in these patients is challenging,[3,86] even when sophisticated customized immobilization and setup techniques are used.[21,87] In a review of 46 patients with gynecologic cancer undergoing IMRT with customized immobilization consisting of upper and lower molds indexed to the treatment table, Haslam et al.[21] compared portal films to simulation films and reported that 20% of the treatment fractions had at least one error greater than 5 mm in magnitude, significantly less, however, than the 59% noted by Huddart et al. using traditional setup and immobilization techniques.[3] Even greater difficulties may exist in setting up obese patients and in patients treated with more comprehensive volumes, including extended-field RT and pelvic–inguinal RT.

In-room IGRT approaches have the potential to improve setup accuracy, reducing the risk of underdosing the target and overdosing nearby normal tissues. Accurate daily patient setup is particularly important with the increasing use of highly conformal IMRT treatment approaches in patients with gynecologic cancer, because of their sharp dose gradients outside the target,[6,88] and is paramount in patients treated with hypofractionated or simultaneous integrated boost approaches.[89–92]

Another important problem that may be addressed with in-room IGRT is internal organ motion. Cervical cancer and other gynecologic tumors have been shown to display considerable interfraction organ motion.[23–29,93]

Tyagi et al. have reported on 10 intact cervical cancer patients undergoing on-line cone beam CT (CBCT) with each fraction.[93] They found that a uniform CTV–PTV margin of 15 mm would have failed to encompass the CTV in 32% of fractions (Table 21-1). The mean volume of CTV missed, however, was small (4 cc). The mean planning margin (across all patients and fractions) required to encompass the CTV was 15 mm.

Intrafraction organ motion, albeit less in magnitude, occurs as well.[26,94] Investigators at Duke University analyzed cervical motion in 10 healthy volunteers with repeat single shot fast spin echo MR at the level of the cervix, with imaging every 6 seconds for 20 minutes.[94] Mean and maximum intrafraction displacements of the cervix in the anterior–posterior and superior–inferior directions were 1.4 mm and 5.1 mm and 3.9 mm and 2.9 mm, respectively. Such motions may adversely impact target coverage and normal tissue sparing, especially when IMRT plans with tight margins are used.[95] In-room IGRT techniques may allow such motions to be detected and managed.

Gynecologic tumors, particularly cervical cancers, unlike many other tumor sites, may regress significantly during the course of EBRT (Figure 21-6).[23–25,96] Lee et al. performed repeat physical examinations on 17 patients with cervical cancer undergoing EBRT and found that the median number of days to achieve a partial and complete response were 21 and 42 days, respectively (Figure 21-7).[25] Investigators at M.D. Anderson Hospital reported a mean regression of 62.3% in 16 patients with cervical cancer by the completion of EBRT, with a range of 20.4% to 87.3%.[96] For 13 women with a greater than 50% response, the average number of days to achieve a partial response was 20. Van de Bunt et al. evaluated 14 patients with cervical cancer with a pretreatment repeat MR after 30 Gy and noted median reductions in the GTV, CTV, and PTV of 46%, 18%, and 9%, respectively.[23] Regression is a serious concern, because highly conformal IMRT plans generated before treatment may be poorly conform midway through treatment, resulting in higher doses to surrounding normal tissues. In-room IGRT technologies open the door to adapting treatment to such changes, improving treatment quality and patient outcomes.

Clinical Applications of In-Room IGRT Technologies

Myriad in-room IGRT technologies have been applied to the treatment of patients with gynecologic cancer. A recent survey found that 55% of respondents have used in-room IGRT techniques in their patients with gynecologic cancer.[97] As shown in Table 21-2, the majority reported using planar-based techniques, particularly electronic portal devices (EPIDs; 28%) and commercial onboard imaging (24%). The percentage of respondents using volumetric-based techniques was also common, notably kilovoltage (kV) and megavoltage (MV) CBCT (19%) and helical tomotherapy (12%).

TABLE 21–1 Patient specific daily uniform margins (in mm) required to encompass the clinical target volume in 10 patients with cervical cancer.

Patient	1	2	3	4	5	6	7	8	9	10	11	12	13	14	15	16	17	18	19	20	21	22	23	24	25	Mean
1	-	11	-	11	12	12	11	12	9	10	8	6	-	11	8	16	6	7	9	9	14	14	15	10	-	10.5
2	42	42	10	10	8	6	6	9	18	18	19	19	17	20	20	20	20	21	22	17	18	17	20	-	-	18.2
3	11	7	10	10	7	10	11	8	14	12	11	12	12	14	15	13	16	10	17	17	10	14	13	13	-	12.0
4	10	32	11	-	35	18	15	11	26	20	26	28	28	13	22	24	27	15	40	31	12	20	37	32	26	23.3
5	12	-	0	30	-	23	-	21	13	23	14	13	22	25	18	17	17	19	17	15	-	-	19	-	19	17.1
6	9	-	0	30	32	31	31	33	34	36	-	33	21	32	32	32	32	25	16	30	32	25	-	-	-	27.3
7	5	7	10	-	7	3	4	5	7	10	7	9	9	5	-	4	5	5	5	6	-	7	-	7	-	6.4
8	13	11	7	-	14	5	15	14	20	-	13	10	15	12	12	-	7	7	-	12	16	-	-	8	9	11.6
9	12	5	13	5	18	18	7	5	16	12	10	7	16	9	10	10	20	5	7	21	3	12	9	12	6	10.4
10	5	7	22	-	22	8	25	11	13	16	13	12	12	10	12	10	7	10	10	9	9	12	10	-	10	12.0
Mean	13.2	15.3	9.2	13.2	17.1	13.4	13.9	12.9	17.0	17.4	13.4	14.9	16.9	15.1	16.6	16.2	15.7	12.4	15.9	16.7	14.3	15.1	17.6	13.7	14.0	14.8

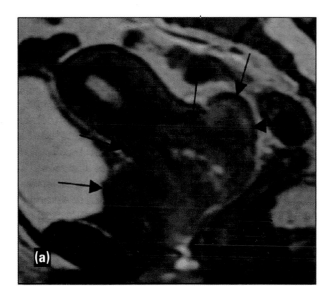

(a)

FIGURE 21-6. Temporal changes of tumor configuration shown on serial magnetic resonance imaging studies (fast spin-echo T2-weighted sagittal images) obtained in a 48-year-old woman with a stage IIB squamous cell carcinoma before treatment (a) and at 21.6 Gy (2.2 weeks) (b) and 45.0 Gy (5 weeks) (c). Reproduced with permission from Mayr et al.[24]

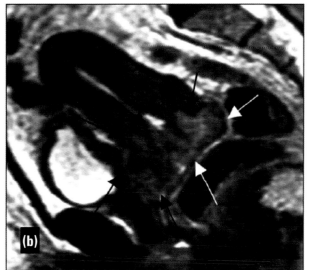

(b)

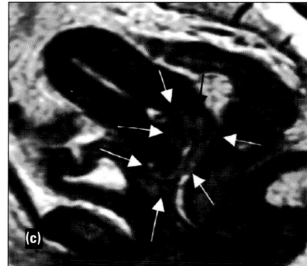

(c)

Albeit less commonly used, ultrasound has long been known to be a useful tool in the treatment of cervical and other gynecologic malignancies, notably to assist the placement of intracavitary devices.[65] However, several groups are now attempting to broaden its role. Davidson and colleagues employed the Restitu System (Resonant Medical, Montreal, Canada) in 35 intracavitary brachytherapy insertions in 21 patients with cervical cancer (Figure 21-8)[67] (see Chapter 21E). Accurate applicator placement was achieved in all patients without a single uterine perforation. Ultrasound during the insertion altered the selection of the tandem length and angle in 49% of patients. Moreover, average insertion times decreased from 34 to 26 minutes and requests for assistance from gynecologic oncologists declined from 38% to 5.7% of procedures.

TABLE 21–2 In-Room Image-Guided Radiation Therapy Technologies Used in Gynecology Patients: Results of a National Survey

Technology	%*
Ultrasound	1%
Video	0.3%
EPID	28%
OBI (kV)	24%
CyberKnife	3%
Novalis	0%
Tomotherapy	12%
CBCT (kV/MV)	19%
CT-on-Rails	1%

*Percentage of survey respondents who reported using a particular IGRT technology in gynecology patients; EPID = electronic portal imaging device; OBI = on-board imaging (commercial gantry-mounted systems); CBCT = cone-beam computed tomography; kV = kilovoltage; MV = megavoltage; CT = computed tomography

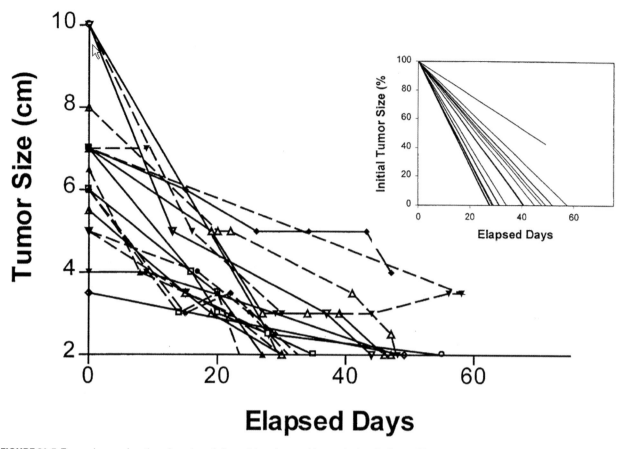

FIGURE 21-7. Tumor size as a function of number of elapsed days (external beam plus brachytherapy) in 17 patients with cervical cancer. Inset shows the initial tumor size normalized to 100%. Reproduced with permission from Lee et al.[25]

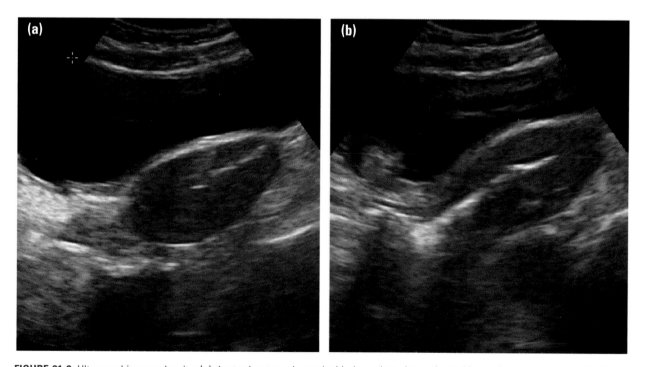

FIGURE 21-8. Ultrasound images showing **(a)** the tandem too advanced with the endouterine cavity pushing against the fundus and **(b)** the repositioned tandem to its optimated location achieved using real-time ultrasound visualization. Reproduced with permission from Davidson et al.[67]

Van Dyk and coworkers utilized transabdominal ultrasound for both applicator insertion and brachytherapy planning in 71 patients with locoregionally advanced cervical cancer (Figure 21-9).[98] All patients were anesthetized before the insertion and applicator position was optimized in the uterus and cervix utilizing real-time ultrasound monitoring. Dwell weights and source positions were manipulated to cover the uterine and cervical dimensions depicted on the ultrasound images. At a minimum follow-up of 2.5 years, local control was achieved in 90% of patients. Significant late bowel toxicity was seen in less than 2% of patients.

The IGRT treatment delivery approach that has received the most attention to date in gynecology patients is planar-based IGRT, particularly EPID-based approaches. In a prospective randomized study of 32 patients with a variety of tumor sites, Michalski and coworkers compared EPID monitoring immediately before treatment versus periodic portal films following treatment and noted significant reductions in setup errors larger than 1 cm, particularly in patients undergoing pelvic RT.[99] In a study of 14 gynecology patients undergoing pelvic irradiation with on-line EPID-based IGRT patient setup, Stroom and colleagues found that 57% of 254 fractions had setup errors larger than 4 mm requiring adjustments (Figure 21-10).[22]

Several more sophisticated planar-based IGRT approaches have been also explored in gynecology patients. Yamamoto et al. evaluated the feasibility of delivering 3D conformal boosts in 10 patients with cervical cancer using the real-time tumor-tracking (RTRT) system, consisting of four sets of diagnostic x-ray tubes and imagers.[100] During treatment, the x-ray systems are used to monitor in real time the location of implanted fiducial markers implanted in the cervix with motion-tracking software. The beam

was "gated" to irradiate when the position of the markers coincides with their planned position. The authors concluded that the appropriate CTV-to-PTV margins in these patients were 6.9 mm, 6.7 mm, and 8.3 mm using the RTRT system. To date, no outcome data have been reported using this novel technology.

Investigators at the Korea Institute of Radiological and Medical Sciences recently reported the outcomes of 30 patients with cervical cancer with isolated para-aortic recurrences treated with a hypofractionated approach (33 Gy to 34 Gy in three fractions) using the CyberKnife system (Accuray Inc, Sunnyvale, CA).[89] Before treatment, all patients had implanted gold fiducial markers in the pedicles of three successive vertebral bodies near the tumor to aid in target localization. All patients also received concomitant chemotherapy and were treated using a custom-made immobilization device to reduce respiratory motion (Figure 21-11A). At a median follow-up of 15 months (range, 2–65 months), the 4-year actuarial local control was 67.4%. Of note, both PTV size and PET response following treatment were correlated with local control. Patients with a PTV 17 cc or less had a significantly better local control than those with a larger PTV (100% vs 34.4%; $P = .009$; Figure 21-11B). In addition, patients with tumors achieving a complete response on a follow-up PET had a higher local control than those with tumors with a partial response or stable disease (90.9% vs 23.7%; $P = .014$). Overall, toxicity was low, with only six patients developing grade 3 or higher acute toxicity, five of which were hematologic. Only one patient developed a severe late toxicity (ureteral stricture).

Sorcini et al. presented their experience using the On-Board Imaging (OBI) system (Varian Medical Systems, Palo Alto, CA) in a variety of tumor sites includ-

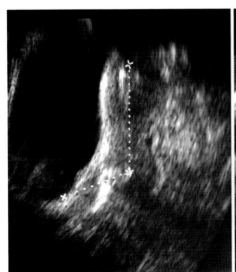
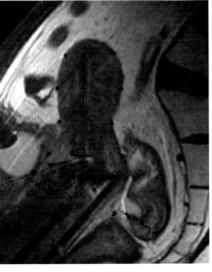

FIGURE 21-9. Sagittal ultrasound image (left) taken at the time of applicator insertion and planning and sagittal magnetic resonance imaging (right) taken after the first fraction of treatment. Size and shape of the cervix and uterus correlate well between the imaging methods. Reproduced with permission from Van Dyk et al.[98]

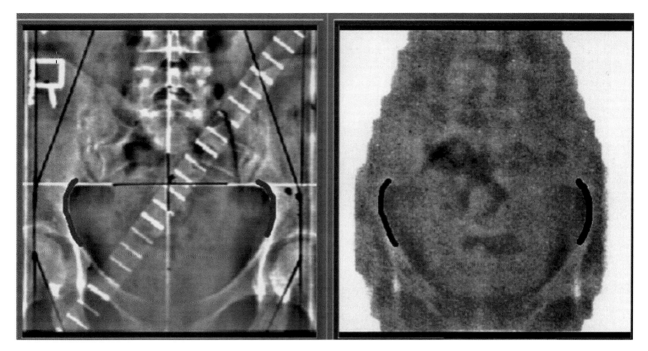

FIGURE 21-10. Illustration of on-line positioning approach in patients with gynecologic cancer using an electronic portal imaging device (EPID). The reference image is shown on the left with a manually drawn contour (gray). In the image on the right, an EPID image is shown on which a similar structure is contoured (black). Cross-correlation image software is used to calculate the required shifts. Reproduced with permission from Stroom et al.[22]

ing gynecologic malignancies.[101] Couch shifts were determined by comparing daily orthogonal films of the patient on the treatment couch with reference films generated at simulation, using a 2D matching algorithm with couch movements made remotely. The entire process added less than 1 minute to treatment. At our institution, gynecology patients are set up daily using the OBI system. In a series of 10 patients with gynecologic cancer, the average shifts observed were 0.03 cm (range, −0.7 cm to 0.8 cm), −0.14 cm (range, −0.9 cm to 0.5 cm), and 0.08 cm (range, −0.5 cm to 0.5 cm) in the anterior–posterior, left–right, and superior–inferior directions, respectively.[102]

Increasing attention has recently turned to the use of volumetric-based IGRT approaches. Several vendors have developed gantry-mounted systems, using either the MV treatment beam itself or kV images generated by gantry-mounted sources. In both approaches, a CBCT is produced from multiple 2D images obtained from

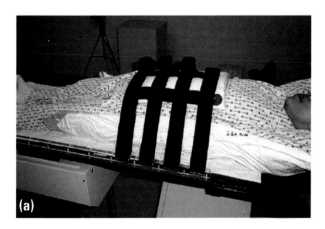

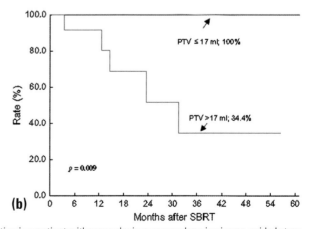

FIGURE 21-11. (a) Custom immobilization device to reduce respiratory motion in a patient with gynecologic cancer undergoing image-guided stereotactic body radiotherapy to an isolated para-aortic lymph node recurrence, using the CyberKnife system. This device consists of a vacuum cradle, four belts, and a small vacuum bag. (b) Local control according to planning target volume (PTV) size in patients with para-aortic lymph node recurrences treated with the CyberKnife system. Sixteen patients had PTVs 17 cc or smaller and 13 patients had PTVs larger than 17 cc. Reproduced with permission from Choi CW et al.[89]

various angles around the patient. McBain et al. presented their initial experience using the Elekta kV CBCT system (Elekta AB, Stockholm, Sweden) in 20 patients with various tumors, including nine patients with pelvic tumors. The authors noted sufficient image quality in all patients to perform setup corrections.[103] Helical tomotherapy (TomoTherapy Inc, Madison, WI) also represents a potential means of providing daily volumetric imaging in these patients.[104]

At the University of California San Diego (UCSD), patients with cervical cancer are treated on a protocol using both planar and volumetric imaging with the OBI system. After the patient is aligned via skin marks, planar images are obtained with couch re-alignment performed remotely for all errors larger than 1 mm. Following treatment delivery, patients then undergo a volumetric kV CBCT, the results of which are reviewed in real time and are used to ensure tumor coverage (see Chapter 21H).

Future Directions

Many exciting possibilities exist to apply IGRT technologies in the treatment of patients with gynecologic cancer. Improved targeting and delivery should increase interest in IMRT, particularly sophisticated IMRT approaches such as dose-painting, to escalate dose to gross disease and/or high-risk areas within the tumor itself.[91,105] Moreover, IGRT technologies will most likely increase the use of hypofractionated treatment regimens, potentially serving as a replacement for brachytherapy in select patients.[90,106,107]

Another exciting potential use of IGRT in patients with gynecologic cancer is adaptive radiotherapy, whereby treatment is altered on the basis of changes occurring *during* treatment. Several groups are actively working in this area, particularly in the treatment of cervical cancer. As noted previously, cervical tumors regress significantly during treatment, and the question arises as to whether adapting to such changes would improve therapy. To explore this question, van de Bunt and coworkers replanned patients with cervical cancer undergoing definitive irradiation after 30 Gy based on repeat MR imaging (Figure 21-12).[23] Replanning significantly improved rectal sparing for all patients. The average rectal volume receiving 95% or more of the prescription dose was 75 cc (range, 20 cc–145 cc) without replanning versus 67 cc (range, 15 cc–106 cc) with replanning (P = .009). Small bowel sparing was also improved in women with bulky (> 30 cc) tumors.

Although this approach may improve normal tissue sparing on the day of replanning, it remains unclear whether there is a similar dosimetric benefit on subsequent days. It is possible that the adapted plan may not prove superior to the original nonadapted plan, because of the high degree of deformation and interfraction motions that occur in these patients. In fact, it is theoretically possible that the adapted plan may be *worse* than the original plan on subsequent days.

To address this question, Lawson et al. studied the impact of midtreatment replanning in a cohort of 10 intact cervical cancer patients undergoing IMRT, using daily CBCT imaging.[108] Overall, replanning significantly improved CTV coverage; the conformity index on remaining treatment days was improved compared with the original nonadapted IMRT plan. Significant reductions were also seen in the V_{45} of the small bowel and rectum. However, no benefit in rectal sparing was observed, and in three patients, rectal irradiation was increased using the adapted plan. These investigators are currently evaluating the dosimetric impact of weekly and daily replanning in a larger cohort.

Apart from *whether* adaptation should be done, the question remains *how* it could be accomplished. Research is currently focused on two main approaches. The first involves the development of high-speed computing techniques for on-line treatment planning and optimization. The UCSD Center for Advanced Radiotherapy Technologies, in collaboration with researchers from the Lawrence Livermore Laboratories and the San Diego Supercomputer Center, have initiated a project known as SCORE (Super-Computing On-line Re-planning Environment; Figure 21-13). The goal of the project is to allow image reconstruction, segmentation, deformation, replanning, and quality assurance to be performed while the patient is on the treatment table (i.e., on-line). Recently, UCSD researchers have shown the feasibility of ultrafast IMRT plan optimization and dose calculation to facilitate on-line replanning.[109,110]

An alternative approach is to develop a "library" of treatment plans before treatment. As envisioned, CBCT images would be obtained during treatment and used to select the most appropriate plan from the library. This plan would then be used to deliver treatment. Known as POLAR (Pre-planned On-Line Adaptive Radiotherapy), this approach is appealing, because all plans could undergo QA evaluation before their use. Multiple questions, however, remain regarding how many plans would be needed, how plans should be generated, and how the selection process should be accomplished. A concern with applying the POLAR approach to patients with cervical cancer is that a large library may be required, because of the degree of interfraction target motion caused by daily changes in rectal and bladder volumes. We are currently evaluating the positional and morphological changes occurring throughout treatment in a large cohort of intact cervical cancer patients. Our hope is to utilize shape modeling techniques to generate a sufficient library of plans, based on the initial CT simulation.

Currently, we are generating several treatment plans before treatment, by simulating patients with both a full and empty bladder, then applying planning margins of

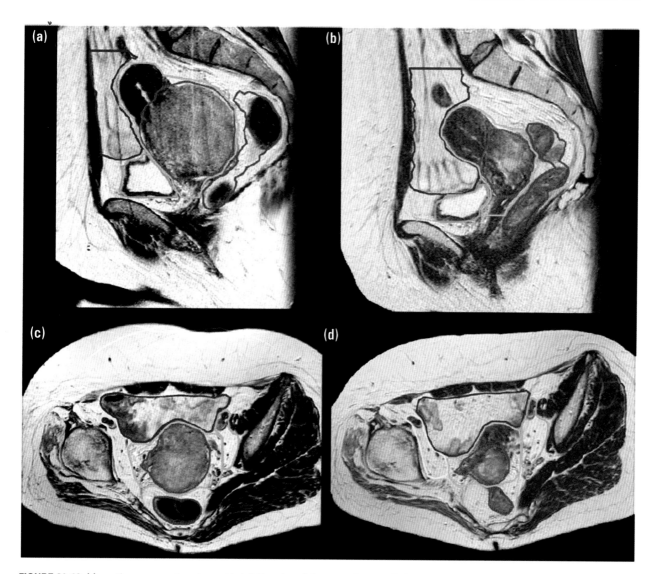

FIGURE 21-12. Magnetic resonance imaging–guided delineation of the target for a cervical cancer patient with bulky disease, illustrating marked tumor regression during external beam irradiation. **(a)** Pretreatment sagittal, **(b)** intratreatment sagittal, **(c)** pretreatment axial, and **(d)** intratreatment axial: Bowel, dark blue; rectum, pink; bladder, orange; primary gross tumor volume, red; primary clinical target volume, light blue; left nodal clinical target volume, green; right nodal clinical target volume, yellow. Reproduced with permission from Van de Bunt et al.[23]

various size. On the day of treatment, a CBCT is obtained (Figure 21-14) and the PTVs from the various plans are cast onto it. The treating physician then selects the plan that best covers the CTV while sparing the surrounding normal tissues. We are currently assessing how often different plans are needed and the ability of trained therapists to select the optimal plan.

Apart from simply adapting the treatment plan to a different PTV, alternative adaptive strategies could involve intensifying treatment in poorly responding patients. Mayr et al. evaluated serial MR imaging in 60 patients with stage IB2–IVB/recurrent cervical cancer undergoing definitive irradiation.[111] All patients underwent MR scans before, as well as at 20 Gy to 25 Gy (early treatment), 45 Gy to 50 Gy (midtreatment), and posttreatment. Outcome was significantly correlated to residual tumor

volume present on the midtreatment scan. The 5-year local control was significantly better in patients with less than 20% residual disease on the midtreatment MR versus 20% or more residual disease (84% vs 22%; $P < .0001$; Figure 21-15). Corresponding 5-year disease-free survival rates were 63% and 20%, respectively ($P = .0005$).

Adaptive RT could, alternatively, be based on physiologic changes. Schwarz and colleagues evaluated 36 cervical cancer patients with serial ^{18}F-FDG PET imaging before, during, and following chemoradiotherapy.[112] Positron emission tomography imaging during treatment was performed on approximately days 16 (early treatment), 33 (midtreatment), and 47 (late treatment), corresponding to the first, third or fourth, and last intracavitary applications. The mean maximum standardized uptake values (SUV_{max}) observed at baseline, early

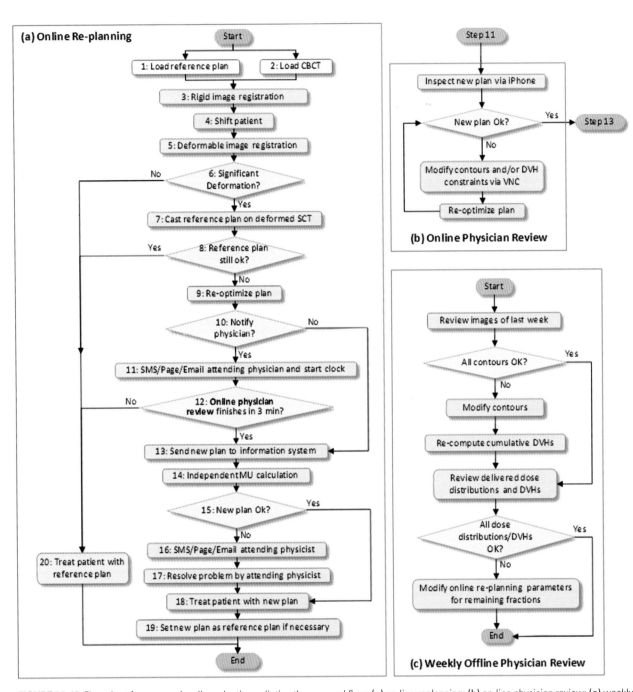

FIGURE 21-13. Flow chart for proposed on-line adaptive radiation therapy workflow: (a) on-line replanning; (b) on-line physician review; (c) weekly off-line physician review. SCT = simulation computed tomography; SMS = short message service; VNC = Virtual Network Computing. Courtesy: Steve Jiang, PhD, University of California San Diego, La Jolla, CA.

treatment, midtreatment, late treatment, and posttreatment were 11.2 (range, 2.1–38), 5.5 (range, 0–25.2), 2.4 (range, 0–5.2), 1.9 (range, 0–5.2) and 0.5 (range, 0–8.3), respectively. Best response based on the PET imaging during treatment were complete (six patients), partial (26 patients), and stable or increased (four patients). Of the six complete responders, one failed locally. Of the 26 partial responders, three recurred locally. No correlation was seen between during treatment response and

local or distant recurrence or survival. However, the overall data set was small and the timing of the PET scans varied considerably. Further work is needed to assess whether a subset of patients at high risk for recurrence could be identified by their metabolic response during treatment.

Adaptive RT approaches are not limited to EBRT. Several groups are exploring the utility of adapting brachytherapy to changes in the tumor based on imaging at each brachytherapy application. Pötter et al. com-

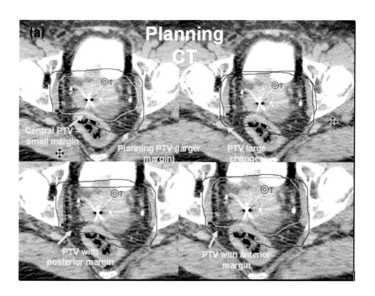

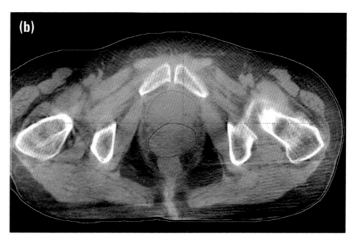

FIGURE 21-14. (a) Planning computed tomography (CT) showing multiple treatment plans generated for a patient undergoing radiotherapy for cervical cancer. (b) Axial kilovoltage cone beam CT image of a patient with cervical cancer in the region of the cervical tumor.

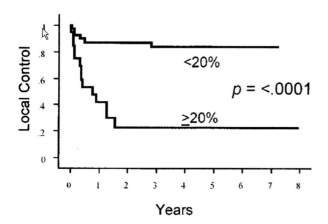

FIGURE 21-15. Local control based on residual disease volume measured on a magnetic resonance imaging study obtained midtreatment (at 45 Gy to 50 Gy) in a series of 60 patients with stage IB2–IVB/recurrent cervical cancer. Reproduced with permission from Mayr NA et al.[111]

pared the benefit of using a new MR scanning at each brachytherapy insertion versus basing all the insertions on a single MR scan.[113] Adapting the plan using new MR scans significantly improved the sparing of normal tissues. As discussed previously, PET has been used for image-guided adaptive brachytherapy, with enticing results suggesting that improvements in patient outcome may be achieved using advanced imaging to adapt brachytherapy plans.[78]

Conclusions

In summary, a vast array of IGRT technologies has been applied in gynecologic cancer to guide target delineation, improve patient setup, and permit adaptation to interfraction changes. These technological advancements are helping shed light on how to optimally deliver radiotherapy for gynecologic malignancies. Subsequent chapters will provide detailed examples of exciting and novel applications of IGRT that will hopefully transform future therapeutic standards.

References

1. Kim RY, McGinnis LS, Spencer SA, et al. Conventional four-field pelvic radiotherapy technique without computed tomography-treatment planning in cancer of the cervix: potential geographic miss and its impact on pelvic control. *Int J Radiat Oncol Biol Phys.* 1995;31:109–112.

2. Finlay MH, Ackerman I, Tirona RG, et al. Use of CT simulation for treatment of cervical cancer to assess the adequacy of lymph node coverage of conventional pelvic fields based on bony landmarks. *Int J Radiat Oncol Biol Phys.* 2006;64:205–209.

3. Huddart RA, Nahum A, Neal A, et al. Accuracy of pelvic radiotherapy: prospective analysis of 90 patients in a randomized trial of blocked versus standard radiotherapy. *Radiother Oncol.* 1996;39:19–29.

4. Datta NR, Srivastava A, Maria Das KJ, et al. Comparative assessment of doses to tumor, rectum, and bladder as evaluated by orthogonal radiographs vs. computer enhanced computed tomography-based intracavitary brachytherapy in cervical cancer. *Brachytherapy.* 2006;5:223–229.

5. Kim RY, Pareek P. Radiography-based treatment planning compared with computed tomography (CT)-based treatment planning for intracavitary brachytherapy in cancer of the cervix: analysis of dose-volume histograms. *Brachytherapy.* 2003;2:200–206.

6. Mell LK, Mehrotra AK, Mundt AJ. Intensity-modulated radiation therapy use in the United States, 2004. *Cancer.* 2005;104:1296–1303.

7. Mell LK, Mundt AJ. Intensity-modulated radiation therapy in gynecologic cancers: growing support, growing acceptance. *Cancer J.* 2008;14:198–199.

8. Mundt AJ, Lujan AE, Rotmensch J, et al. Intensity modulated whole pelvic radiation therapy in women with gynecologic malignancies. *Int J Radiat Oncol Biol Phys.* 2002;52:1330–1337.

9. Mundt AJ, Mell LK, Roeske JC. Preliminary analysis of chronic gastrointestinal toxicity in patients with gynecologic malignancies treated with intensity modulated whole pelvic radiation therapy. *Int J Radiat Oncol Biol Phys.* 2003;56:1354–1360.

10. Chen MF, Tseng CJ, Tseng CC, et al. Adjuvant concurrent chemoradiotherapy with intensity-modulated pelvic radiotherapy after surgery for high-risk, early stage cervical cancer patients. *Cancer J.* 2008;14:200–206.

11. Portelance L, Chao KS, Grigsby PW, et al. Intensity modulated radiation therapy (IMRT) reduces small bowel, rectum, and bladder doses in patients with cervical cancer receiving pelvic and para aortic irradiation. *Int J Radiat Oncol Biol Phys.* 2001;51:261–266.

12. Beriwal S, Gan GN, Heron DE, et al. Early clinical outcome with concurrent chemotherapy and extended-field, intensity-modulated radiation therapy for cervical cancer. *Int J Radiat Oncol Biol Phys.* 2007;68:166–171.

13. Beriwal S, Coon D, Heron DE, et al. Preoperative intensity-modulated radiotherapy and chemotherapy for locally advanced vulvar carcinoma. *Gynecol Oncol.* 2008;109:291–295.

14. Rochet N, Sterzing F, Jensen A, et al. Helical tomotherapy as a new treatment technique for whole abdominal irradiation. *Strahlenther Onkol.* 2008;184:145–149.

15. Small W Jr, Mell LK, Anderson P, et al. Consensus guidelines for delineation of clinical target volume for intensity-modulated pelvic radiotherapy in postoperative treatment of endometrial and cervical cancer. *Int J Radiat Oncol Biol Phys.* 2008;71:428–434.

16. Barillot I, Reynaud-Bougnoux A. The use of MRI in planning radiotherapy for gynaecological tumours. *Cancer Imaging.* 2006;6:100–106.

17. Taylor A, Rockall AG, Reznek RH, et al. Mapping pelvic lymph nodes: guidelines for delineation in intensity-modulated radiotherapy. *Int J Radiat Oncol Biol Phys.* 2005;63:1604–1612.

18. Dimopoulos JC, Schard G, Berger D, et al. Systematic evaluation of MRI findings in different stages of treatment of cervical cancer: potential of MRI on delineation of target, pathoanatomic structures, and organs at risk. *Int J Radiat Oncol Biol Phys.* 2006;64.1380–1388.

19. Viswanathan A, Dimopoulos J, Kirisits C, et al. Computed tomography versus magnetic resonance imaging-based contouring in cervical cancer brachytherapy: results of a prospective trial and preliminary guidelines for standardized contours. *Int J Radiat Oncol Biol Phys.* 2007;68:491–498.

20. Fyles AW, Lim K, Small W, et al. Variability in delineation of clinical target volumes for cervix cancer intensity-modulated pelvic radiotherapy [abstract]. *Int J Radiat Oncol Biol Phys.* 2009;75:S83–S84.

21. Haslam JJ, Lujan AE, Mundt AJ, et al. Setup errors in patients treated with intensity modulated whole pelvic radiation therapy for gynecological malignancies. *Med Dosim.* 2005;30:36–42.

22. Stroom JC, Olofsen-van Acht MJJ, Quint S, et al. On-line setup corrections during radiotherapy of patients with gynecologic tumors. *Int J Radiat Oncol Biol Phys.* 2000;46:499–506.

23. Van de Bunt L, van der Heide UA, Ketelaars M, et al. Conventional, conformal and intensity modulated radiation therapy treatment planning of external beam radiotherapy for cervical cancer: the impact of tumor regression. *Int J Radiat Oncol Biol Phys.* 2006;64:189–196.

24. Mayr NA, Yuh WTC, Taoka T, et al. Serial therapy-induced changes in tumor shape in cervical cancer and their impact on assessing tumor volume and treatment response. *Am J Roentgenol.* 2006;187:65–72.

25. Lee CM, Shrieve DC, Gaffney DK. Rapid involution and mobility of carcinoma of the cervix. *Int J Radiat Oncol Biol Phys.* 2004;58:625–630.

26. Chan P, Dinniwell R, Haider MA, et al. Inter- and intrafractional tumor and organ movement in patients with cervical cancer undergoing radiotherapy: a cinematic-MRI point-of-interest study. *Int J Radiat Oncol Biol Phys.* 2008;70:1507–1515.

27. Huh SJ, Park W, Han Y. Interfractional variation in position of the uterus during radical radiotherapy for cervical cancer. *Radiother Oncol.* 2004;71:73–79.

28. Buchali A, Koswig S, Dinges S, et al. Impact of the filling status of the bladder and rectum on their integral dose distribu-

tion and the movement of the uterus in the treatment planning of gynecological cancer. *Radiother Oncol.* 1999;52:29–34.

29. Kaatee RS, Olofsen MJ, Verstraate MB, et al. Detection of organ movement in cervix cancer patients using a fluoroscopic electronic portal imaging device and radioopaque markers. *Int J Radiat Oncol Biol Phys.* 2002;54:576–583.

30. Simpson DR, Lawson JD, Nath SK, et al. Utilization of advanced imaging technologies for target delineation in radiation oncology. *J Am Coll Radiol.* 2009;6:876–883.

31. Mayr NA, Tali ET, Yuh WT, et al. Cervical cancer: application of MR imaging in radiation therapy. *Radiology.* 1993;189:601–608.

32. Toita T, Kakinohana Y, Shinzato S, et al. Tumor diameter/volume and pelvic node status assessed by magnetic resonance imaging (MRI) for uterine cervical cancer treated with irradiation. *Int J Radiat Oncol Biol Phys.* 1999;43:777–782.

33. Mitchell D, Snyder B, Coakley F, et al. Early invasive cervical cancer: tumor delineation by magnetic resonance imaging, computed tomography, and clinical examination, verified by pathologic results, in the ACRIN6651/GOG 183 Intergroup Study. *J Clin Oncol.* 2006;26:5687–5694.

34. Mayr NA, Yuh WT, Zheng J, et al. Tumor size evaluated by pelvic examination compared with 3-D quantitative analysis in the prediction of outcome for cervical cancer. *Int J Radiat Oncol Biol Phys.* 1997;39:395–404.

35. Kodaira T, Fuwa N, Toita T, et al. Comparison of prognostic value of MRI and FIGO stage among patients with cervical carcinoma treated with radiotherapy. *Int J Radiat Oncol Biol Phys.* 2003;56:769–777.

36. Yang WT, Lam WW, Yu MY, et al. Comparison of dynamic helical CT and dynamic MR imaging in the evaluation of pelvic lymph nodes in cervical carcinoma. *AJR Am J Roentgenol.* 2000;175:759–766.

37. Rockall AG, Sohaib SA, Harisinghani MG, et al. Diagnostic performance of nanoparticle-enhanced magnetic resonance imaging in the diagnosis of lymph node metastases in patients with endometrial and cervical cancer. *J Clin Oncol.* 2005;23:2813–2821.

38. Dinniwell R, Chan P, Czarnota G, et al. Pelvic lymph node topography for radiotherapy treatment planning from ferumoxtran-10 contrast-enhanced magnetic resonance imaging. *Int J Radiat Oncol Biol Phys.* 2009;74:844–851.

39. Will O, Purkayastha S, Chan C, et al. Diagnostic precision of nanoparticle-enhanced MRI for lymph-node metastases: a meta-analysis. *Lancet Oncol.* 2006;7:52–60.

40. Grigsby PW, Siegel BA, Dehdashti F. Lymph node staging by positron emission tomography in patients with carcinoma of the cervix. *J Clin Oncol.* 2001;19:3745–3749.

41. Reinhardt MJ, Ehritt-Braun C, Vogelgesang D, et al. Metastatic lymph nodes in patients with cervical cancer: detection with MR imaging and FDG PET. *Radiology.* 2001;218:776–782.

42. Loft A, Berthelsen AK, Roed H, et al. The diagnostic value of PET/CT scanning in patients with cervical cancer: a prospective study. *Gynecol Oncol.* 2007;106:29–34.

43. Singh AK, Grigsby PW, Dehdashti F, et al. FDG-PET lymph node staging and survival of patients with FIGO stage IIIb cervical carcinoma. *Int J Radiat Oncol Biol Phys.* 2003;56:489–493.

44. Schwarz JK, Siegel BA, Dehdashti F, et al. Association of post-therapy positron emission tomography with tumor response and survival in cervical carcinoma. *JAMA.* 2007;298:2289–2295.

45. Chao A, Chang TC, Ng KK, et al. 18F-FDG PET in the management of endometrial cancer. *Eur J Nucl Med Mol Imaging.* 2006;33:36–44.

46. Lamoreaux WT, Grigsby PW, Dehdashti F, et al. FDG-PET evaluation of vaginal carcinoma. *Int J Radiat Oncol Biol Phys.* 2005;62:733–737.

47. Belhocine T, Thille A, Fridman V, et al. Contribution of whole-body 18-FDG PET imaging in the management of cervical cancer. *Gynecol Oncol.* 2002;87:90–97.

48. Miller TR, Grigsby PW. Measurement of tumor volume by PET to evaluate prognosis in patients with advanced cervical cancer treated by radiation therapy. *Int J Radiat Oncol Biol Phys.* 2002;53:353–359.

49. Lin LL, Yang Z, Mutic S, et al. FDG-PET imaging for the assessment of physiologic volume response during radiotherapy in cervix cancer. *Int J Radiat Oncol Biol Phys.* 2006;65:177–181.

50. Mutic S, Malyapa RS, Grigsby PW, et al. PET-guided IMRT for cervical carcinoma with positive para-aortic lymph nodes-a dose-escalation treatment planning study. *Int J Radiat Oncol Biol Phys.* 2003;55:28–35.

51. Esthappan J, Mutic S, Malyapa RS, et al. Treatment planning guidelines regarding the use of CT/PET-guided IMRT for cervical carcinoma with positive paraaortic lymph nodes. *Int J Radiat Oncol Biol Phys.* 2004;58:1289–1297.

52. Cooper RA, Carrington BM, Loncaster JA, et al. Tumour oxygenation levels correlate with dynamic contrast-enhanced magnetic resonance imaging parameters in carcinoma of the cervix. *Radiother Oncol.* 2000;57:53–59.

53. Okada T, Harada M, Matsuzaki K, et al. Evaluation of female intrapelvic tumors by clinical proton MR spectroscopy. *J Magn Reson Imaging.* 2001;13:912–917.

54. Lapela M, Leskinen-Kallio S, Varpula M, et al. Imaging of uterine carcinoma by carbon-11-methionine and PET. *J Nucl Med.* 1994;35:1618–1623.

55. Torizuka T, Kanno T, Futatsubashi M, et al. Imaging of gynecologic tumors: comparison of 11C-choline PET with 18F-FDG PET. *J Nucl Med.* 2003;44:1051–1056.

56. Dehdashti F, Grigsby PW, Mintun MA, et al. Assessing tumor hypoxia in cervical cancer by positron emission tomography with 60Cu-ATSM: relationship to therapeutic response-a preliminary report. *Int J Radiat Oncol Biol Phys.* 2003;55:1233–1238.

57. Grigsby PW, Malyapa RS, Higashikubo R, et al. Comparison of molecular markers of hypoxia and imaging with 60Cu-ATSM in cancer of the uterine cervix. *Mol Imaging Biol.* 2007;9:278–283.

58. Roeske JC, Lujan A, Reba RC, et al. Incorporation of SPECT bone marrow imaging into intensity modulated whole-pelvic radiation therapy treatment planning for gynecologic malignancies. *Radiother Oncol.* 2005;77:11–17.

59. Mell LK, Liang Y, Bydder M, et al. Functional MRI-guided bone marrow-sparing intensity modulated radiotherapy for pelvic malignancies [abstract]. *Int J Radiat Oncol Biol Phys.* 2009;75:S121.

60. International Commission on Radiation Units and Measurements: ICRU Report 38: Dose and volume specification for reporting intracavitary therapy in gynecology. Bethesda, MD: International Commission on Radiation Units and Measurements; 1985.

61. Wachter-Gerstner N, Wachter S, Reinstadler E, et al. Bladder and rectum dose defined from MRI based treatment planning for cervix cancer brachytherapy: comparison of dose-volume histograms for organ contours and organ wall, comparison with ICRU rectum and bladder reference point. *Radiother Oncol.* 2003;68:269–276.

62. Nguyen TV, Duman I, Petrow P, et al. MRI based treatment planning in cervical cancer brachytherapy: characteristics of the 2 cm³ volume receiving the highest dose in bladder and rectum walls, compared with ICRU reference points. *Radiother Oncol.* 2004;71:S71–S72.

63. Pötter R, Haie-Meder C, Van Limbergen E, et al. Recommendations from gynaecological (GYN) GEC ESTRO working group (II): concepts and terms in 3D image-based treatment planning in cervix cancer brachytherapy-3D dose volume parameters and aspects of 3D image-based anatomy, radiation physics, radiobiology. *Radiother Oncol.* 2006;78:67–77.

64. Kim R, Shen S, Duan J. Image-based three-dimensional treatment planning of intracavitary brachytherapy for cancer of the cervix: dose-volume histograms of the bladder, rectum, sigmoid colon, and small bowel. *Brachytherapy.* 2007;6:187–194.

65. Rotmensch J, Waggoner SE, Quiet C. Ultrasound guidance for placement of difficult intracavitary implants. *Gynecol Oncol.* 1994;54:159–162.

66. Weitmann HD, Knocke TH, Waldhäusl C, et al. Ultrasound-guided interstitial brachytherapy in the treatment of advanced vaginal recurrences from cervical and endometrial carcinoma. *Strahlenther Onkol.* 2006;182:86–95.

67. Davidson MT, Yuen J, D'Souza DP, et al. Optimization of high-dose-rate cervical brachytherapy applicator placement: the benefits of intraoperative ultrasound guidance. *Brachytherapy.* 2008;7:248–253.

68. Viswanathan AN, Erickson BA. Three-dimensional imaging in gynecologic brachytherapy: a survey of the American Brachytherapy Society. *Int J Radiat Oncol Biol Phys.* 2010;76:104–109.

69. Nag S. Controversies and new developments in gynecologic brachytherapy: image-based intracavitary brachytherapy for cervical carcinoma. *Semin Radiat Oncol.* 2006;16:164–167.

70. Dimopoulos JC, Kirisits C, Petric P, et al. The Vienna applicator for combined intracavitary and interstitial brachytherapy of cervical cancer: clinical feasibility and preliminary results. *Int J Radiat Oncol Biol Phys.* 2006;66:83–90.

71. Pötter R, Dimopoulos J, Georg P, et al. Clinical impact of MRI assisted dose volume adaptation and dose escalation in brachytherapy of locally advanced cervix cancer. *Radiother Oncol.* 2007;83:148–155.

72. Haie-Meder C, Pötter R, Van Limbergen E, et al. Recommendations from Gynaecological (GYN) GEC-ESTRO Working Group (I): concepts and terms in 3D image based 3D treatment planning in cervix cancer brachytherapy with emphasis on MRI assessment of GTV and CTV. *Radiother Oncol.* 2005;74: 235–245.

73. Nag S, Cardenes H, Chang S, et al. Proposed guidelines for image-based intracavitary brachytherapy for cervical carcinoma: report from Image-Guided Brachytherapy Working Group. *Int J Radiat Oncol Biol Phys.* 2004;60:1160–1172.

74. Viswanathan AN, Cormack R, Holloway CL, et al. Magnetic resonance-guided interstitial therapy for vaginal recurrence of endometrial cancer. *Int J Radiat Oncol Biol Phys.* 2006;66:91–99.

75. Kim RY, Falkenberg E, Pareek P. Image-based intracavitary brachytherapy in the treatment of inoperable uterine cancer: individual dose specification at specific anatomical sites. *Brachytherapy.* 2005;4:286–290.

76. Mutic S, Grigsby PW, Low DA, et al. PET-guided three-dimensional treatment planning of intracavitary gynecologic implants. *Int J Radiat Oncol Biol Phys.* 2002;52:1104–1110.

77. Malyapa RS, Mutic S, Low DA, et al. Physiologic FDG-PET three-dimensional brachytherapy treatment planning for cervical cancer. *Int J Radiat Oncol Biol Phys.* 2002;54:1140–1146.

78. Lin L, Mutic S, Low D, et al. Adaptive brachytherapy treatment planning for cervical carcinoma using FDG-PET. *Int J Radiat Oncol Biol Phys.* 2007;67:91–96.

79. Pötter R, Van Limbergen E, Wambersie A. Reporting in brachytherapy: dose and volume specification. In: Gerbaulet A, Pötter R, Mazeron JJ, Meertens H, Van Limbergen E, eds. *The GEC-ESTRO Handbook of Brachytherapy.* Brussels, Belgium: ESTRO 2002;155–215.

80. Kirisits C, Pötter R, Lang S, et al. Dose and volume parameters for MRI-based treatment planning in intracavitary brachytherapy for cervical cancer. *Int J Radiat Oncol Biol Phys.* 2005; 62:901–911.

81. Nag S, Gupta N. A simple method of obtaining equivalent doses for use in HDR brachytherapy. *Int J Radiat Oncol Biol Phys.* 2000;46:507–513.

82. Koom WS, Sohn DK, Kim JY, et al. Computed tomography-based high-dose-rate intracavitary brachytherapy for uterine cervical cancer: preliminary demonstration of correlation between dose-volume parameters and rectal mucosal changes observed by flexible sigmoidoscopy. *Int J Radiat Oncol Biol Phys.* 2007;68:1446–1454.

83. Pötter R, Dimopoulos J, Bachtiary B, et al. 3D conformal HDR-brachy- and external beam therapy plus simultaneous cisplatin for high-risk cervical cancer: clinical experience with 3 year follow-up. *Radiother Oncol.* 2006;79:80–86.

84. Berger D, Dimopoulos J, Georg P, et al. Uncertainties in assessment of the vaginal dose for intracavitary brachytherapy of cervical cancer using a tandem-ring applicator. *Int J Radiat Oncol Biol Phys.* 2007;67:1451–1459.

85. Sturdza AE, Berger D, Lang S, et al. Uncertainties in assessing sigmoid dose volume parameters in MRI-guided fractionated HDR brachytherapy [abstract]. *Brachytherapy.* 2008;7:109.

86. Hurksman CW, Remeijer P, Lebesque JV, et al. Setup verification using portal imaging: review of current clinical practice. *Radiother Oncol.* 2001;58:105–120.

87. Olofsen-van Acht M, van den Berg H, Quint S, et al. Reduction of irradiation small bowel volume and accurate patient positioning by use of a belly board device in pelvic radiotherapy of gynecological cancer patients. *Radiother Oncol.* 2001;59: 87–93.

88. Kochanski JD, Mell LK, Roeske JC. Intensity-modulated radiation therapy in gynecologic malignancies: current status and future directions. *Clin Adv Hematol Oncol.* 2006;4:379–386.

89. Choi CW, Cho CK, Yoo SY. Image-guided stereotactic body radiation therapy in patients with isolated para-aortic lymph node metastases from uterine cervical and corpus cancer. *Int J Radiat Oncol Biol Phys.* 2009;74:147–153.

90. Molla M, Escude L, Nouet P, et al. Fractionated stereotactic radiotherapy boost for gynecologic tumors: an alternative to brachytherapy? *Int J Radiat Oncol Biol Phys.* 2005;62:118–124.

91. Taylor A, Powell ME. Conformal and intensity-modulated radiotherapy for cervical cancer. *Clin Oncol (R Coll Radiol).* 2008; 20:417–425.

92. Guerrero M, Li XA, Ma L, et al. Simultaneous integrated intensity-modulated radiotherapy boost for locally advanced gynecologic cancer: radiobiological and dosimetric considerations. *Int J Radiat Oncol Biol Phys.* 2005;62:933–939.

93. Tyagi N, Yashar CM, Lewis JH, et al. Impact of internal organ motion and deformation on target coverage in intact cervical cancer patients undergoing IMRT: a daily cone beam CT study [abstract]. *Int J Radiat Oncol Biol Phys.* 2008;72:S355.

94. Raj KA, Guo P, Marks L, et al. Intrafraction organ motion of the normal cervix [abstract]. *Int J Radiat Oncol Biol Phys.* 2005;63:S220.

95. Lim K, Kelly V, Stewart J, et al. Pelvic radiotherapy for cancer of the cervix: is what you plan actually what you deliver? *Int J Radiat Oncol Biol Phys.* 2009;74:304–312.

96. Beadle BM, Jhingran A, Salehpour M, et al. Cervix regression and motion during the course of external beam chemoradiotherapy for cervical cancer. *Int J Radiat Oncol Biol Phys.* 2009;73:235–241.

97. Simpson DR, Lawson JD, Nath SK, et al. Survey of image-guided radiation therapy use in the United States [abstract]. *Int J Radiat Oncol Biol Phys.* 2009;75:S498.

98. Van Dyk S, Narayan K, Fisher R, et al. Conformal brachytherapy planning for cervical cancer using transabdominal ultrasound. *Int J Radiat Oncol Biol Phys.* 2009;75:64–70.

99. Michalski JM, Graham MV, Bosch WR, et al. Prospective clinical evaluation of an electronic portal imaging device. *Int J Radiat Oncol Biol Phys.* 1996;34:943–951.

100. Yamamoto R, Yonesaka A, Nishioka S, et al. High dose three-dimensional conformal boost (3DCB) using an orthogonal diagnostic x-ray set-up for patients with gynecological malignancy: a new application of real-time tumor-tracking system. *Radiother Oncol.* 2004;73:219–222.

101. Sorcini B, Tilikidis A. Clinical application of image-guided radiotherapy IGRT (on the Varian OBI platform). *Cancer Radiother.* 2006;10:252–257.

102. Lewis JH, Tyagi N, Yashar CM, et al. Impact of daily image guided patient setup on bone marrow sparing in cervical cancer patients undergoing IMRT [abstract]. *Int J Radiat Oncol Biol Phys.* 2008;72:S582.

103. McBain CA, Henry AM, Sykes J, et al. X-ray volumetric imaging in image-guided radiotherapy: the new standard in on-treatment imaging. *Int J Radiat Oncol Biol Phys.* 2006;64: 625–634.

104. Santanam L, Esthappan J, Mutic S, et al. Estimation of setup uncertainty using planar and MVCT imaging for gynecologic malignancies. *Int J Radiat Oncol Biol Phys.* 2008;71:1511–1517.

105. Ahmed RS, Kim RY, Duan J, et al. IMRT dose escalation for positive para-aortic lymph nodes in patients with locally advanced cervical cancer while reducing dose to bone marrow and other organs at risk. *Int J Radiat Oncol Biol Phys.* 2004;60:505–512.

106. Roeske JC, Mundt AJ. A feasibility study of IMRT for the treatment of cervical cancer patients unable to receive intracavitary brachytherapy. *Med Phys.* 2000;27:1382–1383.

107. Duan J, Kim RY, Elassal S, et al. Conventional high-dose-rate brachytherapy with concomitant complementary IMRT boost: a novel approach for improving cervical tumor dose coverage. *Int J Radiat Oncol Biol Phys.* 2008;71:765–771.

108. Lawson JD, Simpson DR, Rose BS, et al. Adaptive radiotherapy in cervical cancer: dosimetric analysis using daily cone-beam CT [abstract]. *Int J Radiat Oncol Biol Phys.* 2009;75:S85–S86.

109. Men C, Gu X, Choi D, et al. GPU-based ultra-fast IMRT plan optimization. *Phys Med Biol.* 2009;54;6565–6573.

110. Gu X, Choi D, Men C, et al. GPU-based ultra-fast dose calculation using a finite size pencil beam model. *Phys Med Biol.* 2009;54:6287–6297.

111. Mayr NA, Taoka T, Yuh WTC, et al. Method and timing of tumor volume measurement for outcome prediction in cervical cancer using magnetic resonance imaging. *Int J Radiat Oncol Biol Phys.* 2002;52:14–22.

112. Schwarz JK, Lin LL, Siegel BA, et al. ^{18}F-fluorodeoxyglucose-positron emission tomography evaluation of early metabolic response during radiation therapy for cervical cancer. *Int J Radiat Oncol Biol Phys.* 2008;72:1502–1507.

113. Pötter R, Fidarova E, Kirisits C, et al. Image-guided adaptive brachytherapy for cervix carcinoma. *Clin Oncol.* 2008;20: 426–432.

MR-Guided Target Delineation in a Patient with Locally Advanced Cervical Cancer Undergoing Brachytherapy

Case Study

Alina Sturdza, MD, Johannes Dimopoulos, MD, Richard Pötter, MD

Patient History

A 35-year-old woman presented with a month history of vaginal bleeding exacerbated by intercourse. Pelvic examination revealed an exophytic tumor extending from the endocervix to the posterior lip of the cervix, between 3 o'clock and 7 o'clock, involving the left distal parametrium, and left and posterior fornix. A pelvic magnetic resonance (MR) scan identified a large cervical mass with a volume of 61 cm3 (5.9 cm × 4.4 cm × 4.7 cm) (Figure 21A-1). Biopsy of the lesion revealed moderately differentiated, infiltrating squamous cell carcinoma.

Computed tomography (CT) of the chest and abdomen and laparoscopic lymph node sampling were performed for staging purposes. The CT revealed the cervical mass and no suspicious lymphadenopathy in the iliac or para-aortic regions. During the laparoscopic lymph node staging, 24 nodes were removed from the obturator and iliac areas bilaterally. All were negative for malignancy. Final clinical staging was IIB (T2bN0M0), according to the International Federation of Gynecology and Obstetrics.

The patient's case was discussed in our multidisciplinary gynecologic oncology conference and the consensus recommendation was for definitive chemoradiation therapy, consisting of pelvic external beam radiation therapy (EBRT; 45 Gy in 1.8-Gy daily fractions) with concurrent chemotherapy (cisplatin, 40 mg/m^2/week) followed by brachytherapy. We elected to use MR to guide target delineation during the brachytherapy phase of her treatment.

Brachytherapy Application

During EBRT, the patient underwent weekly MR scanning as part of an in-house protocol assessing tumor response. At 5 weeks into treatment, the MR revealed residual disease in the cervix, left parametrium, and left fornix (Figure 21A-2). On the basis of these findings and on the clinical examination 1 day before the first application, it was decided to use a combined intracavitary–interstitial applicator to ensure coverage of the uterine cervix and the persistent left parametrial disease. Two applications were planned using 192Ir high dose rate (HDR) brachytherapy with a stepping source afterloading machine (MicroSelectron HDR classic, Nucletron, Veenendaal, The Netherlands). Our brachytherapy approach includes delivery of two fractions per application, at least 12 hours apart. The two applications are done 1 week apart.

On the day of the first application, the patient was brought into the operating room suite. After informed consent was obtained, she received epidural anesthesia and was placed in the lithotomy position. She was then prepped and draped in the usual manner, a Foley catheter was inserted, and her bladder was emptied and then

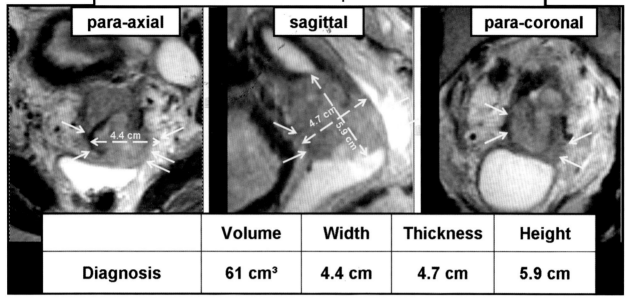

	Volume	Width	Thickness	Height
Diagnosis	61 cm³	4.4 cm	4.7 cm	5.9 cm

FIGURE 21A-1. Magnetic resonance scan at diagnosis demonstrated a bulky endocervical tumor with complete obstruction of the endocervical canal resulting in fluid collection in the intrauterine cavity. (Arrows illustrate the extent of disease at diagnosis; dotted arrows represent the initial measurements of the tumor size.)

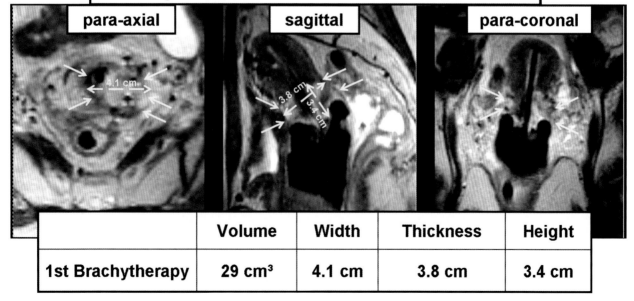

	Volume	Width	Thickness	Height
1st Brachytherapy	29 cm³	4.1 cm	3.8 cm	3.4 cm

FIGURE 21A-2. First brachytherapy magnetic resonance scan (week 5 of external beam radiation therapy demonstrates endocervical tumor response, with significant reduction in tumor volume; however, there is persistent tumor in the left parametrium. (Arrows illustrate the extent of residual disease at first brachytherapy application; dotted arrows represent the measurements of the tumor size at first brachytherapy application.)

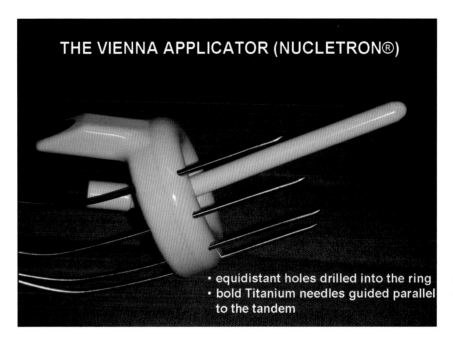

FIGURE 21A-3. The Vienna ring applicator (Nucletron) that allows placement of interstitial needles in patients with residual parametrial involvement (in this case the left parametrium).

filled with 50 mL of saline. Before this application, bowel preparation was performed to achieve an empty sigmoid and rectum.

Examination under anesthesia revealed good regression of the endo- and ectocervical tumor, with persistent disease in the left parametrium and left fornix (as noted on MR). Speculum examination revealed good response of the cervical tumor; however, there was persistent tumor on the ectocervix between 3 o'clock and 7 o'clock and in the left fornix. A modified MR-compatible tandem-ring applicator (Vienna ring applicator Nucletron, Nijmegen, Netherlands) was preferred, allowing placement of interstitial needles to cover the persistent disease in the left parametrium. This applicator includes six to eight holes drilled into the ring allowing a corresponding clockwise representation of the parametrium (Figure 21A-3). The tips of the titanium needles (Acrostak Corp, Winterthur, Switzerland) are made blunt in our mechanical workshop to avoid organ or vessel injuries during needle insertion.

In this patient, an intracavitary–interstitial MR-compatible tandem of 6 cm length and 60° angulation and a ring with a 34-mm diameter were inserted. Four interstitial titanium needles were placed through the ring holes to ensure coverage of the residual mass in the left parametrium. After the insertion of the applicator, vaginal packing with diluted gadolinium (Prohance, dilution 1:10) was performed and a rectal probe (diameter, 10 mm) was inserted into the rectum. Appropriate measures to prevent venous thrombosis and infection were taken for the duration of the implant. Orthogonal x-ray films were performed in the operating room for applicator reconstruction.

Imaging and Target Delineation

The patient was then transferred to the MR suite, which is located in our department in the proximity of the OR, for MR evaluation of the applicator placement in relation to the cervical tumor, the cervix, the uterus, the parametria, and the surrounding normal tissues. Fast spin echo T2-weighted images (TE 96s, TR 4500s) were performed using a pelvic surface coil with a 0.2 T low field system (Magnetom Open-Viva, Siemens AG, Erlangen, Germany), in the transverse (i.e., perpendicular to the body axis), (para)-sagittal, (para)-coronal (parallel to the intrauterine applicator tube), and para-transverse (orthogonal to the intrauterine applicator tube) orientations. The slice thickness was 5 mm, with no interslice gap. Although at brachytherapy the volume of disease had decreased substantially (from 61 cm³ to 29 cm³), this patient was considered to have had insufficient response to treatment because of significant residual disease, also persistent in the left parametrium (Figure 21A-2).

All of the transverse MR scans were transferred to the PLATO treatment planning system (TPS) for contouring (version 14.3, Nucletron, Veenendaal, The Netherlands) via a network connection. The gross tumor volume (GTV), high-risk clinical target volume (HR-CTV), and intermediate-risk clinical target volume (IR-CTV) as well as organs at risk (OARs) were delineated by the radiation oncologists using our current practice and following the recommendations of the GYN GEC-ESTRO working group, based on the MR images at diagnosis, at the time of brachytherapy, and on the clinical examination (under anesthesia).

The GTV encompassed macroscopic tumor extension at time of brachytherapy and is represented by the high-signal-intensity mass (FSE, T2) in cervix–corpus, parametria, vagina, bladder, and rectum. The HR-CTV included the GTV, the whole cervix, and presumed extracervical tumor extension. Pathologic residual tissue(s) as defined by palpable indurations and/or gray zones in parametria, were included in HR-CTV. The IR-CTV encompassed the HR-CTV plus safety margins. These margins are added according to the treatment strategy, tumor size, and tumor regression. In this case, because of moderate response to EBRT, the IR-CTV included the HR-CTV plus a 1-cm margin into the left parametrial residue, into the right parametrium, into the uterine corpus and vagina, and 5 mm both anteriorly between cervix and bladder and posteriorly between cervix and rectum. The OARs (bladder, rectum, sigmoid) were delineated using the outer organ wall. These volumes are outlined in Figure 21A-4 (a and b).

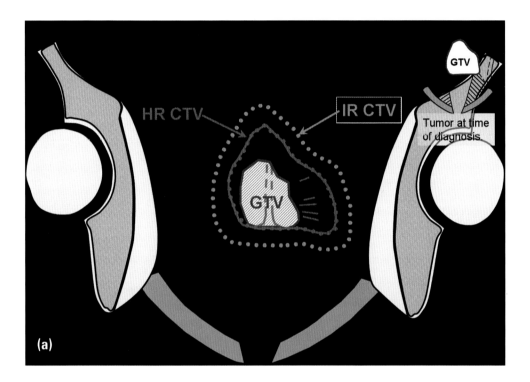

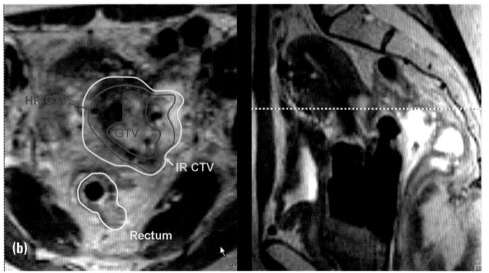

FIGURE 21A-4. Target and organs at risk (OARs) delineation at first magnetic resonance (MR)–guided brachytherapy application. **(a)** Demonstration of volume delineation on a coronal view, using clinical drawings at the time of first brachytherapy (modified after R. Pötter et al.[1]). **(b)** Target and organs at risk (OAR) delineation on MR according to the GEC ESTRO guidelines, axial cut, and the corresponding sagittal level identification (dotted line) on a DICOM viewer software (eFilm, Medical Inc, Toronto, ON).

Treatment Planning

Starting from a standard loading pattern in the tandem-ring applicator and dose normalization to point A, the dose distribution was prescribed and optimized to the HR-CTV by manual loading pattern and dwell time modification, taking into account anatomical positions of OARs. The dose proportion for the needles implanted inside the HR-CTV was individually adapted to cover the target and spare OARs as visualized on the postimplantation MR scans (two were loaded 10%, one 20%, and one was left unloaded). Dosimetric evaluation was performed by visual inspection of isodose lines and by dose–volume histogram (DVH) analysis according to recommendations of the Gynecological GEC-ESTRO Working Group. Cumulative DVHs were calculated for the GTV and HR-CTV. The coverage with the prescribed dose (V_{100}) and the dose that covers 100% and 90% of the GTV and HR-CTV (D_{100}, D_{90}) were evaluated. For OARs, cumulative DVHs were calculated, and the minimum dose to the most irradiated 0.1 cm³, and 2 cm³ ($D_{0.1cc}$ and D_{2cc}) was evaluated. The total dose combining EBRT and brachytherapy was normalized to conventional 2 Gy per fraction using the linear-quadratic model (EQD2). For doses in the target and in the bladder, rectum, and sigmoid an α–β ratio of 10 Gy and 3 Gy, respectively, was used.

For brachytherapy treatment planning and optimization, dose constraints were applied for the D_{90} of HR-CTV and D_{2cc} of OAR. Currently applied total dose constraints (EBRT + BT) are: D_{2cc} (bladder) < 90 Gy, D_{2cc} (rectum, sigmoid) < 75 Gy (< 70 Gy if possible), and a D_{90} (HR-CTV) > 85 Gy (Table 21A-1).

To achieve the target dose constraints, a total dose of 7 Gy was prescribed to the HR-CTV for the first fraction. After the treatment delivery, the patient was transferred to our inpatient unit for an overnight stay. A second fraction of 7 Gy was delivered the second day (after at least 12 hours from the first fraction) and after the position of the applicator in relation to the target and the OAR was verified by a second MR. After irradiation, the gauze and tandem were removed, followed by removal of the ring together with all the needles by a resolute pull. The patient was discharged 24 hours later after clinical examination to exclude bleeding.

A similar procedure to the first MR-guided application took place 1 week later. Contour delineation and planning were adapted to the respective findings (clinical examination and MR) at the second application. Total doses for GTV, HR-CTV, bladder and rectal points, and DVH parameters for OARs are given in Table 21A-1.

Clinical Outcome

Overall, the patient tolerated her EBRT treatment well without any unplanned treatment breaks. She also tolerated both brachytherapy applications without any significant acute sequelae. Regular 3-month follow-up clinical examination and imaging revealed a complete response of the tumor. At 40 months following therapy, the patient remains without disease recurrence on imaging and clinical examination. No significant late side effects have developed.

TABLE 21A–1 Dose–Volume Histogram Parameters for the Four Fractions of Magnetic Resonance–Guided Brachytherapy

Brachytherapy Fraction	1	2	3	4	Total BT Dose, Gy EQD2	Total BT + EB Dose, Gy EQD2
Prescribed dose	7 Gy	7 Gy	7 Gy	7 Gy	39.7	83.9
D_{100} GTV (α/β = 10) EQD2	10.9	10.9	14.5	14.5	50.8	95.1
D_{90} GTV (α/β = 10) EQD2	17.9	17.9	22.9	22.9	81.6	125.8
D_{100} HR CTV (α/β = 10) EQD2	7.5	7.5	9.9	9.9	34.7	79.0
D_{90} HR CTV (α/β = 10) EQD2	12.9	12.9	16.9	16.9	59.6	103.8
Bladder						
ICRU point dose (α/β = 3) EQD2	1.2	1.2	2.5	2.5	7.6	50.8
0.1 cm³ dose (α/β = 3) EQD2	9.4	9.4	14.7	14.7	48.1	91.3
2 cm³ dose (α/β = 3) EQD2	6.5	6.5	9.4	9.4	31.7	74.9
Rectum						
ICRU point dose (α/β = 3) EQD2	5.4	5.4	6.8	6.8	24.3	67.5
0.1 cm³ dose (α/β = 3) EQD2	5.8	5.8	8.0	8.0	27.6	70.8
2 cm³ dose (α/β = 3) EQD2	3.4	3.4	5.6	5.6	18	61.2
Sigmoid						
0.1 cm³ dose (α/β = 3) EQD2	12	12	15.8	15.8	55.6	98.8
2 cm³ dose (α/β = 3) EQD2	7.7	7.7	5.8	5.8	27.1	70.3

Notes. BT = brachytherapy; CTV = clinical target volume; EB = external beam; EQD2 = equivalent dose-2 Gy fractions; GTV = gross tumor volume; ICRU = International Commission on Radiation Units and Measurements.

Our initial clinical experience using MR-guided brachytherapy and CT-based external beam plus simultaneous cisplatin chemotherapy in 48 patients with high-risk cervical cancer was presented earlier.[1–4] Overall, 45 patients (94%) obtained a complete response following treatment. At a median follow-up of 33 months, 27 patients remained free of disease recurrence. Three-year actuarial overall survival and progression-free survival rates were 61% and 51%, respectively. Two patients developed a grade 4 genitourinary sequela, whereas none developed grade 3 or higher gastrointestinal sequelae.

References

1. Potter R, Dimopoulos J, et al. Clinical impact of MRI assisted dose volume adaptation and dose escalation in brachytherapy of locally advanced cervix cancer. *Radiother Oncol.* 2007;83(2): 148–55.
2. Kirisits, C., R. Potter, et al. Dose and volume parameters for MRI-based treatment planning in intracavitary brachytherapy for cervical cancer. *Int J Radiat Oncol Biol Phys.* 2005;62(3):901–11.
3. Dimopoulos, J. C., S. Lang, et al. Dose-volume histogram parameters and local tumor control in magnetic resonance image-guided cervical cancer brachytherapy. *Int J Radiat Oncol Biol Phys* 2009;75(1):56–63.
4. Potter R, Kirisits C, et al. Present status and future of high-precision image guided adaptive brachytherapy for cervix carcinoma. *Acta Oncol.* 2008;47(7):1325–36.

^{18}F-FDG PET-Guided Target Delineation for External Beam Radiotherapy and Intracavitary Brachytherapy Planning in a Patient with Stage IIB Cervical Cancer

Case Study

Perry W. Grigsby, MD

Patient History

A 31-year-old woman presented with bloody vaginal discharge over a period of several weeks. Physical examination was unremarkable except on pelvic examination there was a 5-cm exophytic lesion entirely replacing the cervix with left parametrial extension limited to the medial one third of the pelvis. A cervical biopsy was performed that demonstrated poorly differentiated squamous cell carcinoma.

Imaging evaluation was performed with a whole body ^{18}F-Fluorodeoxyglucose positron emission tomography (^{18}F-FDG PET), which demonstrated a large (58.92 cm^3) cervical mass with markedly increased ^{18}F-FDG uptake (maximum standardized uptake value [SUV$_{max}$], 25.64). There were multiple lymph nodes with moderate to markedly increased ^{18}F-FDG uptake, including a left para-aortic lymph node, an aortocaval lymph node, two lymph nodes at the right common iliac bifurcation, a smaller lymph node at the left common iliac bifurcation, several right internal iliac lymph nodes, and multiple bilateral external iliac lymph nodes. A small focus of moderate ^{18}F-FDG uptake in the left ovary was felt to be physiologic. No distant metastases were noted in the liver, lung, or other sites. No additional imaging studies were

performed. Her tumor was thus staged as a FIGO Stage IIB tumor.

Our consensus recommendation was for concomitant chemoradiation consisting of 6 weekly administrations of cisplatin chemotherapy (40 mg/m^2), intensity-modulated radiation therapy (IMRT) to the pelvis and para-aortic regions, and 6 weekly tandem and ovoid high-dose rate (HDR) intracavitary implants. We elected to use ^{18}F-FDG PET to help guide target delineation for both her external beam and brachytherapy treatments.

Simulation

The patient underwent ^{18}F-FDG PET–computed tomography (CT) simulation. This scan was performed from the diaphragm through the perineum, with the patient positioned supine in an Alpha Cradle immobilization device (Smithers Medical Products, Inc, North Canton, OH). Localization and alignment marks were placed on the patient to minimize setup variability throughout her treatment. To minimize bladder ^{18}F-FDG activity, a Foley catheter was inserted before receiving ^{18}F-FDG. Furosemide (20 mg) was administrated via intravenous (IV) infusion approximately 20 minutes after ^{18}F-FDG injection and the patient also received IV fluids (1000 mL of 0.9% saline) during the imaging.

Imaging and Target Delineation

The PET–CT simulation images were then transferred to an Eclipse Planning System (Varian Medical Systems, Palo Alto, CA) and were registered using point and anatomic matching. The PET–CT images allowed for easy contouring of the metabolically active primary cervix tumor and involved lymph nodes. The ^{18}F-FDG-avid metabolically active tumor, both cervix and PET-positive lymph nodes, were contoured on the PET image. Normal structures were contoured on the CT image.

The primary cervix tumor metabolic target volume (MTV$_{CERVIX}$) was defined as the 40% threshold volume.[1] The PET-positive pelvic and para-aortic lymph nodes were contoured as MTV$_{NODAL}$. The remainder of the common, external, internal iliac, and para-aortic nodal regions were contoured as "vessels," superiorly from the level of the renal vessels and inferiorly to the level of the medial circumflex femoral artery. To create the nodal clinical target volume (CTV$_{NODAL}$), a 7-mm margin was added in all directions to the "vessels" contour excluding the pelvic bones, femoral heads, and vertebral bodies. A 7-mm margin was added uniformly to CTV$_{NODAL}$ to create the final planning target volume (PTV$_{FINAL}$). Figure 21B-1 shows representative contours for MTV$_{CERVIX}$, MTV$_{NODAL}$, and PTV$_{NODAL}$. Normal structures contoured included bladder, rectum (up to the sigmoid colon), spinal cord, kidneys, right and left femoral heads, pelvic bones, and "bowel" (a bag-like structure including small and large intestine).[2]

Treatment Planning

Intensity-modulated RT planning was performed with the Eclipse Planning System (Varian Medical Systems,

Palo Alto, CA). The IMRT prescription was MTV$_{NODAL}$ (60 Gy in 2-Gy fractions), PTV$_{FINAL}$ (50 Gy in 1.67-Gy fractions), and MTV$_{CERVIX}$ (20 Gy in 0.67-Gy fractions). The IMRT plans were optimized to deliver 95% of the prescription dose to 100% of the volume of PTV$_{FINAL}$, while minimizing the volume receiving 110% of the prescription dose (Figure 21B-2). Dose–volume constraints for normal tissues included: less than 40% of bowel to receive 30 Gy, less than 40% of rectum to receive 40 Gy, less than 40% of pelvic bones to receive 40 Gy, and less than 40% of femoral heads to receive 30 Gy.[3]

In addition to the IMRT treatment, the patient received HDR intracavitary brachytherapy delivered in six weekly fractions of 6.5 Gy per fraction to point A using an iridium-192 source (VariSource iX, Varian Medical Systems, Palo Alto, CA) and tandem and ovoid intracavitary applicators. Magnetic resonance image–guided three-dimensional (3D) brachytherapy was performed for the first, third, fifth, and sixth HDR fraction. ^{18}F-FDG PET–CT was performed with the second and fourth HDR fractions. The ^{18}F-FDG PET brachytherapy planning had specific advantages by clearly defining the metabolically active primary cervical tumor in relation to surrounding structures and the brachytherapy implant and allowed for adaptive brachytherapy planning to be performed as the tumor shrank during the course of therapy (Figure 21B-3). The ^{18}F-FDG PET cervical brachytherapy demonstrated the 3D spatial relationship of the cervical tumor to the tandem and ovoid applicators, bladder, and rectum.[4]

Clinical Outcome

The patient tolerated her treatment well without significant acute sequelae. A 3-month posttherapy ^{19}F-FDG-PET–CT scan was performed and demonstrated a complete metabolic response.[5] She has subsequently undergone

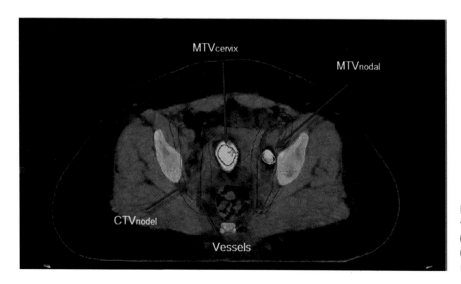

FIGURE 21B-1. Representative contours for the cervix metabolic target volume (MTV$_{CERVIX}$), nodal metabolic target volume (MTV$_{NODAL}$), and nodal clinical target volume (CTV$_{NODAL}$) in our patient.

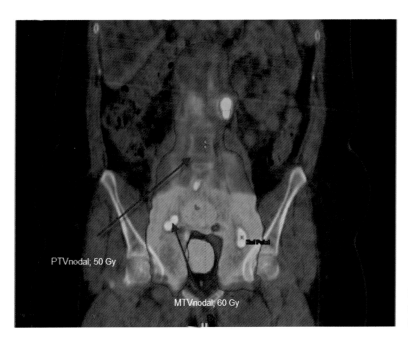

FIGURE 21B-2. Coronal slice through the planning computed tomography scan with colorwash overlay of the external beam isodose distribution.

whole body ^{18}F-FDG PET–CT at 6-month intervals for 18 months and is currently alive without evidence of recurrent cervical cancer.[6] There has been no late toxicity from her therapy.

We have found that ^{18}F-FDG PET imaging is useful in guiding target delineation in patients with cervical carcinoma who are undergoing external beam and brachy-

therapy. At our institution, ^{18}F-FDG PET imaging is now routinely used to guide the extent of the external beam RT portals. Patients who have ^{18}F-FDG PET–positive para-aortic nodal disease have their external beam portals increased to include the para-aortic region. Patients that have no nodal disease or pelvic nodal disease on ^{18}F-FDG PET imaging are treated with a standard pelvic portal.

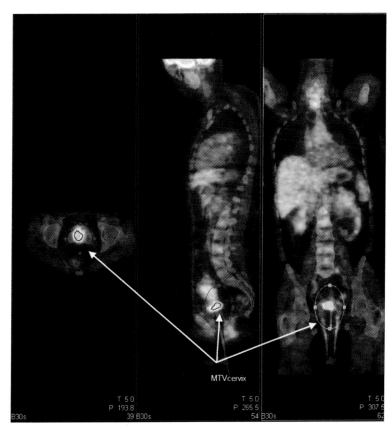

FIGURE 21B-3. Axial, sagittal, and coronal positron emission tomography–computed tomography scans. Brachytherapy planning is performed on the cervix metabolic target volume (MTV_{CERVIX}) as the tumor shrinks during the course of therapy.

As illustrated in the case presented here, ^{18}F-FDG PET can be used to define nodal sites for dose escalation.[3]

We are currently evaluating the role of ^{18}F-FDG PET–based brachytherapy planning.[4,7,8] In our initial report,[7] we demonstrated that incorporating ^{18}F-FDG PET into the brachytherapy planning process was feasible and added information regarding the 3D extent of the tumor volume. In subsequent reports,[4,8] we have evaluated the utility of serial ^{18}F-FDG PET imaging in these patients, noting that repeat ^{18}F-FDG PET imaging improved the tumor coverage particularly in the mid- and last brachytherapy insertions.

References

1. Miller TR, Grigsby PW. Measurement of tumor volume by PET to evaluate prognosis in patients with advanced cervical cancer treated by radiation therapy. *Int J Radiat Oncol Biol Phys.* 2002;53:353–359.
2. Macdhonald DM, Lin LL, Biehl K, et al. Combined intensity-modulated radiation therapy and brachytherapy in the treatment of cervical cancer. *Int J Radiat Oncol Biol Phys.* 2008;71:618–624.
3. Esthappan J, Chaudhari S, Suntanam L, et al. Prospective clinical trial of PET/CT image-guided intensity-modulated radiation therapy for cervical carcinoma with positive para-aortic lymph nodes. *Int J Radiat Oncol Biol Phys.* 2008;72:1134–1139.
4. Lin LL, Mutic S, Low DA, et al. Adaptive brachytherapy treatment planning for cervical cancer using FDG-PET. *Int J Radiat Oncol Biol Phys.* 2007;67:91–96.
5. Schwarz JK, Siegel BA, Dehdashti F, et al. Association of post-therapy positron emission tomography with tumor response and survival in cervical carcinoma. *JAMA.* 2007;298:2289–2295.
6. Brooks RA, Rader JS, Dehdashti F, et al. Surveillance FDG-PET detection of asymptomatic recurrences in patients with cervical cancer. *Gynecol Oncol.* 2009;112:104–109.
7. Malyapa RS, Mutic S, Low DA, et al. Physiologic FDG-PET three dimensional brachytherapy treatment planning for cervical cancer. *Int J Radiat Oncol Biol Phys.* 2002;54:1140–1146.
8. Lin LL, Mutic S, Malyapa RS, et al. Sequential FDG-PET brachytherapy treatment planning in carcinoma of the cervix. *Int J Radiat Oncol Biol Phys.* 2005;63:1494–1501.

^{18}F-FDG PET AND MR-GUIDED TARGET DELINEATION IN A PATIENT WITH STAGE IIIB CERVICAL CANCER

CASE STUDY

JENNIFER F. DE LOS SANTOS, MD, MARK LANGSTON, MD,
JANICE CARLISLE, MED, RICHARD POPPLE, PHD

Patient History

A 51-year-old woman presented with abnormal uterine bleeding. Two years before, the patient was noted to have atypical cells of undetermined significance (ASCUS) on a routine Pap smear and, more recently, noted increasing back and pelvic pain. Pelvic examination revealed an endocervical lesion measuring 4 cm with left greater than right parametrial induration. Colposcopy with biopsies returned positive for carcinoma in situ (CIS). A cold knife cone confirmed the diagnosis of a well- to moderately differentiated squamous cell carcinoma extending to the lateral and deep margins with lymphovascular space invasion.

A computed tomography (CT) scan of the abdomen and pelvis performed for staging purposes demonstrated some mild right hydroureteronephrosis along with a 2.0 cm by 0.9 cm left para-aortic node. A pelvic magnetic resonance (MR) scan revealed increased signal abnormality and thickening of the cervix consistent with cervical carcinoma with extension into the lower uterine segment and right parametrium (Figures 21C-1 and 21C-2). The uterus was prominent, measuring approximately 10 cm by 6 cm by 6 cm with heterogeneous T2 signal throughout, which was felt to be nonspecific. Bilateral iliac lymphadenopathy was noted in the pelvis.

To better clarify the extent of disease, a positron emission tomography (PET) scan was obtained and revealed a hypermetabolic cervical mass with a maximum standardized uptake value (SUV) of 18.1. Uterine involvement was noted and parametrial extension producing right ureteral

obstruction with moderate to severe right hydroureteronephrosis consistent with cervical cancer (Figure 21C-3). Additionally, there was metastatic involvement of bilateral iliac and para-aortic lymph nodes extending cranially to just below the level of the renal veins with maximum SUVs of 7.0 and 4.7, respectively (Figure 21C-4).

The tumor was thus staged as stage IIIB cervical cancer according to the International Federation of Gynecology and Obstetrics (FIGO) staging system. Our consensus

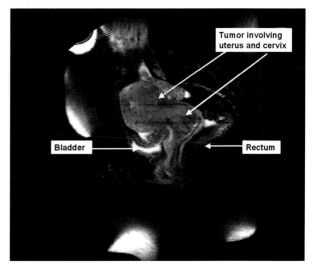

FIGURE 21C-1. Pretreatment sagittal T2-weighted magnetic resonance scan of the pelvis showing the cervical tumor with uterine extension.

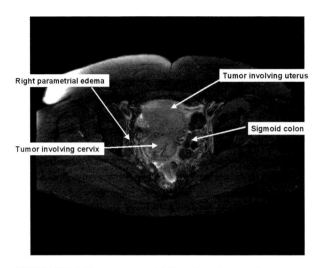

FIGURE 21C-2. Pretreatment axial T2-weighted magnetic resonance scan of the pelvis showing cervical and uterine involvement with right parametrial edema.

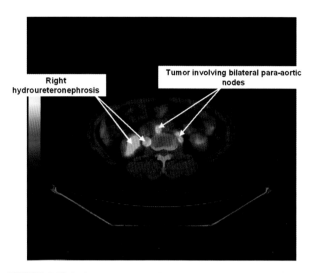

FIGURE 21C-4. Pretreatment positron emission tomography (PET) demonstrating tumor involving bilateral para-aortic nodes.

recommendation was for concomitant definitive chemo-radiotherapy. We elected to treat the patient by using 18F-flourodeoxyglucose (18F-FDG) PET and MR to guide target delineation and in-room megavoltage CT (MVCT) for patient setup and target localization.

Simulation

Before simulation, platinum fiducial markers were placed in the cervix at 6 o'clock and 12 o'clock. On the day of simulation, the patient was brought to our departmental Light Speed CT simulator (GE Healthcare, Waukesha, WI) suite, placed in the supine position with her arms over her head, and immobilized with an overhead arm

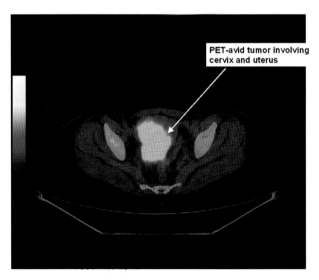

FIGURE 21C-3. Pretreatment positron emission tomography (PET) demonstrating PET-avid tumor involving cervix and uterus.

device and a large cradle (Body Fix, Medical Intelligence, Schwabmünchen, Germany) that extended from her chest to upper thighs. A non–contrast-enhanced simulation scan with a full bladder and a second contrast-enhanced scan with an empty bladder were performed, obtaining axial slices at 2.5-mm increments from her diaphragm to her upper thighs.

Imaging and Target Delineation

Image fusion and contouring were performed with the Eclipse (Varian Medical Systems, Palo Alto, CA) treatment planning system. Both full (primary scan) and empty bladder simulation scans were fused with the pretreatment PET–CT scan and axial T2-weighted and T1 postcontrast pelvic MR, using rigid body registration.

Normal structures contoured included the rectum, bladder, small bowel, femoral heads, and bone marrow. The T1 MR, T2 MR, and the PET images were used to define the gross tumor volume (GTV) in the cervix and uterus and nodes. The PET scan was particularly helpful in defining the extent of disease involving the uterus, as the heterogeneous T2 enhancement of the uterus on MR was felt to be "nonspecific." An internal target volume (ITV) was created from the GTV encompassing positional changes of the tumor on the full and empty bladder scans. The ITV was expanded 2 cm circumferentially and in the cranial–caudal direction to create a planning target volume (PTV_{ITV}). The central clinical target volume (CTV) was defined as the uterus, parametria, upper vagina, and uterosacral ligaments. The central CTV was expanded 1 cm circumferentially and in the cranial–caudal direction to create a $PTV_{Central}$. A nodal CTV encompassing the obturator, internal, external, common iliac, and para-aortic nodes up to the T12–L1 interspace was defined separately and expanded 5 mm to create PTV_{Nodes}. Finally, PET-fused images were used to help delineate gross nodal volumes for the structure GTV_{Nodes} and this volume was expanded 5 mm to create a $PTV_{GTVNodes}$.

Treatment Planning

Intensity-modulated radiation therapy (IMRT) planning was performed for helical tomotherapy delivery using a TomoTherapy Hi-Art System (TomoTherapy Inc, Madison, WI). The PTV_{ITV} was prescribed a dose of 50 Gy in 25 fractions whereas $PTV_{Central}$ and PTV_{Nodes} were prescribed doses of 45 Gy in 25 fractions each. A simultaneous integrated boost for a total dose of 62.5 Gy in 25 fractions was prescribed to gross lymph nodes ($PTV_{GTVNodes}$) in the pelvis and para-aortic chain. The percentage of small bowel receiving 30 Gy or more (V_{30}) was 30%. The V_{22} for the right and left kidneys were 18% each, the V_{20} for the bone marrow was 58%, and mean doses to the bladder and rectum were 45 Gy and 30 Gy, respectively.

Treatment Delivery

Treatment was delivered on the helical tomotherapy unit. Daily MVCT images were obtained with alignment to bone, and were reviewed at least twice weekly to ensure that the GTV + seeds were falling within the PTV_{ITV}. This analysis demonstrated that the patient's GTV consistently fell within PTV_{ITV}. The average beam-on time was approximately 12 minutes and the entire treatment, including pretreatment alignment, took 20 minutes.

Because of the volume of bulky disease present in the uterine fundus, the treatment plan of definitive chemoradiotherapy was modified to include an extrafascial hysterectomy. Immediately after external beam therapy, the patient was taken to the operating room for placement of an after-loading tandem and ovoid for treatment with one high-dose-rate (HDR) brachytherapy treatment. The patient was then brought to the radiation oncology department for CT simulation. The residual GTV (cervix + uterus), bowel, sigmoid colon, rectum, and bladder were contoured. Dose was prescribed in a volume-based fashion ensuring coverage of the GTV with 8 Gy (dose to point A was 11 Gy). Eight weeks later the patient underwent surgery.

Clinical Outcome

The patient tolerated the treatment exceptionally well, experiencing only acute grade 2 gastrointestinal toxicity. She completed her external beam treated within 40 calendar days without unplanned breaks, and received all five cycles of concomitant cisplatin chemotherapy (40 mg/m²).

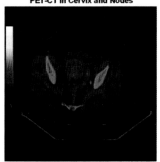
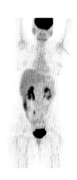

FIGURE 21C-5. Posttreatment, presurgery positron emission tomography demonstrating a complete response in primary tumor and nodes.

A complete clinical response to therapy was noted on pelvic examination 4 weeks posttreatment. A follow-up PET–CT scan obtained 5 weeks posttreatment shown in Figure 21C-5, demonstrated a reduction in maximum SUV in the primary down to a background value of 2.8 from 18.1. A complete radiographic response was also noted in the nodes. She subsequently underwent surgery, and had a complete pathologic response on final pathology. At her most recent follow-up, no significant late toxicities were noted.

Our analysis of MR-guided target delineation in patients with cervical cancer undergoing dose-escalated IMRT to positive para-aortic lymph nodes was published previously.[1] The positive para-aortic lymph nodes identified on MR were contoured as the GTV and the entire para-aortic region was defined as the PTV. Three planning methods were compared: (1) a conventional opposed anterior–posterior (APPA) plan extended field plan, (2) a four-field box extended field plan, and (3) an IMRT plan for the para-aortic region matched to a conventional four-field pelvis plan. With IMRT, the radiation dose to the GTV was escalated from 45 Gy to 60 Gy (2.4 Gy/fraction), whereas the PTV and the whole pelvis fields received 45 Gy. Dose-escalated IMRT matched to a conventional pelvic plan was found to be feasible, with a 95.6% median GTV coverage. This approach was associated with a reduction in the volume of small bowel receiving 45 Gy or higher, compared with the APPA technique, but a level of statistical significance was not reached. Alternatively, the four-field technique for both the pelvis and para-aortic regions resulted in a higher volume of the kidneys receiving 22 Gy or higher.

References

1. Ahmed RS, Kim RY, Duan J, et al. IMRT dose escalation for positive para-aortic lymph nodes in patients with locally advanced cervical cancer while reducing dose to bone marrow and other organs at risk. *Int J Radiat Oncol Biol Phys.* 2004;60:505–512.

Fat Fraction MR and ^{18}F-FDG PET-Guided Active Bone Marrow Delineation in a Patient with Cervical Cancer Treated with Bone Marrow Sparing IMRT

Case Study

Yun Liang, PhD, Loren K. Mell, MD

Patient History

A 27-year-old woman who had not had a Pap smear for 5 years presented with dyspareunia and irregular vaginal bleeding. She was noted to have a 4-cm fungating cervical lesion on pelvic exam. Biopsy demonstrated poorly differentiated squamous cell carcinoma. Pelvic computed tomography (CT) revealed a 5-cm cervical mass with no evidence of hydronephrosis, lymphadenopathy, or bladder invasion. Chest and abdominal CT scans were negative for distant metastases.

The patient underwent an examination under anesthesia, with findings of tumor protruding into but not directly involving the vagina. Proctoscopy showed no invasion into the rectum. Cystoscopy was not performed. Her clinical stage was IB2, according to the International Federation of Gynecology and Obstetrics (FIGO) staging system.

The patient was presented at our multidisciplinary gynecologic oncology tumor board and the consensus recommendation was for radiation therapy (RT) and concurrent chemotherapy (weekly cisplatin, 40 mg/m^2). We elected to treat her with bone marrow (BM)–sparing intensity-modulated RT (IMRT), using fat fraction magnetic resonance (MR) imaging and ^{18}F-flourodeoxyglucose positron emission tomography (^{18}F-FDG PET) to delineate active BM sites within the pelvis.

Simulation

The patient underwent ^{18}FDG PET–CT simulation on our departmental scanner (64-slice Discovery VCT, GE Healthcare, Waukesha, WI; Figure 21D-1). She was simulated with an empty bladder in the supine position, with custom immobilization using a foam cradle to minimize setup variation. Intravenous contrast was administered. Whole body images were obtained with 3.27-mm slice thicknesses and exported to the Eclipse system (Varian Medical Systems, Palo Alto, CA) for treatment planning. The ^{18}FDG PET images confirmed that there was no evidence of lymphadenopathy or distant metastasis.

Imaging and Target Delineation

Bone marrow is comprised of two components: hematopoietically active "red" BM and relatively inactive "yellow" BM. Red BM contains approximately 40% fat, 40%

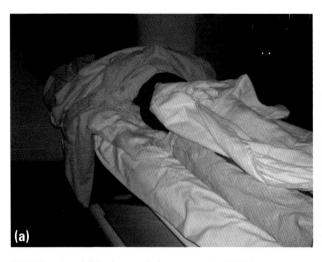
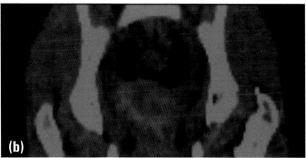

FIGURE 21D-1. (a) Positron emission tomography (PET)/computed tomography (CT) simulation setup. **(b)** Coronal PET–CT image showing a large fluorodeoxyglucose (^{18}F-FDG)-avid cervical mass.

water, and 20% protein, whereas yellow BM contains approximately 80% fat, 15% water, and 5% protein.[1] Red and yellow BM cannot be differentiated on CT but can be differentiated qualitatively using conventional T1- and T2-weighted MR sequences. However, the classic qualitative classification of BM into red and yellow subtypes is an oversimplification. Within red BM, there is considerable heterogeneity in fat content that varies with age and disease status. Quantitative MR techniques can identify gradations within the category of "red" BM, providing greater insight into its characteristics.

We applied a novel imaging method called Iterative Decomposition of water and fat with Echo Asymmetry and Least-squares estimation (IDEAL) to quantify the patient's BM fat fraction. The underlying principle is that the signals from fat and water exhibit resonant frequency/chemical shift differences that can be separated by using multiple measurements taken at different time points following excitation. The so-called T2*-IDEAL protocol combines three-dimensional (3D) gradient echo (GRE) imaging with a multipoint water–fat separation method.[2-4] With T2*-IDEAL, a "complex field map" construct is used to simultaneously estimate both R2* (1/T2*) and local field inhomogeneities with the IDEAL method. T2*-IDEAL also deals with the so-called "ambiguity" problem, whereby signals from fat and water may be incorrectly assigned. The end result is an individualized 3D fat fraction map, as seen in this patient (Figure 21D-2). This patient exhibited a comparatively low mean fat fraction, likely because of her young age.

The simulation PET–CT and MR images were imported and fused using Velocity AI fusion software (Velocity Medical Solutions, Atlanta, GA). Because the goal of image fusion is to register the pelvic bone region, we applied rigid image registration, fusing the PET and MR image with the CT images as a bridge. After image fusion,

the MR fat fraction and ^{18}F-FDG PET SUVbw (standardized uptake values, corrected with body weight) values were quantified within the pelvic bone region defined by CT. Active BM was delineated based on the intersection of regions of low MR fat fraction and high ^{18}F-FDG PET, as red BM is known to be correlated with physiological accumulation of ^{18}F-FDG.[5] The optimal threshold fat fraction and SUV values for defining "active" BM are not known, and were based initially on values from the published literature.[1,5] For this patient, we defined active BM as the intersection between BM with fat fraction less than 40% and SUV greater than 1.2 (Figure 21D-3).

The clinical target volume (CTV) included the tumor and cervix, uterus, parametria, upper half of the vagina, and regional lymph nodes (obturator, presacral, common, internal, and external iliac nodes). The CTV was partitioned into separate subvolumes to apply planning margins. A uniform margin of 15 mm was applied to the cervix, 10 mm to the uterus, and 7 mm to the remainder of the CTV, with the union of these volumes defining the PTV.

In addition to active BM, the bladder, rectum, bowel, and pelvic BM were delineated on the CT as organs at risk (OARs). The rectum was contoured from the anus to the sigmoid flexure, the bowel was contoured from the L4-5 interspace to its lowest extent in the pelvis, and the pelvic BM was contoured from L4 to the ischial tuberosities, including the os coxae, acetabulae, proximal femora, L4-5, and sacrum, as described previously.[6,7]

Treatment Planning

The prescribed dose in this patient was 45 Gy in 1.8-Gy daily fractions to the PTV. Target planning constraints were: (1) greater than 90% of the PTV receives greater than 99% of the prescription dose, (2) greater than 97%

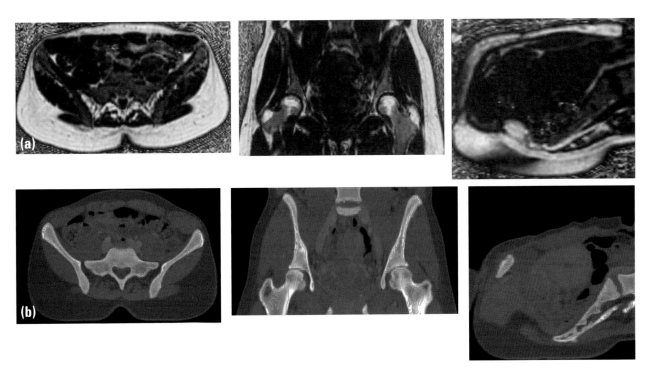

FIGURE 21D-2. (a) Magnetic resonance fat fraction maps of the pelvis shown in axial, coronal, and sagittal views. Lower signal (dark) regions correspond to lower fat content relative to water. **(b)** Pelvic computed tomographs with bone marrow with fat fraction less than 40% overlaid in orange.

of the PTV receives greater than 97% of the prescription dose, (3) less than 10% of the PTV receives greater than 110% of the prescription dose, and (4) maximum dose to the PTV less than 115% of the prescription dose. Based on previous studies,[6,8] normal tissue planning constraints were: (1) active and total pelvic BM: volume receiving greater than 10 Gy (V_{10}) less than 90%; volume receiving greater than 20 Gy (V_{20}) less than 75%; (2) bowel: volume receiving greater than 45 Gy (V_{45}) less than 200 cc;

(3) bladder and rectum: as low as reasonably achievable. The IMRT plan achieved good target coverage and normal tissue sparing (Figures 21D-4 and 21D-5). Active BM V_{10} and V_{20} were 86% and 70%, respectively. The patient was treated with daily on-line kilovoltage cone-beam CT (CBCT) guidance to verify setup and tumor position on a Varian Trilogy linear accelerator (Varian Medical Systems, Palo Alto, CA).

Clinical Outcome

The patient tolerated external beam RT well and received all five planned cycles of chemotherapy. At baseline, her

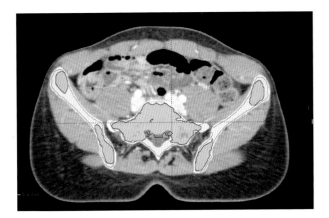

FIGURE 21D-3. Axial slice through the pelvis showing active bone marrow volume (blue) defined by ¹⁸F-fluorodeoxyglucose positron emission tomography and fat fraction magnetic resonance. Active regions are defined as those with standardized uptake value greater than 1.2 and fat fraction less than 40%.

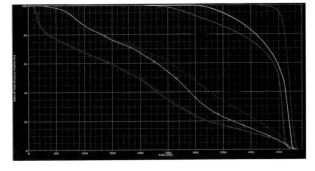

FIGURE 21D-4. Dose–volume histograms for active bone marrow (blue), pelvic bone marrow (orange), bowel (pink), rectum (brown), bladder (yellow), and planning target volume (red).

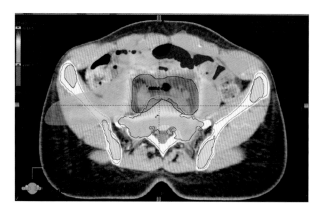

FIGURE 21D-5. Axial view of the pelvis showing isodose regions greater than 20 Gy in colorwash. Active bone marrow volume shown in blue.

white blood cell count, absolute neutrophil count, platelet count, and hemoglobin were $6.5 \times 10^3/\mu L$; $4.4 \times 10^3/\mu L$; $109 \times 10^3/\mu L$; and 10.4 g/dL, respectively. Her nadir values during treatment were $2.2 \times 10^3/\mu L$; $1.7 \times 10^3/\mu L$; $102 \times 10^3/\mu L$; and 10.1 g/dL, respectively, representing Radiation Oncology Group (RTOG) grade 2 leukopenia, grade 1 neutropenia, grade 0 thrombocytopenia, and grade 1 anemia. The patient was transfused two units of packed red blood cells before but not during treatment. She did not require growth factors. She has now gone on to complete her treatment with intracavitary high-dose-rate (HDR) brachytherapy. She will be followed closely for tumor response and possible late treatment sequelae.

References

1. Vogler JB, Murphy WA. Bone marrow imaging. *Radiology.* 1988;168:679–693.
2. Bydder M, Yokoo T, Hamilton G, et al. Relaxation effects in the quantification of fat using gradient echo imaging. *Magn Reson Imaging.* 2008;26:347–359.
3. Yu HZ, McKenzie CA, Shimakawa A, et al. Multiecho reconstruction for simultaneous water-fat decomposition and T2*estimation. *Reson Imaging.* 2007;26(4):1153–1161.
4. Reeder SB, Pineda AR, Wen ZF, et al. Iterative decomposition of water and fat with echo asymmetry and least-squares estimation (IDEAL): application with fast spin-echo imaging. *Magn Reson Med.* 2005;54:636–644.
5. Fan CZ, Hernandez-Pampaloni M, Houseni M, et al. Age-related changes in the metabolic activity and distribution of the red marrow as demonstrated by 2-Deoxy-2-[F-18]fluoro-D-glucose-positron emission tomography. *Mol Imag Biol.* 2007;9:300–307.
6. Roeske JC, Bonta D, Mell LK, et al. A dosimetric analysis of acute gastrointestinal toxicity in women receiving intensity-modulated whole-pelvic radiation therapy. *Radiother Oncol.* 2003;69:201–207.
7. Mell LK, Tiryaki H, Ahn KH, et al. Dosimetric comparison of bone marrow-sparing intensity-modulated radiotherapy versus conventional techniques for treatment of cervical cancer. *Int J Radiat Oncol Biol Phys.* 2008;71:1504–1510.
8. Rose B, Aydogan B, Yeginer M, et al. Normal tissue complication probability modeling of acute hematologic toxicity in cervical cancer patients treated with chemoradiotherapy [abstract]. *Int J Radiat Oncol Biol Phys.* 2010 Apr 16 [Epub ahead of print]

Real-Time Ultrasound-Guided Brachytherapy in a Patient with Cervical Cancer Using the Resonant Restitu System

Case Study

Deidre L. Batchelar, PhD, Melanie T.M. Davidson, PhD,
David P. D'Souza, MD

Patient History

A 77-year-old woman presented with vaginal bleeding, weight loss, and lower abdominal pain. Pelvic examination revealed a friable tumor arising from the cervix extending onto the upper vagina without parametrial involvement. Biopsy was positive for a moderately differentiated adenocarcinoma. The remainder of her physical examination was unremarkable. Radiographic workup included magnetic resonance (MR) imaging of the pelvis, which demonstrated a tumor replacing the cervix and posterior vaginal fornix. Computed tomography (CT) scans of the chest, abdomen, and pelvis were negative for metastatic disease. The patient was thus felt to have, according to the International Federation of Gynecology and Obstetrics (FIGO) staging system, a stage IIA cervical adenocarcinoma.

Our consensus recommendation was for a course of definitive chemoradiotherapy consisting of pelvic external-beam radiotherapy (EBRT; 45 Gy in 25 fractions) with weekly concomitant cisplatin (40 mg/m²) and high-dose-rate (HDR) brachytherapy (28 Gy in four fractions). Our policy is to perform the brachytherapy during the fourth and fifth weeks of treatment, delivering two fractions for each insertion, a minimum of 18 hours apart. Accordingly,

patients are admitted to the hospital for each insertion with the applicators remaining in place overnight.

The first brachytherapy insertion in this patient was performed just before the adoption of routine ultrasound guidance at our institution. Her narrow vagina and small uterus made the insertion technically challenging. Despite the use of uterine sounding to guide the choice of intrauterine tandem length, postinsertion CT revealed that the uterus was perforated at the superior aspect (Figure 21E-1). After careful consideration, it was decided to reduce the prescription dose to 6 Gy for this fraction and not to activate sources in the superior 1.5 cm of the tandem. We elected to perform her second insertion 1 week later using real-time ultrasound guidance.

Intraoperative Procedure

On the day of the second insertion, the patient was taken into the operating room and general anesthetic was administered. She was prepped and draped in the usual manner and placed in the dorsal lithotomy position. A Foley catheter was inserted, 240 cc of saline was instilled into the bladder to provide a sonographic window, and the catheter was clamped. Uterine sounding and cervical

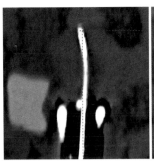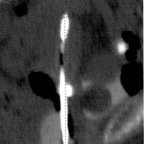

FIGURE 21E-1. Coronal and sagittal computed tomography images of the uterine perforation during the first insertion.

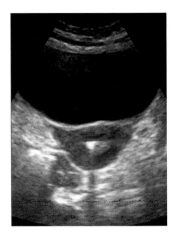

FIGURE 21E-3. An axial ultrasound (US) image demonstrating the central placement of the tandem within the uterine canal. The US probe was swept along the full length of the uterus to ensure that no perforation had occurred.

dilation were monitored in real time with the Restitu Ultrasound System (Resonant Medical, Montreal, Quebec). The choice of tandem angle and length was guided by ultrasound as well as the sounding measurement.

During the tandem insertion, a sagittal view of the midline of the uterus was continuously maintained (Figure 21E-2), allowing visualization of the tandem as it passed through the cervix into the uterus and permitting more effective placement of the tandem within the uterine canal. Once the tandem was positioned, an axial ultrasound sweep of the uterus was performed to confirm the central position of the tandem and verify the position of the tandem tip (Figure 21E-3). The vaginal colpostats and rectal retractor were then inserted and the vagina was packed with gauze. Ultrasound (in both the axial and sagittal planes) was performed to confirm the final, correct, applicator positioning.

Simulation

After recovering from anesthesia, the patient was taken to the CT simulator suite and placed in the supine position.

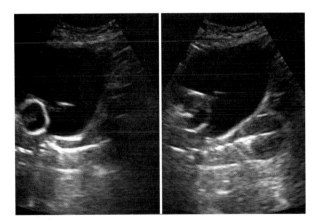

FIGURE 21E-2. Sagittal ultrasound views of the tandem during the second brachytherapy insertion. On the left is the tandem passing through the cervical canal and on the right is an image of the tandem correctly placed within the uterus.

A helical CT scan (3-mm slice thickness and 3-mm table index) from the vaginal introitus to 2 cm to 3 cm superior of the tip of the tandem was acquired on our departmental Brilliance Big Bore CT simulator (Philips Medical Systems, Andover, MA). Before imaging, the patient's bladder was drained via abdominal compression and then dilute contrast (3 cc of 60% Hypaque in 30 cc saline) was instilled in the bladder.

Treatment Planning

Computed tomography does not allow delineation of a clinical target volume (CTV) because of the lack of contrast between diseased and normal tissue in the cervix.[1,2] However, critical organs at risk (OARs; bladder and rectum) can be visualized, and were contoured on the axial slices of the planning CT scan. The applicator and the locations of the points A were then identified on the images. A standard plan, with 7 Gy prescribed to point A, was generated using BrachyVision three-dimensional treatment planning software (Varian Medical Systems Inc, Palo Alto, CA).

Dwell positions and times were manually adjusted to customize the plan to account for the orientation of the vaginal applicator relative to the tandem and the location of the OARs (Figure 21E-4). Conformal avoidance of the OARs was guided by dose–volume histogram (DVH) constraints derived from the American Brachytherapy Society[2] and European Society for Therapeutic Radiology and Oncology[3] guidelines. These provide recommendations for limiting the maximum dose received by a contiguous 2 cm³ volume (D_{2cc}), based on the cumulative DVH for each fraction. The dose constraints combine the EBRT and brachytherapy doses by normalizing the biologically effective dose (BED) for each phase to a 2 Gy per fraction BED (isoeffective dose, EQD2). The EQD2 constraints recommended are defined to be D_{2cc} less than 75 Gy_3 for the rectum and D_{2cc} less than 90 Gy_3 for the bladder (α/β = 3 Gy for OARs), while maintaining an EQD2 at point A of 80 Gy_{10} or greater (α/β = 10 Gy for target).

At the time of the second brachytherapy insertion, residual disease was still clinically evident. Therefore, the objective of this phase of treatment became to deliver at least the intended prescription dose of 7 Gy per fraction rather than to reduce the prescription dose to meet OAR tolerances, as was done at the first insertion. The patient's bladder was positioned in close proximity to the brachytherapy applicators because of the small size of the uterus. As such, only minimal dose shaping could be achieved to avoid this OAR while maintaining prescription dose to point A. As a result, the maximum dose to a contiguous 2 cm^3 of the bladder for EBRT and brachytherapy combined was 108 Gy_3. The EQD2 for the rectum fell within constraints at 68 Gy_3, and the EQD2 at point A was 80 Gy_{10}.

Treatment was delivered using the GammaMed HDR ^{192}Ir stepping source afterloading system (Varian Medical Systems Inc, Palo Alto, CA). The same plan was used for both fractions treated during this second insertion. Before each fraction, the bladder was fully voided via the urinary catheter and 33 cc of sterile water was instilled in the bladder to match the bladder filling on the planning CT.

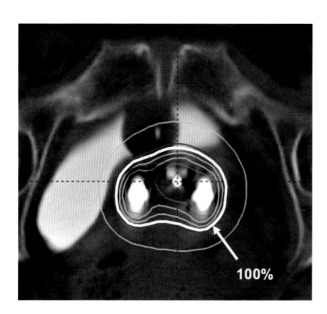

FIGURE 21E-4. An axial display of the dose distribution during the second insertion at the level of the vaginal colpostats. The dose has been sculpted to follow the bladder contour. Because of residual disease, further bladder sparing was not attempted.

Clinical Outcome

The patient tolerated her treatment well with no acute toxicity noted immediately following brachytherapy. Since the completion of treatment, the patient has had regular follow-up visits (initially every 3 months for 2 years, subsequently every 6 months). After achieving a complete response, there has been no evidence of recurrence on regular follow-up assessments (history and physical examination). The last follow-up visit was 28 months following the completion of treatment. She remains free of disease recurrence and has noted no late bladder or rectal sequelae.

Our experience using real-time intraoperative ultrasound guidance in 21 patients with cervical cancer undergoing 35 intracavitary brachytherapy insertions was published earlier.[4] In each patient, cervical dilation, tandem selection, and insertion were guided with the Restitu Ultrasound System. Final tandem position was also confirmed. Computed tomography imaging was used to assess perforation and applicator suitability in all patients. Accurate applicator placement was achieved in each case without a single perforation, compared with a historical institutional perforation rate of 10%. Visualizing patient anatomy during the insertion altered the selection of the tandem length and angle in 49% of cases. Average insertion times decreased from 34 to 26 minutes and requests for assistance from gynecologic oncology declined from 38% to 5.7% of procedures. Of note, ultrasound guidance eliminated repeat insertions because of unfavorable applicator placement, improving department efficiency and quality of patient care.

References

1. Viswanathan AN, Dimopoulos J, Kirisits C, et al. Computed tomography versus magnetic resonance imaging-based contouring in cervical cancer brachytherapy: results of a prospective trial and preliminary guidelines for standardized contours. *Int J Radiat Oncol Biol Phys.* 2007;68:491–498.
2. Nag S, Cardenes H, Chang S, et al. Proposed guidelines for image-based intracavitary brachytherapy for cervical carcinoma: report from the image-guided brachytherapy working group. *Int J Radiat Oncol Biol Phys.* 2004;60:1160–1172.
3. Haie-Meder C, Potter R, Van Limbergen E, et al. Recommendations from the gynecological (GYN) GEC-ESTRO Working Group (I): concepts and terms in 3D image based 3D treatment planning in cervix brachytherapy with emphasis on MRI assessment of GTV and CTV. *Radiother Oncol.* 2005;74:235–245.
4. Davidson MTM, Yuen J, D'Souza DP, et al. Optimization of high-dose-rate cervix brachytherapy applicator placement: the benefits of intraoperative ultrasound guidance. *Brachytherapy.* 2008;7:248–253.

Fractionated Image-Guided Stereotactic Radiotherapy Boost in a Patient with Stage IIB Endometrial Cancer Using the Novalis System

Case Study

Meritxell Mollà, MD, Dolors Linero, DSc, Lluís Escude, DSc, Raymond Miralbell, MD

Patient History

A 61-year-old woman presented with postmenopausal bleeding. Workup included an endometrial biopsy that revealed endometrioid adenocarcinoma. She subsequently underwent a total hysterectomy, bilateral salpingo-oophorectomy, and a pelvic lymphadenectomy. The pathology report showed a grade 1 endometrioid adenocarcinoma invading over half of the myometrium with extension into the cervical stroma but without extrauterine involvement (stage IIB disease).

Our consensus recommendation was for postoperative whole pelvic radiation therapy (RT; total dose, 50.4 Gy) followed by a vaginal vault boost. We elected to deliver the vaginal vault boost with fractionated image-guided stereotactic RT using the Novalis system (BrainLAB AG, Feldkirchen, Germany).

Simulation

The vaginal vault boost was simulated and planned a few days before the completion of the whole pelvic RT phase of treatment. Before simulation, the patient was requested

to void her bladder. An empty bladder was subsequently used at the time of treatment. To further limit target motion and to help to improve the target-defining process in the simulation computed tomography (CT), an endorectal magnetic resonance (MR) probe was used for both simulation and treatment. Sodium phosphate enemas were used to empty the rectum the night before and again 1 to 2 hours before each treatment procedure. To reduce anxiety and prevent or alleviate potential painful rectal spasms during the simulation and treatment, alprazolam 0.5 mg *per os* was prescribed. After inserting the probe into the rectum, 60 mL of air was introduced with a syringe. The inflated probe was then gently pulled down toward the anus. A marker was used to delineate the level of the vaginal cuff.

After the patient was immobilized in a customized vacuum body cast, five to seven metallic infrared (IR) reflecting markers were asymmetrically taped to the skin of the abdomen (Figure 21F-1). These markers were used in conjunction with the ExacTrac system (BrainLAB AG, Feldkirchen, Germany) to accurately reposition the patient for the final high-dose boost. Simulation CT images (TOMOSCAN AV, Philips Medical Systems,

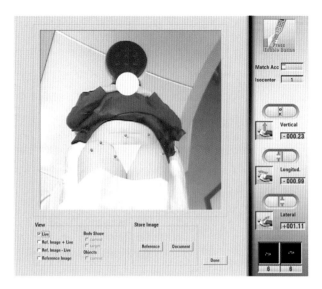

FIGURE 21F-1. Screen view of the patient setup before starting treatment lying in a customized body cast with six infrared reflecting markers taped asymmetrically over the skin of the pelvic–inguinal region.

Andover, MA) were taken in 3-mm increments over the lower pelvic region.

Treatment Planning

Once the planning CT images were transferred to the treatment planning system Brain Scan 5.31 (BrainLAB AG, Feldkirchen, Germany), the target volumes and organs at risk (OARs) were contoured on sequential axial CT slices. The clinical target volume-boost (CTV_{boost}) included the upper 3 cm of the vaginal vault and was expanded uniformly by 9 mm in all directions, generating the boost planning target volume (PTV_{boost}). The OARs considered were the rectum, bladder, small bowel, and femoral heads.

The position of the isocenter with regard to the IR markers was calculated by the planning system. A treatment plan with seven coplanar fields was generated with the following gantry angles: 204°, 255°, 306°, 0°, 51°, 102°, and 153° (Figures 21F-2, 21F-3). A dose of 2×7 Gy to the PTV with a 4-day interval between fractions was prescribed. The following dose constraints were established to optimize the dose distribution: the rectum and the bladder were initially set to receive no more than 50% of the prescribed dose to 50% of the volume, no more than 90% of the dose to 30% of the volume, and a maximum dose of 95%. These values were used as starting points, but often had to be modified according to the results of the calculation cycles to optimize the dose distribution. The treatment plan was evaluated and subsequently accepted. After physician approval, the plan was transferred to the treatment network to make measurements in a phantom to assess the ability of the multileaf collimator (MLC) and linear accelerator to correctly deliver the plan.

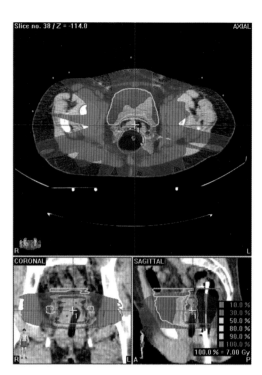

FIGURE 21F-2. Dose distribution of the intensity-modulated radiotherapy plan in the axial, sagittal, and coronal central planes of the planning target volume. Dose distribution is given in percentage values and is displayed in color bands.

Treatment Delivery

Treatment was delivered on a Novalis linear accelerator using 6-MV photon beams. Before each treatment session, the IR markers were placed back on the patient's skin. Their spatial arrangement was detected by a pair of IR cameras to reproduce the same isocenter coordinates when repositioning the patient for daily treatment. During treatment delivery, the IR cameras were used to provide a real-time position monitoring (Figure 21F-4). Each treatment fraction was completed within 45 minutes.

To simulate the repositioning reproducibility, a second CT was performed before the last fraction. The CTV repositioning was checked, first after CT-to-CT fusion of the stereotaxic IR reflecting metallic body markers (to simulate the setup reproducibility with external markers), and second, after CT-to-CT registration of the pelvic bony structures (to simulate for potential further improvement of patients repositioning with pelvic bone registration; Figure 21F-5). This repositioning study was performed for quality assurance purposes and allowed us, in addition, to estimate margins around CTV_{boost} to define an ideal PTV_{boost}.

Clinical Outcome

Treatment was well tolerated, with only grade 1 acute rectal toxicity observed during treatment. No urinary, rectal,

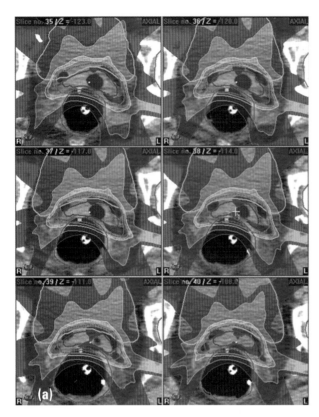

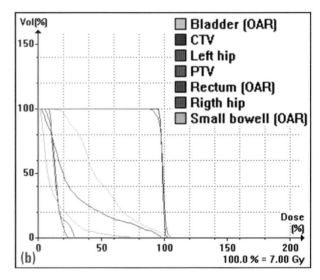

FIGURE 21F-3. Dose distribution in six consecutive computed tomography slices (a) and dose–volume histograms of the clinical target volume, planning target volume, and organs at risk (b). The highlighted isodoses include the 100% (red), 90% (yellow), 80% (green), 50% (light blue), 30% (dark blue), and 10% (purple).

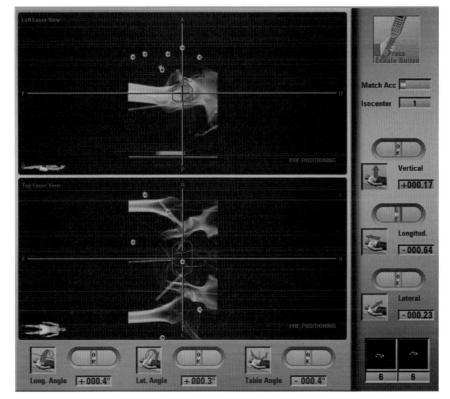

FIGURE 21F-4. Setup reposition control during treatment with the stereotactic infrared-reflecting metallic body markers.

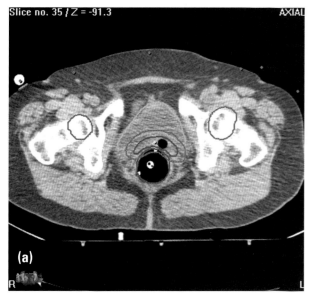

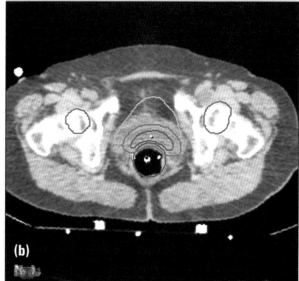

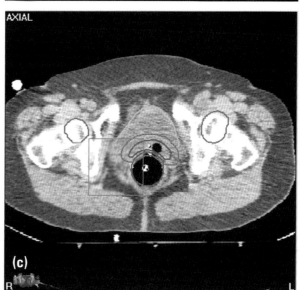

FIGURE 21F-5. Treatment quality assurance of patient repositioning. Simulation-computed tomography (CT) (a) to treatment-CT (b) pelvic bone structures registration at the level of the axial central plane of the planning target volume. The image in the lower right corner (c) displays the fusion of the main image outside the blue square, and the reduced image inside the blue square, for a perfect matching.

or sexual late toxicities have been observed thus far. The patient is free of recurrence at her most recent follow-up more than 5 years after treatment.

Our initial clinical experience using a fractionated stereotactic RT boost in patients with gynecologic cancer was presented earlier.[1] Sixteen patients with either endometrial (n=9) or cervical (n=7) cancers were included. In 14 patients, the CTV included the vaginal vault, the upper vagina, the parametria, or (if not operated) the uterus. In two patients with local relapse, the CTV was defined as the tumor in the vaginal stump. Margins of 6 mm to 10 mm were added to the CTV to generate the PTV. Postoperative patients received 2 × 7 Gy to the PTV with a 4- to 7-day interval between fractions. In the four nonoperated patients, a dose of 5 × 4 Gy was prescribed with 2 to 3 days interval between fractions. Patients were immobilized in a customized vacuum body cast and repositioned using IR-guidance.

Treatments were well tolerated with no patients experiencing severe acute urinary or rectal toxicity. Moreover, no patients developed chronic urinary complaints. One patient treated with a local relapse who previously received pelvic irradiation developed grade 3 rectal bleeding 18 months posttreatment. A second patient with a history of irritable bowel syndrome reported chronic grade 1 abdominal pain. Patients continue to be followed to assess local control and late toxicities.

References

1. Mollà M, Escude L, Nouet P, et al. Fractionated stereotactic radiotherapy boost for gynecologic tumors: an alternative to brachytherapy? *Int J Radiat Oncol Biol Phys.* 2005;62:118–124.

Chapter 21G

Ultrasound-Guided Applicator Placement and Treatment Planning in a Patient with Cervical Cancer Undergoing Brachytherapy

Case Study

David Bernshaw, MB, BS, BMedSci, FRANZCR, FRACP,
Sylvia Van Dyk, Dip App Sci MIR, Kailash Narayan, MB, BS, PhD

Patient History

A 41-year-old woman presented with 4 months of vaginal discharge, as well as intermenstrual and postcoital bleeding. A Pap smear was suggestive of malignancy and she was referred to a gynecologic oncologist. Staging workup included an examination under anaesthesia, which revealed a bulky tumor arising from the cervix with thickening of the left parametrium, consistent with a stage IIB lesion, according to the International Federation of Gynecology and Obstetrics staging system. Biopsy confirmed a moderately differentiated adenocarcinoma.

Radiographic workup included magnetic resonance (MR) imaging, which revealed that the primary lesion was confined to the cervix without uterine or parametrial invasion and measured 4 cm by 4.3 cm by 3 cm. A positron emission tomography (PET)–computed tomography (CT) scan did not show any nodal or other metastasis. The remainder of her workup, including a pretreatment hemoglobin level and blood chemistries, were within normal limits.

The patient was presented at our multidisciplinary tumor board and the consensus recommendation was for external beam pelvic radiation therapy (RT; 40 Gy in 20 fractions) and concomitant cisplatin (40 mg/m^2/week) followed by high-dose-rate (HDR) intracavitary

brachytherapy. We elected to perform her brachytherapy treatments using ultrasound guidance for both applicator insertion and treatment planning.

Imaging and Planning

Intracavitary HDR brachytherapy commenced after completion of her external beam pelvic RT and consisted of four fractions applied twice weekly. Under spinal anaesthesia after perineal preparation with the patient in lithotomy position, the patient was catheterized and her bladder filled with 300 mL to 400 mL sterile 0.9% saline solution. Real-time transabdominal ultrasound (TAUS; Falcon BK-Medical, Hervel, Denmark) with a 2.7 MHz to 5.0 MHz abdominal transducer was used to assist dilation of the cervix and to determine the length of the uterine tandem. The 6.0-cm tandem and small ovoids (Standard Nucletron CT/MR compatible applicators, Nucletron BV, Veenendaal, Netherlands) were inserted under ultrasound guidance. The vaginal spatula was used to displace the anterior rectal wall and the superior aspect of the ovoids was packed to displace the bladder trigone.

With the patient's legs lowered into the treatment position, the TAUS was used to adjust the tandem position and confirm central placement within the uterine cavity.

Measurements of the uterine wall thickness were taken perpendicular to the tandem at 2-cm intervals from the flange to the tip of tandem on the sagittal ultrasound view. The known geometry of the tandem acted as an internal ruler or fiducial marker and enabled verification of placement and measurements. Tandem position and uterine measurements were also verified in the axial plane at the flange and tip of the tandem.

A library plan detailing the applicator geometry was retrieved from the Plato planning system (Nucletron BV, Veenendaal, Netherlands). The initial treatment plan was created by the dosimetrist by modifying the dwell positions and times to conform the isodose lines to the ultrasound-derived anatomic measurements. This plan was printed to scale, assessed on the hard copy of the sagittal ultrasound view of the tandem within the uterus, and reviewed by the radiation oncologist (Figure 21G-1). The data were then transferred to the treatment control system and the first fraction was delivered. After treatment, the patient was taken to the MR scanner with the applicators in situ for imaging. After the scan, the applicator was removed and the patient was allowed to go home.

The implant was reconstructed on the three-dimensional (3D) MR image set on the Plato planning system. The dose, activity, and ultrasound-based dwell weights, dwell positions, and treatment time were entered as treated. The plan was then assessed on the 3D image set. This confirmed that for this patient, the 100% ultrasound-based isodose plan adequately covered the target volume seen on MR (Figure 21G-2).

The concept of a brachytherapy target has evolved over time and is based on the response of initial disease in various tissue compartments to chemoradiation and the imaging of residual disease at the time of brachytherapy. For all patients, the brachytherapy target volume is based

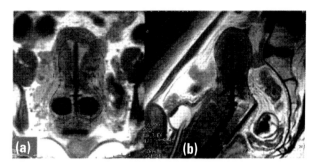

FIGURE 21G-2. (a) Coronal and (b) sagittal view through tandem showing isodose distribution determined with ultrasound measurements.

on the initial (pretreatment) extent of infiltrative disease in the uterine body as seen on MR and PET and the residual disease in the cervix at the time of brachytherapy. Vaginal extension (if present at brachytherapy) is also included. The original extent of disease outside these features is not covered. The prescription isodose is typically shaped to cover the whole cervix containing tumor and the entire body of uterus without a margin. A thin rind of uninvolved uterine fundus is usually spared.

The patient received three further brachytherapy applications under general anaesthesia. Ultrasound was used on each occasion to guide applicator insertion, to reproduce applicator placement, and to measure the cervix and uterine dimensions. These measurements ensured reproducible radiation isodoses during each treatment.

At each insertion, the original isodose plan was assessed on the two-dimensional (2D) ultrasound image. For this patient, as we have found for the majority of our patients treated with this approach, there was no significant change to the target size and shape over the course of brachytherapy, hence, no alteration to the treatment plan. The total combined dose to the target volume was 80 Gy in 2 Gy equivalent dose (EQD_2; $\alpha/\beta = 10$), the total ICRU (International Commission on Radiation Units and Measurements) bladder point dose was 49 Gy (EQD_2), and the total ICRU rectal point dose was 53.5 Gy (EQD_2) delivered over 41 days. The point A dose was 74.5 Gy (EQD_2).

Clinical Outcome

The patient tolerated treatment well without significant acute sequelae. At 3 months, there was no clinical evidence of disease. A repeat PET–CT at 6 months posttreatment demonstrated a complete metabolic response at the primary site, without development of any new sites of disease. At her latest follow-up 2 years posttreatment, she remains disease-free, without any evidence of late gastrointestinal or urinary toxicity. She is sexually active without difficulty. Radiation-induced menopausal symptoms have been managed with hormone replacement

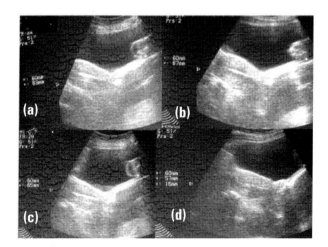

FIGURE 21G-1. Real-time transabdominal ultrasound sagittal view of tandem in uterine canal at (a) fraction 1, (b) fraction 2, (c) fraction 3, and (d) fraction 4. Tandem is identified by "x" measurement. Distance from flange to ICRU-38 bladder reference point identified by "+".

therapy and she continues to use a vaginal cylinder with oestradiol cream twice weekly.

We are satisfied from outcome data already presented[1] that the use of transabdominal ultrasound for applicator insertion and treatment planning is associated with high rates of local control and low levels of late and symptomatic toxicity. In our experience, real-time ultrasound ensures accurate tandem placement for each fraction and can effectively substitute for planning MR.[2] The benefits of incorporating ultrasound into a brachytherapy program are ease of use, accessibility, cost effectiveness, and increased efficiency, particularly in a limited resource set-ting. Use of ultrasound also ensures safe delivery of treatment, makes conformal treatment possible, and has the potential to reduce treatment-related toxicity.

References

1. Narayan K, Fisher RJ, Bernshaw D. Patterns of failure and prognostic factor analyses in locally advanced cervical cancer patients staged by magnetic resonance imaging and treated with curative intent. *Int J Gynecol Cancer.* 2008;18:525–533.
2. van Dyk S, Narayan K, Fisher R, et al. Conformal brachytherapy for cervical cancer using transabdominal ultrasound. *Int J Radiat Oncol Biol Phys.* 2009;75:64–70.

On-Line Planar and Volumetric-Based Patient Setup and Tumor Localization in a Patient with Stage IIB Cervical Cancer Using the Varian Trilogy System

Case Study

Catheryn Yashar, MD, Brent S. Rose, MD, William Yashar, Daniel J. Scanderbeg, PhD

Patient History

A 34-year-old woman presented with 4 months of menometrorrhagia. On examination, she was noted to have an exophytic lesion arising from the ectocervix. Biopsies demonstrated a squamous cell carcinoma and the tumor measured 6 cm both by physical examination and by magnetic resonance (MR) imaging. Metastatic workup was negative for metastases. Her tumor was thus stage IB2, according to the International Federation of Gynecology and Obstetrics (FIGO) staging system.

The patient was presented at our multidisciplinary gynecologic oncology tumor conference and the consensus recommendation was for definitive chemoradiation. We elected to treat her with daily on-line planar and volumetric-based image-guided radiotherapy (RT) using the Trilogy system (Varian Medical Systems, Palo Alto, CA).

Simulation

At her initial consultation, two gold seeds were placed into the cervical tumor at the 10 o'clock and 5 o'clock positions at a depth of approximately 5 mm. On the day of simulation, the patient was asked to evacuate her bowels and to drink sufficiently for a full bladder. She was simulated supine and her lower extremities were immobilized using the Vac Lok system (CIVCO, Kalona, IA). A noncontrast computed tomography (CT) was performed scanning with 2.5-mm slices from T11 thru 4 cm below the ischial tuberosities on our departmental wide-bore CT-simulator (GE Healthcare, Waukesha, WI). A second CT was then obtained after bladder emptying, using intravenous contrast to help delineate the vasculature from the pelvic lymph nodes. An isocenter was chosen and tattoos were placed on the anterior abdominal wall, and on the left and right lateral hips for daily setup. The CT images were transferred to the Eclipse planning station (Varian Medical Systems, Palo Alto, CA) and the two planning CTs were fused.

Treatment Planning

The clinical target volume (CTV) was outlined by the treating physician on the empty bladder scan (planning scan). The CTV consisted of two overlapping volumes, resulting in an internal target volume (ITV). The aortic vessels were outlined starting approximately 7 mm below the L4–L5 interspace (with a 7-mm planning target volume (PTV) expansion, the superior border was located at the L4–L5 interspace). A 5-mm margin around the vessels was used excluding the posterior vertebral body and psoas musculature (Figure 21H-1). The contours were continued inferiorly including the presacral tissues to S3. Below S3, the CTV separated into two distinct structures, right and left. When the fundus of the uterus appeared, it was included medially within the CTV (Figure 21H-2) and included the parametria laterally to the vessels. The border on the uterus was 1 cm, allowing for more movement than is seen with the vessels.

As contouring progressed inferiorly, the rectum and bladder were spared as possible, allowing for at least 1 cm anteriorly and posteriorly on the cervix (Figure 21H-3). If the rectum was noted to be exceptionally full, or if there was intraperitoneal fluid displacing the cervix, patients are asked to return after bowel emptying for resimulation, or are reevaluated after treatment initiation for regression of the intraperitoneal fluid. Neither was necessary in this patient.

The full bladder scan was then fused with the empty bladder scan. The fused scan was then evaluated with empty bladder CTV contours in place, and adjustments were made to the CTV ensuring that targeted tissues remain within the CTV on both scans. Normal tissues were then outlined including the bladder, rectum, sigmoid, other bowel, and pelvic bones (as a surrogate for the pelvic bone marrow), on the empty bladder scan (planning scan).

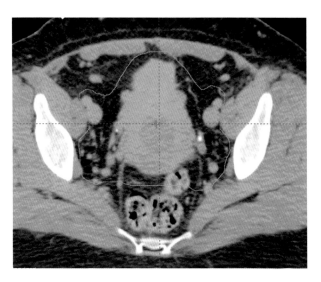

FIGURE 21H-2. The clinical target volume in the midpelvis including the uterine fundus, parametria, and pelvic vessels.

In this patient, there were significant differences in uterine position, cervical position, and the shape of the vasculature between the full bladder and empty bladder scans (Figures 21H-4a–c). Because there was such variation between the full and empty bladder scans, the decision was made to treat the patient with an empty bladder.

An intensity-modulated RT (IMRT) plan was generated to deliver 100% of the prescription dose to 95% of the PTV, sparing the surrounding normal tissues. Bone marrow (BM) constraints included ensuring that the volume of BM receiving 10 Gy or less (V_{10}) and 20 Gy or less (V_{20}) were 90% or less and 75% or less, respectively.

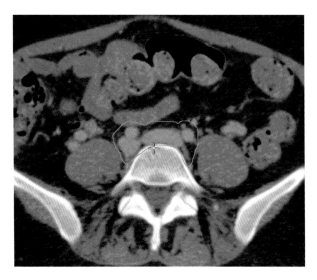

FIGURE 21H-1. The clinical target volume on an axial computed tomography slice in the upper pelvis.

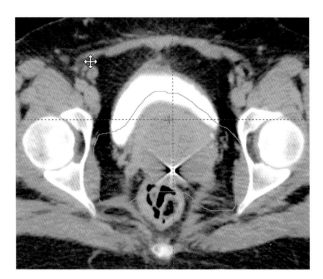

FIGURE 21H-3. The clinical target volume in the lower pelvis including bladder wall and rectal wall anteriorly and posteriorly, respectively. Note the gold seed within the cervix.

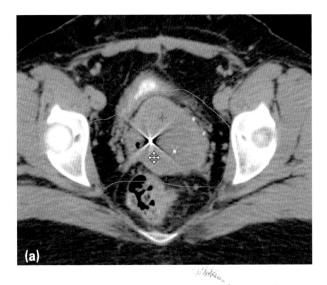

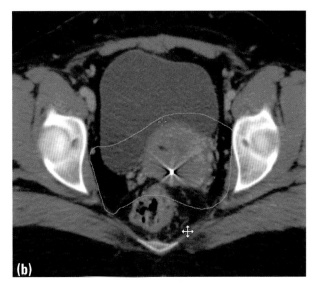

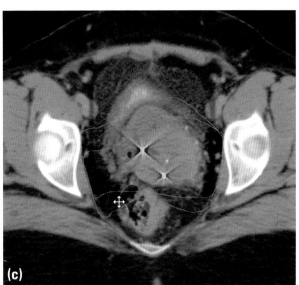

FIGURE 21H-4. Computed tomography scans with empty (a) and full (b) bladder demonstrating cervical movement. The blended scan (c) demonstrates changes in the clinical target volume.

With the Eclipse planning system (Varian Medical Systems, Palo Alto, CA), the pelvic bones and spine were outlined using the autocontour feature, and were cast onto the digitally reconstructed radiograph (DRR) for alignment with the planar images obtained with the onboard imaging. The cone-beam CT (CBCT) isocenter was identical to the treatment isocenter.

Treatment Delivery

Treatment was delivered on a Varian Trilogy linear accelerator equipped with onboard planar and volumetric imaging. The patient was first placed supine on the treatment couch in her customized immobilization device; tattoos were used in conjunction with in-room lasers to align her and to correct for rotation. Onboard planar im-

ages were then performed. Using bony anatomy, the patient position was adjusted to align with bony anatomy contours from the planning DRR as bony anatomy alignment assured nodal anatomy conformed to the IMRT plan. (Figure 21H-5) Planar images of the cervical seeds were not used to calculate patient shifts as with motion of the uterus readjustment of patient position to align the uterus would likely adjust lymph node contours incorrectly.

A CBCT was then performed. The cervix, demarcated by the gold seeds, was evaluated for inclusion within the PTV. If necessary, a shift was made to align the cervix (average is 2 mm at the beginning of treatment but with shrinkage of the cervix shifts became unnecessary; Figures 21H-6a and -6b). Average shifts for the first week were 0.14 cm (0.2 cm to 0.3 cm), second week was 0.0 cm,

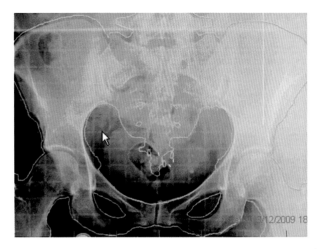

FIGURE 21H-5. Matched planar onboard images with the planning digitally reconstructed radiograph contours.

third week was 0.08 cm (one shift of 0.4 cm), fourth week was 0.0 cm, and fifth week was 0.1 cm (one shift of 0.5 cm). Whenever shifts were made, a repeat CBCT was performed to ensure that nodal regions also remained within the PTV. The IMRT plan was then delivered. When cervical shrinkage was apparent, usually after the initial 3 weeks, the patient was replanned to allow increased sparing of normal tissues.

Clinical Outcome

The patient did well throughout treatment, without significant acute toxicity. She experienced mild nausea during her chemoradiation controlled with antinausea medications. She also experienced mild diarrhea controlled with diet and antidiarrheal medications. After the

completion of external beam irradiation, she underwent five tandem and ring high-dose-rate (HDR) brachytherapy treatments, with visible tumor on the posterior cervix for the initial three implants. To date, she has experienced no long-term RT-related complications and at her most recent examination (5 months posttreatment) is without evidence of recurrent disease.

We have been actively studying the application of planar and volumetric-based image guidance in the treatment of cervical cancer. Reported works include a study quantifying the interfraction and intrafraction cervical motion using onboard images acquired before and after each radiation fraction.[1] Though most movements were small (average 4 mm intrafraction and 6 mm interfraction), the intrafraction mean maximum was 19.1 mm (± 8.57 mm) and interfraction mean maximum was 24.6 mm (± 7.95 mm) suggesting that if one does not account for possible large normal tissue and tumor positional variation, a marginal miss is likely.

One method to account for organ motion currently under investigation at our institution involves creating multiple treatment plans before the start of RT. The different plans correspond to predictable changes in the patient's anatomy that occur with bladder and rectal filling. Before each treatment a CBCT is performed and the plans are cast onto the rigidly registered CBCT. The plan that most closely resembles the patient's anatomy on a given day is then chosen by the physician and delivered. Quantifying the dosimetric implications of this method is an active area of study. In addition, there is parallel research into on-line adaptive periodic replanning to address tumor regression and cervical motion. In a recent study, it was demonstrated that by creating a new plan midway through the IMRT course the mean daily volume

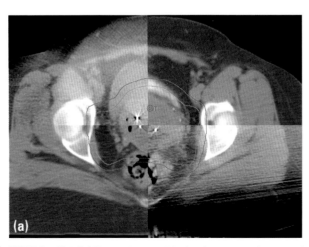
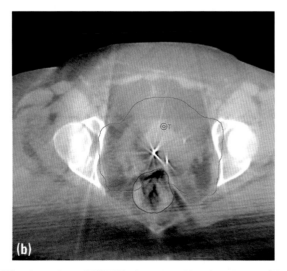

FIGURE 21H-6. (a) Blended image with planning computed tomography (CT) and cone beam CT (CBCT) after onboard imaging alignment (pink and orange lines are cast planning target volume [PTV] and clinical target volume, respectively). **(b)** CBCT with planning PTV cast onto CBCT.

of small bowel and bladder receiving the prescription dose could be reduced by 20% and 16%, respectively.[2] The current study is to identify the optimal timing and frequency of efficient, customized replanning to ensure both tumor coverage and normal tissue sparing.

References

1. Saenz C, Haripotepornkul N, Tang X, et al. Intra- and interfraction movement of the cervix during radiation treatment in cervical cancer patients [abstract]. *Gynecol Oncol.* 2009;112:S47.
2. Lawson JD, Simpson DR, Rose BS, et al. Adaptive radiotherapy in cervical cancer: dosimetric analysis using daily cone-beam CT [abstract]. *Int J Radiat Oncol Biol Phys.* 2009;75:S85–S86.

KV Planar Image-Guided 3DCRT Using a Varian Linear Accelerator in a Patient with Endometrial Adenosarcoma

Case Study

Tracy Bray, MD, Kevin Albuquerque, MD, MS, FRCS

Patient History

A 58-year-old morbidly obese postmenopausal woman presented with a 5-month history of painless vaginal bleeding. She weighed 355 lbs with a body mass index (BMI) of 67 kg/m². Pelvic ultrasound revealed an enlarged heterogeneous uterus with a thick endometrial stripe. A hysteroscopy with dilation and curettage was performed and pathology was consistent with endometrial stromal sarcoma. A chest x-ray revealed no abnormalities.

The patient underwent a total abdominal hysterectomy and bilateral salpingoophorectomy. Pathology demonstrated a 4.5-cm high-grade endometrial adenosarcoma, with no apparent myometrial invasion. The cervix, lower uterine segment, and parametrial tissue were free of tumor; however, an ovarian mass was positive for endometrial adenosarcoma. No lymph nodes were excised. Peritoneal washing cytology was negative for malignancy. The tumor was thus staged as T3ANxM0, stage IIIA, according to the 2002 American Joint Committee on Cancer (AJCC) staging system. Of note, the separate staging schema adopted by the International Federation of Gynecology and Obstetrics (FIGO) for uterine sarcoma would make the stage of this tumor T2ANxM0, stage IIA. The patient's postoperative course was complicated by an abdominal abscess and wound dehiscence necessitating wound vacuum placement.

Our consensus recommendation was for adjuvant pelvic radiotherapy (RT). Because of her body habitus complicating setup verification, and our concern over sparing her abdominal wound, we elected to treat the patient using kilovoltage (kV) image-guided three-dimensional conformal RT (3DCRT) using a Varian 21EX linear accelerator with onboard imaging (OBI) capability (Varian Medical Systems, Palo Alto, CA).

Simulation

The patient's size prohibited the use of an alpha cradle. Instead, a customized thermoplastic lower extremity cradle was used for positioning and immobilization. The cradle was not indexed because of the patient's difficulty mounting the treatment table. She was positioned in the lower extremity cradle with her arms above her head and a vaginal introitus marker was placed by the physician. She was first aligned on the couch using the tracking lasers in the computed tomography (CT) simulation room, with bilateral hips as a reference anatomical landmark. The CT scan origin and setup alignment reference points were marked on the patient's skin; a point on each of her lateral thighs was chosen because it was thought to be most reproducible. Noncontrast images were acquired with a slice thickness of 3 mm using a Philips Big Bore

CT Scanner (Philips, Andover, MA). In preparation for simulation, the patient drank barium sulfate suspension for bowel contrast and water to expand her bladder.

Treatment Planning

Treatment planning was performed with the XiO Treatment Planning System, version 4.5 (Elekta-CMS, St Louis, MO). The clinical target volume (CTV) and organs at risk (OARs) were contoured on individual axial CT slices. The CTV encompassed the upper half of the vaginal cuff and pelvic lymph nodes at risk, including the common iliac, internal and external iliac, presacral, obturator, and parametrial lymph nodes with a 7-mm margin. The OARs consisted of the rectum, bowel, femoral heads, and bladder. A nonuniform margin of 5 mm to 7 mm was added to the CTV to generate the planning target volume (PTV).

The PTV had a prescription dose of 50.4 Gy over 28 fractions. A treatment plan was generated with eight fields, all 45° apart, using a 3DCRT technique. All efforts were made to spare the skin to minimize dose to her surgical wound. The PTV received 97% of the prescription dose to 97% of the volume. The maximum doses to the bladder and rectum were 51.15 Gy and 51.84 Gy, respectively. The maximum doses to the right and left femoral heads were 49.84 Gy and 50.92 Gy, respectively; mean doses were 19.05 Gy and 21.31 Gy, respectively. The maximum dose to the bowel was 51.89 Gy, with a mean dose of 23.52 Gy. Figure 21I-1 shows the dose distribution of 95% of the prescription doses to PTV and the dose–volume histogram (DVH) for the PTV and OARs.

After plan approval, the planning CT image data set, structure contours, and digitally reconstructed radiographs (DRRs) were exported to the Varian 21EX linear accelerator with OBI capability for kV-based image-guided treatment.

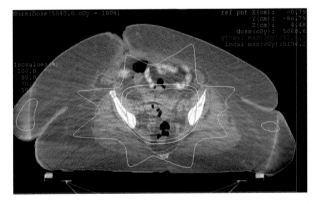

FIGURE 21I-1. Axial slice showing the planning target volume (green) and the clinical target volume (red). Highlighted are the 100%, 90%, 70%, and 50% isodose curves shown in green, yellow, magenta, and brown, respectively.

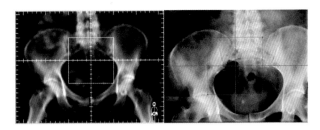

FIGURE 21I-2. Anterior–posterior digitally reconstructed radiographs and corresponding kilovoltage image. Isocenter was shifted 0.8 cm inferiorly, 2.8 cm laterally (left), and 0.4 cm anteriorly.

Treatment Delivery

Each day, the patient was positioned on the treatment couch with her lower extremities in the nonindexed cradle, the same anatomical position during simulation. Tracking lasers, skin markers, and optical distance indicators were used to grossly set up the patient daily. Daily anterior–posterior (AP) and right lateral kV portal images were obtained, and then overlaid with the corresponding DRR to determine translational shifts. Translational setup errors were corrected by shifting the couch in the AP, left–right (LR), and superior–inferior (SI) directions using interactive mode on the OBI software. The lack of reliable skin markers, the necessary use of a nonindexed cradle, and labor involved in adjusting the patient made daily setup erratic. If the decision to use daily kV-based image-guided RT (IGRT) had not been made, her inconsistent setup would warrant using daily megavoltage (MV) portal images to ensure adequate coverage of the CTV thereby increasing dose to the patient.

The value of IGRT in this patient was in minimizing the dose to the patient from MV verification imaging, ensuring adequate coverage of the CTV given her unreliable external markers and guaranteeing minimal dose delivered to her abdominal wound. A representative AP DRR and kV image are shown in Figure 21I-2, demonstrating a significant isocenter offset. A plot of the daily isocenter shifts is shown in Figure 21I-3, summarizing the large, unpredictable shifts required throughout the course of her treatments. The maximum shifts in the superior–inferior, right–left lateral, and anterior–posterior directions were 0.1 cm to -1.3 cm, 6.6 cm to -2.8 cm, and 0.4 cm to -1.0 cm, respectively.

Clinical Outcome

The patient tolerated treatment relatively well. She experienced the anticipated side effects of nausea and diarrhea beginning in the second week of RT. Both of these effects were grade 1 toxicities. She experienced no adverse skin reaction. There were no unplanned treatment interruptions in her course of treatment. The patient was seen most recently 10 months after completion of therapy.

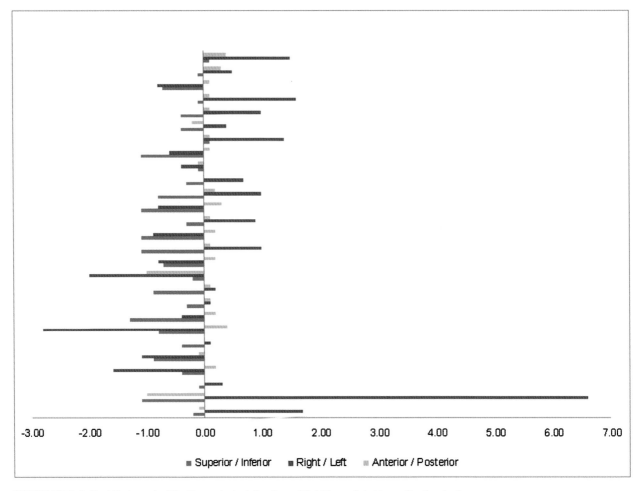

FIGURE 21I-3. Daily shifts in each of the three principal directions. All shifts are listed in centimeters (cm).

Her abdominal wound had healed well and her nausea and diarrhea had completely resolved. She denied any late effects of RT and remains clinically without evidence of disease.

In our experience, of the 28 patients with gynecologic malignancies treated with IGRT for pelvic RT over the past 18 months, 17 had BMIs over 30 and were considered obese. Of these 17 patients, the largest daily shifts in the SI, RL, and AP directions were 2.4 cm, 6.6 cm, and 1.4 cm, respectively. The lateral shifts appeared to be the largest in this obese group of patients.[1]

We are currently reviewing our experience using daily kV-based IGRT in obese patients and will further analyze the impact of greater weight and BMI on setup errors to report this in the near future.

References

1. Bray, TS, Kaczynski A, Albuquerque K, Roeske JC. Image guided radiotherapy for obese patients with gynecological malignancies. Scientific Paper Presentation. RSNA 96th Scientific Assembly. Chicago Nov 2010.

Chapter 22

Lymphoma/Leukemia: Overview

Michael T. Spiotto, MD, PhD, Richard T. Hoppe, MD

Lymphomas are exquisitely radiosensitive cancers. As treatment strategies leading to cure have improved and systemic therapy has more often been included as a component of therapy, both the radiation therapy (RT) volume and dose have been reduced to minimize the risk of late toxicities including secondary cancers. As a result, image-guided RT (IGRT) techniques may not benefit the treatment of lymphomas in the same way as they would with other cancers that require the delivery of high radiation doses to targets intimately associated with normal tissues. However, as increasingly smaller fields and lower doses are used, IGRT techniques promise to plan and to deliver radiation more accurately. Image-guided planning in lymphoma has been aided most by functional imaging, such as positron emission tomography (PET). Similarly, radiation delivery has been improved by techniques to account for respiratory motion and daily setup variations. Thus, IGRT techniques are likely beneficial even in the setting of low-dose, low-volume treatment of disease.

Historical Perspective and Current Treatment Approaches

The use of RT for lymphoma has evolved substantially since its first reported use more than 100 years ago. For limited stage Hodgkin's lymphoma (HL), RT was the first modality to offer cure.[1,2] Until 20 years ago, RT alone was the standard of care for stage I to II HL. With the advent of systemic therapy, abbreviated chemotherapy regimens were combined with limited radiation fields to achieve similar outcomes while avoiding the excessive toxicities associated with either modality alone.[3–6] Furthermore, current investigations are being conducted into reducing the dose further for favorable, early stage HL.[7]

Although similar RT treatment strategies were initially employed for non-Hodgkin's lymphomas (NHLs), the pattern of relapse for NHL differed from that of HL and, consequently, it quickly became apparent that radiation alone would not be sufficient.[8] Whereas patients with HL often relapsed in sites adjacent to the initial sites of disease or just beyond the treatment fields, relapses of NHL were more often systemic or in distant lymph node groups and less predictable. Consequently, systemic therapy for NHL has been employed early and often for many types of early and advanced-stage NHLs.

Currently, RT as a single modality is used for the definitive treatment of stage I to II follicular lymphoma (FL) or early stage diffuse large B-cell lymphoma (DLBCL) in patients who cannot tolerate chemotherapy. In addition, RT alone may be sufficient for stage I to II nodular lymphocyte predominant HL (nLPHL). Finally, RT alone may be sufficient for NHLs arising in some extranodal sites such as primary orbital lymphomas or cutaneous lymphomas including mycosis fungoides or primary cutaneous follicle center lymphoma.

In the 1970s, RT combined with chemotherapy became the mainstay of treatment especially for early stage HL and NHL. For early stage HL, reduced doses of chemotherapy along with limited radiation fields have shown the most promising results.[3–5] By contrast, chemotherapy alone may result in significantly higher recurrence rates compared with combined modality therapy or even RT alone.[9–12] In fact, the excellent outcome for treatment with combined modality therapy utilizing limited radiation fields has been shown in seven trials covering almost 5000 patients. Similarly, reduced-dose chemotherapy with RT has become the standard of care for early stage DLBCL. Two randomized trials have shown that CHOP (cyclophosphamide, doxorubicin, vincristine, and prednisone) chemotherapy combined with radiation resulted in improved failure-free survival (FFS) and overall survival (OS) compared with chemotherapy alone.[13,14] The benefit of combined modality therapy could not be compensated with additional cycles of chemotherapy. In addition, combined modality programs have been shown to be important for early stage mantle cell lymphoma,[15] primary central nervous system (CNS) lymphoma,[16] and mediastinal large B-cell lymphoma.[17]

With advanced lymphomas, chemotherapy is the treatment of choice with radiation held in reserve, or as an adjuvant. For advanced HL, RT for those achieving a complete response (CR) after chemotherapy did not improve FFS.[18] However, patients who achieved only a partial response (PR) to chemotherapy and then received consolidative RT had similar outcomes as those achieving a CR with chemotherapy alone.[19] In addition, RT is an essential component of attenuated chemotherapy regimens for HL such as Stanford V (doxorubicin, mechlorethamine, vincristine, prednisone, bleomycin, vinblastine, and etoposide) where it is administered to bulky sites of disease (> 5 cm) or for splenic involvement.[5] For advanced NHL, RT is beneficial for treatment of bulky sites of disease including both indolent and aggressive subtypes of lymphoma.[20,21]

Radiation therapy also improves the outcomes for relapsed disease after salvage chemotherapy. For relapsed HL, RT may improve outcomes with relapsed early stage disease initially managed with chemotherapy or with combined modality therapy.[22] In addition, RT to involved sites improved FFS and OS in patients undergoing high-dose chemotherapy and stem cell transplants for relapsed HL.[23] For relapsed DLBCL, studies showed improved results with stem cell transplant regimens employing RT to bulky disease sites.[24] Therefore, RT improves the outcomes with early stage, advanced stage, and relapsed HL, as well as NHL.

Involved field RT (IFRT) is currently the standard RT approach for HL and NHL. However, the definition of what constitutes an involved field has evolved substantially in the past two decades. Initially intended as fields that included the entirety of the involved lymphoid regions, as defined by the Ann Arbor criteria, the definition has evolved to exclude those portions of the region that are more distant from the clinically involved nodes, especially in areas that may be associated with significant toxicity. This reduction of field size has been facilitated by the introduction of PET–computed tomography (CT) scanning as a component of the staging workup. Some general guidelines for delineating the involved field that may be used with IGRT techniques are summarized in Table 22-1. Technically, the gross tumor volume (GTV) is defined from the prechemotherapy PET–CT and diagnostic CT as well as a postchemotherapy PET–CT. The GTV includes CT masses that are PET-negative. A separate GTV is delineated for any residual PET-positive areas postchemotherapy for a potential radiation boost. For mediastinal disease or bulky retroperitoneal lymph nodes, the GTV can be reduced in width to include only the involved postchemotherapy volume. When the upper mediastinum is involved, the fields often include the lower supraclavicular regions. The clinical target volume (CTV) extends approximately 2 cm superiorly and

inferiorly along the lymphatic chains, and the planning target volume (PTV) adds an additional 0.5 cm to ensure that the GTV is encompassed by the 95% isodose line.

During simulation and planning, patients with mediastinal disease are immobilized with a face mask with the neck in a neutral position if cervical disease is absent or with neck extended if cervical disease is present. For abdominal disease, patients are positioned with a leg immobilizer and testicular shield, if necessary. For HL and NHL, the commonly used doses are shown in Table 22-1 with doses generally ranging from 30 Gy to 36 Gy depending on treatment strategy. With bulky disease that extends into the lung, the sites of extension may be treated up to 15 Gy. During 3D planning, dose–volume histograms are used to delineate doses to the spinal cord, lung (right, left, and combined), heart, thyroid, and individual breasts for women for supradiaphragmatic fields and the lungs, kidneys, liver, and spinal cord for subdiaphragmatic fields.

Because of the extended field treatments used previously and long-term survival of patients treated for HL, significant information exists regarding the late effects of treatment. Radiation pneumonitis remains a potential complication but may be avoided if the mean lung dose to both lungs remains less than 15 Gy or less than 17 Gy if treating large mediastinal adenopathy. Pericarditis or myocardial dysfunction may be safely avoided if the mean heart dose is less than 20 Gy; however, it is possible that coronary artery disease may develop, especially if the origin of the coronary arteries remains within the high-dose portion of the treatment. Subclinical hypothyroidism occurs in approximately 50% of patients if the majority of the gland is in the treatment field. For treatment below the diaphragm, the kidneys, gonadal tissues, and the spleen are the major organs at risk. Although only a small portion of the kidneys is included in a typical para-aortic field, a significant portion of the left kidney may be included in the splenic field and may become problematic if there is underlying renal disease. In addition, treatment of the spleen predisposes one to gram-positive bacterial sepsis and can be presumptively managed by the appropriate immunizations before radiotherapy. Finally, pelvic RT predisposes women to sterility and gonadal failure. Therefore, women wishing to remain fertile should be offered oophoropexy; however, for women who are older than 30 years, scatter doses may be sufficient to ablate ovarian function even with these procedures, unless the ovaries are positioned well outside the treatment field.

In addition to normal tissue toxicity, radiation also leads to an increased risk of secondary cancers. After treatment of the mediastinum, women aged younger than 20 years have 14-fold increased risk of breast cancer, which may decline to nonsignificant levels after the age of 30 years.[25] Breast tissue receiving less than 4 Gy may not be associated with an increased risk of secondary cancer.[26]

TABLE 22–1 Suggested Guidelines for Involved Field Radiotherapy

Lymphoma	RT Dose	Stage	Chemo-therapy	Single Lung	Both Lungs	Heart	Breast	Kidney
HL	30.6 Gy*	I–IIA (favorable)	Stanford V × 8 wks;	MLD < 17 Gy	MLD < 15 Gy; V15 < 20%	MHD < 10 Gy	V15 < 10%; V4 < 20%	V20 < 30%
			ABVD × 2–4 cycles	MLD < 15 Gy	MLD < 13 Gy; V10 < 20%	MHD < 10 Gy	V15 < 10%; V4 < 20%	V20 < 30%
		Unfavorable I–IIB (nonbulky)	Stanford V × 12 wks;	MLD < 17 Gy	MLD < 15 Gy; V15 < 20%	MHD < 10 Gy	V15 < 10%; V4 < 20%	V20 < 30%
			ABVD × 4–6 cycles	MLD < 15 Gy	MLD < 13 Gy; V10 < 20%	MHD < 10 Gy	V15 < 10%; V4 < 20%	V20 < 30%
		Bulky I–IIA/B	ABVD × 4–6 cycles	MLD < 17 Gy	MLD < 15 Gy; V15 < 40%	MHD < 18 Gy	V10 < 30%; V4 < 50%	V20 < 30%
		Bulky III–IV	ABVD × 6–8 cycles	MLD < 15 Gy	MLD < 13 Gy; V10 < 20%	MHD < 18 Gy	V10 < 30%; V4 < 50%	V20 < 30%
	36 Gy*	Bulky, all stages	Stanford V × 12 wks	MLD < 20 Gy	MLD < 17 Gy; V18 < 40%	MHD < 20 Gy	V18 < 30%; V4 < 50%	V20 < 30%
DLBCL	30 Gy to 40 Gy	I–IIA	R-CHOP × 3–8 cycles	MLD < 17 Gy	MLD < 15 Gy; V15 < 20%	MHD < 10 Gy	V15 < 10%; V4 < 20%	V20 < 30%
	36 Gy	Bulky III–IV	R-CHOP × 6–8 cycles	MLD < 20 Gy	MLD < 17 Gy; V18 < 40%	MHD < 20 Gy	V18 < 30%; V4 < 50%	V20 < 30%
FL	36 Gy	I–IIA		MLD < 17 Gy	MLD < 15 Gy; V15 < 20%	MHD < 10 Gy	V15 < 10%; V4 < 20%	V20 < 30%
	4 Gy	Bulky, III–IV						
Mantle cell lymphoma	36 Gy	I–IIA	R-hyper-CVAD	MLD < 20 Gy	MLD < 17 Gy; V18 < 40%	MHD < 20 Gy	V18 < 30%; V4 < 50%	V20 < 30%

Notes. ABVD = doxorubicin, bleomycin, vincristine, and dacarbazine; DLBCL = diffuse large B cell lymphoma; FL = follicular lymphoma; HL: Hodgkin's lymphoma; MLD = mean lung dose; MHD = mean heart dose; R-CHOP = rituximab, cyclophosphamide, doxorubicin, vincristine, prednisone; R-hyper-CVAD: rituximab, cyclophosphamide, doxorubicin, vincristine, dexamethasone; V4 = volume of normal tissue receiving 4 Gy; V15 = volume of normal tissue receiving 15 Gy; V18 = volume of normal tissue receiving 18 Gy; V20 = volume of normal tissue receiving 20 Gy.
*1.8 Gy per fraction; 1.5 Gy per fraction to 30 Gy if mediastinum treated.

In addition, lung cancer remains a significant concern as doses to the lung greater than 30 Gy have been associated with relative risks of lung cancer of 6.3 to 8.5.[27] The risk for doses less than 30 Gy was not significantly elevated but may be increased for smokers who continue to smoke after RT.

Some investigators are pushing the limits of radiation field reduction by beginning to target only the involved lymph nodes. For involved nodal RT (INRT), the European Organization for Research and Treatment of Cancer (EORTC) has defined the CTV to encompass the prechemotherapy superior to inferior extent of disease combined with the postchemotherapy medial to lateral extent. An additional 1 cm is included for setup margin.[28] Campbell et al. performed a retrospective review of extended field RT (EFRT), IFRT, or INRT (with margins of up to 5 cm beyond the involved nodes) for favorable stage I to IIA HL.[29] Importantly, 95% of the patients received ABVD-type (doxorubicin, bleomycin, vinblastine, and dacarbazine) chemotherapy for only two cycles. Here, INRT was given to nonbulky lymph nodes less than 10 cm. Although the type of RT was given during different eras in time, relapses were similar with all three types of RT: 39% for EFRT, 30% for IFRT, and 31% of INRT.

Interestingly, patients in whom PET scans influenced treatment decisions were excluded from analysis, suggesting that IGRT imaging techniques may further improve INRT delivery.[29] Involved nodal RT may also decrease normal tissue toxicity. Involved nodal RT is currently being tested in an EORTC/Groupe d'Etude des Lymphomes de l'Adulte (GELA) H10 (20051) trial of combined modality therapy for favorable stage I to II HL and it is being compared with IFRT in combined modality therapy in the German Hodgkin Study Group (GHSG) HD17 trial for unfavorable stage I to II HL.

As the field sizes for lymphoma become smaller, it will become even more essential to incorporate image-guided techniques to deliver RT accurately. With INRT, image-guided planning with PET–CT becomes even more essential, as one study showed that the prechemotherapy PET imaging helped pinpoint involved lymph nodes not seen on CT in 36% of patients.[30] Furthermore, Girinsky et al. contend that PET imaging allows the reduction of CTV margins to only 1 cm beyond the GTV.[31] In addition, incorporation of image-guided delivery becomes more relevant when targeting sites are subject to internal motion such as the mediastinum, abdominal nodes, spleen, and/or liver. Finally, because patients with effectively treated lymphoma may have a life expectancy of 40 to 50 years, image-guided techniques to minimize dose to normal structures will help prevent late toxicities and possibly secondary cancers. Therefore, ensuring proper delivery of radiation to limited target volumes is important even with the low doses and limited fields of irradiation that are often adequate for the treatment of lymphoma. Thus, the remainder of this chapter will discuss image-guided techniques to improve the treatment algorithms of lymphoma.

Imaging for Lymphoma

Initially, the imaging studies necessary for the staging of lymphoma included a diagnostic chest x-ray to assess mediastinal lymphadenopathy and lymphangiography (LAG) to assess pelvic or abdominal lymph nodes. These staging procedures had limited sensitivity and specificity and were often technically difficult to perform. Although LAG is effective in evaluating the pelvic and retroperitoneal nodes, it did not provide information regarding the high para-aortic or portahepatic lymph nodes or any of the other abdominal organs, such as the spleen. The implementation of CT superseded these procedures, improving the sensitivity and specificity of detecting abnormal lymph nodes as well as extranodal disease and providing a more comprehensive evaluation of both intrathoracic and intraabdominal sites.

However, the advent of PET imaging has redefined the staging for lymphoma. Computed tomography provides anatomical information, and PET complements staging by providing functional or metabolic information of suspected or unsuspected sites of disease.[32] A meta-analysis of 14 studies comprising 854 patients and 3658 lesions found that the overall sensitivity was 90%, the specificity was 90%, and the overall false-positive rate was 10%.[33] For HL, the sensitivity was 93%, specificity was 87%, and false-negative rate was 13%. For NHL, the sensitivity was 87%, specificity was 87%, and false-negative rate was 11%. Positron emission tomography is useful for detection of disease in the most common types of lymphoma with detection rates of 98% to 100% for DLBCL, FL, HL, and mantle cell lymphoma.[34] However, PET was less reliable for marginal zone lymphoma (67%), peripheral T-cell lymphoma (40%), and bone marrow involvement by any type of lymphoma. Therefore, as summarized in the National Comprehensive Cancer Network (NCCN) guidelines, PET is required for the staging of HL and DLBCL and is recommended for the staging of FL, marginal zone lymphoma, and mantle cell lymphoma.[35,36]

Compared with CT, PET improves the accuracy of staging for lymphoma because it can detect disease in nodes that do not meet size criteria. As shown in Table 22-2, PET more often resulted in the upstaging of patients with HL from 5% to 41% in six studies.[37–41] By contrast, PET much less frequently downstaged patients. In addition, PET upstaged 15% of the cases of aggressive lymphoma and changed treatment plans in 25% of those upstaged.[42] Finally, PET influenced the staging in approximately 45% of patients with stage I to II FL.[43] Among patients

TABLE 22–2 Summary of PET Imaging on the Stage, Prognosis and Radiotherapy Modifications for Lymphoma

Cancer	Study	No. of Patients	PET Only (Total Lesions)	Change in Staging	Upstaged	Downstaged	Change in Treatment	Treatment Escalated	Treatment Reduced
HL	Bangerter et al.[37]	44	11 (128)	14%	12%	2%	14%	11%	2%
	Partridge et al.[40]	44	75 (159)	48%	41%	7%	25%	23%	2%
	Naumann et al.[39]	88	17 patients (80 patients)	20%	13%	8%	18%	10%	8%
	Munker et al.[38]	73		32%	29%	3%			
	Rigacci et al.[41]	186	39	15%	14%	1%	6%	5%	1%
	Stanford (unpublished)	44		5%	5%	0%	11%	11%	0%
DLBCL	Fuertes et al.[42]	40	11 patients	15%	15%	0%	3%	3%	0%
	Sasaki et al.[85]	46	54 (152)	28%			17%		
Indolent NHL	Wirth et al.[43]	42	41 (94)	45%	40%	45%	45%	0%	
	Jerusalem et al.[86]	42	21 (174)	5%	5%	0%	0%		

Notes. DLBCL = diffuse large B-cell lymphoma; HL = Hodgkin's lymphoma; NHL = non-Hodgkin's lymphoma.

with stage I disease, 15% were upstaged to stage II and, importantly, 31% were upstaged to stage III or IV. Without PET, 41% would have been undertreated. The number of patients upstaged by PET is similar to the reported 10-year freedom from relapse (FFR) of 41% to 49%, suggesting that PET may select more appropriate candidates for curative regimens.[44] Therefore, PET provides information essential to staging that is incremental to other diagnostic imaging modalities.

By adding functional criteria to diagnosis, there is a suggestion that PET may also distinguish between different types of NHL by quantitating distinct metabolic signatures. A study from Memorial Sloan Kettering Cancer Center showed that indolent lymphomas generally had lower standard uptake values (SUVs) whereas aggressive lymphomas had higher SUVs.[45] Although the SUVs for aggressive and indolent lymphomas overlapped significantly, SUVs greater than 10 predicted aggressive lymphomas with a specificity of 81%. Furthermore, in this report, no indolent lymphomas had SUVs greater than 13. However, further study into how well hypermetabolic activity correlates with histopathological diagnosis is needed to validate these findings. In addition, PET scans may detect the transformation of an indolent lymphoma into an aggressive lymphoma, because 63% and 50% of transformed lymphomas had SUVs greater than 10 and 13, respectively.[46] Thus, in addition to anatomical information, PET may provide important biological correlates to the histopathological diagnosis of NHL.

Still, the full implications of PET in staging have yet to be fully determined. For example, PET upstages approximately 20% to 40% of patients with HL or NHL. Therefore, as PET may artificially affect overall survival because of stage migration, it will be important to assess whether improved outcomes in clinical trials were attributable to the use of PET to include or to exclude patients or attributable to actual improvements in treatment algorithms. Furthermore, the differences between the resolution and the registration of PET with CT may not always accurately indicate diseased lymph nodes. Finally, because PET cannot distinguish between inflammation, infection, and cancer, the false-positive rates remain uncertain and rarely are PET-positive/CT-negative lymph nodes confirmed by biopsy to actually be involved by lymphoma. Therefore, good clinical judgment is still required to assess the value of PET in the staging of disease and the assessment of treatment response.

Complementing its use in staging, PET imaging during treatment provides valuable information in predicting outcomes for lymphoma (Table 22-3). After ABVD chemotherapy for advanced HL, 25% of patients with PET-positive imaging relapsed versus none of those with PET-negative imaging.[47] After Stanford V chemotherapy for HL, Advani et al. showed that 96% with PET-negative imaging after treatment remained disease-free compared with only 33% with PET-positive imaging.[48] For NHL, 100% of patients with PET-positive imaging and 17% with PET-negative imaging relapsed after chemotherapy.[49] Compared with CT, PET more accurately predicts relapse after treatment.[50-53] Compared with CT, Jerusalem et al. showed that PET had a higher predictive value for relapse (100% for PET versus 42% for CT).[51] Spaepen

TABLE 22–3 Prediction of Postchemotherapy and Interim Chemotherapy PET on Progression-Free Survival

Study	Cancer	No. of Patients	Timing of PET	Chemo	PET Positive, %	Residual With Positive PET (y)	PFS With Negative PET (y)	PFS	PFS With Indeterminant PET (y)
Advani et al.[48]	HL	81	Postchemo	Stanford V	7%	33% (4)	96% (4)		
Zinzani et al.[53]	HL NHL	41 34	Postchemo	ABVD MACOP-B	21%	12.5%	100%		
Jerusalem et al.[51]	HL NHL	19 35	Postchemo	Not stated	11%	0% (1)	86% (1)		
Spaepen et al.[52]	NHL	93	Postchemo	Doxorubicin-based	28%	0% (2)	84% (2)		
Mikhaeel et al.[49]	NHL	49	Postchemo	Majority CHOP	18%	0% (30 mo follow-up)	83% (30 mo follow-up)		
Zinzani et al.[47]	HL	40	2 cycles Postchemo	ABVD × 6	30% 20%	0% 0%	100% 100%	75% 0%	
Gallamini et al.[59]	HL	260	2 cycles	ABVD	20%	12% (2)	95% (2)		
Mikhaeel et al.[58]	NHL	121	2–3 cycles	Majority CHOP	43% positive; 16% MRU	16% (5)	88% (5)	59% (5)	
Hoppe et al.[62]	Relapsed DLBCL	83	Postchemo	HDCT/ASCT	22%	61%	76%		
Castagna et al.[61]	Relapsed HL	24	2 cycles	Salvage chemo	42%	10% (2 y)	93% (2 y)		

Notes. HDCT/ASCT = high-dose chemotherapy/autologous stem cell transplant; HL = Hodgkin's lymphoma; MACOP-B: methotrexate, doxorubicin, cyclophosphamide, vincristine, prednisone, bleomycin; NHL = non-Hodgkin's lymphoma; PET = positron emission tomography.

et al. found that at the completion of therapy, PET was the only diagnostic method to predict relapse in 53% of patients.[52] Positron emission tomography scans had a better negative predictive value as 27% of patients who had a CR by CT relapsed compared with only 4% with a CR by PET.[50] Furthermore, PET scans were a better positive predictive tool as 45% of patients who failed to achieve a CR by PET relapsed compared to only 27% by CT.

Although PET scans are usually negative at the completion of chemotherapy, PET imaging after the first few cycles of chemotherapy may provide earlier and more accurate prognostic information. Iagaru et al. addressed when is the optimal timing for PET scanning during chemotherapy for lymphoma.[54] Although their study reported small numbers, the decrease in hypermetabolic activity was not different after two cycles or after four cycles of chemotherapy. Kostakoglu et al. demonstrated that PET imaging for aggressive lymphomas or HL after just a single cycle of chemotherapy may help to guide treatment decisions.[55] In fact, PET activity after one cycle of chemotherapy had a greater sensitivity (82% vs 45%) and positive predictive value (90% vs 83%) than after the completion of chemotherapy. However, a meta-analysis showed the prognostic value of PET is likely to be more reliable for advanced stage HL compared to NHL.[56] After a few cycles of chemotherapy for advanced stage HL, the sensitivity and specificity for prognosis was 81% and 97%, respectively. By contrast, the results for DLBCL were more heterogeneous (sensitivity = 78%; specificity = 87%) likely because of the inclusion of patients with variable risk factors. Furthermore, the addition of rituximab can increase the false-positive rates of PET scans during or after chemotherapy, which may affect the prognostic value of PET for aggressive NHL.[57] Therefore, with some caveats, early PET imaging may help to determine who might benefit from additional chemotherapy cycles, consolidative RT, or other intensification of treatment. This is the subject of clinical trials.

The scoring of PET imaging after a few cycles of chemotherapy falls into three broad prognostic categories: positive, minimal residual uptake (MRU), or negative. Whereas negative imaging occurs when all abnormal cancer-related uptake disappears, positive imaging refers to persistent or new abnormal areas of hypermetabolic activity. By contrast, MRU refers a focus hypermetabolic activity in previous areas of disease where inflammation could not be differentiated from malignancy. Mikhaeel et al. showed that for aggressive NHL, most commonly treated with CHOP chemotherapy, the 5-year progression-free survival (PFS) was 88%, 59%, and 16% for negative, MRU, and positive imaging on PET, respectively.[58] Similarly for HL, the PFS was 0%, 25%, and 100% with negative, MRU, and positive imaging on PET relapsed after ABVD chemotherapy.[47] No patients with positive imaging on PET after two cycles of chemotherapy

achieved a CR with additional cycles of chemotherapy. By contrast, all patients with MRU imaging achieved a CR after additional cycles of chemotherapy suggesting that there are different prognostic groups that may benefit from different escalations of treatment. Thus, three prognostic groups exist where escalated or reduced therapy should be defined.

Interestingly, PET imaging may also be more predictive than the well-established clinical prognostic indicators for lymphoma. Gallamini et al. have shown that PET-negative imaging after two cycles of ABVD chemotherapy predicted for 95% 2-year FFS regardless of risk status by International Prognostic Score (IPS) scoring.[59,60] Conversely, PET-positive imaging predicted a worse (12%) 2-year FFS for patients with high IPS scores as well as low IPS scores. However, patients with high IPS scores also had more PET-positive disease after two cycles of ABVD compared with patients with low IPS scores (38% vs 12%). Therefore, IPS stratification of high- and low-risk patients may also guide decisions on obtaining PET imaging after the start of chemotherapy in order to adapt treatment protocols.

Finally, PET imaging predicts outcome after salvage chemotherapy for both HL and aggressive lymphoma.[61-64] Negative PET imaging after second line chemotherapy for refractory DLBCL significantly predicted better PFS (HR = 3.4) and OS (HR = 5.4).[62] In this report, IFRT also improved both PFS with both PET-positive and PET-negative disease. Spaepen et al. showed that after one cycle of salvage chemotherapy 83% of patients with negative PET imaging achieved a complete response whereas 86% with positive PET imaging relapsed.[64] Similarly, PET improves the prognostic value for relapsed or refractory HL during salvage chemotherapy. After two cycles of salvage chemotherapy, PET imaging was positive in 42% of patients, and, of these patients, the 2-year PFS was 10%. By contrast, patients with negative PET imaging during salvage chemotherapy had a 2-year PFS of 93%.[61] Therefore, PET may better predict who would remain candidates for stem cell transplant and/or benefit from the addition of RT.

Image-Guided Treatment Planning

Good communication between the radiation oncologist and medical oncologist improves the implementation of PET in treatment planning. Specifically, although PET–CT is important for initial staging, if it is obtained in the treatment position before chemotherapy is initiated, it aids in more accurately defining the target volumes and reducing the amount of normal tissue to be irradiated. Figure 22-1 shows the use of staging PET imaging for the design of mediastinal RT fields after chemotherapy. Furthermore, PET–CT imaging at the completion of chemotherapy aids RT planning by identifying any residual hypermetabolic areas that may be boosted with

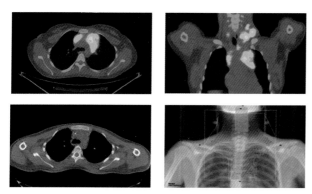

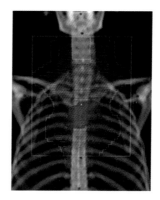

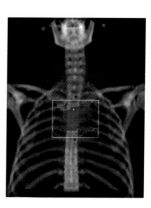

FIGURE 22-1. Use of positron emission tomography (PET) in delineating target volumes for radiotherapy: A 24-year-old woman with stage IIA nodular sclerosis Hodgkin's lymphoma involving the mediastinum and bilateral cervical lymph nodes was imaged with PET–computed tomography (CT) before treatment with Stanford V chemotherapy. The upper-left panel shows an axial PET–CT image showing hypermetabolic activity in the mediastinum. The upper-right panel shows the coronal PET–CT plane with distribution of the involved lymph node areas. The lower-left panel shows the planning CT scan with clinical target volumes (CTVs) outlined in red. Note that the CTV includes only the width of the postchemotherapy lymph node volume. The lower-right panel shows the beam's eye view generated using the prechemotherapy disease based on PET.

FIGURE 22-3. Role of positron emission tomography (PET) imaging in guiding radiotherapy planning for relapsed Hodgkin's lymphoma: The patient in Figure 22-2 was treated with involved-field radiotherapy after high-dose chemotherapy and hematopoietic cell transplant. The left panel shows the beams-eye view of the initial modified mantle field delineated by the pretransplant PET-positive imaging. The modified mantle was treated to 30 Gy. The right panel shows the beams-eye view for cone down field corresponding to the site of relapse. The lymph node areas with residual PET activity after transplant were outlined in blue and used to shape the cone down field, which was treated with an additional 6 Gy. The red volume indicates the targeted mediastinal and cervical lymph nodes.

radiation. Figure 22-2 depicts the PET imaging of a patient with relapsed NHL after stem cell transplant. This residual imaging was used to design boost fields as shown in Figure 22-3. Thus, PET has become the imaging study of choice in guiding RT (see Chapters 22A and 22B).

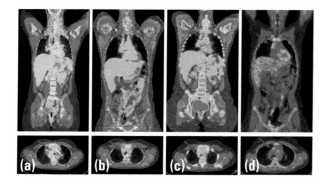

FIGURE 22-2. Role of positron emission tomography (PET) in tracking relapse after initial chemotherapy: (a) Initial staging PET imaging of a 36-year-old patient with stage IIIB nodular sclerosis Hodgkin's lymphoma (NSHL) involving the bilateral cervical, mediastinal, bilateral hilar, and retroperitoneal lymph nodes. (b) Restaging PET imaging after six cycles of ABVD chemotherapy. (c) Surveillance PET imaging showing relapsed NSHL in the mediastinum. (d) Restaging PET imaging after high-dose chemotherapy and autologous hematopoietic cell transplant. Upper rows show the coronal images with extent of disease. Lower rows show axial images at the level of PET-positive relapse. Arrows indicate the area of residual low PET activity after hematopoietic cell transplant.

Positron emission tomography imaging impacts both the selection of patients and areas to target. For FL, 45% of patients became ineligible for RT and 27% required increased RT fields because of PET findings.[43] Furthermore, in HL, Hutchings et al. showed that PET changed the radiation fields in 33% of patients, with field sizes increased by 6% to 51% or decreased by 18% to 30% of the original field.[65] In contrast to chemotherapy, PET imaging during RT may not yield much useful information. Whereas PET imaging during RT may theoretically lead to increased activity secondary to inflammation, Keller et al. showed that PET imaging during RT for aggressive NHL detected a 2.1% decrease in SUV per Gy.[66] Furthermore, the response to radiation detected by PET correlated best with posttreatment response and not the responses during RT, suggesting that interim PET imaging during RT may not predict for radiation sensitivity. Therefore, PET imaging may help in the selection of patients for RT and the definition of areas to target.

As suggested by its importance in staging and prognosis, PET imaging also plays an important role in treatment decisions for lymphoma. However, compared with staging, the impact of initial PET imaging on treatment decisions may not be as pronounced. Although PET changed the stage of patients with HL up to 40% of the time, it only altered treatment in 6% to 25% of these cases. This was more often the case with upstaging of patients, where treatment became more intense 10% to 20% of the time.[37,39–41] By contrast, treatment intensity was lowered only 2% to 3% of the time, even when patients are downstaged. Furthermore, it remains unclear what salvage options are most suitable for patients with PET-positive disease during or after treatment. Sher et al. showed that IFRT converted 69% of PET-positive imaging after chemotherapy to PET-negative imaging.[67] Hoppe et al. showed that IFRT improved PFS of PET-positive disease in relapsed DLBCL after salvage chemotherapy.[62] By contrast, Kahn and coworkers suggested that, after chemotherapy, RT did not salvage residual PET-positive disease in patients with NHL.[68] In this case, 58% of the patients with PET-positive disease relapsed compared with 15% of patients with PET-negative disease. In a separate study of patients with HL, RT was not sufficient to control PET-positive disease after chemotherapy as 63% relapsed with RT compared to 50% without RT.[48] Therefore, more studies are needed to determine what modalities may best combat PET-positive disease that remains during and after chemotherapy.

Positron emission tomography scans have now become an important measure of disease response and, according to the NCCN response criteria, a CR is defined even if masses of any size persist as long as they are PET-negative.[35,36] The addition of PET to International Workshop Criteria for response improved the accuracy in predicting a CR.[69] In fact, one area of difficult clinical judgment is predicting whether residual mediastinal masses after therapy represent remaining cancer or benign scar tissue. Weihrauch and colleagues showed that patients with HL who have residual mediastinal masses after treatment had a 1-year PFS of 95% with PET-negative imaging and 40% with PET-positive imaging.[70] Yet, the role of continued PET imaging for follow-up of lymphoma remains controversial. Although only 2.3% of lymphoma patients had focal positive findings on follow-up PET imaging, 23% of these findings were attributable to causes other than lymphoma.[71] Another study showed that PET scans were 100% sensitive in detecting recurrences yet nearly half of all PET-positive imaging on follow up were false positives.[72] Currently, the NCCN guidelines do not recommend PET imaging for surveillance because of the high risk of false positives and they strongly state that any PET-positive findings require clinical and pathological correlation. Thus, the role of PET in disease surveillance remains unclear and it cannot be recommended.

Image-Guided Treatment Delivery

Three-dimensional (3D) planning for lymphoma is an important aspect for delivering RT. Computed tomography simulation has replaced two-dimensional (2D) treatment planning as it offers the ability to target lymph node regions more consistently while excluding normal tissues. With 2D planning, the design of standard radiation fields varied significantly among radiation oncologists. By contrast, 3D planning allows lymph node regions to be

defined more accurately.[73] In addition, 3D planning provides dose–volume histograms that quantitate more precisely the dose to normal organs and can provide better predictors for late effects. For example, 3D planning has provided better quantification of radiation pneumonitis in patients treated for HL.[74] In general, radiation pneumonitis was a rare event, as only 3% of patients with lymphoma had grade 2 or higher toxicity. However, more than 10% of patients had a V_{20} greater than 36% and all patients with pneumonitis had mean lung doses above 16 Gy.

Lymphomas can also involve sites that are subject to respiratory motion. To compensate for this, active breathing control (ABC) or respiratory gating allows both the reduction of dose to normal tissues and an improvement in the ability of radiation to hit this "moving target." Stromberg and coworkers showed that ABC for modified mantle fields reduced the amount of lung irradiated by 9% to 24% compared with free breathing.[75] Similarly, when one is treating spleen and para-aortic fields, ABC reduced the mean volume of heart irradiated from 26% down to 5%. Although similar results would be expected with respiratory gating, these studies have not yet been reported. Nevertheless, at Stanford, we commonly use respiratory gating to account for organ motion during the delivery of radiation to the spleen. As shown in Figure 22-4, the spleen moves more than 1 cm with breathing. When respiratory gating is used, only 9% of the left kidney remains in the PTV whereas 36% of the left kidney is covered by a PTV used with normal respiration (Figures 22-5 and 22-6). Therefore, methods that account for respiratory

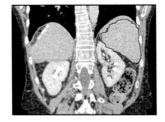
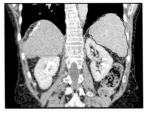
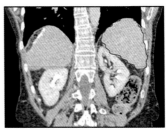

FIGURE 22-4. Movement of the spleen during respiration: Four-dimensional simulation was performed and the spleen was contoured on the 0%, 30%, and 50% phase of the respiratory cycle. The spleen contour for the indicated respiratory phase was overlayed onto the coronal image taken from the 50% phase scan. Note that, compared with the 50% phase, the spleen is displaced by 1.3 cm on the 0% phase. By contrast, the spleen positions for the 30% and 70% phase (not shown) nearly overlap the position for the 50% phase.

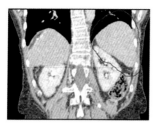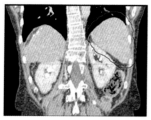

FIGURE 22-5. Accounting for respiratory motion decreases the volume of kidney irradiated with splenic fields: The deviation of the spleen in Figure 22-4 was incorporated into the planning target volume (PTV). On the left panel, the planning target volume (PTV) was expanded by 2 cm in the superior–inferior dimension and 1 cm in the axial direction to account for normal respiration. On the right panel, if radiation is gated between the 30% to 70% phase, the PTV was expanded by 1 cm in all dimensions; 36% or 9% of the kidney overlapped the PTV when no gating or gating was used during radiation, respectively.

motion may better help to guide radiation delivery to hit the target and miss the normal tissues.

Finally, lymphomas involving the abdomen may benefit from cone-beam CT (CBCT) compared with other means of target localization (see Chapter 22E). Boda-Heggemann et al. compared daily CBCT with ultrasound during the irradiation of large target volumes in the abdomen.[76] Of the 15 patients, five had gastric lymphoma and one had bulky abdominal lymphadenopathy. Here, CBCT was superior to skin mark–based positioning by 9 mm to 10 mm and by ultrasound by 5 mm to 7 mm. Thus, techniques to account for respiratory motion and daily imaging may improve the delivery of radiation for certain localizations of lymphoma.

Although few reports describe IGRT delivery for lymphoma only, many of the reports involving helical tomotherapy have included patients with lymphoma.

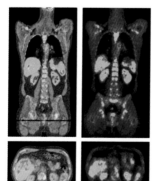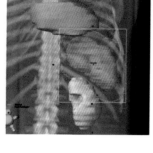

FIGURE 22-6. Using respiratory gating to treat the spleen: A patient with stage IV Hodgkin's lymphoma involving the spleen, liver, and bone marrow was imaged before chemotherapy (upper-left panel) or after 12 weeks of Stanford V chemotherapy (upper-right panel). Note the loss of hypermetabolic activity in the spleen and liver. The lower panel depicts the beam's eye view of the splenic field used with respiratory gating.

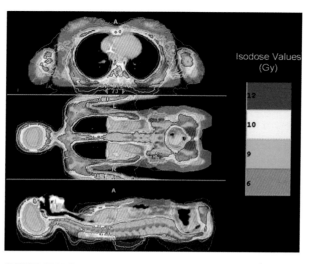

FIGURE 22-7. Color wash shows dose distribution of the first patient treated with targeted total-body irradiation using tomotherapy. Reproduced with permission from Wong JY et al.[78]

A report from Heidelberg describes their experience treating 150 patients with helical tomotherapy including 13 patients with lymphoma.[77] Overall, the mean correction was 6.9 mm per fractionated treatment and the total time on the table was 24.8 minutes. Wong and others employed helical tomotherapy for total marrow irradiation (TMI) in place of total body irradiation during the preparative regimen for multiple myeloma or for acute leukemia patients undergoing stem cell transplant[78] (see Chapter 22D). Figure 22-7 shows the first patient treated with TMI using helical tomotherapy. Interestingly, the median organ dose was 16% to 65% of the target dose and only half of the patients experienced nausea or vomiting. Finally, helical tomotherapy has been used to treat a primary renal lymphoma using daily pretreatment megavoltage (MV) CT imaging to adjust target volumes.[79] Therefore, helical tomotherapy has been used for IGRT of lymphoma and bone marrow irradiation before transplant.

Given the paucity of studies on IGRT for lymphoma, the added benefit of helical tomotherapy may be deduced from the previous work using intensity-modulated radiotherapy (IMRT). Intensity-modulated RT has been used to treat standard nodal fields for lymphoma as well as unique cases such as total scalp irradiation for cutaneous T-cell lymphoma,[80] lymphomas involving the head and neck,[81] or adjacent to critical structures such as the eyes or kidneys.[79,82] Intensity-modulated RT may improve therapy by limiting the amount of normal tissues exposed to high-dose regions. Compared with 3D conformal RT (3DCRT), IMRT for orbital lymphomas significantly decreased the dose to the contralateral lens, orbit, lacrimal gland, and optic chiasm. Compared with opposed anterior–posterior (AP–PA) or four-field 3DCRT for mediastinal masses, IMRT decreased dose to the left anterior descending artery by 50% and was the best technique for heart sparing in five out of six patients.[83] However, the cardiac benefits may be offset by the increased low dose to the breast where the V_{15} for the breast was 60% to 69% compared with 27% to 30% for four-field 3DCRT and 6% to 9% for AP–PA. In addition, although the V_{20} did not significantly differ among the three planning methods, the median lung dose was 1 Gy for AP–PA compared with 6 Gy to 7 Gy for IMRT or four-field 3DCRT. Similarly, Girinsky et al. found that IMRT for mediastinal masses provided greater protection to the heart, coronary arteries, esophagus, and spinal cord at the cost of increasing the volumes of breast and lung receiving low doses of radiation.[84] These low doses to larger volumes of the lungs and breast may theoretically elevate the risk for secondary cancers, and are of special concern for young patients. Therefore, selected IGRT techniques may be a double-edged sword as some short-term toxicities may be minimized at the expense of potential secondary cancers caused by greater volumes of normal tissues receiving lower radiation doses.

Future Directions

Image-guided RT techniques have the potential to improve the outcomes of lymphoma treatment even when low doses of radiation are delivered to small volumes. The use of IGRT techniques to deliver radiation shows promise including the implementation of respiratory gating and helical tomotherapy to better target disease. However, the implementation of imaging techniques such as PET used in IGRT have already improved lymphoma management.

Positron emission tomography is gaining wide acceptance as an assessment of tumor response during treatment and for altering RT planning. Such information will be useful for escalating or reducing therapy to achieve better tumor control or minimize treatment toxicity. The UK RAPID, the EORTC H10 trial, and the GHSG HL16 and HL17 trials are all testing the value of interim PET imaging in defining further therapy in stage I to II HL. For example, in the GHSG HL16 trial, patients who are PET-negative after two cycles of ABVD are randomized to no further therapy or IFRT. Image-guided RT techniques will be even more essential as treatment fields are reduced to target only the involved lymph nodes. In the future, we can expect further studies regarding the value of PET in individualizing treatment for lymphoma. Furthermore, the insights of PET into the biology of lymphoma may yield additional information. Namely, is PET simply more sensitive in detecting residual cancer cells or will it provide us functional and biological information that correlates with its sensitivity or resistance to treatment? Thus, the future of PET in the treatment of lymphoma remains a fascinating area for clinical and basic biological research.

References

1. Kaplan HS. The radical radiotherapy of regionally localized Hodgkin's disease. *Radiology.* 1962;78:553–561.

2. Peters MV. A study of survivals in Hodgkin's disease treated radiologically. *AJR Am R Roentgenol.* 1950;63:299–311.

3. Bonadonna G, Bonfante V, Viviani S, et al. ABVD plus subtotal nodal versus involved-field radiotherapy in early-stage Hodgkin's disease: long-term results. *J Clin Oncol.* 2004;22:2835–2841.

4. Fabian CJ, Mansfield CM, Dahlberg S, et al. Low-dose involved field radiation after chemotherapy in advanced Hodgkin disease. A Southwest Oncology Group randomized study. *Ann Intern Med.* 1994;120:903–912.

5. Horning SJ, Williams J, Bartlett NL, et al. Assessment of the Stanford V regimen and consolidative radiotherapy for bulky and advanced Hodgkin's disease: Eastern Cooperative Oncology Group pilot study E1492. *J Clin Oncol.* 2000;18:972–980.

6. Engert A, Schiller P, Josting A, et al. Involved-field radiotherapy is equally effective and less toxic compared with extended-field radiotherapy after four cycles of chemotherapy in patients with early-stage unfavorable Hodgkin's lymphoma: results of the HD8 trial of the German Hodgkin's Lymphoma Study Group. *J Clin Oncol.* 2003;21:3601–3608.

7. Eich HT, Engenhart-Cabillic R, Hansemann K, et al. Quality control of involved field radiotherapy in patients with early-favorable (HD10) and early-unfavorable (HD11) Hodgkin's lymphoma: an analysis of the German Hodgkin Study Group. *Int J Radiat Oncol Biol Phys.* 2008;71:1419–1424.

8. Sutcliffe SB, Gospodarowicz MK, Bush RS, et al. Role of radiation therapy in localized non-Hodgkin's lymphoma. *Radiother Oncol.* 1985;4:211–223.

9. Biti GP, Cimino G, Cartoni C, et al. Extended-field radiotherapy is superior to MOPP chemotherapy for the treatment of pathologic stage I-IIA Hodgkin's disease: eight-year update of an Italian prospective randomized study. *J Clin Oncol.* 1992;10:378–382.

10. Macdonald DA, Ding K, Gospodarowicz MK, et al. Patterns of disease progression and outcomes in a randomized trial testing ABVD alone for patients with limited-stage Hodgkin lymphoma. *Ann Oncol.* 2007;18:1680–1684.

11. Nachman JB, Sposto R, Herzog P, et al. Randomized comparison of low-dose involved-field radiotherapy and no radiotherapy for children with Hodgkin's disease who achieve a complete response to chemotherapy. *J Clin Oncol.* 2002;20:3765–3771.

12. Thomas J, Ferme C FC, Noordijk M, et al. Six cycles of EBVP followed by 36 Gy involved-field irradiation in favourable supradiaphragmatic clinical stage I-II Hodgkin's lymphoma: the EORTC-GELA strategy in 771 patients. (abstr) *Eur J Haematol.* 2004;73:s65:40.

13. Horning SJ, Weller E, Kim K, et al. Chemotherapy with or without radiotherapy in limited-stage diffuse aggressive non-Hodgkin's lymphoma: Eastern Cooperative Oncology Group study 1484. *J Clin Oncol.* 2004;22:3032–3038.

14. Miller TP, Dahlberg S, Cassady JR, et al. Chemotherapy alone compared with chemotherapy plus radiotherapy for

localized intermediate- and high-grade non-Hodgkin's lymphoma. *N Engl J Med.* 1998;339:21–26.

15. Leitch HA, Gascoyne RD, Chhanabhai M, et al. Limited-stage mantle-cell lymphoma. *Ann Oncol.* 2003;14:1555–1561.

16. Shah SD, Yahalom J, Correa DD, et al. Combined immunochemotherapy with reduced whole-brain radiotherapy for newly diagnosed primary CNS lymphoma. *J Clin Oncol.* 2007;25:4730–4735.

17. Todeschini G, Secchi S, Morra E, et al. Primary mediastinal large B-cell lymphoma (PMLBCL): long-term results from a retrospective multicentre Italian experience in 138 patients treated with CHOP or MACOP-B/VACOP-B. *Br J Cancer.* 2004;90:372–376.

18. Aleman BM, Raemaekers JM, Tirelli U, et al. Involved-field radiotherapy for advanced Hodgkin's lymphoma. *N Engl J Med.* 2003;348:2396–2406.

19. Aleman BM, Raemaekers JM , Tomisic R, et al. Involved-field radiotherapy for patients in partial remission after chemotherapy for advanced Hodgkin's lymphoma. *Int J Radiat Oncol Biol Phys.* 2007;67:19–30.

20. Aviles A, Delgado S, Nambo MJ, et al. Adjuvant radiotherapy to sites of previous bulky disease in patients stage IV diffuse large cell lymphoma. *Int J Radiat Oncol Biol Phys.* 1994;30:799–803.

21. Aviles A, Diaz-Maqueo JC, Sanchez E, et al. Long-term results in patients with low-grade nodular non-Hodgkin's lymphoma. A randomized trial comparing chemotherapy plus radiotherapy with chemotherapy alone. *Acta Oncol.* 1991;30:329–333.

22. Poen JC, Hoppe RT, Horning SJ. High-dose therapy and autologous bone marrow transplantation for relapsed/refractory Hodgkin's disease: the impact of involved field radiotherapy on patterns of failure and survival. *Int J Radiat Oncol Biol Phys.* 1996;36:3–12.

23. Moskowitz CH, Nimer SD, Zelenetz AD, et al. A 2-step comprehensive high-dose chemoradiotherapy second-line program for relapsed and refractory Hodgkin disease: analysis by intent to treat and development of a prognostic model. *Blood.* 2001;97:616–623.

24. Philip T, Guglielmi C, Hagenbeek A, et al. Autologous bone marrow transplantation as compared with salvage chemotherapy in relapses of chemotherapy-sensitive non-Hodgkin's lymphoma. *N Engl J Med.* 1995;333:1540–1545.

25. Dores GM, Metayer C, Curtis RE, et al. Second malignant neoplasms among long-term survivors of Hodgkin's disease: a population-based evaluation over 25 years. *J Clin Oncol.* 2002;20:3484–3494.

26. Travis LB, Hill DA, Dores GM, et al. Breast cancer following radiotherapy and chemotherapy among young women with Hodgkin disease. *JAMA.* 2003;290:465–475.

27. Gilbert ES, Stovall M, Gospodarowicz M, et al. Lung cancer after treatment for Hodgkin's disease: focus on radiation effects. *Radiat Res.* 2003;159:161–173.

28. Girinsky T, Ghalibafian M. Radiotherapy of Hodgkin's lymphoma: indications, new fields, and techniques. *Semin Radiat Oncol.* 2007;17:206–222.

29. Campbell BA, Voss N, Pickles T, et al. Involved-nodal radiation therapy as a component of combination therapy for limited-

30. Girinsky T, Ghalibafian M, Bonniaud G, et al. Is FDG-PET scan in patients with early stage Hodgkin lymphoma of any value in the implementation of the involved-node radiotherapy concept and dose painting? *Radiother Oncol.* 2007;85:178–186.

31. Girinsky T, van der Maazen R, Specht L, et al. Involved-node radiotherapy (INRT) in patients with early Hodgkin lymphoma: concepts and guidelines. *Radiother Oncol.* 2006;79:270–277.

32. Khandani AH, Dunphy CH, Meteesatien P, et al. Glut1 and Glut3 expression in lymphoma and their association with tumor intensity on 18F-fluorodeoxyglucose positron emission tomography. *Nucl Med Commun.* 2009;30:594–601.

33. Isasi CR, Lu P, Blaufox MD. A metaanalysis of 18F-2-deoxy-2-fluoro-D-glucose positron emission tomography in the staging and restaging of patients with lymphoma. *Cancer.* 2005;104:1066–1074.

34. Elstrom R, Guan L, Baker G, et al. Utility of FDG-PET scanning in lymphoma by WHO classification. *Blood.* 2003;101:3875–3876.

35. National Comprehensive Cancer Network. Hodgkin's Disease/Lymphoma. 2009. Available at: http://www.nccn.org/professionals/physician_gls/PDF/hodgkins.pdf. Accessed 15 June 2009.

36. National Comprehensive Cancer Network. Non-Hodgkin's Lymphoma. 2009. Available at: http://www.nccn.org/professionals/physician_gls/PDF/nhl.pdf. Accessed 15 June 2009.

37. Bangerter M, Moog F, Buchmann I, et al. Whole-body 2-[18F]-fluoro-2-deoxy-D-glucose positron emission tomography (FDG-PET) for accurate staging of Hodgkin's disease. *Ann Oncol.* 1998;9:1117–1122.

38. Munker R, Glass J, Griffeth LK, et al. Contribution of PET imaging to the initial staging and prognosis of patients with Hodgkin's disease. *Ann Oncol.* 2004;15:1699–1704.

39. Naumann R, Beuthien-Baumann B, Reiss A, et al. Substantial impact of FDG PET imaging on the therapy decision in patients with early-stage Hodgkin's lymphoma. *Br J Cancer.* 2004;90:620–625.

40. Partridge S, Timothy A, O'Doherty MJ, et al. 2-Fluorine-18-fluoro-2-deoxy-D glucose positron emission tomography in the pretreatment staging of Hodgkin's disease: influence on patient management in a single institution. *Ann Oncol.* 2000;11:1273–1279.

41. Rigacci L, Vitolo U, Nassi L, et al. Positron emission tomography in the staging of patients with Hodgkin's lymphoma. A prospective multicentric study by the Intergruppo Italiano Linfomi. *Ann Hematol.* 2007;86:897–903.

42. Fuertes S, Setoain X, Lopez-Guillermo A, et al. [The value of positron emission tomography/computed tomography (PET/CT) in the staging of diffuse large B-cell lymphoma]. *Med Clin (Barc).* 2007;129:688–693.

43. Wirth A, Foo M, Seymour JF, et al. Impact of [18f] fluorodeoxyglucose positron emission tomography on staging and management of early-stage follicular non-Hodgkin lymphoma. *Int J Radiat Oncol Biol Phys.* 2008;71:213–219.

44. Mac Manus MP, Hoppe RT. Is radiotherapy curative for stage I and II low-grade follicular lymphoma? Results of a long-term

follow-up study of patients treated at Stanford University. *J Clin Oncol.* 1996;14:1282–1290.

45. Schoder H, Noy A, Gonen M, et al. Intensity of 18fluorodeoxyglucose uptake in positron emission tomography distinguishes between indolent and aggressive non-Hodgkin's lymphoma. *J Clin Oncol.* 2005;23:4643–4651.

46. Noy A, Schode Hr, Gonen M, et al. The majority of transformed lymphomas have high standardized uptake values (SUVs) on positron emission tomography (PET) scanning similar to diffuse large B-cell lymphoma (DLBCL). *Ann Oncol.* 2009;20:508–512.

47. Zinzani PL, Tani M, Fanti S, et al. Early positron emission tomography (PET) restaging: a predictive final response in Hodgkin's disease patients. *Ann Oncol.* 2006;17:1296–1300.

48. Advani R, Maeda L, Lavori P, et al. Impact of positive positron emission tomography on prediction of freedom from progression after Stanford V chemotherapy in Hodgkin's disease. *J Clin Oncol.* 2007;25:3902–3907.

49. Mikhaeel NG, Timothy AR, O'Doherty MJ, et al. 18-FDG-PET as a prognostic indicator in the treatment of aggressive non-Hodgkin's lymphoma-comparison with CT. *Leuk Lymphoma.* 2000;39:543–553.

50. de Wit M, Bohuslavizki H, Buchert R, et al. 18FDG-PET following treatment as valid predictor for disease-free survival in Hodgkin's lymphoma. *Ann Oncol.* 2001;12:29–37.

51. Jerusalem G, Beguin Y, Fassotte MF, et al. Whole-body positron emission tomography using 18F-fluorodeoxyglucose for posttreatment evaluation in Hodgkin's disease and non-Hodgkin's lymphoma has higher diagnostic and prognostic value than classical computed tomography scan imaging. *Blood.* 1999;94:429–433.

52. Spaepen K, Stroobants S, Dupont P, et al. Prognostic value of positron emission tomography (PET) with fluorine-18 fluorodeoxyglucose ([18F]FDG) after first-line chemotherapy in non-Hodgkin's lymphoma: is [18F]FDG-PET a valid alternative to conventional diagnostic methods? *J Clin Oncol.* 2001;19:414–419.

53. Zinzani PL, Fanti S, Battista G, et al. Predictive role of positron emission tomography (PET) in the outcome of lymphoma patients. *Br J Cancer.* 2004;91:850–854.

54. Iagaru A, Wang Y, Mari C, et al. (18)F-FDG-PET/CT evaluation of response to treatment in lymphoma: when is the optimal time for the first re-evaluation scan? *Hell J Nucl Med.* 2008;11:153–156.

55. Kostakoglu L, Coleman M, Leonard JP, et al. PET predicts prognosis after 1 cycle of chemotherapy in aggressive lymphoma and Hodgkin's disease. *J Nucl Med.* 2002;43:1018–1027.

56. Terasawa T, Lau J, Bardet S, et al. Fluorine-18-fluorodeoxyglucose positron emission tomography for interim response assessment of advanced-stage Hodgkin's lymphoma and diffuse large B-cell lymphoma: a systematic review. *J Clin Oncol.* 2009;27:1906–1914.

57. Han HS, Escalon MP, Hsiao B, et al. High incidence of false-positive PET scans in patients with aggressive non-Hodgkin's lymphoma treated with rituximab-containing regimens. *Ann Oncol.* 2009;20:309–318.

58. Mikhaeel NG, Hutchings M, Fields PA, et al. FDG-PET after two to three cycles of chemotherapy predicts progression-free

and overall survival in high-grade non-Hodgkin lymphoma. *Ann Oncol.* 2005;16:1514–1523.

59. Gallamini A, Hutchings M, L. Rigacci L, et al. Early interim 2-[18F]fluoro-2-deoxy-D-glucose positron emission tomography is prognostically superior to international prognostic score in advanced-stage Hodgkin's lymphoma: a report from a joint Italian-Danish study. *J Clin Oncol.* 2007;25:3746–3752.

60. Hasenclever D, Diehl V. A prognostic score for advanced Hodgkin's disease. International Prognostic Factors Project on Advanced Hodgkin's Disease. *N Engl J Med.* 1998;339:1506–1514.

61. Castagna L, Bramanti S, Balzarotti M, et al. Predictive value of early 18F-fluorodeoxyglucose positron emission tomography (FDG-PET) during salvage chemotherapy in relapsing/refractory Hodgkin lymphoma (HL) treated with high-dose chemotherapy. *Br J Haematol.* 2009;145:369–372.

62. Hoppe BS, Moskowitz CH, Zhang Z, et al. The role of FDG-PET imaging and involved field radiotherapy in relapsed or refractory diffuse large B-cell lymphoma. *Bone Marrow Transplant.* 2009;43:941–948.

63. Jabbour E, Hosing C, Ayers G, et al. Pretransplant positive positron emission tomography/gallium scans predict poor outcome in patients with recurrent/refractory Hodgkin lymphoma. *Cancer.* 2007;109:2481–2489.

64. Spaepen K, Stroobants S, Dupont P, et al. Prognostic value of pretransplantation positron emission tomography using fluorine 18-fluorodeoxyglucose in patients with aggressive lymphoma treated with high-dose chemotherapy and stem cell transplantation. *Blood.* 2003;102:53–59.

65. Hutchings M, Loft A, Hansen M, et al. Clinical impact of FDG-PET/CT in the planning of radiotherapy for early-stage Hodgkin lymphoma. *Eur J Haematol.* 2007;78:206–212.

66. Keller H, Goda JS, Vines DC, et al. Quantification of local tumor response to fractionated radiation therapy for non-Hodgkin lymphoma using weekly (18)F-FDG PET/CT imaging. *Int J Radiat Oncol Biol Phys.* 2010;76(3):850–858.

67. Sher DJ, Mauch PM, Van Den Abbeele A, et al. Prognostic significance of mid- and post-ABVD PET imaging in Hodgkin's lymphoma: the importance of involved-field radiotherapy. *Ann Oncol.* 2009;20(11):1848–1853.

68. Kahn ST, Flowers C, Lechowicz MJ, et al. Value of PET restaging after chemotherapy for non-Hodgkin's lymphoma: implications for consolidation radiotherapy. *Int J Radiat Oncol Biol Phys.* 2006;66:961–965.

69. Juweid ME, Wiseman GA, Vose JM, et al. Response assessment of aggressive non-Hodgkin's lymphoma by integrated International Workshop Criteria and fluorine 18-fluorodeoxyglucose positron emission tomography. *J Clin Oncol.* 2005;23:4652–4661.

70. Weihrauch MR, Re D, Scheidhauer K, et al. Thoracic positron emission tomography using 18F-fluorodeoxyglucose for the evaluation of residual mediastinal Hodgkin disease. *Blood.* 2001;98:2930–2934.

71. Castellucci P, Nanni C, Farsad M, et al. Potential pitfalls of 18F-FDG PET in a large series of patients treated for malignant lymphoma: prevalence and scan interpretation. *Nucl Med Commun.* 2005;26:689–694.

72. Crocchiolo R, Fallanca F, Giovacchini G, et al. Role of (18)FDG-PET/CT in detecting relapse during follow-up of patients with Hodgkin's lymphoma. *Ann Hematol.* 2009;88(12)1229–1236.

73. Naida JD, Eisbruch A, Schoeppel SL, et al. Analysis of localization errors in the definition of the mantle field using a beam's eye view treatment-planning system. *Int J Radiat Oncol Biol Phys.* 1996;35:377–382.

74. Koh ES, Sun A, Tran TH, et al. Clinical dose-volume histogram analysis in predicting radiation pneumonitis in Hodgkin's lymphoma. *Int J Radiat Oncol Biol Phys.* 2006;66:223–228.

75. Stromberg JS, Sharpe MB, Kim LH, et al. Active breathing control (ABC) for Hodgkin's disease: reduction in normal tissue irradiation with deep inspiration and implications for treatment. *Int J Radiat Oncol Biol Phys.* 2000;48:797–806.

76. Boda-Heggemann J, Mennemeyer P, Wertz H, et al. Accuracy of ultrasound-based image guidance for daily positioning of the upper abdomen: an online comparison with cone beam CT. *Int J Radiat Oncol Biol Phys.* 2009;74:892–897.

77. Sterzing F, Schubert K, Sroka-Perez G, et al. Helical tomotherapy. Experiences of the first 150 patients in Heidelberg. *Strahlenther Onkol.* 2008;184:8–14.

78. Wong JY, Rosenthal J, Liu A, et al. Image-guided total-marrow irradiation using helical tomotherapy in patients with multiple myeloma and acute leukemia undergoing hematopoietic cell transplantation. *Int J Radiat Oncol Biol Phys.* 2009;73:273–279.

79. Renaud J, Yartsev S, Dar AR, et al. Successful treatment of primary renal lymphoma using image guided helical tomotherapy. *Can J Urol.* 2009;16:4639–4647.

80. Samant RS, Fox GW, Gerig LH, et al. Total scalp radiation using image-guided IMRT for progressive cutaneous T cell lymphoma. *Br J Radiol.* 2009;82: 122–125.

81. Tomita N, Kodaira T, Tachibana H, et al. A comparison of radiation treatment plans using IMRT with helical tomotherapy and 3D conformal radiotherapy for nasal natural killer/T-cell lymphoma. *Br J Radiol.* 2009. In press.

82. Goyal S, Cohler A, Camporeale J, et al. Intensity-modulated radiation therapy for orbital lymphoma. *Radiat Med.* 2008; 26:573–581.

83. Nieder C, Schill S, Kneschaurek P, et al. Comparison of three different mediastinal radiotherapy techniques in female patients: impact on heart sparing and dose to the breasts. *Radiother Oncol.* 2007;82:301–307.

84. Girinsky T, Pichenot C, Beaudre A, et al. Is intensity-modulated radiotherapy better than conventional radiation treatment and three-dimensional conformal radiotherapy for mediastinal masses in patients with Hodgkin's disease, and is there a role for beam orientation optimization and dose constraints assigned to virtual volumes? *Int J Radiat Oncol Biol Phys.* 2006;64:218–226.

85. Sasaki M, Kuwabara Y, Koga H, et al. Clinical impact of whole body FDG-PET on the staging and therapeutic decision making for malignant lymphoma. *Ann Nucl Med.* 2002;16:337–345.

86. Jerusalem G, Beguin Y, Najjar F, et al. Positron emission tomography (PET) with 18F-fluorodeoxyglucose (18F-FDG) for the staging of low-grade non-Hodgkin's lymphoma (NHL). *Ann Oncol.* 2001;12:825–830.

PET/CT-Guided Target Delineation in a Patient With Early Stage Hodgkin's Lymphoma

Case Study

Martin Hutchings, PhD, Deborah Schut, BSc, Lena Specht, DMSc, MD

Patient History

A 22-year-old man presented with a nontender cervical lymph node, which remained enlarged four weeks after an upper respiratory tract infection. During the same period, he noticed retrosternal discomfort and some pruritus, but no B symptoms (fever, weight loss, night sweats). Clinical examination showed an excellent general condition and no other abnormal lymph nodes. An excisional biopsy of the enlarged node was performed, and the histological examination revealed classical Hodgkin's lymphoma (HL), nodular sclerosing subtype.

Staging procedures included extensive laboratory tests, bone marrow (BM) biopsy, and a whole-body ^{18}F-fluorodeoxyglucose (^{18}F-FDG) positron emission tomography (PET)–computed tomography (CT) scan. The latter was performed as part of an investigational protocol, and, because the value of PET in HL staging was still somewhat uncertain at that time, the results of the PET were not disclosed to the responsible physicians. The laboratory work showed normal values, except slightly elevated levels of lactate dehydrogenase, alkaline phosphatase, and erythrocyte sedimentation rate. The BM biopsy was normal, and the CT scan revealed lymphoma masses in the mediastinum and the right side of the neck. The patient was thus considered to be in clinical stage IIA with no risk factors.

The initial treatment plan was for two cycles of ABVD (adriamycin, bleomycin, vinblastine, and dacarbazine) followed by radiotherapy (RT) to the initially involved sites (30.6 Gy in 17 fractions plus a 5.4-Gy boost to residual masses after chemotherapy). However, the PET images revealed very intense FDG uptake in the right proximal humerus (Figure 22A-1), and, because this had an important potential impact on the management of the patient, the results of the PET scan were disclosed. There was no history of injury or infection, nor any pain, tenderness, or swelling. In the same anatomical location, magnetic resonance (MR) imaging was highly suspicious for intraosseous involvement (Figure 22A-2). No additional biopsy was considered necessary, and the clinical stage was changed from IIA to IVA.

As a consequence, the patient received full chemotherapy treatment consisting of eight cycles of ABVD. The treatment was well tolerated. Interim ^{18}F-FDG PET–CT (after two cycles of chemotherapy) showed a good reduction in the size of the masses and complete metabolic remission, also in the humerus, and this further indicated an initially malignant involvement of that site. The PET–CT scans after four and eight cycles showed further regression and no pathological ^{18}F-FDG uptake, leaving only a small, PET-negative, residual mass in the mediastinum at the completion of chemotherapy.

At the time of treatment, the standard treatment for this patient would have included RT (36 Gy) to the residual mass only. However, as all known disease sites could be encompassed by reasonable fields, he was offered RT to the initially involved areas plus a boost to the resid-

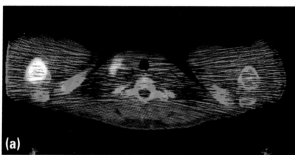

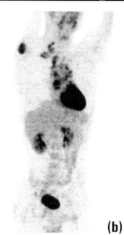

FIGURE 22A-1. Transaxial positron emission tomography (PET)/ computed tomography image showing the high ¹⁸F-fluorodeoxyglucose uptake in the right proximal humerus (a) and an oblique view maximum intensity projection image showing the PET-positive lymphoma masses in the mediastinum, right periclavicular regions, and the right humerus (b).

mimicking the couch of the treatment unit. He was immobilized with a foam cradle extending from shoulders to pelvis. Computed tomography contrast agents were not used for the simulation.

Imaging and Target Delineation

¹⁸F-FDG PET–CT images were imported into the planning workstation. Pretreatment PET images were registered to the planning CT data set. According to the Nordic guidelines, the clinical target volume (CTV) included the tissue volumes that had contained the initially involved areas with a minimum margin of 2 cm, except in the mediastinum and lung hili where a margin of 1 cm laterally was applied (Figure 22A-3). A small internal margin (< 1 cm) accounting for physiological changes such as organ motions was added around the CTV, and the planning treatment volume (PTV) was defined by the outer border of the anatomically adjusted internal margin of the CTV. The tissue volume that had contained the anatomical extent of the primary involvement was defined by an expert radiologist, an expert nuclear medicine physician, and a radiation oncologist, using the PET–CT images from the staging scan. The boost CTV included the residual mass plus a margin of 3 cm, with the same internal margins and PTV definitions.

Treatment Planning

Three-dimensional (3D) conformal RT planning (3DCRT) was performed using the Eclipse software (Varian Medical Systems, Palo Alto, CA) (Figure 22A-4). A dose of 30.6 Gy in 17 fractions was prescribed to the PTV and an additional dose of 5.4 Gy in three fractions to the boost PTV. Both PTVs were treated using anterior–posterior (AP–PA) opposing fields.

ual mass, as described previously. We elected to use the ¹⁸F-FDG PET–CT to aid in optimal target delineation in this patient.

Simulation

The ¹⁸F-FDG PET–CT after completion of chemotherapy was performed as the treatment planning scan, using a General Electric LS Discovery PET–CT scanner (GE Healthcare, Waukesha, WI). He was placed with his arms above his head in the supine position on a flat-top couch

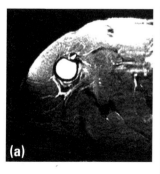

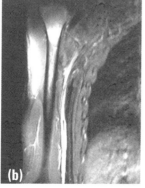

FIGURE 22A-2. Transaxial (a) and coronal (b) T1-weighted magnetic resonance images showing a highly pathological signal in the right proximal humerus.

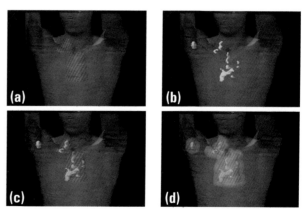

FIGURE 22A-3. Three-dimensional views of the delineations of the clinical target volume as seen on computed tomography (CT) (a), the volume with high ¹⁸F-fluorodeoxyglucose uptake on positron emission tomography (PET) (b), the clinical target volume using both CT and PET information (c), and the planning target volume (d).

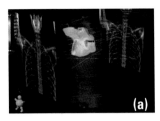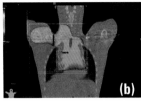

FIGURE 22A-4. Three-dimensional (a) and coronal (b) views of the treatment plan and dose distribution.

Clinical Outcome

The patient tolerated the RT well, with mild soreness of the throat as the only side effect. An ^{18}F-FDG PET–CT 2 months after RT showed a complete remission, which has repeatedly been confirmed by regular follow-up CT scans. Six years after completion of therapy, he remains in good health with no evidence of disease recurrence. So far, he has experienced no late effects of therapy, and fertility is preserved, as he recently had his first child.

Our experience using ^{18}F-FDG PET–CT to guide target delineation in 30 patients with early stage HL undergoing involved field RT (IFRT) was published earlier.[1] All patients underwent ^{18}F-FDG PET–CT before therapy, and IFRT after a short course of ABVD. Involved field RT planning was performed using only the CT data from the ^{18}F-FDG PET–CT scan. Later, the IFRT was performed anew using the ^{18}F-FDG PET–CT data as a basis for contouring. In seven patients, the ^{18}F-FDG PET–CT would have increased the irradiated volume where the volume receiving a minimum of 90% of the target dose was increased by 8% to 87%. ^{18}F-FDG PET–CT would have decreased the volume in two patients where the volume was reduced by 18% and 30%, respectively.

References

1. Hutchings M, Loft A, Hansen M, et al. Clinical impact of FDG-PET/CT in the planning of radiotherapy for early-stage Hodgkin's lymphoma. *Eur J Haematol.* 2007;78:206–212.

^{18}F-FDG PET-Guided Target Delineation in a Patient with Non-Hodgkin's Lymphoma

Case Study

Stephanie Terezakis, MD, Joachim Yahalom, MD

Patient History

An 88-year-old woman presented with left jaw swelling and tenderness after a left molar tooth extraction. A computed tomography (CT) scan of the neck without contrast identified a large mass at the ascending ramus of the left mandible measuring approximately 5 cm by 3 cm. Computed tomography scans of the chest, abdomen, and pelvis revealed no evidence of lymphadenopathy. Her lactate dehydrogenase level was elevated to 624 U/L.

A biopsy of the mass demonstrated diffuse large B cell lymphoma. Immunohistochemical stains were positive for CD20, PAX5, CD10, BCL-2, BCL-6, CD79A, and MUM-1. A fused ^{18}F-fluorodeoxyglucose positron emission tomography (^{18}F-FDG PET) scan and CT scan was performed for staging purposes and demonstrated increased metabolic activity in a left-sided soft tissue mass with bony destruction of the left mandible and parapharyngeal extension measuring 6.3 cm by 6.7 cm, with a maximum standardized uptake value (SUV) of 10.2 (Figure 22B-1).

The patient was begun on systemic chemotherapy with rituximab, cyclophosphamide, doxorubicin, vincristine, and prednisone (R-CHOP). After one cycle, she developed a neutropenic fever secondary to *Klebsiella pneumoniae* bacteremia. Because of her poor performance status, she was unable to tolerate further chemotherapy. Her case was brought to our multidisciplinary lymphoma tumor board. The consensus recommendation was for involved field radiotherapy (RT) because of her advanced age, poor performance status, and limited systemic treatment options. We elected to use ^{18}F-FDG PET scanning to guide target delineation in this patient.

Simulation

The patient was simulated on our departmental PET–CT simulator (GE Discovery/LS scanner, GE Medical Systems, Wausheka, WI). She was placed in the supine position with her neck hyperextended and immobilized in a five-point Aquaplast mask (W F R-Aquaplast Corp, Wyckoff, NJ). She underwent ^{18}F-FDG injection with an activity of 15 mCi (± 10%). The patient was given a first cup of oral contrast (Gastrografin, 25 mL in 1000 mL of Crystal Light) to be consumed over 45 minutes during which the patient was in isolation. A second cup was given immediately before scanning. Iodinated intravenous contrast was also administered immediately before initiation of the spiral CT scan component of simulation. Transaxial 3-mm images were obtained from the top of the skull to her upper thighs.

An isocenter was set using the CT scan information. The PET images were acquired immediately following completion of the CT. The patient was subsequently marked for alignment to define the coordinate system for treatment planning. The CT scan was then automatically coregistered to the PET scan using the Advantage SimMD software available on the GE Discovery ST scanner with rigid body registration.

A nuclear medicine physician performed a diagnostic evaluation of the PET–CT scan with SUV quantitative analysis. A persistent heterogenous mass associated with the left mandible was again identified with an SUV of 11.5. Two new left level II/III cervical lymph nodes demonstrated increased uptake with SUV values of 7.5 and 8.0, but neither met radiographic size criteria for enlargement. These nodes measured only 8 mm and

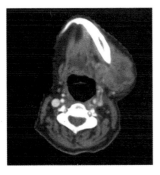
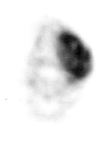

FIGURE 22B-1. Axial computed tomography scan and corresponding axial positron emission tomography scan view of the left neck demonstrating a soft tissue mass with associated bony destruction of the left mandible.

9 mm in greatest dimension, respectively, and had not been identified on the patient's prechemotherapy staging scans.

Imaging and Target Delineation

After automatic registration, the PET window levels were set to a threshold of 40% maximum SUV value for contouring on the fused PET–CT images. The gross tumor volume (GTV) was contoured to include the left mandibular mass as well as the involved left cervical lymph nodes. The clinical target volume (CTV) was designed to encompass a three-dimensional (3D) expansion of 5 mm around the GTV and the clinically uninvolved left neck to encompass levels I through V. The CTV was then expanded in 3D by 8 mm, generating the planning target volume (PTV; Figure 22B-2).

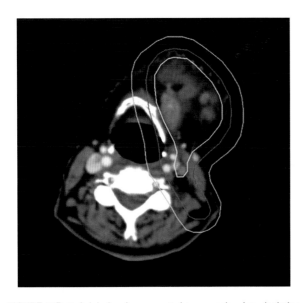

FIGURE 22B-2. Axial planning computed tomography view depicting the gross tumor volume (yellow contour), clinical target volume (pink contour), and planning target volume (blue contour).

Incorporation of PET imaging significantly changed the GTV, which was initially planned using the CT information alone. On the basis of the patient's initial staging studies, the GTV would have included the primary mandibular mass without elective nodal irradiation (Figure 22B-3). The addition of PET enlarged the treated volume and an error in targeting of the tumor volume was avoided.

Treatment Planning

An intensity-modulated radiotherapy (IMRT) plan was generated using our in-house software, the Ported Treatment Planning System. A total dose of 50.4 Gy in 28 fractions was prescribed. Because of tumor bulk and the patient's inability to tolerate chemotherapy, a relatively high total dose was used. The treatment plan consisted of a left lateral, left posterior oblique, right anterior oblique, and two left anterior oblique fields with a 5-mm bolus (Figure 22B-4). Excellent target coverage was achieved with a hot spot of 106% located in the GTV (Figure 22B-5). Because of the extent of local tumor invasion, the left parotid was partially included in the PTV. The right parotid mean dose was kept to 21 Gy.

Clinical Outcome

Treatment was delivered on a 2100 EX (Varian Medical Systems, Palo Alto, CA) equipped with an onboard imager (OBI). Each day, the patient was positioned on the treatment couch in her immobilization device. Before treatment delivery, orthogonal kV x-rays were obtained using the OBI. The bony anatomy from the kV images was matched to the planning digitally reconstructed radiographs (DRRs). On the basis of the daily deviations determined from the software, the couch position was adjusted

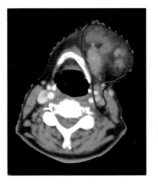
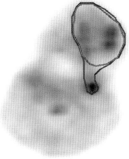

FIGURE 22B-3. Axial computed tomography (CT) scan and corresponding axial positron emission tomography (PET) scan view of the gross tumor volume (GTV). The yellow contour represents the GTV based on CT information alone. The pink contour represents the GTV based on PET–CT information.

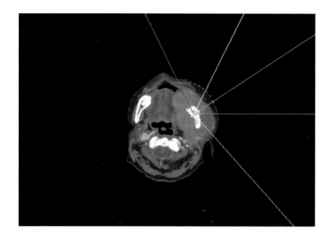

FIGURE 22B-4. Axial computed tomography view depicting the beam arrangement using intensity-modulated radiation therapy; the yellow contour represents the clinical target volume.

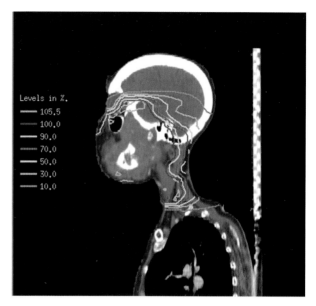

FIGURE 22B-5. Sagittal computed tomography view of the isodose curves generated from an intensity-modulated radiation therapy plan demonstrating 100% coverage of the planning target volume (red).

to ensure that the patient was aligned at the isocenter. The total treatment time, including imaging, verification, and adjustment, was approximately 30 minutes.

The patient had a prophylactic percutaneous endoscopic gastrostomy (PEG) tube placed before initiation of RT. With use of her PEG tube, she was able to maintain her weight throughout the course of treatment. Except for a localized mucosal ulceration in the left buccal mucosa, which required a 3-day treatment break, she tolerated her treatment well. She had a clinically significant treatment response during the course of RT with a decrease in the size of the mass by approximately 50% on visual inspection.

The patient returned to our follow-up clinic 4 weeks posttreatment with evidence of further clinical improvement in the size of her primary mass. She underwent a restaging ^{18}F-FDG PET–CT scan 3 months after completion of RT that demonstrated interval resolution of ^{18}F-FDG

uptake at the site of the primary mass and left neck. Overall, she experienced significant symptomatic improvement with no significant treatment sequelae. Unfortunately, a follow-up ^{18}F-FDG PET–CT surveillance scan 1 year posttreatment demonstrated increased uptake in multiple subcutaneous nodules throughout the abdomen and pelvis (SUVs 7 to 10.5) as well as in the left gluteus muscle (SUV 11.2). Biopsy of an abdominal nodule identified recurrent diffuse large B cell lymphoma. The patient's poor performance status, advanced age, and multiple medical comorbidities precluded her ability to receive effective systemic therapy. Therefore, she is undergoing a course of expectant management and supportive care.

MR-Guided Active Bone Marrow Delineation in a Patient with Acute Pre-T Cell ALL Treated with Intensity Modulated Total Marrow Irradiation

Case Study

Bulent Aydogan, PhD, Mete Yeginer, PhD, Damiano Rondelli, MD

Patient History

A 23-year-old man presented to an outside hospital complaining of night sweats, sore throat, and coldlike symptoms, as well as bilateral cervical adenopathy causing dysphagia. A peripheral blood smear showed an elevated white blood cell count with 80% blasts. Bone marrow (BM) biopsy revealed 90% lymphoid blasts. Flow cytometry analysis of leukemic cells was consistent with the diagnosis of acute pre–T-cell lymphoblastic leukemia.

The patient was referred to our institution for further diagnostic examinations and treatment. Cytogenetic studies performed on marrow cells demonstrated additional material of unknown origin on the short arm of chromosome 19 (present on 60% of the cells). Fluorescent in-situ hybridization studies revealed a deletion of one *ABL1* gene. Computed tomography (CT) scans of the chest, abdomen, and pelvis showed global involvement of the cervical, supraclavicular, mediastinal, periaortic, periilliac, and inguinal lymph nodes.

The patient was treated with a standard pediatric chemotherapy induction protocol for T-cell acute lymphoblastic leukemia (ALL), including daunorubicin, vincristine, methotrexate, prednisone, and PEG-asparaginase. In addition, he received standard central nervous system

(CNS) chemoprophylaxis, consisting of multiple intrathecal infusions of prednisone, cytarabine, and methotrexate. He achieved a complete remission and subsequently also received also consolidative chemotherapy.

Because of poor patient compliance with multiple missed appointments, his maintenance chemotherapy was often delayed, thus greatly increasing the risk of disease relapse. For this reason, we proposed to further consolidate his response with high-dose chemotherapy followed by autologous stem cell transplantation (SCT), without any further chemotherapy. His peripheral blood hematopoietic stem cells were thus collected after mobilization with filgrastim (10 µg/kg over 5 days). A week after stem cell collection, he was admitted to the hospital and started a conditioning regimen with total body irradiation (TBI; 200 cGy twice daily) on days -7, -6, and -5; etoposide at 45 mg/kg on day -4; and cyclophosphamide at 60 mg/kg on days -3 and -2.

Here, we describe a novel alternative treatment approach consisting of magnetic resonance (MR)-guided intensity-modulated total marrow irradiation (IM-TMI) performed on a linear accelerator (Varian Medical Systems, Palo Alto, CA). The rationale of this technique is to use intensity-modulated radiation therapy (IMRT) to target the patient's total BM with MR guidance to identify active BM sites for dose escalation. This approach may potentially improve the efficacy of treatment compared with standard TBI techniques while reducing the risk of serious toxicity.

Simulation

The patient was immobilized in the supine position with a Body Pro-Lok (CIVCO Medical Solution Inc, Kalona, IA) device. A large vacuum body mold was used to immobilize the patient on the indexed Pro-Lok platform with two bridges, one on the chest to reduce the lung motion and another on the thighs to reduce the pelvic and leg motion (Figure 22C-1). Table positions and bridge positions are indexed and a planning CT scan extending from the patient's head to his midfemur was obtained using the department's PQ5000 simulator (Picker Medical Systems, Cleveland, OH).

Imaging and Target Delineation

Magnetic resonance is fast becoming the imaging modality of choice for diagnosing BM disorders. It complements BM biopsies by providing information on the spatial distribution of red, yellow, and diseased marrow. The MR appearance of the bone marrow depends on the presence and proportions of bone, fat, water, and cellular elements. Each of the components gives a proper MR signal and, therefore, displays a specific "brightness." Customarily, for hematological questions, T1-weighted images, T2-weighted fast spin echo, short inversion-time inversion recovery, and short T1 inversion time recovery images with the fat component of the BM being suppressed are produced.[1] Fatty marrow displays a characteristic bright signal in both T1- and T2-weighted images. Red marrow is darker than fatty BM; its signal intensity typically equals that of muscle (Figure 22C-2). Neoplastic marrow

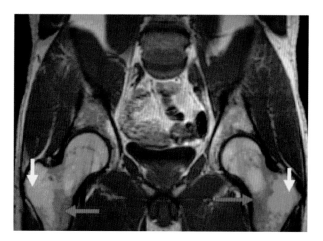

FIGURE 22C-2. T1-weighted coronal pelvis magnetic resonance image showing yellow marrow bright as it is predominantly fatty in consistency (yellow arrows). Normal red marrow is darker than yellow marrow because of the hematopoietic elements (red arrows) but brighter than skeletal muscle, as the marrow still contains some fat.

is also darker than fatty marrow and it is equally or slightly hypointense to red marrow. The major factors responsible for this appearance are increased cellularity and enlarged water content. Figure 22C-3 is the coronal

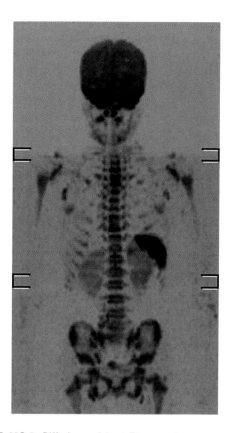

FIGURE 22C-3. Diffusion weighted T1-magnetic resonance image showing red and/or neoplastic marrow in a patient with leukemia.

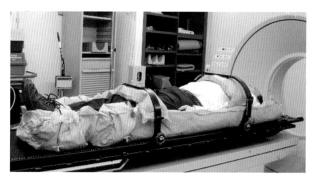

FIGURE 22C-1. Setup for intensity-modulated total marrow irradiation using body Pro-Lok device.

T1-diffusion-weighted MR image showing the red and/or neoplastic bone marrow darker than the yellow marrow in a patient with leukemia.

The clinical treatment volume (CTV) consisted of all the bones in the body from head to midfemur except the forearms and hands (Figure 22C-4). A 3-mm margin is added to form the planning target volume (PTV). The CTV boost consisted of the active BM compartments and was contoured using the diffusion-weighted MR displayed in Figure 22C-2. In this patient, most of the pelvic bones, the upper part of the femur, all of the vertebrae, the majority of the skull, the upper part of the humerus, the sternum, and the clavicles are included in the CTV-boost. Figure 22C-5 displays the CTV boost in the head and neck region, chest, and pelvic regions. Critical organs at risk (OARs) included the lungs, heart, liver, kidneys, brain, eyes, oral cavity, and bowels and were contoured on the axial CT images. A 1-mm gap between the target and the OARs was used to provide more degrees of freedom for the optimization engine.

Treatment Planning

A three-isocenter technique previously developed by our group was employed for the treatment planning in which

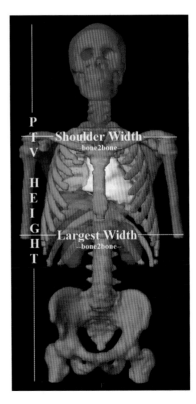

FIGURE 22C-4. Planning target volumes (PTVs) for the three intensity-modulated radiation therapy plans. The head and neck PTV, the chest PTV, and the pelvic PTV are displayed in magenta, orange, and pink, respectively.

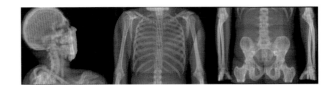

FIGURE 22C-5. Planning target volume boost in the head and neck, chest, and pelvis.

the PTV is divided into three subvolumes (head and neck, chest, and pelvis).[2] The head and neck and the chest volumes are separated at the level of C6. The multileaf collimator (MLC) is rotated by 90° to include the shoulder bones and the humerus in the radiation port when one is treating the chest. The junction between chest and pelvis was at the level of T12 vertebra for this patient. Thus, the kidneys, liver, and bowels were both in the chest and pelvis plans whereas lungs and heart were covered by the chest plan only.

Treatment planning was performed using Eclipse (Varian Medical Systems, Palo Alto, CA). Each of the three subplans consisted of nine fields separated by 40(starting at 0(. The treatment planning of linac-based IM-TMI is a time-consuming process and requires experience. The optimization process can take hours and can converge to a local minimum resulting in unacceptable plan values because of the selection of starting dose volume priorities (DVPs).

To both reduce the subjectivity in optimization process and to obtain acceptable dose distributions within a clinically reasonable time frame, the common dose volume priority (cDVP) method was recently developed by our group.[3] This method employs average priorities derived from a group of similar sized patients as a starting point in the optimization process. Using this method, the average optimization time is reduced from 75 minutes to 45 minutes per plan.

In the patient presented here, treatment optimization took 49 minutes on average per plan. The three plans were then summed to obtain the IM-TMI plan and the fluence map was edited to fine-tune the dose distribution. An additional 75 minutes was required to fine-tune the dose distribution using fluence editing to improve the homogeneity of the dose distribution and to reduce the hot spots in the summed plan.

Traditionally, feathering has been used in radiotherapy to match adjacent fields. Here, we employed electronic feathering using the base plane technique (Varian Medical Systems, Palo Alto, CA). In this technique, one of the adjacent plans is optimized first and then used as the base plan in the optimization of the subsequent plan.[4] The dose distribution of the first plan is thus taken into account to provide an online feathering that results in a more homogeneous dose distribution in the junction regions. We

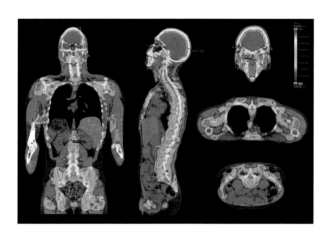

FIGURE 22C-6. Coronal, sagittal, and axial head and neck, chest, and pelvis views of the dose distribution. The 12-Gy (prescription dose) and 16-Gy (boost dose) isodoses are shown in blue and red, respectively.

TABLE 22C–1 Mean Organ at Risk (OAR) Doses With Linac-Based IM-TMI

OAR	Mean Dose, Gy
Lungs	8.0
Heart	7.5
Liver	6.4
Kidneys	6.4
Bowels	7.2
Brain	8.1
Eyes	6.3
Lenses	4.3
Oral cavity	6.0

Note. IM-TMI – intensity-modulated total marrow irradiation.

previously showed that the resultant dose distribution using this technique is very uniform in the junctions and compares well with the measurements.[2]

Figure 22C-6 displays the dose distribution obtained in this study in frontal, sagittal, and axial head and neck, chest, and pelvis views. The 12-Gy isodose (prescription dose) is shown in blue and 16-Gy isodose (boost dose) is shown in red. A PTV coverage of 99% with the prescription dose of 12 Gy, and a PTV-boost coverage of 92% with the prescription dose of 16 Gy was achieved. Mean doses to OARs are listed in the Table 22C-1. The OAR mean organ doses and target coverage shown in Figure 22C-7 demonstrate the successful dose sculpting of desired doses to the targets and a good OAR sparing in this patient. The mean lung dose was 8 Gy, which is well below the reported threshold dose of 9.4 Gy for increased lung complication.[5] Mean OAR doses were observed to increase only slightly (5% to 10%) when simultaneously boosting the active bone marrow to 16 Gy, a 30% escalation.

Clinical Outcome

This patient was treated with our standard TBI protocol. The patient received standard prophylaxis for nausea and vomiting with ondansetron and dexamethasone and for cyclophosphamide toxicity of the bladder with mesna. In addition, he received palifermin for 3 days before TBI to limit the risk of mucositis. A total dose of 12 Gy was delivered using 2-Gy fractions, twice daily. Via a bilateral treatment technique, 18 MV x-rays were delivered at a source–axis distance of 410 cm. A pair of 83% partial lung transmission blocks was used in every fraction to reduce the lung dose to less than 10 Gy. In the future, we plan to treat patients with advanced hematological diseases using the IM-TMI techniques described previously.

Early posttransplant course was characterized by severe mucositis (grade 4) caused by the combined toxicity of chemotherapy and conventional TBI treatment used to treat this patient. The grade 4 mucositis observed required total parental nutrition for 8 days and narcotic analgesics. Stem cell engraftment with recovery of an absolute neutrophil count (ANC) greater than 500/μL and platelet count greater than 20,000/μL occurred on day 10 posttransplant. At 320 days posttransplant, the patient had normal blood counts and remained without evidence of disease recurrence.

We have been exploring the feasibility of linac-based IM-TMI in patients undergoing high-dose chemotherapy and SCT for several years.[3,4] It is well known that TBI causes immunosuppression and importantly also leads to tumor cell kill, augmenting the efficacy of treatment especially in cases where a chemotherapy-resistant cell clones exist. An early study demonstrated a decreased relapse rate in patients in first complete remission undergoing allogeneic SCT when treated with 15.75 Gy compared with those treated with 12 Gy.[6] Clinical studies also reported a 0% recurrence rate with patients with chronic myelogenous leukemia (CML) treated with 15.75 Gy compared with a 25% relapse rate after 12 Gy.[7] However, in both studies, the treatment-related mortality was so high in the 15.75-Gy group that there was no difference in long-term disease-free survival.

We[3,4] and others[8] have shown that IM-TMI can potentially spare surrounding critical organs while achieving a conformal dose delivery to the target BM. Imaging is an integral part of any IMRT procedure and can play an instrumental role in the determination of target and also delivery. The target in hematological malignancies is difficult to define or image. However, it may be reasonable to hypothesize that the active BM is the most important target for the dose escalation in patients with hematological disease, especially in those patients the disease is mostly confined in the BM.

Successful implementation of the IM-TMI technique requires careful consideration of the various biologic, imaging, dosimetric, and treatment delivery issues. It is important to note that it is an experimental treatment technique and its safety and efficacy has to be proven

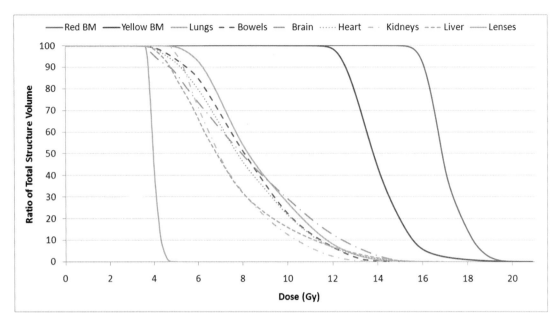

FIGURE 22C-7. Dose–volume histograms obtained in this study demonstrate the dose sculpting to the planning target volume (PTV) boost and to the PTV while reducing the dose to the organs at risk.

through clinical trials before widespread use. To this end, we have designed a prospective phase I clinical trial. Because patients with high-risk acute leukemia have a high relapse rate after allogeneic SCT, new strategies to eliminate the tumor burden before transplantation may be beneficial. We will thus test whether IM-TMI can be safely combined with fludarabine and myeloablative doses of busulfan (FluBu) regimen used before allogeneic SCT. Increasing fractionated doses of IM-TMI will be utilized up to the standard TBI dose (12 Gy) in combination with FluBu and allogeneic SCT. The goal is to establish the safety, tolerability, and transplant-related mortality of this regimen, and to evaluate the how TMI may affect the immune reconstitution post-SCT. Based on these results, we plan to design new clinical trials aimed at investigating the efficacy of higher doses of IM-TMI and chemotherapy-based conditioning regimens in allogeneic SCT.

References

1. Schmidt GP, Schoenberg SO, Reiser MF, Baur-Melnyk A. Whole-body MR imaging of bone marrow. *Eur J Radiol.* 2005;55: 33–40.

2. Wilkie JR, Tiryaki H, Smith BD, et al. Feasibility study for linac-based intensity modulated total marrow irradiation. *Med Phys.* 2008;35:5609–5618.

3. Yeginer M, Aydogan B. Feasibility study of linac-based IMTMI for clinical implementation [abstract]. *Med Phys.* 2009;36:2552.

4. Aydogan B, Mundt AJ, Roeske JC. Linac-based intensity modulated total marrow irradiation (IM-TMI). *Technol Cancer Res Treat.* 2006;5:513–519.

5. Volpe AD, Ferreri AJM, Annaloro C, et al. Lethal pulmonary complications significantly correlate with individually assessed mean lung dose in patients with hematologic malignancies treated with total body irradiation. *Int J Radiat Oncol Biol Phys.* 2002;52:483–488.

6. Clift RA, Buckner CD, FR Appelbaum FR, et al. Allogeneic marrow transplantation in patients with acute myeloid leukemia in first remission: a randomized trial of two irradiation regimens. *Blood.* 1990;76:1867–1871.

7. Clift RA, Buckner CD, Appelbaum FR, et al. Allogeneic marrow transplantation in patients with chronic myeloid leukemia in the chronic phase: a randomized trial of two irradiation regimens. *Blood.* 1991;77:1660–1665.

8. Wong JY, Rosenthal J, Liu A, et al. Image-guided total-marrow irradiation using helical tomotherapy in patients with multiple myeloma and acute leukemia undergoing hematopoietic cell transplantation. *Int J Radiat Oncol Biol Phys.* 2009;73:273–279.

MVCT-Guided Total Marrow Irradiation Using Helical Tomotherapy in a Patient with ALL

Case Study

Jeffrey Y.C. Wong, MD, An Liu, PhD

Patient History

A 60-year-old man presented with fatigue and dyspnea on exertion. A complete blood count showed a white blood cell (WBC) count of $57.8 \times 10^3/\mu L$ (with 95% circulating blasts), a platelet count of $28 \times 10^3/\mu L$, and a hemoglobin level of 9.1 g/dL. Bone marrow biopsy showed precursor B-cell acute lymphoblastic leukemia (ALL) with 95% blasts and poor prognosis cytogenetics. Cerebrospinal fluid (CSF) cytology was negative. Computed tomography (CT) scans of the chest, abdomen, and pelvis were negative.

Induction chemotherapy was initiated with daunorubicin, vincristine, prednisone, and L-asparaginase. Repeat bone marrow biopsy demonstrated no residual leukemic blasts and normal cytogenetics. Repeat CSF cytology was negative. He underwent a second induction therapy of cytarabine, and mitoxantrone followed by consolidation chemotherapy consisting of cyclophosphamide, 6-mercaptopurine, and cytarabine. After identifying a matched-related donor, he was entered on an in-house pilot allogeneic bone marrow transplantation trial using a conditioning regimen of total marrow irradiation (TMI) and the reduced-intensity chemotherapy conditioning of fludarabine and melphalan. We elected to treat him with daily image guidance using helical tomotherapy (Tomotherapy Inc, Madison, WI).

Simulation

The patient was scanned on a large-bore (85-cm) CT simulator with 60-cm field of view (Philips Medical System, Andover, MA). Noncontrast CT scans using 8-mm slices were obtained during normal shallow breathing, inspiration, and expiration phases. The normal shallow breathing CT data set was used for dose calculation and planning. The inspiration and expiration CT data sets were registered to the planning CT to account for changes in organ position during respiration. A body Vac-Lok bag (CIVCO Medical Systems, Kalona, IA) and three thermoplastic masks over the head and shoulders, chest and abdomen were used for immobilization (Figure 22D-1). Esophacat was used to visualize the esophagus for planning purposes. The couch height was set 10 cm below the isocenter of the gantry and the patient was positioned on the couch so that the top of the head was less than 5 cm from the end of the couch. These settings were used to maximize the available couch length for the CT scanning and tomotherapy treatment delivery.

Treatment Planning

Target and avoidance structures were contoured on an Eclipse treatment planning system (Varian Medical Systems, Palo Alto, CA). Avoidance structures contoured included organs at risk: the lungs, heart, kidneys, liver, esophagus, oral cavity, parotid glands, thyroid gland, eyes, lens, optic chiasm, optic nerves, stomach, small bowel, rectum, and bladder. Clinical target volumes (CTVs) included skeletal bone, brain, spleen, testes, and major lymph node chains (cervical, supraclavicular, axillary, mediastinal, para-aortic, pelvic, inguinal, and femoral).

The inspiration and expiration CT data sets were registered to the planning CT so that an internal target volume (ITV) of the ribs, esophagus, kidneys, spleen, and

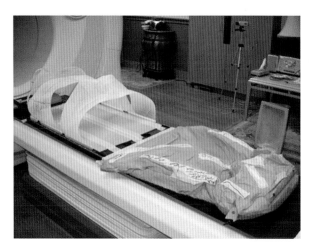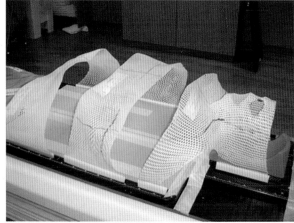

FIGURE 22D-1. Vac-Lok and thermoplastic mask immobilization setup used during simulation and therapy.

liver could be created to account for organ movement during respiration. Additional 5-mm to 10-mm margins were added to the individual CTVs in areas where larger setup uncertainty was observed. These areas included bone in the shoulder regions, lower and upper extremities, and posterior spinous processes. The spinal cord (part of the CTV) was outlined separately to avoid hot spots during planning. The mandible and maxillary bones were excluded per protocol from the CTV in an effort to minimize oral cavity dose and, thus, oral mucositis. Treatment planning images were then transferred to the Hi-Art TomoTherapy treatment planning system.

The helical tomotherapy plan was designed such that a minimum of 85% of the target received the prescribed dose (12 Gy). A jaw size of 2.5 cm, pitch of 0.4, and a modulation factor of 2.5 were used in the treatment planning process. Table 22D-1 shows the optimization settings used in this patient. The final treatment plan

TABLE 22D–1 Optimization Settings Used for Treatment Planning

Clinical Target Volumes	Importance	Max Dose	Max Penalty	DVH Volume	Prescription Dose	Min Dose	Min Penalty
Bone	50	12	1000	85	12	12	300
Brain	10	12	1000	85	11.5	11.5	1
Spinal cord	10	11.5	1000	85	11.5	11.5	10
Lymph nodes	30	12	1000	85	12	12	10
Spleen	10	12	1000	85	12	12	100
Testes	1	11.5	100	85	11.5	11.5	1

Organs at Risk	Importance	Max Dose	Max Penalty	DVH Volume	DVH Dose	DVH Penalty
Bladder	1	12	1	40	6	3
Body	1	12	1	40	10	1
Esophagus	10	10	1	10	3.5	100
Eyes	1	12	1	40	6	1
Heart	1	9.6	1	15	4.8	100
Intestine (bowel)	5	7.2	1	10	3.5	100
Kidneys	3	12	1	20	6	100
Larynx/hHypopharynx	1	10	1	20	6	1
Lens	1	2.5	100	50	2	10
Liver	3	12	1	20	6	10
Lungs	10	10	10	15	4.8	300
Optic Nerve	1	12	1	40	6	1
Oral Cavity	10	10	1	10	3.6	100
Parotids	1	11.2	1	10	5.6	100
Prostate	1	10	1	20	8	1
Rectum	1	10	1	10	3.6	100
Stomach	10	10	10	10	3.6	300
Thyroid	1	10	1	10	4.8	100

Note. DVH = dose–volume histogram.

showed significant sparing of normal organs (Figure 22D-2). Figures 22D-3 and 22D-4 show dose–volume histograms (DVHs) for the CTVs and organs at risk (OARs). Table 22D-2 displays the D_{50} and D_{10} doses for each OAR. From our experience to date, the D_{50} organ doses are reduced to approximately 15% to 65% of the CTV D_{50} dose.[1-3]

Treatment Delivery

Before initiation of treatment, quality assurance (QA) was performed. Film was placed in a tissue-equivalent phantom and exposed to the planned treatment. Film dosimetry was then compared with the treatment plan. In addition, an ion chamber measurement was acquired as a measurement of absolute dose.

For each treatment session, the patient was immobilized in the customized Vac-Lok bag and thermoplastic masks, and aligned to the lasers. Two megavoltage CT (MVCT) scans were then performed and fused to the planning CT. One MVCT scanned from the orbits to the upper thorax and the other scanned from the top of the kidneys to the iliac crest. The couch shifts needed to align the upper scans and lower scans were compared. As per protocol, if the differences between upper and lower scan couch shifts were 1 cm or less in the X, Y, Z directions; the shifts were averaged and treatment initiated. The resultant beam-on time was approximately 42 minutes.

Because the current treatment table on the tomotherapy unit has a maximum travel length of approximately 140 cm, the lower extremities were treated on a conventional linear accelerator through standard anterior–posterior/posterior-anterior (AP–PA) fields because of the lack of sensitive organs in this area. At the time of treatment planning, a radio-opaque marker was placed in the proximal thigh region to define the lower border (50% isodose line) of the tomotherapy plan. The AP–PA fields were gapped to this border at midplane.

The patient received a prescribed dose of 1.5 Gy twice daily on days −7 to −4 with a minimum 6-hour separation between fractions. Fludarabine was administered intravenously (IV) (25 mg/m²/day) from days −7 to −3 and melphalan (140 mg/m² IV) on day −2 followed by hematopoietic stem cell reinfusion on day 0. Supportive care and treatment for prevention of graft-versus-host disease (GVHD; tacrolimus and sirolimus) were given according to institution standard guidelines.

Clinical Outcome

The patient's hospital course was relatively uneventful. He experienced regimen-related grade 2 nausea and vomiting (by National Cancer Institute common toxicity criteria version 3), grade 2 diarrhea, and grade 3 mucositis. The WBC nadir occurred on day 0 and platelet count

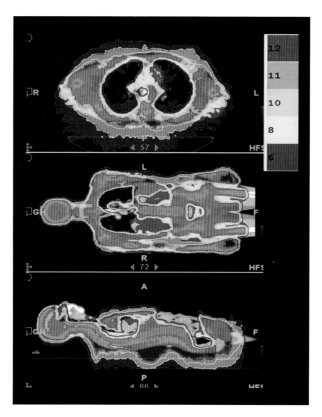

FIGURE 22D-2. Color wash of final treatment plan with doses from 6 Gy to 12 Gy displayed.

nadir on day 2. The first evidence of engraftment was observed at day 11 with platelet counts greater than $20 \times 10^3/$ dL. By day 19, his absolute neutrophil count was greater than 500/dL. He was discharged on day 29 with no evidence of acute GVHD.

He has been followed at least monthly since discharge. Follow-up bone marrow biopsies on days 34, 83, 205, and 345 have continued to show morphologic and cytogenetic complete remission, 100% donor chimerism, and mild decrease in trilineage hematopoiesis. After stopping GVHD prophylaxis, the patient developed mild chronic GVHD with rash and mild elevation of liver transaminases, which resolved after immunosuppressive agents were started. At his most recent follow-up (day 440), he was continuing to do well with no clinical signs of recurrence or GVHD while on tapering doses of immunosuppressants.

The methodology and initial clinical results from two clinical trials using our tomotherapy-based image-guided TMI approach have recently been published.[1-3] In the most recent report,[1] 13 multiple myeloma (MM) patients were treated on an autologous tandem hematopoietic cell transplant (HCT) phase I trial with high-dose melphalan, followed 6 weeks later by TMI. Dose levels were 10 Gy, 12 Gy, 14 Gy, and 16 Gy at 2 Gy delivered once or twice daily. On a separate allogeneic HCT trial, eight patients (five acute myeloid leukemia, one ALL, one non-Hodgkin's

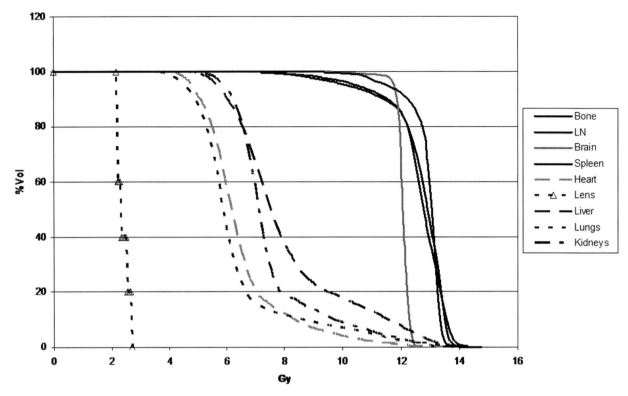

FIGURE 22D-3. Dose–volume histograms (DVHs) for clinical target volume (CTV) target regions (bone, lymph nodes, brain, and spleen). Organs at risk DVHs from right to left are liver, kidneys, heart, lung, and lens, which show significant dose sparing relative to CTV DVHs.

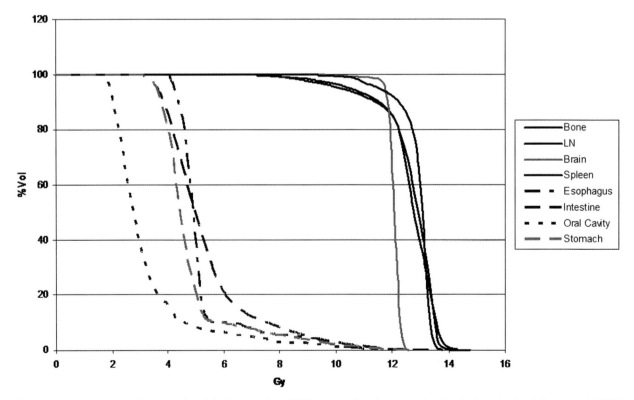

FIGURE 22D-4. Dose–volume histograms for clinical target volume (CTV) target regions (bone, lymph nodes, brain, and spleen). Organs at risk DVHs from right to left are intestine, esophagus, stomach, and oral cavity, which show significant dose sparing relative to CTV DVHs.

TABLE 22D–2 Doses to Normal Organs Using Image-Guided Total Marrow Irradiation

Organs at Risk	D_{50}	D_{10}
Bladder	9.1	12.7
Esophagus	4.9	5.6
Eyes	5.6	8.1
Heart	6.2	8.3
Kidneys	7.1	10.0
Lens	2.4	2.6
Liver	7.6	11.6
Lungs	5.9	8.8
Optic nerve	6.6	12.3
Oral cavity	2.8	4.5
Parotids	5.4	6.5
Rectum	5.3	6.8
Small intestine	5.0	7.5
Stomach	4.4	5.8
Thyroid	5.1	6.0

lymphoma, one MM) were treated with TMI plus total lymphatic irradiation (TLI) plus splenic irradiation to 12 Gy (1.5 Gy twice daily) combined with fludarabine and melphalan (includes case study reported here). For the 13 patients on the tandem autologous HCT trial, grade 1–2 acute toxicities were primarily observed. Six reported no vomiting, nine no mucositis, six no fatigue, and eight no diarrhea. For the eight patients on the allogeneic HCT trial, grade 2–3 nausea, vomiting, mucositis, and diarrhea were observed. No grade 4 nonhematologic toxicity was observed on either trial and all patients engrafted successfully. These initial results are encouraging and compared favorably to standard total body irradiation (TBI) trials. These results also support further evaluation of this approach as a means to escalate targeted TBI dose with acceptable toxicity or to offer TBI-containing regimens to patients unable to tolerate standard TBI regimens.

References

1. Wong JYC, Rosenthal J, Liu A, et al. Image guided total marrow irradiation (TMI) using helical tomotherapy in patients with multiple myeloma and acute leukemia undergoing hematopoietic cell transplantation (HCT). *Int J Radiat Oncol Biol Phys.* 2009;73:273–279.
2. Wong JYC, Liu A, Schultheiss T, et al. Targeted total marrow irradiation using three-dimensional image-guided tomographic intensity-modulated radiation therapy: an alternative to standard total body irradiation. *Biol Blood Marrow Transplant.* 2006;12:306–315.
3. Schultheiss TE, Wong J, Liu A, et al. Image-guided total marrow and total lymphatic irradiation using helical tomotherapy. *Int J Radiat Oncol Biol Phys.* 2007;67:1259–1267.

KV CBCT-Guided IMRT Using the Varian Trilogy System in a Patient with Non-Hodgkin's Lymphoma

Case Study

Loren K. Mell, MD, William Y. Song, PhD

Patient History

A 69-year-old man with a history of stage IV non-Hodgkin's lymphoma (NHL) presented with urinary frequency and nocturia. He was initially diagnosed with NHL 4 years previously, when an enlarged mesenteric lymph node was found incidentally during a laparotomy. The initial pathology showed mixed diffuse large B-cell and high-grade follicular lymphoma, with bone marrow involvement. He received eight cycles of R-CHOP (rituximab, cyclophosphamide, doxorubicin, vincristine, and prednisolone), and later underwent R-ICE (rituximab, ifosfamide, carboplatin, and etoposide) and autologous stem cell transplant for refractory disease.

The patient did well and was without evidence of disease until a follow-up positron emission tomography (PET) scan revealed a 3.5-cm mass anterior to the bladder, with a standardized uptake value (SUV) of 9.6, with no other sites of abnormal uptake. A computed tomography (CT) scan revealed a mass anterior to the bladder (Figure 22E-1). The biopsy was positive for recurrent NHL. The patient was otherwise doing well and had no hematuria, pelvic pain, fevers, night sweats, or weight loss. Physical examination was unremarkable.

The consensus recommendation of our multidisciplinary bone marrow transplant conference was for localized radiation therapy (RT). We elected to treat him with daily kilovoltage (kV) cone-beam CT (CBCT) guidance on a Varian Trilogy linear accelerator (Varian Medical Systems, Palo Alto, CA).

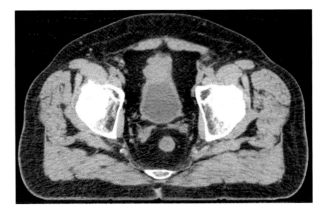

FIGURE 22E-1. Axial computed tomography image illustrating the perivesicular mass anterior to the bladder.

Simulation

The patient underwent CT simulation in the supine position (Figure 22E-1), with custom immobilization using a foam cradle. Whole body images were obtained with 2.5-mm slice thickness on our departmental GE discovery CT simulator (GE Healthcare, Waukesha, WI). No intravenous or oral contrast was administered during simulation.

Treatment Planning

The CT simulation data set was exported to the Eclipse treatment planning system (Varian Medical Systems,

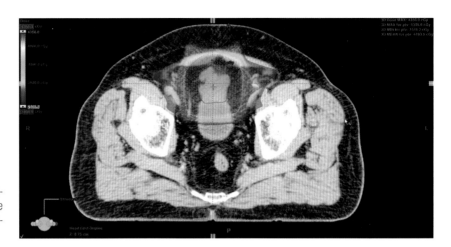

FIGURE 22E-2. Intensity-modulated radiation therapy plan used in this patient. Note that a generous 1.5-cm clinical target volume to planning target volume was used.

Palo Alto, CA). The gross tumor volume (GTV) consisting of the visualized perivesicular mass was delineated on the planning CT and a 15-mm margin was applied to generate the planning target volume (PTV). The following organs at risk (OARs) were also delineated: bladder, rectum, and pelvic bones. A five-field IMRT plan (beam angles: 0°, 51°, 102°, 258°, and 309°) was subsequently generated (Figure 22E-2). The prescription dose was 40 Gy in 2.0-Gy daily fractions delivered to the PTV.

Treatment Delivery

Before each fraction, the patient was instructed to void his bladder. After he was positioned on the treatment table using skin marks, a kV CBCT was obtained for setup verification using the On-Board Imager (Varian Medical Systems, Palo Alto, CA) integrated with the Trilogy linear accelerator. An example CBCT image of the perivesicular mass is shown in Figure 22E-3. A regular "pelvis" protocol was used that includes half-fan mode, 125 kV, 80 mA, 13-ms/frame, and 360° scanning. In this mode, up to

50-cm field-of-view (FOV) can be selected for pelvic visualization. The default setting in our clinic (45 cm FOV) was used in this patient. Shifts were then made each day based on the CBCT scan.

The average daily shifts in the anterior–posterior, superior–inferior, and right–left directions were 0.17 cm (standard deviation [SD] = 0.29 cm), 0.15 cm (SD = 0.19 cm), and 0.17 cm (SD = 0.28 cm), respectively (Figure 22E-4). Corresponding maximum daily shifts were 0.7 cm, 0.6 cm, and 0.8 cm, respectively. During treatment, the tumor mass regressed significantly, with a 74% reduction in volume noted by the last day of treatment (Figure 22E-5). Bladder volumes were fairly consistent with each fraction (Figure 22E-6) and were smaller than at CT simulation, because the patient was specifically instructed to void before each treatment. Image guidance using the CBCT approach added approximately 5 minutes to the patient's daily treatment.

To evaluate the effectiveness of the IGRT procedure implemented for this patient, all GTV contours were drawn and overlaid on the planning CT to estimate the minimum uniform margin that would have encompassed

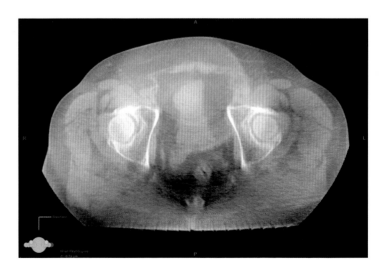

FIGURE 22E-3. A cone-beam computed tomography scan of the pelvis performed before treatment illustrating the perivesicular mass.

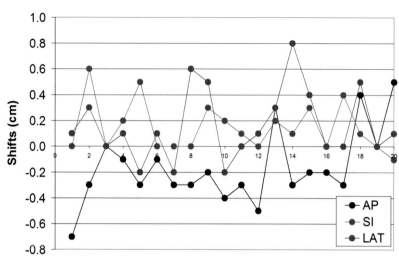

FIGURE 22E-4. Daily shift data based on daily cone-beam computed tomography imaging after alignment was performed to skin marks.

the GTV for each fraction (Figure 22E-7). We estimated that a 10-mm margin would have been sufficient to encompass the GTV throughout the treatment course. Therefore, in retrospect, the 15-mm margin used was adequate. Hypothetically, however, because the 15-mm margin PTV volume was 302 cc and the 10-mm margin PTV volume is 170 cc, if a 10-mm margin had been used, we could have reduced dose to 132 cc of normal tissue.

To evaluate the accuracy of our IGRT procedure, the center-of-mass (COM) of each GTV drawn was calculated and shifted to align with the planning GTV, assuming that the COM alignment represents the perfect image registration for IGRT. The recorded shifts were: mean (SD) of 1.3 mm (1.1 mm), -2.1 mm (2.1 mm), and 0.3 mm (3.9 mm) in left–right (+left), anterior–posterior (+post), and superior–inferior (+sup), respectively. The largest standard deviation occurred, as expected, in the

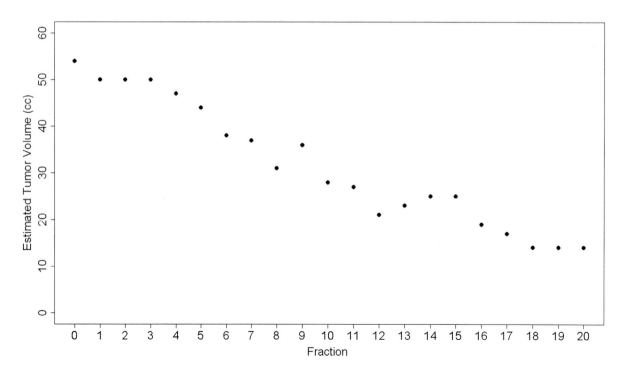

FIGURE 22E-5. Plot of tumor volume over the course of treatment.

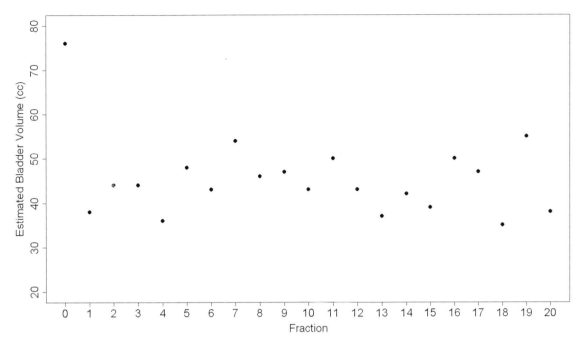

FIGURE 22E-6. Plot of bladder volume over the course of treatment.

superior–inferior direction, because of the poorer image resolution in that direction (i.e., 2.5-mm CT slice thickness). In general, the shifts were minor (< 3 mm), indicating that the quality of image registration performed at each fraction was high and consistent.

Patient Outcome

The patient tolerated treatment well without significant acute complications. He has recently completed treatment and will be undergoing his first follow-up PET–CT scan in 3 months.

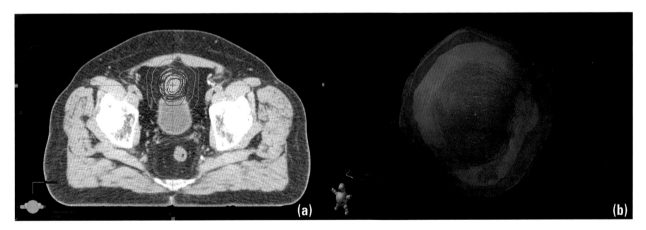

FIGURE 22E-7. (a) Axial view of the pelvic planning computed tomography (CT), with the gross tumor volume contours delineated from the daily cone beam CTs (CBCTs) overlaid (red), along with 1.0 cm (green) and 1.5 cm (cyan) uniform planning margins. The 1.5-cm margin was used for treatment. **(b)** Three-dimensional rendering of daily tumor volumes encompassed by the actual (1.5 cm, green) and theoretical (1.0 cm, cyan) planning target volumes.

Chapter 23

PEDIATRIC TUMORS: OVERVIEW

THOMAS E. MERCHANT, DO, PhD, CHRIS BELTRAN, PhD

Image-guided radiation therapy (IGRT) is broadly defined for children and includes sequential imaging before, during, and after treatment that may be used to improve localization or verify position of the patient, target, and normal tissues. Although relatively new to the field of pediatric radiation oncology, IGRT holds significant promise to increase the precision of radiation therapy (RT) for children and reduce dose to normal tissues. The latter will allow a reduction in the margins required to create the planning target volume (PTV) for most treatment sites.

The process of localizing children for RT has included the use of custom-shaped immobilization devices created from thermoplastic materials or deflatable cushions filled with polystyrene beads. Other unique devices have been constructed according to the requirements of the particular procedure and patient cooperation. In many instances, localization relies on temporary or permanent marking of the skin and, more recently, interstitially placed radiopaque markers.

Conventional kilovoltage (kV) x-ray images may be acquired in the position of treatment using a fluoroscopic RT simulator or computed tomography (CT) scanner configured for radiation simulation. These images are used to document localization of the treatment site and shape treatment fields that conform to the target of interest and avoid adjacent normal tissues. In the simplest form, the treatment field has a shape corresponding to the target, which, along with a defined center and standardized graticule, corresponds to the radiographic bony anatomy and soft tissues.

In the field of pediatric radiation oncology, the classic large and parallel-opposed fields continue to be relevant with examples including whole-abdominal and whole-lung irradiation for Wilms' tumor and Ewing's sarcoma; flank irradiation for Wilms' tumor; mantle, para-aortic-spleen, and pelvic irradiation for Hodgkin's disease (Figure 23-1); cranial irradiation for high-risk leukemia; and total body irradiation (TBI) as a component of stem cell transplantation. Because these fields deploy relatively generous

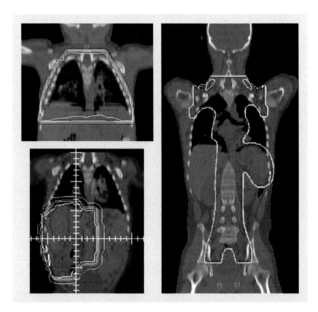

FIGURE 23-1. Examples of large field irradiation in pediatric oncology. Whole-lung irradiation for Wilms' tumor (upper left), flank irradiation for Wilms' tumor (lower left), and mantle, para-aortic, and pelvic irradiation for Hodgkin's disease (right).

margins surrounding the treatment volume, their localization and verification requirements for daily treatment remain minimal.

With the advent of three-dimensional conformal RT (3DCRT) and high-segment-number intensity-modulated RT (IMRT), tomographic arc therapy, and proton beam therapy for children, investigators continue to pursue treatment volume reduction with the aim of limiting collateral dose to normal tissue.[1-3] Institutional and cooperative group studies have been designed for pediatric, central nervous system (CNS), musculoskeletal, and certain solid tumors to systematically reduce the clinical target volume (CTV) margin in prospective study designs. There are a number of poignant examples: for pediatric rhabdomyosarcoma, the margin surrounding gross-residual tumor has been decreased from 1.5 cm to 1.0 cm; for the common pediatric CNS tumors, the CTV margin has been reduced from 2.0 cm to 1.5 cm for medulloblastoma, from 1.0 cm to 0.5 cm for ependymoma, and from 1.0 cm to 0.5 cm for low-grade glioma.[4–10] Although CTV margins have been substantially reduced, little has changed with respect to the PTV margin which is approximately 1.0 cm for musculoskeletal tumors and 0.5 cm for CNS tumors unless rigorous methods of immobilization and verification are utilized.

The process of daily localization and position verification is where pediatric patients may have the most to gain. As the CTV margins become smaller and perhaps less forgiving, the PTV margin becomes increasingly important. Reducing this margin further requires rigorous immobilization and verification, and a better understanding of the subcomponents of the PTV known in the parlance of the International Commission on Radiation Units and Measurements (ICRU) as the internal margin (IM) and setup margin (SM).[11,12] First and foremost, as margins are reduced, the accuracy of the initial targeting and the precision of daily treatment become important because of their impact on disease control. Improving the rigor of daily positioning and verification, which is the fundamental goal of IGRT, may lead to improved disease control even while the target volume margins are reduced.

In past practice, portal images were taken at the beginning and at least once per week to verify the position of the treatment field with respect to bony anatomy. Because of the known variability in day-to-day positioning, patient motion during treatment and changes in anatomy over time were considered, but it was not practical to make real-time changes. With the advent of in-room imaging and its integration with treatment planning systems, it is now feasible to quantitatively evaluate patient positioning and make real-time changes that are verifiable. With the focus on target volume reduction and normal tissue sparing in pediatric radiation oncology, the new question is how to incorporate image-guided therapy in pediatric protocols and ensure that the centers approved for the treatment of children are able to perform image-guided therapy in a reliable manner. The solution is to develop guidelines for pediatric protocols that require in-room imaging in order for patients to receive treatment with reduced target volume margins. The alternative to in-room imaging would be larger target volume margins. To ensure that a particular treatment center is capable of treating with reduced margins, successful completion of a benchmark for immobilization and verification should be required for the treatment center. Similar benchmarks have been developed for the use of IMRT and proton beam therapy in pediatric protocols.[13–14] In addition, specific studies for low-grade glioma and ependymoma require completion of an image registration before acceptance of the patient data.[15]

We have proposed a localization benchmark for pediatric patients that would consist of phantoms containing internal structures that would qualify an institution's preferred method. One phantom would be used for CT simulation, contouring, planning, and digitally reconstructed radiograph (DRR) construction or other items. Another phantom would be used in the treatment room for localization and delivery. Each phantom would contain a removable dosimeter in order to measure the dose delivered by the treatment planning CT unit and the institutional localization method when relevant. Film inserts would also be important to verify accurate spatial delivery of the treatment dose. A localization benchmark for pediatric oncology should be able to quantitatively measure the accuracy of the following localization methods: the imaging of metallic fiducial markers, bone, and soft tissue when possible with the following devices: CT-on-Rails, megavoltage (MV) ports, kV ports, kV cone-beam CT (CBCT), MV CBCT, and ultrasound. In addition, radio frequency transponders, frameless array methods, and surface mapping methods should be allowed for in the localization benchmark.

Image-Guided Target and Tissue Delineation

Targeting

With the exception of classic large field irradiation as described earlier, all treatments in children should be volume-based and target volumes should be defined according to the recommendations of the International Commission on Radiation Units and Measurements reports 50 and 62 with disease-specific margins that are initially empirical and through research refined in phase II or III trials.[11,12] The initial experience with volume-based treatment in the Children's Oncology Group (COG) has been positive with high rates of compliance in CNS and musculoskeletal/solid tumor protocols. The latter have been slower to evolve as they continue to include classic fields or conventional therapy as a treatment option. As newer protocols are developed and ongoing protocols are amended, we will continue our effort to move toward volume-based target definitions.

- gross tumor volume (GTV) – residual tumor and/or tumor bed
- clinical target volume (CTV) – subclinical microscopic disease
- internal target volume (ITV) – temporal variation of the CTV
- planning target volume (PTV) – position uncertainty

The GTV is the first of the target volumes to be contoured, and is defined as the clinically observed tumor. In the realm of IGRT, the GTV is defined with the aid of CT, various magnetic resonance (MR) sequences, and positron emission tomography (PET). These imaging modalities are electronically fused in the treatment planning system where the GTV is contoured.

The next volume to be considered is the CTV, which is an extension of the GTV meant to account for microscopic tumor extension into surrounding tissue. In practice, this margin may also be uniformly added to the GTV; however, the CTV should be anatomically confined and not include structures that are known barriers to the particular disease. At-risk lymph nodes may be included in the CTV. Ideally, the CTV should receive a tumoricidal dose of radiation and all other tissues should be spared. This is not the case in clinical RT because of uncertainties in the position of the CTV and beam delivery.

There are two clinically significant forms of temporal variation in the CTV that may be present during RT. One form is physiological motion of surrounding normal tissues including breathing, cardiac motion, peristalsis, and periodic organ deformation (e.g., bladder, rectum). This type of temporal variation is somewhat regular, always present, and may be predictable or prevented. To account for physiological motion, an IM is added to the CTV to create the ITV. Poignant examples in adult and pediatric patients include lung tumors and neuroblastoma, respectively. The IM can be measured by using four-dimensional (4D) CT, 4D MR, or other imaging modalities that serially measure organ motion. In practice, an ITV is not always required and only the CTV is contoured.

The other form of variation involves changes in shape and volume of the CTV or surrounding tissue. These changes are irregular and cannot be predicted; therefore, they should not be accounted for by the IM. Examples include weight gain or loss and tumor shrinkage or tumor growth. Patients with brainstem glioma are often treated concurrently with steroids, which result in weight gain. Children with craniopharyngioma experience cyst expansion or contraction during treatment. These forms of temporal variation can only be accounted for with adaptive planning.

The last target volume to be considered is the PTV, which is created by adding a SM around the CTV or ITV, accounting for patient setup and machine delivery uncertainties. Setup uncertainty is the day-to-day setup variation that is inherent in fractionated treatment, referred to as interfraction uncertainty, and it also includes the intrafractional motion. Because both the ITV and PTV contain normal tissue and receive the full prescription dose, attempts at safely minimizing them should be requisite in protocols. Reducing the PTV margin is a critical step in reducing dose to normal tissue. Consider a typical brain tumor with a CTV of 33 cc. Increasing the volume by adding a PTV margin of 5 mm would increase the target to 65 cc. In this case, the shell of normal tissue being targeted because of setup uncertainties is as large as the volume considered at risk.

Normal Tissue Tolerances

Investigators in radiation oncology have discussed normal tissue tolerances and hope to achieve a consensus for future guidelines based on published information, institution or cooperative group experience, and contemporary and accepted guidelines. Normal tissue tolerance guidelines are the subject of concern for many investigators who do not treat a substantial number of children and those who are unfamiliar with the concepts driving newer treatment protocols. These concerns often prompt treating physicians to contact investigators asking for recommendations based on limited clinical information. Target volume coverage and protocol aims are compromised when the basis for normal tissue tolerance guidelines are not clear or widely accepted. Further, sufficient data exist for certain tumors to suggest that adhering to normal tissue tolerance guidelines will lower the tumor control probability.

Guidelines for spinal cord and kidney serve as poignant examples. In the era of 3DCRT treatment planning, there is a great opportunity to study normal tissue tolerances based on acquired radiation volumetric data and clinical information (toxicity monitoring, serum chemistry, and hematological data) that are acquired for routine patient management and protocol performance.

Image-Guided Treatment Delivery

Motion Management

The impact of target volume and organ at risk (OAR) motion during treatment delivery is poorly understood in general and in particular for the pediatric patient. Newer methods of RT planning and delivery have increased our ability to study target and normal tissue motion. As these methods reach widespread use, it is imperative that they be implemented in clinical protocols, especially those that seek to reduce target volume margins or that have toxicity reduction as a primary objective.

The CTV and PTV margins used in clinical trials for extracranial tumors have, until recently, deployed margins that were relatively large, thus reducing the requirements for understanding motion during treatment. Newer studies, like those designed for soft tissue and bone sarcomas, reduce clinical target volume margins and allow for a range of PTV margins. This raises the concern about the use of limited margin RT in the setting of significant physiologic motion. It is not clear if there are sufficient resources to study target motion at the cooperative group level. Priority should be given to the study of motion induced by the respiratory excursion, which is known to affect the diaphragm, chest wall, and kidneys.

Immobilization

The process of localizing children for RT has included the use of customized immobilization devices created from thermoplastic materials or deflatable cushions filled with polystyrene beads. Other unique devices have been constructed according to the requirements of the specific procedure and patient cooperation. In many instances, localization relies on temporary or permanent marking on the skin and on rare occasions interstitially placed radio-opaque markers. The latter is becoming increasingly important in proton beam therapy. Investigators in the COG have a longstanding interest in defining PTV margins based on immobilization and localization. This would require that institutions pass an immobilization benchmark to show their level of precision when using such devices. The model would include the image registration benchmark that was implemented for the ACNS0221 study for pediatric low-grade glioma and the requirements mentioned earlier.[15]

Localization and Verification

At a recent meeting of the COG radiation oncology discipline, IGRT was the focus of discussion and there were presentations by experts in cranial and extracranial pediatric localization and verification. Ongoing studies at several of the COG-approved radiation oncology facilities have shown the equivalence between frame-based and frameless stereotaxy for intracranial tumors, the advantages of interstitial radio-opaque markers over anatomic localization and their impact on set-up uncertainty, and the value of daily cone-beam CT (CBCT) in different clinical settings based on the use of anesthesia, positioning, and immobilization devices. A variety of scenarios are envisioned where radiation- and nonradiation-based onboard imaging might be used for localization and verification. Forthcoming data are likely to drive the development of newer PTV and OAR definitions and guidelines in future studies.

Prospective Estimation of Setup Margins

Investigators at St Jude Children's Research Hospital designed a prospective study to estimate the setup margin component of the PTV margin for children treated using 3D CRT or IMRT regardless of treatment site. The study is currently ongoing and employs MV CBCT. Because it has accrued more than 200 children, it is unique in scope and objective among studies in pediatric radiation oncology. Preliminary data from this protocol have been presented that have included more than 10,000 MV CBCT studies.[16]

The protocol deploys an investigational device called the imaging beam line (IBL), which is adapted from the Siemens MV CBCT system (Siemens Medical Solutions, Concord, CA). The IBL replaces the standard tungsten target with a low-Z (carbon) target, removes the flattening

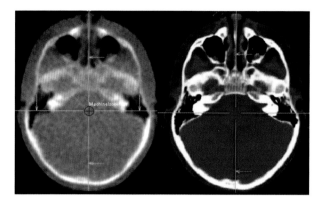

FIGURE 23-2. Axial images of a 5-year-old girl treated in the supine position. The image on the left is a single slice of a 1-cGy imaging beam line cone-beam computed tomography scan. The image on the right is a simulation computed tomography image of the same area.

filter, and the waveguide is detuned to lower the electron energy from 6 MeV to 4 MeV. This results in a mean photon energy of 0.8 MV.[17,18] The dose of the MV CBCT used in the pediatric study is approximately 1 cGy at isocenter, which allows for good contrast of soft bone, water, and lung.[18] Figure 23-2 shows an example of a 1 cGy IBL CBCT image along with the simulation CT. If one considers that an orthogonal pair of portal images would require approximately 2 cGy per image, there is considerable dose reduction with more information.

The protocol specifies imaging with the IBL MV CBCT before each treatment and after every-other-day treatment. The pretreatment imaging will be used to estimate the interfraction uncertainty and the posttreatment imaging will be used to estimate the intrafractional uncertainty. In brief, the imaging studies are automatically registered to the treatment planning CT to generate offsets in X, Y, and Z. These offsets are used to calculate a vector upon which decisions are made to proceed with shifting the patient according to the offset before treatment or attempting to improve alignment of the patient with repeat imaging when the vector exceeds a certain threshold. This threshold is different for body sites versus head and neck or intracranial tumor locations. Although rotational corrections are not performed, these valuable data are recorded for protocol purposes and post hoc analysis to determine the benefit and need for rotational corrections in the future.

Preliminary results, as shown in Table 23-1, suggest that margins as small as 2 mm may be appropriate for patients with brain and head and neck tumors with slightly larger margins for those treated in the prone position compared with supine and for those treated without anesthesia compared with those treated with anesthesia. Similarly, larger margins are required for patients treated at extracranial body sites with differences based on the use of anesthesia versus no anesthesia.

TABLE 23–1 The Required Setup Margins in mm for Various Groups of Pediatric Radiation Therapy Patients Using St Jude Children's Hospital Data: a Standard Geometric Margin Formula[16,23]

Site	Group	Number	Pretreatment Lat	Long	Vert	Posttreatment Lat	Long	Vert
	All	153	3.2	3.9	3.4	1.8	2.0	2.0
	Supine	119	2.8	4.0	3.3	1.4	1.7	1.8
	Prone	34	4.5	3.4	3.8	2.6	2.1	2.2
	GA	70	3.0	3.8	3.4	1.4	1.7	1.5
Head	No GA	83	3.4	3.9	3.4	2.0	2.2	2.2
	Supine with GA	53	2.8	3.8	3.3	1.3	1.7	1.5
	Supine without GA	66	2.8	4.1	3.3	1.5	1.7	2.0
	Prone with GA	17	3.7	3.4	3.1	1.6	1.1	1.6
	Prone without GA	17	5.2	3.1	3.8	3.2	2.7	2.6
	All	47	6.3	5.7	6.6	2.4	3.1	2.7
	Supine	42	6.1	5.7	6.1	2.3	3.1	2.8
Body	Prone	5	8.7	6.3	11.1	3.3	3.2	2.4
	GA	20	4.3	4.7	6.0	1.3	2.6	1.9
	No GA	27	7.4	6.1	7.1	3.0	3.7	3.2

Note. GA = general anesthesia; Lat = Lateral; Long = Longitudinal; Vert = Vertical

Understanding localization and verification uncertainty or setup margin has an important impact on dose to normal tissues. This is especially true for small critical structures adjacent to a high-dose volume or in the gradient of dose. It is possible that even slight motion on the order of millimeters can have a significant effect on the dose to critical structures when one is using highly conformal treatments that include steep gradients. The information generated from this research can be used to determine the biological effect of positional uncertainty.

Uncertainty in dose to targets and critical structures is not limited to setup uncertainty. The internal margin, which forms the ITV, is meant to account for expected motion in tissues resulting from respiration and peristalsis. Four-dimensional CT has been used to demonstrate internal motion of the kidneys and diaphragm caused by breathing. In the setting of treatment for neuroblastoma, one should be able to account for this type of motion when designing treatment volumes or planning beam delivery.

One of the intriguing pieces of information that is embedded in the CBCT data is the projection of organs in different positions as a function of time. The CBCT data used for localization can also be used to quantify respiratory motion. A future application would be to use this motion data to ensure that the ITV is consistent from the day of treatment planning and throughout therapy. It might also be used to establish the efficacy of gated treatment. We are able to obtain each projection image with 0.5 μGy. Figure 23-3 is a set of these projection images when the gantry is near −90, 0, +90 degrees. We are able to collect about two projections per second and 200 projections per CBCT, which includes the full breathing cycle.

Fiducial Markers in Proton Therapy

Investigators at the University of Florida Proton Therapy Institute (UFPTI) studied the impact of setup uncertainties in proton therapy. The objective of their research was to determine the impact of setup uncertainty on proton

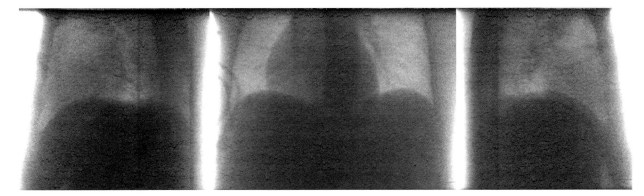

FIGURE 23-3. Multiple, 0.5-μGy imaging beam line (IBL) cone-beam computed tomography projection images. A variety of anatomical structures are visible. These projections may be used for verification of the internal target volume.

therapy, identify ways to minimize uncertainty, and determine other uncertainties relevant to proton planning and delivery.[19] Specific recommendations used to define the PTV for proton therapy have been described in the ICRU Report 78: "for each beam orientation being considered, one would in principle need a separate planning target volume margin with different margins laterally and on the direction of each beam."[20] The approach to proton therapy is distinctly different than for x-ray planning because each beam should be considered its "own plan" because of the 3D properties of the proton beam.

Investigators at UFPTI studied the use of skull metallic fiducial markers and bony anatomical markers for all pediatric CNS proton treatments during 2006 through 2008. The fiducial markers were a component of the imaging verification system called the digital imaging positioning system (DIPS). The DIPS is a two-dimensional registration system[21] that has been used to evaluate translational and rotational uncertainty (Figure 23-4).

The investigators compared and contrasted metallic fiducial to bony anatomic markers. Despite the required semiinvasive procedure and additional logistics to prepare the patient for therapy using metallic fiducials, they were found to be advantageous because they were objective and easy to find and mark on x-ray and digital imaging. For bony anatomy markers (BAMs), the investigators reported that there were no delays when initiating radiation therapy; however, they were potentially less reliable in anesthesia patients and relied on the subjectivity of the radiation therapist.

For reference, BAMs used at UFPTI have included the anterior and posterior clinoid, the anterior and posterior aspects of C-1, the top of the frontal sinus and the hard palate, and the lower tip of the upper incisors. The latter two, hard palate and tip of the upper incisors, were not used for patients who required anesthesia because of interference from endotracheal tubes and laryngeal airways. On the anterior–posterior (AP) or posterior–anterior (PA) radiographs, the left mastoid, right mastoid, left sphenoid wing, and right sphenoid wing were commonly used.

Placement of Fiducial Markers and the DIPS Procedure

Before simulation of CNS patients, the neurosurgeon is required to place four or five noncollinear 1.5 mm by 3.0 mm titanium screws as fiducial markers in the outer table of the skull. Then CT simulation is performed with the fiducial markers in place. For RT planning, the fiducial markers are identified during the treatment planning process and marked in the treatment planning system. The fiducial markers are then confirmed on the DIPS workstation. Typically, the DRRs with the fiducial markers or bony anatomical markers are placed into the digital imaging system of the treatment room before the first fraction of therapy. The in-room steps include daily orthogonal preport kV imaging, which is registered to the DRR. The digital imaging position gives translational shifts, and the patient is repositioned and reimaged. If the shifts are greater than the action level threshold for that particular patient setup (1.0 mm to 3.0 mm), the therapists return to the initial step of preporting with kV imaging. The DIPS is not routinely used for rotational shifts.

In a study conducted at UFPTI, the fiducial markers were taken as the gold standard and the impact of using fiducial markers versus bony anatomy as a setup point was determined. The focus of the research was to determine the value of metallic fiducial makers on setup accuracy and setup time, and the influence of the therapist's experience and interobserver variability, i.e., whether one radiation

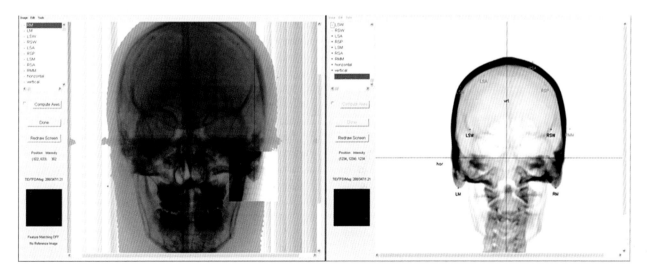

FIGURE 23-4. Orthogonal kilovoltage cranial images using digital imaging positioning system (left) and digitally reconstructed radiographs (right). Common bony anatomic landmarks are indicated on the reconstructed computed tomography image.

therapist marks the patient differently than another. In their initial study, six pediatric patients were treated at the UFPTI, all with fiducial markers. For each patient, BAMs were also identified and followed. More than four BAMs were selected for the lateral and for the AP or PA radiographs. Points were marked first on the DRR and then confirmed on 3D CT images. An orthogonal set of films from the final five treatments were selected for each patient for marking.

Six radiation therapists were selected, each with varying amounts of experience in working with the DIPS. Each radiation therapist was first asked to mark the orthogonal films using the fiducial marker DRRs for the individual patient as a reference. Each therapist was then asked to mark the orthogonal films using bony anatomy DRRs for the same patient as the reference. Each therapist then marked the subsequent patients. The time to mark for fiducials was recorded for three translational vectors for both the fiducials and the bony anatomy. The results of this study showed that the time to mark the patient using bony anatomy took approximately 1 minute 53 seconds whereas the time to mark the patient using fiducial markers was 1 minute 34 seconds. The difference in bony anatomy to fiducial marker setup discrepancy was also found to be larger.

There was a number of problems with this study. A constant relationship was not maintained between bony anatomy regardless of anesthesia and it appeared that any type of airway management obscured the ability to visualize all structures. Bony anatomy points that remain for visualization were more heavily weighted and subject to error. The use of prone positioning was reported to further impact setup using bony anatomy. In summary, given the current margins used for treatment planning in children at their institution, the time difference between marking fiducials and bony anatomy was not meaningfully different. The investigators posed the following questions: How would the findings change with repetition and would it be possible to predict who needed fiducial markers and who did not? Finding answers to these questions remains the goal of current research.

Additional work was conducted by the same investigators to determine the impact of setup error on target coverage in critical structures, including the impact of translational and/or rotational vector setup error on critical structures, and to determine the robustness of proton craniospinal plans and the tangible benefit of fiducial markers. To answer these questions, four craniospinal plans were reviewed. Initial proton craniospinal plans use traditional x-ray margins in the plane perpendicular to the beam axis. The brain was contoured to the foramen magnum including portions of the upper cervical spinal cord. The margin was 1 cm from the brain to aperture edge. The nuchal aspect of the field was custom with a minimum 1 cm from spinal cord to block edge. For the spinal field,

the nerve roots were not specifically contoured; however, a margin of 1.0 cm to 1.2 cm from the lateral aspect of the clip blocks to aperture edge was used based on the current COG study for pediatric medulloblastoma. Proton plans were found to be robust and the margins could be further tightened. In conclusion, the use of fiducial markers does impact daily positioning in some children; however, setup error in proton therapy using classical apertures or perpendicular margins in standard proton planning parameters has minimal impact on target coverage.

Computed Tomography Outside the Treatment Room

Proton therapy delivery at the Paul Scherrer Institute (PSI) employs patient positioning and verification outside the treatment room. This system relies on a semi-automated patient transporter with an attached tabletop docking system to connect the treatment table to both the CT unit and treatment gantry. Patients are prepared outside the treatment room and enter the transport system first docking at the CT unit for verification imaging followed by transfer to the gantry for treatment and then finally exiting the treatment room with the transport system following the same transport path. The transport system movement is controlled by the radiation therapist and the system follows a path using optical guidance (Figure 23-5). The total transport (in and out of the treatment room) is approximately 20 minutes. Daily pretreatment positioning at the CT employs horizontal and vertical scout images, which are compared against reference scout images generated from the treatment planning CT series. No axial CT scan is acquired. There is on-line matching of anatomical landmarks by therapy and physics or physician staff. The matching process may be semiautomated or manual. Offsets for table coordinates at the gantry (translations only) are based on the offsets from the pretreatment imaging. The reported systematic errors are 0.1 mm to 0.6 mm and random errors are 1.2 mm to 2.4 mm.[22] Pretreatment positioning of the patient includes horizontal and vertical digital imaging on the treatment gantry on the first day of treatment, which may require rotation of the gantry and the generated images are compared against the reference DRR.

This is a fully integrated program for patient positioning. Positioning the patient outside the treatment room permits a parallel process with two patients to be performed to increase throughput. This is of particular significance in complex situations and for children who require anesthesia. Complex situations include patients who are immobile or otherwise ill and who require additional setup time and those who have difficult and time-consuming immobilization. In all situations, immobilization of the patient may be performed in advance of entry into the treatment room. For the young child who requires immobilization, the patient transport system

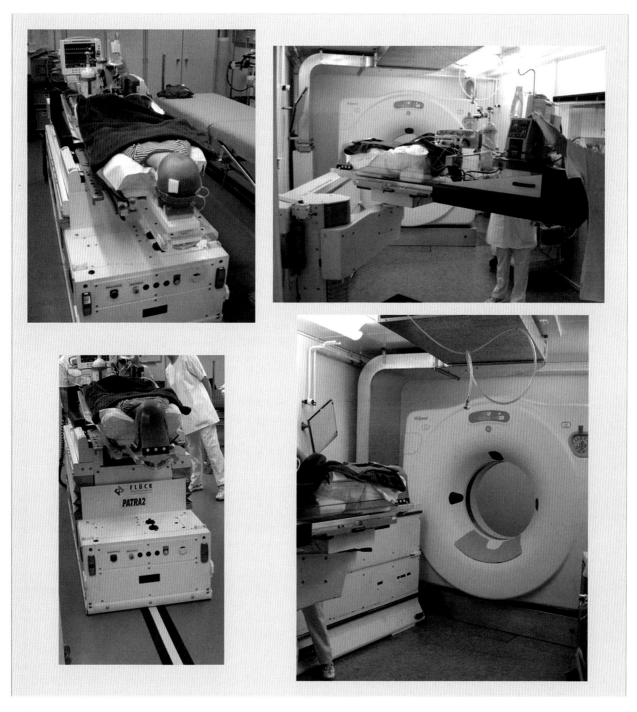

FIGURE 23-5. Patient transport system at the Paul Scherrer Institute. Prone position patient under general anesthesia (upper left), thermoplastic immobilization applied and the transporter begins movement to the computed tomography (CT) room (lower left), robotic arm of CT system lifts patient couch from transporter (upper right), patient about to enter CT ring (lower right).

allows for undisturbed time for the anesthesiologist to prepare the child in a separate room. The child only enters the treatment room when he or she is ready for therapy. The speed of the transport system is the main rate-limiting step. For relatively easy setups, there is no likely time savings; however, the potential time savings depends on the facility layout. There are several vendors who offer such transport systems. Although verification outside the treatment room is feasible and useful, it is not always the optimal tool. Verification outside the treatment room may not meet the present or future opportunities of IGRT or adaptive RT in children.

Conclusions

Image-guided RT is broadly defined for children and may be used to improve localization or verify positioning. Image-guided RT promises to increase the precision of RT for children and reduce dose to normal tissues. The latter will allow a reduction in the margins required to create the PTV for most treatment sites.

References

1. Mansur DB, Klein EE, Maserang BP. Measured peripheral dose in pediatric radiation therapy: a comparison of intensity-modulated and conformal techniques. *Radiother Oncol.* 2007;82: 179–184.

2. Mascarin M, Drigo A, Dassie A, et al. Optimizing cranio-spinal radiotherapy delivery in a pediatric patient affected by sPNET: a case report. *Tumori.* 2010 Mar-Apr; 96(2):316–321.

3. Merchant TE. Proton beam therapy in pediatric oncology. *Cancer J.* 2009;15:298–305.

4. Arndt CA, Stoner JA, Hawkins DS, et al. Vincristine, actinomycin, cyclophosphamide (VAC) vs VAC/V topotecan/cyclophosphamide (TC) for intermediate risk rhabdomyosarcoma (IRRMS), D9803 COG Study. *Proc Am Soc Clin Oncol.* 2009 Nov 1;27(31):5182–5188.

5. Randomized Study of vincristine, dactinomycin and cyclophosphamide (VAC) versus VAC alternating with vincristine and irinotecan (VI) for patients with intermediate-risk rhabdomyosarcoma (RMS). Opened for entry: December 26, 2006. Available at: http://clinicaltrials.gov/ct2/show/NCT00354835. Accessed 22 November 2010.

6. Merchant TE, Kun LE, Krasin MJ, et al. Multi-institution prospective trial of reduced-dose craniospinal irradiation (23.4Gy) followed by conformal posterior fossa (36Gy) and primary site irradiation (55.8Gy) and dose-intensive chemotherapy for average-risk medulloblastoma. *Int J Radiat Oncol Biol Phys.* 2008;70:782–787.

7. Phase III randomized adjuvant study of standard-dose versus reduced-dose craniospinal radiotherapy and posterior fossa boost versus tumor bed boost radiotherapy in combination with chemotherapy comprising vincristine, cisplatin, lomustine, and cyclophosphamide in pediatric patients with newly diagnosed standard-risk medulloblastoma (ACNS0331). Activated September 27, 2004. Available at: http://www.cancer.gov/clinicaltrials/COG-ACNS0331. Accessed 22 November 2010.

8. Merchant TE. Three-dimensional conformal radiation therapy for ependymoma. *Childs Nerv Syst.* 2009 Oct; 25(1):1261–1268.

9. Merchant TE, Kun LE, Wu S, et al. Phase II trial of conformal radiation therapy for pediatric low-grade glioma. *J Clin Oncol.* 2009;27:3598–3604.

10. Phase II study of reduced-field conformal radiotherapy in young patients with low-grade gliomas (ACNS0221). Activated November 28, 2005. Available at: http://www.cancer.gov/ClinicalTrials/COG-ACNS0221. Accessed 22 November 2010.

11. Prescribing, recording, and reporting photon beam therapy, ICRU Report 50. Washington, DC: International Commission on Radiation Units and Measurements; 1993.

12. Prescribing, recording, and reporting photon beam therapy (supplement to ICRU Report 50), ICRU Report 62. Bethesda, MD: International Commission on Radiation Units and Measurements; 1999.

13. NCI Guidelines on the use of IMRT in clinical trials. Available at: http://atc.wustl.edu/home/NCI/NCI_IMRT_Guidelines.html. Accessed 22 November 2010.

14. National Cancer Institute Radiation Research Program [Web page]. Available at: http://www3.cancer.gov/rrp/proton.doc. Accessed 22 November 2010.

15. Quality Assurance Review Center. Image fusion benchmark. Available at: http:www.qarc.org/benchmarks/FusionBenchmarkQuestionnaire.pdf. Accessed 22 November 2010.

16. Beltran C, Pai Panandiker AP, Krasin MJ, et al. Daily Image Guided Localization for Neuroblastoma. *Jour Appl Clin Med Phys.* 2010:11(4)3388.

17. Faddegon BA, Wu V, Pouliot J, et al. Low dose megavoltage cone beam computed tomography with an unflattened 4 MV beam from a carbon target. *Med Phys.* 2008;35:5777–5786.

18. Beltran C, Lukose R, Gangadharan B, et al. Image quality and dosimetric property of an investigational imaging beam line MV-CBCT. *J Appl Clin Med Phys.* 2009;10:3023–3026.

19. Duvvuri SS, Keole SR, Aldana P, et al. Comparison of patient positioning accuracy using fiducial or anatomical markers for proton cranial radiotherapy [abstract]. *Int J Radiat Oncol Biol Phys.* 2008;72:S497.

20. Prescribing, recording and reporting proton-beam therapy, ICRU Report 78. Washington, DC: International Commission on Radiation Units and Measurements; 2007, p 86.

21. Flanz J, Smith A. Technology for proton therapy. *Cancer J.* 2009;15:292–297.

22. Bolsi A, Lomax AJ, Pedroni E, et al. Experiences at the Paul Scherrer Institute with a remote patient positioning procedure for high-throughput proton radiation therapy. *Int J Radiat Oncol Biol Phys.* 2008;71:1581–1590.

23. van Herk M, Remeijer P, Rasch C, et al. The probability of correct target dosage: dose-population histograms for deriving treatment margins in radiotherapy. *Int J Radiat Oncol Biol Phys.* 2000;47:1121–1135.

Optically Guided Frameless SRS Using the Varian Trilogy in a Patient with a Juvenile Pilocytic Astrocytoma

Case Study

Joshua D. Lawson, MD, Jia-Zhu Wang, PhD, Kevin Murphy, MD

Patient History

A 12-year-old boy underwent partial resection of a juvenile pilocytic astrocytoma in 2001 at the age of 6 years; a ventriculoperitoneal shunt was placed at the time. Postoperatively, he received chemotherapy until April 2003 and was then followed with serial magnetic resonance (MR) imaging. In August 2005, he required shunt revision, but otherwise remained largely asymptomatic. On serial imaging, his residual enhancing mass along the anterior–inferior fourth ventricle remained stable until 2006, at which time there was an area of increased enhancement, measuring 10 mm by 12 mm adjacent to the dorsal surface of the medulla.

The patient was seen at that time in the multidisciplinary clinic and there was concern that further growth may result in worsening hydrocephalus. Additional surgery was not thought safe, so a stereotactic radiosurgical (SRS) approach was proposed. After discussion, frameless SRS using real-time image-guided setup was thought the most appealing treatment course for this cooperative pediatric patient with a recurrent juvenile pilocytic astrocytoma.

Simulation

On the day of simulation, a dental mold was made of the child's upper teeth. A fiducial array with a set of four reflective markers (Frameless Array, Varian Medical Systems, Palo Alto, CA) was then attached to the bite block, angled 5° to 10° from horizontal. The patient was then taken to the treatment vault where reseat verification of the bite block was performed, ensuring bite block reproducibility. A helmet with test fiducials was firmly affixed to the patient's head and an optical camera was used to measure the relative positions of the reflective markers to the test fiducials to determine positioning error. The dental mold was removed and replaced 10 times; the variation was less than 0.75 mm.

After confirmation of reproducibility, the patient was taken to our departmental wide-bore multislice computed tomography (CT) simulator (GE Healthcare, Waukesha, WI) and placed in the supine position on a custom head rest. An aquaplast mask was then fabricated with a cut-out to accept the bite block and reflective markers (Figure 23A-1). Transaxial imaging with a slice thickness of 1.25 mm was performed from his vertex to his shoulders. No intravenous or oral contrast was used.

Treatment Planning

The planning CT and diagnostic MR were then transferred to the FastPlan treatment planning system (Varian Medical Systems, Palo Alto, CA) and fused, using initially manual, and then automatic, rigid registration. Visual verification of registration was then done in the axial, coronal, and sagittal planes (Figure 23A-2).

The tumor and organs at risk (OARs) were then contoured. The gross tumor volume (GTV) consisted of all

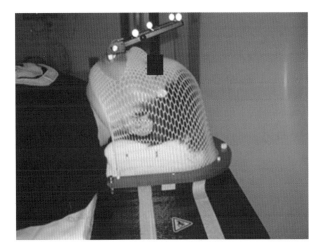

FIGURE 23A-1. Patient immobilized with an aquaplast face mask with a cutout to allow placement of bite block and affixed frameless array. Note that the fiducial array is attached to the bite block at approximately 5° to 10° off horizontal. This improves the detection of the fiducials by the optical camera.

visualized tumor on the MR scan. No expansion was used to create the planning target volume (PTV). The OARs consisted of the optic chiasm, globes, lenses, optic nerves, and brainstem. A single isocenter was then placed manually in the center of the PTV and a 16-mm cone was

used for treatment. Five non-coplanar arcs (table angles: 20°, 55°, 85°, 340°, and 305°) were selected to deliver an optimized treatment plan, with a prescribed PTV dose of 16 Gy to the 90% isodose line (Figure 23A-3). Start and stop angles of each arc were: 60° and 140°, 50° and 130°, 150° and 110°, 220° and 300°, and 230° and 310°, respectively. The doses to normal tissues (chiasm, globes, lens, optic nerves, brainstem, etc.) were reviewed and judged to be acceptable.

After plan approval, the CT image data set, isocenter location, and couch information of each arc were exported to the computer of the camera system (SonArray, Varian Medical Systems, Palo Alto, CA). Anterior–posterior (AP) and right lateral digitally reconstructed radiographs (DRRs) were generated for patient setup.

Treatment Delivery

Before bringing the patient into the vault for treatment, additional quality assurance (QA) was performed by the physics staff. The isocenter pointer was first attached to the linac and the calibration jig was used to check the calibration of the optical camera. The selected cone was then attached to the treatment machine; the Winston-Lutz test was subsequently performed to verify that the cone was aimed at isocenter.

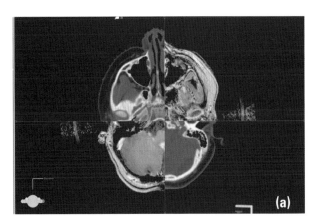

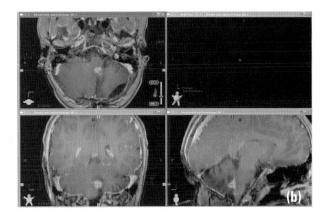

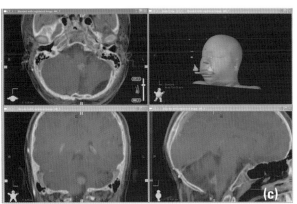

FIGURE 23A-2. Checkerboard (a) (tumor marked by black arrow) and blended (b–c) images of the fused magnetic resonance (MR) and computed tomography (CT) scans showing the adequacy of CT–MR registration.

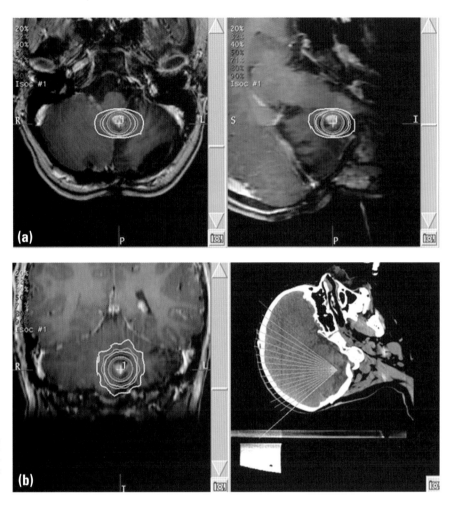

FIGURE 23A-3. Axial, sagittal (a), and coronal (b) images showing dose conformity of the treatment plan and one of the five arcs used for treatment.

The patient was then positioned on the treatment couch, and immobilized in the aquaplast mask with bite block and fiducial array. As additional QA for patient setup, a pair of orthogonal kilovoltage images was taken using the On-Board Imager (OBI) (Varian Medical Systems, Palo Alto, CA). These images were compared with the DRRs to confirm correct patient positioning. To aid in comparing the DRRs and orthogonal films, select bony landmarks in the skull were contoured by the dosimetry staff (Figure 23A-4). In this case, no shifts were required on the treatment machine.

Treatment was delivered on a Varian Trilogy linear accelerator (Varian Medical Systems, Palo Alto, CA) using 6-MV photons at a dose rate of 1000 monitor units per minute. During treatment, the optical camera was used to provide real-time (intrafraction) setup monitoring. If a displacement of more than 0.5 mm were to occur, treatment would be stopped and the patient repositioned. However, no interruptions were required in this case. Before each arc, manual anterior–posterior, lateral, and longitudinal adjustments were made using the optical guidance system to ensure a displacement of less than 0.3

mm. Each arc and couch position additionally underwent anticollision testing before delivery. Finally, all treatment information was double-checked by physics staff before initiation of treatment. Treatment was completed within a 1-hour time slot.

Clinical Outcome

The SRS treatment was well-tolerated, without any significant acute toxicities. The child was able to maintain his normal lifestyle and continued to participate in his usual daily activities. He was seen most recently in follow-up 10 months posttreatment, at which time he remained without complaints and had no neurologic deficits. A follow-up MR image demonstrated a complete radiographic response, with no residual nodular enhancement.

Our initial clinical experience using frameless SRS and stereotactic RT with real-time image-guided setup was recently published.[1] Nine patients, ages ranging from 12 to 19 years (median, 15 years), with a variety of tumors (two juvenile pilocytic astrocytomas, one pontine low-grade glioma, three pituitary adenomas, one metastatic

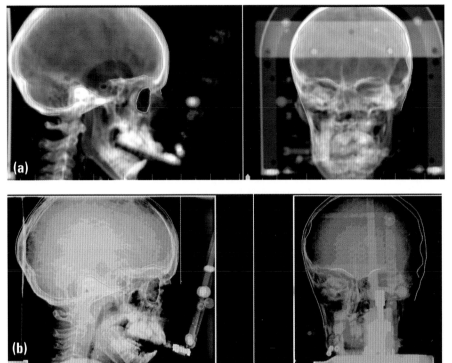

FIGURE 23A-4. On-line patient positioning using the Varian On-Board Imaging (OBI) system. Anterior–posterior (AP) and right lateral digitally reconstructed radiographs (DRRs) with select bony landmarks drawn in green (a) and AP and right lateral orthogonal films obtained using the OBI system (b). Bony landmarks drawn on the DRRs match those seen on the orthogonal films indicating excellent alignment. No shifts are necessary.

medulloblastoma, one acoustic neuroma, and one pineocytoma) were treated on a Varian Trilogy linear accelerator. In all cases, the treatment was well tolerated with no acute toxicity requiring intervention. With a median follow-up of 12 months (range, 3–18 months), no significant delayed RT-related toxicities were seen. Only one patient experienced in-field tumor progression and required repeat surgery. The remaining patients remain controlled locally and are being followed closely for tumor response and potential late toxicities.

Reference

1. Keshavarsi S, Meltzer H, Ben-Haim S, et al. Initial clinical experience with frameless optically guided stereotactic radiosurgery/radiotherapy in pediatric patients. *Child's Nerv Syst.* 2009; 25(7):837–844.

KV Planar Image-Guided Setup Using the Varian Trilogy System in a Patient with an Intracranial Ependymoma

Case Study

Natia Esiashvili, MD, Timothy Fox, PhD

Patient History

A 4-year-old girl presented with escalating headaches, vomiting, and progressive gait ataxia. Magnetic resonance (MR) imaging revealed a heterogeneously enhancing posterior fossa mass centered in the fourth ventricle with minimal extension into the upper cervical spinal canal (Figure 23B-1). No additional lesions were seen in the brain or spine. The patient subsequently underwent a suboccipital craniotomy with resection of the posterior fossa tumor. Pathology was consistent with a World Health Organization grade II ependymoma.

Her postoperative course was complicated with mild symptoms of bulbar dysfunction, which resolved over time. A postoperative MR scan demonstrated a small, nodular enhancement at the ventral aspect of the brainstem, which was difficult to differentiate from a small amount of residual tumor versus postsurgical enhancement. Additional radiographic studies demonstrated no evidence of tumor dissemination in the brain or spine.

A repeat surgery for attempted resection of the suspected residual mass was felt to be associated with a high risk of potential morbidity. After multidisciplinary discussion, a decision was made to not to pursue chemotherapy as the residual enhancement resolved on repeat imaging. Conformal radiation therapy (RT) to the surgical bed, however, was recommended to reduce the risk of tumor recurrence. We elected to treat the patient with intensity-modulated RT (IMRT) with onboard kilovoltage (kV) image guidance using the Trilogy system (Varian Medical Systems, Palo Alto, CA) to optimize daily setup.

Simulation

During simulation, the child was found to be fully cooperative and did not require general anesthesia. She was placed in the supine position and immobilized utilizing a noninvasive system consisting of a thermoplastic mask and head holder. She was scanned with a Lightspeed RT-16 computed tomography (CT) simulator (GE Healthcare, Waukesha, WI) without intravenous or oral contrast. Axial images were obtained with a slice thickness of 1.25 mm, covering the patient's vertex to her shoulders. An isocenter was placed in the posterior fossa, and the mask was marked with chosen coordinates using the laser system.

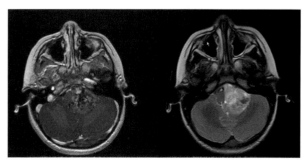

FIGURE 23B-1. T1 postcontrast and T2 sequence magnetic resonance scan demonstrating tumor in posterior fossa.

Treatment Planning

The BrainLAB iPlan Treatment Planning Station (Brain-LAB AG, Feldkirchen, Germany) was utilized for fusing the images from the planning CT and diagnostic MR with rigid registration tools. The registration result was accepted only after careful review of fusion quality in the axial, coronal, and sagittal planes (Figure 23B-2).

The gross tumor volume (GTV) consisted of the residual tumor mass, and the tumor bed was defined on the basis of the initial preoperative MR imaging, taking into account the extent of the disease, as well as postoperative MR findings reflecting the constricted tumor bed. The clinical target volume (CTV) was created by margins added to the GTV to treat subclinical microscopic disease while keeping the volume within anatomically confined spaces as defined by the bony calvarium, falx, and tentorium because there was no evidence of tumor invasion into these structures. The CTV margin did not exceed 1.0 cm in all directions. A planning target volume (PTV) was then generated by adding a 0.3 cm margin to the CTV in three dimensions. Organs at risk (OARs) were contoured separately and included the brainstem, globes, lenses, hypothalamus, pituitary gland, optic nerves, chiasm, cochlea, and temporal lobes.

An IMRT plan was generated using optimization parameters and the dose constraints for achieving the most acceptable target coverage, conformity, homogeneity, and doses in critical structures. Seven coplanar, static, 6-MV photon beams with angles of 204°, 258°, 309°, 0°, 51°, 102°, and 158° were selected to deliver a prescribed PTV dose of 59.4 Gy in 33 fractions to the 100% isodose line (Figure 23B-3). Doses to normal tissues (chiasm, globes, lens, optic nerves, brainstem, etc.) were reviewed and judged acceptable. Anterior–posterior (AP) and right lateral digitally reconstructed radiographs (DRRs) were generated for the patient setup. After plan approval, the CT image data set and isocenter location were exported to the treatment station.

Treatment Delivery

Quality assurance (QA) testing was completed by the physics staff before treatment delivery. On the first day of treatment, the patient was brought to the linac vault and immobilized with the thermoplastic mask. Patient setup QA was completed using the two-dimensional (2D) kV On-Board Imager (OBI; Varian Medical Systems, Palo Alto, CA) with a pair of open-field orthogonal kV images obtained and compared with the reference DRR images, confirming correct patient positioning. Minimal shifts were required as approved by the supervising physician on the first day of treatment (Figure 23B-4). Treatment was delivered on a Varian Trilogy linear accelerator.

The patient continued the prescribed 33 daily fractions of IMRT with daily kV OBI and isocenter shifts carried out by skilled radiation therapists and verified by the treating physician. The kV OBI shifts for this patient were predominantly random and small for the entire course of her treatment.

Clinical Outcome

Overall, the patient tolerated treatment well and completed her entire course without interruption. During the 6-month follow-up period, the patient maintained a complete radiographic response without evidence of tumor local recurrence or dissemination. She also did not experience any significant treatment-related delayed side effects at this relatively short-term observation period. She continues to be closely followed in our clinic.

Our initial clinical experience using onboard kV image-guided setup in 26 pediatric patients was presented

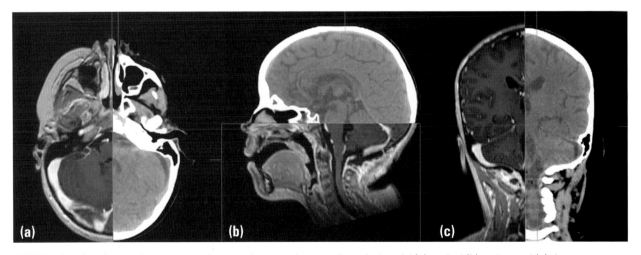

FIGURE 23B-2. Fused magnetic resonance and computed tomography scans shown in the axial (a), sagittal (b), and coronal (c) views.

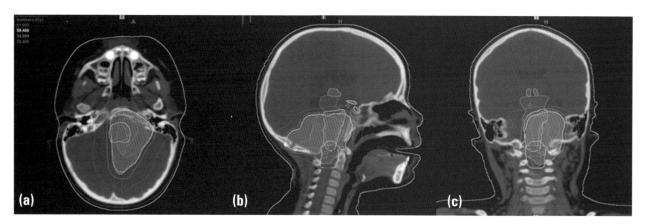

FIGURE 23B-3. Axial (a), sagittal (b), and coronal (c) images showing dose conformity of the intensity-modulated radiation therapy treatment.

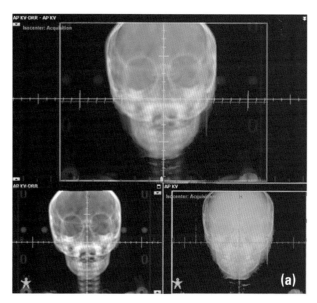

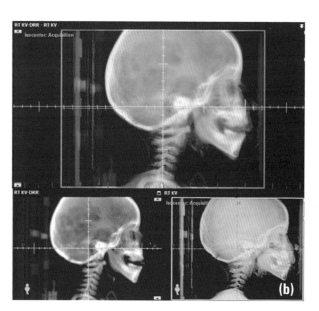

FIGURE 23B-4. Patient setup images using the Varian kilovoltage (kV) On-Board Imaging (OBI) system: (a) Anterior–posterior orthogonal images are obtained using the kV OBI system and shown as blended images with the digitally reconstructed radiographs (DRRs; upper panel) and as separate DRR (lower left panel) and kV radiograph (lower right panel). (b) Similarly, right lateral orthogonal images are obtained with the OBI system and shown as blended images with the DRRs (upper panel) and as separate DRR (lower left panel) and kV radiograph (lower right panel). (c) 2-mm longitudinal and 1-mm lateral shifts were necessary for this acquisition for optimal beam alignment.

Summary: Images (2 Rev) / Couch Corrections (VAR_IEC scale)

	AP KV - RT KV
Status	⊚
Vrt [cm]	0.0
Lng [cm]	-0.2
Lat [cm]	-0.1
Rtn [deg]	0.0

(c)

earlier.[1] Various tumor sites were represented in this study including the brain, head and neck, and thorax. A total of 182 OBI sessions were performed before treatment, with an average session lasting 3.6 minutes. Average shifts were 0.25, 0.23, and 0.12 cm per session in the lateral, longitudinal, and vertical directions, respectively. The average vector shift was 0.45 cm for all patients with the following distribution by anatomical site: brain 0.35 cm, head and neck 0.4 cm, chest 0.02 cm, abdomen 1.1 cm, and pel-

vis 5.7 cm. Calculated offsets for patients treated to each anatomical site were generally random and did not vary during treatment.

Reference

1. Esiashvili N, Fox T, Crocker IR, et al. Kilovoltage image-guided radiotherapy in pediatric tumors. *Int J Radiat Oncol Biol Phys.* 2007;69:S730.

Chapter 24

METASTATIC DISEASE: OVERVIEW

KYLE RUSTHOVEN, MD, BRIAN D. KAVANAGH, MD, MPH

Advances in cytotoxic and molecular targeted therapies have resulted in improved suppression or delayed progression of micrometastatic disease for a variety of solid tumors, in many settings leading to improvements in overall survival. However, measurable metastases remain poorly controlled with systemic therapy alone for most solid tumors. Consequently, there is burgeoning interest in exploring means of safe, effective local therapies directed toward limited sites of metastases in an effort to eradicate them, thereby prolonging the progression-free interval and possibly overall survival of patients.

Several conceptual models of cancer dissemination and progression also support the aggressive treatment of discrete deposits of metastatic disease in selected patients. Perhaps the most popular is the theory of oligometastases,[1] whereby it is hypothesized that there is an intermediate state between early localized cancer and widespread disease. In this context, it is proposed that spatially targeted therapy that eliminates all demonstrable disease will achieve long-term disease control in some patients.

In a more empiric sense, retrospective studies have documented favorable rates of long-term progression-free survival (PFS) and overall survival (OS) in selected patients with limited hepatic metastases from colorectal cancer treated with surgical resection. Fong and coworkers reported 5- and 10-year OS rates of 37% and 22%, respectively, in 1001 patients with limited hepatic metastases from colorectal cancer following surgical resection.[2,3] The most favorable group of patients had negative surgical margins, solitary metastases, tumor size less than 5 cm, a carcinoembryonic antigen (CEA) level of less than 200 ng/mL, a disease-free interval greater than 12 months, node-negative disease, and no evidence of extrahepatic metastases. For this group, the 5-year OS was 60%.

Similarly, Aloia and colleagues compared rates of local control, disease-free survival (DFS), and OS in 180 patients with solitary liver metastases from colorectal cancer treated with radiofrequency ablation (RFA) versus hepatic resection.[4] In this series, 5-year local recurrence-free survival and OS were higher with hepatic resection (92% and 71% vs 60% and 27%, respectively). No differences were observed in the two groups in terms of distant hepatic or systemic recurrences. These findings suggest that effective local therapy is essential in achieving long-term DFS and OS for colorectal cancer patients with hepatic oligometastases.

Large population-based data sets also support the concept of an oligometastatic state in a proportion of patients with metastatic colorectal cancer. An analysis of the Ontario Cancer Registry identified 841 hepatic resections performed for metastatic colorectal cancer from 1996 to 2004.[5] The 5-year survival rate was 43% and was higher when surgery was performed for solitary nodules, at high-volume centers, and in more recent years. Similarly, an analysis of the Surveillance, Epidemiology and End Results (SEER)-Medicare registry identified 7673 patients with colorectal cancer aged 65 years or older with liver metastases.[6] Among them, 833 (6.1%) underwent hepatic resection and 5-year OS in this cohort was 32.8% compared with 10.5% in those not undergoing hepatic resection ($P < .001$). Selection biases likely influenced this type of database to some extent. Regardless, the favorable outcomes observed in at least some patients have encouraged the study of other means of liver tumor ablation, including high-dose radiation therapy (RT),[7] which might be advantageous by virtue of their less-invasive nature.

Similar findings have been observed in patients with lung metastases. The International Lung Metastases Registry (ILMR) analysis documented the survival outcomes of 5206 patients with lung metastases treated with surgical resection.[8] In this study, the 5-, 10-, and 15-year survival rates for patients undergoing complete metastasectomy were 36%, 26%, and 22%, respectively. Incomplete metastasectomy was associated with inferior long-term OS rates of 13% at 5 years and 7% at 10 years. Concordant with the observations in studies of surgery for liver metastases, longer disease-free intervals (> 36 months) and solitary metastases had improved survival. Histology was also an important predictor of survival in the ILMR study. Most patients had either an epithelial primary tumor or a sarcoma. Germ cell tumors represented only a minority of the metastases studied (7%), but were associated with improved survival compared with other primary tumor histologies.

Long-term survival has also been reported for select patients treated with surgery or stereotactic radiosurgery (SRS) for limited brain metastases. For example, Kondziolka and coworkers reviewed the records for 677 patients with brain metastases treated with SRS and identified 44 (6.5%) patients with a survival of at least 4 years.[9] Compared with patients who had a shorter survival after SRS (< 3 months), patients with long-term survival had a higher initial performance status ($P = .01$), fewer brain metastases ($P = .04$), and less extracranial disease ($P < .001$). In a study of patients with non–small cell lung cancer (NSCLC) presenting with synchronous, solitary brain metastases, Flannery et al. reported the long-term outcomes for patients treated with SRS.[10] Five-year survival in this series was 21% in the whole group but was 35% in patients who received definitive therapy (chemoradiation, surgery, or both) for their thoracic disease. In this study, the use of curative-intent therapy in the treatment of thoracic disease and a Karnofsky performance status (KPS) of 90 or higher was associated with improved long-term survival. These data suggest that long-term survival can be achieved in select patients with cerebral metastatic disease in the context of aggressive efforts to eradicate their extracranial disease.

Further clinical evidence supporting the existence of an oligometastatic state of disease can be derived from the patterns of metastatic disease progression. Two studies of patients with limited-burden metastatic NSCLC have demonstrated that progression of existing metastases is the most common pattern of first disease progression, both in the *de novo* and *induced* oligometastatic state. Mehta and colleagues at the University of Chicago analyzed the patterns of progression in 38 patients with stage IIIB or stage IV NSCLC.[11] Among the 17 patients who were eligible for local therapy (with one to four metastases and no pleural effusion), 11 (65%) had no disease progression outside initially involved sites at a median follow-up of 9 months. Similarly, investigators from the University of Colorado analyzed patterns of disease progression in 64 patients with advanced NSCLC after first-line systemic therapy.[12] Among the 34 patients (53%) in this series who were eligible for stereotactic body RT (SBRT; using institutional eligibility criteria) after first-line therapy, first extracranial progression was at sites of initial disease in 68%. Moreover, progression at sites initially involved with disease after first-line therapy occurred at a median of 3 months compared to progression at distant sites, which occurred at a median of 5.7 months. These findings suggest that in the setting of *induced* oligometastases from NSCLC, a limited window may exist during which effective local therapy could be administered and potentially prolong the interval to disease progression.

Although image-guided radiation therapy (IGRT) has been described for the treatment of metastatic and recurrent tumors in multiple sites, the majority of studies using IGRT in these settings have been for treatment of tumors of the lung, liver, spine, and brain. In this chapter, we describe technical and clinical aspects of IGRT, with specific attention to stereotactic hypofractionated treatment techniques in the treatment of limited-burden metastatic and recurrent cancer of the lung, liver, spine, and brain.

Image-Guided Target and Normal Tissue Delineation

Although it is always desirable to minimize radiation-induced normal tissue toxicity, in the treatment of metastatic disease this issue merits especially high priority. Patients in this setting have generally been previously treated with combinations of local and systemic therapy that might have rendered certain organ systems more susceptible to injury.

To enhance the therapeutic ratio, smaller planning target volume (PTV) margins tend to be used to avoid unintended increases in toxicity. This reduction in safety margins, however, increases the risk of tumor underdosing secondary to geographic miss. As a result, precise and accurate imaging to facilitate tumor delineation is required.

Lung

Computed tomography (CT) is currently the reference standard for gross tumor volume (GTV) definition for primary and metastatic tumors of the lung.[13] Slice thicknesses of 3 mm to 5 mm are commonly used for RT treatment planning. Radio-opaque contrast dye can help facilitate planning for mediastinal targets and for targets abutting or invading the great vessels, but is not generally helpful for lesions confined to the lung parenchyma.

Thoracic targets should be contoured using proper visualization parameters. Optimal window and level combinations differ for lung parenchymal versus mediastinal targets. Harris et al. compared the accuracy of volumetric assessment of lung nodules of varying sizes using three different window level (WL) and window width (WW) combinations. Determination of the volume of pulmonary nodules was highly accurate using both the lung setting (WL/WW: -750HU/850HU) and the broad lung setting (WL/WW: -550HU/1350HU), but was inaccurate using the soft tissue setting (WL/WW: +20HU/400HU).[14] Stern and coworkers surveyed thoracic radiologists and found that the mean preferred window and level combination for radiographic evaluation of lung parenchymal targets was WL -600 HU and WW 1500 HU, whereas the preferred window settings for evaluating the mediastinum were WL 40 HU and WW 350 HU.[15]

More recently, ^{18}F-flourodeoxyglucose (^{18}F-FDG) positron emission tomography (PET) and fused PET–CT have been shown to aid target recognition compared with CT alone in studies of patients with NSCLC. Yu and colleagues compared GTV delineation in 43 NSCLC patients as delineated by CT, PET, and integrated PET–CT to the pathologically determined tumor volume after resection.[16] In this study, the correlation coefficient for imaging-determined and pathologically determined tumor size was better for integrated PET–CT than for PET or CT alone. The improved accuracy was most pronounced for determination of lateral tumor extent, in which the correlation coefficient was 0.88 for integrated PET–CT compared with 0.75 for PET and 0.76 for CT. The improved accuracy of tumor delineation with integrated PET–CT was evident for patients both with and without atelectasis. Fitton and others demonstrated that coregistered PET–CT significantly reduced interobserver variability in GTV delineation for tumors involving the hilum, heart, great vessels, pericardium, and mediastinum and for tumors with associated atelectasis.[17] The improved accuracy of integrated PET–CT over CT alone in GTV definition for patients with atelectasis has been confirmed by other investigators.[18]

Preliminary results from studies using PET–CT for treatment planning in NSCLC have empirically confirmed the accuracy of tumor delineation with this technique. Klopp and colleagues retrospectively reviewed the outcomes of PET–CT–based treatment planning for NSCLC and observed out-of-field failure in only 6% when the GTV was limited to only ^{18}F-FDG–avid sites. Moreover, the intensity of ^{18}F-FDG uptake, quantified by standardized uptake value (SUV), was highly predictive of in-field recurrence.[19] These findings suggest that metabolic imaging with PET is not only highly accurate for target delineation but can also be correlated with the biological aggressiveness of the primary tumor (Figure 24-1).

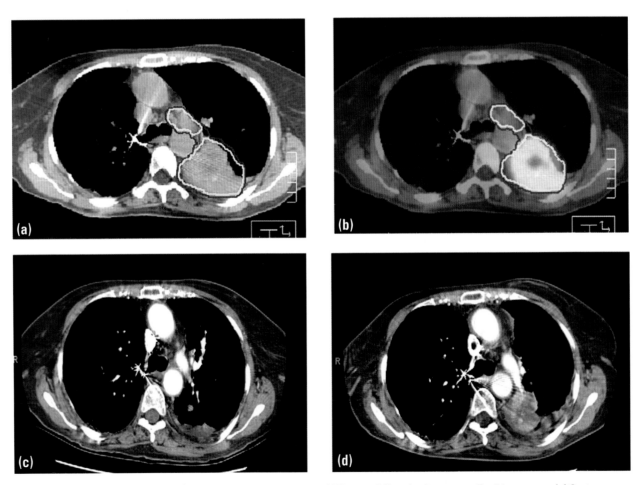

FIGURE 24-1. Positron emission tomography (PET) –computed tomography (CT) target delineation for non–small cell lung cancer. (a) Contours overlaid on the planning CT scan. The treated gross tumor volume is shown in red, and the contoured volumes are shown in green and blue. (b) Overlay of PET and CT images for target delineation. (c) Computed tomography illustrating disease regression at 6 months, and (d) recurrence 11 months posttreatment. Reproduced with permission from Klopp et al.[19]

Given the known improvement in mediastinal and central tumor evaluation with contrast-enhanced CT over non-enhanced CT, recent studies have compared the accuracy of tumor evaluation using contrast-enhanced PET–CT with the standard nonenhanced PET–CT protocol. In one study, contrast-enhanced PET–CT conferred an improvement in staging accuracy over standard PET–CT. Pfannenberg and colleagues demonstrated that contrast-enhanced PET–CT lead to more accurate TNM staging in 8% of patients with NSCLC.[20] The improved accuracy was most pronounced in patients with T4 primary tumors with great vessel invasion.

Modern RT planning software often uses heterogeneity calculations based on tissue density; therefore, the calculation of radiation dose absorption continues to rely on CT-based treatment planning. As such, alternative imaging modalities, such as PET and PET–CT, must be fused to the planning CT scan to help guide treatment planning. PET or PET–CT scans, which are to be used in RT planning, should be performed in the treatment position with immobilization device in place.[21] Moreover, because of breathing-associated tumor motion for tumors of the lung, some investigators have utilized the same respiratory inhibition techniques used during treatment (breath hold) during PET and integrated PET–CT to limit the amplitude of respiratory motion.[22]

Although the accuracy of various imaging modalities has primarily been evaluated in the setting of primary NSCLC, it is assumed that for lung metastases, PET–CT should yield similar benefits in distinguishing tumor from atelectasis. Furthermore, PET–CT can be particularly useful in the setting of recurrent lung cancer after prior RT in distinguishing tumor from the radiation treatment effect.

Liver

Unlike tumors of the lung parenchyma, lesions of the liver are often difficult to distinguish from the surrounding normal hepatic parenchyma. The traditional reference standard for evaluation of liver metastases is CT with and without radio-opaque contrast. Helical image acquisition yields improved detection of hepatic metastases and positive predictive value over axial image acquisition.[23]

After contrast administration, liver imaging is typically performed at two time points, an early hepatic arterial phase and a later portal venous phase. Bader and colleagues performed serial CT scans in 25 healthy volunteers every 2 seconds after contrast administration to evaluate the timing and duration of the arterial and portal venous phases of contrast enhancement.[24] These investigators reported that hepatic arterial enhancement occurred at a mean of 5.4 seconds after aortic enhancement and the mean duration of hepatic arterial phase of enhancement at 8.6 seconds. The mean time to portal venous enhancement in this study was 13.9 seconds after aortic enhancement. Because of the short window

for each phase of enhancement, rapid multidetector CT scanners are necessary for optimal hepatic CT imaging.

Noncontrast imaging remains part of the standard CT evaluation because some hypervascular lesions are better visualized without contrast. Bressler and others reviewed noncontrast and contrast-enhanced liver CT scans in 28 patients with hepatic metastases. In this study, 11 of the 28 lesions were distinguished from the surrounding liver parenchyma (Δ=15 HU) on noncontrast imaging but became isodense and indistinguishable after contrast administration.[25] Similar to lung CT, window level and width settings are also important for optimal liver imaging. Pomerantz and colleagues evaluated the effect of using bone and liver settings on abdominal CT interpretation. In 18 patients with hepatic abnormalities, CT visualization using liver settings (WL/WW +50HU/350HU) led to increased conspicuity or improved lesion characterization in eight (44%) cases, and influenced the final diagnosis in three (17%) relative to image interpretation using standard soft tissue settings (WL/WW +40/400).[26]

Alternative imaging modalities, including magnetic resonance (MR) imaging and integrated PET–CT, have shown promise in the definition of liver metastases. Ward and colleagues compared the accuracy of lesion characterization for 215 metastases using three techniques: dynamic contrast–enhanced thin-section multidetector helical CT, high spatial-resolution 3D dynamic gadolinium-enhanced MR, and super-paramagnetic iron oxide–enhanced MR with optimized gradient-echo sequence.[27] The studies were interpreted by two experienced, blinded radiologists; surgery with histologic examination was the reference standard. For all metastases for both observers, there was no significant difference between MR techniques, but both were significantly more accurate than CT ($P < .01$).

In a multiinstitutional trial, Hammersting et al. compared the accuracy of lesion detection in 169 patients with 302 lesions using liver-specific gadoxetic acid–enhanced MR versus contrast-enhanced biphasic spiral CT.[28] The frequency of correctly detected lesions was significantly higher on gadoxetic acid–enhanced MR compared with CT in the unblinded clinical evaluation. In the blinded reading, however, there was no significant improvement in lesion detection with gadoxetic acid–enhanced MR.

Other investigators have shown no advantage of MR over CT-based target delineation. Braga and associates evaluated 25 patients with 94 operable hepatic lesions with dual phase helical CT and manganese-enhanced MR followed by surgery and histopathologic analysis.[29] In their study, the lesion detection rate was higher with CT ($P = .01$); however, CT was also associated with a higher false-positive rate compared with MR ($P = .06$). The area under the receiver operator curve (ROC) was similar for both CT and MR (0.74 vs 0.72; $P = .751$), indicating similar accuracy for tumor delineation with both techniques.

In a comparison of tumor volume delineation and resultant dose–volume histograms using contrast enhanced CT or MR-based treatment planning, Pech and coworkers reported that tumor volumes as delineated by MR were 181% larger on T1-weighted sequences, 178% larger on gadolinium-enhanced T1-weighted sequences, and 246% larger on T2-weighted sequences compared with the same tumors as delineated by contrast-enhanced CT.[30] The mean dose received by 90% of the tumor volume (D_{90}) according to imaging modality used was 18 Gy for contrast-enhanced CT, 16 Gy for T1-weighted MR, 15.5 Gy for gadolinium-enhanced T1-weighted MR, and 12 Gy for T2-weighted MR. These findings suggest that CT-based target delineation may result in significant underdosing of tumor as visualized on MR. As a result, these authors recommended the routine use of contrast-enhanced T1- and T2-weighted MR for target delineation.

Robinson and others also reported areas of high signal intensity on T2-weighted imaging that were not visible on CT. However, on pathologic analysis, these T2 hyperintense regions did not contain tumor and the cause of the increased T2-signal was not determined.[31] In a similar type of correlative study between radiographic imaging and pathologic findings, Kelsey and colleagues reported a series of 18 patients with primary hepatocellular carcinoma (HCC) who underwent surgical resection of a total of 27 tumors.[32] There was good correlation between the radiographic and pathologic sizes regardless of whether CT or MR was used for preoperative imaging. It was estimated that a PTV using a 0.5-cm or 1.0-cm margin around the radiographic tumor would have encompassed the gross pathologic tumor in 93% and 100% of cases, respectively.

Integrated PET–CT and contrast-enhanced PET–CT have also been utilized to image hepatic metastases. Cantwell et al. compared the lesion detection rate, sensitivity, specificity, accuracy, and area under the ROC using nonenhanced PET–CT, contrast-enhanced PET–CT, and MR in 33 patients with suspected liver metastases from colorectal cancer.[33] The reference standard was pathologic analysis or follow-up imaging of 6 months or greater. The lesion detection rate was significantly higher for MR (95%) and contrast-enhanced PET–CT (91%) compared with nonenhanced PET–CT (74%). The area under the ROC curve was 0.97 for MR, 0.86 for contrast-enhanced PET–CT, and 0.74 for nonenhanced PET–CT. It was concluded that contrast-enhanced PET–CT was superior to nonenhanced PET–CT, but that MR remained the best study for liver lesion characterization in patients with colorectal cancer.

If possible, MR or integrated PET–CT scans used for RT treatment planning should be obtained in the treatment planning position to facilitate accurate fusion with the treatment planning CT images. Similar to lung tumors, lesions of the liver are also affected by breathing-associated tumor motion. Consequently, breath hold techniques of the kind described previously for imaging lung tumors can be advantageous during scan acquisition and radiation treatment.

Spine and Brain

Magnetic resonance is the most sensitive technique for the detection of tumors in the vertebral bodies and epidural space and has replaced invasive methods such as myelography.[34] Computed tomography is less sensitive and accurate than MR, yet many lesions are incidentally detected when CT imaging is performed for other reasons. Buhmann Kirchhoff and colleagues compared the sensitivity and accuracy of high-resolution multidetector CT versus 1.5 Tesla (T) MR in the evaluation of 201 biopsy-confirmed spine metastases.[35] The sensitivity (98.5% vs 66.2%; $P < .001$) and accuracy (98.7% vs 88.8%; $P < .001$) were significantly better with MR. Computed tomography proved less sensitive for the detection of smaller lesions without significant bone destruction. Useful CT WL and WW settings for detection of bone metastases were approximately WL +600 and WW 1600.

Metabolic imaging modalities have also been shown to be sensitive for the detection of spine metastases. Even-Sapir and colleagues described 99% sensitivity and 97% specificity using ^{18}F-FDG PET–CT for the evaluation of skeletal metastases in 44 patients.[36] In this study, integrated PET–CT was associated with improved specificity compared with ^{18}F-FDG PET alone. However, other studies suggest that PET is inferior to anatomic imaging with MR. Schmidt et al. performed a prospective, blinded study comparing whole-body MR (WB-MR) using a 32-channel scanner versus integrated PET–CT for the detection of skeletal metastases.[37] The reference standard was at least 6 months of radiographic follow-up. Sensitivity for detection of bone metastases with WB-MR was 94% compared with 78% with PET–CT. Similarly, diagnostic accuracy was 91% with WB-MR versus 78% with PET–CT.

Technitium-99m (^{99m}Tc) bone scintigraphy is a sensitive modality for detecting blastic osseous metastases, particularly those from prostate, lung, and breast cancer.[38] Some investigators have reported poor sensitivity, however, for spine metastases. Schirrmeister et al. compared bone scintigraphy versus PET in 44 patients with bone metastases from prostate, lung, or thyroid cancer.[39] The sensitivity of bone scan for detection of lesions in the pelvis and spine was only 40% compared with 83% for lesions of the skull, thorax, or extremities. The area under the ROC was 0.99 for PET and 0.64 for bone scintigraphy. In a similar study of 104 patients with metastatic lung cancer, whole body PET exhibited improved accuracy compared with bone scintigraphy for the detection of bone metastases (94% vs 85%; $P < .05$).[40] In contrast, in a pooled analysis of studies comparing PET and bone scintigraphy for the detection of bone metastases from breast cancer, Shie and coworkers reported that both modalities had similar sensitivities for lesion detection. However, PET demonstrated improved specificity, suggesting that it may serve as a better confirmatory test than bone scintigraphy.[41]

Magnetic resonance has also become established as the preferred technique for characterizing brain metastases. Although Taphoorn and others did not observe a difference between CT and MR in this setting,[42] essentially all reported comparative studies since then have favored MR over CT. Davis et al.,[43] Akeson et al.,[44] and Kuhn et al.[45] were among the pioneers in this area. More recently, there has been growing interest in the study of metabolic imaging techniques for brain tumors, particularly for the purpose of differentiating tumor recurrence from post-RT imaging changes. Terakawa and colleagues used PET scanning with l-methyl-(11)C-methionine (^{11}C-MET) in 77 patients who had been previously treated with RT after for metastatic brain tumor (n = 51) or glioma (n = 26).[46] Using tissue and other clinical correlation, the values of each index of ^{11}C-MET PET proved to be higher for tumor recurrence than for radiation necrosis. Among the derived ratios analyzed was the comparison of lesion uptake to contralateral normal frontal-lobe gray matter uptake in terms of the mean and maximum SUV (L/N_{mean} and L/N_{max}). An L/N_{mean} of greater than 1.41 provided the best sensitivity and specificity for metastatic brain tumor (79% and 75%, respectively).

Image-Guided Treatment Delivery

Image guidance can provide accurate target localization before RT and is often accompanied by techniques that minimize intrafraction target motion, especially for the hypofractionated regimens used in SBRT. Image-guided RT for treatment of metastatic or recurrent cancer involving the lungs, liver, spine, and brain have most commonly used planar kilovoltage (kV) x-rays or volumetric CT-based target localization techniques, which will be the focus of the discussion in this chapter.

To account for the component of intrafraction target positional changes, which are most commonly related to breathing-related motion, a variety of respiratory management techniques are available. For sites associated with significant breathing-related tumor motion, specifically the lung and liver, we will briefly discuss methods used to address respiratory motion. A more complete discussion of the management of respiratory motion can be found in Chapter 11.

Lung

Grills et al. analyzed 308 cone-beam CT (CBCT) images obtained in 24 patients undergoing high-dose SBRT.[47] Patients were initially set up using skin marks or a stereotactic frame, and the position was then corrected using CBCT registered to soft tissues. Based on the observed systematic and random errors, a PTV margin on the order of 10 mm in all directions would be required for setup based on skin or frame landmarks only. Setup using CBCT, on the other hand, required PTV margins of approximately 5 mm or less in all directions to account for residual errors after initial setup correction and intrafraction motion (Figure 24-2). Yeung and coworkers have reported quantitatively very similar results in an analysis of patients treated with conventional fractionation, adding that the use of port films allowing alignment to bony landmarks was at best only minimally better than skin marks.[48]

There are numerous means of addressing breathing-related motion. First, there is the use of a broadly encompassing internal target volume (ITV) derived from a "slow scanning" method.[49,50] Here, planning CT scans are acquired with a technique involving a single thin axial slice every 3 to 4 seconds, and, thus, breathing-related tumor motion is represented by the appearance of elongation of the GTV, in this sense generally called an ITV, around which a PTV margin is then added. To this or any planning CT technique, it is easy to add abdominal compression, which can reduce motion by dampening diaphragmatic excursion. Heinzerling and colleagues compared different levels of abdominal compression in lung SBRT patients who had four-dimensional (4D) CT scans without and then with two different intensities of abdominal compression.[51] It was observed that both moderate compression force (mean, 48 N) and high compression force (mean, 91 N) achieved significant reduction in tumor motion, most notably in the superior–inferior direction.

Controlled breath hold techniques can reduce tumor motion to the range of just a few mm,[52,53] but it should be recognized that this technique does not guarantee accurate tumor relocalization based on only skin or bony landmarks. Masi and coworkers analyzed two groups of patients receiving SBRT to lung lesions: group A did not perform any breathing control; group B controlled visually their respiratory cycle and volumes using a commercially available system during the acquisition of planning CT, acquisition of pre-treatment CBCT, and treatment delivery.[54] It was observed that the three-dimensional (3D) tumor breathing displacement (mean ± SD) was significantly higher for group A (14.7 mm ± 9.9 mm) than for group B (4.7 mm ± 3.1 mm). Still, in approximately one third of group B patients, there was a greater than 3 mm difference in tumor position between assessments based on bony landmarks relative to those based on CBCT, emphasizing the need to perform volumetric image guidance when tight margins are used in concert with this breath hold system.

Hoogeman analyzed 44 patients treated with a commercially available tracking system. This system generates a correlative model of tumor motion during the

GTV position pre-correction: Planning CT GTV in Red; Pre-Correction GTV in Green.

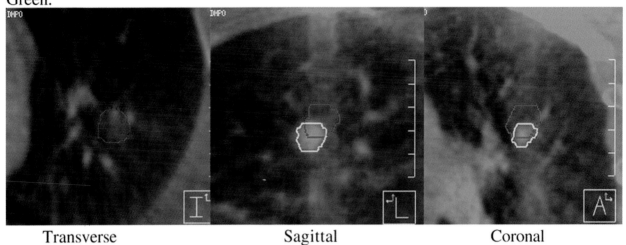

| Transverse | Sagittal | Coronal |

GTV position post-correction: Planning CT GTV in Red; Post-Correction GTV in Blue.

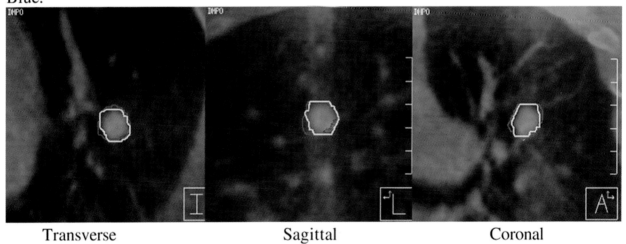

| Transverse | Sagittal | Coronal |

FIGURE 24-2. Illustration of the utility of cone-beam computed tomography to provide on-line corrections for a patient treated in a stereotactic body frame. The upper panel shows the precorrected images with the planning gross tumor volume (GTV) in red and the precorrected GTV in green. Following the positional adjustment of the patient, the corrected images are shown in the lower panel with the planned GTV in red overlapping the corrected GTV shown in light blue. Reproduced with permission from Grills et al.[47]

respiratory cycle with the movement of external fiducial markers and uses the model to drive the linear accelerator in a manner that targets the expected location of the tumor.[55] The results showed that the standard deviation of the residual error between actual tumor location during the breathing cycle, as determined by stereoscopic imaging and expected location according to the model used, is on the order of 1 mm to 2 mm in each axis of motion. An important additional consideration was noted by Nishioka et al.,[56] who observed that in a high percentage of respiratory cycles, there is notable exhale fluctuation that must be considered during the use of systems that

involve tumor tracking or respiratory gating. Case studies focusing on image guidance in patients with lung metastases are provided in Chapters 24F and 24G.

Liver

The accuracy of target localization for liver metastases is similar to the accuracy observed in studies of IGRT for tumors of the lung. Fuss and colleagues evaluated setup accuracy using an ultrasound (US)-based image-guided targeting device to align intensity-modulated RT for 62 patients with upper-abdominal malignancies, including 11 patients with liver metastases. In 15 patients, a control CT was performed after US targeting and the residual error was quantified. The mean vector of residual setup error was 4.6 mm ± 3.4 mm after the correctional shifts determined by US.[57]

Liver target localization using x-ray image guidance has also been shown to be highly accurate. Wurm and colleagues used stereoscopic orthogonal kV X-rays fused to the digitally reconstructed radiographs (DRRs) from the planning CT scan. Internal fiducial markers facilitated the determination of appropriate translational shifts. Verification CT imaging showed that the average marker position deviation from the expected position ranged from 1.5 mm to 4.1 mm, with a median deviation of 2.1 mm.[58] Similarly, Shioyama and colleagues used daily megavoltage (MV) portal imaging aligned to bony anatomy in 20 patients with lung and liver tumors. Reported average setup errors of 2.4 mm ± 0.5 mm, 1.4 mm ± 1.8 mm, and 3.7 mm ± 2.6 mm were seen in the lateral, anterior–posterior (AP), and cranio–caudal (CC) directions, respectively.[59]

Finally, volumetric image guidance using CBCT imaging has shown promising results for daily tumor localization in liver IGRT. Investigators from the Princess Margaret Hospital compared setup errors in liver position using orthogonal MV image pairs and kV CBCT imaging in 13 primary liver tumor patients. Cone-beam CT images were registered with the diaphragm for CC alignment and with the vertebral bodies for lateral and AP alignment.[60] The CBCT was registered to the planning CT to obtain the residual setup error in liver position. Mean random and systematic setup errors after MV orthogonal image guidance were 2.7 mm and 1.1 mm in the CC direction, 2.3 mm and 1.9 mm in the lateral direction, and 3.0 mm and 1.3 mm in the AP direction, respectively. In 33% of cases, liver offsets in at least one direction were greater than 5 mm with orthogonal MV imaging. Setup accuracy was increased with CBCT image guidance, with mean random and systematic setup errors after MV orthogonal image guidance were 0.2 mm in the CC direction, 0 mm in the lateral direction, and 0.2 mm in the AP direction. See Chapters 24H, 24I, and 24J for discussions of using image guidance in patients with liver metastases using various in-room technologies.

Spine and Brain

Image-guided RT for spine metastases is unique in terms of the target volume covered. Unlike metastases to the lung, liver, and brain, the patterns of failure after stereotactic treatment of spine metastases necessitates the inclusion of clinically uninvolved portions of the index vertebral bodies within the clinical target volume (CTV; see Chapters 24D and 24E).

Chang and colleagues identified two specific patterns of failure in a phase I/II trial of three- or five-fraction SBRT for spinal metastases.[61] In this study, the target volume for lesions of the vertebral body included the entire vertebral body from superior to inferior endplate, but did not include the disk or posterior elements. Of the 17 cases of disease progression, eight (47%) occurred in the epidural space and three (18%) occurred in the pedicles immediately posterior to the target volume. It was concluded that there should be routine inclusion of the pedicles and posterior elements in the target volume, with a wide bony margin to account for microscopic disease extension. Similarly, Ryu and others reported an experience using single-fraction SBRT for the treatment of 230 spinal metastases in 177 patients.[62] The pedicles were included in the CTV for lesions confined to the vertebral body, and the posterior elements were included in the CTV in the presence of for gross pedicle involvement.

Because of the routine elective inclusion of clinically uninvolved portions of the vertebral body in the CTV, precise determination of the volume of the index metastasis is less important than for other sites. As noted above, sensitive and accurate imaging modalities for tumor detection, however, remain important to select patients appropriately for spine IGRT. For spine IGRT, precise imaging is also required to delineate the spinal cord, which represents the primary organ at risk. T1- and T2-weighted axial MR is the reference standard for spinal cord delineation. In studies of SBRT for spinal metastases, MR imaging is often fused with the planning CT to facilitate accurate contouring of the spinal cord.[61-63] Because the spinal cord is not fixed within the spinal canal, however, there exists concern about spinal cord movement. Investigators from the University of Virginia evaluated the movement of the thoracic spinal cord during normal respiration.[64] The mean spinal cord motion was 0.5 mm or less at all thoracic levels, ranging up to a maximum of approximately 0.7 mm in either the AP or medial–lateral directions (Figure 24-3). On the basis of these findings, it is reasonable to add a 1-mm margin to the contoured spinal cord to obtain an organ-at-risk volume for RT treatment planning.

A high degree of setup accuracy has been described in the setting of single-fraction and multifraction treatment of spinal metastases. The accuracy of isocenter positioning in these studies is similar for both x-ray- and CBCT-based image-guidance systems.[65-68] Ryu and colleagues evaluated the accuracy of setup accuracy in 10 patients with spinal metastases treated with single-fraction stereotactic boost using stereoscopic localization.[65] Patients were positioned using a combination of infrared, passive marker technology and image fusion of orthogonal kV images with DRRs from the planning CT and translational six-dimensional (6D) shifts. The accuracy of isocenter positioning was measured by image fusion of the DRR and portal images, and was within 1.36 mm ± 0.11 mm. The radiation dose at the isocenter was also evaluated in a phantom using a microion

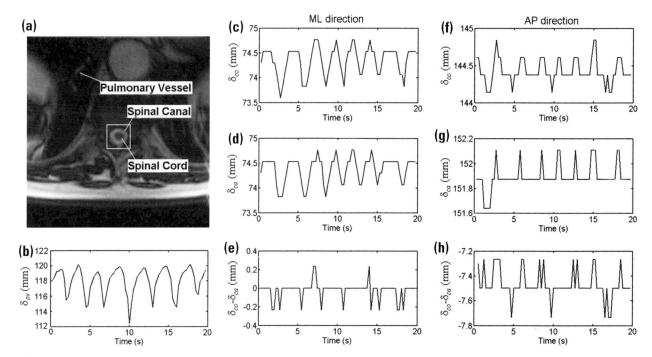

FIGURE 24-3. Example of spinal cord motion. (a) Axial magnetic resonance (MR) image showing the spinal cord, spinal canal, and pulmonary vessel. (b) A motion profile of the pulmonary vessel. (c–h) Motion profiles of the spinal cord, spinal canal, and spinal cord relative to the spinal canal in the medial–lateral and anterior–posterior directions. Reproduced with permission from Cai et al.[64]

chamber and compared with the treatment plan. The average deviation of the measured dose from the estimated dose was only 2%.

Yu and colleagues evaluated setup accuracy using another commercially available stereoscopic system for the treatment of paraspinal metastases in patients with implanted stainless steel fiducials.[66] The mean clinically relevant error was determined to be 0.7 mm ± 0.3 mm. The average treatment delivery precision was 0.3 mm ± 0.1 mm. Yin and coworkers compared setup accuracy using CBCT-based setup compared with conventional two-dimensional (2D) setup using bony markers in 10 patients with liver, lung, and spine metastases.[67] Compared with traditional 2D matching using bony structures, CBCT setup corrected target deviation from 1 mm to 15 mm, with an average of 5 mm. These investigators also evaluated intrafraction motion by comparing pre- and posttreatment radiographic images and found an average deviation of only 2 mm (range, 0 mm to 4 mm) during the 1-hour stereotactic treatments. Letourneau and colleagues evaluated the feasibility of spinal IGRT using a CBCT platform.[68] Image-guided dose placement was assessed using radiochromic film measurements and demonstrated excellent agreement with the treatment plan, with dose delivery within 5% and distance-to-agreement measurements less than 2 mm.

The use of image guidance for target volume recognition in the treatment of primary and metastatic brain tumors is well established. As for the other sites already discussed, technology is now widely available to fuse planning CT scans with other imaging modalities facilitating tumor and normal tissue delineation. Early examples of systems that entered clinical use include the work of Kooy and others,[69] who developed and implemented a method of fusing CT and MR images using a chamfer matching algorithm. Lattanzi and others later described a method involving an initial segmentation of the GTV on planning CT images followed by fusion of these images with MR scans with a point pair matching method.[70] Nowadays, all commercially available planning and delivery systems suitable for cranial SRS or fractionated external beam RT for brain tumors package software that allows for fusion of the planning CT with MR scans to facilitate accurate target volume determination.

Target localization for intracranial treatment can be achieved using two approaches: rigid immobilization with a head frame or "frameless" techniques based on imaging anatomy or other fiducials. Targeting accuracy for the rigid immobilization systems is primarily influenced by the multiple software–hardware interfaces used in this context, and it is discussed in detail in the American Association of Physicists in Medicine (AAPM) Task Group #54 Report.[71]

Because intracranial lesions are poorly visualized on CT and x-ray imaging, in-room IGRT cannot be used to set up directly to the tumor per se. However, because there is negligible movement of the brain within the cranial vault, the bony anatomy of the skull can be used as a stereotactic surrogate for tumor location with the brain parenchyma. Lamba and coworkers compared isocenter alignment errors in an anthropomorphic phantom for both frame-based stereotactic and frameless image-guided alignment.[72] Using the hidden target method, localization errors were comparable for the framed (0.7 mm ± 0.5 mm) and image-guided (0.6 mm ± 0.2 mm) techniques.

Future Directions

Although there remains room for refinement in all of the currently available IGRT systems, there are two major areas of interest in the realm of IGRT that show promise for the future with methods not yet widely implemented clinically. First, there is the notion of IGRT using deformable registration that will not only localize the target but will also account for interfraction shape changes as a result of tumor shrinkage or other causes of tumor contour variability. Brock and colleagues have described an initial effort for using deformable registration in liver IGRT, and the technique appears at least feasible from the standpoint of the amount of time needed for image processing.[73]

The other concept with potential for future clinical implementation is the integration of physiologic imaging into the IGRT process. Feng et al. have reported their pilot experience with the use of pre- and mid-treatment PET scanning to define the initial PTV and subsequently adaptively modified PTV.[74]

It is possible that in the future there might be advances in imaging of a functional nature that would allow real- or near-real-time functional imaging alongside traditional anatomic imaging to guide daily treatment on the basis of not only target relocation but also target modification based on midtreatment response indicators.

References

1. Hellman S, Weichselbaum RR. Oligometastases. *J Clin Oncol.* 1995;13:8–10.
2. Fong Y, Cohen AM, Fortner JG. Liver resection for colorectal metastases. *J Clin Oncol.* 1997;15:938–946.
3. Fong Y, Fortner J, Sun RL. Clinical score for predicting recurrence after hepatic resection for metastatic colorectal cancer: analysis of 1001 consecutive cases. *Ann Surg.* 1999;230:309–318.
4. Aloia TA, Vauthey JN, Loyer EM. Solitary colorectal liver metastasis: resection determines outcome. *Arch Surg.* 2006;141:460–466.
5. Shah SA, Bromberg R, Coates A. Survival after liver resection for colorectal cancer in a large population. *J Am Coll Surg.* 2007;205:676–683.
6. Cummings LC, Payes JD, Cooper GS. Survival after hepatic resection in metastatic colorectal cancer: a population-based study. *Cancer.* 2007;109:718–726.
7. Timmerman RD, Kavanagh BD, Cho LC. Stereotactic body radiation therapy in multiple organ sites. *J Clin Oncol.* 2007;25:947–952.
8. Long-term results of lung metastasectomy: prognostic analyses based on 5206 cases. The International Registry of Lung Metastases. *J Thorac Cardiovasc Surg.* 1997;113:37–49.
9. Kondziolka D, Martin JJ, Flickinger JC. Long-term survivors after gamma knife radiosurgery for brain metastases. *Cancer.* 2005;104:2784–2791.
10. Flannery TW, Suntharalingam M, Regine WF. Long-term survival in patients with synchronous, solitary brain metastasis from non-small-cell lung cancer treated with radiosurgery. *Int J Radiat Oncol Biol Phys.* 2008;72:19–23.
11. Mehta N, Mauer AM, Hellman S. Analysis of further disease progression in metastatic non-small cell lung cancer: implications for locoregional treatment. *Int J Oncol.* 2004;25:1677–1683.
12. Rusthoven KE, Hammerman SF, Kavanagh BD. Is there a role for consolidative stereotactic body radiation therapy following first-line systemic therapy for metastatic lung cancer? A patterns-of-failure analysis. *Acta Oncol.* 2009;48:578–583.
13. Broderick LS, Tarver RD, Conces DJ Jr. Imaging of lung cancer: old and new. *Semin Oncol.* 1997;24:411–418.
14. Harris KM, Adams H, Lloyd DC, et al. The effect on apparent size of simulated pulmonary nodules of using three standard CT window settings. *Clin Radiol.* 1993;47:241–244.
15. Stern EJ, Frank MS, Godwin JD. Chest computed tomography display preferences: survey of thoracic radiologists. *Invest Radiol.* 1995;30:517–521.
16. Yu HM, Liu YF, Hou M. Evaluation of gross tumor size using CT, (18) F-FDG PET, integrated (18) F-FDG PET/CT and pathological analysis in non-small cell lung cancer. *Eur J Radiol.* 2009;72(1):104–113.
17. Fitton I, Steenbackkers RJ, Zijp L. Retrospective attenuation correction of PET data for radiotherapy planning using a free breathing CT. *Radiother Oncol.* 2007;83:42–48.
18. Deniaud-Alexandre E, Touboul E, Lerouge D. Impact of computed tomography and 18F-deoxyglucose coincidence detection emission tomography image fusion for optimization of conformal radiotherapy in non-small-cell lung cancer. *Int J Radiat Oncol Biol Phys.* 2005;63:1432–1441.
19. Klopp AH, Chang JY, Tucker SL. Intrathoracic patterns of failure for non-small-cell lung cancer with positron-emission tomography/computed tomography-defined target delineation. *Int J Radiat Oncol Biol Phys.* 2007;69:1409–1416.
20. Pfannenberg AC, Aschoff P, Brechtel K. Low dose non-enhanced CT versus standard dose contrast-enhanced CT in combined PET/CT protocols for staging and therapy planning in non-small cell lung cancer. *Eur J Nucl Med Mol Imaging.* 2007;34:36–44.
21. Macmanus M, Nestle U, Rosenzweig KE. Use of PET and PET/CT for radiation therapy planning: IAEA expert report 2006–2007. *Radiother Oncol.* 2009;91:85–94.
22. Wurm RE, Gum F, Erbel S. Image guided respiratory gated hypofractionated stereotactic body radiation therapy (H-SBRT) for liver and lung tumors: initial experience. *Acta Oncol.* 2006;45:881–889.

23. Valls C, Lopez E, Guma A, et al. Helical CT versus CT arterial portography in the detection of hepatic metastasis of colorectal carcinoma. *AJR Am J Roentgenol.* 1998;170:1341–1347.

24. Bader TR, Prokesch RW, Grabenwöger F, et al. Timing of the hepatic arterial phase during contrast-enhanced computed tomography of the liver: assessment of normal values in 25 volunteers. *Invest Radiol.* 2000;35:486–492.

25. Bressler EL, Alpern MB, Glazer GM, et al. Hypervascular hepatic metastases: CT evaluation. *Radiology.* 1987;162:49–51.

26. Pomerantz SM, White CS, Krebs TL, et al. Liver and bone window settings for soft-copy interpretation of chest and abdominal CT. *AJR Am J Roentgenol.* 2000;174:311–314.

27. Ward J, Robinson PJ, Guthrie JA, et al. Liver metastases in candidates for hepatic resection: comparison of helical CT and gadolinium- and SPIO-enhanced MR imaging. *Radiology.* 2005; 237:170–180.

28. Hammersting R, Huppertz A, Breuer J, et al. Diagnostic efficacy of gadoxetic acid (Primovist)-enhanced MRI and spiral CT for a therapeutic strategy: comparison with intraoperative and histopathologic findings in focal liver lesions. *Eur Radiol.* 2008;18:457–467.

29. Braga HJ, Choti MA, Lee VS, et al. Liver lesions: manganese-enhanced MR and dual-phase helical CT for preoperative detection and characterization comparison with receiver operating characteristic analysis. *Radiology.* 2002;223:525–531.

30. Pech M, Mohnike K, Wieners G, et al. Radiotherapy of liver metastases. Comparison of target volumes and dose-volume histograms employing CT- or MRI-based treatment planning. *Strahlenther Onkol.* 2008;184:256–261.

31. Robinson DA, McKinstry CS, Steiner RE, et al. Magnetic resonance imaging of the solitary hepatic mass: direct correlation with pathology and computed tomography. *Clin Radiol.* 1987;38:559–568.

32. Kelsey CR, Schefter T, Nash SR, et al. Retrospective clinicopathologic correlation of gross tumor size of hepatocellular carcinoma: implications for stereotactic body radiotherapy. *Am J Clin Oncol.* 2005;28:576–580.

33. Cantwell CP, Setty BN, Holalkere N, et al. Liver lesion detection and characterization in patients with colorectal cancer: a comparison of low radiation dose non-enhanced PET/CT, contrast-enhanced PET/CT, and liver MRI. *J Comput Assist Tomogr.* 2008; 32:738–744.

34. Sze G. Magnetic resonance imaging in the evaluation of spinal tumors. *Cancer.* 1991;67:1229–1241.

35. Buhmann Kirchhoff S, Becker C, Duerr HR, et al. Detection of osseous metastases of the spine: comparison of high resolution multi-detector-CT with MRI. *Eur J Radiol.* 2009;69:567–573.

36. Even-Sapir E, Metser U, Flusser G, et al. Assessment of malignant skeletal disease: initial experience with 18F-fluoride PET/CT and comparison between 18F-fluoride PET and 18F-fluoride PET/CT. *J Nucl Med.* 2004;45:272–278.

37. Schmidt GP, Schoenberg SO, Schmid R, et al. Screening for bone metastases: whole-body MRI using a 32-channel system versus dual-modality PET-CT. *Eur Radiol.* 2007;17:939–949.

38. Osmond JD III, Pendergrass HP, Potsaid MS, et al. Accuracy of 99mTC-diphosphonate bone scans and roentgenograms in the detection of prostate, breast and lung carcinoma metastases. *Am J Roentgenol Radium Ther Nucl Med.* 1975;125:972–977.

39. Schirrmeister H, Guhlmann A, Elsner K, et al. Sensitivity in detecting osseous lesions depends on anatomic localization: planar bone scintigraphy versus 18F PET. *J Nucl Med.* 1999;40:1623–1629.

40. Cheran SK, Herndon JE II, Patz EF Jr, et al. Comparison of whole-body FDG-PET to bone scan for detection of bone metastases in patients with a new diagnosis of lung cancer. *Lung Cancer.* 2004;44:317–325.

41. Shie P, Cardarelli R, Brandon D, et al. Meta-analysis: comparison of F-18 fluorodeoxyglucose-positron emission tomography and bone scintigraphy in the detection of bone metastases in patients with breast cancer. *Clin Nucl Med.* 2008;33:97–101.

42. Taphoorn MJ, Heimans JJ, Kaiser MC, et al. Imaging of brain metastases. Comparison of computerized tomography (CT) and magnetic resonance imaging (MRI). *Neuroradiol.* 1989;31:391–395.

43. Davis PC, Hudgins PA, Peterman SB, et al. Diagnosis of cerebral metastases: double-dose delayed CT vs contrast-enhanced MR imaging. *AJNR Am J Neuroradiol.* 1991;12:293–300.

44. Akeson P, Larsson EM, Kristoffersen DT, et al. Brain metastases–comparison of gadodiamide injection-enhanced MR imaging at standard and high dose, contrast-enhanced CT and non-contrast-enhanced MR imaging. *Acta Radiol.* 1995;36:300–306.

45. Kuhn MJ, Hammer GM, Swenson LC, et al. MRI evaluation of "solitary" brain metastases with triple-dose gadoteridol: comparison with contrast-enhanced CT and conventional-dose gadopentetate dimeglumine MRI studies in the same patients. *Comput Med Imaging Graph.* 1994;18:391–399.

46. Terakawa Y, Tsuyuguchi N, Iwai Y, et al. Diagnostic accuracy of ¹¹C-methionine PET for differentiation of recurrent brain tumors from radiation necrosis after radiotherapy. *J Nucl Med.* 2008;49:694–699.

47. Grills IS, Hugo G, Kestin LL, et al. Image-guided radiotherapy via daily online cone-beam CT substantially reduces margin requirements for stereotactic lung radiotherapy. *Int J Radiat Oncol Biol Phys.* 2008;70:1045–1056.

48. Yeung AR, Li JG, Shi W, et al. Tumor localization using cone-beam CT reduces setup margins in conventionally fractionated radiotherapy for lung tumors. *Int J Radiat Oncol Biol Phys.* 2009;74:1100–1107.

49. Song DY, Benedict SH, Cardinale RM, et al. Stereotactic body radiation therapy of lung tumors: preliminary experience using normal tissue complication probability-based dose limits. *Am J Clin Oncol.* 2005;28:591–596.

50. Schefter TE, Kavanagh BD, Raben D, et al. A phase I trial of SBRT for lung metastases. *Int J Radiat Oncol Biol Phys.* 2006;66(4 Suppl):S120–S127.

51. Heinzerling JH, Anderson JF, Papiez L, et al. Four-dimensional computed tomography scan analysis of tumor and organ motion at varying levels of abdominal compression during stereotactic treatment of lung and liver. *Int J Radiat Oncol Biol Phys.* 2008;70:1571–1578.

52. Cheung PC, Sixel KE, Tirona R, et al. Reproducibility of lung tumor position and reduction of lung mass within the planning

target volume using active breathing control (ABC). *Int J Radiat Oncol Biol Phys.* 2003;57:1437–1442.

53. Koshani R, Balter JM, Hayman JA, et al. Short-term and long-term reproducibility of lung tumor position using active breathing control (ABC). *Int J Radiat Oncol Biol Phys* 2006;65:1553–1559.

54. Masi L, Casamassima F, Menichelli C, et al. On-line image guidance for frameless stereotactic radiotherapy of lung malignancies by cone beam CT: comparison between target localization and alignment on bony anatomy. *Acta Oncol.* 2008;47:1422–1431.

55. Hoogeman M, Prévost JB, Nuyttens J, et al. Clinical accuracy of the respiratory tumor tracking system of the cyberknife: assessment by analysis of log files. *Int J Radiat Oncol Biol Phys.* 2009;74:297–303.

56. Nishioka S, Nishioka T, Kawahara M, et al. Exhale fluctuation in respiratory-gated radiotherapy of the lung: a pitfall of respiratory gating shown in a synchronized internal/external marker recording study. *Radiother Oncol.* 2008;86:69–76.

57. Fuss M, Salter BJ, Cavanaugh SX, et al. Daily ultrasound-based image-guided targeting for radiotherapy of upper abdominal malignancies. *Int J Radiat Oncol Biol Phys.* 2004;59:1245–1256.

58. Wurm RE, Gum F, Erbel S. Image guided respiratory gated hypofractionated stereotactic body radiation therapy (H-SBRT) for liver and lung tumors: initial experience. *Acta Oncol.* 2006;45:881–889.

59. Shioyama Y, Nakamura K, Anai S, et al. Stereotactic radiotherapy for lung and liver tumors using a body cast system: setup accuracy and preliminary clinical outcome. *Radiat Med.* 2005;23:407–413.

60. Hawkins MA, Brock KK, Eccles C, et al. Assessment of residual error in liver position using kV cone-beam computed tomography for liver cancer high-precision radiation therapy. *Int J Radiat Oncol Biol Phys.* 2006;66:610–619.

61. Chang EL, Shiu AS, Mendel E, et al. Phase I/II study of stereotactic body radiotherapy for spinal metastasis and its pattern of failure. *J Neurosurg Spine.* 2007;7:151–160.

62. Ryu S, Jin JY, Jin R, et al. Partial volume tolerance of the spinal cord and complications of single-dose radiosurgery. *Cancer.* 2007;109:628–636.

63. Bilsky MH, Yamada Y, Yenice KM, et al. Intensity-modulated stereotactic radiotherapy of paraspinal tumors: a preliminary report. *Neurosurgery.* 2004;54:823–830.

64. Cai J, Sheng K, Sheehan JP, et al. Evaluation of thoracic spinal cord motion using dynamic MRI. *Radiother Oncol.* 2007;84:279–282.

65. Ryu S, Yin FF, Rock J, et al. Image-guided and intensity-modulated radiosurgery for patients with spinal metastasis. *Cancer.* 2003;97:2013–2018.

66. Yu C, Main W, Taylor D, et al. An anthropomorphic phantom study of the accuracy of Cyberknife spinal radiosurgery. *Neurosurgery.* 2004;55:1138–1149.

67. Yin FF, Wang Z, Yoo S, et al. Integration of cone-beam CT in stereotactic body radiation therapy. *Technol Cancer Res Treat.* 2008;7:133–139.

68. Letourneau D, Wong R, Moseley D, et al. Online planning and delivery technique for radiotherapy of spinal metastases using cone beam CT: image quality and system performance. *Int J Radiat Oncol Biol Phys.* 2007;67:1229–1237.

69. Kooy HM, van Herk M, Barnes PD, et al. Image fusion for stereotactic radiotherapy and radiosurgery treatment planning. *Int J Radiat Oncol Biol Phys.* 1994;28:1229–1234.

70. Lattanzi JP, Fein DA, McNeeley SW, et al. Computed tomography-magnetic resonance image fusion: a clinical evaluation of an innovative approach for improved tumor localization in primary central nervous system lesions. *Radiat Oncol Investig.* 1997;5:195–205.

71. Schell MC, Bova FJ, Larsen DA, et al. Stereotactic radiosurgery: report of Task Group 42 Radiation Therapy. Woodbury, NY: American Institute of Physics; 1995. AAPM report no. 54.

72. Lamba M, Breneman JC, Warnick RE. Evaluation of image-guided positioning for frameless intracranial radiosurgery. *Int J Radiat Oncol Biol Phys.* 2009;74:913–919.

73. Brock KK, Hawkins M, Eccles C, et al. Improving image-guided target localization through deformable registration. *Acta Oncol.* 2008;47:1279–1285.

74. Feng M, Kong FM, Gross M, et al. Using fluorodeoxyglucose positron emission tomography to assess tumor volume during radiotherapy for non-small-cell lung cancer and its potential impact on adaptive dose escalation and normal tissue sparing. *Int J Radiat Oncol Biol Phys.* 2009;73:1228–1234.

KV CBCT-Guided Frameless SRS in a Patient with a Solitary Brain Metastasis Treated on a Varian Linear Accelerator

Case Study

Francesco Fiorica, MD, Francesco Cartei, MD, Stefano Ursino, MD, Sara Fabbri, PhD, Sara Lappi, PhD

Patient History

A 60-year-old man, with a history of a T2N1 non–small cell lung cancer (NSCLC) of the left upper lobe treated with lobectomy and lymph node sampling, presented 7 months posttreatment with left hemiparesis and hypesthesia requiring hospitalization. He was offered but declined adjuvant therapy following his initial surgery.

Radiographic workup included a computed tomography (CT) head scan which revealed a 2-cm lesion in the right lenticular nucleus associated with extensive edema. Metastatic workup, including CT scans of the thorax, abdomen, and pelvis, and positron emission tomography (PET) did not show other metastases. Furthermore, a brain magnetic resonance (MR) scan confirmed the presence of a solitary brain metastasis.

In light of the localized nature of the lesion, surgical excision was proposed. However, the patient refused surgery and, thus, stereotactic radiosurgery (SRS) was recommended. We elected to treat this patient using a frameless SRS approach with cone-beam CT (CBCT) image guidance.

Simulation

The patient was immobilized using the fixator shoulder suppression system (Posi-S, Civco, Kalona, IA) and a thermoplastic mask (Zentec, MT-APUD-3-02, Civco, Kalona, IA; Figure 24A-1a). Orthogonal radiographies on an Acuity simulator (Varian Medical Systems, Palo Alto, CA) were obtained after the mask fabrication.

Before CT acquisition, the reproducibility of the immobilization device was tested by repositioning the patient and reacquiring two orthogonal radiographs (Figure 24A-1b). An off-line review was performed using a coregistration software between the two acquisitions (Figure 24A-1c). Transaxial imaging with a slice thickness of 1.25 mm was performed from the patient's vertex to his shoulders, using to our departmental HiSpeed multislice CT scanner (GE Healthcare, Waukesha, WI) with intravenous contrast.

Treatment Planning

The planning CT and diagnostic MR scans were transferred to our Pinnacle treatment planning system (Philips Medical Systems, Andover, MA) and coregistered, using automatic rigid registration (Normalized Mutual Information algorithm). The registration was verified visually in the three orthogonal planes.

The gross tumor volume (GTV) and organs at risk (OARs) were then contoured, using the contrast-enhanced CT and MR images. No expansion was used to create the planning target volume (PTV). The OARs

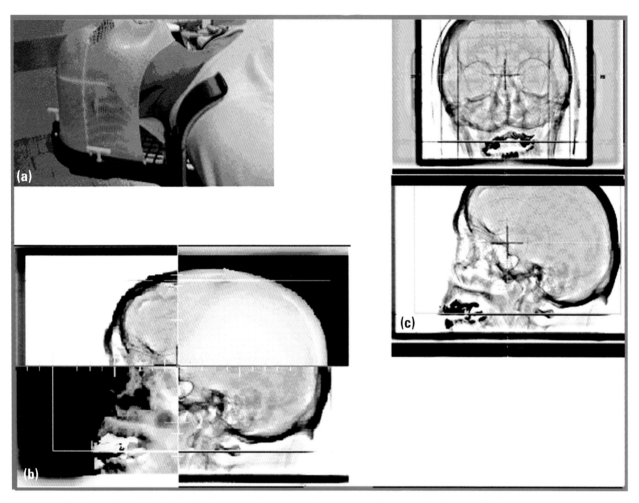

FIGURE 24A-1. Patient immobilized with the fixator shoulder suppression system and a thermoplastic mask (a). After the mask setup and before the computed tomography scan, the patient was repositioned and orthogonal films were obtained (b). The orthogonal films were coregistered and the blended image shows the reproducibility of the patient setup (c).

consisted of the optic chiasm, globes, lenses, optic nerves, and brainstem. A single isocenter was placed automatically in the center of the PTV and non-coplanar dynamic conformal arcs were planned for treatment.

Each arc was conformed to the PTV shape by a multileaf collimator (MLC) (Millennium 120-Leaf, Varian Medical Systems, Palo Alto, CA). Five arcs (table angles: 0°, 0°, 270°, 315°, and 45°; Figure 24A-2a) were selected, with a prescribed PTV dose of 30 Gy to the 80% isodose line in three fractions (Figure 24A-2b). Start and end angles of each arc were: 60° and 160°, 210° and 300°, 190° and 300°, 200° and 300°, and 60° and 160°, respectively.

The doses to normal tissues (chiasm, globes, lens, optic nerves, brainstem, etc.) were reviewed and judged to be acceptable. After plan approval, isocenter location and information of each arc (MLC parameters, jaws, monitor units, couch angles) were exported to the Aria record and verify system (Varian Medical Systems, Palo Alto, CA). The planning CT was also exported as a reference data set to compare with CBCT data to verify the patient's setup.

Treatment Delivery

Treatment was delivered with a 2100 CD linear accelerator (Varian Medical Systems, Palo Alto, CA) equipped with a kilovoltage (kV) On-Board Imager (OBI). Before the patient's first treatment, additional quality assurance (QA) for the verification of the kV-MV isocenters coincidence was performed by the physics staff. For this purpose, a cube phantom with a radio-opaque marker was placed at the linac isocenter and then imaged with the OBI system.

The patient, immobilized with fixator shoulder suppression system and a thermoplastic mask, was aligned using external fiducials. A CBCT was then obtained with the OBI system using a "half-fan" protocol (Figure 24A-3). The volumetric images, acquired during a rotation of 360° in approximately 60 seconds, were matched online with the planning CT (Figure 24A-3). As a first step,

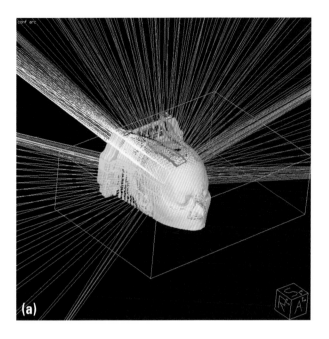

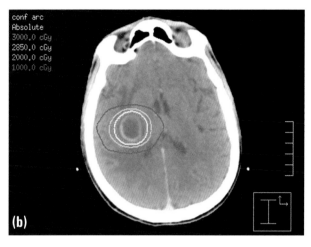

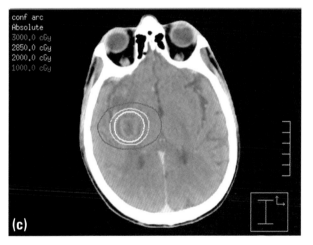

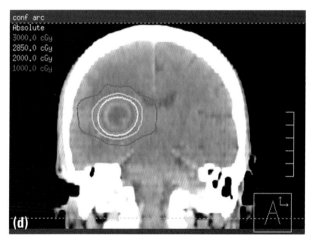

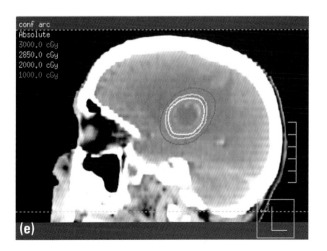

FIGURE 24A-2. A reconstructed image showing the five arcs used for treatment (a) and axial, sagittal, and coronal (b–e) computed tomography images overlaid with isodose curves showing dose conformity of the treatment plan.

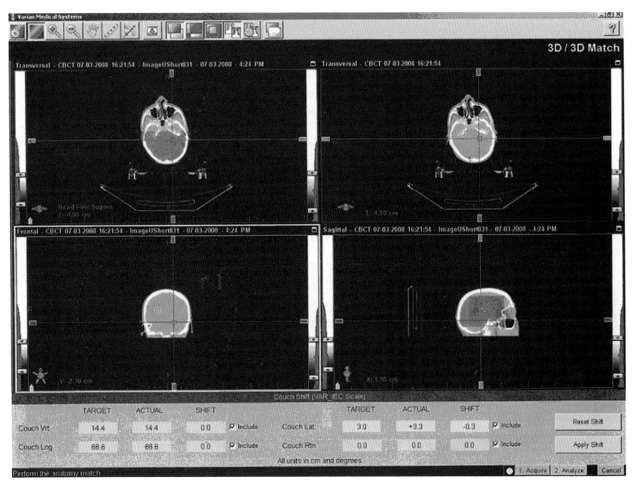

FIGURE 24A-3. On-line patient positioning using the Varian On-Board Imaging system. The cone-beam computed tomography (CT) scan is matched on-line with the planning CT. An automatic registration and a visual check are used and the required corrections are performed.

an automatic registration was performed. The result of the registration was checked visually. The translational errors were minor (< 3 mm) and no rotational errors were detected. The required corrections were performed by automatically moving the treatment couch and a second CBCT was acquired to confirm the correct positioning. As additional QA, the second CBCT was sent to the Pinnacle Planning System (Philips Medical Systems, Andover, MA) to be coregistered with the planning CT as an independent check (Figure 24A-4). Because there was an optimal correspondence between the two data sets of volumetric images, no replanning was performed.

Treatment was delivered using 6-MV photons at a dose rate of 600 monitor units per minute. During treatment, no additional positional verification was performed. Each arc and couch position additionally underwent anticollision testing before delivery. Finally, all treatment information was double-checked by the physics staff before the initiation of treatment. This procedure was repeated in all three fractions and each treatment was completed within a 1-hour time slot.

Clinical Outcome

The treatment was well tolerated, without any significant acute toxicities. The patient was able to maintain his normal lifestyle and usual daily activities. Five months posttreatment, MR demonstrated regression of the treated lesion with a residual nodular enhancement on the axial postcontrast T1-weighted image (Figure 24A-5). However, as seen in Figure 24A-5c, there was no abnormal increment of relative cerebral blood volume in perfusion MR imaging, suggestive of radiation-induced injury. At his most recent follow up, the patient remained without disease recurrence in the brain or significant neurologic sequelae but had developed extracranial disease progression.

Our initial clinical experience utilizing frameless SRS with on-line CBCT image guidance in 12 patients (40 SRS procedures) was presented previously.[1] Before treatment, a CBCT scan was acquired and matched to the planning CT scan aligning bony anatomy and the displacements were corrected on-line. A second CBCT was obtained to confirm repositioning. The average applied shifts were

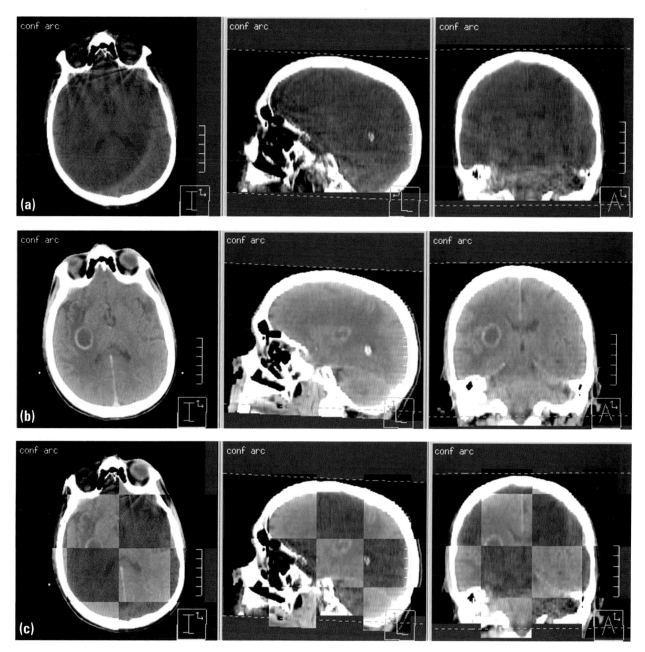

FIGURE 24A-4. After the corrections, a second cone-beam computed tomography (CBCT) scan **(a)** was taken and sent to treatment planning system to be matched with the planning computed tomography (CT) **(b)**. The blended image **(c)** shows an excellent correspondence between the corrected CBCT and planning CT. No replanning was necessary.

0.8 mm ± 1.2 mm, 0.3 mm ± 0.8 mm, and 0.2 mm ± 0.3 mm in the lateral, cranio–caudal and anterior–posterior directions, respectively. The absolute magnitude of the isocenter dislocation was 1.6 mm ± 0.7 mm. The average rotational deviation around the anterior–posterior axis was 0.05° ± 0.64°; no detectable rotational deviations around the other two axes were observed.

Reference

1. Lappi S, Fiorica F, Fabbri S, et al. Frameless hypofractionated stereotactic radiotherapy using cone beam CT image guidance for intra-cranial metastases [abstract]. *Int J Radiat Oncol Biol Phys.* 2008;71(suppl 1):S656.

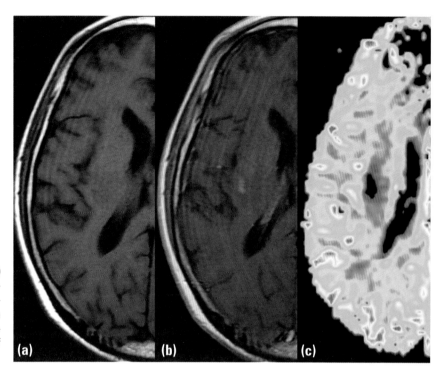

FIGURE 24A-5. Magnetic resonance (MR) scan 6 months after treatment. Axial T1-weighted MR shows no significant abnormalities (a), postcontrast image shows a residual nodular enhancement (b), and perfusion MR shows no abnormal increment of cerebral blood volume (c).

Optically Guided Frameless SRS Using a Single Isocenter Technique in a Breast Cancer Patient with Multiple Brain Metastases Treated on the Varian Trilogy System

Case Study

Joshua D. Lawson, MD, Sameer K. Nath, MD,
Jia-Zhu Wang, PhD, Kevin Murphy, MD

Patient History

A 53-year-old woman with a history of a stage IIIA (T2N2M0) left breast cancer status post–neoadjuvant chemotherapy, breast conserving surgery, and adjuvant radiation therapy (RT) presented with left-sided paresthesias. Magnetic resonance (MR) imaging of the brain revealed multiple brain metastases. No other sites of disease recurrence were noted on physical examination or on restaging radiographic studies.

The patient was treated with whole brain RT (WBRT; 35 Gy in 2.5-Gy daily fractions) and tolerated treatment well. On follow-up MR imaging, however, she was found to have persistence of four enhancing lesions. She was presented at our combined neurosurgery/radiation oncology stereotactic radiosurgery (SRS) conference and the consensus opinion, with consideration of her excellent performance status and absence of other disease sites, was for SRS. We elected to treat her with an optically guided frameless SRS using a single-isocenter technique on a Varian Trilogy linear accelerator (Varian Medical Systems, Palo Alto, CA).

Simulation

On the day of simulation, a customized bite block (a dental mold of the patient's upper teeth) was fabricated. A set of four fiducial markers, angled 5° to 10° from horizontal was then affixed to the bite block (Frameless Array, Varian Medical Systems, Palo Alto, CA). The patient was next taken to the treatment vault where reseat verification of the bite block was performed, ensuring bite block reproducibility. A helmet with test fiducial markers was firmly affixed to the patient's head and an optical camera was used to measure the relative positions of each reflective marker to the test fiducials to determine positioning error. The dental mold was removed and replaced 10 times to estimate the positioning error; an acceptable variation of less than 0.75 mm was confirmed.

After completion of this step, the patient was taken to our departmental wide-bore multislice computed tomography (CT) simulator (GE Healthcare, Waukesha, WI) and placed in the supine position on a custom head rest. An aquaplast mask was then fabricated with a cutout to accept the bite block and reflective markers (Figure 24B-1).

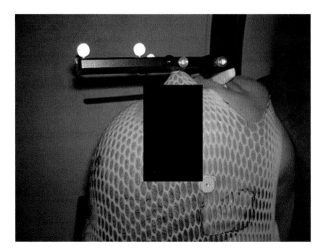

FIGURE 24B-1. Patient immobilized with an aquaplast face mask with a cutout to allow placement of bite block and affixed frameless array. Note that the fiducial array is attached to the bite block at 15° off horizontal, improving the detection of the markers by the optical camera.

Transaxial imaging with a slice thickness of 1.25 mm was performed from her vertex to her shoulders. No intravenous or oral contrast was used. While immobilized in the treatment, the patient next underwent a planning MR using a SRS protocol (fast three-dimensional [3D] volumetric T1 scan, 512 × 512 pixels, 1.5-mm thickness, 26-cm field of view [FOV], no tilt FOV) on our departmental 3-Tesla MR unit (GE Healthcare, Waukesha, WI). The treatment planning MR confirmed the presence

of the four known lesions; however, an additional two lesions were also noted.

Treatment Planning

The planning CT and planning MR scans were transferred to the Varian *FastPlan* Treatment Planning System (Varian Medical Systems, Palo Alto, CA) and fused, using, initially manual, and then automatic, rigid registration to a treatment planning MR scan consisting of approximately 100 T1-weighted axial images of the patient's brain. Visual verification of registration was then done in the axial, coronal, and sagittal planes (Figure 24B-2).

Manual segmentation of the tumor and organs at risk (OARs) was performed. The OARs consisted of the optic chiasm, globes, lenses, optic nerves, and brainstem. The gross tumor volume (GTV) consisted of all visualized tumor on the CT and MR image data sets. A 2-mm GTV to planning target volume (PTV) expansion was used. A single isocenter was placed manually in the center of the brain, independent of the target volumes. Nine intensity-modulated fields were used to target the defined lesions, with gantry angles of 45°, 70°, 75°, 100°, 260°, 275°, 280°, 290°, and 310° (couch angles of 70°, 45°, 0°, 15°, 0°, 305°, 335°, 0°, and 275°, respectively). The prescription dose was 18 Gy to the 98% isodose line, optimized for coverage of each target lesion (Figure 24B-3). Dose–volume histograms (DVHs) were created for each of the target volumes as well as each OAR. The doses

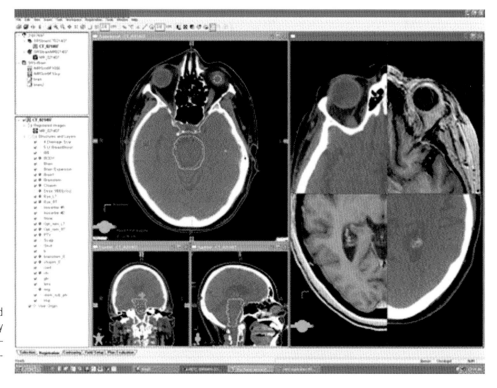

FIGURE 24B-2. A checkerboard image showing the adequacy of the computed tomography–magnetic resonance image registration.

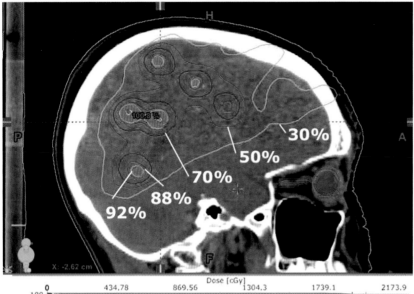

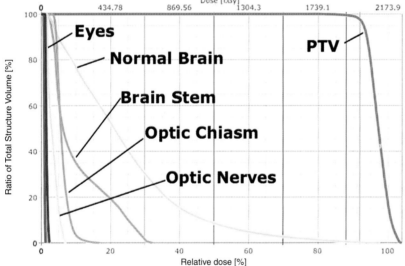

FIGURE 24B-3. Isodose curves and dose–volume histogram results in the treated patient.

to normal tissues (chiasm, globes, lens, optic nerves, brainstem, etc.) and target volumes were reviewed and judged to be acceptable. After plan approval, the CT image data set, isocenter location, and couch information of each field were exported to the computer of the camera system (SonArray, Varian Medical Systems, Palo Alto, CA). Anterior–posterior (AP) and right lateral digitally reconstructed radiographs (DRRs) were generated for patient setup.

Treatment Delivery

Before the patient was brought into the vault for treatment, additional quality assurance (QA) was performed by the physics staff. Manual double-checking of each treatment field calculation was performed. Also, the isocenter pointer was first attached to the linac and the calibration jig was used to check the calibration of the optical camera.

The patient was then positioned on the treatment couch, immobilized in the aquaplast mask with bite block and fiducial array. Further assurance of proper patient positioning was accomplished using the On-Board Imager (OBI; Varian Oncology Systems, Palo Alto, CA) to obtain a set of orthogonal images (Figure 24B-4). Comparison of these images to the DRRs from simulation allowed confirmation of patient positioning. This comparison was aided by the contouring bony landmarks in the skull. In this case, no shifts were required.

Treatment was delivered on a Trilogy linear accelerator (Varian Oncology Systems, Palo Alto, CA) using 6-MV photons at a dose rate of 1000 monitor units per minute. During treatment, the optical camera provides real-time (intrafraction) monitoring of patient position. If a displacement of greater than 0.5 mm were to occur, treatment would be stopped to allow repositioning of the patient. In this case, there were no required treatment

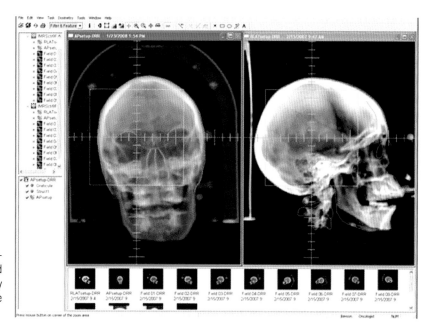

FIGURE 24B-4. Orthogonal digitally reconstructed radiographs (anterior–posterior and right lateral) used for patient positioning. Bony landmarks are contoured in green and aid in the matching process.

interruptions. Before delivery of each treatment field, the optical guidance system was used to make manual adjustments ensuring a displacement of less than 0.3 mm. Each gantry and couch position additionally underwent anticollision testing before delivery. Finally, all treatment information was double-checked by physics staff before initiation of treatment. Treatment was completed within a 1-hour time slot.

Clinical Outcome

The SRS treatment was well-tolerated, without any significant acute toxicities. The patient subsequently initiated capecitabine therapy and was followed for 9 months, at which time a single new right frontal lesion measuring 0.8 cm was noted. She continued to have radiographic control of each of her previously treated lesions, and so received an additional SRS treatment to the new lesion, using a cone-based frameless approach, delivering 18 Gy to the 80% isodose line. Eight months following this second SRS procedure, she again developed a single new lesion, which was treated with a third frame-less SRS procedure. She tolerated this third procedure well and continues to follow up in our clinic, now 20 months since her first treatment.

Our initial experience using an optically guided single-isocenter frameless SRS on a Varian Trilogy in 26 patients (138 lesions) with multiple brain metastases was recently published.[1] Primary tumors were breast (42%), lung (31%), and melanoma (27%). The median prescription dose was 18 Gy and was administered in a single fraction, except in one patient who received 25 Gy in five fractions. Whole-brain RT was given to six patients. At a median follow-up of 3.3 months (range, 0.2–21 months), the 6- and 12-month actuarial survivals were 50% and 38%, respectively. Of 21 patients (116 lesions) evaluable for local control, 6- and 12-month actuarial local control rates were 97% and 83%, respectively. Acute and late grade 3 toxicities occurred in one (4%) and two (8%) patients, respectively. No grade 4 toxicities were observed. The total treatment time and beam-on time ranged from 9.0 to 38.9 minutes (median, 21.0 minutes) and 2.0 to 17.9 minutes (median, 5.4 minutes), respectively.

Reference

1. Murphy KT, Nath SK, Simpson DR, et al. A single-isocenter technique for frameless intensity-modulated stereotactic radiosurgery for multiple brain metastases: clinical experience and outcomes [abstract]. *Int J Radiat Oncol Biol Phys.* 2009;75: 237–238.

Chapter 24C

Image-Guided Single-Fraction IMRT Using a Varian Linear Accelerator in a Patient with a Paraspinal Metastasis

Case Study

Dev R. Puri, MD, Oren Cahlon, MD, Mark H. Bilsky, MD, Yoshiya Yamada, MD

Patient History

A 71-year-old man presented with elevated liver function tests. A computed tomography (CT) scan was performed and identified an extensive, heterogeneously enhancing mass occupying most of the right hepatic lobe. Needle biopsy revealed hepatocellular carcinoma. The tumor was deemed to be unresectable and was treated with hepatic artery embolization.

Four months after diagnosis, the patient complained of mid-back pain and underwent a magnetic resonance (MR) scan of the spine (Figure 24C-1). This demonstrated an expansile lesion involving the left T8 pedicle and left posterolateral vertebral body, with contiguous involvement of the left T8–T9 neural foramen. There was resultant spinal canal compromise and cord displacement but no compression.

The patient's case was discussed at a multidisciplinary tumor board. Upfront surgery versus radiotherapy (RT) were discussed as possible treatment options. The consensus of the tumor board was to proceed with single-fraction intensity-modulated radiotherapy (IMRT). We elected to treat him with an image-guided approach on a linear accelerator (Varian Medical Systems, Palo Alto, CA).

Simulation

For purposes of target localization, six gold seeds were placed around the T8 vertebral body approximately

2 weeks before simulation. On the day of simulation, the patient was immobilized in the Memorial Body Cradle (MBC), which consists of a platform base and four lateral

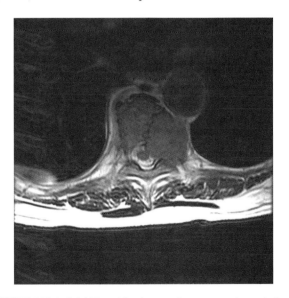

FIGURE 24C-1. Axial T2-weighted magnetic resonance image before treatment shows a focally expansile osseous metastasis involving the left T8 pedicle with contiguous involvement of the posterior and left lateral aspect of the T8 vertebral body with expansion into the left ventral and lateral epidural space. There is mild-to-moderate spinal canal compromise with focal effacement of the thecal sac and spinal cord impingement and displacement without frank spinal cord compression. There is contiguous involvement of the left T8–T9 neural foramen.

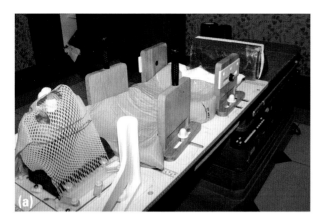
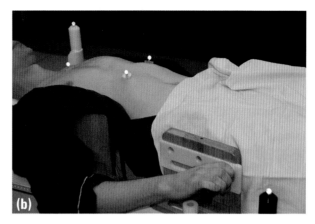

FIGURE 24C-2. The Memorial Body Cradle is a noninvasive device used for immobilization. (**a**) Four sturdy paddles apply pressure to the bony pelvis and rib cage. An Aquaplast face mask is used to improve immobilization for treatments in the cervical or upper thoracic spine. (**b**) Hand grips are adjustable in the superior–inferior direction and allow for improved shoulder reproducibility.

pressure plates that are applied to the bony pelvis (e.g., hips) and ribs under the arms (Figure 24C-2). Adjustable hand grips attached to the hip plates are also used to ensure reproducible upper-body positioning. Unlike patients treated to the cervical and upper thoracic spine, the location of this patient's tumor was caudal enough so that a face mask was not used. An alpha cradle was created to conform to the patient's underside from the shoulders to the buttocks and from the thighs to the ankles. A large roll was placed under the knees.

Once the alpha cradles were fabricated, the patient underwent CT simulation (Philips Medical Systems, Andover, MA) using a 3-mm slice thickness. A preliminary gross tumor volume (GTV) and treatment isocenter were determined from CT images. In addition to the anterior isocenter tattoo, alignment tattoos were placed 12 cm superior and inferior to isocenter. Lateral alignment tattoos were placed on the patient's sides between the rib and hip plates.

Treatment Planning

Directly after CT image acquisition, the patient underwent an MR scan. Magnetic resonance aids in spinal cord localization as well as GTV delineation. The MR was performed with the patient in the treatment position within the MBC and was then fused with the treatment planning CT. More recently, we have replaced MR with a CT myelogram performed 3 to 4 hours before simulation. This enables visualization of the contrast dye in the cerebrospinal fluid (CSF) surrounding the spinal cord on the simulation CT and facilitates delineation of the cord and/or cauda equina. The use of CT myelography instead of MR allows greater treatment planning efficiency, decreased potential for overlay error, and enhanced visualization of critical structures, particularly in the presence of artifact-generating surgical hardware.

The planning target volume (PTV) consisted of a GTV plus a 10-mm uniform margin. However, a reduced margin at the spinal cord interface was required. In cases with vertebral body involvement, we now typically include the entire vertebral body as the clinical target volume (CTV); the PTV is then created by expanding the CTV by 2 mm.

Inverse treatment planning was then used to generate the IMRT plan, with a dose constraint of 1000 cGy to any point along the spinal cord. Using our in-house treatment planning software, an IMRT plan with six equally weighted coplanar treatment beams was generated: one posterior, two right posterior obliques, and three left posterior obliques. These beams were spaced 20° to 30° apart (Figure 24C-3). All six beams had a nominal energy of 6 MV. A total dose of 2100 cGy was prescribed to the 100% isodose line.

Treatment Delivery

On the day of treatment, the MBC was placed on the treatment machine couch and the patient was subsequently positioned within the cradle with therapist assistance. Several pretreatment checks were then performed to ensure proper superior–inferior (SI) placement. The isocenter tattoo was used to confirm that the patient was not displaced more than 1 mm with respect to the MBC in the SI direction. Rotation about the SI axis was checked by inspecting the lateral alignment tattoos relative to lateral room lasers and hip height relative to hip plates. Cushions were placed under the patient's elbows and hands. It is important to note that a patient can release the handgrip and move either arm as the torso remains fixed in place by the lateral plates.

Orthogonal localization images were taken before treatment. The setup coordinates determined at CT simulation were used for the initial setup. In all cases, a correction to the setup is made only if the observed setup error in any direction is greater than 2 mm. More recently,

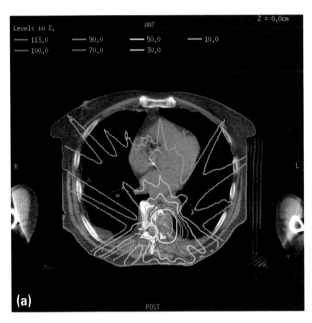
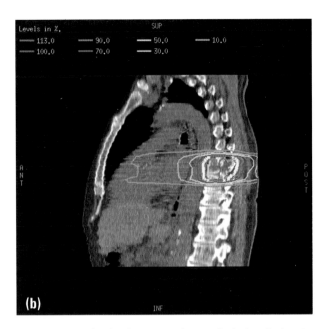

FIGURE 24C-3. Axial (a) and sagittal (b) isodose curves show steep dose gradient between the planning target volume and spinal cord using six-field intensity-modulated radiotherapy plan resulting in less than 50% of the prescribed dose to the cord.

we have also used kilovoltage (kV) cone-beam computed tomography (CBCT) imaging for pretreatment localization. In these cases, a scan length of 50 mm to 60 mm is acquired with a slice thickness of 2 mm (the CBCT scanner cannot scan at the same 3-mm slice thickness as the simulator CT scanner). The positions of the target and other anatomic landmarks are identified on the CT slices, and their stereotactic coordinates are computed in the frame's independent coordinate system. The new coordinates of all landmarks are compared with those from the planning CT study and adjustments are made as for deviations greater than 2 mm.

Once accurate setup was achieved, treatment was delivered using a Varian 2400 CD linear accelerator (Varian Medical Systems, Palo Alto, CA). The total beam-on time was 30 minutes. The patient was on the treatment couch for approximately 2 hours.

Although the results from our immobilization technique have been very encouraging, an inherit limitation to any noninvasive immobilization technique is that it is not possible to ensure that the patient does not move during the treatment. We are now taking the additional measure of monitoring patients with an infrared camera system. Small reflective markers are attached with adhesive tape to the patient's hips and sternum and are tracked during the treatment in a coordinate system referenced to the cradle. These are monitored throughout the treatment and can ensure the patient stays within 2 mm of the treatment position.

Clinical Outcome

The patient tolerated treatment well and had an immediate clinical response. He was pain-free and able to

discontinue narcotic use within 2 weeks after treatment. An MR scan performed 3 months after treatment showed a notable shrinkage of the paraspinal tumor at T8 (Figure 24C-4). Follow-up MR scans 5, 7, and 9 months after treatment revealed no evidence of local progression. He remained free of back pain and off narcotics and did not suffer any RT-related toxicity other than mild fatigue the week after treatment. Ultimately he died of progres-

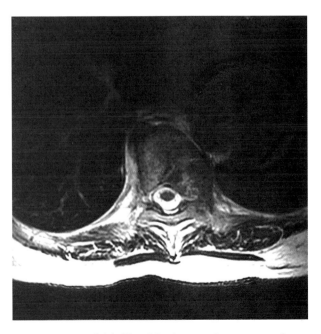

FIGURE 24C-4. Axial T2-weighted magnetic resonance image 3 months after single-fraction image-guided intensity-modulated radiotherapy. Contraction of the T8 vertebral body lesion is noted with significant improvement in the epidural component.

sive systemic disease 10 months after treatment, but, at the time of his death, he remained free of back pain and his imaging studies did not show any local disease progression.

Early clinical reports from our institution in patients with initial or previously irradiated paraspinal masses show an improvement in pain symptoms without significant adverse effects.[1-4] Dosimetric evaluation of the treatment suggests that dose escalation to 24 Gy is possible in paraspinal tumors while respecting cord tolerance and that this dose may result in higher rates of local control compared with less than 24 Gy.[2,3,5] Further investigation is needed to better define cord tolerance in the setting of single-fraction image-guided IMRT.

We have now escalated our single-fraction dose to 24 Gy and recently published our updated experience treating 93 patients with paraspinal tumors with single-fraction doses of 18 Gy to 24 Gy (67 patients received 24 Gy).[2] At a median follow-up of 15 months, the actuarial local control for this cohort was 90% and histologic type was not correlated with outcome. There was, however, a dose-response in this cohort with a statistically significant improvement in local control with a prescribed dose of 24 Gy compared with 18 Gy to 23 Gy ($P = .03$). On the basis of these results, we are currently accruing to a phase 1 dose-escalation protocol investigating the feasibility of using this technique to deliver up to 28 Gy in a single fraction. The maximum point dose allowed to the cord is 14 Gy and to the cauda equina is 16 Gy. The dose constraint on the bowel is 16 Gy.

References

1. Bilsky MH, Yamada Y, Yenice KM, et al. Intensity-modulated stereotactic radiotherapy of paraspinal tumors: a preliminary report. *Neurosurgery.* 2004;54:823–830.
2. Yamada Y, Bilsky MH, Lovelock DM, et al. High-dose, single-fraction, image-guided intensity-modulated radiotherapy for metastatic spinal lesions. *Int J Radiat Oncol Biol Phys.* 2008;71:484–490.
3. Yamada Y, Lovelock DM, Yenice KM, et al. Multifractionated image-guided and stereotactic intensity-modulated radiotherapy of paraspinal tumors: a preliminary report. *Int J Radiat Oncol Biol Phys.* 2005;62:53–61.
4. Wright JL, Lovelock DM, Bilsky MH, et al. Clinical outcomes after reirradiation of paraspinal tumors. *Am J Clin Oncol.* 2006; 29:495–502.
5. Yenice KM, Lovelock DM, Hunt MA, et al. CT image-guided intensity-modulated therapy for paraspinal tumors using stereotactic immobilization. *Int J Radiat Oncol Biol Phys.* 2003;55:583–593.

KV Planar Image-Guided Frameless SRS in a Patient with a Cervical Spine Metastasis Treated Using the CyberKnife System

Case Study

Peter C. Gerszten, MD, Steven A. Burton, MD, Cihat Ozhasoglu, PhD

Patient History

A 24-year-old man with a history of a mediastinal germ cell tumor presented with neck pain, progressive weakness, and numbness in both upper extremities. A magnetic resonance (MR) scan revealed a C7 lesion with a collapse of the vertebral body and significant spinal canal and neural foraminal compromise (Figure 24D-1). The patient's pain was uncontrolled despite oral hydromorphone. On physical examination, he was found to have bilateral diminished sensation in a C8 nerve root distribution, as well as bilateral triceps and hand grasp weakness.

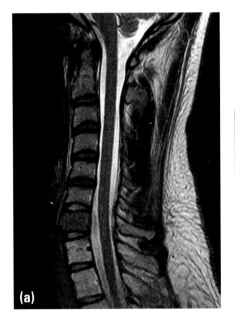
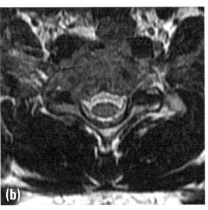

FIGURE 24D-1. Magnetic resonance study with gadolinium enhancement revealing the C7 vertebral body metastasis on (a) sagittal and (b) axial views.

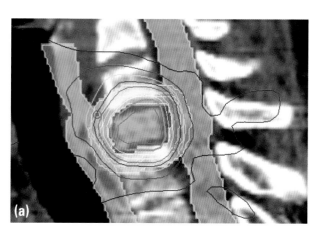
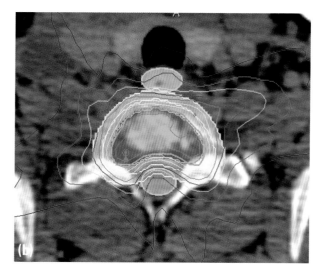

FIGURE 24D-2. Sagittal (a) and axial (b) images of the isodose lines of the treatment plan. This plan was designed to treat the tumor with a prescribed dose of 17 Gy to the edge of the tumor in a single fraction with a maximum tumor dose of 21.25 Gy. The tumor volume was 9.2 cm³ and the spinal cord received a maximum dose of 8.5 Gy. Note the conformality of the isodose lines around the target, minimizing dose to the spinal cord.

Severely diminished range of motion of his cervical spine because of mechanical pain was also noted.

The patient was referred by his medical oncologist for neurosurgical and radiation oncology consultation. At the time of referral, he was found to have a large right malignant pleural effusion and progressive systemic disease. Open surgery for neural element decompression and fixation was felt to be associated with an unacceptably high risk, and a stereotactic radiosurgical (SRS) approach was proposed. We elected to treat the patient with frameless image-guided SRS using the CyberKnife System (Accuray Inc, Sunnyvale, CA).

Simulation

On the day of simulation, six 0.8 mm by 5 mm gold fiducial markers (Alpha-Omega Services, Bellflower, CA) were percutaneously implanted into the vertebral pedicles immediately above and below the C7 level in the department of radiology as a "same-day surgery" outpatient procedure. Following fiducial implantation, the patient was taken directly to the radiation oncology department for computed tomography (CT) simulation. He was placed in supine position in a conformal Vac-Lok bag (CIVCO, Kalona, IA). Transaxial CT imaging was performed using a Lightspeed scanner (GE Healthcare, Waukesha, WI) with a slice thickness of 1.25 mm. The scan was performed from his skull base to T9 using intravenous contrast.

Treatment Planning

The planning CT was then transferred to the Accuray InView workstation. The C7 vertebral body tumor and

organs at risk (OARs) were contoured jointly by the neurosurgeon and the radiation oncologist. The gross tumor volume (GTV) consisted of all visualized tumor on the enhanced planning CT scan as well as the diagnostic MR, including the entire vertebral body and both pedicles. No expansion was used to create a planning target volume (PTV). The OARs included the spinal cord, both lungs, and the esophagus. A treatment dose of 17 Gy was prescribed to the 80% isodose line, with a maximum dose to the spinal cord of 8.5 Gy (Figures 24D-2 and 24D-3).

A conformal nonisocentric treatment plan consisting of 148 beams was generated using inverse planning. Because of the proximity of the lesion to the cord, two cone sizes (10 mm and 15 mm) were selected. Use of the smaller collimator (10 mm) allowed the posterior aspect of the lesion close to the cord to be covered sufficiently by the prescription dose while the larger collimator was used to deliver most of the dose to the portion of the tumor away from the cord (anterior part of the tumor). In general, a CyberKnife plan is considered acceptable if the prescription dose covers 80% of the tumor volume. The prescription isodose line shown in orange in Figure 24D-2 covered 87% of the tumor volume in this patient.

Treatment Delivery

On the day of treatment, the patient was immobilized in the same rigid fixation device as used during CT simulation and was further positioned on the treatment couch by using diagnostic near-real-time x-ray imaging. Digitally reconstructed radiographs (DRRs) were generated for patient setup (Figure 24D-4).

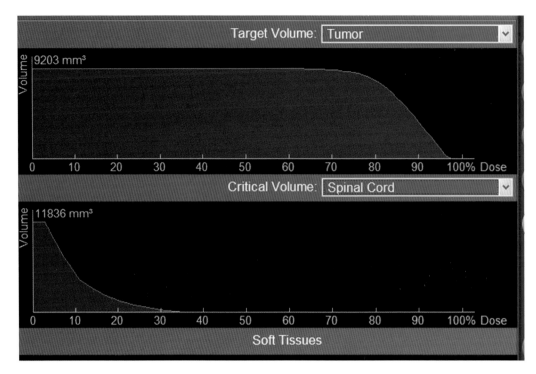

FIGURE 24D-3. The dose–volume histogram of the treatment plan demonstrating dose received by the tumor as well as the spinal cord.

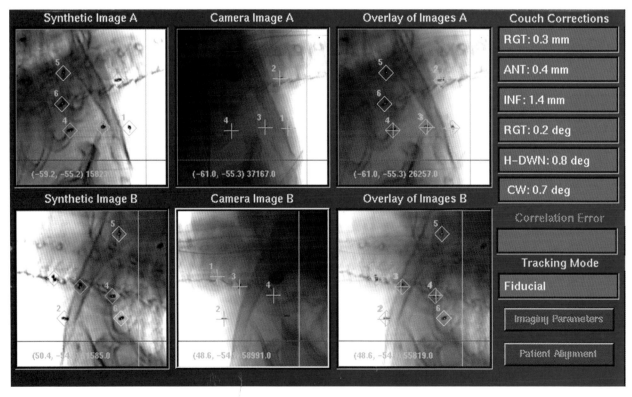

FIGURE 24D-4. A screen capture of the CyberKnife console computer taken during treatment. The synthetic images are digitally reconstructed radiographs (DRRs) generated from the patient's computed tomography scan. The "diamonds" in the DRRs indicate the position of the gold markers. The camera images are the near-real-time x-ray images taken during the treatment. The green crosses in these images depict the positions of the gold fiducial markers as determined by real-time automatic image-processing algorithm. "Couch corrections" indicate the required couch adjustments to set up the patient exactly as he was scanned. Note that these corrections are six-dimensional (three translations and three rotations).

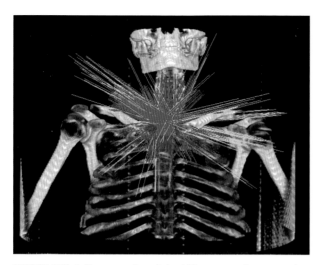

FIGURE 24D-5. Demonstration of the 148 treatment beams used to deliver the radiosurgery treatment. Beams with non-zero dose are shown in cyan.

The SRS treatment was delivered using 6-MV photons at a dose rate of 400 monitor units (MU) per minute. A total of 148 beams was used to deliver the treatment dose (Figure 24D-5). Two orthogonal near-real-time diagnostic x-ray images were obtained after every four beams (approximately every 2 minutes) and compared with DRRs to determine the patient position throughout the treatment. The robot automatically adjusted the radiation beam to compensate for patient movement (Figure 24D-6), which averaged approximately 1.5 mm. Treatment was completed in 67 minutes.

Clinical Outcome

The SRS treatment was well tolerated, without any significant acute or subacute toxicity. The patient reported significant improvement in his symptoms within several weeks of the treatment. A follow-up MR scan performed 7 weeks after treatment demonstrated no tumor progression, and open surgical intervention was thus successfully avoided.

Our clinical experience using the CyberKnife system in the treatment of patients with metastatic spinal tumors was recently published.[1] A cohort of 500 cases of spinal metastases treated with frameless image-guided SRS was reviewed. Lesion location included 73 cervical, 212 thoracic, 112 lumbar, and 103 sacral. Tumor volumes ranged from 0.20 cc to 264 cc (mean, 46 cc). Maximum intratumoral doses ranged from 12.5 Gy to 25 Gy (mean, 20 Gy). Long-term pain improvement was seen in 290 of 336 cases (86%) presenting with pain. Long-term tumor control was noted in 90% of lesions treated with SRS as a primary treatment and in 88% of lesions treated for radiographic tumor progression. Twenty-seven of 32 patients (84%) presenting with a progressive neurologic deficit experienced at least some clinical improvement following treatment.

Reference

1. Gerszten PC, Burton SA, Ozhasoglu C, et al. Radiosurgery for spinal metastases: clinical experience in 500 cases from a single institution. *Spine.* 2007;32:193–199.

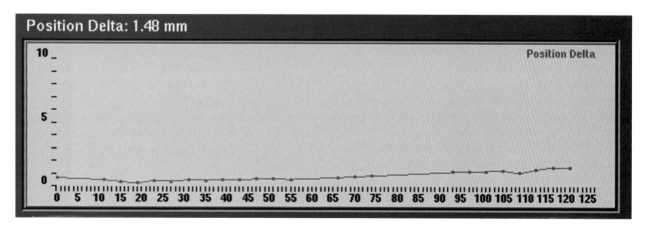

FIGURE 24D-6. "Position delta" is the deviation of the patient's position during treatment from the planning computed tomography position. The vertical axis shows the deviation in millimeters, and the horizontal axis indicated the beam number. The patient moved only a few millimeters throughout the treatment, which is typical of most spine treatments.

KV CT-Guided SBRT Using the Varian CT-on-Rails System in a Patient with a Solitary Spine Metastasis

Case Study

QUYNH-NHU NGUYEN, MD, ALMON SHIU, PhD, ERIC L. CHANG, MD

Patient History

A 41-year-old man presented with complaints of mid-back pain and lower extremity weakness. A magnetic resonance (MR) scan revealed a metastatic lesion involving the body and pedicles of the T8 vertebral body, extending into the soft tissues and epidural space compressing the cord. Further radiographic studies including an abdominal–pelvic computed tomography (CT) scan revealed a 4.3 cm right renal mass, felt to represent the primary tumor. The patient underwent vertebrectomy and decompression of T8 with placement of an expandable titanium cage from T7 to T9 for stabilization. He subsequently received neoadjuvant bevacizumab followed by a radical nephrectomy; pathology review confirmed the diagnosis of renal cell carcinoma.

The patient was discussed at the multidisciplinary spine conference and our consensus recommendation was for stereotactic body radiotherapy (SBRT) to sterilize residual microscopic disease. We elected to treat him on our CT-on-Rails system using volumetric image guidance.

Simulation

To minimize intrafraction movement and vertebral body movement associated with breathing, the patient was placed in a supine position and immobilized using a stere-

otactic body frame system (SBFS; Integra Radionics, Burlington, MA), consisting of a carbon fiber base plate, whole body vacuum system, plastic fixation sheet, stereotactic localizer, and target-positioning frame. The patient was placed straight and supine on the vacuum cushion with his arms above his head resting on an arm-supporting device. A plastic fixation sheet was placed on top of the patient and vacuum sealed.

The T8 vertebral body was localized under fluoroscopy on a conventional simulator (Simulix-MC, Oldelft, Fairfax, VA) with anterior–posterior (AP) and lateral films as shown in Figure 24E-1. The center of the T8 vertebral body was marked on the patient and the body frame was used for positioning the patient during the planning CT scan.

The patient was then taken to the diagnostic imaging suite for intrathecal contrast administration to delineate the spinal cord. In the afternoon, he was brought to our CT-on-Rails suite, placed supine in the stereotactic body-fix frame with the plastic fixation sheet. The CT myelogram images were then acquired using the EXaCT targeting system (Varian Medical Systems, Palo Alto, CA) as shown in Figure 24E-2a. The EXaCT system integrates a high-speed CT scan on rails (GE Healthcare, Waukesha, WI) and a 21 EX linear accelerator (Varian Medical Systems, Palo Alto, CA) equipped with a Millenium 120 multileaf collimator in addition to 6-MV and 18-MV photon

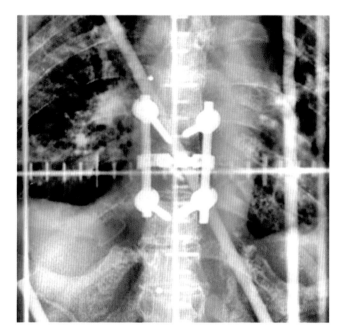
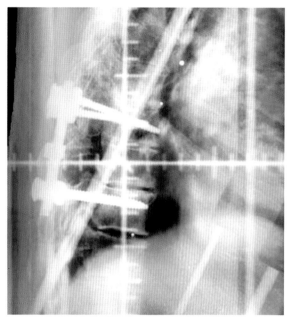

FIGURE 24E-1. Anterior–posterior (left) and right lateral (right) simulation films. These films are used to identify the correct location of the vertebrae to be scanned on the CT-on-Rails unit.

energies. We have augmented the capabilities of our EXaCT by incorporating a 6-dimensional robotic couch top (HexaPOD, Elekta/Medical Intelligence Medizintechnik GmbH, Schwabmünchen, Germany) to replace the existing treatment couch top on our EXaCT as shown in Figure 24E-2b. The advantages of this system are that the couch top can be leveled to remove the sagging caused by patient's weight and can be swung into treatment with the linear accelerator or for CT scanning without moving the patient because the couch is shared between the two machines. The patient was scanned from T5 to T10 with 2-mm slice thickness.

Treatment Planning

Treatment planning was performed using inverse-planning intensity-modulated radiotherapy (IMRT) software (P³IMRT, Philips Medical Systems, Andover, MA). The gross target volume (GTV) included any gross disease delineated by MR scan. The clinical target volume (CTV) included the involved vertebral body and a bony margin on the posterior elements and pedicles. The CTV was expanded by 2 mm to generate the planning target volume (PTV). Organs at risk (OARs) included the spinal cord, kidneys, and small bowel. The treatment

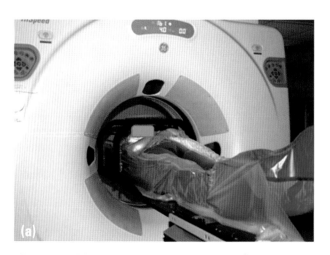
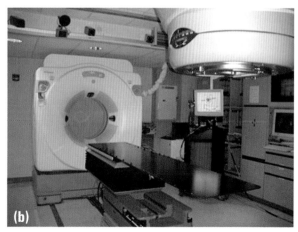

FIGURE 24E-2. (a) Patient undergoing imaging on the CT-on-Rails unit. (b)The EXaCT system, the treatment couch with 6-dimensional robotic couch-top is shared between the GE Hi-Speed CT scanner and Varian EX Linac 6/18MV with Millenium 120 multileaf collimator (60 leaves 40 cm × 40 cm).

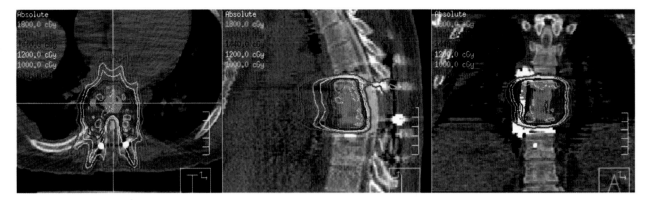

FIGURE 24E-3. Axial, sagittal, and coronal isodose distributions overlaid on the planning computed tomography scan illustrating the intensity-modulated radiation therapy plan used in this patient. A high degree of dose conformity is achieved limiting the volume of normal tissue irradiated.

plan consisted of nine coplanar beams using both 6- and 18-MV photon beams to deliver 16 Gy to the CTV in a single fraction. The isodose distributions for the final plan are shown in Figure 24E-3.

Treatment Delivery

Before treatment, the patient was set up using the stereotactic body immobilization system, and the CT scan repeated on the ExaCT system with the same 2-mm slice thickness as the planning CT. An in-house 3-dimensional rigid body image registration program was used to detect daily patient translation and rotation. The couch-top was rotated back to linac position and the body positioning frame with five infrared markers was attached to the proper index position as shown in Figure 24E-4. The updated isocenter coordinates including the pitch rotational corrections were manually entered into HexaPOD control software, which drives the movement of the 6D robotic couch-top so that the target isocenter correctly coincides with the linac radiation isocenter. The final verification of the treatment position, by the radiation oncologist, was based on the comparison of orthogonal portal images with the digitally reconstructed radiographs generated from the planning CT image (Figure 24E-5). The total treatment time was approximately 1 to 2 hours.

Clinical Outcome

The patient tolerated treatment well without any significant acute toxicities. He reported a decrease in pain at 3 months that was durable at 24 months. A follow-up MR scan performed 6 months after SBRT and showed no evidence of recurrence. At his most recent follow up 24 months after treatment, there was no evidence of recurrence.

Our initial clinical experience using volumetric-based setup in patients with metastatic spinal tumors treated

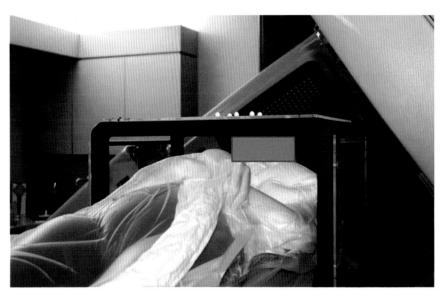

FIGURE 24E-4. The body positioning frame with five infrared markers is attached to the proper index position on the couch top. The physicist inputs the updated isocenter position into the 6-dimensional robotic couch control software. The three infrared cameras are tracking five reflected markers to position the desired target isocenter to coincide with the linac radiation isocenter.

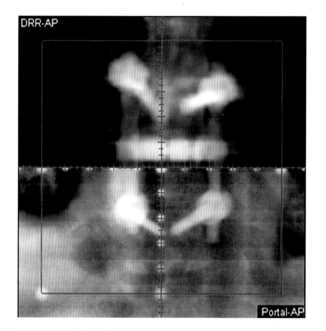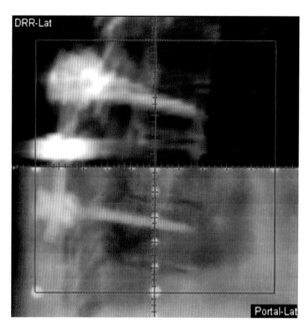

FIGURE 24E-5. Coregistration of treatment planning digitally reconstructed radiographs (anterior–posterior [left] and right lateral [right]) with pre-treatment orthogonal portal film for final verification before treatment delivery.

with SBRT on our CT-on-Rails system was published earlier.[1] In that phase I/II trial, 63 patients with 74 spinal metastases were enrolled. Thirty-two received five 6-Gy fractions, with the total dose reduced to ensure a maximum cumulative spinal cord dose of 10 Gy or less. All subsequent patients received three 9-Gy fractions (maximum cumulative cord dose ≤ 9 Gy). The majority of patients had tumors in the thoracic (58.1%) or lumbar (33.8%) spine. The most common primary tumors were renal cell, breast, sarcoma, and lung. Fifty-one patients underwent irradiation of a solitary site, whereas 12 received treatment to two sites. At a median follow-up of 21.3 months (range, 0.9–49.6 months), the 1-year actuarial local control of all irradiated sites was 84%. Three patients experienced grade 3 acute toxicities: one nausea, emesis, and diarrhea; one dysphagia; and one noncardiac chest pain. No patients developed grade 3 or higher subacute or late treatment toxicities.

Reference

1. Chang EL, Shiu AS, Mendel E, et al. Phase I/II study of stereotactic body radiotherapy for spinal metastasis and its pattern of failure. *J Neurosurg Spine.* 2007;7:151–160.

MVCT-Guided Simultaneous Multitarget Hypofractionated Radiotherapy Using Helical Tomotherapy in a Patient with Multiple Lung Metastases

Case Study

Chul-Seung Kay, MD, Ji-Yoon Kim, MD, Young-Nam Kang, PhD

Patient History

A 60-year-old man, with a history of a hard palate adenoid cystic carcinoma, presented with multiple lung metastases on a routine follow-up chest x-ray. Five years previously, his adenoid cystic tumor was treated with surgery alone without adjuvant radiotherapy (RT) or chemotherapy. A computed tomography (CT) scan of the chest confirmed the presence of bilateral metastases.

The patient received six cycles of chemotherapy and was noted to have stable disease. However, the following year, he was noted to again have progressive disease on follow-up chest x-ray and chest CT, with four nodules in the right upper lobe (RUL) and the left upper (LUL) and lower (LLL) lobes ranging in size from 0.8 cm to 3.4 cm. The largest lesion was present in the LLL. His forced expiratory volume in 1 second (FEV_1) and carbon monoxide diffusing capacity (DLCO) were 87.1% and 81.8% of predicted, respectively.

The patient refused chemotherapy and surgical resection. Because of his favorable pulmonary function profile and limited number of pulmonary lesions, we elected to treat him with image-guided simultaneous multitarget hypofractionated RT using helical tomotherapy (Tomo-Therapy Inc, Madison, WI).

Simulation

After the patient was trained to breathe shallowly, he was immobilized in the supine position for simulation and treatment using the BodyFix system (Medical Intelligence, GmbH, Schwabmunchen, Germany). This system compresses the abdomen with low pressure using foil to minimize respiratory-induced motion of the tumors and internal organs (Figure 24F-1a). Fiducial markers were placed on three points of the patient's body surface as references for planning and for each treatment. Two series of CT scans were then obtained, one in inspiration and the other in expiration to track the motion of the tumors and internal organs, respectively (Figure 24F-1B). Both scans were performed on the TSX-101A scanner (Toshiba,

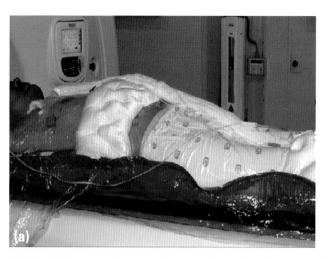
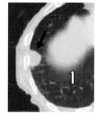
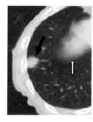
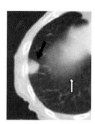
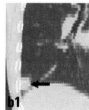
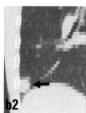
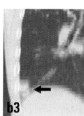

FIGURE 24F-1. (a) Patient immobilization with the BodyFix system, which compresses the abdomen with a low-pressure foil minimizing respiratory-induced motion of the tumors and internal organs. Three fiducial markers were placed on the skin surface to indicate reference points. The patient was instructed to breathe shallowly and avoid deep breaths. (b) The two series computed tomography (CT) scan composed of inspiratory and expiratory phases illustrating differences in the shape and location of tumor (black arrow) and organs at risk (white arrow indicates liver) in same table position. The internal target volume was defined as the superposition of the gross tumor volumes on the axial image of the planning CT.

Tokyo, Japan). The extent of CT scans was from the supraclavicular fossa to the upper abdomen as the patient had no extrathoracic metastasis by pretomotherapy evaluation.

Treatment Planning

Simulation CT images were then transferred to the Pinnacle (v 8.0) planning station (Philips Medical Systems, Andover, MA). Contours of tumors and organs at risk (OARs) were outlined using lung and mediastinal windows of the CT scans, respectively. The internal target volume (ITV) was defined as superposition of each visible tumor on the two series of CT scans. The planning target volume (PTV) margin around the ITV was 1 cm in the RUL and LUL tumors and 1.5 cm in two LLL tumors. Our experience has shown that the respiratory movement of lung tumors varies on the basis of location. The upper lobe tumor's movement is generally less than that of the lower lobe tumor. The 1-cm PTV expansion is thought to be sufficient in the upper lobe tumors but a larger margin (1.5 cm) is necessary in the lower lobe tumors. The OARs consisted of the right lung, left lung, esophagus, heart, spinal cord, liver, stomach, and spleen.

Treatment planning was performed using the Tomotherapy Hi Art planning software (Tomotherapy Inc, Madison, WI) after obtaining the images and contours from the Pinnacle system. Total doses of 53 Gy and 50 Gy to the 95% isodose line encompassing the ITV and PTV of the largest lesion and 43 Gy and 40 Gy to ITV and PTV of the other three small lesions were prescribed in 10 fractions. To optimize the treatment plan, we used a 2.5-cm field width, 0.3 pitch, and 2.0 modulation factor and tried to achieve the lowest dose to the smallest volume

of each OAR without compromising dose homogeneity within each target. The mean lung dose was 18.5 Gy in the left lung and 11.5 Gy in the right lung. The percentage of lung volume receiving more than 25 Gy (V_{25}) was 23% in the left lung and 7.5% in the right lung. The isodose curves distribution and dose–volume histogram (DVH) of the optimized treatment plan are shown in Figure 24F-2.

Treatment Delivery

Before each treatment, we performed a megavoltage CT (MVCT) scan on the TomoTherapy unit. The displacement of tumors and internal organs from their original position on simulation CT was automatically or manually corrected online in three axes (x, y, and z) and rotation (Figure 24F-3). After corrections were made, we confirmed that the 95% isodose line encompassed all four tumors on the MVCT (Figure 24F-4) and then started the treatment. On average, 25 minutes was required to deliver each treatment including MVCT and on-line correction. During treatment, the patient was allowed to breathe shallowly but prohibited to breathe deeply. The treatment was delivered once daily over 2 weeks.

Clinical Outcome

The patient tolerated his treatment well without significant acute toxicity. At 3 months posttreatment, a partial response was seen (Figure 24F-5). One year later, the patient had achieved a complete response on both chest CT and whole body positron emission tomography. During the follow-up period, the patient did not develop any

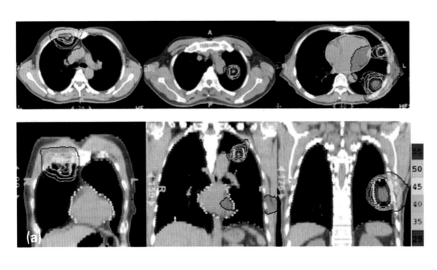

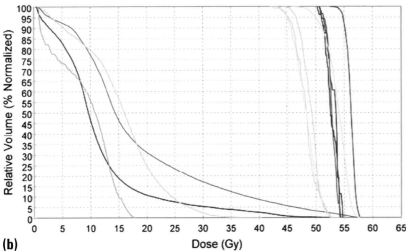

FIGURE 24F-2. (a) The optimized treatment plan with isodose lines superimposed on the planning computed tomography scan. The following isodose lines are shown: 55 Gy, 50 Gy, 45 Gy, 40 Gy, 35 Gy, and 25 Gy. **(b)** Dose–volume histograms illustrate a homogeneous dose distribution to the internal target volumes (ITVs) and planning target volumes (PTVs). The L-shape lines of organs at risk express the lowest achievable dose to the smallest volume of tissues. (ITV in left upper lobe ITV ━━━ in LUL, ▬▬▬ in RUL, ▬▬▬ the largest in LLL, ▬▬▬ in LLL; (LUL), in right upper lobe PTV ▬▬▬ in LUL, ▬▬▬ in RUL, ▬▬▬ the largest in LLL, ▬▬▬ in LLL; (RUL), the largest in left lower lobe OAR ▬▬▬ lt lung; ▬▬▬ rt lung; ▬▬▬ heart; ▬━━━ spinal cord. (LLL), in LLL; PTV in LUL, in RUL, the largest in LLL, in LLL; left lung; right lung; heart; spinal cord.)

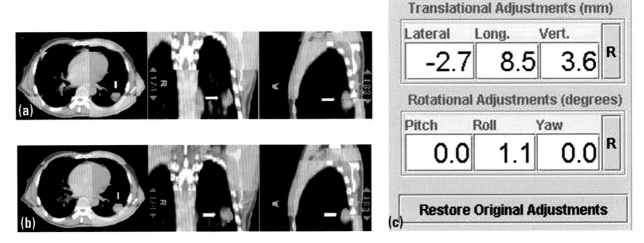

FIGURE 24F-3. On-line correction was performed using image fusion of the planning computed tomography (CT; black and white) and the megavoltage CT (yellow). The displacement of tumor (white arrow) and internal organs corrected after adjustment. **(a)** Precorrection (or preregistration) fusion images (axial, coronal, and sagittal). **(b)** Postcorrection (or postregistration) fusion images (axial, coronal and sagittal). **(c)** The displacement was −2.7 mm, 8.5 mm, 3.6 mm, and 1.1° in x, y, and z axes and rotation. It is not possible to determine or adjust displacement of pitch and yaw in the present version of the software.

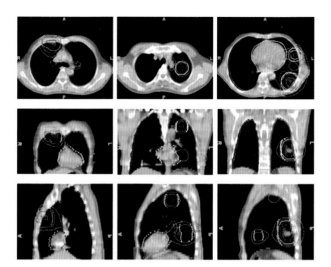

FIGURE 24F-4. Confirmation that the 95% isodose line encompassed all gross tumors on the megavoltage computed tomography scan before the initiation of each fraction.

significant late toxicities. Approximately 3 months following treatment, he was noted to have grade 1 pneumonitis. However, he never became symptomatic and did not require medications or interruptions in his activities of daily living. His latest FEV_1 and DLCO were, respectively, 93.7% and 77.7% of predicted value. Ultimately, he survived more than 2 years posttreatment.

Our initial clinical experience of image-guided simultaneous multitarget radiotherapy in patients with lung metastases using helical tomotherapy was recently pre-sented.[1-5] Thirty-two patients with an average of five pulmonary lesions (range, 1–15) were included. The majority (81%) received chemotherapy before treatment and four patients had previous chest RT. The median prescription dose to the gross tumor volume and PTV were 50 Gy ± 5.99 Gy and 40 Gy ± 7.03 Gy, respectively. Before each treatment, target position and isodose distributions were checked using MVCT scanning. The median follow-up of 30 evaluable patients was 6 months (range, 1–13 months). The rates of complete and partial responses were 3.3% and 46.7% at 1 month and 15.6% and 36.7% at 3 months, respectively. Radiation pneumonitis was seen in 10 patients (33.3%), but all cases were either grade 1 or 2.

References

1. Kay C, Jang J, Bae S, et al. Clinical experience of simultaneous multi-target irradiation using tomotherapy in pulmonary metastasis [abstract]. *Int J Radiat Oncol Biol Phys.* 2008;69:S529–S530.
2. Kim J, Kay C, Kim Y, et al. Helical tomotherapy for simultaneous multitarget radiotherapy for pulmonary metastasis. *Int J Radiat Biol Phys* 2009;75:703–710
3. Park H, Kim K, Park S, et al. Early CT findings of tomotheapy induced radiation pneumonitis after treatment of lung malignancy. *Am J Roentgenol* 2009;193:W209–W213
4. Yamazaki H. Response to "Helical tomotherapy for simultaneous multitarget radiotherapy for pulmonary metastasis." *Int J Radiat Biol Phys* 2010;76:1276
5. Kay C. In reply to Dr. Yamazaki. *Int J Radiat Biol Phys* 2010;76:1276–1277

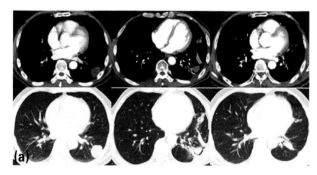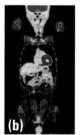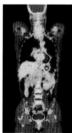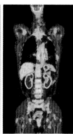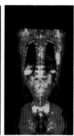

FIGURE 24F-5. (a) Preradiotherapy computed tomography (CT) scan shows a 3.4-cm left lower lobe (LLL) tumor and its size decreased on CT scan 3 months posttreatment. The adjacent radiation pneumonitis (grade 1) is evident. The LLL tumor was no longer seen on a CT scan of 1 year posttreatment. The other small tumors in right upper lobe, left upper lobe, and LLL had also completely regressed. **(b)** Positron emission tomography–CT 1 year posttreatment revealing no abnormal metabolic uptake.

KV Planar Image-Guided SBRT Using the CyberKnife System in a Renal Cell Carcinoma Patient with Multiple Pulmonary Metastases

Case Study

Fahed Fayad, MD, William T. Brown, MD, James M. Hevezi, PhD, Xiadong Wu, PhD, Irene Monterroso, MS, James G. Schwade, MD

Patient History

A 56-year-old man with a history of a left nephrectomy for a 10-cm stage II renal cell carcinoma 2 years previously presented with multiple bilateral lung metastases on routine follow-up examination. He subsequently underwent a medial sternotomy with wedge resections of four nodules, two in the right and the other two in the left lung. The pathology was consistent with renal cell carcinoma. One year later, he was found to have a new metastasis in the right lower lobe and underwent a thoracotomy and wedge resection. The following year, a follow-up computed tomography (CT) scan demonstrated multiple metastatic lesions in both lungs.

Because of his multiple previous thoracotomies, surgery was deemed no longer feasible and the patient was referred for definitive radiotherapy (RT). A review of his serial CT scans revealed enlargement of a left lung 2 cm by 2.5 cm by 2.5 cm nodule in close proximity to the aortic arch. Positron emission tomography (PET) demonstrated increased 18F-fluorodeoxyglucose (^{18}F-FDG) uptake in this lesion (Figure 24G-1). The other lesions remained stable on serial scans. We thus elected to treat the enlarging lesion with image-guided stereotactic body RT (SBRT) using the CyberKnife (Accuray Inc, Sunnyvale, CA).

Simulation

Approximately 1 week before simulation, the patient was sent for placement of a single gold fiducial marker in the center of the tumor under CT guidance using preloaded needles introduced transthoracically. The use of a single marker reduces the risk of pneumothorax that may occur with the placement of multiple fiducials. An interval of 5 to 7 days between marker placement and the planning CT scan allows edema to subside and the fiducial marker to stabilize, minimizing fiducial migration. Presently, we are using a fiducial-less technique (Xsight Lung, Accuray Inc, Sunnyvale, CA) for selective cases where the tumors can be well visualized by the x-ray tracking images.

On the day of simulation, the patient was placed in the supine position and imaged on our departmental CT-simulator. A thin-slice CT scan of the chest (1.5-mm con-

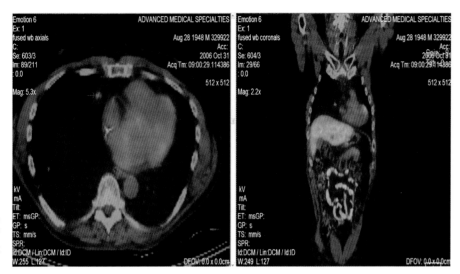

FIGURE 24G-1. Positron emission tomography–computed tomography scan of the patient before the initial treatment demonstrating the left lung lesion.

tiguous axial slices) was obtained with contrast while the patient held his breath full expiration.

Treatment Planning

The CT data set was sent to the MultiPlan treatment planning workstation (Accuray Inc, Sunnyvale, CA). The gross tumor volume (GTV) was defined as the visualized lesion on the planning CT scan using a lung window. The clinical target volume (CTV) included the GTV plus a 3-mm margin in all directions. An additional 2-mm margin was added to the CTV to generate the planning target volume (PTV). The spinal cord, heart, esophagus, proximal

bronchus, ipsilateral brachial plexus, trachea, and whole lung were designated as organs at risk (OARs). The OARs were contoured on the planning station and the ray tracing algorithm was used for lung heterogeneity correction. A total dose of 26 Gy was prescribed to the 70% isodose line to be delivered in three fractions (one fraction of 10 Gy and two fractions of 8 Gy; Figure 24G-2). The fraction size was decreased on the last two treatments based on concerns over potential toxicity.

The plan was evaluated to ensure a minimum number of beams was used while preserving the dose conformity surrounding the lesion, and minimizing the dose to the nearby OARs. An additional check was performed to

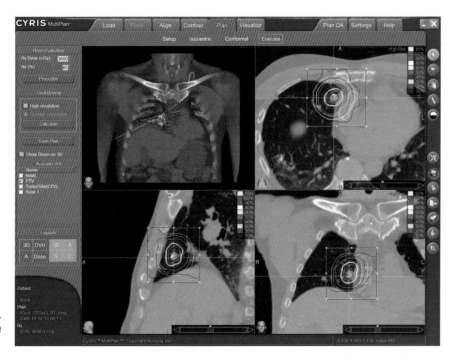

FIGURE 24G-2. CyberKnife (Accuray Inc, Sunnyvale, CA) treatment plan for the treated lesion.

evaluate "hot spots" away from the target by expanding the dose calculation matrix in all three dimensions.

When acceptable, the radiation oncologist and the thoracic surgeon approved the plan and the plan was sent to the treatment console for delivery. Because only a single fiducial was used for the Synchrony Respiratory Tracking System (Accuray Inc, Sunnyvale, CA), patient rotational alignment was not obtained from this plan. Instead, an additional "dummy" plan was produced using the XSight Spine algorithm (Accuray Inc, Sunnyvale, CA), allowing rotational and translational information to be obtained for patient setup on the treatment couch. This plan was sent to the treatment console and used solely to align the patient for the Synchrony treatment course to follow. Once the patient alignment had been achieved, the Xsight Spine setup plan was abandoned and the Synchrony plan was loaded on the treatment console, the respiratory tracking model was established, and the treatment began. Synchrony, an optic and radiographic motion monitoring system for real-time tumor tracking, allows for frequent updates to the respiratory model during treatment (before each beam delivery, if chosen), a technique unique to this motion-tracking algorithm.

Treatment Delivery

The CyberKnife Robotic Radiosurgery System consists of a compact linear accelerator manipulated by a robot capable of moving with six degrees of freedom, two orthogonally placed x-ray units for radiographic three-dimensional (3D) target localization, and, as described above, the Synchrony tracking system. Radio-opaque fiducial markers implanted in the tumor and light-emitting diodes (LED) placed on the patient's chest were used for target tracking. During treatment delivery, the respiratory tracking system first establishes a mathematical model correlating the respiratory motion of the LED tracked by an infrared camera array, and the tumor motion monitored through the internal markers by the x-ray sources. The real-time tracking instruction is then sent to the main computer to guide the robotic linear accelerator to deliver a beam to the tumor as it moves with the patient's breathing cycle.

The patient was fitted with a Velcro vest and positioned supine on the treatment couch. The LEDs were attached to the vest and the optic scanner was used to assist in following respiration externally. The computer analyzed each image, identified the fiducial, and, when a synchronization between the robotic movement of the linear accelerator and respiratory motion of the patient was achieved, the beam was turned on. Each treatment took about 45 minutes to an hour.

Clinical Outcome

The patient tolerated his treatment well without significant acute sequelae. Although follow-up scans revealed excellent control of this treated lesion, the patient was subsequently noted to develop both new lung and brain metastases. Over the following 5 years, he received 14 further CyberKnife treatments (12 to the lungs and two to the brain; Table 24G-1). Of note, his pulmonary function on serial testing remained relatively stable (Table 24G-2).

On his most recent CT scan, new pulmonary lesions were noted that were stable on chemotherapy (Figure 24G-3). Repeat scans will be obtained and, if enlargement is noted, then the patient will be considered for additional treatment by CyberKnife.

TABLE 24G–1 Treatment Dates, Tumor Location, Volume, Dose, Number of Fractions and Biologically Equivalent Dose

Date	Location	Volume, cc	Dose, Gy	Col, mm	Fractions, No.	IDL, %	Beams, No.	BED 10 Gy
9/04	LUL	4.7	26	30	3	70	92	49
11/04	LUL	4.3	30	15	2	58	87	75
4/05	CNS	0.36	18	7.5	1	70	106	100
9/05	CNS	0.19	18	7.5	1	70	91	100
12/06	RUL	3.3	36	20	3	65	111	26
12/06	LUL	1.7	36	20	3	70	120	26
1/07	RUL	2.8	45	25	3	65	68	112
3/07	RUL	0.7	32	25	4	65	71	57
5/07	LUL	4.8	30	15	3	68	90	60
7/07	RLL	6.4	30	15	3	60	77	60
3/08	LUL	8.14	30	15	3	80	157	60
3/08	LLL	3.6	30	25	3	65	110	60
4/08	RLL	1.7	30	25	3	67	115	60
2/09	LLL	7.18	30	25	3	70	84	60
4/09	CNS	0.75	18	7.5	1	63	136	100

Note. BED = biologically equivalent dose; CNS = central nervous system; Col = collimator; IDL = isodose line; LLL = left lower lobe; LUL = left upper lobe; RLL = right lower lobe; RUL = right upper lobe.

TABLE 24G–2 Pulmonary Function Studies

1/11/07 Spirometry	Pred	Actual	%Ref	3/4/08 Pred	Actual	%Ref	1/15/09 Pred	Actual	%Ref	8/3/09 Pred	Actual	%Ref
FVC, L	5.1	4.7	92	5.06	5.06	75	5.04	5.04	67	4.9	3.33	68
FEV$_1$, L	4.09	3.69	90	3.90	3.90	83	3.87	2.70	70	3.7	2.46	65
FEV$_1$/FEC, %	79	79	100	78	86	110	78	80	102	78	74	95
FEF 25%–75%, L/sec	4.09	3.53	86	3.62	3.84	106	3.58	2.36	66	3.54	1.67	47
FEF 50%, L/sec	4.99	5.46	110	4.81	4.90	102	3.0	4.77	64	4.67	2.37	51
FEF 75%, L/sec	1.92	1.18	62	1.83	1.51	83	1.81	0.89	49	1.75	0.52	30
FIVC, L	9.40	4.56	89		3.70			3.32			3.14	
DLCO, mL/minute	20.5	25.1	82	18.9	29.27	65	29.2	18.91	65	28.9	11	38

Note. DLCO = diffusion capacity of the lung for carbon monoxide; FEC = forced expiratory capacity; FEF = forced expiratory flow; FEV$_1$ = forced expiratory volume in 1 second; FIVC = forced inspiratory vital capacity; FVC = forced vital capacity; %ref = percent reference; Pred = predicted.

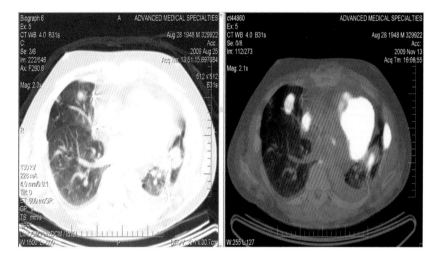

FIGURE 24G-3. Appearance of treated lesion (red arrow) on follow-up positron emission tomography–computed tomography scan showing durable local control. Note the adjacent new metastatic lesion described in the text.

KV Planar Image-Guided SBRT Using the Novalis System in an Ovarian Cancer Patient with Liver Metastases

Case Study

Alan W. Katz, MD, MPH, Praveena Cheruvu, MD, Michael C. Schell, PhD, Abraham Philip, CMD, Michael T. Milano, MD, PhD

Patient History

A 76-year-old woman with a history of ovarian cancer presented with multiple progressive liver metastases on follow-up imaging. Her oncologic history dates back more than 25 years when she was diagnosed with an ovarian granulosa cell tumor and was treated with an abdominal hysterectomy and bilateral salpingo-oophorectomy. She did well until approximately 10 years ago when she developed a pelvic recurrence, which was treated with surgical resection. Over the subsequent intervening years, she has suffered multiple recurrences that have been treated with further surgery and multiple chemotherapeutic regimens.

A recent follow-up computed tomography (CT) scan revealed progressive liver involvement with no disease seen outside the liver. A large heterogeneous mass measuring 9.4 cm by 7.6 cm was located near the dome of the liver, with an adjacent satellite lesion measuring 2.2 cm by 1.8 cm. A third, 1.2-cm lesion was seen inferiorly in the right lobe. These lesions were considered refractory to chemotherapy, so a course of stereotactic body radiation therapy (SBRT) was recommended. We elected to treat her with daily image guidance using the Novalis system (BrainLAB AG, Feldkirchen, Germany).

Simulation

Patient immobilization for simulation and treatment was accomplished using the ExacTrac patient positioning platform (BrainLAB AG, Feldkirchen, Germany), consisting of a Vak-Lok vacuum cushion (CIVCO, Kalona, IA) for initial positioning, and seven infrared reflecting body fiducial markers placed on the patient's skin over the thorax and abdomen (Figure 24H-1). A planning CT scan of the patient was then obtained on our High Speed Advantage CT (GE Healthcare, Waukesha, WI) using an end-expiratory breath hold technique. Axial images of the liver were obtained with slice thickness of 3 mm. No intravenous or oral contrast was used.

Treatment Planning

The planning and contrast-enhanced diagnostic CT scans of the abdomen were transferred to the BrainScan Treatment Planning System (BrainLAB AG, Feldkirchen, Germany) and fused using automatic registration. Verification of registration was done in the axial, coronal, and sagittal planes.

The tumors and organs at risk (OARs) were subsequently contoured. Because of the small size of the third

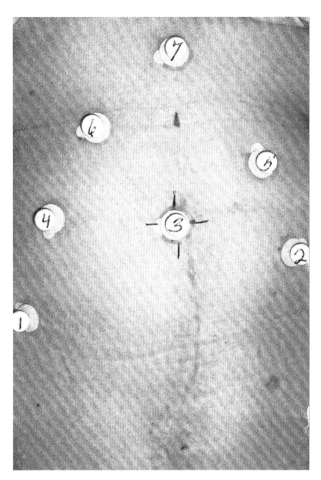

FIGURE 24H-1. Placement of infrared body fiducial markers at simulation.

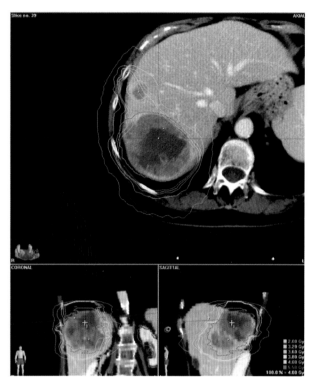

FIGURE 24H-2. Treatment plan showing coverage of the planning target volume by the 80% isodose line.

lesion, as well as its inferior location, it was decided to treat only the two larger dome lesions. A gross tumor volume (GTV) was drawn for each tumor. The clinical target volume (CTV) consisted of the GTV with no expansion. The planning target volume (PTV) was designed to include the GTV with 7 mm of lateral and anterior–posterior margin and 10 mm of superior–inferior margin. Treatment was prescribed to the 100% isodose line, with 80% isodose line covering the PTV (Figure 24H-2). The OARs included the liver, kidneys, stomach, bowel, and spinal cord.

Two isocenters were used to treat the larger lesion and one isocenter for the smaller lesion. Six coplanar arcs were selected to deliver an optimized treatment plan, with a prescribed dose of 40 Gy in 10 fractions. Start and stop angles of each arc were 190° and 250°, 280° and 320°, 160° and 180°, 190° and 260°, 290° and 350°, and 280° and 20°, respectively. A dose–volume histogram (DVH) was calculated for all of the irradiated OARs. For the liver, a volume of at least 1000 cc tumor-free liver was required and the dose to 60% of this volume was not to exceed 30 Gy.

Treatment Delivery

Before treatment, additional quality assurance (QA) was performed by the physics staff. Accuracy of the dose delivery occurs by minimizing the Target Registration Error (TRE) in the ExacTrac 6D System. The TRE is reduced through optimization of the Body Marker Array (BMA) by (1) centering the BMA over the target, (2) placing each body marker over the largest feasible area on firm skin, and (3) avoiding body marker alignments in each infrared camera's field of view.

Immediately before the first treatment, a CT scan was acquired with the patient in the treatment immobilization apparatus with the optimized BMA. The planning CT was fused with the pretreatment CT by fusing the BMA pairs. The target in the pretreatment scan was reviewed for alignment within the planning isodose distributions by the treating radiation oncologist and a dosimetrist or physicist. Only after the patient pretreatment CT scans aligned with the prescribed dose delivery did the actual treatment proceed.

Treatment was delivered on the Novalis system using 6-MV photons at a dose rate of 480 monitor units per minute. Respiratory gating was accomplished using shallow breathing. During treatment, infrared cameras were used to provide real-time monitoring by the radiation therapist. The beam was turned off for displacement exceeding 3 mm in any axial dimension. The beam was

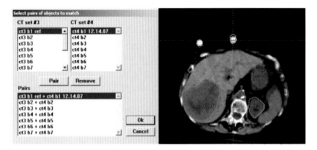

FIGURE 24H-3. Verification computed tomography (CT) scan fused with planning CT scan using fiducial markers as reference.

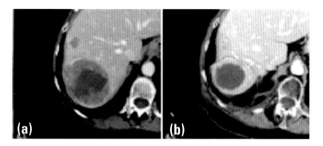

FIGURE 24H-4. Fusion of planning computed tomography (CT) scan (a) with follow-up CT scan (b) showing treatment response.

not turned on until all displacements in the axial dimensions were less than 2 mm.

Assessment of patient positioning and tumor localization was verified with repeat CT scans following every third fraction. Verification scans were fused to initial planning scan using the fiducial markers as reference (Figure 24H-3). Isodose coverage of each PTV was evaluated and approved before delivery of the next fraction.

Clinical Outcome

Treatment was well tolerated without any significant acute sequelae. The patient was able to participate in her daily activities with no interruptions. At her 4-month follow up, she remained without complaints. An abdominal CT abdomen revealed very good response; the largest lesion measured 5.4 cm (previously 9.4 cm × 7.6 cm). The previously seen satellite lesion measuring 2.2 cm by 1.8 cm was replaced by a 6-mm cyst without any nodular or focal enhancement consistent with complete response (Figure 24H-4). However, the third lesion at the tip of the inferior right lobe, not included in the previous SBRT treatment, had increased in size from 1.2 cm to 2.2 cm, consistent with progressive disease. We therefore offered her a second course of SBRT. One isocenter was used to deliver a dose of 30 Gy at 6 Gy per fraction using 6-MV photons. She completed her second SBRT course without complaints.

She was seen most recently 10 months posttreatment, at which time she remained without complaints and maintains her normal lifestyle. A CT scan of the abdomen demonstrated continued shrinkage of the largest mass, now 4 cm by 3 cm, no change in the 6-mm cyst, and complete radiological response of the third lesion.

Our clinical experience using image-guided SBRT in patients with liver metastases using the Novalis system was published earlier.[1] The outcome of a total of 69 patients with 174 metastases was reviewed. The median number of lesions irradiated was 2.5 (range, 1–6) with a median diameter of 2.7 cm (range, 0.6 cm–12.2 cm). Dose per fraction ranged from 2 Gy to 6 Gy, with a median total dose of 48 Gy (range, 30 Gy–55 Gy).

At a median follow-up of 14.5 months, the 10- and 20-month actuarial in-field local control rates of irradiated lesions were 76% and 57%, respectively. The median overall survival of the entire group was 14.5 months. Six- and 12-month actuarial progressive-free survival rates were 46% and 24%, respectively. No patient experienced grade 3 or higher toxicity.

Reference

1. Katz AW, Carey-Simpson M, Muhs AG, et al. Hypofractionated stereotactic body radiation therapy (SBRT) for limited hepatic metastases. *Int J Radiat Oncol Biol Phys.* 2007;67:793–798.

Electronic Portal Cine Imaging During Single-Fraction SBRT Using a Varian Linear Accelerator in a Breast Cancer Patient with a Liver Metastasis

Case Study

Christopher F. Serago, PhD, Laura A. Vallow, MD,
Ricardo Paz-Fumagalli, MD, Siyong Kim, PhD,
Ashley A. Gale, MS, Wilza L. Magalhaes, CMD

Patient History

A 69-year-old woman with a history of metastatic breast cancer presented with a solitary liver metastasis on follow-up imaging. Her oncologic history dates back 3 years previously when she presented with numerous lesions involving the liver, left breast, and left axilla. Biopsy of the breast mass revealed infiltrating ductal carcinoma, estrogen and progesterone receptor–negative, human epithelial growth factor receptor 2–positive disease.

She was initially treated with carboplatin, taxol, and herceptin for four cycles and achieved a partial response. She then received vinorelbine and herceptin and subsequently herceptin as a single agent. A solitary cerebellar brain metastasis was noted and treated with stereotactic radiosurgery. Subsequent follow-up imaging revealed complete resolution of disease in all metastatic sites.

The patient continued to do well until a recent follow-up magnetic resonance (MR) scan of her abdomen revealed a 2.8-cm enhancing mass in segment VI of the right lobe of the liver. Positron emission tomography (PET) performed at the same time correlated with this finding showing no other areas of increased uptake.

The patient was asymptomatic with good performance status and normal liver function tests.

After multidisciplinary discussion, our consensus recommendation was to enroll the patient on our in-house clinical trial of stereotactic body radiotherapy (SBRT) for liver metastases. We elected to use electronic portal imaging in the cine mode during treatment to evaluate interfraction motion.

Simulation

Before simulation, the patient had four gold fiducial seeds (1.2 mm × 3 mm) implanted by an interventional radiologist into the liver metastatic lesion under ultrasound guidance. On the day of simulation, the patient was immobilized in the supine position using a BodyFIX vacuum bag (Elekta AB, Stockholm, Sweden). A respiratory-gated computed tomography (CT) simulation was performed with the patient free-breathing normal respiration. Her average respiratory cycle time was 4.4 seconds. Ten CT images per respiratory cycle with a 1.25-mm slice thickness and spacing were acquired with a wide-bore multi-slice LightSpeed scanner (GE Healthcare, Waukesha, WI).

The four-dimensional CT (4DCT) images were reviewed at the time of simulation and the segment of the patient's respiratory cycle showing the minimal range of motion was selected for treatment. The CT images, which were binned within the selected segment of the respiratory cycle, were averaged and the average CT data set was exported to the treatment planning system. Also evaluated at the time of simulation was the range of motion of the implanted fiducial seeds. For this patient, an 8.8-mm range of motion was observed implying a similar range of motion of the liver and the targeted lesion.

Treatment Planning

Treatment planning was performed using Pinnacle software (Philips Medical Systems, Andover, MA). Magnetic resonance was used to assist contouring and images were fused to the CT simulation data set. Contours of the gross tumor volume (GTV), liver, spinal cord, gallbladder, small bowel, and both kidneys were drawn by the treating radiation oncologist. Digitally reconstructed radiographs (DRRs) were created for verification use before treatment. The fiducial seeds were highlighted on the DRRs for ease of comparison with future images planned for the treatment session.

This patient was treated according to an institutional review board–approved dose escalation protocol. A total dose of 15 Gy was prescribed to the 95% isodose line. Six conformal non-coplanar 6-MV photon beams were used shaped by 5-mm multileaf collimator leaves. The maximum dose to the liver was 16.3 Gy, with a mean dose of 1.5 Gy. The targeted lesion was located directly adjacent to the right kidney. The maximum dose to the right kidney was 12.7 Gy, with a mean dose of 0.7 Gy. Doses to the other critical structures were as follows: left kidney: maximum 3.7 Gy, mean 0.2 Gy; spinal cord: maximum 2.0 Gy, mean 0.4 Gy; gallbladder: maximum 14.9 Gy, mean 3.7 Gy; and small bowel: maximum 0.3 Gy.

Treatment Delivery

The patient' simulation position was reproduced on the linear accelerator treatment couch with the aid of the previously fabricated immobilization device. Treatment was delivered on a Clinac iX (Varian Medical Systems, Palo Alto, CA). The patient was instructed to breathe normally. Her respirations were monitored and the radiation beam-on was synchronized to her breathing using the Real-Time Position Management Respiratory Gating System (Varian Medical Systems, Palo Alto, CA).

Anterior–posterior (AP) and right lateral gated kilovoltage (kV) images were taken before treatment and compared with DRRs to verify the patient position. Adjustments to the patient position were made so the treatment isocenter was aligned within 2 mm of the planned position. The upper pair of images of Figure 24I-1 shows the AP DRR and acquired kV image.

Cine images of the treatment fields were continuously acquired during treatment. Physical interference of the treatment couch with the electronic portal imaging device (EPID; Varian Medical Systems, Palo Alto, CA) prevented cine imaging for two of the six treatment beams. The lower pair of images in Figure 24I-1 illustrates a comparison of a single cine image with the corresponding DRR for beams 1–3. For beams 1–3 in Figure 24I-1, 35 cine images were acquired, the number depending on the total number of monitor units for the particular beam. The position of the fiducial seed as seen in the cine images was compared with the planned position of the seed in the DRR and differences or displacements of the seed position were measured on each cine image. For beams 1–3, the mean displacement of the fiducial seeds was 1.7 mm (0.4 mm standard deviation) and the maximum displacement was 2.5 mm.

Table 24I-1 shows a summary of the measured displacements of the fiducial seeds for all the treatment beams for which cine images were acquired. For all four beams, the measured mean displacement was 2.2 mm (1.0 mm standard deviation) and the maximum displacement was

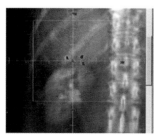
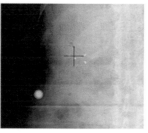

DRR-kV image match

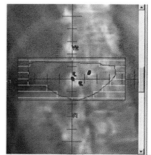
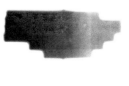

DRR-cine image match

FIGURE 24I-1. Digitally reconstructed radiograph (DRR)–kV pair, and a DRR–cine image pair for treatment beams 1–3.

TABLE 24I–1 Measured Displacements of Fiducial Seeds Acquired From Each Treatment Beam's Cine Image, and the Maximum Movement of the Fiducial Seeds During the Four-Dimensional Computed Tomography Simulation

Beam	1-3	1-2	1-6	1-5	All beams
Number cine frames	35	58	42	62	197
Mean displacement	1.7 mm	2.5 mm	1.0 mm	3.0 mm	2.2 mm
Standard deviation	0.4 mm	0.2 mm	0.7 mm	0.6 mm	1.0 mm
Max. displacement	2.5 mm	2.9 mm	3.8 mm	4.5 mm	4.5 mm
Max Movement 4D CT		8.8 mm			

4.5 mm. When compared with the maximum movement of the fiducial seeds during the 4DCT simulation of 8.8 mm, the maximum movement of 4.5 mm with respiratory-gated treatment represented a reduction of motion of almost 50%. We found the use of cine imaging to be an effective tool for evaluation of the efficacy of respiratory gating for this patient.

Clinical Outcome

The SBRT procedure was tolerated well. The week following the procedure, the patient did experience 2 days of grade 3 right upper quadrant abdominal pain, which resolved completely. She was evaluated every 2 weeks per protocol with no treatment-related toxicity.

Magnetic resonance follow-up 3 months after treatment revealed decrease in the size and enhancement of the treated lesion. Unfortunately, the MR scan 5 months posttreatment revealed multiple subcentimeter liver metastases. The patient went on to receive lapatinib and capecitabine and at most recent documented follow-up 8 months following SBRT, her liver disease continued to progress although she remained asymptomatic aside from grade 1 fatigue.

Our initial clinical experience using electronic portal imaging in the cine mode during SBRT in patients with liver metastases was reported earlier.[1] Four patients on our in-house dose escalation SBRT trial had gold seeds placed in or near the liver metastases before treatment. Each patient underwent 4DCT simulation with respiratory motion data acquired simultaneously. Before treatment, patients were positioned with gated kV x-ray image guidance. Digitally reconstructed radiographs were created for each static field showing the expected position of the seed markers. During treatment, continuous cine images were acquired and positions of the seeds on cine images were compared with expected positions on the DRRs.

The average maximum seed displacement during CT simulation without gating was 11.1 mm (range, 8.8 mm–13.2 mm). During respiratory-gated treatment, the average displacement was 5.9 mm (range, 4.5 mm–9.4 mm). The mean displacement of the seeds during treatment was 2.2 mm. These results suggest that cine imaging during treatment may be an effective tool to evaluate interfraction position of implanted seeds in patients with liver metastases.

Reference

1. Serago CF, Vallow LA, Paz-Fumagalli R, et al. Electronic portal cine imaging of implanted marker seeds during respiratory-gated treatment to evaluate interfraction movement for stereotactic body radiotherapy of liver metastases [abstract]. *Int J Radiat Oncol Biol Phys.* 2008;72:S543–S544.

KV CBCT-Guided SBRT Using the Elekta Synergy System in a Breast Cancer Patient with Multiple Liver Metastases

Case Study

Franco Casamassima, MD, Laura Masi, PhD, Katia Pasciuti, PhD, Claudia Menichelli, MD, I. Bonucci, MD, Raffaella Doro, PhD, Elena D'Imporzano, MD

Patient History

A 74-year-old woman with a history of a stage T1N1 estrogen receptor (ER)–positive left breast cancer presented with an elevated Ca 15.3 level of 70.6 U/mL on a routine follow-up visit. Her breast cancer was diagnosed 9 years previously and was treated with a radical mastectomy followed by adjuvant chemo-hormonal therapy.

Restaging radiographic studies including contrast-enhanced total body computed tomography (CT), bone scintigraphy, and a liver ultrasound revealed two liver lesions in segments IV and VII. ^{18}F-fluorodeoxyglucose positron emission tomography (^{18}F-FDG PET) was only positive in the segment VII lesion, with a standardized uptake value (SUV) of 10.7. Ultrasound-guided fine needle biopsy was performed for this lesion; pathology was consistent with her prior ER-positive breast cancer.

In light of her disease recurrence limited to the liver, our consensus recommendation was for stereotactic body radiation therapy (SBRT). We elected to treat her with kilovoltage (kV) cone-beam CT (CBCT)–guided SBRT on an Elekta Synergy system (Elekta AB, Stockholm, Sweden).

Simulation

Seven days before the planning CT scan, two gold fiducial markers were implanted under CT guidance within the larger liver lesion. The use of fiducials was introduced in our liver SBRT patients to facilitate image guidance using kV CBCT. The 7-day interval between implantation and simulation is considered sufficient to ensure stability of the fiducials within the liver.

All CT data sets used for planning purposes were acquired on a Lightspeed multislice scanner (GE Healthcare, Waukesha, WI) in helical mode with a 2.5-mm thickness including the whole liver and kidneys volume, for a total of 96 contiguous axial images for each data set.

Before the planning CT acquisition, the patient received breath coaching based on an internal protocol introduced into our clinical practice for lung and liver SBRT.[1,2] The patient checked the regularity of her respiratory pattern as displayed on the monitor of the Active Breathing Coordinator (ABC) computerized spirometer system (Elekta AB, Stockholm, Sweden). As a first step, she was trained to maintain a reproducible and regular breathing cycle reducing her maximum breathing volume to the lowest physiologically tolerable level (Figure 24J-1a; shallow breathing). To simulate the extreme phases of this shallow breathing cycle for planning purposes, two CT data sets were acquired in breath hold, setting respectively the ABC threshold level at the minimum volume (end-exhale), and the maximum shallow volume (end-inhale; Figure 24J-1b). During treatment delivery the patient was instructed to maintain her shallow breathing cycle both

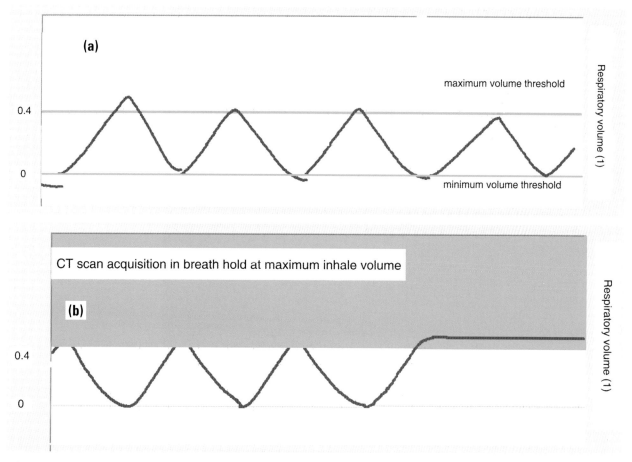

FIGURE 24J-1. Breathing pattern as displayed by the Active Breathing Control monitor. (a) Shallow regular free breathing. (b) Breath hold at maximum volume (end-inhale) for computed tomography scan acquisition.

for CBCT acquisition and for dose delivery, which were performed in free breathing. The adopted ABC protocol has the aim to ensure the reproducibility of the individual breathing pattern between the simulation session and the IGRT session, reducing the liver maximum breathing excursion.

The end-exhale CT data set was synchronized with the contrast-enhanced triphasic CT scan acquisition, in order to correspond to the portal phase (75 seconds after contrast injection). For the end-inhale data set, an extra contrast boost was administered and images acquired after 70 seconds.

Treatment Planning

For each of the treated lesions, two gross tumor volumes (GTVs) were delineated on the end-exhale and end-inhale data sets, encompassing the visible tumors using a window width of 400 HU and a level of 40 HU. When imaging artifacts were present because of the fiducials' high density, the ^{18}F-FDG PET images, previously registered with the planning CT, were used to guide target delineation (Figures 24J-2a and -2b). Moreover, in the end-inhale

CT data sets, even after additional contrast, enhancement was partially diminished.

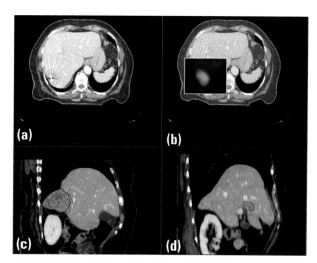

(a) (b)

(c) (d)

FIGURE 24J-2. (a) Computed tomography image artifacts attributable to the presence of the high-density fiducials. (b) Corresponding positron emission tomography image fusion used to guide contouring. (c) Sagittal view of the VII segment lesion in exhale (red); the fused inhale contour is also shown (blue). (d) Sagittal view of the IV segment lesion in exhale (red); the fused inhale contour is also shown (blue).

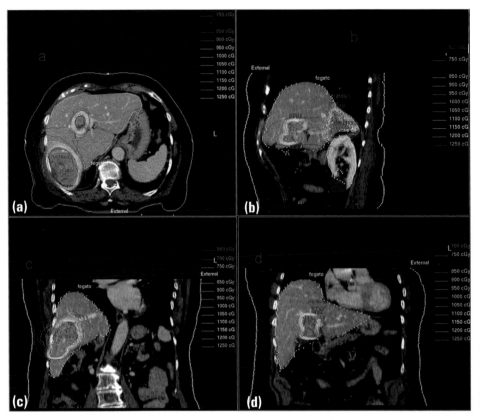

FIGURE 24J-3. Isodose distributions overlaid on computed tomography for the two treated lesions in axial (a), sagittal (b), and coronal views (c and d).

Although the contouring physician checked the correspondence in shape and size of the inhale and exhale GTV contours in each axial view, a nonperfect coherence was observed between the volumes delineated in the two breathing phases. For the larger lesion (lesion 1), it measured 85 cm³ in exhale and 78 cm³ in inhale, whereas the second lesion (lesion 2) was 4.1 cm³ in exhale and 3.5 cm³ in inhale (Figure 24F-2c and -2d). The fiducials were also manually delineated in both breathing phases. The tumor breathing excursion was evaluated as GTV displacement between expiration and inspiration and as a quality check compared with the fiducials displacement between these two phases. The cranio–caudal respiratory excursion was 13 mm for lesion 1, 11 mm for lesion 2, and 10 mm for both fiducials.

An internal target volume (ITV) was created for each lesion encompassing the inhale and exhale GTV; a uniform 4-mm margin was then added to the ITV to generate a PTV accounting for residual positioning uncertainties after on-line image-guided corrections. This margin was based on the alignment results obtained on 30 postcorrection and posttreatment CBCTs acquired for 11 previously treated patients. A contour encompassing the inhale and exhale positions of each fiducial marker was also created to be used as a guide for alignment by CBCT.

A treatment plan was created using ERGO++ treatment planning software (Elekta AB, Stockholm, Sweden) consisting of a dynamic conformal arc technique with two isocenters (one for each lesion; Figure 24J-3). Six arcs of 30° each, were planned for each isocenter with the leaves of a dynamic multileaf collimator (MLC; 5-mm leaf width) conforming to each PTV. A total dose of 30 Gy in three fractions was prescribed to the 67% isodose (44.78 Gy at the isocenter) for both lesions, requiring a conformity index for this isodose of no more than 1.5. Organ-at-risk (OAR) dose constraints were as follows: at least 700 cm³ of healthy (uninvolved) liver must receive less than 15 Gy, and no more than 35% of the combined kidney volume could receive 15 Gy or more.

To meet the above prescriptions and constraints, a negative margin (–2 mm) was chosen for MLC conformation around the PTV. We obtained a conformity index of 1.51 for both lesions and OAR constraints were easily achieved.

Treatment Delivery

Cone beam CT acquisition before each fraction and for each isocenter was performed in free-breathing following the ABC protocol, with the patient observing her respiratory pattern on the ABC monitor.

For image guidance purposes, the CBCT image was aligned with the CT planning images using Elekta XVI software (Elekta AB, Stockholm, Sweden), in two steps: (1) an automatic registration based on the vertebrae was performed (bony alignment) using a chamfer matching

FIGURE 24J-4. Cone-beam computed tomography images showing fiducials (axial, coronal, and sagittal view) aligned inside the corresponding contours delineated on planning CT and enveloping the two breathing positions.

algorithm, and (2) a physician checked the alignment of the fiducials on the CBCT scan, with the corresponding enveloping contours delineated on the planning CT and manual corrections were performed (Figure 24J-4). A maximum difference of 3.8 mm was detected between bone- and fiducial-based alignment. Generally, the vertebrae position is not a good surrogate for tumor position in liver SBRT, even when breathing motion is simulated in the planning session and ABC is employed. The overall time required for IGRT and treatment delivery in this patient was approximately 20 minutes.

Clinical Outcome

The hypofractionated SBRT treatment was well tolerated without any appreciable treatment-related symptoms. All parameters of liver functionality were in the range of normality during, and for the 2 months after, the end of treatment. The Ca 15.3 value dropped to 31 U/mL 1 month after treatment, and has remained stable up to the most recent follow-up.

A CT scan acquired 2 months after treatment showed complete disappearance of the smaller lesion and substantial reduction in the size of the larger lesion. The larger lesion also developed a central necrotic area circumscribed by a contrast-enhancing ring (probably arterialized liver parenchyma; Figure 24J-5a). In an ^{18}F-FDG PET scan obtained at the same time, the treated lesions appeared as "cold areas" (Figure 24J-5b). The patient remains free of any significant chronic sequelae.

Our initial clinical experience using kV CBCT-guided hypofractionated SBRT in 48 patients with liver tumors (33 metastatic, 15 primary) was recently presented.[3] Eligibility included four lesions or fewer, diameter 6 cm or less, controlled extrahepatic primary, no other sites of progressive disease, normal liver function, and a Karnofsky performance status of 80 or higher. The GTV was delineated on two CT data sets acquired at the end of inspiration and expiration and was used to define an ITV. Thirty Gy to 36 Gy in three consecutive fractions was prescribed to the 90% isodose level. Cone beam CT was used before each treatment for setup and target localization.

At a median follow-up of 8.2 months, five recurrences were noted within the irradiated area and 14 new lesions developed in the liver. Of nine patients with follow-up PET, one achieved a complete response and six visually reduced uptake. Overall, survival at 6 and 12 months was 81% and 58%, respectively. No acute toxicity was observed, except for transient nausea. Ulceration on gastric and duodenal mucosa occurred in two patients 3 months following treatment, but has resolved.

References

1. Masi L, Casamassima F, Menichelli C, et al. On-line image guidance for frameless stereotactic radiotherapy of lung malignancies by cone beam CT: comparison between target localization and alignment on bony anatomy. *Acta Oncol.* 2008;47:1422–1431.
2. Masi L, Casamassima F, Menichelli C, et al. Efficacy of patient training by a computerized spirometer to reduce respiratory target motion in lung and liver malignancies SRT. *Int J Radiat Oncol Biol Phys.* 2008;72 Supplement:S607.
3. Casamassima F, Masi L, Menichelli C, et al. IGRT stereotactic hypofractionated radiotherapy for treatment of focal liver malignancies. *Int J Radiat Oncol Biol Phys.* 2008;72 Supple-ment:S277.

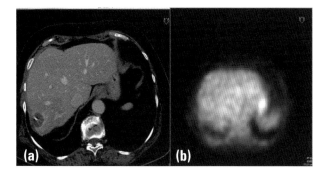

FIGURE 24J-5. Two months after the end of treatment: (a) triphasic contrast-enhanced computed tomography scan; (b) ^{18}F-fluorodeoxyglucose positron emission tomography scan.

KV CT-Guided SBRT in a Hepatocellular Carcinoma Patient with a Solitary Lung Metastasis Treated with Voluntary Breath Hold and Beam Switching on a CT-on-Rails System

Case Study

Hiroshi Onishi, MD, Masayuki Araya, MD, Kan Marino, MD, Takafumi Komiyama, MD, Kengo Kuriyama, MD, Ryo Saito, MD, Shinichi Aoki, MD, Yoshiyasu Maehata, MD, Tsutomu Araki, MD

Patient History

A 73-year-old man with a history of hepatocellular carcinoma (HCC) presented with a solitary 4-cm pulmonary nodule in the left lung (Figure 24K-1). This lesion was considered to represent a metastasis from his primary HCC which was treated the year before with surgical resection. Workup included a positron emission tomography (PET) scan, which demonstrated increased ^{18}F-fluorodeoxyglucose (^{18}F-FDG) uptake in the lung nodule. No other abnormalities were noted in lung, liver, or other sites. His serum alpha-fetoprotein (AFP) level was markedly elevated (125 μg/L).

The patient was advised to undergo surgical resection. However, he refused and we recommended treatment with stereotactic body radiotherapy (SBRT). We elected to treat him with image-guided SBRT using a CT-on-Rails system.

Simulation

To reproduce and maintain tumor position during treatment, the patient was trained in the procedure of voluntary self-breath-holding in the inspiration phase using a simple respiratory indicator (Figure 24K-2) that we developed in 2005[1] and has been commercially available in Japan. This indicator was named "Abches" (Apex Medical, Tokyo, Japan), as it comprises two arms for measurement of the levels of the abdominal and chest walls. An indicator of respiratory phase is obtained from mechanical movement of the two arms. In our experience, the average (±1 standard deviation) maximum difference in tumor position from three computed tomography (CT) series of 80 patients under voluntary self-breath-hold using the Abches was 1.8 mm ± 1.4 mm cranio–caudally, 1.4 mm ± 1.1 mm antero–posteriorly, and 1.0 mm ± 0.7 mm in a right–left direction. The merits of breath hold at the

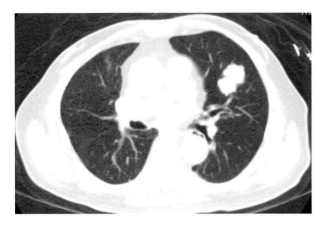

FIGURE 24K-1. Computed tomography image of the left lung nodule.

inspiration phase include a reduction in irradiation of the normal lung and better time efficiency than breath hold in the expiration phase.

Precise reproducibility of tumor position in this patient under voluntary self-breath-hold using the Abches was measured. Computed tomography images (Hi-Speed DX/I; GE Yokogawa Medical Systems, Tokyo, Japan) were obtained with a 2-mm slice thickness in the vicinity of the tumor under one breath hold, and the CT was repeated three times at intervals of 3 minutes. Maximum differences in three-dimensional tumor position in the three CT series were measured on the monitor using customized application software installed on the CT unit. As a result of the measurement for this patient, the maximum differences in tumor position were 1.5 mm cranio–caudally,

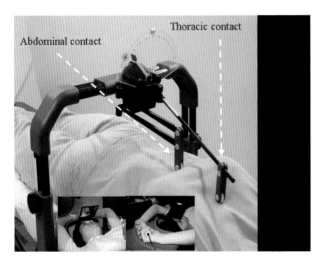

FIGURE 24K-2. The Abches, a simple respiratory indicator that comprises two arms for measurement of levels of the abdominal and chest walls. An indicator of respiratory phase is converted from the movements of the two arms. The Abches includes a mirror and a switch for the patient. The mirror allows the patient to visualize the level indicator easily.

1.2 mm antero–posteriorly, and 0.7 mm in a right–left direction.

Treatment Planning

A chest CT under voluntary self-breath-hold using the Abches was performed and a plan was generated using the 3D treatment-planning computer (FOCUS version 3.2; Elekta-CMS, Maryland Heights, MO). The planning target volume (PTV) was defined as the gross tumor volume (GTV) plus an internal target volume (ITV) that summed the maximum differences in tumor position measured previously. An additional margin of 5 mm was added to compensate for intrasession reproducibility and to provide a safety margin. Because tumor position was adjusted to the planned position before each session using the CT-on-Rails unit, setup error was almost negligible.[2] Elective nodal irradiation to the hilar and mediastinal regions was not delivered.

Ten different non-coplanar static beams were used in this patient. The isocenter was set at center of GTV. The radiation port was delivered using a dynamic sliding window technique with 5-mm-thick multileaves at the isocenter, adjusted with a 5-mm margin around the border of the PTV. A total dose of 60 Gy in 10 fractions over 5 days (6–7 hours between each daily fraction) at the minimum dose point in the PTV was delivered using 6-MV x-rays. Dose was calculated using a superposition algorithm with heterogeneity corrections. Target delineations and isodose lines overlaid on a CT image are shown in Figure 24K-3. According to the linear-quadratic model, the biologically effective dose (BED; α/β = 10 Gy) at the isocenter was approximately 120 Gy.

Treatment Delivery

The SBRT treatments were delivered using a unit comprising a linear accelerator (linac) (EXL-15DP; Mitsubishi Electric, Tokyo, Japan) coupled to a self-moving gantry-CT scanner (Hi-Speed DX/I; GE Yokogawa Medical Systems, Tokyo, Japan) sharing a common couch (Figure 24K-4), the so called "CT-on-Rails." The center of the CT image was aligned with the isocenter of the linac when the couch was rotated 180°. During scanning, the CT-gantry moved along rails on the floor. Accuracy of matching between the linac isocenter and CT image center was within 0.5 mm.[1] A patient-handheld switch was connected directly to the console box of the linac (Figure 24K-4), enabling the patient to turn the radiation beam on and off during a term designated by the radiation technologist. The patient was instructed to turn the switch on only during breath hold using Abches.

A flowchart of the irradiation process is shown in Figure 24K-5. Before each fraction, the beam isocenter was visually adjusted with in-room CT images of 2-mm

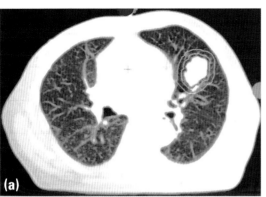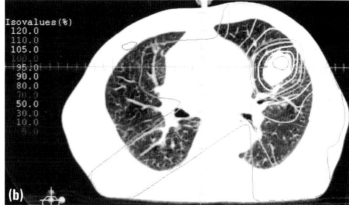

FIGURE 24K-3. Target delineations **(a)** and isodose (%) lines **(b)** overlaid on an axial computed tomography image. Inner, middle, and outer lines on **(a)** correspond to the gross tumor volume (GTV), internal target volume (ITV), and planning target volume (PTV), respectively. The isodose lines on **(b)** present relative dose of the maximum in the PTV.

thickness taken under voluntary self-breath-hold using Abches to correspond to the planned isocenter. A signal indicating readiness to start irradiation was given by a radiation technologist when alignment was obtained. Irradiation was started only when both switches for the patient and console of the linac were turned on. Actual switching of the radiation beam was delayed less than 0.1 second relative to switching by the patient. The patient determined the breath-holding time and controlled the beam delivery. With this voluntary self-breath-holding approach, the radiation beam was turned on and off repeatedly by the handheld switch connected to the linac console box until the full dose was obtained. Radiation technologists were able stop irradiation whenever necessary.

Tumor position during each treatment session was complementarily verified with an electronic portal-imaging device. Electronic portal images (EPIs) were almost real-time and taken every 2 seconds during irradiation. Whenever the tumor was visually determined to move beyond the PTV on EPI, the radiation technologist turned off the

radiation beam. The average treatment time including patient setup, adjustment of the isocenter, and irradiation (6 Gy) was approximately 30 minutes.

Clinical Outcome

Treatment was completed smoothly without any significant acute toxicity. Two months posttreatment his serum AFP had normalized. By 4 months, the metastatic tumor had completely disappeared. No acute or chronic adverse reactions were encountered. At present, 22 months after treatment, the patient remains alive with no evidence of disease or any chronic sequelae (Figure 24K-6).

Our experience using this novel treatment approach in 35 patients with stage I lung cancer was presented earlier.[3] Twenty-three patients (66%) were considered medically inoperable because of chronic obstructive lung disease and/or advanced age. All patients received 60 Gy in 10 fractions (over 5–8 days) and were treated with voluntary breath hold and beam switching using the Abches device on a CT-on-Rails system. Overall, complete and partial responses were noted in 23% and 71% of patients, respectively. At a median follow-up of 13 months, two patients (6%) developed local progression. Five (14%) failed distantly and/or in regional lymph nodes. The 2-year overall survival in the entire group was 58%. Greater than grade 2 pulmonary sequelae were noted in three (9%) patients. A more detailed description of our treatment approach has been published earlier.[4]

References

1. Onishi H, Marino K, Sano N, et al. A simple and efficient irradiation system for a lung tumor with small internal margin: patient's self-breath-hold using a newly developed respiratory indicator (Abches) and self-turning radiation-beam on and off. *Int J Radiat Oncol Biol Phys.* 2006;66:S462.

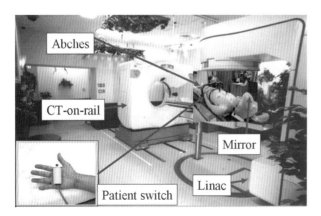

FIGURE 24K-4. Photograph of the treatment room and a scene of image-guided stereotactic body radiotherapy in collaboration with patient voluntary self-breath-hold using Abches and beam-switching.

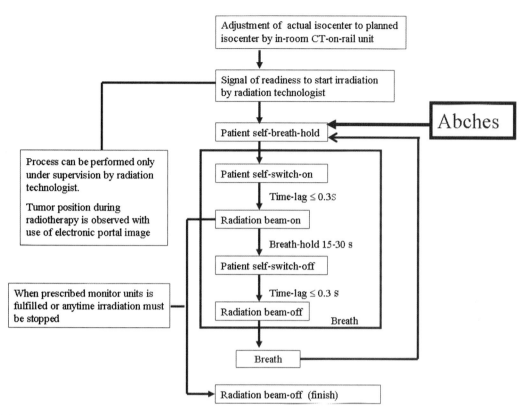

FIGURE 24K-5. Flowchart of the irradiation process.

2. Kuriyama K, Onishi H, Komiyama T, et al. A new irradiation unit constructed of self-moving gantry-CT and linac. *Int J Radiat Oncol Biol Phys.* 2003;55:428–435.

3. Onishi H, Kuriyama K, Komiyama T, et al. Clinical outcomes of stereotactic radiotherapy for stage I non-small cell lung cancer using a novel irradiation technique: patient self-controlled breath-hold and beam switching using a combination of a linear accelerator and CT scanner. *Lung Cancer.* 2004;45:45–55.

4. Onishi H, Kuriyama K, Komiyama T, et al. A new irradiation system for lung cancer combining linear accelerator, computed tomography, patient self-breath-holding, and patient-directed beam-control without respiratory monitoring devices. *Int J Radiat Oncol Biol Phys.* 2003;56:14–20.

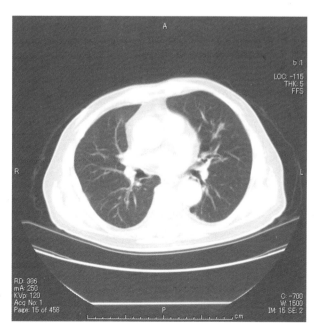

FIGURE 24K-6. Metastatic tumor in the left lung has completely disappeared and no acute or chronic adverse reactions were encountered.

Chapter 25

ADAPTIVE IGRT: A PHYSICIAN'S PERSPECTIVE

DANIEL R. SIMPSON, MD, SAMEER K. NATH, MD, BRENT S. ROSE, MD, LOREN K. MELL, MD, JOSHUA D. LAWSON, MD, ARNO J. MUNDT, MD

Image-guided radiation therapy (IGRT) currently consists of myriad technologies focused on augmenting tumor delineation and improving patient setup and target localization.[1] These technologies hold considerable promise to improve the quality of radiation therapy (RT) planning and delivery and patient outcomes by increasing tumor control and reducing toxicity.

In the future, however, the concept of IGRT will most likely be broadened to include the use of imaging to identify *changes* in tumors and surrounding normal tissues that can be adapted to during treatment. This so-called adaptive IGRT approach will transform RT from a static process, whereby treatment plans are generated based on the state of the tumor and patient before treatment and then delivered over a number of days or weeks, into a dynamic one, with treatment based on the state of the tumor and patient during treatment and adapted as needed.

What changes could form the basis of an adaptive IGRT approach? Two broad categories exist: morphologic and functional. The former includes changes in the size and/or shape of tumors and normal tissues; the latter consists of changes in the physiology or biology of tumors and normal tissues. Morphologic changes are readily detected by a variety of conventional radiologic approaches, including computed tomography (CT) and magnetic resonance (MR) imaging, but also by novel in-room IGRT technologies including megavoltage (MV) CT (MVCT) and cone-beam CT (CBCT). In contrast, functional changes are at present only detected outside the treatment room using advanced radiologic imaging including positron emission tomography (PET) and functional MR (fMR) imaging. However, as described in Chapter 13 "Emerging In-Room IGRT Technologies," such techniques may one day also be available in the treatment vault.

Both morphologic and functional changes represent appealing bases for adaptive IGRT. Most attention to date has been focused on adapting to morphologic changes. Adapting to a regressing tumor is perhaps the most intuitive of all adaptive IGRT strategies, because of the potential to improve normal tissue sparing and escalate dose to areas of residual disease. Such approaches have long been practiced by radiation oncologists, for example in patients with bulky Hodgkin's lymphoma. Equally important, however, is adapting treatment in cases of tumor enlargement, because of either tumor progression or pseudo-progression (edema, intratumoral bleeding, etc.). This is particularly important when highly conformal techniques, such as intensity-modulated RT (IMRT), are used, because of the risk of underdosing the tumor.

A different rationale exists for adapting to functional changes. Functional imaging may identify tumors or subregions within tumors (such as hypoxic areas) that may benefit from higher-than-conventional doses. Conversely, functional imaging may help identify tumors requiring lower-than-conventional doses, thereby reducing the risk of serious toxicity without compromising tumor control. Moreover, functional changes in normal tissues may allow the modification of treatment plans during the course of therapy, potentially reducing the risk of treatment-related sequelae.

Should one adapt to changes in tumors or normal tissues identified during treatment? The answer to this important question will only be provided by carefully designed, prospective clinical trials in which the volume and dose of radiation is varied on the basis of morphologic and/or functional changes. Several centers have already initiated such trials, predominantly adapting treatment to morphologic changes. Hopefully, in the coming years, more clinical trials will be launched evaluating the benefits and risks of adaptive IGRT. These trials are truly important for only if an appreciable gain in tumor control or reduced toxicities are realized will the added time, expense, and increased manpower requirements of adaptive IGRT be acceptable.

The purpose of this chapter is to provide the reader with a site-by-site overview of the variety of morphologic and functional changes observed with imaging during a course of RT, representing potential bases for adaptive IGRT. Attention is focused on studies evaluating the impact of such changes on the quality of treatment and the potential benefits of adapting to them.

Finally, published and ongoing clinical protocols evaluating adaptive IGRT will also be reviewed. Note that technical issues of adaptive IGRT, including novel automated segmentation and deformable registration algorithms, will not be discussed here but are instead the subject of the following chapter "Adaptive IGRT: A Physicist's Perspective."

Morphologic Changes

Morphologic changes have been identified in tumors of nearly every disease site. Many studies have used conventional radiographic imaging, notably CT and MR. However, literature is emerging examining morphologic changes identified by novel in-room IGRT technologies, including MVCT and CBCT. These studies are particularly interesting because of the potential for more frequent, even daily, on-line imaging. The majority of these studies have found that tumors can change significantly in size and/or shape during the course of RT, including ones previously believed to change little or not at all.

Central Nervous System

Central nervous system (CNS) tumors, particularly high-grade gliomas, have traditionally been thought to change little during treatment. However, recent evidence with the use of serial MR scanning throughout RT has questioned this belief. Investigators at the University of Michigan have presented a series of reports of serial MR scans in a cohort of high-grade glioma patients undergoing three-dimensional (3D) conformal RT (3DCRT).[2–4] In their initial study, Tsien and colleagues evaluated 19 patients with high-grade glioma with T1-weighted contrast-enhanced and T2-weighted and fluid-attenuated inversion recovery imaging performed 1 to 2 weeks before RT, during RT (weeks 1 and 3), and posttreatment.[2] Changes observed at week 3 compared with pre-RT were as follows: two patients had a 50% or greater decrease in the gross tumor volume (GTV), 12 showed a slight decrease in rim enhancement or a change in cystic characteristics, two demonstrated no changes, and three were noted to have an increase in the GTV. Both patients with a 50% or greater decrease in the GTV had grade 3 tumors (Figure 25-1), whereas all three with an increase had grade 4 tumors. The median increase in GTV was 11.7 cc (range, 9.8 cc–21.3 cc), resulting in a decrease in the planning target volume (PTV) receiving 95% of the prescription dose ($V_{95\%}$) in all three patients.

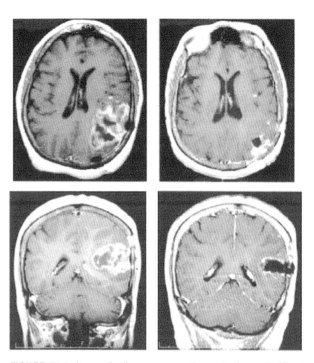

FIGURE 25-1. An anaplastic astrocytoma demonstrating a significant tumor response on magnetic resonance imaging performed during week 3 of a course of fractionated three-dimensional conformal radiotherapy. Reproduced with permission from Tsien et al.[2]

Head and Neck

It has long been known that morphologic changes occur in patients with head and neck cancers and their tumors during treatment. It is therefore commonplace to resimulate and replan patients with significant weight loss and/or reductions in tumor volume. The increasing availability of in-room imaging, notably volumetric imaging techniques including MV and kilovoltage (kV) CBCT, has further increased awareness of these changes and their impact on treatment, particularly when highly conformal approaches are used.

Investigators at the M.D. Anderson Cancer Center performed serial conventional CT scans on 14 patients with locally advanced head and neck cancer undergoing definitive RT using an in-room CT-on-Rails system.[5] All patients underwent three CT scans each week. By the last day of treatment, the median overall reduction in the GTV was 69.5%, with comparable reductions seen in the primary tumors and involved lymph nodes. On average, the GTV decreased at a rate of 0.2 cm³ per treatment day (Figure 25-2), with a median percentage decrease of 1.8% per treatment day. Others have noted the great majority of tumor shrinkage occurs during the first 2 weeks of therapy, with minimal continued shrinkage beyond that time.[6]

Recent data suggest that overall tumor response and regression rates during RT may vary between head and neck patients. Ricchetti and colleagues evaluated 45 bulky

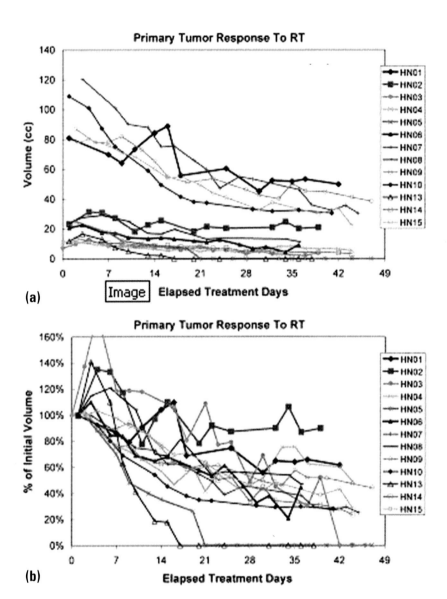

(a)

(b)

FIGURE 25-2. Gross tumor volume changes seen in patients with head and neck cancer undergoing serial computed tomography imaging, as a function of initial volume **(a)** and percentage initial volume **(b)**. Reproduced with permission from Barker et al.[5]

lymph nodes in 17 patients with oropharyngeal carcinoma using weekly conventional CT imaging.[7] Mean nodal volumes at week 4 and at the completion of RT were 53.1% and 37.2% of the initial volumes, respectively. However, lymph nodes characterized as solid regressed more rapidly than those characterized as hypodense. Mean nodal volumes assessed at week 4 for the solid and hypodense lymph nodes were 33.1% and 78.0% of the mean initial volumes ($P < .001$), respectively. Moreover, of the 20 hypodense nodes, 10 (50%) demonstrated enlargement at some point during the RT course. None of the 25 solid lymph nodes demonstrated enlargement during treatment.

Serial imaging of patients with head and neck cancer during treatment has also provided valuable insight into changes that occur in surrounding normal tissues, in particular the parotid glands.[5,8–12] Lee and coworkers performed daily MVCT scans on 10 patients with head and neck cancer using helical tomotherapy.[9] On average, the

parotid glands decreased in size by 21.3% by the end of treatment, at a median rate of 0.7% per day. Barker and colleagues reported a mean reduction in parotid size of 0.19 cm³ per treatment day in 14 patients with head and neck cancer.[5] Han et al. noted average parotid volumes on the first and last treatment days in five patients with nasopharyngeal cancer of 20.5 cm³ and 13.2 cm³, respectively.[10]

The regression of bulky head and neck tumors as well as patient weight loss appear to also result in positional shifts of the parotid glands, typically bringing them into the high-dose region. Lee et al. analyzed parotid displacements in 10 patients undergoing daily MVCT imaging and noted that they move medially during treatment, with mean overall displacements of 5.26 mm, with an average shift of 0.22 mm per day.[9] Kuo and colleagues performed repeat CT simulations at 41.4 Gy in 10 patients with locally advanced head and neck cancer and noted that the parotids were consistently displaced laterally because of

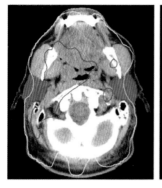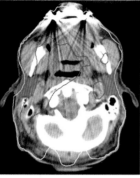

FIGURE 25-3. Comparison of dose distributions in a patient with head and neck cancer based on the initial planning computed tomography (CT) scan (left) and a repeat CT scan obtained at the 27th treatment fraction (right). Weight loss, parotid gland shrinkage, and parotid gland center-of-volume medial displacement all contribute to an increase in parotid gland mean dose. Red denotes 63 Gy and yellow 26 Gy. Reproduced with permission from O'Daniel et al.[11]

bulky cervical nodes; however, with regression of these nodes, the parotids shifted medially.[13]

The dosimetric impact of morphologic and positional changes in the tumor and normal tissues in patients with head and neck cancer have been analyzed by several investigators, with decrements noted in target coverage and sparing of normal tissues, particularly the parotid glands. O'Daniel and colleagues evaluated 11 patients with head and neck cancer with twice weekly in-room scans performed using a CT-on-Rails system.[11] As shown in Figure 25-3, patient weight loss, parotid gland shrinkage, and migration all contributed to higher-than-planned parotid doses. Others have noted increased doses to both the parotid glands and the spinal cord in patients with nasopharyngeal cancer using daily MVCT imaging.[10]

An important question is whether adapting to morphologic changes would mitigate their adverse effects on the treatment plan. To answer this question, investigators at the University of California San Francisco reviewed 13 patients with head and neck cancer who underwent repeat simulation during treatment because of significant tumor shrinkage and/or weight loss.[12] A new (adapted) treatment plan was generated and used for the remainder of treatment. A hybrid plan was generated for each patient by applying the beam configurations of the initial plan to the anatomy of the second plan. When comparing replanning with not replanning, the hybrid plan (without replanning) was associated with reduced target coverage and increased doses to normal tissues. Without replanning, doses to 95% of the PTV and the clinical target volume (CTV) were reduced in 92% of patients, by 0.8 Gy to 6.3 Gy and 0.2 Gy to 7.4 Gy, respectively. Moreover, the maximum dose to the spinal cord was increased in all patients and the maximum brainstem dose was increased in 85% of patients. The benefit of replanning is illustrated in an example case in Figure 25-4.

Kuo and colleagues performed a similar analysis in 10 nasopharyngeal cancer patients undergoing repeat CT simulation at 45 Gy and found that replanning reduced the dose to the bilateral parotid glands.[13] The mean dose reductions to the left and right parotid glands were 2.95 Gy ± 1.16 Gy and 3.23 Gy ± 1.37 Gy, respectively. In contrast, others have reported that replanning based on tumor regression did not result in improved sparing of the surrounding normal tissues.[14]

Lung

Lung cancer is another tumor site in which morphologic changes have long been known to occur during RT.

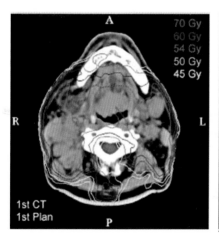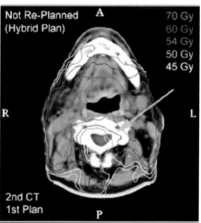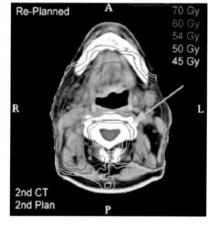

FIGURE 25-4. The dosimetric impact of replanning in a patient with stage T2N2c base-of-tongue cancer. The top image is from the planning computed tomography (CT) scan with superimposed isodose lines from the initial treatment plan. The middle image is from the repeat CT simulation and shows isodose lines obtained without replanning. The bottom image illustrates the same slice in the repeat CT scan but with isodose lines obtained by replanning. The second scan was obtained after 22 fractions and a 12% weight loss. The turquoise arrows demonstrate increased spinal cord dose without replanning. Reproduced with permission from Hansen et al.[12]

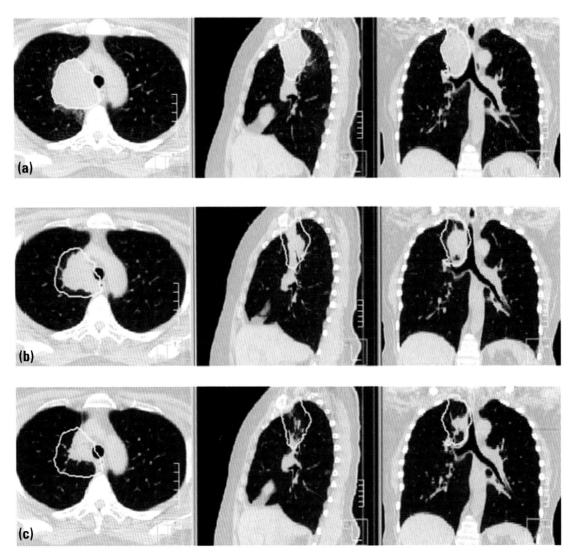

FIGURE 25-5. Example of a patient with lung cancer with continuous tumor reduction during treatment: **(a)** initial gross tumor volume (GTV); **(b)** first repeat scan, with initial contour in yellow, showing a 41.6% volume reduction; and **(c)** second repeat scan, with initial contour in yellow, showing a 70.8% volume reduction. Reproduced with permission from Fox et al.[18]

However, recognition of the magnitude of such changes has grown in recent years because of the proliferation of in-room IGRT volumetric imaging technologies.[15,16] Interestingly, morphologic changes are evident even using two-dimensional (2D) planar imaging. Erridge and coworkers treated 25 patients with non–small cell lung cancer (NSCLC) with 3DCRT. Orthogonal MV images were taken throughout the 6 to 7 week treatment course using an electronic portal imaging device (EPID).[17] In 40% of patients, the projected area of the tumor regressed by more than 20% in at least one projection.

More recently, multiple investigators have quantified morphologic changes in NSCLC patients undergoing RT using volumetric imaging approaches. Investigators at Johns Hopkins performed pretreatment and midtreatment (at 30 Gy and 50 Gy, respectively) CT scans in 22 patients with stage I–III NSCLC (Figure 25-5).[18] Mean GTV reduction was 24.7% on the first scan and 44.3% comparing the second scan with the pretreatment scan. Of note, the largest volume change occurred early in the treatment course (< 30 Gy), with subsequent changes considerably smaller.

Morphologic changes in patients with NSCLC undergoing RT have also been evaluated using four-dimensional (4D) CT (4DCT).[19–21] Haasbeek and colleagues evaluated tumor volume changes in a cohort of patients with early stage lung cancer undergoing stereotactic body RT (SBRT) with a repeat 4DCT scan a mean of 6.6 days after the first treatment fraction.[19] Overall, 25% of patients were noted to have an increase in the PTV; however, the magnitude of this increase was small, ranging from 0.1% to 7.6%. In 21 patients with NSCLC undergoing fractionated RT, Spoelstra et al. performed 4DCT (after 15 fractions) and noted mean reductions in the internal target volume (ITV) of 34 cm³.[21] The mean overall PTV reduction was 55.6 cm³. In six patients, an enlargement of the ITV was noted, with three increasing greater than 5% (6%, 21%, and 47%). These increases translated into corresponding PTV increases of 2%, 4%, and 39%, respectively.

The clinical implementation of in-room volumetric IGRT imaging has provided increased insight into morphologic changes in patients with lung cancer, because of the feasibility of more frequent imaging. Woodford and coworkers noted an average GTV change of −38%, over a course of fractionated RT in 17 patients with NSCLC.[22] The mean volume decrease per day was −0.79% (range, −0.24% to −1.65%). Ramsey and colleagues evaluated seven patients with NSCLC undergoing helical tomotherapy and noted that the GTV in these patients decreased by 60% to 80% by the end of treatment.[23] Siker and others found that the initial GTV in 10 of 25 patients with NSCLC undergoing daily helical tomotherapy decreased by greater than 25%.[24]

Several investigators have assessed the potential benefits of adapting to morphologic changes in patients with lung cancer. Woodford and coworkers found that adaptive replanning based on serial MVCT images was beneficial in some but not all patients studied.[22] Patients benefiting from replanning included those with global linear decreases in their tumor volumes as well as those displaying an initial plateau then a rapid decrease in GTV size. In two patients with a global linear decrease, the optimal times for replanning were at 16 Gy and 20 Gy. In a patient with an initial plateau followed by a rapid decrease in the GTV, frequent replanning early during the treatment course was the best approach. Patients with variable changes or no clear decrease in the GTV did not benefit from replanning. This latter group comprised four of 17 (24%) patients studied. These results suggest that whereas adaptive IGRT may be dosimetrically beneficial in some patients with lung cancer, others may not benefit or only minimally so. The development of accurate predictive models may aid in identifying the best candidates for adaptation early in their treatment course.[25]

Limited data are available assessing morphologic changes in other thoracic tumors and the potential dosimetric benefit of adapting to them. Investigators at the London Regional Cancer Center recently reported imaging changes during treatment in a patient with unresectable mesothelioma and bulky mediastinal lymph nodes.[26] Based on daily MVCT imaging, the primary lesion and regional lymph nodes were noted to regress by 16.2% and 32.5%, respectively. Adapting to a smaller GTV and reducing the PTV to 4 mm after 22 fractions, the mean lung dose could have been reduced by 19.4%. Moreover, normal tissue sparing would have permitted dose escalation from 60 Gy to a total dose of 70.5 Gy, potentially improving tumor control.

Gastrointestinal Tract

Few studies have been presented evaluating morphologic changes in gastrointestinal (GI) tumors using CT, MR, or in-room volumetric imaging. Moreover, no analyses have been performed evaluating the impact of such changes on the treatment plan or the potential of adapting treatment to such changes.

Investigators at the University of Leuven evaluated 15 patients with locally advanced rectal cancer with several MR scans performed before treatment, after 10 fractions, and before surgery.[27] Significant tumor volume reductions were seen at each time point: 27.1 cm³ (pretreatment), 13.4 cm³ (after 10 fractions), and 6.7 cm³ (presurgery).

Hawkins and colleagues[28] evaluated the use of CBCT-based adaptive plan for 14 patients with esophageal cancer. For each patient, two plans were created: a conventional plan based on the simulation CT and an adaptive plan based on a composite PTV acquired from CBCTs on days 1 through 4 (PTV_1). In addition, a composite PTV based on CBCTs acquired during weeks 2 through 6 (PTV_2) was created. The adaptive plan provided adequate target coverage, with a 95% prescription isodose for PTV_1 = 95.6% ± 4% and the PTV_2 = 96.8% ± 4.1%. In terms of normal tissues, the adaptive plan reduced the lung V_{20} (15.6 Gy vs 10.2 Gy), as well as the mean dose to the heart (26.9 Gy vs 20.7 Gy) and lungs (9.1 Gy vs 6.8 Gy) compared with the conventional plan.

Only one study to date has been published evaluating a GI tumor undergoing RT with daily in-room volumetric imaging. Li and colleagues evaluated changes in position and shape of the pancreas in a single patient undergoing RT and daily MVCT imaging using helical tomotherapy.[29] As seen in Figure 25-6, significant deformations and positional changes were observed throughout treatment.

Breast

Breast cancer is an example of a tumor site in which little or no morphologic changes are thought to occur throughout a course of RT. This is most likely because of the preponderance of early stage patients who are treated with adjuvant RT following breast-conserving surgery. However, even in these patients, evidence exists suggesting that a variety of morphologic changes occur in the lumpectomy cavity.

Oh and colleagues evaluated 30 patients with early stage breast cancer with 31 tumors using conventional CT scans performed before and prior to 40 Gy.[30] Significant changes in cavity size were observed, with reductions seen in 94.7% of the 31 cavities. The mean lumpectomy cavity volumes pre-RT and at 40 Gy were 32.1 cm³ and 25.1 cm³, respectively ($P < .0001$), a mean reduction of 22.5% (Figures 25-7 and 25-8). Of note,

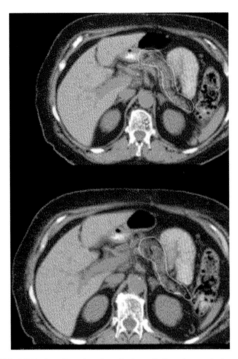

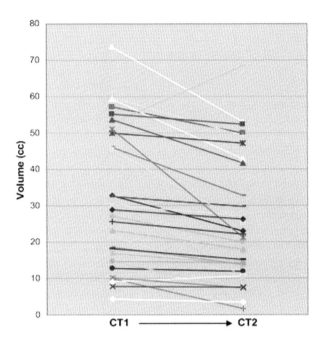

FIGURE 25-6. Interfractional variation of the size and shape of the pancreas observed in a patient with pancreatic cancer undergoing RT and daily megavoltage computed tomography imaging. Two pancreas contours from two treatment days (green and blue) are compared with the planning contour (yellow). Reproduced with permission by Li et al.[28]

FIGURE 25-7. Changes in the lumpectomy cavity volume during whole breast irradiation. Each line represents the change of a single patient's excision cavity before (left) and after (right) whole breast irradiation. The average change was −22.5%. CT1 = first computed tomography scan; CT2 = second computed tomography scan. Reproduced with permission from Oh et al.[30]

no appreciable change was observed in the irradiated breasts, with mean breast volumes pre-RT and at 40 Gy of 774 cm³ and 761 cm³, a mean reduction of only 0.11%. Others have noted volume reductions of greater than

20% of lumpectomy cavities in 16 of 20 patients undergoing serial conventional CT scans during treatment.[31]

Harris and colleagues performed serial conventional CT scans (pre-RT and during the last week of treatment)

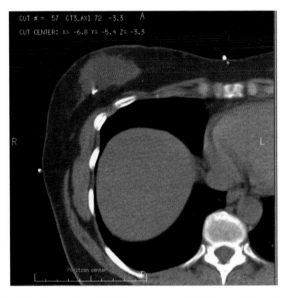

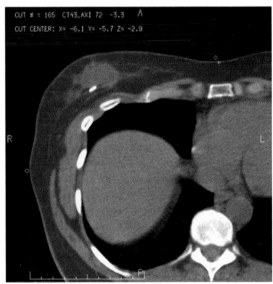

FIGURE 25-8. Comparison of the lumpectomy cavity before and after whole breast irradiation in a representative patient. Over the course of treatment, the seroma appears to have been contracted and replaced with a soft tissue density. Subsequently, the surgical clip has moved in the medial direction. Reproduced with permission from Oh et al.[30]

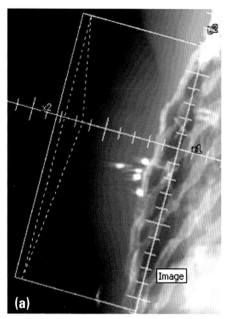
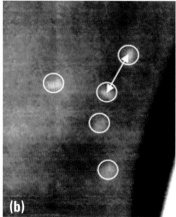
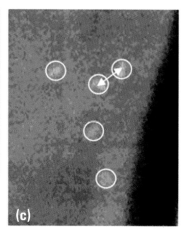

FIGURE 25-9. Left anterior oblique digitally reconstructed radiograph **(a)** in a patient with breast cancer from a computed tomography (CT) scan performed before treatment and portal images of fiducial markers acquired 8 **(b)** and 10 **(c)** days after the CT scan. Implanted fiducial markers are shown as circles. The change in the most superior marker is seen. Reproduced with permission by Harris et al.[32]

and EPID images (on treatment day 1 and between 4 and 13 subsequent treatment days) in 11 early stage patients undergoing adjuvant whole breast irradiation.[32] All had multiple surgical clips sewn into the lumpectomy cavity at the time of surgery. Three patients had significant lumpectomy volume reductions and deformations. In one patient with a large lumpectomy specimen and resulting seroma, the lumpectomy cavity decreased 47% by treatment day 1 and by 65% by the end of treatment. A second patient with a small lumpectomy cavity was noted to have marked deformations in the cavity shape (Figure 25-9). Similar reductions were observed by Vicini et al. of 18 patients with breast cancer presenting with large initial cavity volumes and seromas undergoing accelerated partial breast 3DCRT.[33]

In a cohort of 102 patients with early stage breast cancer undergoing breast conserving therapy, Yang et al. performed a planning CT scan and a repeat CT before the final boost to evaluate changes in the seroma volumes.[34] Ten women also underwent multiple CBCT scans during treatment. The mean reduction in the seroma volume between the two conventional CT scans was 54% ($P < .001$). A significant linear reduction in seroma volume was noted in the 10 patients with multiple CBCT scans up to 8 weeks postsurgery. Of note, an *inverse* relationship between seroma reduction per week and the number of RT fractions was observed, suggesting that RT may hinder resolution of seromas.

Morphologic changes in the lumpectomy cavity raise concerns regarding the use of pretreatment CT imaging in designing the boost treatment. Significant changes in

the cavity could result in excess dose to the lung, ribs, or heart.[31] In a series of 40 patients with early stage breast cancer, Nichols and colleagues found significant reductions in the lumpectomy cavity volume in all women assessed with an initial planning CT and a repeat CT at 37.8 Gy to 41.4 Gy.[35] In women with a 25% or greater reduction, replanning based on the second CT scan significantly reduced the volume of breast tissue irradiated by the 90% isodose line (median difference, 119 cc). Overall, 25 patients had clinically relevant changes in their boost plans, with 13 requiring a lower electron energy and 11 a smaller cone size.

Limited data are available evaluating imaging changes in patients with breast cancer undergoing adjuvant brachytherapy. Rice and coworkers evaluated 34 patients with breast cancer treated using Mammosite intracavitary brachytherapy (Hologic, Bedford, MA).[36] In patients undergoing Mammosite therapy, the optimal balloon-to-skin distance (BSD) is 7 mm or greater, with a minimum acceptable BSD of 5 mm. The initial minimum BSD in the 34 patients studied was 7 mm or greater and 5 mm and 6.9 mm in 32 and 2 patients, respectively. However, serial CT imaging revealed that the BSD decreased in 79% of women by 1 mm to 7.7 mm. In four, the BSD increased. Of particular note, in 53% of patients with an initial BSD of 7 mm to 12 mm, the BSD decreased to less than 7 mm by the final day of treatment and to less than 5 mm in 13%.

Genitourinary

Multiple studies have been published evaluating morphologic changes occurring in patients with genitourinary cancer throughout a course of RT, particularly patients with prostate or bladder cancer. Most demonstrate that a variety of morphologic changes occur during RT in these patients.

In one of the first studies of its kind, Roeske and co-workers performed weekly conventional CT scans on 10 patients with prostate cancer undergoing definitive RT.[37] The average prostate and seminal vesicle volumes were 56 cm^3 (range, 30 cm^3–115 cm^3) and 17.5 cm^3 (range, 3.4 cm^3–34.2 cm^3), respectively. Throughout treatment, no significant differences were seen in the prostate volumes, but large variations were seen in the volume of the seminal vesicles. Moreover, large variations were also seen in the volume of the bladder and rectum, with a trend toward decreasing bladder and rectal volumes over time. In a study of 17 patients with prostate cancer undergoing three repeat CT scans during treatment, Antolak et al. combined the prostate and seminal vesicles into a single structure and noted relatively large variations in their volume on subsequent scans in select patients, caused by deformations induced by changes in the bladder and rectal volumes.[38]

Deurloo and colleagues examined 19 patients with prostate cancer with eight to 12 repeat CT scans during a 7- to 8-week course of 3DCRT.[39] Comparing GTVs throughout treatment, a nonsignificant average decrease was noted of –0.05 cm^3 per day. However, considerable variations were noted in the shape of these tissues, the largest occurring at the tip of the seminal vesicles and the smallest along the right and left sides of the prostate. The standard deviation of these deformations at the tip of the seminal vesicles, along the right and left sides of the prostate, and elsewhere were 2 mm, 1 mm, and 1.5 mm, respectively. Deformations observed in a representative patient are illustrated in Figure 25-10. Others have noted similar results in patients assessed with serial CT scans during treatment.[40]

Investigators at the Princess Margaret Hospital performed serial MR scans (once at simulation and then randomly during treatment) in a cohort of 25 patients with early stage prostate cancer undergoing RT with implanted fiducial markers.[41] During RT, the prostate volume decreased by 0.5% per fraction ($P = .03$) and the fiducial markers in-migrated by 0.05 mm per fraction ($P < .05$). Deformation was also noted, particularly in men with a history of a transurethral resection. In a study of 22 patients with prostate cancer with implanted electromagnetic transponders undergoing daily CBCT imaging, King and colleagues reported an initial enlargement of the prostate volume (mean increase, 2.3%) by treatment day 7.[42] However, by the end of treatment, the mean prostate volume decreased by 12.6%.

Morphologic changes in patients with prostate cancer may negatively impact both target coverage and normal tissue sparing. Wu and colleagues examined the dosimet-ric impact of such changes in a patient undergoing RT assessed by daily CBCT imaging.[43] Although the overall volume of the prostate and seminal vesicles changed little, large deformations were noted in both the anterior portion of the prostate and the seminal vesicles because of changes in the rectal and bladder volumes, leading to underdosage of the target (Figure 25-11). To assess the benefit of replanning in this patient, the authors compared the original IMRT plan based on the planning CT, the original IMRT plan cast onto the CBCT (unadapted plan), and a reoptimized IMRT plan based on the CBCT (adapted plan). The adapted plan resulted in significant improvements in target coverage, with comparable conformity seen compared with the original plan based on the planning CT scan. Interestingly, results were mixed regarding normal tissue sparing, with improvements seen in rectal sparing but not in bladder sparing (Figure 25-12).

Most attention has been focused on men with intact prostate cancer; however, morphologic changes also have been described in the postoperative setting. Craig and colleagues assessed the potential dosimetric benefit of an adaptive approach in six patients undergoing postprostatectomy IMRT using daily CBCT imaging.[44] A CTV was contoured on the planning CT and on the CBCT obtained following fractions 1 through 4. An ITV was then generated by a union of these five CTVs and expanded (6 mm in the anterior–posterior and superior–inferior directions and 5 mm in the left–right direction) creating an adapted PTV. Compared with the average nonadapted PTV used to treat these patients with a PTV expansion of 5 mm to 14 mm, the adapted PTV was significantly smaller (256 cc vs 352 cc; $P < .001$), particularly in the anterior-posterior and superior–inferior directions. Moreover, based on CBCT images obtained on days 10, 20, and 30, plans based on the adapted PTV resulted in significantly lower mean doses to the bilateral femoral heads, bladder, rectum, and penile bulb. No differences were seen in CTV coverage between the adapted and nonadapted plans.

A growing volume of literature is also focused on morphologic changes seen in patients with bladder cancer undergoing RT. In fact, multiple investigators have evaluated changes in the bladder (size, shape, position) and tumors in patients with bladder cancer undergoing definitive RT, using a variety of imaging techniques including conventional CT,[45–51] EPID,[48,52] and CBCT.[52–55]

Muren and coworkers evaluated 20 patients undergoing definitive RT with weekly conventional CT scans and EPID images.[48] Bladder volumes based on planning CT scans were consistently larger than those based on the repeat CT scans, with average volumes on the planning and repeat scans of 206 cm^3 and 143 cm^3, respectively. The ratio of average repeat CT–based bladder volumes to planning CT–based bladder volumes was 0.70, but considerable variability existed. Overall, the repeat CT–based

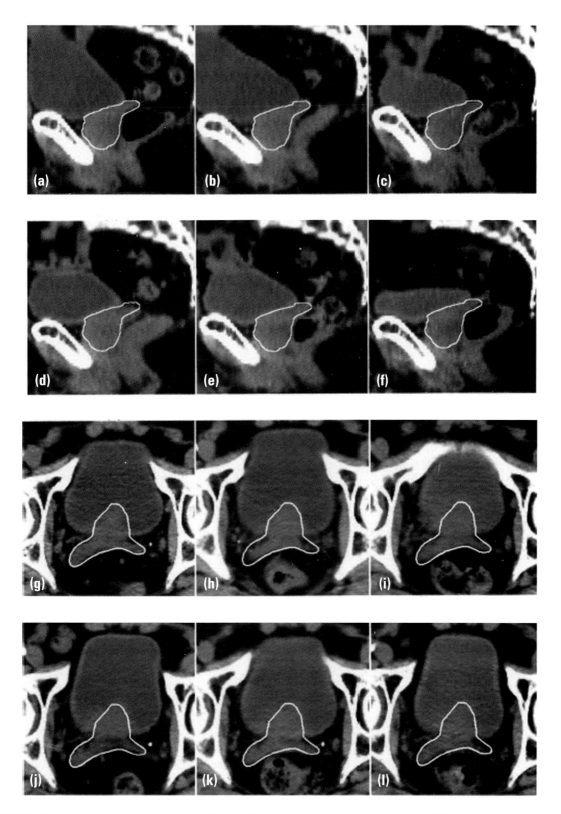

FIGURE 25-10. Sagittal (a–f) and transverse slices (g–i) of the planning and repeat computed tomography (CT) scans performed during definitive radiotherapy (RT) in a patient with prostate cancer. The gross tumor volume (GTV) of the repeat scans is registered onto the GTV of the planning CT scan. The white contour represents the prostate and seminal vesicles from the planning CT, which was overlaid on all other scans. (a,g) Planning CT scan. (b–f, h–i) Repeat CT scans of weeks 1, 2, 4, 6, and 8 of treatment. Even though the bladder and rectum changed significantly, the shape of the prostate and seminal vesicles changed little during the course of RT. Only in (d,h) is some deformation of the seminal vesicles visible. Reproduced with permission by Deurloo et al.[38]

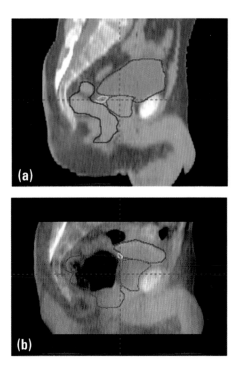

FIGURE 25-11. The planning computed tomography (CT) **(a)** and cone-beam CT **(b)** of a patient with prostate cancer with large organ deformations during radiotherapy. Contours include the prostate (red), seminal vesicles (green), rectum (brown), and bladder (blue). Reproduced with permission by Wu et al.[42]

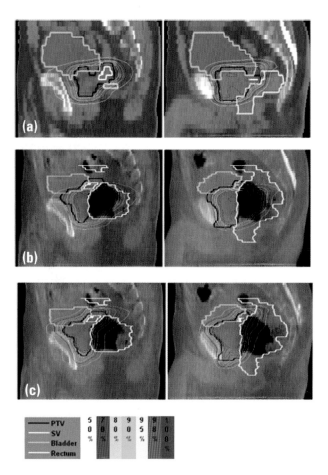

FIGURE 25-12. Dose distributions of the original planning computed tomography plan **(a)**, unadapted plan **(b)**, and adapted plan **(c)** in a patient with prostate cancer with large organ deformations. Reproduced with permission by Wu et al.[42]

bladder volumes were larger than the planning CT–based volumes on 19 scans in eight patients. Considerable variety also existed in the bladder shape, with displacements as large as 29 mm to 36 mm in the superior, left, anterior, and posterior bladder walls (Figure 25-13).

In a similar study, Pos and colleagues evaluated 17 patients undergoing definitive RT with weekly conventional CT scans.[47] Unlike other investigators who noted relatively stable bladder volumes during treatment in the majority of patients,[45,49] bladder volumes varied considerably week to week, with a weekly difference relative to the planning CT ranging from –84% to +129%. Average bladder volumes decreased with increasing radiation dose, measuring 206 cm³ on the planning CT and then 159 cm³, 123 cm³, 131 cm³, and 97 cm³ on subsequent weeks.

More recently, several investigators have evaluated changes in bladder size, position and shape using CBCT.[52–55] Using daily CBCT imaging, Yee et al. evaluated 10 patients with bladder cancer undergoing RT and, consistent with the previously mentioned reports, the mean bladder volumes were found to be consistently smaller than those obtained at simulation.[54] The mean bladder volumes obtained at simulation and during treatment were 156.8 cm³ and 131.1 cm³, respectively. Considerable deformations were also seen in the bladder, particular along the anterior bladder wall. In contrast, others have noted considerably smaller changes in 20 patients with

bladder cancer evaluated with pretreatment conventional CT versus CBCT and EPID imaging daily during week 1 and then weekly thereafter.[52] Most (75%) of the patients studied had consistent bladder volumes throughout treatment. In 11 of 16 patients in whom bladder volumes were calculated during treatment, no significant differences were seen between volumes based on the planning CT and those on the CBCT scans. In fact, a significant difference was seen in only one patient.

Pos and colleagues evaluated changes in bladder tumors in 21 patients undergoing partial bladder irradiation and serial conventional CT imaging.[55] The mean GTV measured 40 cm³, ranging from 4 cm³ to 100 cm³. Fourteen patients exhibited a significant decrease in the GTV during RT; no significant changes were noted in six patients and one patient showed an increase in GTV size. Overall, the GTV decreased on average 0.09 cm³ per day. In addition, the GTV changed markedly in shape.

Many of these same investigators have analyzed the dosimetric implications of changes observed in patients with bladder cancer undergoing definitive RT.

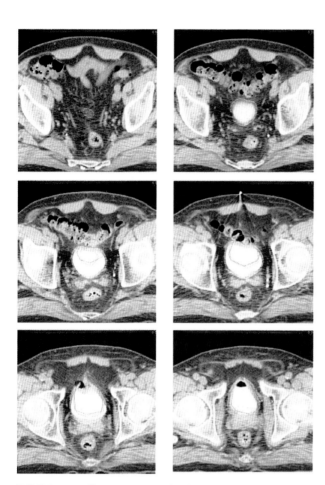

FIGURE 25-13. Six repeat conventional computed tomography (CT) scans in a patient with early stage bladder cancer undergoing definitive radiotherapy (RT) were acquired during treatment and registered to the planning CT scan. The contours of the bladder in the registered, repeat scans are shown superimposed on the planning CT scan. A loop of intestine displaced the bladder posterior at the time of the planning CT scan. Reproduced with permission from Muren et al.[48]

Unsurprisingly, given the small variations throughout treatment in the patients studied, Henry et al. found that in 93.5% of imaged fractions the CTV based on the daily CBCT was encompassed completely by the PTV based on the planning CT scan.[52]

Others, however, have noted that alterations in bladder size, position, and shape occurring during treatment have an adverse impact on target coverage and normal tissue sparing in patients with bladder cancer.[46–48,54] Yee et al. reported that the mean CBCT-based PTV outside the planning CT–based PTV was 47.35 cm[3].[54] The mean CBCT-based bladder volume extending outside the planning CT–based PTV was 4.18 cm[3]. Pos and coworkers noted that in 65% of patients studied part of the CTV extended outside the planning CT–based PTV at least one time during RT.[47] Incomplete coverage of the bladder occurred more commonly in the cranial aspect of the bladder than in the caudal aspect. In only 12 patients

(71%), the GTV received 95% of the prescribed dose on weekly scans.

Gynecology

Cervical cancer is among the most radiosensitive tumors treated with RT and it is well known that marked morphologic changes occur even early on during treatment.[56] Over the years, multiple investigators have quantified regression rates in patients undergoing definitive irradiation using a variety of imaging approaches, including CT[57] and MR.[58–66] All have demonstrated marked rates of regression in these women. Many have also noted significant changes in the size and shape of surrounding normal tissues.

Investigators at M.D. Anderson Cancer Center performed weekly conventional CT scans in 16 patients with cervical cancer undergoing RT.[53] The average cervical tumor volumes before treatment and after 45 Gy were 97.0 cc and 31.9 cc, respectively, a mean reduction of 62.3%. Median time to a 50% reduction in tumor size was 20 days (range, 7–34 days). Of note, the uterus changed little in size throughout treatment although significant positional changes were observed. However, in three women, the uterus decreased markedly in volume after the expulsion of intrauterine blood and/or fluid.

Because of its superior soft tissue imaging capabilities, multiple investigators have evaluated cervical cancer patients with serial MR scans. Mayr et al. performed MR scans before the start of RT, at 2 to 2.5 weeks, at 4 to 5 weeks, and following completion of RT in 60 patients with cervical cancer undergoing definitive RT.[65] The median tumor volume before treatment, at 2 to 2.5 weeks, at 4 to 5 weeks, and following RT were 54 cc, 31 cc, 7 cc, and 0 cc, respectively.

Others have reported significant regression rates based on serial MR scanning, ranging from 46% to 71%,[61,62,66] depending on the time point assessed. Van de Bunt and colleagues performed a repeat MR scan after 30 Gy in 14 patients and noted a median tumor volume of 39 cm[3] compared with a median pretreatment volume of 71 cm[3] (Figure 25-14).[61] Noh et al. reported pretreatment and midtreatment (week 4) tumor volumes of 20.8 cm[3] and 9.2 cm[3], respectively.[62] Of note, the magnitude of regression may vary greatly between patients. Zahra and colleagues performed serial MR scans during treatment in 13 patients and reported a median regression of 71% but a relatively wide range (35% to 100%).[66] Mayr and others observed a median regression rate of 1.8% per Gy; however, the range of regression rates was also high (0.3% to 3.6% per Gy).[64]

Several investigators have also evaluated morphologic changes in cervical tumors occurring during the brachytherapy portion of treatment. Dimopoulos and colleagues performed repeat MR scans before each brachytherapy insertion in a series of 49 patients with cervical cancer.[67]

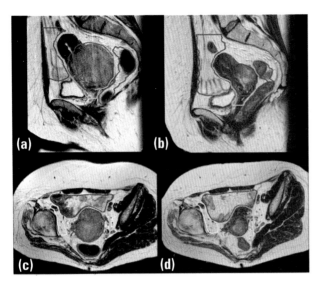

FIGURE 25-14. Example of marked regression seen in a cervical tumor in a patient with cervical cancer undergoing definitive irradiation. Magnetic resonance images include (a) pretreatment sagittal, (b) intratreatment sagittal, (c) pretreatment axial, and (d) intratreatment axial: bowel, dark blue; rectum, pink; bladder, orange; primary gross tumor volume, red; primary clinical target volume, light blue; left nodal clinical target volume, green; right nodal clinical target volume, yellow. Note also significant deformations and positional changes of the uterus, bladder, and rectum. Reproduced with permission from Van de Bunt et al.[60]

The median volumes of the cervical tumor at the first and last insertions were 16 cm³ and 8 cm³, respectively, illustrating that continued regression occurs during this phase of treatment.

Serial imaging studies in patients with cervical cancer undergoing RT have also provided insight into morphologic changes in surrounding organs and structures. Huh et al. quantified changes in uterine shape and position in 66 patients with cervical cancer undergoing RT with MR imaging performed before and 3 to 4 weeks into RT.[58] Significant changes in the cervical and uterine canal length and the angle of the cervix and corpus were noted. Of 44 ante-flexed uteruses, five became retro-flexed. Changes were more pronounced in women aged younger than 60 years, suggesting increased organ motion and deformation in younger women. Marked day-to-day deformations of the uterus and cervix have also been seen with the use of weekly MR scans[68] and daily in-room MVCT imaging.[28] Serial imaging studies have also demonstrated marked changes in the size and shape of the rectum, sigmoid, and bladder during RT.[68,69]

Increasing interest has been focused in recent years on the potential impact of the observed changes in the size, shape, and position of tumors and surrounding structures and organs in patients with cervical cancer undergoing definitive RT, particularly when one is using highly conformal techniques. Lim and coworkers evaluated the

dosimetric impact of tumor regression and deformations in a series of 20 patients with locally advanced cervical cancer undergoing weekly MR scans.[63] Various plans were generated based on the pretreatment MR and their resultant target coverage during treatment was assessed. The mean GTV D_{98} was reduced in patients planned with a small-margin IMRT plan (5 mm CTV–PTV expansion); however, although statistically significant, the difference was quite modest (5017 cGy versus 4987 cGy). Moreover, although again statistically significant, the mean CTV D_{98} decreased from 4920 cGy to 4865 cGy. The accumulated GTV dose was 95% or greater of the prescription dose in all patients and the accumulated CTV dose was 95% or greater of the prescription dose in all but one patient in whom the uterus became increasingly anteverted as the tumor regressed.

A less favorable result was reported by Tyagi and colleagues at the University of California San Diego using daily CBCT imaging.[70] In each patient, the CTV defined on the planning CT was cast onto each CBCT and modified to reflect changes in tumor size, shape, and position. Individual CTVs were then cast back onto the planning CT and treatment plans with various PTV margins were generated. Using a 5-mm margin, the percentage of treatment fractions and the average CTV *not* covered by the prescription dose were 95.4% and 20.3 cc, respectively. Even with generous margins (2 cm), the percentage of fractions not covered by the prescription dose was nearly 20%. However, the absolute volume of target underdosed was quite small.

Recently, multiple investigators have explored the potential role of adapting to morphologic changes in the tumor and normal tissues in patients with cervical cancer, both during external beam RT and intracavitary brachytherapy. Van de Bunt and colleagues evaluated 14 patients with cervical cancer with MR scans before and at 30 Gy.[61] Comparing IMRT plans generated based on the pretreatment and midtreatment MR scans, the midtreatment-based IMRT plan significantly improved the sparing of the rectum. Although no overall benefit was seen in terms of bladder and bowel sparing, in a subgroup of five patients with substantial regression of the GTV (> 20 cc), repeat IMRT planning improved sparing of the bowel.

To assess the impact of midtreatment adaptation on the overall treatment course, Lawson and coworkers performed a dosimetric study in 10 patients with locally advanced cervical cancer undergoing daily in-room CBCT.[71] Using 1-cm planning margins, two IMRT plans were generated: one based on the simulation CT and the second on a midtreatment CBCT. These two plans were then used to simulate an adaptive and nonadaptive approach. The nonadaptive approach used only the simulation-based plan and the adaptive plan used the midtreatment-based plan throughout the remainder of the treatment. Overall, the adaptive approach improved the CTV V_{100} and conformity index compared with the nonadaptive approach. Moreover, better sparing of the bladder and small bowel were achieved with the adaptive approach. In contrast, mixed results were seen in terms of rectal sparing, with three patients having no change, four with improved sparing, and three with worse sparing.

The potential benefit of weekly adaptation has been explored in two recent reports. Kerkhoff and colleagues evaluated 11 patients with cervical cancer with weekly MR imaging during external beam RT.[68] The initial median CTV was 232 cc. Beginning in week 2, smaller median CTVs were seen: 199 cc (week 2), 188 (week 3), and 172 cc (week 4). Overall, repeat planning based on the weekly MR scans significantly improved the sparing of normal tissues.

Stewart and others evaluated a potential adaptive IGRT strategy using weekly MR scans in 33 patients with locally advanced cervical cancer.[72] An initial IMRT plan using 3-mm CTV–PTV margins was generated based on a pretreatment MR and cast on the weekly MR scans. If the accumulated D_{98} of the GTV or CTV fell below 49 Gy or 47 Gy, respectively, a new IMRT plan was generated. Overall, 17 women (52%) required at least one new plan. The number of patients requiring one, two, or three repeat plans were 11, 4, and 2, respectively. Using this approach, all patients met the desired GTV and CTV accumulated doses; however, without this approach, eight of 33 would not have. Normal tissue sparing was maintained for all organs except for the sigmoid colon.

Lymphoma

Although lymphomas are among the most radiosensitive of all tumors and it has long been commonplace to resimulate patients during a course of RT because of significant tumor regression, little data exist quantifying morphologic changes during treatment in these patients or the potential dosimetric benefits of adapting treatment to such changes. Renaud and colleagues described the potential use of adaptive IGRT in a patient with bulky abdominal non-Hodgkin's lymphoma treated on a helical tomotherapy unit undergoing daily MVCT imaging.[73] Over the course of treatment, the GTV reduced by 50.6%. Adapting to the smaller GTV and reducing the PTV margins from 15 mm to 10 mm after 12 fractions would have significantly improved the sparing of surrounding normal tissues, including the liver, spinal cord, and colon. Overall, the mean liver and spinal cord doses could have been reduced by 3.8 Gy and 4 Gy, respectively.

Pediatrics

Data regarding morphologic changes in irradiated pediatric tumors and the potential benefits of adapting to them are extremely scarce. Beltran et al. at St Jude Children's Research Hospital evaluated changes in 10 patients with pediatric craniopharyngioma (median age, 8.4 years) us-

ing weekly MR scans during a course of fractionated RT.[74] The mean GTV size at baseline was 12.9 cc. The mean maximal change in the GTV was 28.4% (range, –24.8% to 82.0%) or 4.1 cc (range, –1.6 cc to 15.9 cc). Replanning based on the weekly MR scans compared with no replanning improved the tumor control probability from 90.8% to 95.7% and the D_{95} from 52.1% to 54.3%. However, no changes in the normal tissue complication probabilities or the D_{50} or D_5 were noted for the following normal structures: cochlea, hippocampus, pituitary, optic chiasm, and brainstem.

Functional Changes

Data assessing functional changes in tumors and normal tissues during RT are more limited than data assessing morphologic changes. However, in recent years, serial functional imaging has been performed in a variety of tumor sites using various advanced imaging techniques including PET and novel MR approaches. These studies provide valuable insight into biologic and physiologic changes occurring during RT which may, like morphologic changes, serve as potential bases for adaptation.

Central Nervous System

Tsien and coworkers at the University of Michigan evaluated the prognostic significance of early quantitative changes in signal intensity in the contrast-enhancing tumor rim and nonenhancing core in patients with high-grade glioma using serial MR scans.[3] Regional T1-weighted signal intensity changes in both the contrast-enhancing core and the nonenhancing core were observed in all patients during weeks 1 and 3. Imaging parameters including signal intensity changes after weeks 1 to 2, weeks 3 to 4, and 1 month after the completion of RT were all predictive of overall survival on univariate analysis. However, only the signal intensity change in the nonenhancing core 1 month posttreatment remained significant on multivariate analysis after controlling for patient age, performance status, and extent of surgery.

Cao et al. assessed changes in the blood–tumor barrier (BTB) and the blood–brain barrier (BBB) in 16 patients with high-grade glioma undergoing 3DCRT and MR scans before, during, and following treatment.[4] A gadolinium-diethylene triamine pentaacetic acid (Gd-DTPA) uptake index was analyzed in all patients with respect to the tumor and RT dose received. In the nonenhancing tumor region, contrast uptake increased significantly after doses as low as 10 Gy, and reached a maximum after 30 Gy. In the initially contrast-enhanced tumor region, contrast uptake decreased over the treatment course. Healthy brain tissue showed only nonsignificant changes during RT. These results suggest an opening of the BTB early during RT.

Investigators at the University of Iowa recently reported the results of MR spectroscopic imaging in 11 patients with malignant glioma performed before and during week 3 of external beam RT.[75] Eight patients exhibited a reduction in tumor activity during RT compared with baseline; two patients showed minimal changes and one patient exhibited increased activity. At a median follow-up of 5 months, five patients with the greatest reduction in tumor activity had clinically stable disease, whereas three of four patients with minimal or increased changes developed tumor progression.

Head and Neck

Limited data are available evaluating functional changes in head and neck tumors during a course of RT. Hentschel and coworkers performed serial ^{18}F-FDG PET scans on 23 patients with locally advanced head and neck cancer undergoing RT.[76] Scans were performed before treatment and at the end of weeks 2, 4, and 6. A steady decline in median maximum standardized uptake value (SUV_{MAX}) levels was seen throughout treatment: 15.2 (before treatment), 10.2 (week 2), 6.5 (week 4), and 6.4 (week 6). Two different groups of patients were identified: group A (10 patients) displayed a continuous decline in SUV_{MAX} and group B (13 patients) displayed an increase of SUV_{MAX} on at least one subsequent scan.[76] Using a source-to-background segmentation method, an enlargement in the PET-defined GTV was noted: 9.3 cm[3] (before treatment), 12.4 cm[3] (week 2), 14.0 cm[3] (week 4), and 17.9 cm[3] (week 6). In contrast, other investigators using a gradient-based segmentation approach have noted a continuous decline in PET-defined GTV through treatment.[15]

More recently, attention has begun to focus on other PET tracers. Lee and colleagues performed serial ^{18}F-misonidazole (^{18}F-FMISO) PET–CT scans to identify and monitor hypoxic subregions in 20 patients with head and neck cancer undergoing definitive RT.[77] ^{18}F-FMISO scans were performed beforeand after 4 weeks of treatment. Pretreatment ^{18}F-FMISO imaging revealed hypoxic subregions in 18 patients, in either the primary or involved neck nodes. In 16 patients, these regions completely resolved on the midtreatment scan. At a median follow-up of 36 months, none of the patients (including both with residual hypoxic regions at 4 weeks) developed a local recurrence. One patient experienced a regional or distant failure but had no detectable residual hypoxia on the midtreatment scan.

Serial functional imaging data are also available for normal tissues in patients with head and neck cancer undergoing RT. Saito and coworkers performed serial CT perfusion studies of the parotid glands in 10 patients with head and neck cancer.[78] Perfusion parameters studies included mean parotid blood flow (BF), blood volume (BV), mean transit time (MTT), and capillary permeability (CP). By the end of treatment, significant increases were seen in BF (265.3%), BV (194%), and CP (184%); however, no differences were seen in MTT. Of note, increased BF, BV, and CP were noted in patients devel-

oping xerostomia compared with those not developing xerostomia; however, these differences did not reach statistical significance.

Lung

Several investigators have assessed changes in patients with NSCLC using serial ^{18}F-FDG PET-CT scans during treatment.[79-83] To date, most attention has been focused on assessing volumetric changes using PET instead of assessing functional characteristics. Gillham and others performed ^{18}F-FDG PET before treatment and at 50 Gy to 60 Gy in a cohort of 10 patients with inoperable NSCLC.[79] Comparing these two time points, the mean PTV reduced in size by 20%. Sethi et al. from Loyola University repeated a ^{18}F-FDG PET–CT scan at 40 Gy to 50 Gy in 12 patients with locally advanced NSCLC and noted average reductions in the GTV and PTV of 79.2% and 70.0%, respectively.[82] Investigators at the University of Michigan performed ^{18}F-FDG PET–CT scans before and at 40 Gy to 50 Gy in a series of 14 ^{18}F-FDG-avid tumors undergoing fractionated RT (Figure 25-15).[81] The mean decrease in the GTV-based imaging on CT and PET were –26% (range, 15% to –75%) and –44% (range, 10% to –100%).

Yuan and coworkers performed ventilation and perfusion single photon emission computed tomography (SPECT) imaging before and during RT in 40 patients with stage I–III NSCLC.[84] All patients demonstrated functional deficits (ventilation, perfusion, or both) before treatment in the primary tumor with or without additional involvement of the adjacent lung. By 45 Gy, ventilation and perfusion deficits improved significantly in 37.5% and 35% of patients, respectively.

Several investigators have performed dosimetric studies assessing the potential benefits of adapting the RT plan based on serial PET imaging in the patients with NSCLC. Feng and colleagues performed repeat ^{18}F-FDG PET–CT scans at 40 Gy to 50 Gy in 14 ^{18}F-FDG-avid patients and found that designing boosts based on the repeat scan allowed dose escalation of 20 Gy to 100 Gy (mean, 58 Gy) and reductions in the normal tissue complication probability (NTCP) in five of six patients with small-volume residual disease.[81] Similarly, others have found that repeat ^{18}F-FDG PET–CT scanning and replanning allowed significant improvements in target coverage and normal tissue sparing in 12 patients with locally advanced NSCLC.[82] Overall, mean lung volumes receiving 20 Gy or more (V_{20}) were reduced by 15.5%. The NTCP rates were reduced in all normal tissues including the lungs, esophagus, heart, and spinal cord. Kong and colleagues found that adaptive IGRT plans based on ^{18}F-FDG PET–CT images performed at 45 Gy allowed significant dose escalation in all 52 patients studied, without significant increases in doses to the esophagus, heart, spinal cord, and normal lungs.[83]

Gillham and colleagues reported less-favorable results in 10 patients with inoperable NSCLC undergoing a

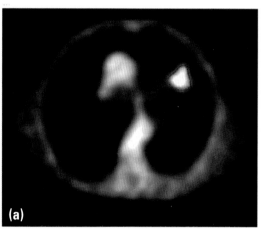 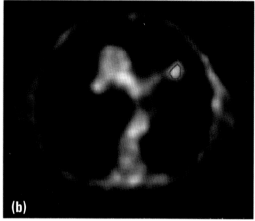

FIGURE 25-15. Example of the change in the positron emission tomography tumor volume between pretreatment (a) and after 40 Gy to 50 Gy during the course of radiation therapy (b) in a patient with non–small cell lung cancer. Reproduced with permission from Feng et al.[81]

midtreatment ^{18}F-FDG PET–CT (at 40 Gy–50 Gy) for planning of the final PTV boost.[79] Delivery of the planned prescription dose (78 Gy) was possible in only four of 10 patients using the initial PTV. However, despite median PTV reductions of 18% on the midtreatment ^{18}F-FDG PET–CT, the total planned dose still could not be delivered without exceeding predefined normal tissue constraints.

Gastrointestinal Tract

Multiple studies have been performed evaluating functional changes in a variety of GI tumors during a course of RT, in particular rectal cancer using PET.[27,85–88] The majority identify changes that may form the basis of an adaptive IGRT approach. To date, however, no trials have been presented exploring the potential benefit of adapting to such changes.

In 33 patients with locally advanced rectal cancer treated with concomitant chemoradiotherapy, Cascini and coworkers preformed serial ^{18}F-FDG PET scans (pretreatment, day 12, and presurgery).[85] A progressive reduction in glucose metabolism was noted when comparing the three time points. Excluding one patient who achieved a complete metabolic response (CMR) on day 12 and nine patients with a CMR presurgery, the median maximum standard uptake value (SUV_{MAX}) pretreatment, on day 12, and presurgery were 11.2, 6.0, and 2.7, respectively. Mean SUV values similarly decreased at each time point. Roels and colleagues performed serial ^{18}F-FDG PET scans (pretreatment, after 10 RT fractions, and presurgery) in 15 patients with locally advanced rectal cancer undergoing chemoradiotherapy.[27] The mean tumor size based on PET imaging pretreatment, after 10 fractions, and presurgery were 18.3 cm³, 11.4 cm³, and 4.9 cm³, respectively.

Janssen and colleagues reported a comparable study in 30 patients with locally advanced rectal cancer, but performed ^{18}F-FDG PET–CT scanning twice during RT (on day 8 and day 15).[88] Consistent with the results of Cascini et al.,[85] progressive declines in the mean and maximum SUV levels were seen at each time point. Mean SUV levels presurgery, day 8, day 15, and presurgery were 8.3, 7.1, 5.7, and 2.6, respectively. Corresponding median SUV_{MAX} levels were 16.3, 13.4, 10.4, and 5.4, respectively. Of note, only four patients exhibited increased SUV uptake in the surrounding normal tissues, consistent with RT-induced inflammation.

Wieder and associates assessed patients with locally advanced rectal cancer undergoing chemoradiation with PET imaging using ^{18}F-deoxyfluorothymidine (^{18}F-FLT).[87] Scans were performed pretreatment, 2 weeks after initiating chemoradiation, and preoperatively. Mean ^{18}F-FLT uptake was 4.2 SUV pretreatment and decreased to 2.9 two weeks after initiating treatment ($P = .005$). The preoperative scan demonstrated a further decrease in the mean ^{18}F-FLT uptake to 1.9 SUV ($P = .005$).

Considerably less data are available evaluating imaging changes in other GI tumors. Wieder and colleagues assessed 38 patients with locally advanced esophageal cancer undergoing preoperative chemoradiation with ^{18}F-FDG PET scans before 2 weeks of treatment (38 patients), after 2 weeks of initiating RT (27 patients), and presurgery (38 patients).[89] Mean ^{18}F-FDG SUV levels decreased significantly throughout and following treatment: 9.3 ± 2.8 (pretreatment), 5.7 ± 1.9 (after 2 weeks of RT), and 3.3 ± 1.1 (presurgery).

Gynecology

Several investigators have performed serial functional imaging studies in patients with cervical cancer during both external beam RT and brachytherapy. In a series of 36 stage IB1–IIIB patients, Schwarz et al. performed serial ^{18}F-FDG PET scans before and at three time points during external beam RT (early, ~day 16; mid-, ~day 32; and late, ~day 47).[90] The average volumes before, and at the early, mid-, and late treatment timepoints were 96 cm³, 51 cm³, 11 cm³, and 6 cm³, respectively. Corresponding median SUV_{MAX} levels were 11.2, 5.5, 2.4, and 1.9, respectively. The median times to reach a 50% reduction in volume and in SUV_{MAX} level were 16.1 and 15.8 days, respectively. Yoon and associates performed ¹⁸F-FDG PET–CT scans before and at 45 Gy and noted significant reductions in the volume and SUV_{MAX} of involved pelvic and para-aortic lymph nodes in 21 patients with cervical cancer.[91] Pretreatment and midtreatment nodal volumes were 2.5 cm³ and 0.8 cm³, respectively. Corresponding SUV_{MAX} levels were 4.9 and 0.6, respectively. Of note, 33 of the 42 nodal volumes evaluated experienced a complete metabolic response during treatment.

Magnetic resonance approaches have also demonstrated physiologic changes in patients with cervical cancer undergoing RT. Zahra and others performed dynamic contrast-enhanced MR (DCE-MR) scans in 13 women undergoing definitive RT and noted increased tumor perfusion early during treatment, which returned to baseline by the completion of therapy.[66] Others have similarly noted marked changes in tumor perfusion during treatment of cervical cancer using DCE-MR.[92–94]

Mell et al. have used serial MR fat fraction (FF) maps in 10 patients with pelvic malignancies (six cervical cancer, four anal cancer), to quantify changes in bone marrow FF resulting from chemoradiotherapy (Figure 25-16).[95] The mean baseline (n = 10), midtreatment (n = 7), and posttreatment (n=6) pelvic bone marrow FFs were 48%, 58%, and 67%, respectively, corresponding to a significant increase in FF during treatment in each patient ($P < .05$).

Limited data are available evaluating the potential benefit of adaptive IGRT based on functional imaging in patients with gynecologic cancers. Investigators at Washington University have explored the potential benefit of basing each brachytherapy plan on repeat ¹⁸F-FDG PET imaging performed before each insertion.[96] In a cohort of 11 patients, improved target coverage and higher point A doses were achieved using this technique. No benefit was seen in terms of normal tissue sparing.

Adaptive IGRT Clinical Studies

Multiple investigators have initiated adaptive IGRT protocols in recent years in a wide number of tumor sites. In the following section, published and ongoing adaptive IGRT clinical trials are reviewed and discussed. In addition, potential new trials will be described, based on both morphologic and functional changes.

Central Nervous System

The variety of morphologic and functional changes described earlier in CNS tumors provides support for a number of potential adaptive IGRT strategies. Particularly interesting is adaptation of the RT treatment based on functional changes identified early in the treatment course. However, to date, no adaptive IGRT trials have been presented in these patients.

Head and Neck

Considerable interest is focused on the development of adaptive IGRT trials in patients with head and neck cancer, based predominantly on morphologic changes. Investigators at the M.D. Anderson Cancer Center have recently launched a prospective adaptive IGRT trial in patients with localized head and neck cancer.[97,98] In this study, patients with locally advanced oropharyngeal cancer undergo daily CT imaging using the EXaCT CT-on-Rails system (Varian Medical Systems, Palo Alto, CA). Each week, volumetric images are assessed off-line and when significant changes or trends occur, a new (adapted) treatment plan is generated. To date, 16 patients have been enrolled. All received at least one replan and

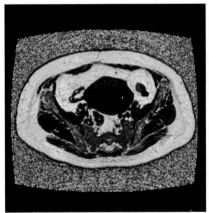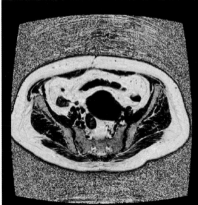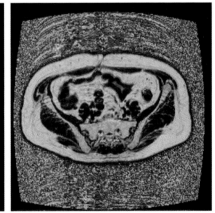

FIGURE 25-16. Serial axial slices through the pelvis of an IDEAL magnetic resonance fat fraction (FF). Map in a patient with cervical cancer treated with cisplatin and pelvic radiotherapy (45 Gy). Left: pretreatment. Middle: week 3 (midtreatment). Right: week 6 (posttreatment). Note the change from low to high signal within the ilium and sacrum, indicating an increased FF.

four received two replans. The median trigger point for the first replan was at the 17th fraction, at which point the bilateral parotid volumes had shrunk by 17% and the combined CTVs had shrunk by 5%. For the four patients requiring two replans, the median trigger point for the first replan was at the ninth fraction and for the second replan at the 20th fraction, at which point the bilateral parotid volumes and the CTVs had shrunk by 20% and 8%, respectively. In one patient receiving two replans, the GTV increased by 50% between the planning CT and treatment day 1 requiring immediate replanning. Compared with non-replanning, the use of one adaptive replan was able to reduce the mean parotid dose in 11 of 13 evaluable patients. Second replanning failed to reduce the mean parotid dose further. Additional patients are currently being accrued.

The results of the M.D. Anderson trial and other subsequent adaptive IGRT protocols in patients with head and neck cancer based on morphologic changes during treatment are important for they address not only the potential benefits of adaptation, but also its risks. A major concern with adapting treatment to a regressing tumor is the potential for adversely impacting tumor control by inadvertently underdosing areas of subclinical disease that would have received full dose if adaptation had not been performed. This is a valid concern because many head and neck cancers are highly infiltrative. It should be noted that only carefully designed, prospective analyses of the patterns of failure of patients using this approach will adequately address this concern.

An even more complicated issue is whether it would be beneficial to adapt the radiation dose to imaging changes in patients with head and neck cancer. One potential approach might be to escalate dose in select high-risk patients, based on either morphologic or functional changes. Conversely, one might explore de-escalating dose in low-risk patients. However, to date, no studies have successfully identified morphologic or functional changes in head and neck tumors that could be used as a basis for dose adaptation.

Lung

Lung cancer represents a highly appealing site for adaptive IGRT, based on both morphologic and functional changes. However, few investigators to date have explored the potential benefit of adaptation in these patients. In a cohort of 21 patients with NSCLC undergoing definitive RT, Spoelstra and colleagues performed repeat 4D CT imaging after the first 15 fractions.[21] Modifications of treatment plans were performed if any one of the following criteria was met: a dosimetric miss, defined as a 5% reduction of the PTV included within the 95% isodose volume; reduction in PTV observed in patients whose initial V_{20} was greater than 35%; or unacceptable rise in the critical

organ dose. However, the criteria for replanning were met only once, in a patient with a significant reduction in GTV size. In all 20 other patients, no need for replanning occurred. The authors pointed out that the use of more conformal techniques, including IMRT, could have yielded a greater percentage of patients requiring replanning.

It should be noted that lung cancer, like head and neck cancer, is an infiltrative tumor and, thus, concerns exist regarding adapting the treatment to a regressing tumor volume, because of the risk of inadvertently underdosing areas of subclinical disease spread. As in other sites, this issue will only be addressed by carefully designed, prospective clinical trials with detailed patterns of failure analyses.

Breast

Only one adaptive IGRT clinical trial in patients with breast cancer has been proposed.[99] As envisioned, patients would undergo daily CT imaging, contours of the target and normal tissues would be generated by registering the CT of the day with the planning CT, the new contours would be modified as needed, beam or segment apertures would be adjusted, dose distributions of the new contours would be computed, weights of the new apertures would be optimized and dose–volume histograms would be computed and compared, and treatment would be delivered. This proposed process was evaluated using a series of patients with breast cancer treated with accelerated partial breast irradiation with daily CT imaging on a CT-on-Rails system. The greatest benefit was seen in patients with large breast deformations. The minimum dose and D_{95} for the lumpectomy cavities were increased by up to 35% and 15%, respectively. The times required to complete the online replanning ranged from 7 to 10 minutes.

Gastrointestinal

To date, no trials exploring adaptive IGRT have been presented or proposed in GI tumors. One particularly appealing strategy might be to adapt treatment volumes and/or dose based on the imaging response. Unfortunately, to date, poor correlations have been found between imaging changes and tumor response and patient outcome in most GI tumors. In patients with rectal cancer, morphologic changes based on MR have been poorly correlated with histopathologic response.[27] Similarly, correlations between midtreatment PET response and pathologic tumor response have revealed mixed results in patients with rectal cancer undergoing chemoradiation. In two studies,[85,88] significant differences were seen in midtreatment SUV levels between responders and nonresponders. In contrast, Rosenberg et al.[86] using ^{18}F-FDG PET and Wieder et al.[87] using ^{18}F-FLT PET imaging did not report a significant correlation between SUV levels and histopathologic response.

The most favorable results have been seen in patients with esophageal cancer, where early metabolic changes after 2 weeks of initiating RT have been correlated with histopathologic response and overall survival. In a study by Wieder and colleagues, responders (< 10% viable tumor cells) had an average SUV decrease of 44% ± 15% versus 21% ±14% in nonresponders.[89] Mean overall survivals in patients with less than 30% SUV decrease was 18 months versus 38 months in patients with 30% or greater SUV decrease on the midtreatment ^{18}F-FDG PET scan.

Genitourinary

Multiple investigators have explored a variety of adaptive IGRT strategies in prostate cancer, particularly off-line approaches. Yan and coworkers at William Beaumont Hospital have used serial imaging early on during treatment to gain knowledge of the individual patient setup and organ motion to alter the treatment plan. As initially conceived, treatment is initiated with a population-based margins and setup errors are measured daily using EPID imaging.[100,101] Systemic and random errors and the time-dependent drift of treatment setup are then predicted.[102] Yan and colleagues reported that this strategy could be used to modify treatment margins and the total prescribed dose.[103] Setup errors were estimated at the 95% confidence level with nine or fewer EPID images. Moreover, a significant percentage of patients could have their dose safely increased because of the use of smaller margins. In a separate report, Yan et al. applied this approach prospectively to a cohort of 20 patients and reported that the average number of treatment days to confidently predict the setup error was 6.[102]

More recently, volumetric imaging has been introduced into the Beaumont adaptive RT process.[104] Based on the planning CT simulation, an initial treatment plan is generated with a 1-cm generic CTV–PTV margin. On each of the first four treatment days, EPID and CT scans are acquired before or after treatment. Confidence-limited PTV margins are generated based on each patient's setup inaccuracies and internal organ motion. Rectal and bladder constraints are used to determine the individual patient's total dose, ranging from 70.2 Gy to 79.2 Gy.

Vargas and colleagues used this approach to treat a cohort of 441 T1–3 patients with prostate cancer.[105] At a median follow-up of 1.6 years, grade 2 chronic rectal toxicity was seen in 10% of patients; 3% developed grade 3 chronic rectal toxicity. No difference was noted between dose levels, supporting the adaptive process. Brabbins and others evaluated chronic toxicities in 280 men followed for a minimum of 1 year using this treatment approach and noted no differences in toxicity rates between higher- and lower-dose groups.[104]

Nuver and colleagues proposed a similar off-line adaptive RT approach but incorporated knowledge of changes in the rectal volume as well.[106] In a cohort of 19 patients

with prostate cancer, four conventional CT scans were obtained in week 1, two during week 2 (at the beginning and end), and once weekly thereafter. The planning scan and scans obtained during week 1 were then used to construct average volumes of the prostate and seminal vesicles as well as the rectum. This approach was found capable of reducing the average CTV–PTV expansion to 7 mm without decreasing target coverage.

Nijkamp and coworkers have further refined this off-line adaptive IGRT approach by incorporating in-room kV CBCT imaging as well as dietary measures and laxative medications to improve image quality and reduce internal organ motions.[107] In a cohort of 20 patients with prostate cancer undergoing definitive RT treated with a generic 10-mm CTV–PTV margin, CBCT scans were obtained during the first six fractions and used to generate an average prostate CTV (CTV_{AVG}). The CTV_{AVG} was then expanded by 7 mm to create an average prostate PTV (PTV_{AVG}). The CBCT scans were used to generate an average rectal volume ($RECT_{AVG}$). A new treatment plan was then developed and target coverage was then assessed by analyzing CBCT scans obtained weekly. Overall, in 96% of the follow-up CBCT scans, the CTV as determined on the CBCT was within the PTV_{AVG}. In one patient, the prostate extended outside the original target volume because of the resolution of a lymphocele present at simulation. In another patient, large changes in the rectal volume led to deformations in the seminal vesicles resulting in poor coverage. No outcome data are yet available in patients treated with this novel approach.

Several investigators have explored different adaptive IGRT strategies in patients with bladder cancer undergoing definitive RT.[55,108,109] In a series of 21 patients, Pos and colleagues performed a pretreatment conventional CT and generated a PTV consisting of the GTV plus 2 cm (PTV_{CONV}).[55] During week 1, five daily conventional CT scans were obtained. During week 2, a volume encompassing the GTV on the planning CT and five week-1 CT scans was generated (adaptive GTV, GTV_{ART}) and expanded in 3D generating the PTV_{ART} (Figure 25-17). A new adaptive treatment plan based on the PTV_{ART} was delivered beginning in week 3 and coverage of the GTV_{ART} was assessed with repeat CT imaging. Overall, the GTV_{ART} was adequately covered on 94.5% of the repeat CT scans. Using this adaptive approach, the treatment volume was significantly decreased reducing the volume of surrounding normal tissues irradiated. Average PTV_{ART} and PTV_{CONV} were 228 cm³ ± 84 cm³ and 382 cm³ ± 129 cm³, respectively. Albeit promising, no clinical data have been published evaluating the outcome of these patients. Using a similar approach, Foroudi and colleagues noted an improvement in CTV coverage, with a minimum CTV dose improving from 60.1% to 94.7%.[109]

An alternative adaptive IGRT approach has been proposed by Burridge and coworkers.[108] In a planning study,

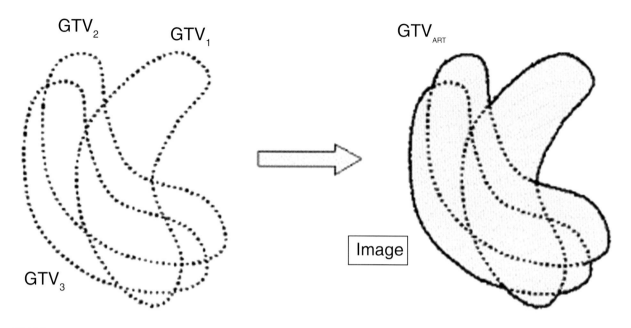

FIGURE 25-17. Illustration of the construction of the adaptive radiation therapy gross tumor volume (GTV_{ART}). Reproduced with permission from Pos et al.[55]

20 patients with bladder cancer undergoing definitive RT (52.5 Gy in 20 fractions) underwent serial CBCT scans during treatment. Three treatment plans with different PTVs were then generated: plan 1 (the delivered plan) had a PTV consisting of the bladder on the planning CT scan plus a 15-mm margin; plan 2 reduced the PTV margin in the superior direction to 10 mm; and plan 3 reduced the PTV margin in the superior direction to 5 mm. The three PTVs were then cast on the individual CBCT scans to assess coverage of the "anatomy of the day." The selected PTV had to encompass the whole bladder visualized on the CBCT with a minimum of 2 mm, accounting for potential intrafractional motion. If the daily CBCT was of insufficient quality, the original PTV (with a 15-mm margin) was selected. Overall, the majority of the patients would have benefited from this adaptive IGRT strategy, with reduced PTV margins possible on 58.1% of CBCTs analyzed. The average volume of small bowel that would have been spared was 31 cm³ ± 23 cm³, with the largest volume (76 cm³) seen in one patient that had a systematically smaller bladder on all CBCT scans.

Gynecology

The large number of morphologic and functional changes identified in patients with gynecologic cancer provides a strong rationale for developing adaptive IGRT protocols in these patients, particularly those with cervical cancer. Yashar and colleagues at the University of California San Diego have recently launched a prospective adaptive IGRT in patients with cervical cancer undergoing definitive IMRT.[110] In this study, four different IMRT plans are generated before treatment. The primary plan includes a 0.7-cm

CTV–PTV margin. The other three plans have varying CTV–PTV margins around the primary tumor. One designed for patients with anterior displacement of the cervix has an additional 1 cm anteriorly but reduces the posterior margin to 0 cm. A second plan designed for patients with a posterior displacement of the cervix has an additional 1 cm posteriorly but reduces the anterior margin to 0 cm. A third plan includes an additional 1 cm *both* anteriorly and posteriorly. On the day of treatment, a CBCT is obtained with the four different PTVs superimposed on it. The physician chooses the plan that irradiates the anatomy of the day while best sparing the surrounding normal tissues.[110]

An adaptive brachytherapy protocol in patients with cervical cancer has been ongoing for many years at the University of Vienna. Before each implant, patients undergo an MR with a MR-compatible applicator in place,[111,112] with brachytherapy plan based on the current tumor volume. In a recent report, Potter and coworkers compared the outcome and toxicity of 72 patients treated with adaptive brachytherapy compared with 73 previously treated patients at their center.[111] Overall, the 3-year actuarial local control rates of nonadaptive and adaptive patients were 82% and 89%, respectively. A trend toward better local control was seen when using the adaptive approach in tumors greater than 5 cm (82% vs 64%; $P = .09$). Improvements were seen in 3-year pelvic control and overall survival. In women with tumors greater than 5 cm, the 3-year pelvic control rates with and without adaptive brachytherapy were 90% and 71% ($P = .05$), respectively. Corresponding 3-year overall survival rates were 58% and 28% ($P = .003$), respectively. Significant reductions were also seen in terms of late rectal and bladder toxicity (10% in nonadaptive patients versus 2% in adaptive patients).

As in other tumor sites, valid concerns exist regarding adapting the treatment volume to a regressing tumor, because of the risks of potentially underdosing subclinical disease. However, most of the adaptive protocols in gynecologic cancer patients to date have explored reducing dose to normal tissues, such as the bladder and rectum, and not reducing dose to surrounding normal tissues that may harbor subclinical disease. However, only carefully designed trials with detailed patterns of failure analyses will address this important question.

Other potential adaptive IGRT approaches in patients with gynecologic cancer could involve other aspects of RT, in particular the dose delivered. This concept is supported by data correlating tumor regression with tumor control and patent survival. Mayr and coworkers reported that women with a residual tumor volume of 20% or greater at 40 Gy to 50 Gy had an inferior 5-year actuarial local tumor control (53% vs 97%; $P < .001$) compared with those with a residual volume of less than 20%.[64] Corresponding 5-year disease-specific survival rates were 50% and 72%, respectively ($P = .009$). The rate of shrinkage during RT was also correlated with both local tumor control and patient survival. One could envision a trial escalating dose in patients with significant residual disease at 40 Gy to 50 Gy. However, to date, no such trials have been initiated.

Conclusions

This review illustrates that a great variety of changes occur in tumors and normal tissues in nearly all tumor sites during a course of RT. However, these studies likely only "scratch the surface," and provide a glimpse into the changes that tumors truly undergo. Many tumors have not been assessed to date during treatment and the available data even in the sites studied remain relatively limited. This is not surprising for until recently one rarely looked for changes. Now changes seem to be identified whenever and wherever one looks. In the coming years, many new studies will appear in other tumor sites elucidating further morphologic and functional changes, not only in tumors, but also in surrounding normal tissues undergoing RT.

As more and more changes are identified, the question will quickly turn from whether changes occur to whether one should adapt to them by altering the volume irradiated and/or the dose prescribed. In some sites, prospective clinical studies are now underway assessing a variety of adaptive IGRT approaches. The results of these studies will provide valuable insight into both the feasibility and clinical benefit of adaptive IGRT.

References

1. Mell LK, Jiang SB, Pawlicki T, Mundt AJ. Image-guided radiation therapy. In: *Principles and Practice of Radiation Oncology.* Halperin E, Perez C, Brady L, eds. Baltimore, MD: Lippincott Williams & Wilkins; 2008: 263–299.
2. Tsien C, Gomez-Hassan D, Ten Haken RK, et al. Evaluating changes in tumor volume using magnetic resonance imaging during the course of radiotherapy treatment of high-grade gliomas: implications for conformal dose-escalation studies. *Int J Radiat Oncol Biol Phys.* 2005;62:328–332.
3. Tsien C, Gomez-Hassan D, Chenevert TL, et al. Predicting outcome of patients with high-grade gliomas after radiotherapy using quantitative analysis of T1-weighted magnetic resonance imaging. *Int J Radiat Oncol Biol Phys.* 2007;67:1476–1483.
4. Cao Y, Tsien C, Shen Z, et al. Use of magnetic resonance imaging to assess blood-brain/blood-glioma barrier opening during conformal radiotherapy. *J Clin Oncol.* 2005;23:4127–4136.
5. Barker JL Jr, Garden AS, Ang KK, et al. Quantification of volumetric and geometric changes occurring during fractionated radiotherapy for head-and-neck cancer using an integrated CT/linear accelerator system. *Int J Radiat Oncol Biol Phys.* 2004;59:960–970.
6. Michaud AL, Yang CC, Cui J, et al. Image guidance is most critical in the first two weeks for patients treated by radiation therapy for head and neck cancer: implications for adaptive radiotherapy [abstract]. *Int J Radiat Oncol Biol Phys.* 2009;75:599.
7. Ricchetti F, Wu B, McNutt T, et al. Volumetric change of positive lymph nodes during IMRT for HPV-associated oropharyngeal SCC [abstract]. *Int J Radiat Oncol Biol Phys.* 2009;75:S403.
8. Thomas OC, Ricchetti F, Wu B, et al. Evaluating parotid gland shrinkage during IMRT for oropharyngeal SCC [abstract]. *Int J Radiat Oncol Biol Phys.* 2009;75:S411.
9. Lee C, Langen KM, Lu W, et al. Evaluation of geometric changes of parotid glands during head and neck cancer radiotherapy using daily MVCT and automatic deformable registration. *Radiother Oncol.* 2008;89:81–88.
10. Han C, Chen YJ, Liu A, et al. Actual dose variation of parotid glands and spinal cord for nasopharyngeal cancer patients during radiotherapy. *Int J Radiat Oncol Biol Phys.* 2008;70:1256–1262.
11. O'Daniel JC, Garden AS, Schwartz DL, et al. Parotid gland dose in intensity-modulated radiotherapy for head and neck cancer: is what you plan what you get? *Int J Radiat Oncol Biol Phys.* 2007;69:1290–1296.
12. Hansen EK, Bucci MK, Quivey JQ, et al. Repeat CT imaging and replanning during the course of IMRT for head-and-neck cancer. *Int J Radiat Oncol Biol Phys.* 2006;64:355–362.
13. Kuo YC, Wu TH, Chung TS, et al. Effect of regression of enlarged neck lymph nodes on radiation doses received by parotid glands during intensity-modulated radiotherapy for head and neck cancer. *Am J Clin Oncol.* 2006;29:600–605.
14. Geets X, Tomsej M, Lee JA, et al. Adaptive biological image-guided IMRT with anatomic and functional imaging in pharyngo-laryngeal tumors: impact on target volume delineation and dose distribution using helical tomotherapy. *Radiother Oncol.* 2007;85:105–115.

15. Simpson DR, Lawson JD, Nath SK, et al. Survey of image-guided radiation therapy use in the United States [abstract]. *Int J Radiat Oncol Biol Phys.* 2009;75:S498.

16. Purdie TG, Bissonnette JP, Franks K, et al. Cone-beam computed tomography for on-line image guidance of lung stereotactic radiotherapy: localization, verification and intrafraction tumor position. *Int J Radiat Oncol Biol Phys.* 2007;68:243–252.

17. Erridge SC, Seppenwoolde Y, Muller SH, et al. Portal imaging to assess setup errors, tumor motion and tumor shrinkage during conformal radiotherapy of non-small cell lung cancer. *Radiother Oncol.* 2003;66:75–85.

18. Fox J, Ford E, Redmond K, et al. Quantification of tumor volume changes during radiotherapy for non small-cell lung cancer. *Int J Radiat Oncol Biol Phys.* 2009;74:341–348.

19. Haasbeek CJA, Lagerwaard FJ, Cuipers JP, et al. Is adaptive treatment planning required for stereotactic radiotherapy of stage I non-small-cell lung cancer? *Int J Radiat Oncol Biol Phys.* 2007;67:1370–1374.

20. Mohammed N, Glide-Hurst C, Kestin L, et al. Assessment of radiographic regression, intrafraction and interfraction motion of primary lung tumors and regional lymph nodes during treatment: implications for adaptive image-guided radiotherapy [abstract]. *Int J Radiat Oncol Biol Phys.* 2009;75:S635.

21. Spoelstra FO, Pantarotto JR, van Sornsen de Koste JR, et al. Role of adaptive radiotherapy during concomitant chemoradiotherapy for lung cancer: analysis of data from a prospective clinical trial. *Int J Radiat Oncol Biol Phys.* 2009;75(4):1092–1097.

22. Woodford C, Yartsev S, Dar AR, et al. Adaptive radiotherapy planning on decreasing gross tumor volumes as seen on megavoltage computed tomography images. *Int J Radiat Oncol Biol Phys.* 2007;69:1316–1322.

23. Ramsey CR, Langen KM, Kupelian PA, et al. A technique for adaptive image-guided helical tomotherapy for lung cancer. *Int J Radiat Oncol Biol Phys.* 2006;64:1237–1244.

24. Siker ML, Tome WA, Mehta MP. Tumor volume changes on serial imaging with megavoltage CT for non-small-cell lung cancer during intensity-modulated radiotherapy: how reliable, consistent and meaningful is the effect? *Int J Radiat Oncol Biol Phys.* 2006;66:135–141.

25. Siebert RM, Ramsey CR, Hines JW et al. A model for predicting lung cancer response to therapy. *Int J Radiat Oncol Biol Phys.* 2007;67:601–609.

26. Renaud J, Yartsev S, Dar AR, et al. Adaptive radiation therapy for localized mesothelioma with mediastinal metastasis using helical tomotherapy. *Med Dosim.* 2009;34:233–242.

27. Roels S, Slagmolen P, Nuyts J, et al. Biological image-guided radiotherapy in rectal cancer: challenges and pitfalls. *Int J Radiat Oncol Biol Phys.* 1. 2009;75(3):782–790.

28. Hawkins MA, Brooks C, Hansen VN, et al. Cone beam computed tomography-derived adaptive radiotherapy for radical treatment of esophageal cancer. *Int J Radiat Oncol Biol Phys.* 2010;77(2):378–383.

29. Li XA, Qi XS, Pitterle M, et al. Interfractional variation in patient setup and anatomic change assessed by daily computed tomography. *Int J Radiat Oncol Biol Phys.* 2007;68:581–591.

30. Oh KS, Kong FM, Griffith KA, et al. Planning the breast tumor bed boost: changes in the excision cavity volume and surgical scar location after breast-conserving surgery and whole-breast irradiation. *Int J Radiat Oncol Biol Phys.* 2006;66:680–686.

31. Jacobson G, Betts V, Smith B. Change in volume of lumpectomy cavity during external-beam irradiation of the intact breast. *Int J Radiat Oncol Biol Phys.* 2006;65:1161–1164.

32. Harris EJ, Donovan EM, Yarnold JR, et al. Characterization of target volume changes during breast radiotherapy using implanted fiducial markers and portal imaging. *Int J Radiat Oncol Biol Phys.* 2009;73:958–966.

33. Vicini FA, Remouchamps V, Wallace M, et al. Ongoing clinical experience utilizing 3D conformal external beam radiotherapy to deliver partial-breast irradiation in patients with early-stage breast cancer treated with breast-conserving therapy. *Int J Radiat Oncol Biol Phys.* 2003;57:1247–1253.

34. Yang Z, Chen J, Guo X, et al. Evaluation of the accuracy of tumor bed boost using clips-cased electron fields in early-stage breast cancer patients receiving breast conservative surgery [abstract]. *Int J Radiat Oncol Biol Phys.* 2009;75:S213.

35. Nichols EM, Marter KM, Flannery TW, et al. Small field boost re-planning after lumpectomy shrinkage in early stage breast cancer: is it necessary [abstract]? *Int J Radiat Oncol Biol Phys.* 2009;75:S212.

36. Rice BK, Torre TG, Walker J, et al. Resolution of breast edema over the course of MammoSite partial breast radiation treatment can cause decreased skin sparing [abstract]. *Int J Radiat Oncol Biol Phys.* 2009;75:S205.

37. Roeske JC, Forman JD, Mesina CF, et al. Evaluation of changes in the size and location of the prostate, seminal vesicles, bladder, and rectum during a course of external beam radiation therapy. *Int J Radiat Oncol Biol Phys.* 1995;33:1321–1329.

38. Antolak JA, Rosen II, Childress CH, et al. Prostate target volume variations during a course of radiotherapy. *Int J Radiat Oncol Biol Phys.* 1998;42:661–672.

39. Deurloo KEI, Steenbakkers RJHM, Zijp LJ, et al. Quantification of shape variation of prostate and seminal vesicles during external beam radiotherapy. *Int J Radiat Oncol Biol Phys.* 2005;61:228–238.

40. Van der wielen GJ, Mutanga TF, Incrocci L, et al. Deformation of prostate and seminal vesicles relative to intraprostatic fiducial markers. *Int J Radiat Oncol Biol Phys.* 2008;72:1604–1611.

41. Nichol AM, Brick KK, Lockwood GA, et al. A magnetic resonance imaging study of prostate deformation relative to implanted gold fiducial markers. *Int J Radiat Oncol Biol Phys.* 2007;67:48–56.

42. King BL, Butler WM, Reed JL, et al. Electromagnetic transponders indicate size fluctuation during the course of external beam radiation therapy. *Int J Radiat Oncol Biol Phys.* 2009;75:S331.

43. Wu QJ, Thongpiew D, Wang Z, et al. On-line re-optimization of prostate IMRT plans for adaptive radiation therapy. *Phys Med Biol.* 2008;53:673–691.

44. Craig T, Chu W, Odedra D, et al. Potential benefit of adaptive radiation therapy following prostatectomy. *Int J Radiat Oncol Biol Phys.* 2009;75:S645.

45. Redpath AT, Muren LP. CT-guided intensity-modulated radiotherapy for bladder cancer: isocentre shifts, margins and their impact on target dose. *Radiother Oncol.* 2006;81:276–283.

46. Fokdal L, Honore H, Hoyer M, et al. Impact of changes in bladder and rectal filling volume on organ motion and dose distribution of the bladder in radiotherapy for urinary bladder cancer. *Int J Radiat Oncol Biol Phys.* 2004;59:436–444.

47. Pos FJ, Koedooder K, Hulshof MCC, et al. Influence of bladder and rectal volume on spatial variability of a bladder tumor during radical radiotherapy. *Int J Radiat Oncol Biol Phys.* 2003;55:835–841.

48. Muren LP, Smaaland R, Dahl O. Organ motion, set-up variation and treatment margins in radical radiotherapy of urinary bladder cancer. *Radiother Oncol.* 2003;69:291–304.

49. Meijer GJ, Rasch C, Remeijer P, et al. Three-dimensional analysis of delineation errors, setup errors, and organ motion during radiotherapy of bladder cancer. *Int J Radiat Oncol Biol Phys.* 2003;55:1277–1287.

50. Harris SJ, Buchanan RB. An audit and evaluation of bladder movements during radical radiotherapy. *Clin Oncol (R Coll Radiol).* 1998;10:262–264.

51. Turner SL, Swindell R, Bowl N, et al. Bladder movement during radiation therapy for bladder cancer: implications for treatment planning. *Int J Radiat Oncol Biol Phys.* 1997;39:355–360.

52. Henry AM, Stratford J, McCarthy C, et al. X-ray volume imaging in bladder radiotherapy verification. *Int J Radiat Oncol Biol Phys.* 2006;64:1174–1178.

53. Lotz HT, Pos FJ, Hulshof MCC, et al. Tumor motion and deformation during external radiotherapy of bladder cancer. *Int J Radiat Oncol Biol Phys.* 2006;64:1551–1558.

54. Yee D, Parliament M, Rathee S, et al. Cone beam CT imaging analysis of interfractional variations in bladder volume and position during radiotherapy for bladder cancer. *Int J Radiat Oncol Biol Phys.* 1. 2010;76(4):1045–1053.

55. Pos FJ, Hulshof M, Lebesque J, et al. Adaptive radiotherapy for invasive bladder cancer: a feasibility study. *Int J Radiat Oncol Biol Phys.* 2006;64:862–868.

56. Lee CM, Shrieve DC, Gaffney DK. Rapid involution and mobility of carcinoma of the cervix. *Int J Radiat Oncol Biol Phys.* 2004;58:625–630.

57. Beadle BM, Jhingran A, Salehpour M, et al. Cervix regression and motion during the course of external beam chemoradiation for cervical cancer. *Int J Radiat Oncol Biol Phys.* 2009;73:235–241.

58. Huh SJ, Park W, Han Y. Inter-fractional variation in position of the uterus during radical radiotherapy for cervical cancer. *Radiother Oncol.* 2004;71:73–79.

59. Hatano K, Sekiya Y, Araki H, et al. Evaluation of the therapeutic effect of radiotherapy on cervical cancer using magnetic resonance imaging. *Int J Radiat Oncol Biol Phys.* 1999;45:639–644.

60. Ohara K, Oki A, Tanaka YO, et al. Early determination of uterine cervical squamous cell carcinoma radioresponse identifies high and low response tumors. *Int J Radiat Oncol Biol Phys.* 2006;64:1179–1182.

61. van de Bunt L, van der Heide UA, Ketelaars M, et al. Conventional, conformal, and intensity-modulated radiation therapy treatment planning or external beam radiotherapy for cervical cancer: the impact of tumor regression. *Int J Radiat Oncol Biol Phys.* 2006;64:189–196.

62. Noh J, Park W, Huh S, et al. Correlation between tumor volume response to radiotherapy and expression of biological markers in patients with cervical squamous cell carcinoma [abstract]. *Int J Radiat Oncol Biol Phys.* 2008;72:S354.

63. Lim K, Kelly V, Stewart J, et al. Pelvic radiotherapy for cancer of the cervix: is what you plan actually what you deliver? *Int J Radiat Oncol Biol Phys.* 2009;74:304–312.

64. Mayr NA, Wang JZ, Lo SS, et al. Translating response during therapy into ultimate treatment outcome: a personalized 4-dimensional MRI tumor volumetric regression approach in cervical cancer. *Int J Radiat Oncol Biol Phys.* 1. 2010;76(3):719–727.

65. Mayr NA, Magnotta VA, Ehrhardt JC, et al. Usefulness of tumor volumetry by magnetic resonance imaging in assessing response to radiation therapy in carcinoma of the uterine cervix. *Int J Radiat Oncol Biol Phys.* 1996;35:915–924.

66. Zahra MA, Tan LT, Priest AN, et al. Semiquantitative and quantitative contrast-enhanced magnetic resonance imaging measurements predict radiation response in cervix cancer. *Int J Radiat Oncol Biol Phys.* 2009;74:766–773.

67. Dimopoulos JCA, Schirl G, Baldinger A, et al. MRI assessment of cervical cancer for adaptive radiotherapy. *Strahlenther Onkol.* 2009;85:282–287.

68. Kerkhoff EM, Raaymakers BW, van der Heide UA, et al. On-line MRI guidance for healthy tissue sparing in patients with cervical cancer: an IMRT planning study. *Radiother Oncol.* 2008;88:241–249.

69. van de Bunt L, Jurgenliemk-Schulz IM, de Kort GAP, et al. Motion and deformation of the target volumes during IMRT for cervical cancer: what margins do we need? *Radiother Oncol.* 2008;88:233–240.

70. Tyagi N, Yashar CM, Lewis JH, et al. Impact of internal organ motion and deformation on target coverage in intact cervical cancer patients undergoing IMRT: a daily cone-beam CT study [abstract]. *Int J Radiat Oncol Biol Phys.* 2008;72:S355.

71. Lawson JD, Simpson DR, Rose BS, et al. Adaptive radiotherapy in cervical cancer: dosimetric analysis using daily cone-beam CT [abstract]. *Int J Radiat Oncol Biol Phys.* 2009;75:S85–S86.

72. Stewart JMP, Lim K, Brock KK, et al. Automated weekly online replanning for IMRT of cervix cancer [abstract]. *Int J Radiat Oncol Biol Phys.* 2008;72:S18.

73. Renaud J, Yartsev S, Dar AR, et al. Successful treatment of primary renal lymphoma using image-guided helical tomotherapy. *Can J Urol.* 2009;16:4639–4647.

74. Beltran C, Naik M, Merchant TE. The role of adaptive radiotherapy in pediatric craniopharyngioma [abstract]. *Int J Radiat Oncol Biol Phys.* 2009;75:S511.

75. Muruganandham M, Bayouth JE, Anderson CM, et al. 3D-MR spectroscopic imaging assessment of metabolic status of malignant gliomas during external beam radiation therapy: preliminary results [abstract]. *Int J Radiat Oncol Biol Phys.* 2009;75:S228–S229.

76. Hentschel M, Appold S, Schreiber A, et al. Serial FDG-PET on patients with head and neck cancer: implications for radiation therapy. *Int J Radiat Biol.* 2009;85:796–804.

77. Lee N, Nehmeh S, Schoder H, et al. Prospective trial incorporating pre-mid-treatment [18F]-misonidazole positron

emission tomography for head-and-neck cancer patients undergoing concurrent chemoradiotherapy. *Int J Radiat Oncol Biol Phys.* 2009;75:101–108.

78. Saito N, Sakai O, Lee RJ, et al. Assessing CT perfusion changes of salivary glands during head and neck radiotherapy [abstract]. *Int J Radiat Oncol Biol Phys.* 2009;75:S430.

79. Gillham C, Zips D, Ponisch F, et al. Additional PET/CT in week 5-6 of radiotherapy for patients with stage III non-small cell lung cancer as a means of dose escalation planning? *Radiother Oncol.* 2008;88:335–341.

80. Kong FMS, Frey KA, Quint LE, et al. A pilot study of [^{18}F]-fluorodeoxyglucose positron emission tomography scans during and after radiation-based therapy in patients with non-small-cell lung cancer. *J Clin Oncol.* 2007;25:3116–3126.

81. Feng M. Kong FM, Gross M, et al. Using fluorodeoxyglucose positron emission tomography to assess tumor volume during radiotherapy for non-small-cell lung cancer and its potential impact on adaptive dose escalation and normal tissue sparing. *Int J Radiat Oncol Biol Phys.* 2009;73:1228–1234.

82. Sethi A, Dombrowski J, Hong R, et al. PET/CT guided adaptive radiotherapy of locally advanced non-small cell lung cancer [abstract]. *Int J Radiat Oncol Biol Phys.* 2007;66:S250–S251.

83. Kong F, Ten Haken RK, Gross M, et al. FDG-PET/CT during radiation therapy to predict survival and guide individualized adaptive dose escalation in patients with non-small-cell lung cancer [abstract]. *Int J Radiat Oncol Biol Phys.* 2009;75:S35.

84. Yuan S, Frey KA, Gross MD, et al. The additional value of V/Q SPECT over Q SPECT alone for pulmonary function mapping before, during and after radiotherapy in patients with non-small cell lung cancer [abstract]. *Int J Radiat Oncol Biol Phys.* 2009;75:S448.

85. Cascini GL, Avallone A, Delrio P, et al. ^{18}F-FDG PET is an early predictor of pathologic tumor response to preoperative radio-chemotherapy in locally advanced rectal cancer. *J Nucl Med.* 2006;47:1241–1248.

86. Rosenberg R, Hermann K, Gertler R, et al. The predictive value of metabolic response to preoperative radiochemotherapy in locally advanced rectal cancer measured by PET/CT. *Int J Colorectal Dis.* 2009;24:191–200.

87. Wieder HA, Geinitiz H, Rosenberg R, et al. PET imaging with [^{18}F]3'-deoxy-3'-fluorothymidine for prediction of response to neoadjuvant treatment in patients with rectal cancer. *Eur J Nucl Med Mol Imaging.* 2007;34:878–883.

88. Janssen MHM, Ollers M, Riedl RG, et al. Accurate prediction of pathological rectal tumor response after two weeks of preoperative radiochemotherapy using ^{18}F-fluorodeoxyglucose-positron emission tomography-computed tomography imaging. *Int J Radiat Oncol Biol Phys.* 2010;77(2):392–399.

89. Wieder HA, Brucher BLDM, Zimmerman F, et al. Time course of tumor metabolic activity during chemoradiotherapy of esophageal squamous cell carcinoma and response to treatment. *J Clin Oncol.* 2004;22:900–908.

90. Schwarz JK, Lin LL, Siegel BA, et al. ^{18}F-fluorodeoxyglucose-positron emission tomography evaluation of early metabolic response during radiation therapy for cervical cancer. *Int J Radiat Oncol Biol Phys.* 2008;72:1502–1507.

91. Yoon M, Nam T, Ahn S, et al. Lymph node response on ^{18}F-fluorodeoxyglucose positron emission tomography during

radiation therapy in carcinoma of the cervix with positive pelvic or para-aortic lymph nodes [abstract]. *Int J Radiat Oncol Biol Phys.* 2009;75:S363.

92. Yuh WTC, Zhang D, Montbello JF, et al. Enhancing outcome prediction in cervical cancer: a multivariate approach with hypoxia-related parameters [abstract]. *Int J Radiat Oncol Biol Phys.* 2009;75:S17.

93. Mayr NA, Wang JZ, Zhang D, et al. Temporal changes in tumor perfusion pattern during the radiation therapy course and their clinical significance in cervical cancer [abstract]. *Int J Radiat Oncol Biol Phys.* 2009;75:S17.

94. Semple SI, Harry VN, Parkin DE, et al. A combined pharmacokinetic and radiologic assessment of dynamic contrast-enhanced magnetic resonance imaging predicts response to chemoradiation in locally advanced cervical cancer. *Int J Radiat Oncol Biol Phys.* 2009;75:611–617.

95. Mell LK, Liang Y, Bydder M, White G, Lawson J, Yashar C, Mundt AJ, Bydder GM. Functional MRI-guided bone marrow-sparing intensity modulated radiotherapy for pelvic malignancies [abstract]. *Int J Radiat Oncol Biol Phys.* 2009; 75:S121.

96. Lin LL, Mutic S, Low DA, et al. Adaptive brachytherapy treatment planning for cervical cancer using FDG-PET. *Int J Radiat Oncol Biol Phys.* 2007;67:91–96.

97. Schwartz DL, Garden AS, Tong S, et al. Clinical experience with in-room CT-guided adaptive radiotherapy for head and neck cancer [abstract]. *Int J Radiat Oncol Biol Phys.* 2008;72:S389.

98. Schwartz D, Ang K, Chronowski G, et al. Prospective experience with CT-guided adaptive radiotherapy for head-and-neck cancer [abstract]. *Int J Radiat Oncol Biol Phys.* 2009;75:S72.

99. Li X, Ahunbay E, Godley A, et al. An online replanning technique for breast adaptive radiation therapy [abstract]. *Int J Radiat Oncol Biol Phys.* 2009;75:S71.

100. Yan D, Wong J, Vicini F, et al. Adaptive modification of treatment planning to minimize the deleterious effects of treatment setup errors. *Int J Radiat Oncol Biol Phys.* 1997;38:197–206.

101. Yan D, Ziaja E, Jaffray D, et al. The use of adaptive radiation therapy to reduce setup errors: a prospective clinical study. *Int J Radiat Oncol Biol Phys.* 1998;41:715–720.

102. Brabbins D, Martinez A, Yan D, et al. A dose-escalation trial with the adaptive radiotherapy process as a delivery system in localized prostate cancer: analysis of chronic toxicity. *Int J Radiat Oncol Biol Phys.* 2005;61:400–408.

103. Yan D, Wong J, Gustafson G, et al. A new model for "accept or reject" strategies in off-line and on-line megavoltage treatment evaluation. *Int J Radiat Oncol Biol Phys.* 1995;31:943–952.

104. Brabbins D, Martinez A, Yan D, et al. A dose-escalation trial with the adaptive radiotherapy process as a delivery system in localized prostate cancer: analysis of chronic toxicity. *Int J Radiat Oncol Biol Phys.* 2005;61:400–408.

105. Vargas C, Yan D, Kestin LL, et al. Phase II dose escalation study of image-guided adaptive radiotherapy for préstate cancer: use of dose-volume constraints to achieve rectal isotoxicity. *Int J Radiat Oncol Biol Phys.* 2005;63:141–149.

106. Nuver TT, Hoogeman MS, Remeijer P, et al. An adaptive off-line procedure for radiotherapy of prostate cancer. *Int J Radiat Oncol Biol Phys.* 2007;67:1559–1567.

107. Nijkamp J, Pos FJ, Nuver TT, et al. Adaptive radiotherapy for prostate cancer using kilovoltage cone-beam computed

tomography: first clinical results. *Int J Radiat Oncol Biol Phys.* 2008;70:75–82.

108. Burridge N, Amer A, Marchant T, et al. Online adaptive radiotherapy of the bladder: small bowel irradiated-volume reduction. *Int J Radiat Oncol Biol Phys.* 2006;66:892–897.

109. Foroudi F, Wong J, Haworth A, et al. Offline adaptive radiotherapy for bladder cancer using cone beam computed tomography. *J Med Imaging Radiation Oncol.* 2009;53:226–233.

110. Catherine Yashar, MD, personal communication.

111. Potter R, Kirisits C, Fidarova EF, et al. Present status and future of high-precision image-guided adaptive brachytherapy for cervix carcinoma. *Acta Oncol.* 2008;47:1325–1336.

112. Potter R, Dimopoulos J, Georg P, et al. Clinical impact of MRI-assisted dose volume adaptation and dose escalation in brachytherapy of locally advanced cervix cancer. *Radiother Oncol.* 2007;83:148–155.

Chapter 26

ADAPTIVE IGRT: A PHYSICIST'S PERSPECTIVE

MATTHEW A. QUINN, PhD, JOHN C. ROESKE, PhD

Modern image-guided radiotherapy (IGRT) comes on the heels of other recent advances in the field including three-dimensional conformal radiation therapy (3DCRT) and intensity-modulated radiation therapy (IMRT). The highly conformal dose distributions afforded by these approaches demand a precise knowledge of tumor and normal tissue position through imaging. This desire for imaging, along with the development of high-quality in-room imaging devices, has resulted in an initial IGRT paradigm in which patients may be repositioned on the treatment table to bring them into better alignment with their planned positioning. Alternatively, treatment may be postponed and replanned if good alignment is not possible.

As technology further improves, it will become possible to do much more than simply reposition the patient on the treatment table. Although the phrase "image-guided" implies spatial location, advances in computing and imaging will turn IGRT into a process that is concerned with time as well. Treatment plans will be designed to incorporate regular or irregular intrafraction motion, and will be easy to adapt to anatomic changes over the course of therapy. Highly conformal doses will be delivered with much more confidence, as changes in anatomy that produce underdosing to the tumor, or overdosing to normal tissue can be monitored and corrected.

There are a number of technological developments that are necessary for adaptive treatment planning. Many of these technologies are used clinically or exist in various stages of development. The first requirement for adaptive planning is to have imaging techniques that are available in the treatment room, can scan a patient quickly, have good resolution, and can be used to perform dose calculations. Cone-beam computed tomography (CBCT) is widely implemented, but there are still questions about its ability to stand in for a conventional planning computed tomography (CT). Next, fast computer processing is necessary to reconstruct images, perform deformable registration,

and automatically segment patient images. Developing these tools will make radiotherapy (RT) departments much more efficient at planning all patients, even without regard to adaptive therapy. They will also provide a much better means for tracking the doses that patients have received throughout the course of treatment. Finally, fast dose calculations and plan optimization algorithms must be implemented to provide deliverable treatment plans from in-room images. Related algorithms and workflows for implementing these plans, responding to intrafraction motion, and providing reliable quality assurance (QA) procedures are also necessary.

The future of adaptive IGRT is very bright. A variety of different technologies are coming together to provide all members of the radiation oncology team much more flexibility in the approach to treatment planning and delivery. In this chapter we describe these technologies, and where they may lead us. However, it will be the flexibility provided by these approaches that drives the next wave of innovation in RT.

Imaging

Part of the interest in adaptive planning is attributable to the availability of patient imaging in the treatment room. With the advent of technologies such as CBCT, megavoltage CT (MVCT), and CT-on-Rails, clinicians now have the ability to obtain three-dimensional (3D) images of patients on a daily basis. Various studies have documented the need to correct for patient setup errors and organ motion, as well as possibly adapt treatment. The ability for these in-room technologies to provide images suitable for adaptive planning varies widely depending on the nature of their use.

Megavoltage Computed Tomography

Megavoltage CT and MV CBCT imaging are obvious possibilities for adaptive treatment because they make use of the MV beam that is used for patient treatment. Morin et al. have demonstrated that dose calculations on MV CT scans corrected for cupping effects are feasible.[1] They used corrected MV CT scans to compare the dose to structures in patients with head and neck cancer versus the dose calculated from the same plan on a kilovoltage (kV) CT. Contours for the MV CT were obtained from fused kV CT images. The calculations produced dose–volume histograms (DVH) that were nearly identical for the two imaging modalities.

Despite this promise, MV CT images provide poorer image resolution compared with kV CT images. It is therefore difficult to delineate soft tissues with MV CT, and kV imaging remains the standard for contouring and planning. Thomas et al. have studied the feasibility of using MV CT images for adaptive treatment planning, and found that for various sites throughout the body (prostate, head and neck, and lung) MV CT is largely inadequate for such purposes.[2] Structures contoured on MV CT were significantly smaller (65%–75%) than the same structures contoured on kV CT images. Song et al. studied the variability between contours drawn on MV CT versus kV CT in patients with prostate caner and found consistently larger prostate volumes, and larger interobserver volume variability with MV CT images (Figure 26-1).[3] The average prostate contour volume for the five patients studied was 54.1 cc ± 8.6 cc for kV CT and 59.9 cc ± 14.8 cc for MV CT.

Although MV CT images are able to reveal changes in patient positioning, they do not offer enough resolution to design treatments. Given the interest in obtaining these images to capture changes in the position, volume, and shape of soft tissues, it remains to be seen the extent to which MV CT will play a role in adaptive planning going forward. However, one important use of MV CT is for cases in which metallic implants are present. These implants cause streaking artifacts in kV CT images, which can cause errors in dose calculations. Such streaking artifacts are reduced in MV CT, as was shown by Holly et al. for brachytherapy patients with metallic hip prostheses.[4] In their case study, a patient was imaged using MV CT after the streak artifacts (caused by metallic hip prostheses) on the kV CT images limited the ability to visualize the prostate and surrounding normal tissues. The MV CT showed no streaking artifacts, and was used to delineate those organs (Figure 26-2).

Kilovoltage Computed Tomography

Cone-beam CT using kV x-rays appears to be the most promising imaging technology for adaptive radiotherapy. Several manufacturers have already incorporated CBCT systems into their linac systems. These imagers are widely used for imaging patients before treatment to correct for

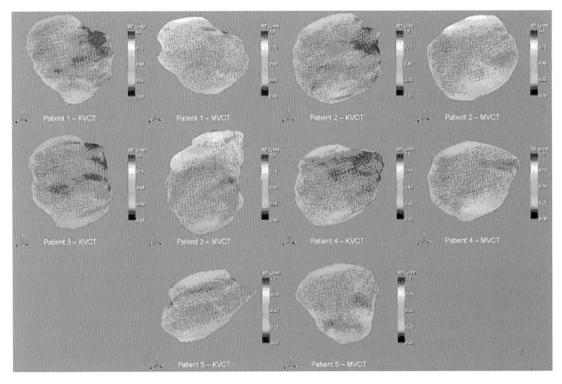

FIGURE 26-1. Standard deviation of contours from an interobserver study mapped onto average prostate surfaces for kilovoltage computed tomography (kV CT) and megavoltage (MV) CT images. Cooler colors indicate better contour agreement between observers. Reproduced with permission from Song et al.[3]

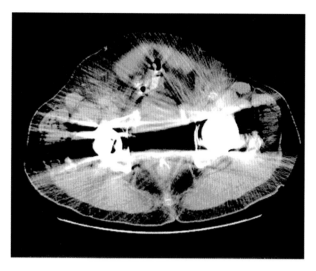 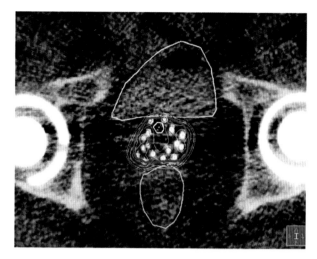

FIGURE 26-2. Streak artifacts from a kilovoltage computed tomography (kV CT) scan of a patient with double hip prostheses (top). A planning megavoltage (MV) CT scan of same patient without these artifacts is shown below. Contours on MV CT include bladder (yellow), rectum (blue), prostate (red), and isodose lines. Reproduced with permission from Holly et al.[4]

changes in patient setup, and after treatment to verify patient position. Because images are produced with kV x-rays, the image quality is superior to MV imaging, and may possibly be used in place of a conventional CT scanner. Yoo and Yin have demonstrated the feasibility of using CBCT to perform dose calculations that are similar to conventional CT results.[5] They found that despite Hounsfield unit (HU) differences of up to 200 HU between CT and CBCT, dose calculation results for the two imaging modalities were within 1% to 3% of each other. Their study examined phantom calculations, as well as patient with brain, lung, or prostate cancers calculations.

Ding and coworkers performed a similar study that also inquired into the ability of CBCT to reproduce CT dose results for a midtreatment replan of a patient with head and neck cancer.[6] They observed that the original CBCT calculated dose to the gross tumor volume (GTV), lymph nodes, parotid glands, and spinal cord matched the original CT calculated dose within 0% to 3%. The dose to these structures after a midtreatment replan also agreed within 0% to 3%. Additional results for CBCT versus conventional CT for two patients with prostate cancer showed calculated doses to the planning target volume (PTV), prostate, rectum, bladder, and other structures that agreed within 0% to 1.7%.

Rong et al. examined CBCT for planning different sites throughout the body. Using a phantom to simulate the head, lungs, and abdomen and pelvis they reported that CBCT plans agreed with CT plans to within 2%.[7] These results were obtained using a HU to electron density (ED) calibration curve for each particular site. Various other groups have reported using CBCT for delineating soft tissues in addition to bony anatomy.[8-11] This is a critical

feature of any imaging modality to be used for adaptive planning, and is what makes CBCT quite promising relative to other imaging techniques.

Foroudi et al. compared the contours drawn by four radiation oncologists for a clinical target volume (CTV; including the whole bladder, tumor bed, proximal urethra, and extra-vesical extension) and rectum in four patients with bladder cancer.[8] They observed that the contoured volumes had an average conformity index (overlapping contour volume divided by total contour volume) between observers of 0.79 for conventional CT and 0.75 for CBCT for the CTV, and agreement of 0.80 and 0.74 for the rectum. The difference in maximum contour variability between observers was also similar for the two modalities. These results indicate that the variability in structures contoured on CBCT by different observers is nearly the same as if they were contoured on the planning CT scan. Showalter and coworkers showed that bladder and rectum borders were able to be defined in 94% of prostatectomy patients using CBCT.[9] Letourneau and colleagues have used CBCT images to create online plans for bone metastasis in the spine.[10] Al-Halabi et al. have used CBCT for planning patients with cervical cancer receiving high-dose-rate (HDR) brachytherapy.[11]

In addition to 3D planning, it is worth considering the possibility of using CBCT to perform four-dimensional (4D) planning. Bissonnette and coworkers showed that 4D CBCT is able to accurately reproduce lung tumor motion seen in planning 4DCT scans.[12] In this study, patients with stage I non–small cell lung cancer receiving stereotactic body RT (SBRT) in three fractions were scanned with a conventional 4DCT scanner to create a planning scan. For each fraction, they received a 4D CBCT on the treatment table. The extent of tumor motion seen in the 4D CBCT agreed with the motion seen in conventional 4DCT to within 1 mm in all directions for patients without abdominal compression. These results illustrate that it is feasible to utilize 4D planning techniques with CBCT. Future adaptive treatments will be able to adjust for intrafraction tumor and healthy tissue motion, which may change on a day-to-day basis.

Various groups have also shown the feasibility of using CBCT with soft tissue registration algorithms for patients with prostate, cancer, as well as automatic contour propagation in patients with prostate, head or neck cancers.[13–16] Using these techniques with CBCT is important because they are necessary for any adaptive planning strategy.

Processing

The engine driving the discussion of adaptive planning is the efficient manipulation of patient images and calculated dose matrices. Obtaining multiple scans is of little use if they are unable to be processed within appropriate treatment timescales. For example, current computation speeds allow for deformable registration or autosegmentation of two full CT scans (512 × 512 × ~50 pixels) in approximately 5 minutes.[17] As this is being written, with the aid of graphics processing unit (GPU) technology, this time is being reduced to a few seconds. Gu et al.[18] have demonstrated the ability to perform GPU-based deformable registration in approximately 10 seconds. It is not inappropriate to think that, shortly, the ability to process images and make treatment decisions will be available in near real time.

Deformable Registration

Image registration is the process of obtaining and applying a coordinate transformation between two or more data sets. The purpose of this transformation is to align these image sets as closely as possible. The most straightforward method of image registration is to simply translate one image in the x, y, and z dimensions until it best matches the other. This method is currently employed by linacs with onboard imaging systems. Manual and automated methods are quick and can be used to provide corrections for simple patient translations, accounting for most daily setup errors.

Because internal anatomical variations are often more complicated than simple translations, a more sophisticated approach must be taken to account for changes in anatomy. Methods that allow each voxel in an image to be shifted independently are known as deformable registration methods (Figure 26-3). Because of this freedom to manipulate each voxel, deformable registration can incorporate changes such as tumor shrinkage, bladder and rectum filling, and patient weight loss. Most often one of two methods is used: either spline warping[14,20–22] or optical flow warping.[17,23,24]

Spline warping is a technique for deforming images that utilizes a series of polynomial functions to act as local deforming forces.[14] These polynomials are defined between the points of a grid that overlays the images of interest. The initial grid size and spacing is chosen by the investigator, and is typically much coarser than the image itself. Transformation vectors between the moving and atlas images are computed at the vertices of the mesh grid.[14] The polynomial spline functions are used to create interpolated values for the transformation between the mesh grid points. B-splines in particular are a popular choice because they are defined between adjacent mesh grid points ensuring only a local effect, and because they provide smooth values between grid points.[20,21] Generally a multiresolution approach is used, in which a series of mesh grids with increasing resolution is used. Such an approach helps to speed calculations and avoid incorrect local solutions while providing a high-resolution image registration.

Optical flow techniques or diffusion techniques such as the Demon's algorithm are other widely used methods for performing deformable registration.[17,23,24] These

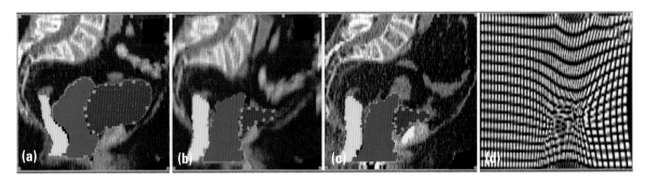

FIGURE 26-3. Fluid-landmark method deformable registration between images **(a)** and **(c)** using rectum (yellow), vagina/uterus (blue), and bladder (red). Results of the registration are shown in image **(b)**. Image **(d)** shows the deformation field obtained from the registration. Reproduced with permission from Christensen et al.[19]

methods work by treating the moving (defined as the image being deformed) and the reference image voxels as fluids that flow from one to another.[23] Voxels with similar intensities are made to attract one another, while voxels with differing intensities repel each other. The equation governing the optical flow is:

$$v \, \text{grad}(S) = M - S. \qquad (1)$$

In this equation, M is the voxel intensity value in the moving image, S is the voxel value in the stationary image, and grad(S) is the gradient of the stationary image. Here, v is the displacement vector that connects a voxel in M with a corresponding voxel in S. Therefore, the voxels in M are shifted according to the displacement vector v for each voxel. The optical flow between this new image and the image S is computed, and the process is repeated until a convergence criterion is satisfied.[24]

Autosegmentation

Autosegmentation is the process of automatically contouring relevant structures on patient images.[25-33] This is an essential component of any future adaptive radiotherapy system. Currently, physician-drawn contours take a significant amount of time to produce.[34] Such a time commitment makes even weekly imaging and replanning a burden, and makes real-time replanning virtually impossible. Implementing an automatic procedure to contour structures is therefore highly desirable for both initial planning and subsequent adaptive planning. There is a wide range of techniques for autosegmentation, from brute force intensity-based algorithms[25-28] to methods that take into account the expected size and location of anatomical structures[29-34] (Figure 26-4).

Intensity-based methods rely on the pixel values in an image to make a decision about the edges of a structure. Edge detection is generally done by searching for minima in the image gradient, or inflection points in the second derivative of the image.[25,26] Often the edges detected by these methods are not closed, and, therefore, need to be further processed to make closed contours. Region growing methods use the intensity values of pixels surrounding a seed pixel, which may be chosen manually or automatically.[27,28] Surrounding pixels are added to the region by comparing their intensity values to the mean intensity value of the region. If the surrounding pixels are within a chosen threshold they are added to the region, otherwise they are excluded. These methods can be computed quickly and are very generally applicable; however, they are susceptible to failure in the presence of excess image noise.

Better autosegmentation results are obtained by more advanced methods, which incorporate information about structures expected to be present in an image. The image features and algorithms used vary widely. Feature-based methods start by sorting images into gross categories (bone, tissue, air/lung) and then progress to specific structures (such as the femoral heads).[29] Models for the shapes and locations of internal organs are used to generate initial contours. These initial contours are then refined using the pixel intensity value methods such as flood filling and geometric models for the expected structure shapes.

Deformable methods parameterize structures as triangular surface meshes.[30] The mesh is created from landmark points in the structure, which are determined by creating meshes on training data sets. Refinement of the mesh is performed by minimizing the internal and external energies of the mesh. These parameters are formulated

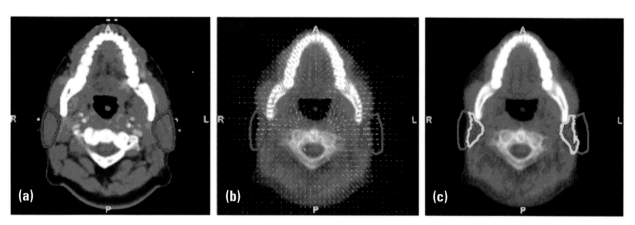

FIGURE 26-4. Image sequence illustrating a technique for generating automatic contours in a patient that has experienced weight loss during the course of treatment. Image **(a)** is the initial kilovoltage (kV) planning computed tomography (CT) image with manually drawn parotid gland contours. Image **(b)** is a later megavoltage (MV) CT image with original contours overlaid. Arrows indicate the shift in voxels from the original image to the latter image, obtained by a deformable registration. Image **(c)** is the MV CT with new contours (yellow) created from the deformable registration results and the original contours (red). Reproduced with permission from Lee et al.[31]

to correspond to, respectively, the overall shape of the mesh with respect to a model shape, and the agreement of the mesh with the structure boundary. The benefit of this type of method is that it balances fitting the volume and boundary of a structure, so that it avoids being misled by spurious or missing information from one of these features.

Atlas-based autosegmentation is another promising method for contour generation.[32,33] Contours on an image set are derived from contours drawn on previous images (atlases). The adjusted contours are obtained by performing a deformable registration between the new and previous image sets. The deformation field determining the registration between the two images is used to warp the atlas contours to fit the new image. Beyond the deformation field, models may take into account parameters such as the shape of or placement between structures to provide a better fit. A benefit of the atlas-based approach is that a library of atlases may be built up from previously treated patients. It may be possible to search the library for the atlas that best fits the current patient, based on patient size or other features. It is also possible to search through the library for the best structure-by-structure match to the current patient. For example, the bladder contour may be derived from one patient in the library while the rectum is taken from another. With sufficient patient volume, a large library may be built up providing an atlas that will fit the current patient well.

Hoggarth et al. have shown that atlas-based autocontouring programs can provide contours that agree reasonably well with physician-drawn contours.[34] They used a commercially available program, ABAS (Elekta/CMS Inc, Maryland Heights, MO), to autocontour the CT scans of 10 patients receiving multifraction HDR brachytherapy. Contours of the bladder, rectum, and sigmoid were drawn on the first scan and were deformed to the subsequent scans by ABAS. Separately, a physician contoured these structures on the same data sets. The ABAS-generated contours were then compared with physician-drawn contours using the Dice Similarity Coefficient (DSC) as a metric. Values close to 1 indicate good agreement, whereas values closer to 0 indicate poor agreement. Median values of the DSC were 0.90 for bladder and 0.73 for rectum. The agreement between contours was the best for the middle of the structures, and was lower for the superior and inferior edges. Dose–volume histograms were calculated for manual and ABAS-generated contours. The mean doses for each type of contouring were very similar, with an average of the mean bladder doses of 1.763 Gy (ABAS) versus 1.764 Gy (manual) and mean rectum doses of 1.513 Gy (ABAS) versus 1.459Gy (manual).

In addition to the possibility of performing real-time adaptive planning, these programs may save physicians a great deal of time by performing the bulk of the initial contouring. Comsia and colleagues have shown that the time saved can be one half hour or more per patient, even for unoptimized cases.[35] Their study examined 18 patients with gynecologic cancer divided into three groups according to body habitus. One patient from each group was chosen as the atlas, and had CTV, rectum, and bladder contours drawn by a physician. The ABAS program was used to generate these contours from the atlas onto the remaining patients in each group. The automaticalsly generatcd contours were then edited by a physician and the time to re-edit was recorded. The mean re-editing time was approximately 30 minutes. This combined with the processing time of approximately 5 minutes was a substantial time savings compared with the typical contouring time of between 60 and 90 minutes.

Real-Time Adaptive Planning

Innovations in imaging, computing, and delivery systems are leading toward the ability to replan a patient as he or she is on the treatment table. In the future, the process of imaging, obtaining new contours, adjusting the plan, and calculating the patient dose will likely take only a minute or two. Still under consideration are the methods by which the plans will be quickly adapted to the images of the day. Generally, any strategy must incorporate two elements: the change in size and position of the linac aperture, and the change in segment weights for IMRT plans. Until a full real-time plan is able to be generated in a reasonable amount of time, other methods must be used to provide adaptation.

Offline Calculations

With the current technology, some amount of offline processing is done to generate treatment plans ahead of time that will account for changes in patient anatomy (Figure 26-5). Basic methods to implement a "plan of the day" generate multiple plans before treatment, or make assumptions about the position of patient anatomy. Depending on the site, the focus may be on random or systematic patient setup errors, organ or tumor motion, or patient weight loss. Methods that use a plan of the day compute different plans for different predicted patient setups or changes in anatomy.[36,37] The changes in anatomy may be based on measured organ motions, or the deformation matrices from a deformable registration. The images of the day are compared with these different predicted scenarios, and the plan corresponding to the closest match of the current patient anatomy is then used. Methods that attempt to incorporate organ motion may take into account the extremes of organ motion seen in previous studies, or create an average of organ motion from several previous image sets.[38–41] These methods can provide an improvement over not adapting the plan at all, but fall short of performing a full replan and dose calculation based on the daily CT.

3D Conformal

GTV Volume: 19 cc

Tumor Motion: 0.9 cm SI, 0.4 cm AP, 0.1 cm ML.

4D Union

37 cc

4D Adaptive IGRT

25 cc

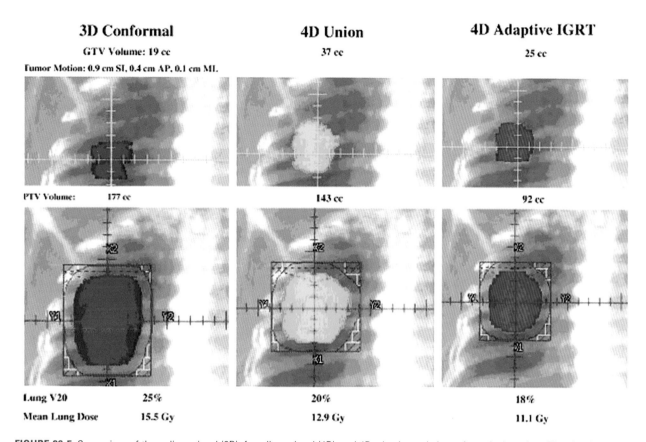

PTV Volume: 177 cc   143 cc   92 cc

	3D Conformal	4D Union	4D Adaptive IGRT
Lung V20	25%	20%	18%
Mean Lung Dose	15.5 Gy	12.9 Gy	11.1 Gy

FIGURE 26-5. Comparison of three-dimensional (3D), four-dimensional (4D), and 4D adaptive techniques for a single patient. The planning target volume (PTV), lung volume receiving 20 Gy (V_{20}), and mean lung dose are smallest for the adaptive technique. Reproduced with permission from Harsolia et al.[42]

Online Replanning
Methods to Reshape the Beam Aperture

The segment aperture morphing (SAM) method relies on the contours of the PTV from a previous image and the image of the day.[43] By using the contour points and leaf segment control points, it calculates the multileaf collimator (MLC) leaf pattern shifts to change the aperture opening to match the new PTV shape and position. The SAM method can be implemented in conjunction with a segment reoptimization algorithm to provide a new IMRT treatment plan. Because the SAM relies on having contours on the image of the day, its use as a real-time replanning scheme depends on the ease of generating contours of the PTV on the new image. Ahunbay et al. demonstrated that recontouring the PTV for patients with prostate cancer takes approximately 2 minutes.[43] In this case, the SAM process may be feasible, but going forward it is desirable to incorporate autosegmentation into the process.

A more complex approach is the direct aperture deformation (DAD) method.[44] It uses the deformation field from a deformable registration to shift the aperture. The daily CT scan is deformed to the planning CT scan to produce the deformation field. Next the deformation vectors from the voxels inside the PTV are projected onto the treatment plane. These projection vectors are summed in the treatment plane to create a 2D deformation field that is used to morph the aperture. This method works very quickly (< 30 s), and does not require recontouring. The time necessary to implement this strategy is that required to perform a deformable registration of the two image sets. Feng and coworkers showed that, for patients with prostate cancer, the results from a DAD replan are nearly identical to those when one is performing a full dose recalculation.[44]

The most advanced methods of reshaping the beam aperture include motion-tracking capabilities. These methods are designed to continuously follow the tumor in real time throughout the course of treatment. Some rely on predicted motion patterns, using neural networks or other models to estimate tumor trajectories.[45] Given an external surrogate's speed and position, these systems predict where the tumor will be some time in the future. This can allow a leaf sequence that minimizes the tracking error to be implemented. Some methods rely on a 4DCT correlated breathing signal.[46] This dose rate–regulated tracking (DRRT) system increases or decreases the dose rate being delivered as the breathing rate increases or decreases.

The leaf sequences are delivered at a different time, and the dose rate is changed to deliver the leaf sequences in the same phase of the breathing cycle that they are planned. Other methods to reshape the beam aperture utilize intrafraction fluoroscopic images.[47,48] These methods use image processing software to continuously track a tumor and adjust the MLC leaves to follow it. Still others use radio frequency (RF)–based motion-tracking implants.[49] These methods track a tumor in real time using RF beacons implanted into a tumor. The beacons can provide the position of the tumor in real time throughout the course of treatment. Leaf sequences for phased tumor location are defined and delivered, with beam gating possible for unexpected tumor motion.

Most of these are still in the research phase, and have yet to be implemented clinically. Each method has its own benefits and drawbacks, but the basic tradeoff seems to be that better monitoring requires more invasive procedures such as surgically implanted beacons. Methods that use less-involved tumor position monitoring must accept more uncertainty in the real-time tumor position, or rely on motion surrogates such as an external breathing signal. It is very likely that planning and delivery systems will need to be able to handle multiple types of methods for real-time tumor tracking.

Plan Optimization Methods

Several groups have put forward methods to adjust segment weights for IMRT plans.[43–51] These may be used with static replanning, but they are often created with the goal of dynamically adjusting the treatment plan in response to intrafraction tumor or patient motion. Some approaches are more sophisticated than others, and include monitoring and adjustment of the dose delivered throughout the treatment fraction.

The segment weight optimization (SWO) routine was used by Ahunbay et al. in conjunction with their SAM method for adjusting the machine aperture size.[43] It reoptimizes the planned segment weights by performing a quadratic programming search over the state space of an objective function. The SWO can be performed quickly because it uses the segment dose distributions that were calculated by the planning system for the original plan. Ahunbay et al. have shown the plans generated by the SAM–SWO method to be similar to fully reoptimized plans for patients with prostate cancer. Men et al. have implemented a similar scheme to the SWO using a GPU calculation instead of a central processing unit calculation.[50] They are able to obtain reoptimized plans in a few seconds or even fractions of a second, depending on the plan complexity.

Yi et al. have created a system that combines a preprogrammed leaf sequence with a dose rate modification engine to create the DRRT.[46] This method was developed to deliver treatments for patients with lung cancer. The preprogrammed plan is delivered in synchronization

with an external breathing surrogate signal. If the patient is breathing faster or slower than the simulated breathing rate, the leaf sequences and delivered dose rate can be sped up or slowed down. Agreement between the planned breathing signal and actual breathing signal is done every 0.1 s. Tests of this method in a phantom have shown tracking errors of less than 1 mm, and 97% gamma-index agreement (3% and 2 mm distance to agreement).

If performed quickly enough, reoptimization can be done in response to intrafraction motion. Real-time plan reoptimization has been demonstrated by Lu et al.[51] Their motion adaptive optimization method calculates the accumulated dose delivered during the treatment and the future projected dose based on anticipated motion. The dose to be delivered in each sequence is then reoptimized to deliver an isodose distribution as close to the stationary plan as possible. Calculations are completed within 100 ms, allowing use in conventional IMRT or tomotherapy IMRT delivery.

Adaptive Planning in the Future

Recent advances in the technology used to plan and deliver RT treatments point to great changes in what these treatments will look like in the future. Many of the tools for IGRT and adaptive planning already exist, but as stand-alone components. The first wave of improvement to IGRT and adaptive treatment will be to integrate imaging, deformable registration, autosegmentation, planning, and delivery systems so that they work seamlessly with each other. Each of these steps may still require a sizeable amount of human intervention or oversight, but their integration will make adaptive planning much more feasible.

The use of GPU approaches for dose calculations, deformable registration, and plan optimization will make these tasks efficient enough to implement in daily interfraction or intrafraction settings. It may be possible for daily adaptive planning to be done automatically and with minimal supervision. There will be a need for guidelines determining what levels of deviation from the original plan can be implemented without more substantial review from either physicians or physicists. Methods for performing QA on individual components such as deformable registration and autocontouring, as well as on the entire adaptive planning system, need to be developed. Quality assurance for deformable registration and autosegmentation can be performed using phantom studies,[52–55] by comparing results with those from other algorithms,[56,57] or, in the case of autosegmentation, comparing with manual contours.[58–60] Currently, there are no guidelines indicating what performance standards are sufficient. Quality assurance for changes to leaf sequences may be checked by measurement, but because of the desire to implement these changes during

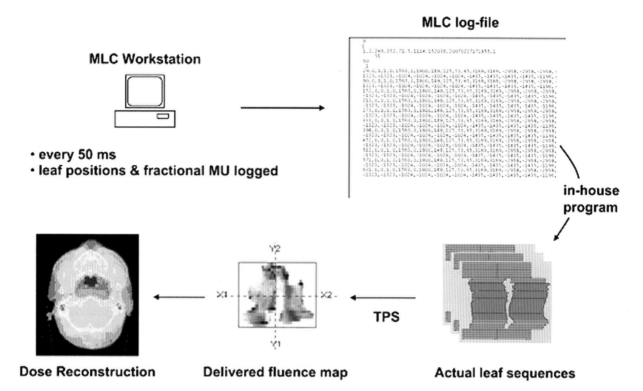

MLC log-file

MLC Workstation

• **every 50 ms**
• **leaf positions & fractional MU logged**

in-house program

Dose Reconstruction   **Delivered fluence map**   **TPS**   **Actual leaf sequences**

FIGURE 26-6. Workflow of dose reconstruction method using the multileaf collimator (MLC) log file. Log files are used to generate a delivered fluence map for each leaf sequence. The dose from each leaf sequence is then added together to provide a reconstruction of the total dose delivered throughout the course of one fraction. Reproduced with permission from Lee et al.[61]

treatment, it may also be desirable to use MLC log files to compare the dose actually delivered with the planned dose (Figure 26-6).

Technological advances in processing images will also assist in the initial planning phase. Autosegmentation programs will be able to contour normal structures on patient planning scans and, in certain cases, the GTV and CTV. Advances in informatics may also make a clinic's database one of the most important tools for designing more effective treatments. By incorporating the scans and plans of the patients with similar anatomies and diagnosis as the current patient, physicians will be able to evaluate dose distributions and outcomes to make treatment-related decisions based on these data. Moreover, the important question of whether one should attempt to adapt treatment in certain disease sites may also be answered.

The recent advances associated with in-room imaging, image processing, autosegmentation, and GPU-based computation have started to find their way into RT clinics. In certain cases, they have already proven themselves valuable tools for improving patient care. Using them in an integrated fashion will provide substantial progress in responding to changes in tumor size and patient anatomy. In a short amount of time, the delivery of radiation for cancer therapy will be a fully dynamic process that may provide even better patient outcomes.

References

1. Morin O, Chen J, Aubin M, et al. Dose calculation using megavoltage cone-beam CT. *Int J Radiat Oncol Biol Phys.* 2007;67:1201–1210.
2. Thomas SR, Haradat H, Vonk DT, et al. Can MVCT be used for adaptive radiotherapy? A feasibility study. *Int J Radiat Oncol Biol Phys.* 2007;69:S653.
3. Song W, Chiu B, Bauman G, et al. Prostate contouring uncertainty in megavoltage computed tomography images acquired with a helical tomotherapy unit during image-guided radiation therapy. *Int J Radiat Oncol Biol Phys.* 2006;65:595–607.
4. Holly R, Myrehaug S, Kamran A, et al. High-dose-rate prostate brachytherapy in a patient with bilateral hip prostheses planned using megavoltage computed tomography images acquired with a helical tomotherapy unit. *Brachytherapy.* 2009;8:70–73.
5. Yoo S, Yin FF. Dosimetric feasibility of cone beam CT-based treatment planning compared to CT-based treatment planning. *Int J Radiat Oncol Biol Phys.* 2006;66:1553–1561.
6. Ding G, Duggan D, Coffey C, et al. A study on adaptive IMRT treatment planning using kV cone beam CT. *Radiother Oncol.* 2007;85:116–125.
7. Rong Y, Smilowitz J, Tewatia D, et al. Dose calculation on kV cone beam CT images: an investigation of the HU-density

conversion stability and dose accuracy using the site-specific calibration. *Med Dos.* 2010;35(3):195–207.

8. Foroudi F, Haworth A, Pangehel A. Inter-observer variability of clinical target volume delineation for bladder cancer using CT and cone beam-CT. *J Med Imaging Radiat Oncol.* 2009;53:100–106.

9. Showalter T, Nawaz A, Xiao Y, et al. A cone beam CT-based study for clinical target definition using pelvic anatomy during postprostatectomy radiotherapy. *Int J Radiat Oncol Biol Phys.* 2008;70:431–436.

10. Letourneau D, Wong R, Moseley D, et al. Online planning and delivery technique for radiotherapy of spinal metastases using cone-beam CT: image quality and system performance. *Int J Radiat Oncol Biol Phys.* 2007;67:1229–1237.

11. Al-Halabi H, Portelance L, Duclos M, et al. Cone beam CT-based three-dimensional planning in high-dose-rate brachytherapy for cervical cancer. *Int J Radiat Oncol Biol Phys* 2010:77(4):1092–1097.

12. Bissonnette JP, Purdie TG, Higgins JA, et al. Cone-beam computed tomographic image guidance for lung cancer radiation therapy. *Int J Radiat Oncol Biol Phys.* 2009;73:927–934.

13. Smitsmans M, DeBois J, Sonke JJ, et al. Automatic prostate localization on cone beam CT scans for high precision image-guided radiotherapy. *Int J Radiat Oncol Biol Phys.* 2005;63: 975–984.

14. Xie Y, Chao M, Lee P, Xing L. Feature based rectal contour propagation from planning CT to cone beam CT. *Med Phys.* 2008;35:4450–4459.

15. Chao M, Li T, Schreidmann E, et al. Automated contour mapping with a regional deformable model. *Int J Radiat Oncol Biol Phys.* 2008;70:590–608.

16. Zhang T, Chi Y, Meldolesi E, Yan D. Automatic delineation of on-line head and neck computed tomography images: toward on-line adaptive radiotherapy. *Int J Radiat Oncol Biol Phys.* 2007;68:522–530.

17. Wang H, Garden A, Zhang L, et al. Performance evaluation of automatic anatomy segmentation algorithm on repeat or four-dimensional computed tomography images using deformable image registration method. *Int J Radiat Oncol Biol Phys.* 2008;72:210–219.

18. Gu X, Pan H, Lian Y, et al. Implementation and evaluation of various demons deformable image registration algorithms on a GPU. *Phys Med Biol.* 2010;55:207–219.

19. Christensen G, Carlson B, Chao C, et al. Image-based dose planning of intracavitary brachytherapy: registration of serial-imaging studies using deformable anatomic templates. *Int J Radiat Oncol Biol Phys.* 2001;51:227–243.

20. Greene W, Chelikani S, Purushothaman K, et al. Constrained non-rigid registration for use in image-guided adaptive radiotherapy. *Med Image Anal.* 2009;13:809–817.

21. Wenckebach T, Lamecker H, Hege H. Capturing anatomical shape variability using B-spline registration. *Inf Process Med Imaging.* 2005;19:578–590.

22. Coselmon M, Balter J, McShan D, et al. Mutual information based CT registration of the lung at exhale and inhale breathing states using thin-plate splines. *Med Phys.* 2006;31:2942–2948.

23. Thirion J. Image matching as a diffusion process: an analogy with Maxwell's demons. *Med Image Anal.* 1998;2:243–260.

24. Yang D, Li H, Low D, et al. A fast inverse consistent deformable image registration method based on symmetric optical flow computation. *Phys Med Biol.* 2008;53:6143–6165.

25. Letourneau D, Kaus M, Wong R, et al. Semiautomatic vertebrae visualization, detection, and identification for online palliative radiotherapy of bone metastases of the spine. *Med Phys.* 2008;35:367–376.

26. Yan J, Zhao B, Wang L, et al. Marker-controlled watershed for lymphoma segmentation in sequential CT images. *Med Phys.* 2006;33:2452–2460.

27. Day E, Betler J, Parda D, et al. A region growing method for tumor volume segmentation on PET images for rectal and anal cancer patients. *Med Phys.* 2009;36:4349–4358.

28. Frimmel H, Nappi J, and Yoshida H. Centerline-based colon segmentation for CT colonography. *Med Phys.* 2005;32:2665–2672.

29. Huyskens D, Maingon P, Vanuytsel L, et al. A qualitative and a quantitative analysis of an auto-segmentation module for prostate cancer. *Radiother Oncol.* 2009;90:337–345.

30. Pekar V, McNutt T, Kaus M. Automated model-based organ delineation for radiotherapy planning in prostatic region. *Int J Radiat Oncol Biol Phys.* 2004;60:973–980.

31. Lee C, Langen K, Lu W, et al. Assessment of parotid gland dose changes during head and neck cancer radiotherapy using daily megavoltage computed tomography and deformable image registration. *Int J Radiat Oncol Biol Phys.* 2008;71:1563–1571.

32. Hardisty M, Gordon L, Argawal P, et al. Quantitative characterization of metastatic disease in the spine. Part 1. Semiautomated segmentation using atlas-based deformable registration and the level set method. *Med Phys.* 2007;34:3127–3134.

33. Klein S, van der Heide U, Lips I, et al. Automatic segmentation of the prostate in 3D MR images by atlas matching using localized mutual information. *Med Phys.* 2008;34:1407–1417.

34. Hoggarth M, Quinn M, Comsia N, et al. Use of autosegmentation software to contour normal tissues in multi-fractional HDR brachytherapy for cervical cancer. *Int J Radiat Oncol Biol Phys.* 2009;75:S655.

35. Comsia N, Hoggarth M, Albuquerque K, et al. An evaluation of autosegmentation software in contouring clinical target volume and normal tissue in postoperative endometrial cancer patients. *Int J Radiat Oncol Biol Phys.* 2009;75:S651.

36. Yan D, Wong J, Vicini F, et al. Adaptive modification of treatment planning to minimize the deleterious effects of treatment setup errors. *Int J Radiat Oncol Biol Phys.* 1997;58:197–206.

37. Thongphiew D, Wu Q, Lee W, et al. Comparison of online IGRT techniques for prostate IMRT treatment: adaptive vs repositioning correction. *Med Phys.* 2009;36:1651–1662.

38. McShan D, Kessler M, Vineberg K, Fraass B. Inverse plan optimization accounting for random geometric uncertainties with a multiple instance geometry approximation. *Med Phys.* 2006; 33:1510–1521.

39. Foroudi F, Wong J, Haworth A, et al. Offline adaptive radiotherapy for bladder cancer using cone beam computed tomography. *J Med Imaging Radiat Oncol.* 2009;53:226–233.

40. Nuver T, Hoogeman M, Remeijer P, et al. An adaptive off line procedure for radiotherapy of prostate cancer. *J Med Imaging Radiat Oncol.* 2007;67:1559–1567.

41. Guide-Hurst C, Hugo G, Liang J, Yan D. A simplified method of four-dimensional dose accumulation using the mean patient density representation. *Med Phys.* 2008;35:5269–5277.

42. Harsolia A, Hugo G, Kestin L, et al. Dosimetric advantages of four-dimensional adaptive image-guided radiotherapy for lung tumors using online cone-beam computed tomography. *Int J Radiat Oncol Biol Phys.* 2008;70:582–589.

43. Ahunbay E, Peng C, Chen G, et al. An on line replanning scheme for interfractional variations. *Med Phys.* 2008;35:3607–3615.

44. Feng Y, Castro-Pareja C, Shekhar R, Yu C. Direct aperture deformation: an interfraction image guidance strategy. *Med Phys.* 2006;33:4490–4498.

45. Goodband J, Haas O, Mills J. A comparison of neural network approaches for on-line prediction in IGRT. *Med Phys.* 2008;35:1113–1122.

46. Yi B, Han-Oh S, Lerma F, et al. Real-time tumor tracking with preprogrammed dynamic multileaf collimator motion and adaptive dose-rate regulation. *Med Phys.* 2008;35:3955–3962.

47. Shirato H, Shimizu S, Kitamura K, et al. Four-dimensional treatment planning and fluoroscopic real-time tumor tracking radiotherapy for moving tumor. *Int J Radiat Oncol Biol Phys.* 2000;48:435–442.

48. Mestrovic A, Nichol A, Clark B, Otto K. Integration of on-line imaging, plan adaptation and radiation delivery: proof of concept using digital tomosynthesis. *Phys Med Biol.* 2009;54:3803–3819.

49. Li J, Jin L, Pollack A, et al. Gains from real-time tracking of prostate motion during external beam radiation therapy. *Int J Radiat Oncol Biol Phys.* 2009;75:1613–1620.

50. Men C, Gu X, Choi D, et al. GPU-based ultrafast IMRT plan optimization. *Phys Med Biol.* 2009;54:6565–6573.

51. Lu W, Chen M, Ruchala K, et al. Real-time motion-adaptive-optimization (MAO) in TomoTherapy. *Phys Med Biol.* 2009;54:4373–4398.

52. Sharpe M, Brock K. Quality assurance of serial 3D image registration, fusion, and segmentation. *Int J Radiat Oncol Biol Phys.* 2008;71:S33–S37.

53. Mutic S, Dempsey J, Bosch W, et al. Multimodality image registration quality assurance for conformal three-dimensional treatment planning. *Int J Radiat Oncol Biol Phys.* 2001;51:255–260.

54. Moore C, Liney G, Beavis A. Quality assurance of registration of CT and MRI data sets for treatment planning of radiotherapy for head and neck cancers. *J Appl Clin Med Phys.* 2004;5:25–35.

55. Lavely W, Scarfone C, Cevikalp H, et al. Phantom validation of coregistration of PET and CT for image-guided radiotherapy. *Med Phys.* 2004;31:1083–1092.

56. Castadot P, Lee J, Parraga A, et al. Comparison of 12 deformable registration strategies in adaptive radiation therapy for the treatment of head and neck tumors. *Radiother Oncol.* 2008;89:1–12.

57. Ezhil M, Choi B, Starkschall G, et al. Comparison of rigid and adaptive methods of propagating gross tumor volume through respiratory phases of four-dimensional computed tomography image data set. *Int J Radiat Oncol Biol Phys.* 2008;71:290–296.

58. Boldea V, Sharp G, Jiang S, Sarrut D. 4D-CT lung motion estimation with deformable registration: quantification of motion nonlinearity and hysteresis. *Med Phys.* 2008;35:1008–1018.

59. Pevsner A, Davis B, Joshi S, et al. Evaluation of an automated deformable image matching method for quantifying lung motion in respiration-correlated CT images. *Med Phys.* 2006;33:369–376.

60. Reed V, Woodward W, Zhang L, et al. Automatic segmentation of whole breast using atlas approach and deformable image registration. *Int J Radiat Oncol Biol Phys.* 2009;73:1493–1500.

61. Lee L, Le QT, Xing L. Retrospective IMRT dose reconstruction based on cone-beam CT and MLC log-file. *Int J Radiat Oncol Biol Phys.* 2008;70:634–644.

Chapter 27

ECONOMIC ANALYSIS OF IGRT

ANDRE KONSKI, MD, MBA

Image-guided radiation therapy (IGRT) is another in a long line of technologic advancements designed to improve the therapeutic ratio to radiotherapy (RT) between normal and cancerous tissues. As mentioned throughout this text, RT has evolved from aligning treatment fields to external landmarks on patients to using sophisticated imaging devices such as kilovoltage (kV) and megavoltage (MV) cone-beam computed tomography (CBCT). The basis for the introduction of these new technologies into clinical practice is the hypotheses that improvements in outcomes can occur by using more sophisticated imaging to locate and align patients; the margins needed to account for various uncertainties could be diminished resulting in less radiation dose to normal structures with fewer acute and late side effects. In addition, better targeting would also potentially improve outcomes by improved cell killing, local control, and disease-free survival. These points have been eloquently elucidated elsewhere in this text, in other symposia, and in other publications.[1–5]

Implementation of these advances in the clinic is not subject to the same safety and efficacy requirements as required of the pharmaceutical companies when new drugs are introduced into clinical practice. Machine manufacturers are only required to prove safety in a device that provides similar treatment to an already approved device.[6,7] Radiation oncologists have moved from using low-energy orthovoltage treatment machines to cobalt machines to finally MV linear accelerators without the need to compare outcomes of treatment using one machine compared with another. An evidence-based review comparing three-dimensional conformal radiation therapy (3DCRT) with conventional RT reported no difference in overall or disease-free survival but found that patients treated with 3DCRT experienced less toxicity and, therefore, improved quality of life.[8] In addition, there have been only a few studies that have randomized patients with head and neck cancer or breast cancer to receive either 3DCRT or intensity-modulated radiation therapy (IMRT).[9,10]

Randomized trials comparing the two are very difficult currently because of the belief among clinicians that IMRT is superior to 3DCRT in the prevention of normal tissue toxicity. In addition, IMRT has the added potential to deliver higher radiation doses with the hope of improved tumor control with similar or lower toxicity. Likewise, it may be difficult to compare via a randomized clinical trial outcomes of patients treated with image-guided IMRT (IG-IMRT) versus IMRT without image guidance because of the beliefs that IG-IMRT is superior to IMRT. A comparison of IG-IMRT and IMRT in the treatment of patients with prostate cancer was recently published. Although not a randomized comparison, 25 patients treated at the University of California, San Francisco (UCSF) and the National University Hospital in Singapore were treated with or without IG-IMRT. Patients treated at UCSF were treated with the placement of fiducials within the prostate whereas those treated in Singapore did not have implanted fiducials. The planning target volumes (PTVs) differed between the two institutions with smaller margins used at UCSF. Patients treated with IG-IMRT experienced less Radiation Therapy Oncology Group (RTOG) grade 2 acute rectal (13% vs 80%; $P = .004$) and bladder (13% vs 60%; $P = .014$) toxicity than those treated without IG-IMRT.[11]

In addition, RT has come under the microscope in the United States for an increasing share of health care expenditures. Intensity-modulated RT has been used with increasing frequency in the treatment of many malignancies because of the potential to spare normal tissue from unwanted radiation while improving the conformality of the radiation dose around the tumor. Intensity-modulated RT requires additional work from all members of the radiation oncology team, including physicians to contour the organs at risk, dosimetrists to create plans that optimize treatment to the PTV while minimizing radiation dose to the normal structures, and physicists who are charged with performing the quality assurance of the plans. This increases cost to the depart-

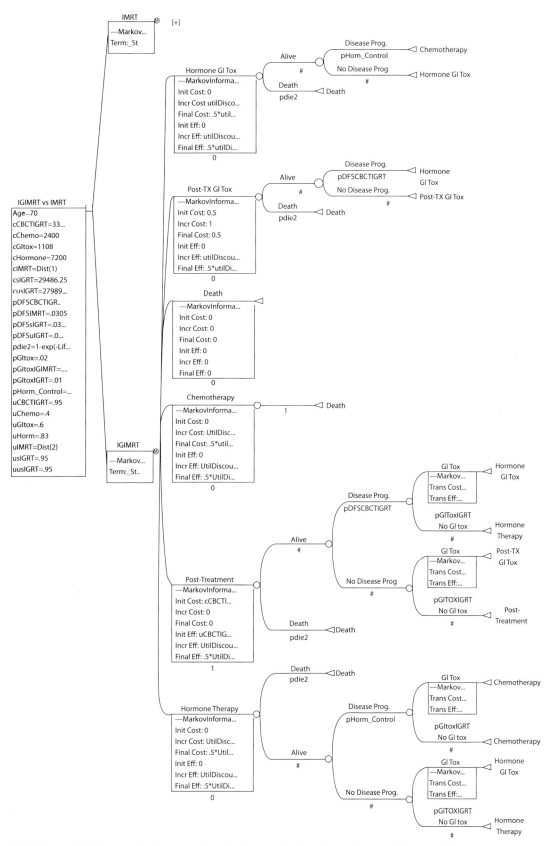

FIGURE 27-1. A Markov model of an economic analysis comparing intensity-modulated radiotherapy (IMRT) to image-guided IMRT in the treatment of a 70-year-old man with adenocarcinoma of the prostate treated to 80 Gy in 2-Gy fractions.

ment as well as health care payers because IMRT is reimbursed at a higher rate compared with standard 3DCRT. Mills and coworkers have recently published a framework for measuring both costs and outcomes for novel IGRT technologies.[12] This methodology may be expensive to implement because of the cost of the equipment necessary to capture all of the data needed to perform the calculations. Economic models have also been used to evaluate cost-effectiveness of various treatments.[13–17] Similar techniques could also be employed to compare IG-IMRT with IMRT.

Figure 27-1 is a Markov model of an economic analysis comparing IMRT with IG-IMRT in the treatment of a 70-year-old man with adenocarcinoma of the prostate treated to 80 Gy in 2-Gy fractions. The top portion, which is collapsed to facilitate presentation, represents treatment with IMRT while the bottom portion of the tree represents IG-IMRT. Daily ultrasound guidance, stereoscopic imaging with the use of fiducial markers, and CBCT were the IG-IMRT treatments tested in this model. The model and procedures used for evaluating treatment are exactly the same as in previous publications except for the evaluation of gastrointestinal toxicity (GI Tox) in the posttreatment state.[15–17] Patients enter the posttreatment state where they could or could not experience a GI Tox, which they would experience only once during their lifetime. Likewise, patients could experience a GI Tox if they had a biochemical recurrence receiving hormone therapy. Patients becoming hormone refractory would not have the opportunity to have GI Tox because they had only 1 year of life to live. Patients with GI Tox would have an increased expense resulting from treatment of the toxicity as well as have a decrease in quality of life or utility because of the toxicity. It was assumed the patient would be treated at an outpatient free-standing center.

Table 27-1 lists the 2009 relative value units (RVUs) used to calculate the cost of treatment assuming 40 treatments. A consultation code was not included because each patient would have a consultation with a radiation oncologist before initiating treatment and would not differ across each treatment arm. The 2009 conversion factor of $36.0666 was multiplied by the total RVUs to arrive at the total cost of treatment. Table 27-2 lists the variable and ranges used in the sensitivity analysis used to inform the model. It was assumed patients would have an improvement in quality of life or utility by using the IG-IMRT but it was not assumed that an improvement in freedom from biochemical failure (FFBF) would be experienced as a result of the IG-IMRT. There are no data to support an improvement in FFBF and the possibility exists for worse outcome with the use of smaller margins around the tumor. Chung and colleagues only reported a reduction in toxicity and did not report FFBF as it is too early to do so.[11] Patients experiencing GI toxicity would

TABLE 27–1 2009 Relative Value Units (RVUs) used to Calculate Cost of Initial Treatment

CPT Code	Description	Quantity	RVU
77263	Treatment plan	1	4.38
77014	CT treatment planning	1	5.4
77280	Simple simulation (verification simulation)	1	5.26
77290	Complex simulation	1	15.14
77300	Dosimetry	5	1.88
77301	IMRT	1	66.13
77334	Treatment devices	6	4.15
77336	Continuing medical physics	8	1.26
77418	IMRT treatment	40	13.01
77427	Weekly treatment management	8	5.32
77470	Special treatment procedure	1	4.71
77695	Ultrasound guidance	40	1.88
For stereoscopic guidance			
55876	Interstitial insertion of fiducials	1	3.11
77421	Stereoscopic guidance	40	2.84
For CBCT			
77014	CT guidance	40	5.4

Note. CBCT = cone-beam computed tomography; CT = computed tomography; CPT = current procedural terminology; IMRT = intensity-modulated radiotherapy.

have a negative utility for the year they are in that state. A Markov termination condition of 10 years was used and patients would spend 1 year in each state before transitioning to another state.

Table 27-3 shows the expected mean costs comparing IMRT without image guidance with ultrasound-based IG-IMRT, IG-IMRT using fiducials, and CBCT-based IG-IMRT. The expected mean cost of IG-IMRT delivered with CBCT is the highest with IMRT without image guidance having the lowest expected mean cost. The quality-adjusted life years (QALYs) did not differ among the different forms of IG-IMRT. It was assumed that the QALYs would be similar for each IG-IMRT method because there are no data comparing one method of IG-IMRT to another. In a sensitivity analysis of CBCT-based IG-IMRT, IGRT was found to be superior to IMRT if the utility of patients undergoing IG-IMRT was greater than 0.927, if the yearly probability of disease progression was less than 0.046, if the utility of IMRT was less than 0.934, if the cost of the CBCT was less than $42,000, if the yearly probability of GI Tox was less than 0.056, and if the yearly probability of progression of patients receiving IMRT was greater than 0.015.

In this example, IG-IMRT using ultrasound, fiducials, or CBCT would be considered cost-effective compared with IMRT without image guidance under the assumptions used to inform this model. As in all economic analyses, the results are only as good as the data used to inform the model. Image-guided IMRT may not be cost-effective if future studies find patients treated with IG-IMRT have worse local control or survival because of the smaller margins used or if they did not experience improvements in quality of life.

TABLE 27–2 Variables Used to Inform Markov Model

Variable	Value	Range
Pdie2	Probability of dying obtained from life tables	None
Cost of IMRT	$25,548	$20,000–70,000
Cost of ultrasound IG-IMRT	$28,260	$20,000–70,000
Cost of stereoscopic IG-IMRT	$29,757	$20,000–70,000
Cost of CBCT IG-IMRT	$33,338	$20,000–70,000
Cost of hormone therapy	$7200	
Cost of chemotherapy	$24,000	
Cost of treating GI toxicity	$1200	$1,108–1,374
Utility of IMRT	.909	0.8–0.99
Utility of ultrasound IG-IMRT	.95	0.8–0.99
Utility of stereoscopic IG-IMRT	.95	0.8–0.99
Utility of CBCT IG-IMRT	.95	0.8–0.99
Utility of hormone therapy	.83	0.5–0.99
Utility of chemotherapy	.4	0.5–0.99
Utility of GI toxicity	−.3	−0.1−−0.3
Yearly probability of GI toxicity after IMRT	.02	0.01–0.1
Yearly probability of GI toxicity after IG-IMRT	.01	0.01–0.1
Yearly probability of progression after IRMT	.0305	0.01–0.1
Yearly probability of progression after ultrasound IGRT	.0305	0.01–0.1
Yearly probability of progression after stereotactic IG-IMRT	.0305	0.01–0.1
Yearly probability of progression after CBCT IG-IMRT	.0305	0.01–0.1
Yearly probability of progression after hormone therapy	.13	

Note. CBCT = cone-beam computed tomography; GI = gastrointestinal; IMRT = intensity-modulated radiotherapy; IG = image-guided.

TABLE 27–3 Results of Cost-Effectiveness Analysis Comparing IMRT to Different Forms of IG-IMRT

Modality	Expected Mean Cost	Outcome in Quality Adjusted Life-Years (QALYs)	Cost-Effectiveness Ratio ($/QALY)
IMRT	$30,361	6.76	
Ultrasound IG-IMRT	$32,995	7.14	$6931/QALY
Stereoscopic IG-IMRT	$34,492	7.14	$14,244/QALY
CBCT IG-IMRT	$38,073	7.14	$23,369/QALY

Note. CBCT = cone-beam computed tomography; IG = image-guided; IMRT = intensity-modulated radiation therapy.

References

1. Grau C, Muren LP, Hoyer M, et al. Image-guided adaptive radiotherapy - integration of biology and technology to improve clinical outcome. *Acta Oncol.* 2008;47:1182–1185.
2. Rit S, Wolthaus J, van Herk M, et al. On-the-fly motion-compensated cone-beam CT using an a priori motion model. *Med Image Comput Comput Assist Interv Int Conf Med Image Comput Comput Assist Interv.* 2008;11:729–736.
3. Smitsmans MH, Pos FJ, de Bois J, et al. The influence of a dietary protocol on cone beam CT-guided radiotherapy for prostate cancer patients. *Int J Radiat Oncol Biol Phys.* 2008;71:1279–1286.
4. Sonke JJ, Lebesque J, van Herk M. Variability of four-dimensional computed tomography patient models. *Int J Radiat Oncol Biol Phys.* 2008;70:590–598.
5. Van Herk M. Will IGRT live up to its promise? *Acta Oncol.* 2008;47:1186–1187.
6. Wallner PE, Konski A. A changing paradigm in the study and adoption of emerging health care technologies: coverage with evidence development. *J Am Coll Radiol.* 2008;5:1125–1129.
7. Wallner PE, Konski A. The impact of technology on health care cost and policy development. *Semin Radiat Oncol.* 2008;18:194–200.
8. Morris DE, Emami B, Mauch PM, et al. Evidence-based review of three-dimensional conformal radiotherapy for localized prostate cancer: an ASTRO outcomes initiative. *Int J Radiat Oncol Biol Phys.* 2005;62:3–19.
9. Pignol JP, Olivotto I, Rakovitch E, et al. A multicenter randomized trial of breast intensity-modulated radiation therapy to reduce acute radiation dermatitis. *J Clin Oncol.* 2008;26:2085–2092.
10. Kam MK, Leung SF, Zee B, et al. Prospective randomized study of intensity-modulated radiotherapy on salivary gland function in early-stage nasopharyngeal carcinoma patients. *J Clin Oncol.* 2007;25:4873–4879.
11. Chung HT, Xia P, Chan LW, et al. Does image-guided radiotherapy improve toxicity profile in whole pelvic-treated high-risk prostate cancer? Comparison between IG-IMRT and IMRT. *Int J Radiat Oncol Biol Phys.* 2009;73:53–60.
12. Mills MD, Spanos WJ, Esterhay RJ. Considerations of cost-effectiveness for new radiation oncology technologies. *J Am Coll Radiol.* 2006;3:278–288.
13. Lee JH, Glick HA, Hayman JA, et al. Decision-analytic model and cost-effectiveness evaluation of postmastectomy radiation therapy in high-risk premenopausal breast cancer patients. *J Clin Oncol.* 2002;20:2713–2725.
14. Ng AK, Kuntz KM, Mauch PM, et al. Costs and effectiveness of staging and treatment options in early-stage Hodgkin's disease. *Int J Radiat Oncol Biol Phys.* 2001;50:979–989.

15. Konski A, Speier W, Hanlon A, et al. Is proton beam therapy cost effective in the treatment of adenocarcinoma of the prostate? *J Clin Oncol.* 2007;25:3603–3608.

16. Konski A, Watkins-Bruner D, Brereton H, et al. Long-term hormone therapy and radiation is cost-effective for patients with locally advanced prostate carcinoma. *Cancer.* 2006;106:51–57.

17. Konski A, Watkins-Bruner D, Feigenberg S, et al. Using decision analysis to determine the cost-effectiveness of intensity-modulated radiation therapy in the treatment of intermediate risk prostate cancer. *Int J Radiat Oncol Biol Phys.* 2006;66: 408–415.

Chapter 28

IGRT: A CAUTIONARY NOTE

BAHMAN EMAMI, MD

A radiation oncologist is an integral member of the multidisciplinary team managing patients with cancer and is responsible for the evaluation, staging, treatment decision-making, planning, and delivery of radiation either alone or in combination with other modalities. Imaging is an essential tool in every step of the process. Therefore, in a broad sense, one can state that "imaging is guiding our therapy." However, there is a recent emergence of a new buzzword, "image-guided radiotherapy" (IGRT). The new concept under this buzzword is the use of information obtained from images in the process of radiotherapy (RT; Figure 28-1).[1] However, one should note that the concept is not new. Some form of image guidance has always existed, probably dating back to when the first kilovoltage (kV) units were used for both imaging and treatment.

Currently, there is no consensus on the definition of IGRT. The Radiation Therapy Oncology Group (RTOG) research plan of 2002–2006 defines IGRT as referring broadly to "treatment delivery using modern imaging methods, such as computed tomography (CT), magnetic resonance imaging (MRI), positron emission tomography (PET), and ultrasound, in target and non-target structures and in RT definition, design and delivery. . . ." The authors further continue, "IGRT includes, but is not limited to, 3-dimensional conformal RT (3DCRT), intensity modulated RT (IMRT), stereotactic radiosurgery, stereotactic RT, and brachytherapy, etc."

Reemergence of this concept has resulted in an avalanche of manuscripts by physicists, dosimetrists, and physicians trying to be part of this bandwagon with the perceived claim of possession of state-of-the-art technology and providing better patient care. The latter is used as surrogate for an improved therapeutic ratio that has yet to be proven. One cannot underestimate the huge marketing potential of IGRT. Thus, as with every new emerging technology and in spite of its commercial frenzy, one needs to learn "to use it and not to abuse it." The intention of this chapter is to point out some, not all, potential benefits and shortcomings of IGRT, and will focus only on the physician's involvement in the process of IGRT.

As mentioned previously, the concept of IGRT is not new. So why has its reawakening gained so much attention? Ling et al.[2] have stated at least three reasons: First, the precise dose distribution produced by IMRT is less forgiving in terms of treatment uncertainties. Second, the availability of on-line electronic portal imaging devices has lead to improved understanding of treatment uncertainties, and of the need for strategies reducing them. The third reason is the development and commercial availability of advanced on-line imaging technologies, particularly cone-beam CT (CBCT) systems using kV x-ray sources. More simply, the emergence of 3DCRT and IMRT has highlighted the potential uncertainties in current practice of RT and IGRT and has the perceived potential to help radiation oncologists better understand uncertainties and to develop strategies to reduce them, thus improving patient outcomes.

To start with, we are obligated to know what the uncertainties are. Moreover, it is also important to understand the magnitude of these uncertainties as well as to appreciate their influence on the outcome of the treatment. With this information, we need to develop strategies for a meaningful intervention to reduce the level of uncertainties and most importantly to verify that the process has resulted in improved patient outcome. The magnitude of uncertainties has been studied in every organ by various methodologies during the past decade, albeit some of them are clinically meaningless, such as motion of prostate during respiration. Others can be clinically important but cannot be helped by current IGRT technology, such as moment-to-moment control of the rectal content (gas or feces) during day-to-day treatment of localized prostate cancer (random errors).

In general, the practice of RT consists of identification of tissues involved by cancer, construction of a plan to deliver the desired dose to predetermined tissues both cancerous and noncancerous, and, finally, delivery and execution of the plan. A review of the available literature reveals that there are uncertainties in each of these steps. It is generally agreed that there are two types of

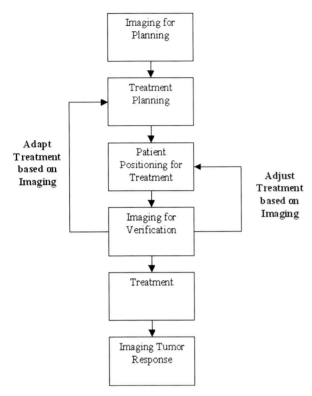

FIGURE 28-1. Illustration of the use of imaging in the radiotherapy treatment chain. Adapted from Evans.[1]

uncertainties: systematic and random. Systematic uncertainties are attributable to differences between snapshot imaging during simulation and actual anatomies during the treatment. Random uncertainties are the day-to-day deviations from the average target position of the simulation. It is also agreed that systematic uncertainties are clinically more important.

Target Delineation

This review will follow the recommendations of the International Commission of Units and Measurements (ICRU) in which the target volumes are designated as the gross tumor volume (GTV), the clinical target volume (CTV), and the planning target volume (PTV). We will begin with the identification and delineation of the GTV, its associated uncertainties, and how imaging can help.

Computed tomography imaging has traditionally been, and continues to be, the mainstay of delineating the GTV. It also has been helpful in estimation of dose prediction. Other modalities such as PET, MR imaging, and ultrasound have also been used for delineation of the GTV. An important consideration is that radiation oncologists are not formally trained to interpret images from CT scans or any other imaging modalities. The same is true for medical physicists, dosimetrists, and radiation therapists who definitely are not trained in the interpre-

tation of the images in a way required for IGRT. Even in the specialty of radiology, separate expertise exists for the interpretation of various modalities such as CT and MR. Moreover, interpretation of each modality is subspecialized according to anatomical region of the body. On the other hand, diagnostic radiologists are less concerned about the precise boundaries of tumor that is needed in GTV delineation.

The process of GTV delineation, which is mostly manual, has serious limitations of which one needs to be aware. In most instances, the anatomical image contains no functional information. Use of PET and its fusion in the RT planning system, which nowadays has become very popular, has its own limitations and uncertainties, which will be discussed later. The "snapshot" anatomy of the planning image may not be completely indicative of the anatomy during treatment. The changes may be caused by a patient's weight loss or the positional difference between simulation and treatment. As discussed previously, these will result in so-called systematic errors. The issue of inter- and intraobserver variation and the lack of realistic consensus on delineation of the involved tissues with the disease and how to separate them from uninvolved tissues is still an unsolved problem in RT. Changes of tumor volume (both in terms of size and shape) caused by response to treatment are another real issue, which is often ignored. Because of the lack of proper training by radiation oncologists and/or inadequate resolution of our imaging modalities, fiducial markers, either external or internal, have been used as surrogates for soft tissue changes. However, the exact correlation of these markers to the changes of the tumor or other organs is far from certain.

In the treatment of thoracic tumors, intra- and interfraction variations may also occur as a result of motion such as breathing and cardiac cycle. Therefore, the problem of motion is also added to previously mentioned difficulties. The choice of modality and the methodology of image acquisition in the presence of motion can have a significant impact on images,[3] which has not been fully recognized, nor has a standard solution been implemented. Although an attempt has been made to solve this problem (using respiratory gating, four-dimensional [4D] planning and delivery), treatment errors still occur because the single or infused snapshot of the breathing distribution can hardly be indicative of real changes during the course of treatment. A detailed analysis of the volumetric uncertainties in RT can be found in Hamilton and Ebert.[4]

The use of PET and its infusion to treatment planning systems has gained wide popularity. One should be aware that all of the issues described previously for CT are even more pertinent to PET.[5] Use of an arbitrary standard uptake value (SUV), such as 2.5, or the use of an arbitrary percentage point of the maximum SUV has not provided a real solution to GTV delineation problems. Although technology has been developed to obtain sharp edges for every SUV, at least for one site (lung cancer),[6] there is no information on the relationship between these SUVs and the real pathology of the tumor for precise delineation of boundaries of involved tissues.

Radiation oncologists still, therefore, rely on traditional margins for microscopic extensions to create the CTV. However, there is a dearth of information on pathological verifications of CTV margins used in RT. The effort by Girard et al.[7] was probably the only attempt to study and pathologically verify the margin to adequately address the microscopic extension of tumor in lung cancer. Nevertheless, even in that study, connecting the information obtained from paraffin-fixed samples of tissues under the microscope to the real tumor inside the moving lung tissue represents a quantum leap of faith. So, at least up to this moment, there is no imaging modality or process to aid radiation oncologists in the delineation of or in devising strategies to correct the uncertainties of the CTV.

In summary, it is difficult to imagine that a radiation oncologist, who is not trained for and does not have a clear knowledge of the exact tumor boundaries, which vary with the imaging used, and with intra- and interobserver interpretation, and may change during RT and even during a single variable breathing cycle, will have the confidence of using these images for correction of few millimeter uncertainties, which is desired by physicists and promoted by manufacturers of IGRT.

Sources of uncertainties in delineating the PTV are setup accuracy and organ motion. Both of these can cause systematic and/or random errors. The goal of IGRT in this effort is to minimize the PTV margins, thereby reducing the irradiated volume and sparing more uninvolved normal structures. This, in turn, has been taken as a surrogate for reduction in radiation-induced complications. The last goal has yet to be clinically proven. The role of IGRT in correction of setup inaccuracies and uncertainties falls vastly in the domain of medical physics and is beyond discussion of this chapter.

However, organ motion is an issue in which the physician is directly involved. Organ or tumor motion can be caused by respiration or by nonrespiratory elements. The former has been a focus of intense attention and research and, therefore, will be discussed. It is a general belief that if one can reduce tumor motion caused by breathing during the course of radiation, one can reduce the PTV and, therefore, reduce the volume of lung receiving a high dose. Over the past two decades many different methods have been devised to reduce respiratory motion during the course of radiation (Table 28-1). In spite of numerous publications on the merits on each one of these methods, none of them has gained universal use for the simple reason that each of the methods has been applicable to a very limited number of patients in the hands of that specific investigator. Moreover, most of these techniques result

TABLE 28–1 Respiratory Motion Management Strategies

Image-guided radiation therapy
How to limit motion:
A. Simple techniques
   • Patient immobilization: molds, casts, etc.
   • Breath control by patient instruction
   • Abdominal compression
B. Complex techniques
   • Deep inspiration breathing training
   • Active breathing control (ABC)
   • Target tracking
      a. Gated radiotherapy
      b. Real-time tumor tracking

in significantly longer times that patients must remain on the treatment table and, therefore, add more potential uncertainties.

One of these methods, which has gained considerable attention, is tumor tracking, either by gated RT or by real-time tumor tracking. Real-time tumor tracking has not been possible because of lack of adequate soft tissue and tumor resolution by the mentioned modalities, which has been discussed extensively earlier. Therefore, radiation oncologists have used radio-opaque markers, either intratumoral or external, as a surrogate for evaluating motion. Placing intratumoral markers has a long history of practice in tumors such as the cervix. However, the fact that cervix does not have significant motion during radiation and the object of correction of motion nowadays is cancers of the lung and upper abdomen, one should seriously reconsider placing intratumoral opaque markers in a centrally located lung cancer in a patient with poor pulmonary function or intratumoral markers in patients with liver tumors or pancreatic cancer.

The RT process has inherent uncertainties aside from imaging,[8] which are far greater than the attempted correction of a few millimeters of random errors by some of the current IGRT techniques. Thus, the use of internal markers in treatment of prostate cancer appears to be "gilding the lily" for the happiness of radiotherapists. No clinically meaningful, real-life benefit has been shown from this practice. Thus, in the most current situation, tumor tracking or gating usually refers to the use of an external surrogate for tumor position to guide the radiation. Numerous publications in the literature have pointed out that external surrogate markers may or may not have any correlation with the motion of internal organs.[9,10] One is reminded of the old story of a fellow who lost his keys a mile away but looked for them under a streetlight because there was light at that location.

Gated RT for pulmonary and upper-abdominal malignancies has another insurmountable problem. At most institutions, the signals from external surrogate markers (usually placed on the skin) are used to bin the CT into the various phases of respiration. A decision is then made to choose one of these phases and perform planning and radiation delivery specifically during that phase of respiration. It would have been fine and dandy if a patient with lung cancer with poor pulmonary function would have a very uniform and exact respiratory cycle all the time and the external surrogates would directly and unambiguously represent tumor motion. Unfortunately none of these are the case. The pattern of respiration changes from patient to patient, and from day to day during treatment. One can hardly expect to use one snapshot of the respiratory signal for the entire 6 weeks of therapy. It has been suggested that radiation therapists should obtain three to five series of these correlated studies in the first 5 days of treatment (irrespective of cost, time, and resource utilization) and use this as a model for the rest of treatment, ignoring the changes that can happen in patients breathing or the tumor status during the 6 or 7 weeks of treatment. Unless one decides to do the entire process of these correlative studies before every treatment, the current approach has inherent significant flaws.

Treatment Delivery

The ideal method of delivery is that the anatomy and tumor (location, position, and volume) would remain the same throughout the course and every day of treatment exactly the same as the original perfect plan that was initially constructed. For many obvious reasons, this will not be the case. Systematic and random errors have long been recognized to various degrees by radiation oncologists and others, and, over the past several decades, some remedies have been proposed for salvage. However, the recent surge of technology and advancement of IMRT is focused on better identifying and attempting to solve these problems through the use of IGRT. With this noble goal and with the "force" of marketing, radiation oncologists have been under the avalanche of technologies. Every one of these technologies and methodologies has the inherent problem of low resolution of soft tissues (i.e., CT), problems of using surrogate markers (as discussed before), issues of who will interpret the images (lack of specialized training on any of them), and expense and resource utilization in many departments. More importantly, none of these technologies, which are currently flooding the exhibition halls of American Society for Radiation Oncology (ASTRO) and Radiological Society of North America (RSNA) conferences, have been clinically verified. It is claimed that the use of these technologies and expected benefits to patients is a "no brainer" such as the "apple pie" and "motherhood" argument, but most often in publications promoting IGRT, the study design is such that the conclusion has preceded or replaced the hypothesis. It is argued that when technology is involved, there is no need for validation of presumed benefits or randomized trials to show the efficacy. Often the comparison of the use of cobalt versus the linac has been cited. In my opinion, this comparison is irrelevant.

Clinical Issues

The hypothesis behind gated RT for the treatment of lung cancer is to reduce the PTV margin and, therefore, by reducing volume of uninvolved normal lung, one can reduce the potential complication rate (pneumonitis) and possibly attempt dose escalation (Figure 28-2).[11] Although on the surface this hypothesis appears to be attractive and quasiscientific, in real life it has many serious flaws. First of all, dose escalation is not an open-ended proposal. There is adequate information in the literature in the era of chemoradiotherapy that the current highest safe dose is set at 74 Gy.[12] Beyond that dose there are problems with serious complications such as hemorrhage and bronchial fistula. More importantly, by reducing normal uninvolved lung from the high dose of radiation, in addition to the fact that it has the risk of missing microscopic tumor cells (because of lack of knowledge on CTV), one cannot potentially reduce radiation-induced complications such as radiation pneumonitis. It is well known that in IMRT the energy deposited from x-rays simply does not disappear but rather is deposited in other areas and, therefore, the integral dose in IMRT is higher than with 3DCRT. Thus, there is obviously an increased volume of normal tissue that receives less than prescribed dose—the so-called "low dose volume." Current literature[13] points out that in radiation-induced complications of the lung, namely pneumonitis, low dose areas are equally and possibly even more important in their development. Thus, both goals of the IGRT hypotheses in treatment of lung cancer appear to be on shaky grounds.

Adaptive IGRT is probably one of the real advantages of new technology, namely through the use of onboard imaging. Although use of IGRT for random errors appears to be too much noise for too little gain (if any), detection of the changes during 7 weeks of RT as a result of treatment or patient condition and adjusting the plan according to major changes is most likely to benefit the patient and improve patient care. Thus, changes detected by imaging and replanning most likely will benefit patients. However, one has to be cognizant that this issue may not be as straightforward as it sounds. In real life, more often than not, tumor shrinkage is not uniform, spheric, and concentric. Therefore it is mandatory to rescan, replan, and re-execute. Because it is not practical to rescan and replan on a day-to-day basis, we need to determine which frequencies are suitable for which disease site for proper use for adaptive IGRT and to conduct a properly designed study to verify its merit in improvement of the therapeutic ratio.

In summary, I will utilize my IGRT equipment to study major changes during the 6- or 7-week course of RT and to adjust my treatment plan via replanning if there is a major change in the volume—either tumor

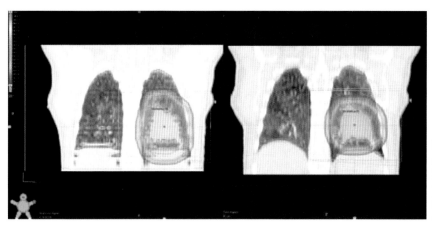

FIGURE 28-2. Colorwash overlay of the high dose region for non-gated (left) and gated (right) treatment delivery. Note the reduction in the volume of normal lung irradiated. Reprinted with permission from Huntzinger *et al.*[11]

shrinkage or progression. I will not rely on IGRT to correct my few-millimeter random errors on a day-to-day basis. Until the time comes that oncological imaging technology clearly depicts the exact boundaries of the GTV and CTV, which are pathologically verified, I will still rely on my experience and currently practiced tradition of adding the GTV and CTV while I am treating patients.

References

1. Evans PM. Anatomical imaging for radiotherapy. *Phys Med Biol.* 2008;53:R151–R191.
2. Ling CC, Yorke E, Fuks Z. From IMRT to IGRT: Frontierland or neverland? *Radiother Oncol.* 2006; 78:119–122.
3. Vedam SS, Keall PJ, Kini VR, et al. Acquiring a four-dimensional computed tomography dataset using an external respiratory signal. *Phys Med Biol.* 2003;48(1):45–62.
4. Hamilton CS, Ebert MA. Volumetric uncertainties in radiotherapy. *Clin Oncol.* 2005;17:456–464.
5. Christian N, Lee JA, Bol A, et al. The limitation of PET imaging for biological adaptive-IMRT assessed in animal models. *Radiother Oncol.* 2009;91:101–106.
6. Hong R, Halama J, Bova D, et al. Correlation of PET standard uptake value and CT window-level thresholds for target delineation in CT-based radiation treatment planning. *Int J Radiat Oncol Biol Phys.* 2007;67(3):720–726.
7. Girard P, Antoine M, Larrouy A, et al. Evaluation of microscopic tumor extension in non-small-cell lung cancer for three-dimensional conformal radiotherapy planning. *Int J Radiat Oncol Biol Phys.* 2000;48(4):1015–1024.
8. Amols H. Personal communication; March 28, 2008.
9. Beddar AS, Kainz K, Briere TM, et al. Correlation between internal fiducial tumor motion and external marker motion for liver tumors imaged with 4D-CT. *Int J Radiat Oncol Biol Phys.* 2007;67:630–638.
10. Berbeco RI, Nishioka S, Shirato H, et al. Residual motion of lung tumours in gated radiotherapy with external respiratory surrogates. *Phys Med Biol.* 2005;50:3655–3667.
11. Huntzinger C, Munro P. Johnson S, et al. Dynamic targeting image-guided radiotherapy. *Med Dosim.* 2006;31(2):113–125.
12. Rosenman JG, Halle JS, Socinski MA. High-dose conformal radiotherapy for treatment of stage IIIA/IIIB non-small-cell lung cancer: technical issues and results of a phase III trial. *Int J Radiat Oncol Biol Phys.* 2002;54(2):348–356.
13. Wang S, Liao Z, Wei X, et al. Analysis of clinical and dosimetric factors associated with treatment-related pneumonitis (TRP) in patients with non-small-cell lung cancer (NSCLC) treated with concurrent chemotherapy and three-dimensional conformal radiotherapy (3D-CRT). *Int J Radiat Oncol Biol Phys.* 2006;66(5):1399–1407.

INDEX

Note: Page numbers followed by f refer to figures; page numbers followed by t refer to tables.